Lecture Notes in Computer Science   11765

More information about this series at http://www.springer.com/series/7412

Dinggang Shen · Tianming Liu ·
Terry M. Peters · Lawrence H. Staib ·
Caroline Essert · Sean Zhou ·
Pew-Thian Yap · Ali Khan (Eds.)

Medical Image Computing and Computer Assisted Intervention – MICCAI 2019

22nd International Conference
Shenzhen, China, October 13–17, 2019
Proceedings, Part II

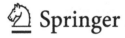 Springer

Editors
Dinggang Shen
University of North Carolina
at Chapel Hill
Chapel Hill, NC, USA

Terry M. Peters ⓘ
Western University
London, ON, Canada

Caroline Essert ⓘ
University of Strasbourg
Illkirch, France

Pew-Thian Yap
University of North Carolina
at Chapel Hill
Chapel Hill, NC, USA

Tianming Liu
University of Georgia
Athens, GA, USA

Lawrence H. Staib ⓘ
Yale University
New Haven, CT, USA

Sean Zhou
United Imaging Intelligence
Shanghai, China

Ali Khan
Western University
London, ON, Canada

ISSN 0302-9743   ISSN 1611-3349 (electronic)
Lecture Notes in Computer Science
ISBN 978-3-030-32244-1   ISBN 978-3-030-32245-8 (eBook)
https://doi.org/10.1007/978-3-030-32245-8

LNCS Sublibrary: SL6 – Image Processing, Computer Vision, Pattern Recognition, and Graphics

This Springer imprint is published by the registered company Springer Nature Switzerland AG
The registered company address is: Gewerbestrasse 11, 6330 Cham, Switzerland

Preface

We are pleased to present the proceedings for the 22nd International Conference on Medical Image Computing and Computer-Assisted Intervention (MICCAI), which was held at the InterContinental Hotel, Shenzhen, China, October 13–17, 2019. The conference also featured 34 workshops, 13 tutorials, and 22 challenges held on October 13 or 17. MICCAI 2019 had an approximately 63% increase in submissions and accepted papers compared with MICCAI 2018. These papers, which comprise six volumes of *Lecture Notes in Computer Science* (LNCS) proceedings, were selected after a thorough double-blind peer-review process. Following the example set by the previous program chairs of MICCAI 2018 and 2017, we employed Microsoft's Conference Managing Toolkit (CMT) for paper submissions and double-blind peer-reviews, and the Toronto Paper Matching System (TPMS) to assist with automatic paper assignment to area chairs and reviewers.

From 2625 original intentions to submit, 1809 full submissions were received and sent out to peer-review. Of these, 63% were considered as pure Medical Image Computing (MIC), 5% as pure Computer-Assisted Interventions (CAI), and 32% as both MIC and CAI. The MICCAI 2019 Program Committee (PC) comprised 69 area chairs, with 25 from the Americas, 21 from Europe, and 23 from Asia/Pacific/Middle East. Each area chair was assigned ~25 manuscripts, with up to 15 suggested potential reviewers using TPMS scoring and self-declared research areas. Subsequently, over 1200 invited reviewers were asked to bid for the papers for which they had been suggested. Final reviewer allocations via CMT took account of PC suggestions, reviewer bidding, and TPMS scores, finally allocating 5–6 papers per reviewer. Based on the double-blinded reviews, 306 papers (17%) were accepted immediately, and 920 papers (51%) were rejected, with the remainder being sent for rebuttal. These decisions were confirmed by the area chairs. During the rebuttal phase, two additional area chairs were assigned to each rebuttal paper using CMT and TPMS scores, who then independently scored them to accept or reject, based on the reviews, rebuttal, and manuscript, resulting in clear paper decisions using majority voting. This process resulted in the acceptance of further 234 papers for an overall acceptance rate of 30%. Regional PC teleconferences were held in late June to confirm the final results and collect PC feedback on the peer-review process.

For the MICCAI 2019 proceedings, 538 accepted papers have been organized in six volumes as follows:

Part I, LNCS Volume 11764: Optical Imaging; Endoscopy; Microscopy
Part II, LNCS Volume 11765: Image Segmentation; Image Registration; Cardiovascular Imaging; Growth, Development, Atrophy, and Progression
Part III, LNCS Volume 11766: Neuroimage Reconstruction and Synthesis; Neuroimage Segmentation; Diffusion-Weighted Magnetic Resonance Imaging; Functional Neuroimaging (fMRI); Miscellaneous Neuroimaging

Part IV, LNCS Volume 11767: Shape; Prediction; Detection and Localization; Machine Learning; Computer-Aided Diagnosis; Image Reconstruction and Synthesis

Part V, LNCS Volume 11768: Computer-Assisted Interventions; MIC Meets CAI

Part VI, LNCS Volume 11769: Computed Tomography; X-ray Imaging

We would like to thank everyone who contributed to the success of MICCAI 2019 and the quality of its proceedings, particularly the MICCAI Society for support, insightful comments, and providing funding for Kitty Wong to be the ongoing Conference System Manager. Given the increase in workload for this year's meeting, the Program Committee simply could not have functioned effectively without her, and she will provide ongoing oversight of the review process for future MICCAI conferences. Without the dedication and support of all of the organizers of the workshops, tutorials, and challenges, under the guidance of Kenji Suzuki, together with satellite event chairs Hongen Liao, Qian Wang, Luping Zhou, Hayit Greenspan, and Bram van Ginneken, none of these peripheral events would have been feasible.

Also, the Industry Forum (led by Xiaodong Tao and Yiqiang Zhan), the Industry Session (led by Sean Zhou), as well as the Doctoral Symposium (led by Junzhou Huang and Dajiang Zhu) brought new events to MICCAI 2019. The publication chairs, Li Wang and Gang Li, undertook the onerous task of assembling the camera-ready proceedings for publication by Springer.

Behind the scenes, MICCAI secretariat personnel, Janette Wallace and Johanne Langford, kept a close eye on logistics and budgets, while Doris Lam and her team from Momentous Asia, this year's Professional Conference Organization, along with the Local Organizing Committee chair, Dong Ni (together with Jing Qin, Qianjin Feng, Dong Liang, Xiaoying Tang), handled the website and local organization. The Student Travel Award Committee chaired by Huiguang He, Jun Shi, and Xi Jiang evaluated numerous applications, including awards for undergraduate students, which is new in the history of MICCAI. We also thank our sponsors for their financial support and presence on site. We are especially grateful to all members of the Program Committee for their diligent work in the reviewer assignments and final paper selection, as well as the reviewers for their support during the entire process. Finally, and most importantly, we thank all authors, co-authors, students/postdocs, and supervisors, for submitting and presenting their high-quality work that made MICCAI 2019 a greatly enjoyable, informative, and successful event. We are indebted to those reviewers and PC members who helped us resolve issues relating to last-minute missing reviews. Overall, we thank all of the authors and attendees for making MICCAI 2019 a spectacular success. We look forward to seeing you in Lima, Peru at MICCAI 2020!

October 2019

Dinggang Shen
Tianming Liu
Terry M. Peters
Lawrence H. Staib
Caroline Essert
Sean Zhou
Pew-Thian Yap
Ali Khan

Organization

General Chairs

Dinggang Shen   The University of North Carolina at Chapel Hill, USA
Tianming Liu   The University of Georgia, USA

Program Executive

Terry Peters   Robarts Research Institute, Western University, Canada
Lawrence H. Staib   Yale University, USA
Sean Zhou   United Imaging Intelligence (UII), China
Caroline Essert   University of Strasbourg, France
Pew-Thian Yap   The University of North Carolina at Chapel Hill, USA
Ali Khan   Robarts Research Institute, Western University, Canada

Submissions Manager

Kitty Wong   Robarts Research Institute, Western University, Canada

Workshops/Challenges/Tutorial Chairs

Kenji Suzuki   Illinois Institute of Technology, USA
Hayit Greenspan   Tel Aviv University, Israel
Bram van Ginneken   Radboud University Medical Center, The Netherlands
Qian Wang   Shanghai Jiao Tong University, China
Luping Zhou   The University of Sydney, Australia
Hongen Liao   Tsinghua University, China

MICCAI Society, Board of Directors

Leo Joskowicz (President)   The Hebrew University of Jerusalem, Israel
Stephen Aylward   Kitware, Inc., NY, USA
  (Treasurer)
Josien Pluim (Secretary)   Eindhoven University of Technology, The Netherlands
Wiro Niessen   Erasmus Medical Centre, The Netherlands
  (Past President)
Marleen de Bruijne   Erasmus Medical Centre, The Netherlands
                              and University of Copenhagen, Denmark
Hervé Delinguette   Inria, Sophia Antipolis, France
Caroline Essert   University of Strasbourg, France
Alejandro Frangi   University of Leeds, UK
Lena Maier-Hein   German Cancer Research Center, Germany

Shuo Li   Western University, London, Canada
Tianming Liu   University of Georgia, USA
Anne Martel   University of Toronto, Canada
Daniel Racoceanu   Pontifical Catholic University of Peru, Peru
Julia Schnabel   King's College, London, UK
Guoyan Zheng   Institute for Surgical Technology & Biomechanics,
                                     Switzerland
Kevin Zhou   Chinese Academy of Sciences, China

Industry Forum

Xiaodong Tao   iFLYTEK Health, China
Yiqiang Zhan   United Imaging Intelligence (UII), China

Publication Committee

Gang Li   The University of North Carolina at Chapel Hill, USA
Li Wang   The University of North Carolina at Chapel Hill, USA

Finance Committee

Dong Ni   Shenzhen University, China
Janette Wallace   Robarts Research Institute, Western University, Canada
Stephen Aylward   Kitware, Inc., USA

Local Organization Chairs

Dong Ni   Shenzhen University, China
Jing Qin   The Hong Kong Polytechnic University, SAR China
Qianjin Feng   Southern Medical University, China
Dong Liang   Shenzhen Institutes of Advanced Technology,
                                     Chinese Academy of Sciences, China
Xiaoying Tang   Southern University of Science and Technology, China

Sponsors and Publicity Liaison

Kevin Zhou   Institute of Computing Technology, Chinese Academy
                                     of Sciences, China
Hongen Liao   Tsinghua University, China
Wenjian Qin   Shenzhen Institutes of Advanced Technology,
                                     Chinese Academy of Sciences, China

Keynote Lectures Chairs

Max Viergever	University Medical Center Utrecht, The Netherlands
Kensaku Mori	Nagoya University, Japan
Gözde Ünal	Istanbul Technical University, Turkey

Student Travel Award Committee

Huiguang He	Institute of Automation, Chinese Academy of Sciences, China
Jun Shi	Shanghai University, China
Xi Jiang	University of Electronic Science and Technology of China, China

Student Activities Liaison

Julia Schnabel	King's College London, UK
Caroline Essert	University of Strasbourg, France
Dimitris Metaxas	Rutgers University, USA
MICCAI Student Board Members	

Area Chairs

Purang Abolmaesumi	The University of British Columbia, Canada
Shadi Albarqouni	The Technical University of Munich (TUM), Germany
Elsa Angelini	Imperial College London, UK
Suyash Awate	Indian Institute of Technology (IIT) Bombay, India
Ulas Bagci	University of Central Florida (UCF), USA
Kayhan Batmanghelich	University of Pittsburgh, USA
Christian Baumgartner	Swiss Federal Institute of Technology Zurich, Switzerland
Ismail Ben Ayed	Ecole de Technologie Superieure (ETS), Canada
Weidong Cai	The University of Sydney, Australia
Xiaohuan Cao	United Imaging Intelligence (UII), China
Elvis Chen	Robarts Research Institute, Western University, Canada
Xinjian Chen	Soochow University, China
Jian Cheng	Beihang University, China
Jun Cheng	Cixi Institute of Biomedical Engineering, Chinese Academy of Sciences, China
Veronika Cheplygina	Eindhoven University of Technology, The Netherlands
Elena De Momi	Politecnico di Milano, Italy
Ayman El-Baz	University of Louisville, USA
Aaron Fenster	Robarts Research Institute, Western University, USA
Moti Freiman	Philips Healthcare, The Netherlands
Yue Gao	Tsinghua University, China

Daoqiang Zhang　　　　　Nanjing University of Aeronautics and Astronautics,
　　　　　　　　　　　　　China
Miaomiao Zhang　　　　　Washington University in St. Louis, USA
Tuo Zhang　　　　　　　　Northwestern Polytechnical University, China
Guoyan Zheng　　　　　　Shanghai Jiao Tong University, China
S. Kevin Zhou　　　　　　Institute of Computing Technology, Chinese Academy
　　　　　　　　　　　　　of Sciences, China
Dajiang Zhu　　　　　　　The University of Texas at Arlington, USA

Reviewers

Abdi, Amir
Abduljabbar, Khalid
Adeli, Ehsan
Aganj, Iman
Aggarwal, Priya
Agrawal, Praful
Ahmad, Ola
Ahmad, Sahar
Ahn, Euijoon
Akbar, Shazia
Akhondi-Asl, Alireza
Akram, Saad
Al-Kadi, Omar
Alansary, Amir
Alghamdi, Hanan
Ali, Sharib
Allan, Maximilian
Amiri, Mina
Anton, Esther
Anwar, Syed
Armin, Mohammad
Audigier, Chloe
Aviles-Rivero, Angelica
Awan, Ruqayya
Awate, Suyash
Aydogan, Dogu
Azizi, Shekoofeh
Bai, Junjie
Bai, Wenjia
Balbastre, Yaël
Balsiger, Fabian
Banerjee, Abhirup
Bano, Sophia

Barbu, Adrian
Bardosi, Zoltan
Bateson, Mathilde
Bathula, Deepti
Batmanghelich, Kayhan
Baumgartner, Christian
Baur, Christoph
Baxter, John
Bayramoglu, Neslihan
Becker, Benjamin
Behnami, Delaram
Beig, Niha
Belyaev, Mikhail
Benkarim, Oualid
Bentaieb, Aicha
Bernal, Jose
Beyeler, Michael
Bhatia, Parmeet
Bhole, Chetan
Bhushan, Chitresh
Bi, Lei
Bian, Cheng
Bilinski, Piotr
Bise, Ryoma
Bnouni, Nesrine
Bo, Wang
Bodenstedt, Sebastian
Bogunovic, Hrvoje
Bozorgtabar, Behzad
Bragman, Felix
Braman, Nathaniel
Bridge, Christopher
Broaddus, Coleman

Bron, Esther
Brooks, Rupert
Bruijne, Marleen
Bühler, Katja
Bui, Duc
Burlutskiy, Nikolay
Burwinkel, Hendrik
Bustin, Aurelien
Cabeen, Ryan
Cai, Hongmin
Cai, Jinzheng
Cai, Yunliang
Camino, Acner
Cao, Jiezhang
Cao, Qing
Cao, Tian
Carapella, Valentina
Cardenes, Ruben
Cardoso, M.
Carolus, Heike
Castro, Daniel
Cattin, Philippe
Chabanas, Matthieu
Chaddad, Ahmad
Chaitanya, Krishna
Chakraborty, Jayasree
Chakraborty, Rudrasis
Chang, Ken
Chang, Violeta
Charaborty, Tapabrata
Chatelain, Pierre
Chatterjee, Sudhanya
Chen, Alvin
Chen, Antong
Chen, Cameron
Chen, Chao
Chen, Chen
Chen, Elvis
Chen, Fang
Chen, Fei
Chen, Geng
Chen, Hanbo
Chen, Hao
Chen, Jia-Wei
Chen, Jialei
Chen, Jianxu

Chen, Jie
Chen, Jingyun
Chen, Lei
Chen, Liang
Chen, Min
Chen, Pingjun
Chen, Qingchao
Chen, Xiao
Chen, Xiaoran
Chen, Xin
Chen, Xuejin
Chen, Yang
Chen, Yuanyuan
Chen, Yuncong
Chen, Zhiqiang
Chen, Zhixiang
Cheng, Jun
Cheng, Li
Cheng, Yuan
Cheng, Yupeng
Cheriet, Farida
Chong, Minqi
Choo, Jaegul
Christiaens, Daan
Christodoulidis, Argyrios
Christodoulidis, Stergios
Chung, Ai
Çiçek, Özgün
Cid, Yashin
Clarkson, Matthew
Clough, James
Collins, Toby
Commowick, Olivier
Conze, Pierre-Henri
Cootes, Timothy
Correia, Teresa
Coulon, Olivier
Coupé, Pierrick
Courtecuisse, Hadrien
Craley, Jeffrey
Crimi, Alessandro
Cury, Claire
D'souza, Niharika
Dai, Hang
Dalca, Adrian
Das, Abhijit

Das, Dhritiman
Deeba, Farah
Dekhil, Omar
Demiray, Beatrice
Deniz, Cem
Depeursinge, Adrien
Desrosiers, Christian
Dewey, Blake
Dey, Raunak
Dhamala, Jwala
Ding, Meng
Distergoft, Alexander
Dobrenkii, Anton
Dolz, Jose
Dong, Liang
Dong, Mengjin
Dong, Nanqing
Dong, Xiao
Dong, Yanni
Dou, Qi
Du, Changde
Du, Lei
Du, Shaoyi
Duan, Dingna
Duan, Lixin
Dubost, Florian
Duchateau, Nicolas
Duncan, James
Duong, Luc
Dvornek, Nicha
Dzyubachyk, Oleh
Eaton-Rosen, Zach
Ebner, Michael
Ebrahimi, Mehran
Edwards, Philip
Egger, Bernhard
Eguizabal, Alma
Einarsson, Gudmundur
Ekin, Ahmet
Elazab, Ahmed
Elhabian, Shireen
Elmogy, Mohammed
Eltanboly, Ahmed
Erdt, Marius
Ernst, Floris
Esposito, Marco

Esteban, Oscar
Fan, Jingfan
Fan, Xin
Fan, Yong
Fan, Yonghui
Fang, Xi
Farag, Aly
Farzi, Mohsen
Fauser, Johannes
Fawaz, Hassan
Fedorov, Andrey
Fehri, Hamid
Feng, Chiyu
Feng, Jun
Feng, Xinyang
Feng, Yuan
Fenster, Aaron
Ferrante, Enzo
Feydy, Jean
Fischer, Lukas
Fischer, Peter
Fishbaugh, James
Fletcher, Tom
Flores, Kevin
Forestier, Germain
Forkert, Nils
Fotouhi, Javad
Fountoukidou, Tatiana
Franz, Alfred
Frau-Pascual, Aina
Freysinger, Wolfgang
Fripp, Jurgen
Fu, Huazhu
Funka-Lea, Gareth
Funke, Isabel
Funke, Jan
Fürnstahl, Philipp
Furukawa, Ryo
Gahm, Jin
Galassi, Francesca
Galdran, Adrian
Gan, Yu
Gao, Fei
Gao, Mingchen
Gao, Siyuan
Gao, Zhifan

Huang, Weilin
Huang, Xiaolei
Huang, Yawen
Huang, Yixing
Huang, Yufang
Huang, Zhongwei
Huaulmé, Arnaud
Huisman, Henkjan
Huo, Xing
Huo, Yuankai
Husch, Andreas
Hussein, Sarfaraz
Hutter, Jana
Hwang, Seong
Icke, Ilknur
Igwe, Kay
Ingalhalikar, Madhura
Irmakci, Ismail
Ivashchenko, Oleksandra
Izadyyazdanabadi, Mohammadhassan
Jafari, Mohammad
Jäger, Paul
Jamaludin, Amir
Janatka, Mirek
Jaouen, Vincent
Jarayathne, Uditha
Javadi, Golara
Javer, Avelino
Jensen, Todd
Ji, Zexuan
Jia, Haozhe
Jiang, Jue
Jiang, Steve
Jiang, Tingting
Jiang, Weixiong
Jiang, Xi
Jiao, Jianbo
Jiao, Jieqing
Jiao, Zhicheng
Jie, Biao
Jin, Dakai
Jin, Taisong
Jin, Yueming
John, Rogers
Joshi, Anand
Joshi, Shantanu

Jud, Christoph
Jung, Kyu-Hwan
Jungo, Alain
Kadkhodamohammadi, Abdolrahim
Kakileti, Siva
Kamnitsas, Konstantinos
Kang, Eunsong
Kao, Po-Yu
Kapoor, Ankur
Karani, Neerav
Karayumak, Suheyla
Kazi, Anees
Kerrien, Erwan
Kervadec, Hoel
Khalifa, Fahmi
Khalili, Nadieh
Khallaghi, Siavash
Khalvati, Farzad
Khan, Hassan
Khanal, Bishesh
Khansari, Maziyar
Khosravan, Naji
Kia, Seyed
Kikinis, Ron
Kim, Geena
Kim, Hosung
Kim, Hyo-Eun
Kim, Jae-Hun
Kim, Jinman
Kim, Jinyoung
Kim, Minjeong
Kim, Namkug
Kim, Seong
Kim, Young-Ho
Kitasaka, Takayuki
Klein, Stefan
Klinder, Tobias
Kolli, Kranthi
Kong, Bin
Kong, Xiang-Zhen
Konukoglu, Ender
Koo, Bongjin
Koohbanani, Navid
Kopriva, Ivica
Kose, Kivanc
Koutsoumpa, Christina

Kozinski, Mateusz
Krebs, Julian
Krishnan, Anithapriya
Krishnaswamy, Pavitra
Krivov, Egor
Kruggel, Frithjof
Krupinski, Elizabeth
Kuang, Hulin
Kügler, David
Kuijper, Arjan
Kulkarni, Prachi
Kumar, Arun
Kumar, Ashnil
Kumar, Kuldeep
Kumar, Neeraj
Kumar, Nitin
Kumaradevan, Punithakumar
Kunz, Manuela
Kunze, Holger
Kuo, Weicheng
Kurc, Tahsin
Kurmann, Thomas
Kwak, Jin
Kwon, Yongchan
Laadhari, Aymen
Ladikos, Alexander
Lalonde, Rodney
Lamata, Pablo
Langs, Georg
Lartizien, Carole
Lasso, Andras
Lau, Felix
Laura, Cristina
Le, Ngan
Ledig, Christian
Lee, Hansang
Lee, Hyekyoung
Lee, Jong-Hwan
Lee, Kyong
Lee, Minho
Lee, Soochahn
Léger, Étienne
Leger, Stefan
Lei, Baiying
Lekadir, Karim
Lenga, Matthias

Leow, Wee
Lessmann, Nikolas
Li, Annan
Li, Bin
Li, Fuhai
Li, Gang
Li, Guoshi
Li, Hongwei
Li, Hongying
Li, Huiqi
Li, Jian
Li, Jianning
Li, Ke
Li, Minli
Li, Quanzheng
Li, Rongjian
Li, Shaohua
Li, Shulong
Li, Shuyu
Li, Wenqi
Li, Xiang
Li, Xianjun
Li, Xiaojie
Li, Xiaomeng
Li, Xiaoxiao
Li, Xiuli
Li, Yang
Li, Yuexiang
Li, Zhang
Li, Zhi-Cheng
Li, Zhiyuan
Li, Zhjin
Lian, Chunfeng
Liang, Jianming
Liang, Shanshan
Liang, Yudong
Liao, Ruizhi
Liao, Xiangyun
Licandro, Roxane
Lin, Hongxiang
Lin, Lanfen
Lin, Muqing
Lindner, Claudia
Lippert, Christoph
Lisowska, Aneta
Litjens, Geert

Liu, Bin
Liu, Daochang
Liu, Dong
Liu, Dongnan
Liu, Fang
Liu, Feihong
Liu, Feng
Liu, Hong
Liu, Hui
Liu, Jianfei
Liu, Jiang
Liu, Jin
Liu, Jing
Liu, Jundong
Liu, Kefei
Liu, Li
Liu, Mingxia
Liu, Na
Liu, Peng
Liu, Shenghua
Liu, Siqi
Liu, Siyuan
Liu, Tianming
Liu, Tiffany
Liu, Xianglong
Liu, Yixun
Liu, Yong
Liu, Yue
Liu, Zhe
Loddo, Andrea
Lopes, Daniel
Lorenzi, Marco
Lou, Bin
Lu, Allen
Lu, Donghuan
Lu, Jiwen
Lu, Le
Lu, Weijia
Lu, Yao
Lu, Yueh-Hsun
Luo, Gongning
Luo, Jie
Lv, Jinglei
Lyu, Ilwoo
Lyu, Junyan
Ma, Benteng

Ma, Burton
Ma, Da
Ma, Kai
Ma, Xuelin
Mahapatra, Dwarikanath
Mahdavi, Sara
Mahmoud, Ali
Maicas, Gabriel
Maier-Hein, Klaus
Maier, Andreas
Makrogiannis, Sokratis
Malandain, Grégoire
Malik, Bilal
Malpani, Anand
Mancini, Matteo
Manhart, Michael
Manjon, Jose
Mansoor, Awais
Mao, Yunxiang
Martel, Anne
Martinez-Torteya, Antonio
Mathai, Tejas
Mato, David
Mcclelland, Jamie
Mcleod, Jonathan
Medrano-Gracia, Pau
Mehta, Ronak
Meier, Raphael
Melbourne, Andrew
Meng, Qingjie
Meng, Xianjing
Meng, Yu
Menze, Bjoern
Mi, Liang
Miao, Shun
Michielse, Stijn
Midya, Abhishek
Milchenko, Mikhail
Min, Zhe
Miyamoto, Tadashi
Mo, Yuanhan
Molina, Rafael
Montillo, Albert
Moradi, Mehdi
Moreno, Rodrigo
Mortazi, Aliasghar

Mozaffari, Mohammad
Muetzel, Ryan
Müller, Henning
Muñoz-Barrutia, Arrate
Munsell, Brent
Nadeem, Saad
Nahlawi, Layan
Nandakumar, Naresh
Nardi, Giacomo
Neila, Pablo
Ni, Dong
Nichols, Thomas
Nickisch, Hannes
Nie, Dong
Nie, Jingxin
Nie, Weizhi
Niethammer, Marc
Nigam, Aditya
Ning, Lipeng
Niu, Shuaicheng
Niu, Sijie
Noble, Jack
Noblet, Vincent
Novo, Jorge
O'donnell, Thomas
Obeid, Mohammad
Oda, Hirohisa
Oda, Masahiro
Odry, Benjamin
Oeltze-Jafra, Steffen
Oksuz, Ilkay
Oliveira, Marcelo
Oliver, Arnau
Oñativia, Jon
Onofrey, John
Orasanu, Eliza
Orihuela-Espina, Felipe
Orlando, Jose
Osmanlioglu, Yusuf
Otalora, Sebastian
Pace, Danielle
Pagador, J.
Pai, Akshay
Pan, Yongsheng
Pang, Shumao
Papiez, Bartlomiej

Parajuli, Nripesh
Park, Hyunjin
Park, Jongchan
Park, Sanghyun
Park, Seung-Jong
Paschali, Magdalini
Paul, Angshuman
Payer, Christian
Pei, Yuru
Peng, Jialin
Peng, Tingying
Pennec, Xavier
Perdomo, Oscar
Pereira, Sérgio
Pérez-Carrasco, Jose-Antonio
Pesteie, Mehran
Peter, Loic
Peters, Jorg
Petitjean, Caroline
Pezold, Simon
Pfeiffer, Micha
Phellan, Renzo
Phophalia, Ashish
Pisharady, Pramod
Playout, Clement
Pluim, Josien
Pohl, Kilian
Portenier, Tiziano
Pouch, Alison
Prasanna, Prateek
Prevost, Raphael
Ps, Viswanath
Pujades, Sergi
Qi, Xin
Qian, Zhen
Qiang, Yan
Qiao, Lishan
Qiao, Yuchuan
Qin, Chen
Qin, Wenjian
Qirong, Bu
Qiu, Wu
Qu, Liangqiong
Raamana, Pradeep
Rabbani, Hossein
Rackerseder, Julia

Rad, Reza
Rafii-Tari, Hedyeh
Rajpoot, Kashif
Ramachandram, Dhanesh
Ran, Lingyan
Raniga, Parnesh
Rashwan, Hatem
Rathore, Saima
Ratnarajah, Nagulan
Raval, Mehul
Ravikumar, Nishant
Raviprakash, Harish
Raza, Shan
Reaungamornrat, Surreerat
Rekik, Islem
Remeseiro, Beatriz
Rempfler, Markus
Ren, Jian
Ren, Xuhua
Ren, Yudan
Reyes-Aldasoro, Constantino
Reyes, Mauricio
Riedel, Brandalyn
Rieke, Nicola
Risser, Laurent
Rittner, Leticia
Rivera, Diego
Ro, Yong
Robinson, Emma
Robinson, Robert
Rodas, Nicolas
Rodrigues, Rafael
Rohr, Karl
Roohani, Yusuf
Roszkowiak, Lukasz
Roth, Holger
Rouco, José
Roy, Abhijit
Ruijters, Danny
Rusu, Mirabela
Rutter, Erica
S., Sharath
Sabuncu, Mert
Sachse, Frank
Safta, Wiem
Saha, Monjoy

Saha, Pramit
Sahu, Manish
Samani, Abbas
Samek, Wojciech
Sánchez-Margallo, Francisco
Sánchez-Margallo, Juan
Sankaran, Sethuraman
Sanroma, Gerard
Sao, Anil
Sarhan, Mhd
Sarikaya, Duygu
Sarker, Md.
Sato, Imari
Saut, Olivier
Savardi, Mattia
Savitha, Ramasamy
Scarpa, Fabio
Scheinost, Dustin
Scherf, Nico
Schirmer, Markus
Schlaefer, Alexander
Schmid, Jerome
Schnabel, Julia
Schultz, Thomas
Schwartz, Ernst
Sdika, Michael
Sedai, Suman
Sekou, Taibou
Sekuboyina, Anjany
Selvan, Raghavendra
Semedo, Carla
Senouf, Ortal
Seoud, Lama
Sermesant, Maxime
Serrano, Carmen
Sethi, Amit
Shaban, Muhammad
Shaffie, Ahmed
Shah, Meet
Shalaby, Ahmed
Shamir, Reuben
Shan, Hongming
Shao, Yeqin
Sharma, Harshita
Shehata, Mohamed
Shen, Haocheng

Shen, Li
Shen, Mali
Shen, Yiru
Sheng, Ke
Shi, Bibo
Shi, Jun
Shi, Kuangyu
Shi, Xiaoshuang
Shi, Yonggang
Shi, Yonghong
Shigwan, Saurabh
Shin, Hoo-Chang
Shin, Jitae
Shontz, Suzanne
Signoroni, Alberto
Siless, Viviana
Silva, Carlos
Silva, Wilson
Simonovsky, Martin
Simson, Walter
Sinclair, Matthew
Singh, Vivek
Soans, Rajath
Sohel, Ferdous
Sokooti, Hessam
Soliman, Ahmed
Sommen, Fons
Sommer, Stefan
Song, Ming
Song, Yang
Sotiras, Aristeidis
Sparks, Rachel
Spiclin, Ziga
St-Jean, Samuel
Steinbach, Peter
Stern, Darko
Stimpel, Bernhard
Strait, Justin
Studholme, Colin
Styner, Martin
Su, Hai
Su, Yun-Hsuan
Subramanian, Vaishnavi
Subsol, Gérard
Sudre, Carole
Suk, Heung-Il

Sun, Jian
Sun, Li
Sun, Tao
Sung, Kyunghyun
Suter, Yannick
Tajbakhsh, Nima
Tan, Chaowei
Tan, Jiaxing
Tan, Wenjun
Tang, Min
Tang, Sheng
Tang, Thomas
Tang, Xiaoying
Tang, Youbao
Tang, Yuxing
Tang, Zhenyu
Tanner, Christine
Tanno, Ryutaro
Tao, Qian
Tarroni, Giacomo
Tasdizen, Tolga
Thung, Kim
Tian, Jiang
Tian, Yun
Toews, Matthew
Tong, Yubing
Topsakal, Oguzhan
Torosdagli, Neslisah
Toussaint, Nicolas
Troccaz, Jocelyne
Trzcinski, Tomasz
Tulder, Gijs
Tustison, Nick
Tuysuzoglu, Ahmet
Ukwatta, Eranga
Unberath, Mathias
Ungi, Tamas
Upadhyay, Uddeshya
Urschler, Martin
Uslu, Fatmatulzehra
Uyanik, Ilyas
Vaillant, Régis
Vakalopoulou, Maria
Valindria, Vanya
Varela, Marta
Varsavsky, Thomas

Vedula, S.
Vedula, Sanketh
Veeraraghavan, Harini
Vega, Roberto
Veni, Gopalkrishna
Verma, Ujjwal
Vetter, Thomas
Vialard, Francois-Xavier
Villard, Pierre-Frederic
Villarini, Barbara
Virga, Salvatore
Vishnevskiy, Valery
Viswanath, Satish
Vlontzos, Athanasios
Vogl, Wolf-Dieter
Voigt, Ingmar
Vos, Bob
Vrtovec, Tomaz
Wang, Bo
Wang, Changmiao
Wang, Chengjia
Wang, Chunliang
Wang, Dadong
Wang, Guotai
Wang, Haifeng
Wang, Haoqian
Wang, Hongkai
Wang, Hongzhi
Wang, Hua
Wang, Huan
Wang, Jiazhuo
Wang, Jingwen
Wang, Jun
Wang, Junyan
Wang, Kuanquan
Wang, Kun
Wang, Lei
Wang, Li
Wang, Liansheng
Wang, Manning
Wang, Mingliang
Wang, Nizhuan
Wang, Pei
Wang, Puyang
Wang, Ruixuan
Wang, Shanshan

Wang, Sheng
Wang, Shuai
Wang, Wenzhe
Wang, Xiangxue
Wang, Xiaosong
Wang, Xuchu
Wang, Yalin
Wang, Yan
Wang, Yaping
Wang, Yuanjun
Wang, Ze
Wang, Zhe
Wang, Zhinuo
Wang, Zhiwei
Wang, Zilei
Weber, Jonathan
Wee, Chong-Yaw
Weese, Jürgen
Wei, Benzheng
Wei, Dong
Wei, Donglai
Wei, Dongming
Weigert, Martin
Wein, Wolfgang
Wels, Michael
Wemmert, Cédric
Werner, Rene
Wesierski, Daniel
Williams, Bryan
Williams, Jacqueline
Williams, Travis
Williamson, Tom
Wilms, Matthias
Wiskin, James
Wittek, Adam
Wollmann, Thomas
Wolterink, Jelmer
Wong, Ken
Woo, Jonghye
Wu, Guoqing
Wu, Ji
Wu, Jian
Wu, Jiong
Wu, Pengxiang
Wu, Xi
Wu, Ye

Wu, Yicheng
Wuerfl, Tobias
Xi, Xiaoming
Xia, Jing
Xia, Wenfeng
Xiao, Deqiang
Xiao, Yiming
Xie, Hai
Xie, Hongtao
Xie, Jianyang
Xie, Long
Xie, Weidi
Xie, Yiting
Xie, Yuanpu
Xie, Yutong
Xing, Fuyong
Xiong, Tao
Xu, Chenchu
Xu, Jiaofeng
Xu, Jun
Xu, Kele
Xu, Rui
Xu, Ting
Xu, Yan
Xu, Yongchao
Xu, Zheng
Xu, Zhenlin
Xu, Zhoubing
Xu, Ziyue
Xue, Jie
Xue, Wufeng
Xue, Yuan
Yahya, Faridah
Yan, Chenggang
Yan, Ke
Yan, Weizheng
Yan, Yu
Yan, Yuguang
Yan, Zhennan
Yang, Guang
Yang, Guanyu
Yang, Hao-Yu
Yang, Jie
Yang, Lin
Yang, Shan
Yang, Xiao

Yang, Xiaohui
Yang, Xin
Yao, Dongren
Yao, Jianhua
Yao, Jiawen
Ye, Chuyang
Ye, Jong
Ye, Menglong
Ye, Xujiong
Yi, Jingru
Yi, Xin
Ying, Shihui
Yoo, Youngjin
Yousefi, Bardia
Yousefi, Sahar
Yu, Jinhua
Yu, Kai
Yu, Lequan
Yu, Renping
Yu, Weichuan
Yushkevich, Paul
Zanjani, Farhad
Zenati, Marco
Zeng, Dong
Zeng, Guodong
Zettinig, Oliver
Zhan, Liang
Zhang, Baochang
Zhang, Chuncheng
Zhang, Dongqing
Zhang, Fan
Zhang, Haichong
Zhang, Han
Zhang, Haopeng
Zhang, Heye
Zhang, Jianpeng
Zhang, Jiong
Zhang, Jun
Zhang, Le
Zhang, Lichi
Zhang, Mingli
Zhang, Pengyue
Zhang, Pin
Zhang, Qiang
Zhang, Rongzhao
Zhang, Shengping

Zhang, Shu
Zhang, Songze
Zhang, Tianyang
Zhang, Tong
Zhang, Wei
Zhang, Wen
Zhang, Wenlu
Zhang, Xiang
Zhang, Xin
Zhang, Yi
Zhang, Yifan
Zhang, Yizhe
Zhang, Yong
Zhang, Yongqin
Zhang, You
Zhang, Yu
Zhang, Yue
Zhang, Yueyi
Zhang, Yungeng
Zhang, Yunyan
Zhang, Yuyao
Zhang, Zizhao
Zhao, Haifeng
Zhao, Jun
Zhao, Qingyu
Zhao, Rongchang
Zhao, Shijie
Zhao, Shiwan
Zhao, Tengda
Zhao, Wei
Zhao, Yitian
Zhao, Yiyuan

Zhao, Yu
Zhao, Zijian
Zheng, Shenhai
Zheng, Yalin
Zheng, Yinqiang
Zhong, Zichun
Zhou, Bo
Zhou, Jianlong
Zhou, Luping
Zhou, Niyun
Zhou, S.
Zhou, Shoujun
Zhou, Tao
Zhou, Wenjin
Zhou, Yuyin
Zhou, Zhiguo
Zhu, Hancan
Zhu, Junjie
Zhu, Qikui
Zhu, Weifang
Zhu, Wentao
Zhu, Xiaofeng
Zhu, Xinliang
Zhu, Yingying
Zhu, Yuemin
Zhu, Zhuotun
Zhuang, Xiahai
Zia, Aneeq
Zimmer, Veronika
Zolgharni, Massoud
Zou, Ju
Zuluaga, Maria

Accepted MICCAI 2019 Papers

By Region of First Author

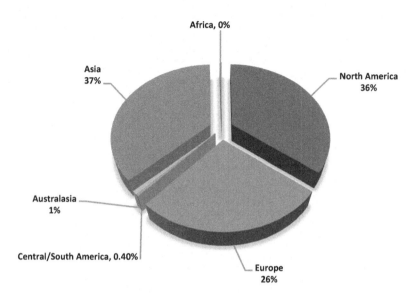

By Technical Keyword

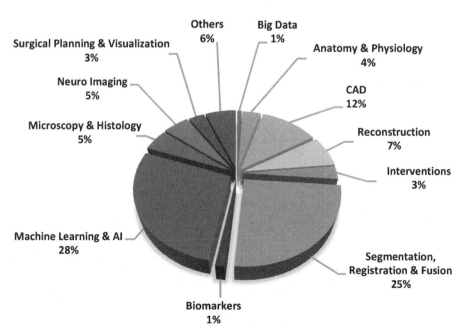

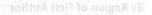
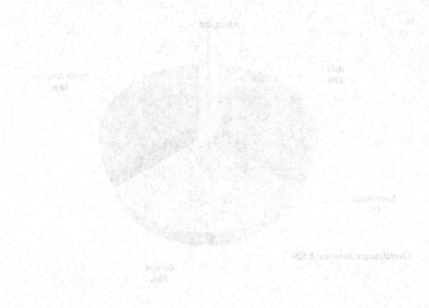
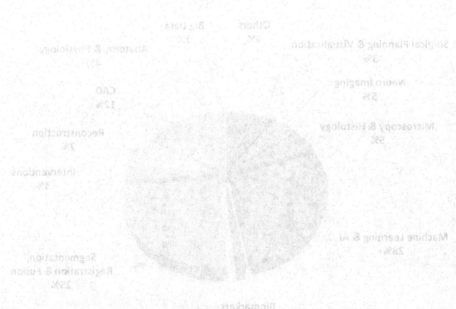

Awards Presented at MICCAI 2018, Granada, Spain

MICCAI Society Enduring Impact Award: The Enduring Impact Award is the highest award of the MICCAI Society. It is a career award for continued excellence in the MICCAI research field. The 2018 Enduring Impact Award was presented to Sandy Wells, Brigham and Women's Hospital/Harvard Medical School, USA.

MICCAI Society Fellowships: MICCAI Fellowships are bestowed annually on a small number of senior members of the society in recognition of substantial scientific contributions to the MICCAI research field and service to the MICCAI community. In 2018, fellowships were awarded to:

- Pierre Jannin (Université de Rennes, France)
- Anne Martel (University of Toronto, Canada)
- Julia Schnabel (King's College London, UK)

Medical Image Analysis Journal Award Sponsored by Elsevier: Jianyu Lin, for his paper entitled "Dual-modality Endoscopic Probe for Tissue Surface Shape Reconstruction and Hyperspectral Imaging Enabled by Deep Neural Networks," authored by Jianyu Lin, Neil T. Clancy, Ji Qi, Yang Hu, Taran Tatla, Danail Stoyanov, Lena Maier-Hein, and Daniel S. Elson.

Best Paper in *International Journal of Computer-Assisted Radiology and Surgery* (IJCARS) journal: Arash Pourtaherian for his paper entitled "Robust and Semantic Needle Detection in 3D Ultrasound Using Orthogonal-Plane Convolutional Neural Networks," authored by Arash Pourtaherian, Farhad Ghazvinian Zanjani, Svitlana Zinger, Nenad Mihajlovic, Gary C. Ng, Hendrikus H. M. Korsten, and Peter H. N. de With.

Young Scientist Publication Impact Award: MICCAI papers by a young scientist from the past 5 years were eligible for this award. It is made to a researcher whose work had an impact on the MICCAI field in terms of citations, secondary citations, subsequent publications, h-index. The 2018 Young Scientist Publication Impact Award was given to Holger R Roth: "A New 2.5D Representation for Lymph Node Detection Using Random Sets of Deep Convolutional Neural Network Observations" authored by Holger R. Roth, Le Lu, Ari Seff, Kevin M. Cherry, Joanne Hoffman, Shijun Wang, Jiamin Liu, Evrim Turkbey, and Ronald M. Summers.

MICCAI Young Scientist Awards: The Young Scientist Awards are stimulation prizes awarded for the best first authors of MICCAI contributions in distinct subject areas. The nominees had to be full-time students at a recognized university at, or within, two years prior to submission. The 2018 MICCAI Young Scientist Awards were given to:

- Erik J. Bekkers for the paper entitled: "Roto-Translation Covariant Convolutional Networks for Medical Image Analysis"
- Bastian Bier for the paper entitled: "X-ray-transform Invariant Anatomical Landmark Detection for Pelvic Trauma Surgery"

- Yuanhan Mo for his paper entitled: "The Deep Poincaré Map: A Novel Approach for Left Ventricle Segmentation"
- Tanya Nair for the paper entitled: "Exploring Uncertainty Measures in Deep Networks for Multiple Sclerosis Lesion Detection and Segmentation"
- Yue Zhang for the paper entitled: "Task-Driven Generative Modeling for Unsupervised Domain Adaptation: Application to X-ray Image Segmentation"

Contents – Part II

Image Registration

Cardiovascular Imaging

Image Segmentation

Searching Learning Strategy with Reinforcement Learning for 3D Medical Image Segmentation

Dong Yang, Holger Roth, Ziyue Xu, Fausto Milletari, Ling Zhang, and Daguang Xu[✉]

NVIDIA, Bethesda, USA
daguangx@nvidia.com

Abstract. Deep neural network (DNN) based approaches have been widely investigated and deployed in medical image analysis. For example, fully convolutional neural networks (FCN) achieve the state-of-the-art performance in several applications of 2D/3D medical image segmentation. Even the baseline neural network models (U-Net, V-Net, etc.) have been proven to be very effective and efficient when the training process is set up properly. Nevertheless, to fully exploit the potentials of neural networks, we propose an automated searching approach for the optimal training strategy with reinforcement learning. The proposed approach can be utilized for tuning hyper-parameters, and selecting necessary data augmentation with certain probabilities. The proposed approach is validated on several tasks of 3D medical image segmentation. The performance of the baseline model is boosted after searching, and it can achieve comparable accuracy to other manually-tuned state-of-the-art segmentation approaches.

1 Introduction

Medical image segmentation plays an important role in research and clinical practice and is necessary for tasks such as disease diagnosis, treatment planning, guidance, and surgery. Researchers have been developing various automated and semi-automated approaches for 2D/3D medical image segmentation. Among the prevailing approaches, deep neural networks (DNNs) have been successfully deployed for image/volume segmentation during past few years [3]. Deep neural networks are capable to not only achieve state-of-the-art accuracy at inference but also to deliver results in a quick and efficient manner due to readily available GPU-accelerated computing routines. So far, many baseline neural network models [10,11,13] have been created and validated for various segmentation applications. However, training such models requires careful design of the work-flow, and setup of data augmentation, learning rate, loss functions, optimizer and so on. To achieve state-of-the-art performance, the model hyper-parameters need to be well-tuned, based either on extensive experimentation and grid parameter search or heuristics stemming from specific domain knowledge and expertise.

© Springer Nature Switzerland AG 2019
D. Shen et al. (Eds.): MICCAI 2019, LNCS 11765, pp. 3–11, 2019.
https://doi.org/10.1007/978-3-030-32245-8_1

Recent works indicate that the full potential of current state-of-the-art network models may not yet be well-explored. For instance, the winning solution of the *Medical Decathlon Challenge* [1, 6] (consisting of ten 3D image segmentation tasks) is using ensembles of 2D/3D U-Net only, and elaborate engineering designs. The argument raised by such work is that the potentials of the successful baseline models may be neglected. This argument cannot be easily confirmed since the theoretical explanation of deep neural network has not been well-established. Therefore, although the current research trend is to develop elaborate and powerful 3D segmentation network models (within GPU memory limit), it is also very important to pay attentions to the details of model training.

Automatic Machine Learning (AutoML) has been recently proposed to automatically search the best learning approaches and minimize human interaction at the same time. Different approaches [7–9, 12, 16, 17] have been introduced in computer vision to search for the best neural network architecture for image analysis and scene understanding tasks. Unlike specifically designed networks (e.g. ResNet [5]), the often peculiar neural architectures resulting from the automatic search process can achieve state-of-the-art performance for tasks at hand.

Since 3D segmentation is very expensive to train, efficient 3D architecture search is extremely difficult to attain. Instead, a more feasible task is represented by hyper-parameter searching which still plays a central role on the test-time performance. In this work, we propose a reinforcement learning-based approach to search the best training strategy of deep neural networks for a specific 3D medical image segmentation task. Training strategies include the learning rate, data augmentation strategies, data pre-processing, etc. In the proposed framework, an additional recurrent neural network (RNN) - the controller - is trained to generate hyper-parameters of the training strategies. The reward signal supplied during training to our RL-based controller is the validation accuracy of segmentation network. The RNN is trained with the reward and observation (the previous set of training strategies). Finally, the best strategy is generated once the searching process is done.

2   Related Work

In machine learning, the hyper-parameter optimization has been studies for years, and several approaches have been developed such as grid search, Bayesian optimization, random search and so on [2]. The main idea of grid search and random search is using brute force to enumerate possible hyper-parameter combinations in order to determine the one with the best validation accuracy. They can be naturally implemented in parallel. However, in practice, such approaches only work well within a low-dimensional searching space and they becomes extremely impractical once the searching space is large with a high dimension. Bayesian optimization like *Gaussian Processes* (GP) normally generate better results in fewer steps comparing with the "brute-force" approaches because the feedback from each training process is actually used for updating posterior functions, and generating the next parameter settings for searching. On the other hand, it requires the definition of a prior function to describe the behaviors of the objective, and the final performance relies heavily on the choice of this prior.

Recently, researchers proposed reinforcement learning (RL) based approaches for neural architecture searching [12,16,17]. In principle, a RNN-based agent/policy collects the information (reward, state) from the environment, update the weights within itself, and creates the next potential neural architectures for validation. The searching objectives are the parameters of the convolutional kernels, and how they are connected one-by-one. The validation output is utilized as the reward to update the agent/policy. The RL related approaches fit such scenario since there is no ground truth for the neural architectures with the best validation performance. In order to avoid the request of huge amounts of GPU hours, researchers also investigated more efficient ways to conduct neural architecture search. The progressive neural architecture search introduced a new way to construct new neural architecture on the fly during training [8]. Furthermore, the differentiable architecture search presented a searching strategy through learning a weighted sum of potential components, and finalizing a discrete architecture with arg max operations. However, there might be an unexpected gap between the "continuous" and discretized architectures in specific applications. In addition, the differentiable architecture search requires to load all possible neural components during training, which potentially takes a lot of GPU memory, especially in 3D image processing. Alternatively, RL based approaches can be applied to the tasks of optimizing other parts of neural network model training, such as data augmentation policies [4] and design of loss functions [15] in order to bypass some limitations of differentiable architecture search.

3   Methodology

In this section, we firstly introduce the definition of the searching space in our framework and then describe the RNN controller, and how the searching procedure is achieved using RL. The proposed approach is inspired by the work "auto-augment" [4]. We expand its original idea and apply our extended version to 3D medical image segmentation.

3.1   Searching Space Definition

The upper-bound performance of a machine learning model is always directly limited by the hyper-parameter setup during training. For example, the learning rate for weight updates is critical for achieving decent performance in most deep learning applications. The conventional way to determine hyper-parameters is to use domain knowledge and necessary heuristics. However, some of the hyper-parameters are often highly related to the dataset itself, which may not be easily understood by humans. Thus, we propose to automatically search within certain hyper-parameter spaces, to ease the burden for setting those numbers.

In our setting, given a parameter λ, the maximum value λ_{max} and minimum value λ_{min} are required. Then the range between λ_{max} and λ_{min} is mapped to $[0, 1]$. The floating number λ^* is the searching target with the optimal performance. For a set of hyper-parameters $\Lambda = \{\lambda_1, \lambda_2, ...\}$, the searching objective is $\Lambda^* = \{\lambda_1^*, \lambda_2^*, ...\}$. Each λ_i^* may not be optimal for that specific parameter, since greedy-type searching algorithms may lead to sub-optimal performance. Therefore, it is necessary to search for all the hyper-parameter jointly.

Firstly, we consider the parameters for data augmentation, which is an important component for training neural networks in 3D medical image segmentation as it increases the robustness of the models and avoids overfitting [6]. Augmentation includes image sharpening, image smoothing, adding Gaussian noise, contrast adjustment, and random shift of intensity range, etc. We assign a probability value p_i to each augmentation approach to determine how likely the corresponding augmentation will occur. During training, a random number $r_i \in (0, 1)$ for the ith augmentation approach is generated at each iteration. If $r_i \geq a$, the augmentation is executed; if $r_i < a$, this augmentation will not be conducted. In this way, we can have information about the relative importance between different augmentation approaches according to the specific dataset or application. Secondly, we found the learning rate α is also critical for medical image segmentation. Sometimes, large network models favor a large α for activation, and small datasets prefer small α. Once α_{max} and α_{min} are determined, the searching range of α is set and mapped to $(0, 1)$. Similar treatment can be applied to any possible hyperparameters in the training process for optimization. Moreover, unlike other approaches, we search for the optimal hyper-parameters in the high-dimensional continuous space instead of discrete space.

Algorithm 1. RL based training strategy searching

Result: Optimal training strategy C^*, given a dataset D
1 Set MAX_EPOCH $= 1000$, EPOCH $= 0$;
2 Random initialization $C_1, C_2, C_3, \cdots$;
3 Launch training jobs $T(C_1), T(C_2), T(C_3), \cdots$;
4 **while** EPOCH $<$ MAX_EPOCH **do**
5 $\quad$ Collect validation accuracy $V_i = T(C_i)$ from a finished job;
6 $\quad$ Update weights of RNN controller;
7 $\quad$ Generate a new training strategy C_j;
8 $\quad$ Launch a training job $T(C_j)$;
9 $\quad$ EPOCH $=$ EPOCH $+ 1$;
10 **end**

3.2 RL Based Searching Approach

Because there is no ground truth for the optimal validation accuracy, RL fits the scenario to derive the optimal training strategy/configuration C given specific dataset D. Our searching approach is shown in Algorithm 1. During the process, an RNN-based job controller H is created for communicating with different launched jobs. In the beginning, H launches n training jobs with randomly

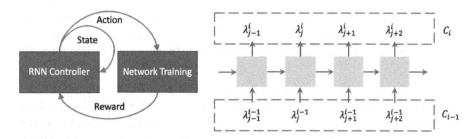

Fig. 1. Left: the communication between training jobs and RNN controller H. The RNN controller provides the action and state for next step, and network training produces a reward for H. Right: previous training strategy C_{i-1} is the input of H, and output is the next strategy C_i after updating the weights.

initialized training configurations C_i. C_i can be defined as a vector, and each element is sampled from one dimension of the aforementioned searching space. Also, C_i is sufficient to accomplish each training job T. After training, the validation accuracy $V = T(C_i)$ is returned to H for updating the weights of the RNN in controller, and generating a new strategy C for future training epochs.

Our framework is shown in Fig. 1. For the RL setting, the reward is the validation accuracy, the action is the newly generated C_i, environment observation/state is C_{i-1} from the last step, and the policy is the RNN job controller H. H is a basic recurrent unit with one hidden layer. And the input nodes (observation) and output nodes (action) of H share the same quantity. Each output node produces two-channel outputs after softmax activation. Then the first channel of the output is fed to the next step as action after mapping back to the original searching space. The *Proximal Policy Optimization* (PPO) is adopted to train the RNN cells in H [14]. The loss function is as follows.

$$\theta \leftarrow \theta + \gamma r \nabla_\theta \ln H (C_i | C_{i-1}, \theta) \tag{1}$$

Here, θ represents the weights in RNN. During training, the reward r is utilized to update the weights using gradient back-propagation. To train the RNN controller, we use RMSprop as the optimizer with a learning rate γ of 0.1.

4 Experimental Evaluation

Datasets. The medical decathlon challenge (MSD) provides ten different tasks on 3D CT/MR image segmentation [1]. Datasets of task02 (left atrium segmentation), task06 (lung tumor segmentation), task07 (pancreas and tumor segmentation), and task09 (spleen segmentation) are used with our own random split for training/validation. For task02, 16 MR volumes for training, 4 for validation. For task06, 50 CT volumes for training, 13 for validation. For task07, 224 CT volumes for training, 57 for validation. And for task09, 32 CT volumes for training, 9 for validation. We re-sample both the images and labels into the isotropic resolution 1.0 mm. The voxel intensities of the images are normalized to the range [0, 1] according to the following input ranges: 5th and 95th percentile of overall voxel intensities for MRI and −1000 and 1000 Hounsfield units for CT.

Implementation. Our baseline model follows the work the 2D-3D hybrid network proposed in [10], but without the *PSP* component. The pre-trained ResNet-50 (on ImageNet) possesses a powerful capability for feature extraction as the encoder. And the 3D decoder network with *DenseBlock* provides smooth 3D predictions. The input of the network are $96 \times 96 \times 96$ patches, randomly cropped from the re-sampled images during training. Meanwhile, the validation step follows the scanning window scheme with a small overlap (one quarter of a patch). By default, all training jobs use the Adam optimizer, and the Dice loss is used for gradient computing [11]. The validation accuracy is measured with the Dice's score after scanning window. Our method is implemented with TensorFlow and trained on NVIDIA V100 GPUs with 16 GB memory.

Firstly, we compare the proposed approach with the local searching approaches, shown in Table 1. The hill climbing algorithm is a classical greedy search technique. It is more efficient than grid or random search if the initial position is properly set. We implemented two versions: discrete searching and continuous searching. The discrete version assumes the searching space is discrete with fixed dimension, and step size at each move is fixed. In our setting, the dimension of the searching space for one parameter is 100, and the step size is 0.01. At each move, the target value cannot go above 1.0 or below 0.0. The continuous version uses an adaptive step. If the moving direction improves the value, the step size will be multiplied by 1.1, otherwise, it will be divided by 1.1. The searching space has to be positive for the continuous version. Both versions stop when the local minimum is reached after convergence.

To save searching time, we start the searching process from a pre-trained model trained after 500 epochs without any augmentation or parameter searching. In Table 1, "no augmentation" indicates the performance of the pre-trained model. In our proposed approach, each job fine-tunes the pre-trained model with 200 epochs with its training strategy. To make a fair comparison, the initial status before searching is set to 0.5 for all parameters to search (the searching space for learning rate is [0.01, 0.0001]). After searching, our approach outperforms other baseline approaches according to the overall Dice's score in the validation dataset in the tested applications. The maximum epoch number in our approach is set as 400, which takes circa 24 h to finish searching with 32 GPUs running in parallel. The baseline approach normally takes longer time because of the large searching space and small step size being employed.

Secondly, we conduct another experiment with three different datasets to validate the effectiveness of our proposed approach for the models trained from scratch. "Routine" means all the searched parameters are fixed as 0.5 (learning rate is set as 0.0001), and the model is trained from scratch. Our proposed approach searches from the same setting as "routine". The maximum epoch number is 100 in our approach. And the entire searching procedure takes about

Table 1. Performance comparison with baseline approaches and our proposed approach. The validation accuracy is the overall average Dice's score among different subjects and classes.

MSD task02		MSD task09	
Method	Validation acc.	Method	Validation acc.
No augmentation	0.88	No augmentation	0.87
Discrete hill climbing	0.90	Discrete hill climbing	0.90
Continuous hill climbing	0.90	Continuous hill climbing	0.92
Proposed approach	**0.92**	Proposed approach	**0.92**

48 h with 50 GPUs. All training jobs are trained with 800 epochs. We can see that the models after searching work better, and the fixed parameter is clearly not optimal for these applications. From the resulting parameters after the search, we can see clearly that each application has a preference for different augmentations or hyper-parameters. For instance, the task09 is the spleen segmentation in CT. According to CT imaging quality, the training strategy containing a random intensity scale shift would perform better. The similar conclusion can be achieved from other CT datasets (e.g. task06, task07). For MRI segmentation, the image sharpening is preferable as can be seen from the resulting training strategy. The reason might be that the MRI quality varies a lot, and sharpening operation can strengthen the region-of-interest, especially the boundary regions.

Table 2. Performance comparison of models training from scratch with or without using our proposed approach. The validation accuracy is the overall average Dice's score among different subjects and classes.

MSD task06		MSD task07		MSD task09	
Method	Validation acc.	Method	Validation acc.	Method	Validation acc.
Routine	0.383	Routine	0.491	Routine	0.957
Proposed	**0.449**	Proposed	**0.519**	Proposed	**0.960**

The same task, task09, is used in both, the first and second experiment. From the Tables 1 and 2, we can see training from scratch with augmentation could achieve a higher Dice's score compared with the one fine-tuned from a "no-augmentation" model. This suggests that the found data augmentation strategy is effective when applied to training from scratch.

5   Conclusions

In this paper, we proposed a RL-based searching approach to optimize the training strategy for 3D medical image segmentation. The proposed approach has been validated on several segmentation tasks with clear effectiveness. It also possesses large potentials to be applied for general machine learning problems. For example, the heuristic parts of any learning algorithm can be easily determined after optimization or searching, given a specific medical imaging application. Moreover, extending the single-value reward function to a multi-dimensional reward function could be studied as the future direction.

References

1. Medical decathlon challenge (2018). http://medicaldecathlon.com
2. Bergstra, J.S., Bardenet, R., Bengio, Y., Kégl, B.: Algorithms for hyper-parameter optimization. In: Advances in Neural Information Processing Systems, pp. 2546–2554 (2011)
3. Choy, G., et al.: Current applications and future impact of machine learning in radiology. Radiology **288**(2), 318–328 (2018). https://doi.org/10.1148/radiol.2018171820
4. Cubuk, E.D., Zoph, B., Mane, D., Vasudevan, V., Le, Q.V.: Autoaugment: learning augmentation policies from data. arXiv preprint arXiv:1805.09501 (2018)
5. He, K., Zhang, X., Ren, S., Sun, J.: Deep residual learning for image recognition. In: Proceedings of the IEEE Conference on Computer Vision and Pattern Recognition, pp. 770–778 (2016). https://doi.org/10.1109/cvpr.2016.90
6. Isensee, F., et al.: nnU-Net: self-adapting framework for U-Net-based medical image segmentation. arXiv preprint arXiv:1809.10486 (2018)
7. Liu, C., et al.: Auto-DeepLab: hierarchical neural architecture search for semantic image segmentation. arXiv preprint arXiv:1901.02985 (2019)
8. Liu, C., et al.: Progressive neural architecture search. In: Ferrari, V., Hebert, M., Sminchisescu, C., Weiss, Y. (eds.) ECCV 2018. LNCS, vol. 11205, pp. 19–35. Springer, Cham (2018). https://doi.org/10.1007/978-3-030-01246-5_2
9. Liu, H., Simonyan, K., Yang, Y.: DARTS: differentiable architecture search. arXiv preprint arXiv:1806.09055 (2018)
10. Liu, S., et al.: 3D anisotropic hybrid network: transferring convolutional features from 2D images to 3D anisotropic volumes. In: Frangi, A.F., Schnabel, J.A., Davatzikos, C., Alberola-López, C., Fichtinger, G. (eds.) MICCAI 2018. LNCS, vol. 11071, pp. 851–858. Springer, Cham (2018). https://doi.org/10.1007/978-3-030-00934-2_94
11. Milletari, F., Navab, N., Ahmadi, S.A.: V-Net: fully convolutional neural networks for volumetric medical image segmentation. In: 2016 Fourth International Conference on 3D Vision (3DV), pp. 565–571. IEEE (2016). https://doi.org/10.1109/3dv.2016.79
12. Pham, H., Guan, M., Zoph, B., Le, Q., Dean, J.: Efficient neural architecture search via parameter sharing. In: International Conference on Machine Learning, pp. 4092–4101 (2018)
13. Ronneberger, O., Fischer, P., Brox, T.: U-Net: convolutional networks for biomedical image segmentation. In: Navab, N., Hornegger, J., Wells, W.M., Frangi, A.F. (eds.) MICCAI 2015. LNCS, vol. 9351, pp. 234–241. Springer, Cham (2015). https://doi.org/10.1007/978-3-319-24574-4_28
14. Schulman, J., Wolski, F., Dhariwal, P., Radford, A., Klimov, O.: Proximal policy optimization algorithms. arXiv preprint arXiv:1707.06347 (2017)

15. Xu, H., Zhang, H., Hu, Z., Liang, X., Salakhutdinov, R., Xing, E.: AutoLoss: learning discrete schedules for alternate optimization. arXiv preprint arXiv:1810.02442 (2018)
16. Zoph, B., Le, Q.V.: Neural architecture search with reinforcement learning. arXiv preprint arXiv:1611.01578 (2016)
17. Zoph, B., Vasudevan, V., Shlens, J., Le, Q.V.: Learning transferable architectures for scalable image recognition. In: Proceedings of the IEEE Conference on Computer Vision and Pattern Recognition, pp. 8697–8710 (2018). https://doi.org/10.1109/cvpr.2018.00907

Comparative Evaluation of Hand-Engineered and Deep-Learned Features for Neonatal Hip Bone Segmentation in Ultrasound

Houssam El-Hariri[1][(✉)], Kishore Mulpuri[2], Antony Hodgson[3], and Rafeef Garbi[1]

[1] Department of Electrical and Computer Engineering,
University of British Columbia, Vancouver, BC, Canada
houssam@ece.ubc.ca
[2] Department of Orthopedic Surgery, BC Children's Hospital,
Vancouver, BC, Canada
[3] Department of Mechanical Engineering, University of British Columbia,
Vancouver, BC, Canada

Abstract. Developmental dysplasia of the hip (DDH) is one of the most common congenital disorders seen in newborns. Undetected cases may lead to serious consequences including limping, leg length discrepancy, pain, osteoarthritis, disability, and total hip replacement. Diagnosis typically relies on ultrasound (US) screening of the infant hip between 0–4 months of age. An inexpensive and safe non-ionizing modality, US imaging enables measurement of DDH metrics based on hip bone features such as the α angle. Though DDH assessment remains mostly a manual process in clinical practice, notorious for its significant operator variability, a number of automated measurement methods were recently proposed. These computational methods rely on highly engineered, hand-crafted features most notable of which are phase-based bone image features. Though promising, especially as they were shown to significantly reduce user variability, challenges remain with regards to robustness, as well as generalizability to new data. To improve bone localization, from which the metrics are calculated, we first build upon recent phase-based feature extraction by applying spatial anatomical priors to eliminate false positives and accurately segment the ilium and acetabulum contour. Second, we propose the use of deep-learned features, using the popular U-Net with single and multi-channel inputs. We observe superior performance of deep-learned features compared to the enhanced engineered features including shadow peak and confidence-weighted phase symmetry. We present quantitative evaluation on extensive data from two clinical datasets collected with two different ultrasound probes as part of a study we performed on a cohort of 103 pediatric patients.

D. Shen et al. (Eds.): MICCAI 2019, LNCS 11765, pp. 12–20, 2019.
https://doi.org/10.1007/978-3-030-32245-8_2

1 Introduction

Developmental dysplasia of the hip (DDH) is one of the most common disorders seen in newborns, with prevalence up to about 3% [3], and incidence up to about 7.5% in some populations, ranging widely between populations [4]. Undetected or late cases lead to serious consequences for the patient and family including limping, leg length discrepancy, pain, frequent operations, osteoarthritis, disability, and total hip replacement. Traditionally, the standard metric for clinical diagnosis is the α angle, defined as the angle between the vertical cortex of the ilium and acetabular roof, measured from a coronal ultrasound image of the hip. More recently, three-dimensional (3D) US has been proposed as an alternative to two-dimensional (2D) US for more reproducible DDH measurement [5,8]. Typically, a prerequisite for extracting DDH metrics such as the α angle is accurate segmentation of the ilium and acetabulum bone surfaces. Manual annotation of bone surfaces is laborious and time consuming, particularly in 3D data, as well as error-prone potentially affecting DDH diagnosis. Therefore, accurate, robust, and efficient automatic segmentation is crucial.

Several works have explored automatic segmentation in neonatal hip ultrasound for DDH diagnosis, which presents unique challenges due to the partially cartilaginous composition of neonatal bone. Hand-engineered phase features were proposed, of which a prominent example is the confidence-weighted structured phase symmetry (CSPS) feature proposed by Quader et al. [9]. CSPS combined SPS, an orientation-independent variant of phase symmetry (PS) designed to segment non-planar bone structures, with bone shadowing features reducing soft tissue false positives. Quader incorporated this method into an automated system for α_{3D} angle measurement and showed much improved reproducibility over the analogous α_{2D} angle [8]. More recently, Pandey et al. [6] proposed Shadow Peak (SP), a simplified method that uses only bone shadowing features to segment bone, and has shown certain improvements in accuracy and speed over CSPS in a limited study. Though promising, these methods still rely on highly engineered hand-crafted features hence challenges remain with regards to robustness and generalizability to new data, as we later show.

Data-driven methods have also been proposed for this task. In [2], Hareendranathan et al. proposed using superpixel classification with a deep Convolutional Neural Network (CNN) and reported a Hausdorff distance of $2.1 \pm 0.9\,\mathrm{mm}$ between contours. Zhang et al. [12] proposed a neural network based on Mask R-CNN and compared to the popular architectures FCN-32s and U-Net but they reported very poor Dice scores of 0.386 for their network, compared to 0.049 with U-Net and 0.223 with FCN-32s (we note that their results contradict our own tests and findings, as will be presented later).

Our goal is to improve DDH measurement reliability in ultrasound, and towards this end a crucial prerequisite is accurate bone localization. In this paper, we test the hypothesis that deep-learned features can localize bone more accurately than current state-of-the-art phase- and shadow-based features for this task, and whether this technique performs equally well when applied to different ultrasound probes. We first build upon recent phase-based feature extraction by applying spatial anatomical priors to eliminate false positives and accurately segment the ilium and acetabulum bone surface contour. Second, we propose the use of deep-learned features, using U-Net with single and multi-channel inputs. We present quantitative evaluation on extensive data from two clinical datasets collected with two different ultrasound probes as part of a clinical study we performed on a cohort of 103 pediatric patients.

2 Methods

2.1 Data Acquisition

With all required research ethics board approvals in place, we collected data from 84 neonates with an Ultrasonix 4DL14-5/38 3D ultrasound probe (BK Ultrasound, Richmond, BC, Canada). Inclusion criteria required participants to be between 0–4 months chronological age and suspected of having DDH, which constituted having family history of DDH, being born breech, or with Caesarean section. We excluded infants with other congenital defects. Our imaging protocol included scanning both hips of each patient, with each hip scanned multiple times, for a total of 1,775 3D US volumes. Each volume included on average 214 2D coronal slices for a total of 379,364 coronal slices. Volumes were collected at multiple depths (40–52 mm) and were of resolution 0.16 mm/voxel. In addition to this main dataset, we collected data of 19 neonates from another patient group using a Clarius L7 wireless portable probe (Clarius Mobile Health, Burnaby, BC), which comprised 72 2D US coronal scans. This dataset was also collected at variable depths (40–70 mm). Both datasets were collected by experienced ultrasound technicians.

2.2 Hand-Crafted Features

We include CSPS and SP in our comparisons given their consistently good performance on neonatal hip ultrasound [6,9]. Both methods tend to localize hip bone surfaces well but suffer from significant false positive responses at soft tissue, e.g. labrum and other irrelevant bone structures like the femur. To improve performance we incorporate the spatial prior that the ilium and acetabulum are a continuous bone structure that always appears as the most medial (or deepest with respect to the probe) and superior bone in the image.

To apply this spatial prior, we start with the observation that SP only detects one structure along each vertical scan line, which due to its high acoustic impedance is likely to be bone. The hip bone is the most superior connected component of the SP segmentation. To find this region, we first define the set of k regions $CC = \{CC_1, ..., CC_i, ..., CC_k\}$ obtained by applying connected component analysis to the SP binary segmentation mask, with 8-connectivity test in 2D and 26-connectivity in 3D. We further define the corresponding set of their centroids $C = \{c_1, ..., c_i, ..., c_k\}$, with $c_i = (x_i, y_i)$, and the corresponding set of x-components of the centroids $X = \{x_1, ..., x_i, ..., x_k\}$. We find the hip contour

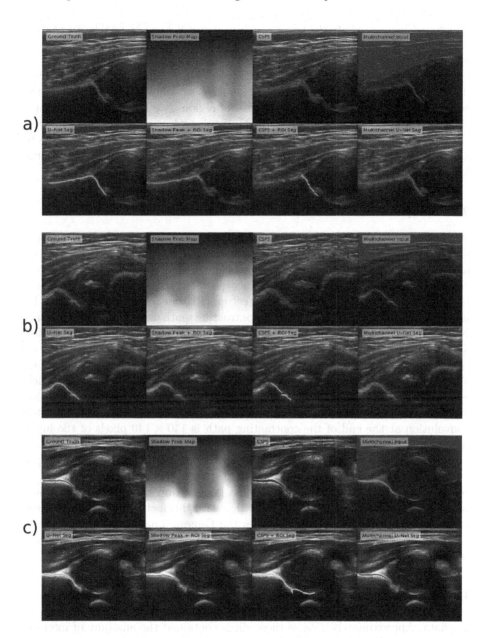

Fig. 1. Example segmentation results. (a, b) different segmentation techniques including Shadow Peak, Phase Symmetry, and U-Net applied to Ultrasonix test data. (c) the same techniques applied to Clarius test data. Some common failures with CSPS shown here are false positives at muscles, pulvinar fat, labrum, and femur; under-segmented ilium; and fragmented segmentation. With SP, the acetabulum is often under-segmented as shown here. U-Net segmentation is more accurate and closely matches the ground truth.

region as CC_{xmin}, where the index $xmin = argmin(X)$. The final segmentation with SP is obtained by converting this connected region CC_{xmin} to a binary mask.

For CSPS, we first threshold the CSPS map to obtain a binary mask. Similarly, we apply connected component analysis to obtain a set of connected regions. To find the hip bone from this set of regions, we leverage the segmentation previously obtained from SP of the hip bone, CC_{xmin}, as a region-of-interest (RoI), and use it to find the CSPS region with most overlap. We convert this to a binary mask, and to eliminate any soft tissue connected to the bone, we only keep the most medial (deepest) pixel along each scan line.

2.3 Deep Learned Features

Architecture. We use the U-Net architecture for our task of segmenting the ilium and acetabulum [10]. We choose U-Net for its proven performance on medical image data, ability to train on very few training samples, and for direct comparison with a recent paper that has attempted to use U-Net for DDH segmentation [12]. As in the original architecture [10], our implementation includes nine convolution blocks, five in the contracting path and four corresponding blocks in the expanding path. Each block is made up of six layers in the following order: conv3x3-batchnorm-ReLU-conv3x3-batchnorm-ReLU, in contrast to the original architecture which did not include batch normalization layers. We use stride 1 for the 3x3 convolutions. We use max pooling with 2x2 kernels and stride 2 in the contracting path, and corresponding transposed convolution layers in the expanding path. With this configuration, the receptive field of the convolution at the end of the contracting path is 140×140 pixels of the input image whose size is 250×250. The number of feature maps in the nine blocks is 64-128-256-512-1024-512-256-128-64. We explore training U-Net with two types of inputs: (1) Raw B-mode image data, and (2) a multi-channel input based on results from several recent papers [1,11] on bone segmentation that have shown much improved accuracy of bone localization with this method. In our implementation, the multi-channel input includes the B-mode image, the corresponding SPS, and shadow confidence map features in the R, G, B channels, respectively (see Fig. 1).

U-Net Training. To prepare data, we start with 231,384 coronal slices, obtained with the Ultrasonix probe from 59 neonate scans as potential training data. Approximately 25% of these slices contained the anatomy of interest, so we filter out all other slices with a recently proposed recurrent neural network (RNN) scan adequacy architecture [7]. We randomly select 500 such adequate slices, from which a trained user manually labelled the ilium and acetabulum bone contour. To aid with this manual training data labelling step, whose reproducibility is known to be low, we overlaid the PS features on the B-mode image to help guide the user while allowing flexibility to deviate from PS features should the user deem suitable. Further we allow the user to reject inadequate slices not detected by the RNN from the training set. In summary, we end up with 439 adequate, labelled samples in our training set from the Ultrasonix set. We intentionally did not include Clarius samples in the training set to test generalizability of U-Net on different domains. We subsequently dilate the manually traced contours as originally proposed by Villa to alleviate the class imbalance problem [11], the imbalance between the number of contour and background pixels, converting our bone contour to a ribbon-like structure. We train U-Net on both B-mode input only, as well as the multi-channel input. We select Dice loss, Adam optimizer, two-slice batch size, with learning rate of 0.0001 over 30 epochs, and resize the input images to 250×250.

2.4   Evaluation Scheme

We contrasted segmentation accuracy of five methods: original CSPS (with naive thresholding), CSPS after applying the RoI prior, SP with RoI prior, U-Net with only B-mode input, and U-Net with multi-channel input data. Our first test set was prepared from 880 3D ultrasound volumes (from 25 neonate patients) using the Ultrasonix 4DL14-5/38 probe, not overlapping with patients in the training set. Similar to the training data, we filtered inadequate slices with the RNN approach, randomly selected a subset of adequate slices, on which the same user manually delineated the contours. A final total of 103 labelled samples constituted this primary test set. We also prepared a secondary test set using data from the Clarius L7 probe, constituting 72 2D US images from a different pool of 19 neonates.

Following segmentation using the contrasted methods, we performed simple post-processing to convert the output segmentation map output of U-Net to a crisp contour. Specifically, we threshold the probability map at 0.5, skeletonize, and prune the resulting binary mask to generate a contour. We use classification metrics as well as distance metrics to assess segmentation accuracy, specifically, the Dice-Sorensen Coefficient, Jaccard Index, Precision, and Recall. Since these metrics were designed for blob-type segmentation, we first dilated the contours, dilating both ground truth and test masks by the same amount. We applied distance metrics directly to the extracted contours, including the Hausdorff Distance and Vertical Root Mean Square Error (VRMSE), defined as the root mean squared vertical distance between the ground truth and test contours at every scan line that contains both contours.

3   Results and Discussion

Quantitative results for both the Ultrasonix and Clarius probe datasets are summarized in Table 1. Across all evaluation metrics, the B-mode U-Net and multi-channel U-Net appeared to be virtually tied for best performance, and appeared to perform well consistently as evident by the reduced standard deviations. CSPS suffered from significant soft tissue false positives despite its use of shadow features, which explains its high recall but low precision rates, but we observe that precision was much improved after applying the RoI, with a small drop in recall.

To evaluate generalizability, we tested our model trained only on the Ultrasonix data on a secondary test set from obtained with the Clarius probe. We saw a similar pattern on this secondary Clarius set, with U-Net and multichannel U-Net outperforming the other methods. Although not directly comparable, as the Clarius dataset was comprised of only 2D US optimal coronal images of the infant hip, whereas the Ultrasonix dataset is 3D and contained coronal slices away from the optimal central slice, these results still provides some evidence that U-Net is likely capable of generalizing to image data from probes not included in the training set.

We show exemplar qualitative results on both Ultrasonix and Clarius data in Fig. 1. To extract the α angle, it is crucial for the segmentation algorithm to accurately delineate the ilium-acetabulum vertex, and enough of the ilium and acetabulum surfaces surrounding it, while simultaneously not capturing any false positive soft tissue or unrelated bone such as the femur. It is subsequently crucial to reduce outliers and carefully assess failure cases beyond mere aggregate quantitative measures comparisons such as those in Table 1. For CSPS, common failure cases included soft tissue false positives; completely missing the ilium when rotated at certain angles; as well as fragmented contour, as shown in Fig. 1. Similarly, SP often missed the acetabulum due to weak shadow in that

Table 1. Mean (and standard deviation) segmentation accuracy of five methods we tested on the primary and secondary datasets. From left to right: (1) Shadow Peak with RoI spatial prior, (2) Confidence-Weighted Structured Phase Symmetry with naive thresholding, (3) Confidence-Weighted Structured Phase Symmetry with RoI spatial prior, (4) U-Net with B-mode input, (5) U-Net with multi-channel input. Best performers along each row are bolded.

	SP+RoI	CSPS	CSPS+RoI	U-Net	MC U-Net
Ultrasonix					
Jaccard	0.61 (0.13)	0.28 (0.14)	0.70 (0.16)	0.76 (0.10)	**0.77 (0.11)**
Dice-Sorensen	0.75 (0.12)	0.42 (0.16)	0.81 (0.14)	**0.86 (0.07)**	0.86 (0.08)
Precision	0.79 (0.12)	0.30 (0.15)	0.86 (0.11)	**0.89 (0.07)**	0.89 (0.07)
Recall	0.71 (0.14)	0.82 (0.11)	0.78 (0.17)	**0.85 (0.10)**	0.85 (0.11)
Hausdorff (mm)	4.41 (3.04)	21.89 (9.7)	3.06 (3.1)	**1.60 (1.67)**	1.91 (2.17)
VRMSE (mm)	0.35 (0.32)	5.45 (4.96)	0.37 (0.61)	0.21 (0.07)	**0.20 (0.07)**
Clarius					
Jaccard	0.58 (0.08)	0.34 (0.09)	0.69 (0.14)	0.85 (0.07)	**0.86 (0.06)**
Dice-Sorensen	0.73 (0.06)	0.51 (0.10)	0.81 (0.10)	**0.92 (0.04)**	0.92 (0.04)
Precision	0.88 (0.04)	0.35 (0.09)	0.72 (0.15)	0.92 (0.07)	**0.94 (0.05)**
Recall	0.64 (0.09)	0.93 (0.06)	**0.95 (0.05)**	0.93 (0.03)	0.91 (0.05)
Hausdorff (mm)	5.79 (1.92)	25.68 (3.54)	5.65 (4.55)	2.34 (4.79)	**1.09 (0.90)**
VRMSE (mm)	0.33 (0.12)	2.42 (3.27)	0.33 (0.12)	0.22 (0.10)	**0.20 (0.07)**

region (Fig. 1). In contrast, U-Net rarely detected false positive soft tissue, and consistently and accurately segmented the full ilium and acetabulum contour. Errors were mainly due to slightly under- or over-segmenting the ilium or acetabulum at the superior and inferior extremities of the contour. Along each scan line, we observe that U-Net very accurately segmented the bone contours as is reflected in the negligible VRMSE errors observed on our clinical dataset.

In contrast to recent papers reporting improved results by fusing phase symmetry and shadow features within multi-channel deep learning networks [1,11], we did not observe significant improvements in our main dataset. However, an apparent improvement in Hausdorff Distance indicates slight improvement on the secondary test set, and this is consistent with qualitative observations as we observed that multi-channel U-Net is sometimes more robust to soft tissue false positives. Comparing to the closest literature, we observed on the primary test set improved mean Hausdorff distance of 1.60 ± 1.67 mm and VRMSE of 0.20 ± 0.07 mm compared to Hareendranathan's 2.1 ± 0.9 mm and 1.8 ± 0.7 mm with the superpixel classification method [2]. Further we report much improved mean Dice score of 0.88 on our primary test set, compared to Zhang's [12] scores of 0.386 for their proposed architecture, and Dice of 0.049 with their implementation of U-Net.

With regards to computational complexity, we had about 15 million parameters in our U-Net implementation. When tested on 250×250 2D coronal US slices, on a machine with Intel Core i-7 (4.0 GHz, 6 core) processor and NVIDIA Titan Xp GPU, we logged run times of 0.007 s for Shadow Peak, 0.155 s for CSPS, and 0.003 s for U-Net.

4   Conclusions

We proposed a deep-learned feature based approach for bone segmentation in neonatal hip ultrasound. We showed this method improved accuracy and speed over current techniques in the literature, and more importantly, reduced outliers and failure rates associated with automated DDH assessment from US. Results on a secondary dataset show that U-Net is robust to domain shifts such as images from a probe that produces significantly different images, and that using a multi-channel input may improve robustness further. We expect such improved results to contribute to a more streamlined clinical translation and to higher reliability, potentially improving patient screening and outcomes. Future work will focus on evaluating the effect of our improved segmentation on α angle reproducibility, and correlating effects on clinical outcomes as part of a longitudinal clinical study. Our clinical study is continuing and we expect to pool data from multiple collaborating centres, allowing us to collect more varied data from a bigger patient population and from more probes. Ultimately, our plan is to build a completely 3D US imaging based solution for DDH assessment.

Acknowledgement. This work was funded by the Natural Sciences and Engineering Research Council (grant no. CHRP 478466-15), the Canadian Institutes of Health

Research (grant no. CPG-140180), and the Institute for Computing, Information, and Cognitive Systems (ICICS) at UBC. We would also like to thank NVIDIA Corporation for supporting our research through their GPU Grant Program by donating the GeForce Titan Xp.

References

1. Alsinan, A.Z., Patel, V.M., Hacihaliloglu, I.: Automatic segmentation of bone surfaces from ultrasound using a filter-layer-guided CNN. Int. J. Comput. Assist. Radiol. Surg. **14**, 775–783 (2019)
2. Hareendranathan, A.R., et al.: Toward automatic diagnosis of hip dysplasia from 2D ultrasound. In: Proceedings of International Symposium on Biomedical Imaging, pp. 982–985 (2017)
3. Jackson, J., Runge, M., Nye, N.: Common questions about developmental dysplasia of the hip. Am. Fam. Physician **90**(12), 843–850 (2014)
4. Loder, R.T., Skopelja, E.N.: The epidemiology and demographics of hip dysplasia. ISRN Orthop. **2011**, 1–46 (2011)
5. Mostofi, E., et al.: Reliability of 2D and 3D ultrasound for infant hip dysplasia in the hands of novice users. Eur. Radiol. **29**(3), 1489–1495 (2019)
6. Pandey, P., Quader, N., Mulpuri, K., Guy, P., Garbi, R., Hodgson, A.J.: Shadow peak: accurate real-time bone segmentation for ultrasound and developmental dysplasia of the hip. In: 19th Annual Meeting of the International Society for Computer Assisted Orthopaedic Surgery, New York (2019)
7. Paserin, O., Mulpuri, K., Cooper, A., Hodgson, A.J., Garbi, R.: Real time RNN based 3D ultrasound scan adequacy for developmental dysplasia of the hip. In: Frangi, A.F., Schnabel, J.A., Davatzikos, C., Alberola-López, C., Fichtinger, G. (eds.) MICCAI 2018. LNCS, vol. 11070, pp. 365–373. Springer, Cham (2018). https://doi.org/10.1007/978-3-030-00928-1_42
8. Quader, N., Hodgson, A., Mulpuri, K., Cooper, A., Abugharbieh, R.: Towards reliable automatic characterization of neonatal hip dysplasia from 3D ultrasound images. In: Ourselin, S., Joskowicz, L., Sabuncu, M.R., Unal, G., Wells, W. (eds.) MICCAI 2016. LNCS, vol. 9900, pp. 602–609. Springer, Cham (2016). https://doi.org/10.1007/978-3-319-46720-7_70
9. Quader, N., Hodgson, A., Mulpuri, K., Savage, T., Abugharbieh, R.: Automatic assessment of developmental dysplasia of the hip. In: Proceedings of International Symposium on Biomedical Imaging, 13–16 July 2015 (2015)
10. Ronneberger, O., Fischer, P., Brox, T.: U-Net: convolutional networks for biomedical image segmentation. In: Navab, N., Hornegger, J., Wells, W.M., Frangi, A.F. (eds.) MICCAI 2015. LNCS, vol. 9351, pp. 234–241. Springer, Cham (2015). https://doi.org/10.1007/978-3-319-24574-4_28
11. Villa, M., Dardenne, G., Nasan, M., Letissier, H., Hamitouche, C., Stindel, E.: FCN-based approach for the automatic segmentation of bone surfaces in ultrasound images. Int. J. Comput. Assist. Radiol. Surg. **13**(11), 1707–1716 (2018)
12. Zhang, Z., Tang, M., Cobzas, D., Zonoobi, D., Jagersand, M., Jaremko, J.L.: End-to-end detection-segmentation network with ROI convolution. In: Proceedings of International Symposium on Biomedical Imaging (ISBI), April 2018, pp. 1509–1512 (2018)

Unsupervised Quality Control of Image Segmentation Based on Bayesian Learning

Benoît Audelan$^{(\boxtimes)}$ and Hervé Delingette

Université Côte d'Azur, Inria, Epione Project-Team, Sophia Antipolis, France
benoit.audelan@inria.fr

Abstract. Assessing the quality of segmentations on an image database is required as many downstream clinical applications are based on segmentation results. For large databases, this quality assessment becomes tedious for a human expert and therefore some automation of this task is necessary. In this paper, we introduce a novel unsupervised approach to assist the quality control of image segmentations by measuring their adequacy with segmentations produced by a generic probabilistic model. To this end, we introduce a new segmentation model combining intensity and a spatial prior defined through a combination of spatially smooth kernels. The tractability of the approach is obtained by solving a type-II maximum likelihood which directly estimates hyperparameters. Assessing the quality of the segmentation with respect to the probabilistic model allows to detect the most challenging cases inside a dataset. This approach was evaluated on the BRATS 2017 and ACDC datasets showing its relevance for quality control assessment.

Keywords: Quality control · Image segmentation · Bayesian learning

1 Introduction

Quality control of image segmentation is an important task since it impacts the decisions that clinicians or other downstream algorithms can make about the patient. In the case of an automatic pipeline used in a clinical routine, it is therefore of great importance to be able to detect the possible failed segmentations. Many segmentation algorithms follow a supervised learning approach, learning the segmentation task on databases where images and ground truth are jointly available. The main challenges are thus to verify the quality of ground truth segmentations but also to monitor the application of a segmentation algorithm on images for which no ground truth is available. Despite its relevance, the quality control of segmentation has been relatively little studied. In [11], a framework to detect failures in cardiac segmentation based on shape and intensity features has been proposed. A more generic feature based approach has also

Electronic supplementary material The online version of this chapter (https://doi.org/10.1007/978-3-030-32245-8_3) contains supplementary material, which is available to authorized users.

D. Shen et al. (Eds.): MICCAI 2019, LNCS 11765, pp. 21–29, 2019.
https://doi.org/10.1007/978-3-030-32245-8_3

been explored in [4] where Dice coefficients are predicted by an SVM regressor. Reverse Classification Accuracy (RCA) was proposed in [10], assuming the availability of a subset ground truth dataset. In that case, the proposed segmentation on a new image is compared to the predicted segmentations based on this subset of reference images, which can result in rejection if discrepancies are too large. This approach was further investigated by [8] on larger databases where they showed the ability to isolate segmentations of poor quality but pointed out the relatively long computation time as a bottleneck. In [7] the authors propose a neural network to directly predict the Dice coefficient. Finally, another deep learning-based approach was introduced in [9] where the uncertainty in the produced segmentation is correlated with its quality.

These methods allow to detect poor segmentations in the absence of ground truth ones but have also some limitations. They are all supervised meaning that they require a subset of segmented data to be considered as "representative ground truth", the size of this subset being potentially large for deep learning-based methods which somewhat defies its purpose. Furthermore, some methods lack interpretability as one may not know why a segmentation has failed.

In this paper, we propose a novel unsupervised approach to automated quality control by comparing segmentations S produced by an algorithm or a human rater to a generic model of segmentation M instead of an arbitrary selected subset of segmentations. This allows to remove the bias related to the subset selection and to monitor the quality of segmentations when few or even no other segmentations are available from a database. In addition, it provides visually interpretable results which could be used for manual corrections of poor cases. To assess the quality of a given segmentation S, we propose to fit a probabilistic generative segmentation model M making simple intensity and smoothness assumptions. The underlying hypothesis is that explainable segmentations correspond to clearly visible boundaries in the image which is well captured by M. On the contrary, segmentations far from M are categorized as challenging as they would require other priors than intensity and smoothness to be explained. These difficult cases can be highlighted by comparing the adequacies between M and S inside a same dataset.

We use a Bayesian framework to estimate automatically all parameters of the segmentation model where the prior probability of a voxel label is defined as a generalized linear model of spatially smooth kernels. Parameter estimation is performed by a sparsity inducing prior for the automatic selection of the number of components of Student mixtures, by solving *type-II maximum likelihood* for controlling the coefficient shrinkage and by performing model selection for the choice of kernels. We show on two public databases, ACDC and BRATS 2017, that our approach is able to monitor the quality of ground truth segmentations but also to indicate the potential performances of segmentations on test data (in the absence of ground truth).

2   Probabilistic Segmentation Framework

Given a segmentation S on an image I, our objective is to produce a smooth contour or surface M close to S which is mostly aligned with visible contours in the image. The estimated segmentation M should not be seen as a surrogate ground truth, but only as a comparison tool. The adequacy between S and M gives an estimate of the quality of the segmentation S.

We consider a binary image segmentation problem on image I made of N voxels having intensity $I_n \in \mathbb{R}$, $n = 1, \ldots, N$. We introduce for each voxel a binary hidden random variable $Z_n \in \{0,1\}$ with $Z_n = 1$ if voxel n belongs to the structure of interest.

Appearance models of the foreground and background regions of S are defined respectively by the two image likelihoods $p(I_n|Z_n = 1, \theta_I^1)$ and $p(I_n|Z_n = 0, \theta_I^0)$ where θ_I^0, θ_I^1 are parameters governing those models. In this paper, we consider generic parametric appearance models as variational mixtures of Student-t distributions [1]. The Student-t unlike Gaussian distributions lead to robust mean and covariance estimates and variational Bayesian methods allow to select automatically the number of components. We introduce the appearance probability ratio $r_n(I, \theta_I^0, \theta_I^1) \triangleq p(I_n|Z_n = 1, \theta_I^1)/\left(p(I_n|Z_n = 0, \theta_I^0) + p(I_n|Z_n = 1, \theta_I^1)\right)$ which is the posterior label probability with non-informative prior $(p(Z_n = 1) = 0.5)$.

Classical label priors in the literature are based on discrete formulations such as Markov random fields that are relying on labels of neighboring voxels. In this paper, we propose a novel continuous label prior framework defined through a generalized linear model of spatially smooth functions. This approach allows a Bayesian estimation of its parameters $\mathbf{W}$ and produces by construction continuous posterior label distributions. More precisely, the prior probability $p(Z_n = 1)$ is defined as a Bernouilli distribution whose parameter depends on a *spatially random* function $p(Z_n = 1|\mathbf{W}) = \sigma\left(\sum_{l=1}^{L} \Phi_l(\mathbf{x}_n)w_l\right)$ where $\mathbf{x}_n \in \mathbb{R}^d$ is the voxel position in an image of dimension d and $\sigma(u)$ is the sigmoid function $\sigma(u) = 1/(1 + \exp(-u))$. The basis $\{\Phi_l(\mathbf{x})\}$ are L functions of space, typically radial basis functions, and $w_l \in \mathbf{W}$ are weights considered as random variables. Thus the prior probabilities of two geometrically close voxels will be related to each other through the smoothness of the function $f(\mathbf{x}_n) = \sum_{l=1}^{L} \Phi_l(\mathbf{x}_n)w_l$.

The smoothness of the label prior $\sigma(f(\mathbf{x}_n))$ depends on the choice of the L basis functions $\Phi_l(\mathbf{x}_n)$. The weight vector $\mathbf{W} = (w_1, \ldots, w_L)^T$ is equipped with a zero mean Gaussian prior parameterized by the diagonal precision matrix $\alpha\mathbf{I}$: $p(\mathbf{W}) = \mathcal{N}(0, \alpha^{-1}\mathbf{I})$. Experiments have shown that sharing the same precision α across the weights w_l improves the model stability. Finally, a non-informative prior is chosen for α, $p(\alpha) \propto 1$. The graphical model of the segmentation framework is shown in Fig. 1a.

Once the distribution on $\mathbf{W}$ is known, the prior $p(Z_n = 1)$ can be computed by marginalizing over the weights $\int_{-\infty}^{+\infty} \sigma(\boldsymbol{\Phi}_n\mathbf{W})\, p(\mathbf{W})\, d\mathbf{W}$ writing $\boldsymbol{\Phi}_n = (\Phi_1(\mathbf{x}_n), \ldots, \Phi_L(\mathbf{x}_n))$. It is approximated by $\sum_{l=1}^{L} \Phi_l(\mathbf{x}_n)\boldsymbol{\mu}_l^\star$, where $\boldsymbol{\mu}^\star$ is the mode of $\mathbf{W}$. The posterior label probability $p(Z_n = 1|I, \mathbf{W})$, combining prior and intensity likelihoods, is obtained through Eq. 1:

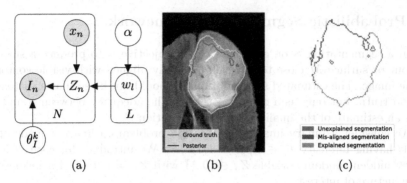

(a)   (b)   (c)

Fig. 1. Graphical model of the framework (a). Study of the ground truth of the BRATS 2017 challenge with a case of possible under segmentation (b and c).

$$p(Z_n = 1|I, \mathbf{W}) = \frac{r_n(I, \theta_I^0, \theta_I^1)p(Z_n = 1)}{r_n(I, \theta_I^0, \theta_I^1)p(Z_n = 1) + (1 - r_n(I, \theta_I^0, \theta_I^1))p(Z_n = 0)} \quad (1)$$

Finally, the maximum a posteriori estimate of the segmented structure is obtained as the isosurface $p(Z_n = 1|I, \mathbf{W}) = 0.5$. To estimate prior and hyperprior parameters, we propose to maximize the following log joint probability:

$$\log p(I, \mathbf{W}, \alpha, \theta_I) = \log p(I|\theta_I, \mathbf{W})p(\mathbf{W}|\alpha)p(\alpha)$$
$$= \sum_{n=1}^{N} \log \left(\sum_{k=0}^{1} p(I_n|\theta_I^k, Z_n = k)p(Z_n = k|\mathbf{W}) \right) - \frac{1}{2}\alpha\mathbf{W}^T\mathbf{W} + \frac{L}{2}\log \alpha$$
$$(2)$$

3   Bayesian Learning of Prior Parameters

As the final objective is the quality control of the given segmentation S, it is of little interest to work with the whole image and computationally inefficient. We thus restrict the analysis inside a narrow band of width typically between 8 and 30 voxels defined around the boundaries of the foreground region of S.

The method starts with the estimation of the appearance probability ratio r_n for each voxel n. Two variational mixture models of Student-t distributions are fitted, one for the foreground region of S and the other for the background, following the approach of [1]. The sparsity inducing Dirichlet prior over the mixture proportions allows to automatically select the appropriate number of components. Once r_n are known, the problem reduces to estimate the weights $\mathbf{W}$ and the precision α in Eq. 2. Setting $y_n = \boldsymbol{\Phi}_n\mathbf{W}$, the sum in Eq. 2 can be indeed rewritten as $\sum_{n=1}^{N} \log [r_n\sigma(y_n) + (1 - r_n)(1 - \sigma(y_n))] + \text{cst}$.

To learn the parameters of the model, we adopt a *type-II maximum likelihood* approach, based on the maximization of the *marginal log likelihood* $\mathcal{L}(\alpha) = \log p(I, \alpha) = \log \int P(I, \mathbf{W}, \alpha)d\mathbf{W}$. The idea is to marginalize out the weight variables such that the maximization is performed only on the precision variable.

The marginal log likelihood is intractable but can be approximated through the Laplace approximation of Eq. 2: $\log p(I, \mathbf{W}, \alpha) \approx \log p(I|\boldsymbol{\mu}^\star) + \log p(\boldsymbol{\mu}^\star|\alpha) - \frac{1}{2}(\mathbf{W} - \boldsymbol{\mu}^\star)^T(\boldsymbol{\Sigma}^\star)^{-1}(\mathbf{W} - \boldsymbol{\mu}^\star)$ which corresponds to the following approximation of the posterior probability of the weights: $q(\mathbf{W}) = \mathcal{N}(\boldsymbol{\mu}^\star, \boldsymbol{\Sigma}^\star) \approx p(\mathbf{W}|I)$.

The computation of the Laplace approximation requires to find the mode $\boldsymbol{\mu}^\star$ of Eq. 2 and to compute the Hessian matrix at the mode. This is done through a Gauss-Newton optimization formulated as an iterative reweighted least squares. This leads to the following expression of the covariance $\boldsymbol{\Sigma}^\star = (\boldsymbol{\Phi}^T \mathbf{B} \boldsymbol{\Phi} + \alpha \mathbf{I})^{-1}$ where $\mathbf{B} = \text{diag}\left(g_1''\left(\sum_i w_i \Phi_i^1\right), \cdots, g_L''\left(\sum_i w_i \Phi_i^L\right)\right)$ is a diagonal matrix, g_n being the function defined as $g_n(x) = \log[r_n\sigma(x) + (1 - r_n)\sigma(1 - x)]$.

The algorithm alternates between estimating the mean $\boldsymbol{\mu}^\star$ and the covariance $\boldsymbol{\Sigma}^\star$ and updating the precision parameter α through Eq. 3, obtained by taking the derivatives of $\mathcal{L}(\alpha)$ with respect to α, following the approach of [5].

$$\alpha_{new} = \frac{L - \alpha_{old}\,\text{Tr}\,(\boldsymbol{\Sigma}^\star)}{\boldsymbol{\mu}^{\star T}\boldsymbol{\mu}^\star} \tag{3}$$

The sketch of the algorithm is provided in Algorithm 1.

Algorithm 1. Bayesian Learning algorithm for segmentation

  - Define the basis functions and compute their values on the narrow band
  - **while** *not converged* **do**
       1) Recompute $\boldsymbol{\Sigma}^\star$ and $\boldsymbol{\mu}^\star$ from the Laplace approximation
       2) Re-estimate α following Eq. 3
  end

The choice of the basis functions Φ_l controls the smoothness of the prior. In the remainder, we use a dictionary of Gaussian bases centered on a regular staggered grid. The key parameters are the spacing between the bases centers, the standard deviations and the position of the origin basis. In practice, model selection is performed by selecting among different basis settings the one that gives the lowest average distance between the segmentation S and the segmentation obtained by thresholding the prior probability map at the level 0.5.

It has been experimentally assessed that the convergence rate of Algorithm 1 is high and even a few iterations give acceptable results. Nevertheless, to guarantee a reasonable computation time, large images are split into overlapping patches where Algorithm 1 is performed independently. This approach produces good results since each basis only interacts with very few neighboring bases. The bases from all patches are then combined in the whole image, but bases lying on overlapping regions are weighted with bicubic (resp. tricubic) spline functions for 2D (resp. 3D) images. This approach still leads to a generalized linear model $\sigma(\boldsymbol{\Phi}_n \mathbf{W})$ with C^1 continuity between isoprobability surfaces from neighboring patches.

Once the probabilistic model is fitted, a new segmentation M is generated by thresholding the posterior $p(Z_n|I_n, \mathbf{W})$ at the level 0.5. Two metrics are extracted to measure the adequacy of S with M: the Dice coefficient (DC) $E_D = 2|M \cap S|/(|S| + |M|)$ and the average asymmetric surface error (ASE) $E_S = d(S, M) = \frac{1}{\partial S} \sum_{x \in \partial S} \min_{y \in \partial M} d(x, y)$ where ∂ denotes the segmentation surface. We discard the metric $d(M, S)$ as being uninformative since M is not a surrogate ground truth.

4   Results

4.1   Quality Control of Ground Truth Segmentations

We demonstrate the ability of our algorithm to highlight challenging cases on 285 3D MR segmentations of whole brain tumor from the training set of the BRATS 2017 challenge [6]. The 4 modalities (T1, T1c, T2 and T2 FLAIR) are combined in a multivariate variational mixtures of Student-t distributions with 7 initial components to learn the appearance models of the foreground and background regions defined by the ground truth. Then the posterior is computed using Algorithm 1. The distribution of the ASE over the whole dataset (Fig. 2) allows to isolate a dozen of cases at the right tail of the distribution. The case 2c is thus clearly more challenging than the case 2b taken from the left tail. Indeed, the ground truth contour in Fig. 2c is more irregular and could be even questioned because of the very weak intensity variations in some regions (indicated by the arrows). It was maybe extracted through thresholding instead of being manually drawn. This hypothesis is plausible as a thresholding step might have been included in the annotation process [3,6]. Further examples can be seen in the supplementary material. Note that depending on the segmentation task, samples with abnormally low ASE could also be suspicious. Moreover, the average signed distance error gives some indication about the behavior of the segmentation rater. Large negative (resp. positive) average errors probably indicate under (resp. over) segmentations in comparison with M. This is shown in Fig. 1b for under segmentation and Fig. 2d for over segmentation. This could be useful to detect rater biases and to improve their delineation performances.

To further enhance the visualisation and interpretability of the results, we can categorize the voxels belonging to the ground truth surface depending on the value of the posterior map at their location and their distance to the isosurface ∂M (Fig. 1c). Explained segmentation are voxels in a neighborhood of 4 mm around ∂M and with a posterior value below 0.9 or above 0.1, for which there is an agreement between the rater and our segmentation model. Mis-aligned segmentations are voxels close to ∂M but with a posterior value above 0.9 or below 0.1 possibly corresponding to a small deviation of the rater around the visible boundary. Finally, voxels that are far from ∂M with a posterior value also above 0.9 or below 0.1 correspond to regions not explained by the probabilistic model and for which a visual review might be worthy.

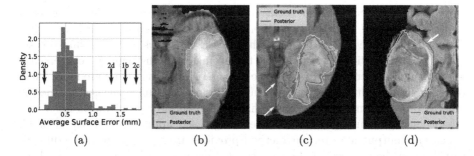

Fig. 2. Study of the BRATS 2017 challenge training set. Distribution of the ASE (a). Example of a segmentation explained by the model (b), of a case with regions not explained by the model (c), and with possible over segmentation (d), all shown in FLAIR modality.

4.2 Quality Control of Predicted Segmentations

Our algorithm can be of great interest in situations where segmentations are generated by algorithms in the absence of ground truth. For instance, we consider predicted segmentations given by a convolutional neural network (CNN) on 46 test images of the BRATS 2017 challenge as illustrated in Fig. 3. The Dice score computed between the predicted segmentation S and the one obtained by thresholding the posterior map, M, is then compared to the true value obtained by uploading the prediction on the evaluation website of the challenge. Correlations for 3 different tumor compartments are all above 0.69 with few outliers. These results are satisfactory considering that no regression model was learned unlike for example what was proposed in [4].

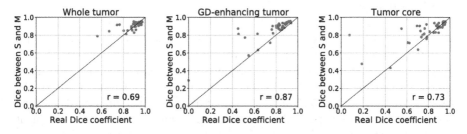

Fig. 3. Real Dice coefficient versus Dice score between the prediction S of the CNN and the probabilistic segmentation M exhibiting good correlation.

We further investigated our algorithm on MR cardiac images from the training set of the ACDC challenge [2]. We evaluate the quality of predicted left-ventricular myocardium segmentations given by a CNN for 100 subjects for which ground truth is available at 2 time points. Each slice is processed individually in 2D due to the large inter-slices distance (1797 slices in total). A good correlation is again observed between the two Dice scores, the first computed between S and M and the other between S and the ground truth (Fig. 4a). Figure 4b illustrates a difficult case whereas Fig. 4c shows a well explained case.

Our probabilistic approach is able to automatically distinguish between easy and difficult segmentation cases. Since large segmentation errors are more likely to occur in difficult images rather than easy ones, our unsupervised method is able to provide hints for the cases that are potentially problematic for a segmentation algorithm. Compared to learning-based approach such as [4] or [7] which only output a score, our method provides an explanation of the difficulties through the analysis of the posterior (as highlighted by arrows in Fig. 4b).

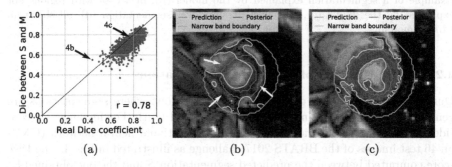

Fig. 4. Study of predicted segmentations by a CNN on the ACDC dataset. Real Dice versus Dice score between the prediction S and the probabilistic segmentation M (a). Posterior for an ambiguous case (b) and an easier one (c).

5   Conclusion

We presented a novel method for quality control assessment of ground truth or predicted segmentations using a Bayesian framework. Our method relies on a generic segmentation model which produces contours of variable smoothness aligned with visible boundaries in the image. Bayesian inference leads to the estimation of all (hyper)parameters without resorting to supervised learning from a subset of data as performed in prior works. Furthermore, the assessment of each segmentation is interpretable. The approach was shown to be a useful tool for quality control assessment for small databases and can indicate the potential performances of segmentations on test data.

Acknowledgements. This work was partially funded by the French government, through the UCA^{JEDI} "Investments in the Future" project managed by the National Research Agency (ANR) with the reference number ANR-15-IDEX-01 and supported by the Inria Sophia Antipolis - Méditerranée, "NEF" computation cluster.

References

1. Archambeau, C., Verleysen, M.: Robust Bayesian clustering. Neural Netw. **20**(1), 129–138 (2007)
2. Bernard, O., Lalande, A., et al.: Deep learning techniques for automatic MRI cardiac multi-structures segmentation and diagnosis: is the problem solved? IEEE Trans. Med. Imaging **37**(11), 2514–2525 (2018)
3. Jakab, A.: Segmenting brain tumors with the slicer 3D software (2012). http://www2.imm.dtu.dk/projects/BRATS2012/Jakab_TumorSegmentation_Manual.pdf. Accessed 16 July 2019
4. Kohlberger, T., Singh, V., Alvino, C., Bahlmann, C., Grady, L.: Evaluating segmentation error without ground truth. In: Ayache, N., Delingette, H., Golland, P., Mori, K. (eds.) MICCAI 2012. LNCS, vol. 7510, pp. 528–536. Springer, Heidelberg (2012). https://doi.org/10.1007/978-3-642-33415-3_65
5. MacKay, D.J.: Bayesian interpolation. Neural Comput. **4**, 415–447 (1991)
6. Menze, B.H., Jakab, A., et al.: The multimodal brain tumor image segmentation benchmark (BRATS). IEEE Trans. Med. Imaging **34**(10), 1993–2024 (2015)
7. Robinson, R., et al.: Real-time prediction of segmentation quality. In: Frangi, A.F., Schnabel, J.A., Davatzikos, C., Alberola-López, C., Fichtinger, G. (eds.) MICCAI 2018. LNCS, vol. 11073, pp. 578–585. Springer, Cham (2018). https://doi.org/10.1007/978-3-030-00937-3_66
8. Robinson, R., Valindria, V.V., et al.: Automated quality control in image segmentation: application to the UK biobank cardiovascular magnetic resonance imaging study. J. Cardiovasc. Magn. Reson. **21**(1), 18 (2019)
9. Roy, A.G., Conjeti, S., et al.: Bayesian QuickNAT: model uncertainty in deep whole-brain segmentation for structure-wise quality control. NeuroImage **195**, 11–22 (2019)
10. Valindria, V.V., Lavdas, I., et al.: Reverse classification accuracy: predicting segmentation performance in the absence of ground truth. IEEE Trans. Med. Imaging **36**(8), 1597–1606 (2017)
11. Xu, Y., Berman, D.S., et al.: Automated quality control for segmentation of myocardial perfusion SPECT. J. Nucl. Med. **50**(9), 1418–1426 (2009)

One Network to Segment Them All: A General, Lightweight System for Accurate 3D Medical Image Segmentation

Mathias Perslev[1]([envelope]), Erik Bjørnager Dam[1,2], Akshay Pai[1,2], and Christian Igel[1]

[1] Department of Computer Science, University of Copenhagen, Copenhagen, Denmark
map@di.ku.dk
[2] Cerebriu A/S, Copenhagen, Denmark

Abstract. Many recent medical segmentation systems rely on powerful deep learning models to solve highly specific tasks. To maximize performance, it is standard practice to evaluate numerous pipelines with varying model topologies, optimization parameters, pre- & postprocessing steps, and even model cascades. It is often not clear how the resulting pipeline transfers to different tasks.

We propose a simple and thoroughly evaluated deep learning framework for segmentation of arbitrary medical image volumes. The system requires no task-specific information, no human interaction and is based on a fixed model topology and a fixed hyperparameter set, eliminating the process of model selection and its inherent tendency to cause method-level over-fitting. The system is available in open source and does not require deep learning expertise to use. Without task-specific modifications, the system performed better than or similar to highly specialized deep learning methods across 3 separate segmentation tasks. In addition, it ranked 5-th and 6-th in the first and second round of the 2018 Medical Segmentation Decathlon comprising another 10 tasks.

The system relies on *multi-planar* data augmentation which facilitates the application of a single 2D architecture based on the familiar U-Net. Multi-planar training combines the parameter efficiency of a 2D fully convolutional neural network with a systematic train- and test-time augmentation scheme, which allows the 2D model to learn a representation of the 3D image volume that fosters generalization.

1 Introduction

More and more systems for medical image segmentation rely on deep learning (DL). However, most publications on this topic report performance improvements for a particular segmentation task and imaging modality and use a

Electronic supplementary material The online version of this chapter (https://doi.org/10.1007/978-3-030-32245-8_4) contains supplementary material, which is available to authorized users.

specialized processing pipeline adapted through hyperparameter tuning. This makes it difficult to generalize the obtained results and bears the risk that the reported findings are artifacts. In line with the idea behind the 2018 Medical Segmentation Decathlon (MSD)[1] [1], a challenge evaluating the generalisability of machine learning based segmentation algorithms, we argue that new segmentation systems should be evaluated across many different data cohorts and maybe even tasks. This reduces the risk of unintentional method overfitting and may help to gain more general insights about, for example, superior model architectures and learning methods for particular problem classes. This does not only contribute to our basic understanding of the segmentation algorithms, but also to the clinical acceptance and applicability of the systems – even if the generality could come at the cost of not reaching state-of-the-art performance on each individual cohort or task.

A DL segmentation framework that works across a wide range of tasks and in which the individual components and hyperparameters are sufficiently understood allows to automate the task-specific adaptations. This is a prerequisite for being useful for practitioners who are not experts in DL. Big compute clusters offer a way to design systems that provide accurate segmentations for a variety of tasks and do not require tuning by DL experts. If compute resources are not limited, automatic model and hyperparameter selection can be implemented. Given new training data, the systems tests a large variety of segmentation algorithms and, for each algorithm, explores the space of the required hyperparameters. While this approach may produce powerful systems, and was employed to variable extents by top-performing MSD submissions, we argue that it has crucial drawbacks. First, it comes with a risk of automated method overfitting, even if the data is handled carefully. Second, the approach may be prohibitive in clinical practice (and for many scientific institutions) when there is simply no access to sufficient (data regulations compliant) compute resources.

This paper presents an open-source system for medical volume segmentation that addresses all the issues outlined above. It relies on a single neural network of fixed architecture that (1) showed very good performance across a variety of diverse segmentation tasks, (2) can be trained efficiently without DL expert knowledge, large amounts of data, and compute clusters, and (3) does not need large resources when deployed. The system architecture is a 2D U-Net [2,3] variant. The decisive feature of our approach lies in extensive data augmentation, in particular by rotating the input volume before presenting slices to the fully convolutional network. Because of the latter, we refer to our approach as *multi-planar* U-Net training (*MPUnet*). We present a thorough evaluation of our system on a total of 13 different 3D segmentation tasks, including 10 from MSD, on which it obtains high accuracies – often reaching state-of-the-art performance from even highly specialized DL-based methods.

---

[1] http://medicaldecathlon.com.

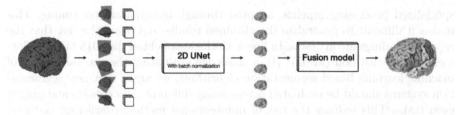

Fig. 1. Model overview. In the inference phase, the input volume (left) is sampled on 2D isotropic grids along multiple view axes. The model predicts a full volume along each axis and maps the predictions into the original image space. A fusion model combines the 6 proposed segmentation volumes into a single final segmentation.

2   Method

At the heart of our system lies a 2D U-net [2] modified slightly to **(1)** include batch normalization layers [4] intervening each double convolution- and up-convolution block and **(2)** use nearest-neighbor up-sampling followed by convolution to implement up-convolutions [5]. Basic network topology and hyper-parameters can bet set to their default choices as done in all experiments in this paper, see Table S.1 in the supplementary material for an overview. Compared to [2], the number of filters has been increased by a factor of $\sqrt{2}$, see supplementary Table S.6 for details. As a result, the model has ≈ 62 million parameters. While one would assume that the size of the model is a crucial hyperparameter, we kept the model architecture the same for all tasks. For each task, only the filters in the first layer were resized according to the number C of input channels and the number of output units was set to the number of classes K.

The decisive feature of our multi-planar U-Net training (*MPUnet*) is the generation of the inputs at training and test time, which is done by sampling from multiple planes of random orientation spanning the image volume. That is, the network must learn to segment the input seen from different views, see Fig. 1.

The model $f(x; \theta)$ takes as input multi-channel 2D image slices of size $w \times h$, $x \in \mathbb{R}^{w \times h \times C}$, and outputs a probabilistic segmentation map $P \in \mathbb{R}^{w \times h \times K}$ for K classes. Prior to training we define a set $V = \{v_1, v_2, ..., v_i\}$ of i randomly sampled unit vectors in $\mathbb{R}^3$. The set defines the axes through the image volume along which we sample 2D inputs to the model, visualized in Fig. 2. We re-sample the set V until all pairs of vectors have an angle of at least 60° between them. A sampled set of planar axes is shown in Fig. 2(a). Note that the model could also be fit using a set of fixed, predefined planes, but we found no performance gain in doing so, even if the fixed set included the standard planes. We use $i = 6$ for all reported evaluations. This number was chosen based on prior experiments in which we observed monotonically improving performance with the inclusion of additional planes and $i = 6$ providing a good balance between accuracy and computation, see supplementary Table S.2.

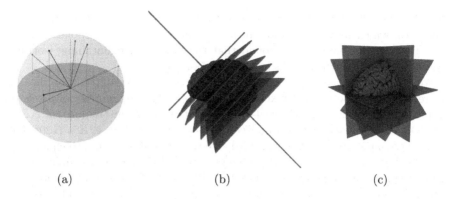

(a)   (b)   (c)

Fig. 2. (a) Visualization of a set V of sampled view axis unit vectors. (b) Illustration of images sampled along one view. (c) Illustration of multiple images sampled along multiple unique views.

During training, the model is provided batches of images randomly sampled from the i planes in V without supplying information about the corresponding axis. During inference, the model predicts along each plane producing a set of i segmentation volumes $\mathbf{P} = \{P_v \in \mathbb{R}^{w \times h \times d \times K} \mid v \in V\}$. Each P_v is mapped to the input image space to obtain point correspondence by assigning to each voxel in the input image the value of its nearest predicted point in P_v. Distances are computed in physical coordinates.

At test-time, the learned invariance to orientation is exploited by segmenting the entire volume from each view. This results in several candidate segmentations for each subject, which are combined by a linear fusion model, see Fig. 1. We map $\mathbf{P}$ to a single probabilistic segmentation by a weighted sum of the per-class and per-view softmax-scores. For all $w \cdot h \cdot d$ voxels x in $\mathbf{P}$ and each class $k \in \{1, ..., K\}$, the *fusion model* $f_{\text{fusion}} : \mathbb{R}^{|V| \times K} \to \mathbb{R}^K$ calculates $z(x)_k = \sum_{n=1}^{|V|} W_{n,k} \cdot p_{n,x,k} + \beta_k$. Here $p_{n,x,k}$ denotes the probability of class k at voxel x as predicted by segmentation P_n. The $W \in \mathbb{R}^{|V| \times K}$ weighs the probabilities of each class as predicted from each view and $\beta \in \mathbb{R}^K$ are bias parameters, which can adjust the overall tendency to predict a given class. The parameters of f_{fusion} are learned from the validation data. The model scales the predictions according to which views do well on each class, motivated by the fact that different target classes may appear in different shapes and levels of recognizability when seen from the different directions in V.

Isotropic Image Sampling. Interpolation is needed to sample image planes not aligned with the original voxel grid. We use tri-linear and nearest-neighbour interpolation to sample the image and label map, respectively. We take advantage of the necessity for interpolation by sampling images on isotropic grids in the physical scanner space, oriented according to the patient's position in the scanner. This ensures that the model always operates on images in which the shapes of anatomical structures are maintained across scanners and acquisition protocols. Note that this approach may lead to over- or under-sampling along some axes, which may lead to loss of image information or interpolation artefacts. Empirically, however, we found that the benefit of maintaining isotropy outweighed potential drawbacks of interpolation.

We must define a set of parameters restricting the sampling. Specifically, we are free to choose (1) the pixel dimensions, $q \in \mathbb{Z}^+$ (the number of pixels to sample for each image), (2) the real-space extent of the image (in mm), $m \in \mathbb{R}^+$, and (3) the real-space distance between consecutive voxels, $r \in \mathbb{R}^+$. Note that two of these parameters define the third. We restrict our sampling to equal q, m and r for both image dimensions producing squared images. We sample images within a sphere of diameter m centered at the origin of the scanner coordinate system. We employ a simple heuristic that attempts to pick q, m and r so that (1) the training is computable on our GPUs with batch sizes of at least 8, (2) r approximately matches the resolution of the images along their highest resolution axis and (3) the sampled images span the entirety of the relevant volume of all images in the dataset. When this is not possible, the requirements are prioritized in the given order, with 1 having highest priority. Note that 3 becomes less important with increasing numbers of planes as voxels missed in one plane are likely to be included in some of the others.

Augmentation. Processing the input image from different views has the same effect as applying affine transformations to the 3D input and presenting the transformed images to a (single-view) network. Thus, at the heart the MPUnet is a U-Net with extensive, systematic affine data augmentation. On top of the multi-view sampling, we also employ non-linear transformations to further augment the training data. We apply the Random Elastic Deformations algorithm [6] to each sampled image in a batch with a probability of 1/3. The elasticity constants σ and deformation intensity multipliers α are sampled uniformly from $[20, 30]$ and $[100, 500]$, respectively. This generates augmented images with high variability in terms of both deformation strength and smoothness.

The augmented images do not always display anatomically plausible structures. Yet, they often significantly improve the generalization especially when training on small datasets or tasks involving pathologies of highly variable shape. However, we weigh the loss-contribution from augmented images by 1/3 in order to optimize primarily over true images.

Pre- and Post-processing. Our model uses a minimum of image processing outside of the network itself. We restrain from applying any post-processing of the model's output, because post-processing is typically highly task-specific. We only apply an image- and channel-wise outlier-robust pre-possessing that scales intensity values according to the median and inter-quartile range computed over all non-background voxels. Background voxels are defined by having intensities less than or equal to the first percentile of the intensity distribution.

Implementation. The MPUnet is available as open-source. The fully autonomous implementation makes the MPUnet applicable also for users with limited

Table 1. Performance of the MPUnet across thirteen segmentation tasks. The shown F1 (dice) scores are mean values computed across all non-background per-class F1 scores. For the 10 MSD datasets evaluation was performed by the challenge organisers on non-publicly available test-sets. For MICCAI and HarP, evaluation was performed over three trials. Five fold cross-validation was used for OAI. The 'Classes' column include the background class, which is not included when computing the F1 scores. The 'Size' column gives the total dataset size. Note that the F1 standard deviations for tasks 8, 9 & 10 are not yet published by the challenge organizers. We refer to http://medicaldecathlon.com/results.html for a detailed comparison of our results (team CerebriuDIKU) with those of other challenge participants.

Dataset	Modality	Segmentation target(s)	Classes	Size	F1 score
MICCAI	MRI	Whole-Brain	135	35	0.74 ± 0.03
HarP	MRI	L+R Hippocampus	3	135	0.85 ± 0.03
OAI	MRI	Knee Cartilages	7	176	0.87 ± 0.06
2018 Medical Segmentation Decathlon					
Task 1	MRI	Brain Tumours	4	750	0.60 ± 0.24
Task 2	MRI	Cardiac, Left Atrium	2	30	0.89 ± 0.09
Task 3	CT	Liver & Tumour	2	201	0.76 ± 0.18
Task 4	MRI	Hippocampus ROI	2	394	0.89 ± 0.04
Task 5	MRI	Prostate	3	48	0.78 ± 0.10
Task 6	CT	Lung Tumours	2	96	0.59 ± 0.23
Task 7	CT	Pancreas & Tumour	3	420	0.48 ± 0.21
Task 8	CT	Hepatic Ves. & Tumour	3	443	0.49
Task 9	CT	Spleen	2	61	0.95
Task 10	CT	Colon Cancer	2	190	0.28

deep learning expertise and/or compute resources. A command line interface supports fixed split or cross-validation training and evaluation on arbitrary images. Any non-constant hyperparameter can automatically be inferred from the training data. See the GitHub repository at https://github.com/perslev/MultiPlanarUNet for a user guide.

3 Experiments and Results

We applied the MPUNet without task-specific modifications to a total of 13 segmentation tasks. Ten of those datasets were part of the 2018 MSD challenge, described in detail and sourced on the challenge's website. The remaining three datasets were the MICCAI 2012 Multi-Atlas Challenge (MICCAI) dataset [7], the EADC-ADNI Harmonized Hippocampal Protocol (HarP) dataset [8] and a knee MRI dataset from the Osteoarthritis Initiative (OAI) [9]. The evaluation covers healthy and pathological anatomical structures, mono- and multi-modal MR and CT, and various acquisition protocols. The mean per-class F1 (dice) scores of the MPUNet are reported in Table 1. Note that in MSD tumour segmentation tasks 3 & 7 both organ and tumour are segmented, and the mean F1 for those tasks is lifted by the performance on the organ and decreased by the performance on the tumour. We refer to the supplementary Table S.4 for detailed per-class scores for the ten MSD tasks.

The MPUnet reached state-of-the-art performance for DL methods on the three non-challenge datasets (MICCAI, HaRP and OAI) despite comparable methods being developed and tuned specifically to the cohorts and tasks. On MICCAI, with a mean F1 of 0.74 the MPUnet compares similar to the 0.74 obtained in [10] using a 2D multi-scale CNN on brain-extracted images and 0.75 obtained in [11] using a combination of a multi-scale 2D CNN, 3D patch-based CNN, a spatial information encoder network and a probabilistic atlas also on brain-extracted images. With a mean F1 of 0.85 on HaRP, the MPUnet compares favorable to 0.78–0.83 (depending on subject disease state) reported in [12]. On OAI, with a mean F1 of 0.87, the MPUnet gets near the 0.88/0.89 (baseline/follow-up) obtained in [13] using a task-specific pipeline including 2D- and 3D U-nets along with multiple statistical shape model refinement steps. However, the comparison cannot be directly made as [13] worked on a smaller subset of the OAI data and predicted only 4 classes while we distinguished 7.

The MPUnet ranked 5th and 6th place in the first and second phases of the Medical Segmentation Decathlon respectively, in most cases comparing unfavorable only to significantly more compute intensive systems (see below).[2]

The question arises how the performance of a 2D U-net with multi-planar augmentation compares to a U-net with 3D convolutions. Such 3D models are computationally demanding and typically need – in our experience – large training datasets to achieve proper generalization. While we are not making the claim that the MPUnet is universally superior to 3D models, we did find the MPUnet to outperform a 3D U-net of comparable topology, learning and augmentation procedure across multiple tasks including one for which the 3D model had sufficient spatial extent to operate on the entire input volume at once. We refer to the supplementary Table S.5 for details. We also found the MPUnet superior to both single 2D U-Nets trained on individual planes as well as ensembles of separate 2D U-Nets trained on different planes, see Tables S.2 & S.3 and Fig. S.1 in the supplementary material.

4   Discussion and Conclusions

The empirical evaluation over 13 segmentation tasks showed that multi-planar augmentation provides a simple mechanism for obtaining accurate segmentation models without hyperparameter tuning. With no task-specific modifications the MPUnet performs well across many non-pathological tissues imaged with various MR and CT protocols, in spite of the target compartments varying drastically

---

[2] For comparison, the median F1 scores over all 10 tasks of the best five phase 1 submissions were 0.74, 0.67, 0.69, 0.66, and (our method) 0.69. Note that the official ranking was based on a more rigorous statistical analysis.

in number, physical size, shape- and spatial distributions, as well as contrast to the surrounding tissues. Also the accuracies on the more difficult pathological targets are favorable compared to most other MSD contesters.

The MSD winning algorithm [14] relied on selecting a suitable model topology and/or cascade from an ensemble of candidates through cross-validation. In contrast to this and other top-ranking participants, we were interested to develop a task-agnostic segmentation system based on a single architecture and learning procedure that makes the system lightweight and easily transferable to clinical settings with limited compute resources.

That the MPUnet can be applied 'as is' across many tasks with high performance and its robustness against overfitting can be attributed to both the fully convolutional network approach, which is already known to generalize well, and our multi-planar augmentation framework. The latter allows us to apply a single 2D model with fixed hyperparameters, resulting in a fully autonomous segmentation system of low computational complexity. Multi-planar training improves the generalization performance in several ways: **(1)** Sampling from multiple planes allows for a huge number of anatomically relevant images augmenting the training data; **(2)** Exposing a 2D model to multiple planes takes the 3D nature of the input into account while maintaining the statistical and computational efficiency of 2D kernels; **(3)** The systematic augmentation scheme allows test time augmentation to be performed, which increases the performance through variance reduction if errors across views are uncorrelated for a given subject (visualized in supplementary Fig. S.2). This makes the MPUnet an open source alternative to 3D fully convolutional neural networks.

Acknowledgements. We would like to thank both Microsoft and NVIDIA for providing computational resources on the Azure platform for this project.

References

1. Simpson, A.L., et al.: A large annotated medical image dataset for the development and evaluation of segmentation algorithms. CoRR abs/1902.09063 (2019)
2. Ronneberger, O., Fischer, P., Brox, T.: U-Net: convolutional networks for biomedical image segmentation. In: Navab, N., Hornegger, J., Wells, W.M., Frangi, A.F. (eds.) MICCAI 2015. LNCS, vol. 9351, pp. 234–241. Springer, Cham (2015). https://doi.org/10.1007/978-3-319-24574-4_28
3. Louring Koch, T., Perslev, M., Igel, C., Brand, S.S.: Accurate segmentation of dental panoramic radiographs with U-Nets. In: International Symposium on Biomedical Imaging (ISBI). IEEE (2019)
4. Ioffe, S., Szegedy, C.: Batch normalization: accelerating deep network training by reducing internal covariate shift. In: International Conference on Machine Learning (ICML), pp. 448–456. PMLR (2015)
5. Odena, A., Dumoulin, V., Olah, C.: Deconvolution and checkerboard artifacts. Distill (2016)
6. Simard, P.Y., Steinkraus, D., Platt, J.: Best practices for convolutional neural networks applied to visual document analysis. In: International Conference on Document Analysis and Recognition (ICDAR). IEEE (2003)

7. Marcus, D.S., Wang, T.H., Parker, J., Csernansky, J.G., Morris, J.C., Buckner, R.L.: Open access series of imaging studies (OASIS): cross-sectional MRI data in young, middle aged, nondemented, and demented older adults. J. Cogn. Neurosci. **19**(9), 1498–1507 (2007)

8. Boccardi, M., et al.: Training labels for hippocampal segmentation based on the EADC-ADNI harmonized hippocampal protocol. Alzheimer's Dementia **11**(2), 175–183 (2015)

9. Dam, E., Lillholm, M., Marques, J., Nielsen, M.: Automatic segmentation of high- and low-field knee MRIs using knee image quantification with data from the osteoarthritis initiative. J. Med. Imaging **2**(2), 024001 (2015)

10. Moeskops, P., Viergever, M.A., Mendrik, A.M., de Vries, L.S., Benders, M.J.N.L., Isgum, I.: Automatic segmentation of MR brain images with a convolutional neural network. IEEE Trans. Med. Imaging **35**(5), 1252–1261 (2016)

11. Ganaye, P., Sdika, M., Benoit-Cattin, H.: Towards integrating spatial localization in convolutional neural networks for brain image segmentation. In: International Symposium on Biomedical Imaging (ISBI), pp. 621–625. IEEE (2018)

12. Roy, A.G., Conjeti, S., Navab, N., Wachinger, C.: QuickNAT: segmenting MRI neuroanatomy in 20 seconds. CoRR arXiv:1801.04161 (2018)

13. Ambellan, F., Tack, A., Ehlke, M., Zachow, S.: Automated segmentation of knee bone and cartilage combining statistical shape knowledge and convolutional neural networks: data from the osteoarthritis initiative. Med. Image Anal. **52**, 109–118 (2019). OAI-ZIB dataset (supplementary material)

14. Isensee, F., et al.: nnU-Net: self-adapting framework for U-Net-based medical image segmentation. CoRR arXiv:1809.10486 (2018)

'Project & Excite' Modules
for Segmentation of Volumetric
Medical Scans

Anne-Marie Rickmann[1,2(✉)], Abhijit Guha Roy[1,2], Ignacio Sarasua[1],
Nassir Navab[2,3], and Christian Wachinger[1]

[1] Artificial Intelligence in Medical Imaging (AI-Med), KJP, LMU München,
Munich, Germany
`a.rickmann@tum.de`
[2] Computer Aided Medical Procedures, Technische Universität München,
Munich, Germany
[3] Computer Aided Medical Procedures, Johns Hopkins University, Baltimore, USA

Abstract. Fully Convolutional Neural Networks (F-CNNs) achieve
state-of-the-art performance for image segmentation in medical imaging.
Recently, squeeze and excitation (SE) modules and variations thereof
have been introduced to recalibrate feature maps channel- and spatial-
wise, which can boost performance while only minimally increasing
model complexity. So far, the development of SE has focused on 2D
images. In this paper, we propose 'Project & Excite' (PE) modules that
base upon the ideas of SE and extend them to operating on 3D volumetric images. 'Project & Excite' does not perform global average pooling,
but squeezes feature maps along different slices of a tensor separately to
retain more spatial information that is subsequently used in the excitation step. We demonstrate that PE modules can be easily integrated in
3D U-Net, boosting performance by 5% Dice points, while only increasing
the model complexity by 2%. We evaluate the PE module on two challenging tasks, whole-brain segmentation of MRI scans and whole-body
segmentation of CT scans. Code: https://github.com/ai-med/squeeze_
and_excitation.

1 Introduction

Fully convolutional neural networks (F-CNNs) have been widely adopted for
semantic image segmentation in computer vision [4] and medical imaging [5]. As
computer vision tasks mainly deal with 2D natural images, most of the architectural innovations have focused towards 2D CNNs. These innovations are often
not applicable for processing volumetric medical scans like CT, MRI and PET.
For segmentation, 2D F-CNNs were used to segment 3D medical scans slice-wise.
In such an approach the contextual information from adjacent slices remains

---

A.-M. Rickmann, A.G. Roy and I. Sarasua—Have contributed equally.

© Springer Nature Switzerland AG 2019
D. Shen et al. (Eds.): MICCAI 2019, LNCS 11765, pp. 39–47, 2019.
https://doi.org/10.1007/978-3-030-32245-8_5

unexplored, which might lead to imperfect segmentations, especially if the target class is small. Hence, the natural choice of segmenting 3D scans would be to use 3D F-CNN architectures. However, there exist some practical challenges in using 3D F-CNNs: (i) 3D F-CNNs require large amount of GPU RAM space for training, and (ii) the number of weight parameters are much higher than for its 2D counter-part, which can make the models prone to over-fitting with limited training data. Although the first issue can be effectively addressed using recent GPU clusters, the second issue still remains. This problem is prominent in medical applications, where training data is commonly very limited. To overcome the problem of over-fitting, 3D F-CNNs are carefully engineered for a task to minimize the model complexity by reducing the number of convolutional layers or by decreasing the number of channels per convolutional layer. Although this might aid training models with limited data, the exploratory capacity of the 3D F-CNN gets limited. In such a scenario, it is necessary to ensure that the learnable parameters within the F-CNN are maximally utilized to solve the task at hand. Recently, a computational module termed 'Squeeze and Excite' (SE) block [2] has been introduced to recalibrate CNN feature maps, which boosts the performance while increasing model complexity marginally. This is performed by modeling the interdependencies between the channels of feature maps, and learning to provide attention on specific channels depending on the task. They demonstrated the ease of inclusion of such modules into existing CNN architectures, providing boost in performance with fractional increase in learnable parameters. This idea was also extended to medical image segmentation [7], where it was demonstrated that such light-weight blocks can be a better architectural choice than extra convolutional layers. Although, SE blocks were customarily designed for 2D architectures, they have recently been extended to 3D F-CNNS to aid volumetric segmentation [10]. In this paper, we propose the

'Project & Excite' (PE) module, a new computational block custom-made to recalibrate 3D F-CNNs. Zhu et al. [10] directly extended the concept of SE to 3D by averaging the 4D tensor over all spatial dimensions to generate a channel descriptor for recalibration. We hypothesize that removing all spatial information leads to a loss of relevant information, particularly for segmentation, where we need to exactly localize anatomical structures. In contrast, we aim at preserving the spatial information

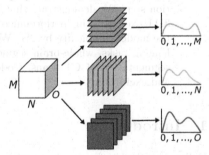

Fig. 1. Projections in 'PE' block

without any excess model complexity or FLOP operations, which is relevant for fine-grained volumetric segmentation. We draw our inspiration from traditional tensor slicing techniques, by averaging along the three principle axes of the tensor as indicated in Fig. 1. We term this operation the 'Projection' operation. By this, we get three projection-vectors indicating the relevance of the slices along the three axes. A spatial location is important if all the corresponding slices associated with it provide higher estimates. So, instead of learning the dependencies of the scalar values across the channels as in [10], we learn the dependencies of these projection-vectors across the channels for excitation. Also, PE blocks provide a global receptive field to the network at every stage. Our contributions are: (i) we propose a new computational block termed 'Project & Excite' for recalibration of 3D F-CNNs, (ii) we demonstrate that our proposed PE blocks can easily be integrated into any F-CNN boosting the segmentation performance, especially for small target classes, (iii) we demonstrate that PE blocks minimally increase the model complexity in contrast to using more convolutional layers, while providing much higher segmentation accuracy, substantiating its effectiveness in recalibration.

2 Methods

'Squeeze & Excite' (SE) blocks $\mathbf{F}_{se}(\cdot)$ take a feature map $\mathbf{U}$ as input and recalibrate it to $\hat{\mathbf{U}} = \mathbf{F}_{se}(\mathbf{U})$. Let $\hat{\mathbf{U}} \in \mathbb{R}^{H \times W \times D \times C}$, with height H, width W, depth D, and number of channels C. Commonly, SE blocks are placed after every encoder and decoder blocks of an F-CNN. In this section, we detail the extension of SE to 3D F-CNNs and our proposed 'Project & Excite' blocks.

3D 'Squeeze & Excite' Module: This 3D SE block [10], that can be termed channel SE (cSE) module, is a direct extension of the 2D SE blocks proposed in [2] to a 3D version. The transformation $\mathbf{F}_{se}(\cdot)$ is divided into the squeeze operation $\mathbf{F}_{sq}(\cdot)$ and excite operation $\mathbf{F}_{ex}(\cdot)$. The squeeze operation $\mathbf{F}_{sq}(\cdot)$ performs a global average pooling operation that squeezes the spatial content of the input $\mathbf{U}$ into a scalar value per channel $\mathbf{z} \in \mathbb{R}^C$. The excitation operation $\mathbf{F}_{ex}(\cdot)$ takes in $\mathbf{z}$ and adaptively learns the inter-channel dependencies by using two fully-connected layers. The operations are defined as:

$$z_c = \mathbf{F}_{sq}(\mathbf{u}_c) = \frac{1}{H}\frac{1}{W}\frac{1}{D}\sum_{i=1}^{H}\sum_{j=1}^{W}\sum_{k=1}^{D}\mathbf{u}_c(i,j,k), \tag{1}$$

$$\hat{\mathbf{z}} = \mathbf{F}_{ex}(\mathbf{z},\mathbf{W}) = \sigma(\mathbf{W}_2\delta(\mathbf{W}_1\mathbf{z})), \tag{2}$$

with δ denoting the ReLU nonlinearity, σ the sigmoid layer, $\mathbf{W}_1 \in \mathbb{R}^{\frac{C}{r} \times C}$ and $\mathbf{W}_2 \in \mathbb{R}^{C \times \frac{C}{r}}$ the weights of the fully-connected layers and r is the channel reduction factor similar to [2]. The output of the 3D cSE module is defined by a channel-wise multiplication of $\mathbf{U}$ with $\hat{\mathbf{z}}$. The cth channel of $\hat{\mathbf{U}}$ is defined as: $\hat{\mathbf{u}}_c = \mathbf{F}_{ex}(\mathbf{F}_{sq}(\mathbf{u}_c))\mathbf{u}_c = \hat{z}_c\mathbf{u}_c$.

3D 'Project & Excite' Module: The 3D cSE module squeezes spatial information of a volumetric feature map into one scalar value per channel. Especially in the first/last layers of a typical architecture, these feature maps have a high spatial extent. Our hypothesis is that a volumetric input of large size holds relevant spatial information which might not be properly captured by

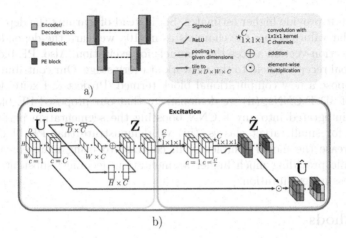

Fig. 2. (a) Typical U-net based F-CNN with PE blocks placed after each block. (b) Illustration of the proposed 'Project & Excite' block. Projection operation, with 3 different pooling operations and Excitation operation with 2 convolutional layers and recalibration of the feature map.

a global pooling operation. Hence, we introduce the 'Project & Excite' module that retains more of the valuable spatial information within our proposed *projection operation instead of spatial squeeze operation*. This follows the excite operation, which learns inter-dependencies between the projections across the different channels. Thus, it combines spatial and channel context for recalibration. The architectural details of the 'PE' block are illustrated in Fig. 2. The projection operation $\mathbf{F}_{pr}(\cdot)$ is separated into three projection operations ($\mathbf{F}_{pr_H}(\cdot)$, $\mathbf{F}_{pr_W}(\cdot)$, $\mathbf{F}_{pr_D}(\cdot)$) along the spatial dimensions with outputs $\mathbf{z}_{h_c} \in \mathbb{R}^{C \times H}$, $\mathbf{z}_{w_c} \in \mathbb{R}^{C \times W}$ and $\mathbf{z}_{d_c} \in \mathbb{R}^{C \times D}$. The projection operations are done by average pooling defined as:

$$\mathbf{z}_{h_c}(i) = \mathbf{F}_{pr_H}(\mathbf{u}_c) = \frac{1}{W}\frac{1}{D}\sum_{j=1}^{W}\sum_{k=1}^{D} \mathbf{u}_c(i,j,k), \quad i \in \{1, \ldots, H\} \qquad (3)$$

$$\mathbf{z}_{w_c}(j) = \mathbf{F}_{pr_W}(\mathbf{u}_c) = \frac{1}{H}\frac{1}{D}\sum_{i=1}^{H}\sum_{k=1}^{D} \mathbf{u}_c(i,j,k), \quad j \in \{1, \ldots, W\} \qquad (4)$$

$$\mathbf{z}_{d_c}(k) = \mathbf{F}_{pr_D}(\mathbf{u}_c) = \frac{1}{H}\frac{1}{W}\sum_{i=1}^{H}\sum_{j=1}^{W} \mathbf{u}_c(i,j,k), \quad k \in \{1, \ldots, D\}. \qquad (5)$$

The outputs $\mathbf{z}_c$ are tiled to the shape $H \times W \times D \times C$ and added to obtain $\mathbf{Z}$, which is then fed to the excitation operation $\mathbf{F}_{ex}(\cdot)$, which is defined by two convolutional layers followed by a ReLU and sigmoid activation respectively. The convolutional layers have kernel size $1 \times 1 \times 1$, to aid modelling of channel dependencies. The first layer reduces the number of channels by r, and the second layer brings the channel dimension back to the original size. The excite operation is defined as:

$$\hat{\mathbf{U}} = \hat{\mathbf{Z}} \odot \mathbf{U} = \mathbf{F}_{ex}(\mathbf{Z}) \odot \mathbf{U} = \sigma(\mathbf{V}_2 \star \delta(\mathbf{V}_1 \star \mathbf{Z})) \odot \mathbf{U}, \qquad (6)$$

where $\star$ describes the convolution operation, $\odot$ indicates point-wise multiplication, $\mathbf{V}_1 \in \mathbb{R}^{1 \times 1 \times 1 \times \frac{C}{r}}$ and $\mathbf{V}_2 \in \mathbb{R}^{1 \times 1 \times 1 \times C}$ the convolution weights, σ the sigmoid and δ the ReLU activation function. The final output of the PE block $\hat{\mathbf{U}}$ is obtained by an element-wise multiplication of the feature map $\mathbf{U}$ and $\hat{\mathbf{Z}}$.

3 Experimental Setup

Datasets: For evaluation, we choose two challenging 3D segmentation tasks. (i) *Whole-brain segmentation of MRI T1 scans:* For this task, we use the Multi-Atlas Labelling Challenge (MALC) dataset [3]. It consists of 30 T1 MRI volumes of the brain. We segment the brain volumes into 32 cortical and subcortical structures. 15 scans were used for training, 3 scans for validation and the remaining 12 scans for testing. Manual segmentations for MALC were provided by Neuromorphometrics, Inc. (ii) *Whole-body segmentation of contrast enhanced CT scans:* For this task, we use the Visceral dataset [8]. The gold corpus of the dataset has 20 annotated scans. We perform 5-fold cross-validation. One scan from the test fold was kept as validation set. We segment 14 organs from thorax and abdomen. Both datasets have common challenges w.r.t the limited amount of training scans and severe class-imbalance across the target classes.

Training Setup: We choose 3D U-Net [1] architecture for our experimental purposes. We train with whole 3D scans, for which we slightly modified the 3D U-Net architecture to ensure proper trainability. Our design consists of 3 encoder and 3 decoder blocks, with only the first two encoders performing downsampling, and the last two decoders performing upsampling. Each encoder/decoder consists of 2 convolutional layers with kernel size $3 \times 3 \times 3$. Further, the number of output channels at every encoder/decoder block was reduced to half of original size used in 3D U-Net to keep the model complexity low. For example, the two convolutions in encoder 1 have number of channels $\{16, 32\}$ instead of $\{32, 64\}$ and so on. We performed preliminary experiments to conclude that this architecture was the best for our application.

Training Parameters: Due to the large and variable dimensions of the input volumes we chose a batch size of 1 for training purpose. As low batch sizes make training unstable with Batch normalization layers, we use Instance normalization [9] instead which is agnostic to batch size. Optimization was done using SGD with momentum of 0.9. The learning rate was initially set to 0.1 and was reduced by a factor of 10 when validation loss plateaued. Data augmentation using elastic deformations and random rotations was performed on the training set. We used a combined Cross Entropy and Dice loss with the Cross Entropy loss being weighted using median frequency balancing to tackle the high class imbalance, similar to [6].

4   Experimental Results and Discussions

Position of 'PE' Blocks: In this section, we investigate the positions at which our proposed 'Project & Excite' (PE) blocks need to be placed within the 3D U-Net architecture. We explored 6 possibilities by placing them after every encoder block (P1), after every decoder block (P2), after the bottleneck block (P3), after both encoder and decoder blocks (P4), after each encoder block and bottleneck (P5), and finally after all the blocks (P6). We present the results of all these configurations in Table 1 and compared against having no 'PE' blocks. We observed that placing the blocks after every encoder, decoder and bottleneck provided the best accuracy, boosting by 4% Dice points. Also, we observed that placing it after encoder and bottleneck blocks improves the Dice score by 2% points, whereas placing it after decoder blocks does not effect the performance. We conclude that 'PE' blocks are most effective in encoder and bottleneck positions of F-CNN. In the following experiments, we place the 'PE' blocks after every encoder, decoder and bottleneck blocks.

Table 1. Mean Dice score on MALC dataset due to placement of 'PE' blocks within 3D U-Net architecture.

	Position of 'PE' block			
	Encoders	Bottleneck	Decoders	Mean Dice ± std
3D U-Net	✗	✗	✗	0.802 ± 0.171
P1	✓	✗	✗	0.828 ± 0.111
P2	✗	✗	✓	0.796 ± 0.215
P3	✗	✓	✗	0.822 ± 0.144
P4	✓	✗	✓	0.819 ± 0.159
P5	✓	✓	✗	0.818 ± 0.156
P6	✓	✓	✓	**0.843 ± 0.079**

Model Complexity: Here we investigate the increase of model complexity due to addition of 'PE' blocks within 3D U-Net architecture. We compare the PE blocks with 3D cSE blocks complexity-wise and report them in Table 2. We present results on MALC dataset. We observe that both PE blocks and cSE blocks cause the same fraction of 1.97% increase in model complexity, whereas PE blocks provide a 2% higher boost in performance at the same expense. One might think that this boost in performance is due to the added complexity, which might also be gained by adding more convolutional layers. We investigated this matter by conducting two more experiments. First, we added an extra encoder and decoder block within the architecture. This immensely increased the model complexity by almost 40% and we observed a drop in Dice performance. One possible reason might be due to over-fitting given the limited data samples and sudden increase in model complexity. So, next we only added two additional convolutional layers at the second encoder and second decoder to make sure that the increase in model complexity is only marginal ($\sim$4%), not risking over-fitting.

Table 2. Mean Dice vs model complexity measured in number of trainable parameters

	Dice	Complexity
3D-UNet [1]	0.802	$5.57 \cdot 10^6$
+3D cSE [10]	0.825	+1.97%
+PE	**0.843**	+1.97%
+Encoder/Decoder	0.779	+39.7%
+2 conv layers	0.826	+3.97%

Table 3. Comparison of 3D U-Net with 3D cSE and our proposed PE block. Mean Dice scores for selected classes of both datasets. WM stands for white matter, GM for grey matter and R for right.

	MALC dataset					
	Mean Dice ± std	WM	GM	Inf. Lat. Vent	Amygdala	Accumbens
3D U-Net [1]	0.802 ± 0.171	0.906	0.887	0.242	0.761	0.483
3D cSE [2, 10]	0.825 ± 0.119	0.907	0.888	0.403	0.761	0.704
Project & Excite	**0.843** ± 0.079	**0.916**	**0.899**	**0.604**	**0.789**	**0.735**
	Visceral dataset					
	Mean Dice ± std	Liver	R. Lung	R. Kidney	Trachea	Sternum
3D U-Net [1]	0.810 ± 0.137	0.922	0.965	0.907	0.815	0.438
3D cSE [2, 10]	0.797 ± 0.168	0.930	0.966	0.919	0.491	0.427
Project & Excite	**0.846** ± 0.095	0.931	0.966	**0.929**	**0.845**	**0.699**

Here, we did observe a boost in performance similar to cSE with double the increase in parameters, but still failed to match the performance of our PE blocks. Thus, we can conclude that PE blocks are in fact more effective than simply adding convolutional layers.

Segmentation Results: We present the results of whole-brain segmentation and whole-body segmentation in Table 3. We compared 'PE' blocks to the 3D channel SE (cSE) blocks [10] and the baseline 3D U-Net. The placement of the cSE blocks in the architecture was kept identical to ours. For brain segmentation, we observe the overall mean Dice score by using 3D cSE increases by 2% Dice points, whereas our proposed 'PE' blocks lead to an increase of 4% Dice points, substantiating its efficacy. For whole body segmentation, the mean Dice score by using 3D cSE even decreases by 1%, while, when using PE blocks, it increases by 3.5%. Further, we explored the impact of PE blocks on some selected structures. Firstly, we selected bigger structures, white and grey matter for brain segmentation, and liver and right lung for whole-body segmentation. The boost in Dice score for white and grey matter was very marginal by using either cSE or PE blocks ranging within 1% Dice points. For liver and right lung the performance using cSE or PE blocks is comparable to the baseline 3D U-Net. Next, we analyze some smaller structures, namely inferior lateral ventricles, amygdala and accumbens for brain segmentation, and right kidney, trachea and sternum for whole body segmentation, which are difficult to segment. We observe an immense boost in performance using PE blocks in these structures ranging between 3–36% Dice points, while using cSE blocks even leads to decreasing performance for trachea and sternum. In Fig. 3, we present visualizations of the segmentation performance of PE models in comparison to baseline 3D U-Net and 3D cSE models. In the top row, white arrows indicate the region of left inferior lateral ventricle, which was missed by both 3D U-Net and 3D csE models. Our proposed PE model, however, was able to segment this very small structure. In

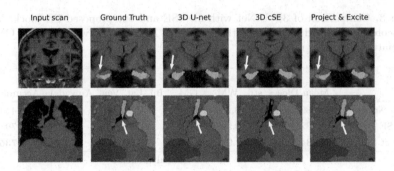

Fig. 3. Input scans, manual segmentation and results for 3D U-Net, 3D cSE and our PE model, for both datasets. White arrows point to the structures where our PE model improved the performance.

the bottom row, white arrows point to the bifurcation of the trachea, where the 3D U-Net is oversegmenting the right lung and 3D cSE model is missing the trachea completely. In conclusion, we observed similar trends in both, whole-brain and whole-body segmentation, demonstrating the efficacy of PE blocks for segmentation of small structures in 3D scans.

5   Conclusion

We propose 'Project & Excite', a light-weight recalibration module that can be easily integrated within any 3D F-CNN architectures and boosts segmentation performance while increasing model complexity by a small fraction. We demonstrated that PE blocks can be an attractive alternative to adding more convolutional layers in 3D F-CNNs, especially in situations where training data and GPU resource is limited. We exhibited the effectiveness of 'PE' blocks by conducting experiments on two challenging tasks of whole-brain and whole-body segmentation.

Acknowledgements. This research was partially supported by the Bavarian State Ministry of Science and the Arts in the framework of the Centre Digitisation.Bavaria (ZD.B). We thank NVIDIA corporation for GPU donation.

References

1. Çiçek, Ö., Abdulkadir, A., Lienkamp, S.S., Brox, T., Ronneberger, O.: 3D U-Net: learning dense volumetric segmentation from sparse annotation. In: Ourselin, S., Joskowicz, L., Sabuncu, M.R., Unal, G., Wells, W. (eds.) MICCAI 2016. LNCS, vol. 9901, pp. 424–432. Springer, Cham (2016). https://doi.org/10.1007/978-3-319-46723-8_49
2. Hu, J., Shen, L., Sun, G.: Squeeze-and-excitation networks. In: The IEEE Conference on Computer Vision and Pattern Recognition (CVPR), June 2018

3. Landman, B., Warfield, S.: MICCAI 2012 workshop on multi-atlas labeling. In: Medical Image Computing and Computer Assisted Intervention Conference (2012)
4. Long, J., Shelhamer, E., Darrell, T.: Fully convolutional networks for semantic segmentation. In: The IEEE Conference on Computer Vision and Pattern Recognition (CVPR), June 2015
5. Ronneberger, O., Fischer, P., Brox, T.: U-Net: convolutional networks for biomedical image segmentation. In: Navab, N., Hornegger, J., Wells, W.M., Frangi, A.F. (eds.) MICCAI 2015. LNCS, vol. 9351, pp. 234–241. Springer, Cham (2015). https://doi.org/10.1007/978-3-319-24574-4_28
6. Roy, A.G., Conjeti, S., Sheet, D., Katouzian, A., Navab, N., Wachinger, C.: Error corrective boosting for learning fully convolutional networks with limited data. In: Descoteaux, M., Maier-Hein, L., Franz, A., Jannin, P., Collins, D.L., Duchesne, S. (eds.) MICCAI 2017. LNCS, vol. 10435, pp. 231–239. Springer, Cham (2017). https://doi.org/10.1007/978-3-319-66179-7_27
7. Roy, A.G., Navab, N., Wachinger, C.: Recalibrating fully convolutional networks with spatial and channel "squeeze and excitation" blocks. IEEE TMI **38**(2), 540–549 (2019)
8. Jimenez-del Toro, O., et al.: Cloud-based evaluation of anatomical structure segmentation and landmark detection algorithms: visceral anatomy benchmarks. IEEE TMI **35**(11), 2459–2475 (2016)
9. Ulyanov, D., Vedaldi, A., Lempitsky, V.: Improved texture networks: maximizing quality and diversity in feed-forward stylization and texture synthesis. In: CVPR, pp. 6924–6932 (2017)
10. Zhu, W., et al.: AnatomyNet: deep learning for fast and fully automated whole-volume segmentation of head and neck anatomy. Med. Phys. **46**(2), 576–589 (2019)

Assessing Reliability and Challenges of Uncertainty Estimations for Medical Image Segmentation

Alain Jungo[✉] and Mauricio Reyes

Insel Data Science Center, Inselspital, Bern University Hospital,
University of Bern, Bern, Switzerland
alain.jungo@artorg.unibe.ch

Abstract. Despite the recent improvements in overall accuracy, deep learning systems still exhibit low levels of robustness. Detecting possible failures is critical for a successful clinical integration of these systems, where each data point corresponds to an individual patient. Uncertainty measures are a promising direction to improve failure detection since they provide a measure of a system's confidence. Although many uncertainty estimation methods have been proposed for deep learning, little is known on their benefits and current challenges for medical image segmentation. Therefore, we report results of evaluating common voxel-wise uncertainty measures with respect to their reliability, and limitations on two medical image segmentation datasets. Results show that current uncertainty methods perform similarly and although they are well-calibrated at the dataset level, they tend to be miscalibrated at subject-level. Therefore, the reliability of uncertainty estimates is compromised, highlighting the importance of developing subject-wise uncertainty estimations. Additionally, among the benchmarked methods, we found auxiliary networks to be a valid alternative to common uncertainty methods since they can be applied to any previously trained segmentation model.

Keywords: Uncertainty · Segmentation · Deep learning

1 Introduction

Deep learning-based methods have led to impressive improvements in medical image segmentation over the past years. For many tasks, the performance is comparable to human-level performance, or even surpasses it [11]. Nonetheless, despite improvements in accuracy, the robustness aspects of these systems call for significant improvements for a successful clinical integration of these technologies, where each data point corresponds to an individual patient. This highlights

Electronic supplementary material The online version of this chapter (https:// doi.org/10.1007/978-3-030-32245-8_6) contains supplementary material, which is available to authorized users.

the importance of having mechanisms to effectively monitor computer results in order to detect and react on system's failures at the patient level. Among others, uncertainty measures are a promising direction since uncertainties can provide information as to how confident the system was on performing a given task on a given patient. This information in turn can be used to leverage the decision-making process of a user, as well as to enable time-effective corrections of computer results by for instance, focusing on areas of high uncertainty.

Different approaches have been proposed to quantify uncertainties in deep learning models. Among the most popular approaches are: (a) Bayesian uncertainty estimation via test-time dropout [5], (b) aleatoric uncertainty estimation via a second network output [9], and (c) uncertainty estimation via ensembling of networks [10]. In medical image segmentation, uncertainty measures are of interest at three levels. The first, most fine-grained level, is the voxel[1]-wise uncertainty, which provides a measure of uncertainty for the predicted class of each voxel. This level of uncertainty is especially useful for the interaction with humans, be it by providing additional information to foster comprehensibility or as guidance for correction tasks. The second level is the uncertainty at the level of a segmented instance (or object). Nair et al. [12] and Graham et al. [6] used instance-level uncertainty to reduce the false discovery rate of brain lesions and cells, respectively. In both approaches voxel-wise uncertainties were aggregated to obtain an instance-wise uncertainty. Similarly, Eaton-Rosen et al. [4] aggregated voxel-wise uncertainties of brain tumor segmentations to obtain confidence intervals for tumor volumes. The third level is the subject-level uncertainty, which informs us whether the segmentation task was successful (e.g., above a certain metric). Having information about success or failure would be sufficient for many tasks, e.g., high-throughput analysis or selection of cases for expert review. As proposed by Jungo et al. [8], task-specific aggregation of the voxel-wise uncertainties could be used to obtain subject-level uncertainties. In contrast, DeVries et al. [3] and Robinson et al. [13], proposed an auxiliary neural network that predicts segmentation performance at the subject-level. A current challenge to use these latter type of approaches is that considerable large training datasets are necessary in practice to ensure their reliability [3].

In order to better understand the benefits and current challenges in uncertainty estimation for medical image segmentation, we evaluated common uncertainty measures with respect to their reliability, their benefit, and limitations[2]. Additionally, we analyzed the requirements for uncertainties in medical image segmentation and we make practical recommendations for their evaluation.

2   Material and Methods

2.1   Data

We selected two publicly available, and distinct datasets for the experiments. The first dataset is the brain tumor segmentation (BraTS) challenge dataset

---

[1] For simplicity, we use *voxel* even if it could be a two-dimensional image.

[2] Code available at https://github.com/alainjungo/reliability-challenges-uncertainty.

2018 [1] consisting of 265 subjects. Each subject features four magnetic resonance images (T1-weighted, T1-weighted post-contrast, T2-weighted, FLAIR)
of a size of $240 \times 240 \times 155$ isotropic (1 mm^3) voxels. We split the dataset into
100 training, 25 validation, and 160 testing subjects, combined the three tumor
sub-compartment labels to segment the whole tumor, and performed a z-score
intensity normalization ($\mu = 0, \sigma = 1$) on each subject and image individually.
The second dataset is the international skin imaging collaboration (ISIC) lesion
segmentation dataset 2017 [2] consisting of 2000 training, 150 validation, and
600 testing images. We resized the color images to a size of 256×192 pixels and
normalized the intensities to the range $[0, 1]$.

2.2 Experimental Setting

Our aim is to evaluate the reliability of uncertainty measures for deep learning-
based segmentation of medical images. Rather than building a specific fine-tuned,
top-performing segmentation model, we used a U-Net-like architecture [14] due
to its popularity, simplicity, and to minimize architectural influences on the
outcomes[3]. The architecture consists of four pooling/upsampling steps and has
dropout regularization ($p = 0.05$) and batch normalization after each convolution. We used a common training scheme consisting of a cross-entropy loss with
Adam optimizer (learning rate: 10^{-4}), and applied early stopping with respect
to the validation set Dice coefficient. Any adaptation to this architecture and
training scheme was performed to fit the needs of each studied uncertainty approach.

2.3 Uncertainty Methods

We evaluated the following five different uncertainty measures:

Baseline Uncertainty: Softmax Entropy. Although the softmax output of a
model is arguably a probability measure [5], we considered it as reference comparison as it is implicitly generated by segmentation networks. We named this strat-
egy *baseline*. We used the normalized entropy $H = -\sum_{c \in \mathcal{C}} p_c log(p_c)/log(|\mathcal{C}|) \in [0, 1]$
as a measure of uncertainty, where p_c is the softmax output for class c and $\mathcal{C}$ is
the set of classes ($\mathcal{C} = \{0, 1\}$ in our case).

MC Dropout. Test time dropout can be viewed as an approximation of a
Bayesian neural network [5]. T stochastic network samples can be interpreted as
Monte-Carlo samples of the posterior distribution of the network's weights and
result in a class probability of $p_c = 1/T \sum_{t=1}^{T} p_{t,c}$. We employed the normalized
entropy of these probabilities as a measure of uncertainty. For the experiments,
we used $T = 20$ and considered two different dropout layer positioning strategies.
First, we applied MC dropout on the base model (see Sect. 2.2), which uses
minimal dropout ($p = 0.05$) after each convolution. Second, we applied more

---

[3] We also conducted experiments with a DenseNet-like architecture with no notable
differences in the outcome and therefore omit it here for space and clarity reasons.

prominent dropout ($p = 0.5$) at the center positions (i.e., before pooling and after upsampling, similar to [12]). Accordingly, we name these two strategies as *baseline+MC* and *center+MC*.

Aleatoric Uncertainty. In contrast to the model uncertainty (captured by e.g. MC dropout), the aleatoric uncertainty is said to capture noise inherent in the observation [9]. It is obtained by defining a network f with two outputs $[\hat{x}, \sigma^2] = f(x)$ and input x, where the outputs $\hat{x}$ and σ^2 are the mean and variance of the logits perturbed with Gaussian noise. The aleatoric loss optimizes both outputs simultaneously by MC sampling (ten samples in our case) of the perturbed logits. We used $\hat{x}$ for the class predictions and the variance σ^2 as a measure of uncertainty. We normalized the variance to $[0, 1]$ over all predictions.

Ensembles. Another way of quantifying uncertainties is by ensembling multiple models [10]. We combined the class probabilities of each network k by the average $p_c = 1/K \sum_{k=1}^{K} p_{k,c}$ over all $K = 10$ networks and used the normalized entropy as uncertainty measure. The individual networks share the same architecture (see Sect. 2.2) but were trained on different subsets (90%) of the training dataset and different random initialization to enforce variability.

Auxiliary Network. Inspired by [3,13], where an auxiliary network is used to predict segmentation performance at the subject-level, we apply an auxiliary network to predict voxel-wise uncertainties of the segmentation model by learning from the segmentation errors (i.e., false positives and false negatives). For the experiments, we considered two opposing types of auxiliary networks. The first one, named *auxiliary feat.*, consists of three consecutive 1×1 convolution layers cascaded after the last feature maps of the segmentation network. The second auxiliary network, named *auxiliary segm.*, is a completely independent network (same U-Net as described in Sect. 2.2) that uses as input the original images and the segmentation masks produced by the segmentation model (generated by five-fold cross-validation). We normalized the output uncertainty subject-wise to $[0, 1]$ for comparability purposes.

2.4 Assessing Quality of Uncertainties

We adopted three metrics to evaluate the quality of uncertainties. Additionally, we computed the Dice coefficient to also verify segmentation performance as uncertainty methods typically link both tasks.

Calibration. Model calibration is important when not only the predicted class but also its corresponding confidence is of interest. In this regards, calibration has been used as a surrogate to asses the reliability of uncertainties [9]. A model is said to be perfectly calibrated if its predictions $f(x)$ with confidence p do occur with a fraction p of the time ($P(y = 1|f(x) = p) = p$ for the binary case). Meaning for example that for 100 predictions with a confidence of 0.7, 70 predictions are expected to be correct [7]. We assessed calibration of uncertainties by reliability diagrams and expected calibration error (ECE) [7]. Reliability diagrams show the deviation of the perfect calibration by plotting the binned predicted confidences against the accuracy obtained for each bin (fraction of positives). The ECE is defined as the absolute error of these bins (i.e., the gap between confidence and accuracy) weighted by the number of samples in the bins, where a lower ECE (close to zero) indicates a better calibration. In our experiments, we used a bin size of ten and used the model output probabilities as confidence. For methods not providing segmentation probabilities but direct segmentation uncertainty estimates (i.e., auxiliary and aleatoric), we translated the uncertainties by $y(1 - 0.5q) + (1 - y)(0.5q)$ to confidences, where $y \in \{0, 1\}$ is the segmentation label and $q \in [0, 1]$ is the normalized uncertainty.

Uncertainty-Error Overlap. In a practical setting, perfect calibration of a model is impossible [7]. Often, segmentation tasks do not require perfect calibration but it would be sufficient for a model to be uncertain where it makes mistakes and certain where it is correct. To assess this condition, we used the overlap (determined by the Dice coefficient) between the segmentation error and the thresholded uncertainty, termed *uncertainty-error overlap* (*U-E*). This metric is not influenced by the true negatives from background areas, which are typically enormous in medical image segmentation. It is therefore an alternative for the ECE, which includes foreground as well as background areas.

Corrections. Motivated by previous works using uncertainty estimations, we assessed the quality of uncertainties by evaluating their benefit to correct segmentations. We define TPU, TNU, FPU, FNU as uncertainty in the true positives (TP), true negatives (TP), false positives (FP), and false negatives (FN). A beneficial correction is said to improve the Dice coefficient, hence, to benefit from removal of false positives, the relation $FPU(TP) > TPU(TP+FP+FN)$ needs to be satisfied (for the accuracy $FPU > TPU$ is sufficient). Similarly, in order to benefit from adding voxels (i.e., correct false negatives), the relation $FNU(TP + FP + FN) > TNU(TP)$, needs to be satisfied. However, the latter relation is not practically applicable due to large backgrounds and thus typically large TNU. Since voxel-wise corrections (as opposed to instance-wise corrections) might be more harmful than beneficial, we calculated the proportion of subjects that fulfill the benefit condition for false positive removal, BnF, as means of comparison to other methods.

3   Results

Figure 1 compares the calibration at the dataset level (i.e., all voxels in the dataset) with the calibration at the subject level (i.e., voxels of one subject). It shows the miscalibration that can occur at subject level (S1 and S2) while the calibration at dataset level is good. We found approximately 28%/46% underconfident and 32%/18% overconfident calibrations for the subjects of the BraTS/ISIC dataset. This underlines the special caution needed when using the calibration-based metrics (e.g., ECE) at the dataset level, as it can lead to misperception on the actual calibration quality of a model, and hence, the reliability of

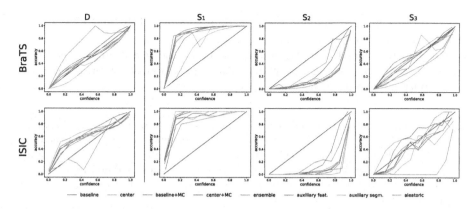

Fig. 1. Calibration at the dataset level (D) compared to the (mis)calibration at the subject level (S1, S2, S3) for the different uncertainty methods. S1, S2, S3 correspond to exemplary subjects for which the models are underconfident (S1), overconfident (S2), and well-calibrated (S3). Rows correspond to results on the BRATS and ISIC datasets.

its uncertainty estimations. Noticeable is also the agreement among the uncertainty methods at subject-level, suggesting only little benefit in selecting one uncertainty method over another.

In Table 1, we report for BraTS and the ISIC dataset the following metrics: average subject-level ECE (dataset-level ECE in supplementary material A), uncertainty-error overlap (U-E), proportion of correction-benefiting test subjects (BnF), and Dice coefficient. For a fair comparison, we selected the best-performing threshold for each method whenever the metric required an uncertainty threshold (i.e., U-E and BnF). Overall for both datasets, no uncertainty method outperforms and stands out over the others. Particularly, the *aleatoric* method and methods with large dropout (*center/+MC*) yield worst performance. The *aleatoric* method fails to produce uncertainty at the locations of segmentation errors (i.e., low U-E) and is therefore unable to improve segmentation results through corrections, whereas the large dropout mainly negatively affects segmentation performance and ECE. The results further show that MC dropout (*baseline+MC* and *center+MC*) typically improves ECE, U-E, and Dice coefficient over the non-MC versions (*baseline* and *center*), but larger amounts of dropout (*baseline<center* and *baseline+MC<center+MC*) results in worse performances, which suggests using MC dropout in the regimes where the benefit with respect to the uncertainty is minimal compared to standard softmax. We could confirm this finding through intermediate dropout strategies (see supplementary material B). We also observe good performances of the auxiliary networks, which are typically well-calibrated and profit from a good segmentation performance of their segmentation network (i.e., *baseline* model). In regards to the metrics, we note that low ECE values stem from large amount of low-confident background areas that positively affects the ECE. This also explains the lower ECE values for the BraTS dataset, which contains more background (even with applied brain mask) than the ISIC dataset, due to the additional

image dimension. Additionally, the BnF only considers TPU and FPU uncertainties and is therefore favorable for methods with low precision (more FP typically yields more FPU). We found this to be the reason for the bad correction performance of the ensemble on the BraTS dataset, even though the uncertainty-error overlap was good.

Table 1. Performances of the different uncertainties with respect to expected calibration error (ECE), uncertainty-error overlap (U-E), proportion of correction-benefiting test subjects (BnF), and Dice coefficient. Values are presented as *mean (rank)*. Standard deviation is omitted due to marginal differences. Upwards and downwards arrow indicate desired higher and lower metric values, respectively. Horizontal separation group types of uncertainty methods.

	BraTS				ISIC			
	ECE % ↓	U-E ↑	BnF ↑	Dice ↑	ECE % ↓	U-E ↑	BnF ↑	Dice ↑
Baseline	0.925 (4)	0.432 (2)	0.39 (3)	0.874 (2)	7.256 (4)	0.424 (4)	0.26 (4)	0.814 (3)
Center	1.758 (7)	0.409 (5)	**0.5** (1)	0.866 (5)	9.415 (8)	0.411 (6)	0.27 (3)	0.78 (6)
Baseline+MC	**0.9** (1)	**0.433** (1)	0.36 (4)	0.874 (2)	7.36 (5)	0.428 (3)	0.24 (5)	0.813 (4)
Center+MC	1.233 (6)	**0.433** (1)	0.27 (6)	0.868 (4)	8.766 (7)	0.428 (3)	0.17 (6)	0.794 (5)
Ensemble	0.919 (2)	**0.433** (1)	0.32 (5)	**0.879** (1)	**7.131** (1)	0.431 (2)	0.31 (2)	**0.831** (1)
Auxiliary feat	0.923 (3)	0.427 (3)	0.48 (2)	0.874 (2)	7.216 (3)	0.421 (5)	**0.33** (1)	0.814 (3)
Auxiliary segm	0.925 (4)	0.412 (4)	0.48 (2)	0.874 (2)	7.212 (2)	**0.433** (1)	0.27 (3)	0.814 (3)
Aleatoric	1.134 (5)	0.054 (6)	0.06 (7)	0.872 (3)	7.837 (6)	0.058 (7)	0.12 (7)	0.82 (2)

4   Discussion

The results show that although current voxel-wise uncertainty measures are rather well-calibrated at the dataset level (i.e., all voxels in the dataset) they tend to fail at the subject level (Fig. 1). This observation is to be expected since subject-level calibration errors (under- or overcalibration) can average out at the dataset level. Based on the proposed calibration-based metric, no overall best uncertainty measure was found among the studied methods. From our experiments we can conclude that methods that aggregate voxel-wise uncertainty to provide subject-level estimations are not reliable enough to be used as a mechanism to detect failed segmentations. We thus conclude on the importance of developing subject-level uncertainty estimation in medical image segmentation that can cope with the issue of High-Dimension-Low-Sample-Size (HDLSS) to ensure their reliability in practice.

Unsurprisingly, the ensemble method yields rank-wise the most reliable results (Table 1) and would typically be a good choice (if the resources allow it). The results also revealed that methods based on MC dropout are heavily dependent on the influence of dropout on the segmentation performance. In contrast, auxiliary networks turned out to be a promising alternative to existing uncertainty measures. They perform comparable to other methods but have the benefit of being applicable to any high-performing segmentation network not optimized to predict reliable uncertainty estimates. No significant differences were found between using *auxiliary feat.* and *auxiliary segm.*. Through a sensitivity analysis performed over all studied uncertainty methods (see supplementary material C), we could confirm our observations that different uncertainty estimation methods yield different levels of precision and recall. Furthermore, we observed that when using current uncertainty methods for correcting segmentations, a maximum benefit can be attained when preferring a combination of low precision segmentation models and uncertainty-based false positive removal.

Our evaluation has several limitations worth mentioning. First, although the experiments were performed on two typical and distinctive datasets, they feature large structures to segment. The findings reported herein may differ for other datasets, especially if these consists of very small structures to be segmented. Second, the assessment of the uncertainty is influenced by the segmentation performance. Even though we succeeded in building similarly performing models, their differences cannot be fully decoupled and neglected when analyzing the uncertainty.

Overall, we aim with these results to point to the existing challenges for a reliable utilization of voxel-wise uncertainties in medical image segmentation, and foster the development of subject/patient-level uncertainty estimation approaches under the condition of HDLSS. We recommend that utilization of uncertainty methods ideally need to be coupled with an assessment of model calibration at the subject/patient-level. Proposed conditions, along with the threshold-free ECE metric can be adopted to test whether uncertainty estimations can be of benefit for a given task.

Acknowledgments. This work was supported by the Swiss National Foundation by grant number 169607. The authors thank Fabian Balsiger for the valuable discussions.

References

1. Bakas, S., et al.: Identifying the best machine learning algorithms for brain tumor segmentation, progression assessment, and overall survival prediction in the BRATS challenge. arXiv preprint arXiv:1811.02629 (2018)
2. Codella, N.C., et al.: Skin lesion analysis toward melanoma detection: a challenge at the 2017 international symposium on biomedical imaging (isbi), hosted by the international skin imaging collaboration (isic). In: ISBI, pp. 168–172. IEEE (2018)
3. DeVries, T., Taylor, G.W.: Leveraging uncertainty estimates for predicting segmentation quality. arXiv preprint arXiv:1807.00502 (2018)
4. Eaton-Rosen, Z., Bragman, F., Bisdas, S., Ourselin, S., Cardoso, M.J.: Towards safe deep learning: accurately quantifying biomarker uncertainty in neural network predictions. In: Frangi, A.F., Schnabel, J.A., Davatzikos, C., Alberola-López, C., Fichtinger, G. (eds.) MICCAI 2018. LNCS, vol. 11070, pp. 691–699. Springer, Cham (2018). https://doi.org/10.1007/978-3-030-00928-1_78
5. Gal, Y., Ghahramani, Z.: Dropout as a bayesian approximation: representing model uncertainty in deep learning. In: ICML, pp. 1050–1059 (2016)

6. Graham, S., et al.: Mild-net: minimal information loss dilated network for gland instance segmentation in colon histology images. Med. Image Anal. **52**, 199–211 (2019)
7. Guo, C., Pleiss, G., Sun, Y., Weinberger, K.Q.: On calibration of modern neural networks. In: ICML, pp. 1321–1330. JMLR. org (2017)
8. Jungo, A., et al.: Uncertainty-driven sanity check: application to postoperative brain tumor cavity segmentation. MIDL (2018)
9. Kendall, A., Gal, Y.: What uncertainties do we need in bayesian deep learning for computer vision? In: NIPS, pp. 5574–5584 (2017)
10. Lakshminarayanan, B., Pritzel, A., Blundell, C.: Simple and scalable predictive uncertainty estimation using deep ensembles. In: NIPS, pp. 6402–6413 (2017)
11. Litjens, G., et al.: A survey on deep learning in medical image analysis. Med. Image Anal. **42**, 60–88 (2017)
12. Nair, T., Precup, D., Arnold, D.L., Arbel, T.: Exploring uncertainty measures in deep networks for multiple sclerosis lesion detection and segmentation. In: Frangi, A.F., Schnabel, J.A., Davatzikos, C., Alberola-López, C., Fichtinger, G. (eds.) MICCAI 2018. LNCS, vol. 11070, pp. 655–663. Springer, Cham (2018). https://doi.org/10.1007/978-3-030-00928-1_74
13. Robinson, R., et al.: Real-time prediction of segmentation quality. In: Frangi, A.F., Schnabel, J.A., Davatzikos, C., Alberola-López, C., Fichtinger, G. (eds.) MICCAI 2018. LNCS, vol. 11073, pp. 578–585. Springer, Cham (2018). https://doi.org/10.1007/978-3-030-00937-3_66
14. Ronneberger, O., Fischer, P., Brox, T.: U-Net: convolutional networks for biomedical image segmentation. In: Navab, N., Hornegger, J., Wells, W.M., Frangi, A.F. (eds.) MICCAI 2015. LNCS, vol. 9351, pp. 234–241. Springer, Cham (2015). https://doi.org/10.1007/978-3-319-24574-4_28

Learning Cross-Modal Deep Representations for Multi-Modal MR Image Segmentation

Cheng Li[1], Hui Sun[1], Zaiyi Liu[2], Meiyun Wang[3], Hairong Zheng[1],
and Shanshan Wang[1(✉)]

[1] Paul C. Lauterbur Research Center for Biomedical Imaging,
Shenzhen Institutes of Advanced Technology,
Chinese Academy of Sciences, Shenzhen, Guangdong, China
sophiasswang@hotmail.com
[2] Department of Radiology, Guangdong General Hospital,
Guangdong Academy of Medical Sciences, Guangzhou, Guangdong, China
[3] Department of Medical Imaging, Henan Provincial People's Hospital,
Zhengzhou, Henan, China

Abstract. Multi-modal magnetic resonance imaging (MRI) is essential in clinics for comprehensive diagnosis and surgical planning. Nevertheless, the segmentation of multi-modal MR images tends to be time-consuming and challenging. Convolutional neural network (CNN)-based multi-modal MR image analysis commonly proceeds with multiple downsampling streams fused at one or several layers. Although inspiring performance has been achieved, the feature fusion is usually conducted through simple summation or concatenation without optimization. In this work, we propose a supervised image fusion method to selectively fuse the useful information from different modalities and suppress the respective noise signals. Specifically, an attention block is introduced as guidance for the information selection. From the different modalities, one modality that contributes most to the results is selected as the master modality, which supervises the information selection of the other assistant modalities. The effectiveness of the proposed method is confirmed through breast mass segmentation in MR images of two modalities and better segmentation results are achieved compared to the state-of-the-art methods.

Keywords: Supervised feature fusion · Multi-modal image segmentation · Spatial attention

1 Introduction

Multi-modal magnetic resonance imaging (MRI) is an essential tool in clinics for the screening and diagnosis of different diseases including breast cancer, prostate

---

C. Li and H. Sun—These authors contributed equally to this work.

© Springer Nature Switzerland AG 2019
D. Shen et al. (Eds.): MICCAI 2019, LNCS 11765, pp. 57–65, 2019.
https://doi.org/10.1007/978-3-030-32245-8_7

cancer, and neurodegenerative disorders. The combination of different imaging modalities can overcome the limitations of the individual modalities. In breast cancer screening, for example, while contrast-enhanced MRI possesses high sensitivity in detecting breast lesions, T2-weighted MRI is effective in reducing false-positive results [1,2]. Considering different MRI modalities is thus important for the acquisition of accurate lesion information. Lesion segmentation of MR images is a critical step in the process for the following diagnosis and surgical planning. Manual segmentation is both time-consuming and error-prone. Therefore, the development of automatic and reliable algorithms is of high clinical values.

Learning-based methods, especially those based on convolutional neural networks (CNNs), have seen rapid development in medical image analysis in the last decade [3]. CNNs were originally proposed for the task of image-level classification. The intuitive application of CNNs to image segmentation, which is a pixel-level classification task, was conducted by classifying each pixel in a sliding window manner (R-CNN) [4]. Fully convolutional neural networks (FCNs) were designed later to avoid the cumbersome and memory-intensive R-CNN approach [5]. FCNs segment the input image directly by generating heatmap output. Following FCNs, U-Net was proposed specifically for biomedical image segmentation [6], which is the current baseline network for various medical image segmentation tasks and is the inspiration of many subsequent works.

A critical issue regarding multi-modal image segmentation is the fusion of information from the different imaging modalities. CNN-based multi-modal image fusion can be realized through early fusion, late fusion, and multi-layer fusion. Early fusion happens at the input stage or low-level feature stages [7,8]. This strategy may fail to achieve the expected information compensation, especially when the different modal images have complex relationships. Late fusion refers to the fusion of high-level and high-abstract features, and multi-stream networks are commonly utilized in this case with each stream processing images from one modality. Late fusion has been demonstrated to generate better segmentation results than direct early fusion [9,10]. Nevertheless, multi-layer fusion should be a more generalized strategy. Multi-layer fusion was first proposed for RGB-D image segmentation where FuseNet was designed to incorporate depth information into RGB images [11]. Further network optimization over FuseNet confirmed that multi-layer fusion was a more effective approach [12]. Multi-layer fusion has also been successfully applied to multi-modal medical image segmentation [13]. Although inspiring results have been achieved, the feature fusion was conducted through direct pixel-wise summation or channel-wise concatenation. Without supervision and selection, the fusion process may introduce irrelevant signals and noise signals to the final outputs.

In this study, we propose a novel multi-stream CNN-based feature fusion network for the processing of multi-modal MR images. In accordance with real clinical situations, we pick one MR modality that contributes most to the final segmentation results as the master modality, and the other modalities are treated as assistant modalities. Inspired by the knowledge distillation concept [14], where a teacher network supervises the training of a student network, our master modal

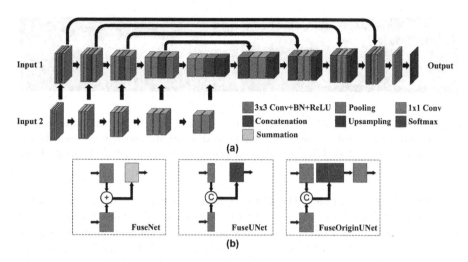

Fig. 1. Baseline network architecture. The overall network structure (a) and the implementation details of the modality fusion by the three networks (b). (Color figure online)

network stream supervises the training of the assistant modal network streams. In detail, we adopt an attention block to extract the supervision information from the master modality and utilize this supervision information to select useful information from both the master modality and the assistant modalities. The effectiveness of the proposed method is evaluated through the mass segmentation in breast MR images of two modalities. Segmentation of breast mass structures is a challenging task, as the masses have a large range of sizes and shapes, especially for spiculated masses that have ill-defined borders. The results show that our method can achieve the best performance compared to existing feature fusion strategies.

2 Methodology

Breast MRI Dataset. The breast MR images were collected using an Achieva 1.5T system (Philips Healthcare, Best, Netherlands) with a four-channel phased-array breast coil. All acquisitions of 313 patients in the prone position were conducted between 2011 and 2017. Two MRI sequences were applied. Axial T2-weighted (T2W) images (TR/TE = 3400 ms/90 ms, FOV = 336 mm × 336 mm, section thickness = 1 mm) with fat suppression were obtained before the injection of contrast medium. After the intravenous injection of 0.3 mL/kg of gado-diamide (BeiLu Pharmaceutical, Beijing, China), axial fat-suppressed contrast-enhanced T1-weighted (T1C) images were collected (TR/TE = 5.2 ms/2.3 ms, FOV = 336 mm × 336 mm, section thickness = 1 mm, and flip angle = 15°). Since manual segmentation of the breast masses in 3D multi-modal MR images is very difficult and time-consuming, only the central slices with the largest cross-section areas were labelled by two experienced radiologists in this retrospective study.

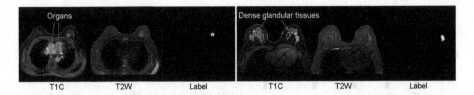

Fig. 2. Example breast MR images when T1C images highlight irrelevant regions (organs or dense glandular tissues) and T2W can distinguish these regions from the targeted breast masses. Label images are the manual segmentation results. (Color figure online)

A Better Feature Fusion Baseline Network Architecture. Our baseline model is built from FuseNet [11] with two major modifications. First, FuseNet was proposed for the analysis of natural images. The encoder part of FuseNet adopted the VGG 16-layer model for the convenience of utilizing ImageNet pre-trained network parameters. To better adapt to medical image processing, we build a FuseNet-like network architecture based on U-Net, named FuseOrigin-UNet (Fig. 1). Second, in FuseNet, the feature fusion of different imaging modalities was realized by pixel-wise summation, which could preserve the VGG 16-layer model after introducing the feature fusion module. In FuseOriginUNet, a channel-wise concatenation is implemented instead. To make the overall network lightweight, we half the convolution kernels for each layer in the encoder part compared to U-Net and achieve the final baseline model FuseUNet (Fig. 1). The experiments show that FuseUNet achieves better performance compared to both FuseNet and FuseOriginUNet.

Supervised Cross-Modal Deep Representation Learning. Different imaging modalities contain different sorts of useful information for the targeted task. For breast MR images, the T1C modality has a high sensitivity and a relatively low specificity in detecting breast masses. Two examples are shown in Fig. 2. It can be observed that the T1C image highlights not only the breast mass area but also the irrelevant regions, such as the organs and the dense glandular tissues. In this case, T2W images are important in distinguishing the true masses from all the enhanced areas. Accordingly, the two imaging modalities are treated differently in the proposed method. T1C is chosen as the master modality having a greater impact on the results. T2W is regarded as the assistant modality complementing the information of the master modality.

Inspired by the knowledge distillation between teacher–student networks [14], we propose a supervised master–assistant cross-modal learning framework (Fig. 3a). The master modality generates supervision information that modulates the learning of the assistant modality. Enlightened by the activation-based attention transfer strategies [15], a spatial attention (SA) block is designed to extract the supervision information (Fig. 3b). The input of the block is the features from the master modal stream and the output, which is a weight heatmap, is utilized to guide the information selection for both the master and the assistant modalities.

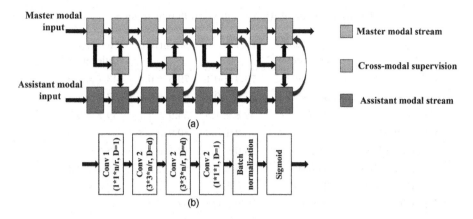

Fig. 3. The encoder section of the proposed master–assistant cross-modal learning network (a) and the cross-modal supervision learning module (n is the input feature number, r is a reduction factor, and D is the atrous rate of dilated convolutions) (b). (Color figure online)

Implementation Details. Five-fold cross-validation experiments were conducted. All the images along with the label images were resized to 256×256 and intensity normalized. No further data processing or augmentation was applied. The models were implemented with PyTorch on a NVIDIA TITAN Xp GPU (12G) with batch size of 4. ADAM with AMSGRAD was applied to train the models. The step decay learning rate strategy was used with an initial learning rate of 1e-4 that was decreased by half every 30 epochs. The hyperparameters in the SA module were set as $r = 16$ and $d = 4$. To tackle the widely recognized class-imbalance problem in medical image analysis, a loss function combining cross-entropy loss and Dice loss was adopted:

$$
\begin{aligned}
L &= L_{Dice} + \alpha \times L_{CE} \\
&= (1 - \frac{2\sum_{i=1}^{N} p_i y_i + \varepsilon}{\sum_{i=1}^{N} p_i + \sum_{i=1}^{N} y_i + \varepsilon}) + \alpha \times (-\frac{1}{N}(y_i \sum_{i=1}^{N} p_i + (1 - y_i) \sum_{i=1}^{N}(1 - p_i)))
\end{aligned}
\tag{1}
$$

where L is the loss function utilized, L_{Dice} is the Dice loss, L_{CE} is the cross-entropy loss, N is the total number of pixels in the image, $y_i \in \{0, 1\}$ is the manual segmentation label of the ith pixel in the image where 0 refers to the background and 1 refers to the foreground, $p_i \in [0, 1]$ is the corresponding predicted probability of the ith pixel belonging to the foreground class, $\varepsilon = 1.0$ is a constant to keep the numerical stability, and $\alpha = 1.0$ is a weight constant to control the tradeoff between the two losses.

Three metrics were utilized to quantify the segmentation performance, the Dice similarity coefficient, sensitivity, and relative area difference. Three independent experiments were run, and the results are presented as ($mean \pm s.d.$).

Table 1. Segmentation results of different models.

Models	Number of parameters*	Dice#	Sensitivity#	Relative area difference#
U-Net (T1C)	34.5M	73.3 ± 0.1	79.5 ± 0.8	43.7 ± 1.9
U-Net + SA (T1C)	34.7M	75.8 ± 0.2	82.6 ± 0.5	33.9 ± 2.2
FuseNet	29.4M	52.8 ± 1.5	54.9 ± 2.7	49.2 ± 2.7
FuseNetConcate	74.0M	73.2 ± 0.3	80.9 ± 0.8	41.8 ± 1.3
FuseOriginUNet	56.2M	75.0 ± 0.5	82.1 ± 0.5	38.0 ± 4.4
EarlyFuseUNet	34.5M	74.4 ± 0.2	81.4 ± 1.0	38.1 ± 4.8
LateFuseUNet	**25.1M**	73.8 ± 0.1	81.4 ± 1.7	39.3 ± 4.1
FuseUNet	26.7M	74.9 ± 0.2	82.2 ± 0.4	37.9 ± 2.5
FuseUNet + SA	26.8M	76.3 ± 0.2	83.4 ± 0.4	32.4 ± 0.8
Proposed	26.7M	**77.6 ± 0.3**	**84.4 ± 0.7**	**30.9 ± 1.6**

* M–millions. # Values in percentage.

3   Results and Discussion

Table 1 lists the quantitative segmentation results of the different networks. It can be concluded that compared to the pixel-wise summation strategy used in FuseNet, multi-modal feature fusion by channel-wise concatenation (FuseNet-Concate) is more effective. Adopting the U-Net blocks (FuseOriginUNet) leads to further performance enhancement. Moreover, the lightweight FuseUNet achieves a comparable or even superior level of segmentation accuracy with only half of the parameters used by FuseOriginUNet. U-Net trained solely on T1C presents worse performance than all the two-modal U-Net based networks, suggesting

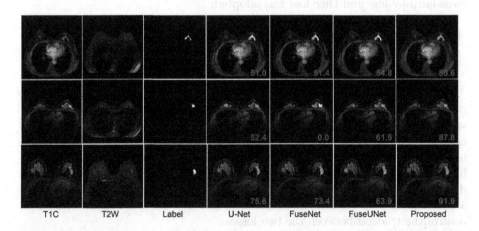

Fig. 4. Example results of the different networks. White lines indicate the boundaries of the manual segmentation labels. Green lines are the boundaries of the network segmentation results. The value in each image is the Dice similarity coefficient (%). (Color figure online)

that T2W images provided useful complementary information for the segmentation task. For the two-modal U-Net based networks, multilayer fusion of FuseNet is more effective than both early fusion (EarlyFuseUNet) and late fusion (Late-FuseUNet). Introducing our SA block to both U-Net (U-Net + SA) and Fuse-UNet (FuseUNet + SA) before each pooling layer elevates segmentation performance. Finally, our proposed supervised cross-modal deep representation learning method generates the best segmentation results reflected by all three metrics.

The segmentation results of several examples are given in Fig. 4. Overall, models utilizing two modal inputs are more effective than the single-modal U-Net. Except in the last example, the improved baseline model FuseUNet achieves a higher Dice similarity coefficient than FuseNet. The proposed method consistently achieves much better results than the existing methods with decreased false negatives (first example) and decreased false positives (second and third examples).

To demonstrate the mechanism behind the improved performance brought by the proposed method, the SA maps of all five down-sampling blocks are visualized. One example is presented in Fig. 5. It is clear from Fig. 5 that the T1C modal stream in both the proposed method and the FuseUNet + SA model was able to localize the mass regions through implementing the SA modules (red arrows in Fig. 5). The T2W modal stream could hardly find the interesting areas and even highlighted the regions that were irrelevant for the task (blue arrows in Fig. 5). Therefore, it is reasonable and necessary to apply the T1C attention maps to the information selection of T2W. For situations where different modalities generate images with similar sensitivites, our network architecture can still be utilized with an accordinly designed supervision information extraction strategy. The main idea regarding the supervised feature fusion of different imaging modalities should always be beneficial.

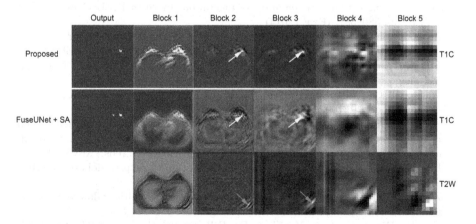

Fig. 5. SA maps of the proposed method and the FuseUNet + SA model. Blocks 1–5 refer to the attention maps generated at the five blocks before the respective pooling layers. T1C and T2W refer to the feature maps generated by the T1C modal stream and the T2W modal stream. (Color figure online)

4   Conclusion

In this work, we presented a novel network for the segmentation of multi-modal MR images. Inspired by the knowledge distillation and attention transfer strategies, a supervised cross-modal deep representation learning method was designed that selectively fused the useful information from the different modalities and suppressed the respective noise signals. Results on an in-vivo breast MR image dataset of two modalities confirmed the effectiveness of the proposed method. The proposed method is extendable to different medical image segmentation scenarios and will be investigated in the future.

Acknowledgements. This research was partially supported by the National Natural Science Foundation of China (61601450, 61871371, 81830056), Science and Technology Planning Project of Guangdong Province (2017B020227012, 2018B010109009), the Basic Research Program of Shenzhen (JCYJ20180507182400762), and Youth Innovation Promotion Association Program of Chinese Academy of Sciences (2019351).

References

1. Heywang-Köbrunner, S.H., Viehweg, P., Heinig, A., Küchler, C.: Contrast-enhanced MRI of the breast: accuracy, value, controversies, solutions. Eur. J. Radiol. **24**(2), 94–108 (1997)
2. Westra, C., Dialani, V., Mehta, T.S., Eisenberg, R.L.: Using T2-weighted sequences to more accurately characterize breast masses seen on MRI. Am. J. Roentgenol. **202**(3), 183–190 (2014)
3. Litjens, G., et al.: A survery on deep learning in medical image analysis. Med. Image Anal. **42**, 60–88 (2017)
4. Girshick, R., Donahue, J., Darrell, T., Malik, J.: Rich feature hierarchies for accurate object detection and semantic segmentation. In: 2014 IEEE Conference on CVPR, pp. 580–587. IEEE (2014)
5. Long, J., Shelhamer, E., Darrell, T.: Fully convolutional networks for semantic segmentation. In: 2015 IEEE Conference on CVPR, pp. 3431–3440. IEEE (2015)
6. Ronneberger, O., Fischer, P., Brox, T.: U-Net: convolutional networks for biomedical image segmentation. In: Navab, N., Hornegger, J., Wells, W.M., Frangi, A.F. (eds.) MICCAI 2015. LNCS, vol. 9351, pp. 234–241. Springer, Cham (2015). https://doi.org/10.1007/978-3-319-24574-4_28
7. Zhou, C., Ding, C., Lu, Z., Wang, X., Tao, D.: One-pass multi-task convolutional neural networks for efficient brain tumor segmentation. In: Frangi, A.F., Schnabel, J.A., Davatzikos, C., Alberola-López, C., Fichtinger, G. (eds.) MICCAI 2018. LNCS, vol. 11072, pp. 637–645. Springer, Cham (2018). https://doi.org/10.1007/978-3-030-00931-1_73
8. Zhang, W., et al.: Deep convolutional neural networks for multi-modality isointense infant brain image segmentation. Neuroimage **108**, 214–224 (2015)
9. Nie, D., Wnag, L., Gao, Y., Shen, D.: Fully convolutional networks for multi-modality isointense infant brain image segmentation. In: IEEE 13th ISBI, pp. 1342–1345. IEEE (2016)

10. Pinto, A., et al.: Enhancing clinical MRI perfusion maps with data-driven maps of complementary nature for lesion outcome prediction. In: Frangi, A.F., Schnabel, J.A., Davatzikos, C., Alberola-López, C., Fichtinger, G. (eds.) MICCAI 2018. LNCS, vol. 11072, pp. 107–115. Springer, Cham (2018). https://doi.org/10.1007/978-3-030-00931-1_13

11. Hazirbas, C., Ma, L., Domokos, C., Cremers, D.: FuseNet: incorporating depth into semantic segmentation via fusion-based CNN architecture. In: Lai, S.-H., Lepetit, V., Nishino, K., Sato, Y. (eds.) ACCV 2016. LNCS, vol. 10111, pp. 213–228. Springer, Cham (2017). https://doi.org/10.1007/978-3-319-54181-5_14

12. Chen, H., Li, Y.: Progressively complementarity-aware fusion network for RGB-D salient object detection. In: 2018 IEEE Conference on CVPR, pp. 3051–3060. IEEE (2018)

13. Dolz, J., Gopinath, K., Yuan, J., Lombaert, H., Desrosiers, C., Ayed, I.B.: HyperDense-Net: a hyper-densely connected CNN for multi-modal image segmentation. IEEE Trans. Med. Imaging **38**(5), 1116–1126 (2018)

14. Hinton, G., Vinyals, O., Dean, J.: Distilling the knowledge in a neural network. arXiv:1503.02531, pp. 1–9 (2015)

15. Zagoruyko, S., Komodakis, N.: Paying more attention to attention: improving the performance of convolutional neural networks via attention transfer. In: 5th ICLR, pp. 1–13. Microtome Publishing (2017)

Extreme Points Derived Confidence Map as a Cue for Class-Agnostic Interactive Segmentation Using Deep Neural Network

Shadab Khan[1]([✉]), Ahmed H. Shahin[1,2], Javier Villafruela[1], Jianbing Shen[1], and Ling Shao[1]

[1] Inception Institute of Artificial Intelligence, Al Bustan Offices, Abu Dhabi, UAE
skhanshadab@gmail.com, ahmedhshahen@gmail.com, fruela@gmail.com,
shenjianbingcg@gmail.com, ling.shao@inceptioniai.org
[2] Center for Informatics Sciences, Nile University, Giza, Egypt

Abstract. To automate the process of segmenting an anatomy of interest, we can learn a model from previously annotated data. The learning-based approach uses annotations to train a model that tries to emulate the expert labeling on a new data set. While tremendous progress has been made using such approaches, labeling of medical images remains a time-consuming and expensive task. In this paper, we evaluate the utility of extreme points in learning to segment. Specifically, we propose a novel approach to compute a confidence map from extreme points that quantitatively encodes the priors derived from extreme points. We use the confidence map as a cue to train a deep neural network based on ResNet-101 and PSP module to develop a class-agnostic segmentation model that outperforms state-of-the-art method that employs extreme points as a cue. Further, we evaluate a realistic use-case by using our model to generate training data for supervised learning (U-Net) and observed that U-Net performs comparably when trained with either the generated data or the ground truth data. These findings suggest that models trained using cues can be used to generate reliable training data. Our code is publicly available (https://github.com/ahmedshahin9/AssistedAnnotator).

1 Introduction

Deep neural networks have enabled tremendous progress in medical image segmentation. This progress has been greatly enabled by the large quantity of annotated data. Supervised techniques trained with large annotated data, have accomplished outstanding results on many segmentation tasks. However, the annotations need to cover the inter- and intra-patient variability, tissue heterogeneity, as well as lack of consistency between imaging scanners, operators, and annotators. As a result, image labeling is slow, expensive, and subject to availability of annotation experts (clinicians), which varies widely across the world.

S. Khan and A. H. Shahin—Equal contribution.

© Springer Nature Switzerland AG 2019
D. Shen et al. (Eds.): MICCAI 2019, LNCS 11765, pp. 66–73, 2019.
https://doi.org/10.1007/978-3-030-32245-8_8

To address this issue, techniques that can employ cues such as image label, scribbles, bounding box, and more recently, extreme points, (Fig. 1) have been used to enable weakly supervised training with results that are comparable to those obtained using ground truth pixel-level segmentation [1,5–7,10]. Learnt models that produce pixel-level segmentation from user-provided cues can then be used to significantly accelerate the annotation process. This approach has the advantage of exploiting existing annotations as a prior knowledge to enable the annotation of a new related data set. In this paper, we evaluate the utility of extreme points as a cue for medical image segmentation. Extreme points can be labeled more quickly than bounding boxes ($\sim$7.2 s vs $\sim$34.5 s), as shown by a recent study [6], and implicitly provide more information to the learning models as they lie on the object of interest.

We explore a novel algorithm to encode information from extreme points and generate a confidence map to guide the neural networks in understanding where the object lies within the extremities defined by the extreme points. The training data is augmented with confidence map to train a model that produces accurate segmentation, using confidence map and image as input. Further, we present an algorithm for fast computation of distance of points from a line segment that allows us to generate confidence maps during training and keeps the memory footprint low. We tested our approach against the state-of-the-art method in employing extreme points as a cue [5] under identical and unbiased settings and found that our approach improves the segmentation performance for all organ categories in the multi-class SegTHOR data set [12]. We also evaluated the algorithm under a use-case scenario (labeling a new data set) and found that supervised training using segmentation produced by our approach performs well compared to when the ground truth segmentation were used for training.

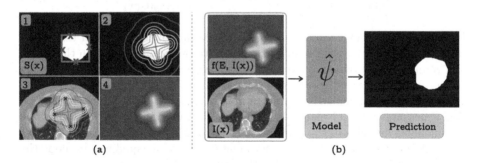

Fig. 1. (a) Extreme points ('x') and bounding box(red) shown on a given segmentation $S(x)$ (1), which was used to compute the confidence map (CM) $f(E, I(x))$ (4) as shown. The CM produces iso-contours with negative curvature, this is desired as explained in Sect. 2. (3) shows iso-contours overlaid on the image, where boundary of segmented region has been shown in blue and user-clicked extreme points as 'x' markers. (b) For inference, a confidence map computed using extreme points is input to the model. (Color figure online)

2   Methods

Given an image $I(x) \in \Omega; x \in \mathbb{R}^2$ and the four extreme points $E = x_1, x_2, x_3, x_4$; $x_i \in \mathbb{R}^2$, we aim to compute a segmentation $S(x)$ of the image, such that $S : \Omega \mapsto \{0, 1\}$. This is accomplished using a segmentation map $\psi : \Omega \mapsto \Omega$. In a supervised learning setting, an approximate map $(\hat{\psi})$ is learnt using a set of training pairs $\{(I(x), S(x))_i; i \in [1, N]\}$, with cardinality N. In our approach, we propose to learn $(\hat{\psi})$ using an augmented training set $\{(f(E, x), I(x), S(x))_i\}$, where $f(E, x) : \Omega \mapsto \Omega$ is a function that assigns a confidence score to every point in the image domain. Our objective is to develop a class-agnostic $(\hat{\psi})$ that can segment a region-of-interest using the points in E as a cue.

To accomplish this, we propose to exploit the following cues: (i) The extreme points form line segments $\overline{x_1 x_2}$ and $\overline{x_3 x_4}$ respectively that have a point of intersection, denoted as c, (ii) $\overline{x_1 x_2}$, $\overline{x_3 x_4}$, and c are likely to lie on region-of-interest (RoI), (iii) Points in Ω away from c, $\overline{x_1 x_2}$ or $\overline{x_3 x_4}$ are less likely to lie on RoI. We formulate $f(E, x)$ to take into account this prior information while assigning a RoI-membership confidence score to each point in Ω.

Before explaining our generalized formulation for $f(E, x)$, we consider a simpler case where two assumptions are made: (i)$\overline{x_1 x_2} \perp \overline{x_3 x_4}$, (ii) c bisects $\overline{x_1 x_2}$, and $\overline{x_3 x_4}$. In this scenario, assuming that the lengths of $\overline{x_1 x_2}$ and $\overline{x_3 x_4}$ can be used to approximate the measure of spread of the RoI (variance along $\overline{x_1 x_2}$ and $\overline{x_3 x_4}$), the following formulae allow us to incorporate the priors with one exception (explained ahead):

$$d_1(x) = min \odot \{R^{-1}(x - c)\Lambda^{-\frac{1}{2}}\}, \qquad d_2(x) = \{(x - c)^T S^{-1}(x - c)\}^{\frac{1}{2}} \quad (1)$$

$$d_3(x) = \begin{cases} 1 \text{ if } d_2(x) \leqslant \tau \\ 0 \text{ if } d_2(x) > \tau \end{cases}, \qquad f(E, x) = \frac{d_3(x)}{1 + d_1(x)d_2(x)} \quad (2)$$

In the equations above, $min\odot$ is an element-wise minimum taken over the resulting vector, S is the covariance matrix of the data (foreground pixels in the $S(x)$), and R and Λ are obtained by decomposing S as: $S = R\Lambda R^T$, where R represents the rotation matrix that rotates the standard axes into alignment with $\overline{x_1 x_2}$ and $\overline{x_3 x_4}$, Λ is the diagonalized covariance matrix, and τ is a threshold. In Eq. (1), $d_1(x)$ measures an equivalent of Chebyshev distance, and $d_2(x)$ measures the Mahalonobis distance in the coordinate frame of $\overline{x_1 x_2}$ and $\overline{x_3 x_4}$. Figure 1 shows $d_1(x), d_2(x), d_3(x)$, and $z(x)$. This formulation places an equal weight along the line $\overrightarrow{x_1 x_2}$, which is a departure from the priors.

To overcome this limitation, we use the following formulae:

$$d_{\overline{x_1 x_2}}(x) = \frac{dist(x, \overline{x_1 x_2})}{\sigma_{\overline{x_1 x_2}}}, \qquad d_{\overline{x_3 x_4}}(x) = \frac{dist(x, \overline{x_3 x_4})}{\sigma_{\overline{x_3 x_4}}} \quad (3)$$

$$\hat{d}_1(x) = min\{d_{\overline{x_1 x_2}}(x), d_{\overline{x_3 x_4}}(x)\}, \quad \hat{d}_2(x) = \{d_{\overline{x_1 x_2}}(x)^2 + d_{\overline{x_3 x_4}}(x)^2\}^{\frac{1}{2}} \quad (4)$$

$$f(E, x) = \frac{1}{1 + \hat{d}_1(x)\hat{d}_2(x)} \quad (5)$$

where $dist(x, \overline{x_1 x_2})$ is the distance of point x from line segment $\overline{x_1 x_2}$ and $\sigma_{\overline{x_1 x_2}}$ approximates the variance along $\overline{x_1 x_2}$. Equation (1) is a special case of Eq. (4), when x_1 and x_2 are at $\pm\infty$, x_3 and x_4 are at $\pm\infty$, and $\overline{x_1 x_2} \perp \overline{x_3 x_4}$. By including $f(E, x)$ with $I(x)$ and $S(x)$ we create an augmented data-set that is used for computing $(\hat{\psi})$.

3 Implementation

3.1 Model and Data Set

We use a deep neural network with ResNet-101 architecture [3] to approximate $(\hat{\psi})$, with a few changes. The fully-connected layers and the final two max-pool layers at the end of the ResNet-101 architecture are removed and atrous convolution is added in the final two layers. Lastly, a Pyramid Scene Parsing (PSP) [13] module is incorporated at the last stage to introduce global context. To experiment with medical images where multiple organs have been annotated, we chose SegTHOR data set [12]. SegTHOR data set comprises annotated CT images of heart, aorta, trachea and esophagus. The soft tissue in heart, aorta and esophagus have a closely matching dynamic range in Hounsfield Units(HU) and therefore present challenging conditions for testing segmentation performance.

3.2 Data Pre-processing and Model Setting

SegTHOR comprises CT scans of 40 patients, acquired with 0.9–1.37 mm in-plane (512×512 field-of-view) and 2–3.7 mm out-of-plane resolution resulting in 150–284 slices per patient. Heart, trachea, esophagus, and aorta were annotated in a total of 7390 slices. To create our training data, 4 extreme points were deduced for each organ in all annotated slices using ground truth segmentation. The input to the neural network was a resized crop of the anatomy with dimensions 512×512. To create the input to the neural network, a bounding box of dimensions $w \times h$ was calculated using the extreme points. Next, using $b = max(w, h)$, we calculated a zoom factor z, such that $z = b_m/b$, where b_m is a random number in [350,400]. This approach of calculating z ensures that approximately 45–60% pixels seen by the network belong to the anatomy of interest. Images were windowed (−200, 250) and intensity normalized before input to the network.

We used the implementation of ResNet-101 and PSP module provided by [2] and [5]. The network was initialized using pre-trained weights for a 4-channel version provided by [5]. We fine-tuned the network using a learning rate of 1e-7, batch size $= 14$, Adam optimizer [4] ($\beta_1 = 0.90$, $\beta_2 = 0.99$), L2-regularization ($\alpha = $5e-4) and loss function set to weighted cross entropy. Data augmentation in the form of random scaling (0.9–1.1), rotation (−30° to +30°), and horizontal flip was used. Data was split at patient-level into 60/20/20 splits for training, validation, and test respectively. Training loop was executed for 100 epochs, and model selection was done by evaluating validation set performance. To report results, the best model was tested on test set only once.

3.3 Confidence Map ($f(E, x)$)

Computing $f(E, x)$ requires evaluating distance of each point in Ω from the line segments $\overline{x_1 x_2}$ and $\overline{x_3 x_4}$. This is non-trivial if Ω is large. A time-efficient solution was obtained by implementing calculation of distance from line segments for all points in Ω as follows (Fig. 2):

Algorithm 1. Compute distance of points in image from line segment ($\mathbf{D}_{\overline{x_1 x_2}}$)

1: Calculate x_-, x_+, and y_-, y_+ as the extent of image size
2: Create 2D arrays $\mathbf{X}$ and $\mathbf{Y}$ as: $\mathbf{X}, \mathbf{Y} \leftarrow meshgrid(x_-, x_+, y_-, y_+)$
3: $\mathbf{X} = \mathbf{X} - c$; $\mathbf{Y} = \mathbf{Y} - c$
4: $x_1 = x_1 - c$; $x_2 = x_2 - c$
5: Calculate unit vector along $\overline{x_1 x_2}$ as: $cos(\theta)\hat{i} + sin(\theta)\hat{j}$
6: $\mathbf{X}^{rot} \leftarrow \mathbf{X}cos(\theta) - \mathbf{Y}sin(\theta)$; $\mathbf{Y}^{rot} \leftarrow \mathbf{X}sin(\theta) + \mathbf{Y}cos(\theta)$
7: $x_{1i}^{rot} \leftarrow x_{1i}cos(\theta) - x_{1j}sin(\theta)$; $x_{1j}^{rot} \leftarrow 0$; x_1^{rot} lies along $1\hat{i} + 0\hat{j}$
8: $x_1^{rot} = (x_{1i}^{rot}, 0)$; similarly calculate x_2^{rot}
9: $\mathbf{D}_{x_1} = \sqrt{(\mathbf{X}^{rot} - x_{1i}^{rot})^2 + (\mathbf{Y}^{rot})^2}$; similarly calculate $\mathbf{D}_{x_2}$
10: $\mathbf{D}_p = \left| \mathbf{Y}^{rot} \right|$
11: $\mathbf{M}_{x_1} = \mathbf{X}^{rot} < x_{1i}^{rot}$; $\mathbf{M}_{x_2} = \mathbf{X}^{rot} > x_{2i}^{rot}$; $\mathbf{M}_p = \neg \mathbf{M}_{x_1} \wedge \neg \mathbf{M}_{x_2}$
12: $\mathbf{D}_{\overline{x_1 x_2}} = \mathbf{M}_{x_1}\mathbf{D}_{x_1} + \mathbf{M}_{x_2}\mathbf{D}_{x_2} + \mathbf{M}_p\mathbf{D}_p$
13: $\mathbf{M}_R = \mathbf{X}^{rot} > 0$; $\mathbf{M}_L = \mathbf{X}^{rot} \leq 0$ # Right and left mask
14: $\sigma_L = \left| x_{1i}^{rot} \right|$; $\sigma_R = \left| x_{2i}^{rot} \right|$ # Approximation to right and left variance
15: $\mathbf{\Sigma} = \sigma_R \mathbf{M}_R + \sigma_L \mathbf{M}_L$
16: $\mathbf{D}_{\overline{x_1 x_2}} = \mathbf{D}_{\overline{x_1 x_2}} / \mathbf{\Sigma}$

Above, $meshgrid()$ is a computer program, boldface letters are 2D arrays, rot refers to 'rotated', and all $\mathbf{M}$'s are 2D boolean arrays. This algorithm can be implemented without using any loops in Python and can be used to generate confidence maps during training itself. On a CPU equipped with 2.2 GHz Intel Xeon 5120 processor, it took 88 ms to compute $\mathbf{D}_{\overline{x_1 x_2}}$ for an image size 512×512. Figure 2 helps explain the algorithm. The confidence map $f(E, x)$ was incorporated into the input as an extra channel passed to the neural network.

4 Results

4.1 Our Approach and Baseline

In testing the performance of our approach, our objective was to evaluate how to best encode information from the 4 extreme points for class-agnostic segmentation. We evaluated our model's performance on unseen data by evaluating mean Dice overlap score on ~20% of the patients from SegTHOR, the model was not exposed to any slice from this set at any time during training or validation. For baseline comparison, we also fine-tuned a state-of-the-art pre-trained model [5] with hyper-parameter, data pre-processing steps, and all other settings identical to the one used to test our model. The baseline model places Gaussians at the

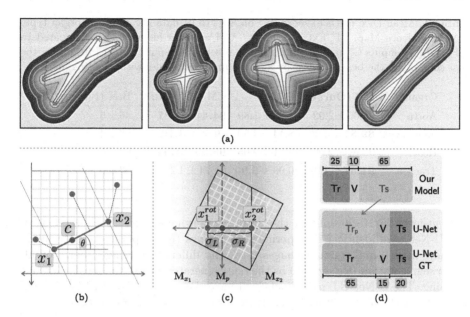

Fig. 2. (a) Iso-contour plots are shown overlaid on the computed confidence map for a few different object shapes. For visualization, we set the area outside last contour to a gray intensity, blue line shows the boundary of the object, and red 'x' markers are the extreme points. We draw attention to how the iso-contour lines flex and bend to retain the negative curvature characteristic across varying object shapes. (b) and (c) help explain Algorithm 1, and (d) shows how the CHAOS data was split for reporting results in Sect. 4.2, where Tr=Train, V=Val, Ts=Test, and numbers ('65', '25', etc) show the %. 'U-Net GT' was trained using ground truth segmentation, and 'U-Net' was trained using segmentation produced by our model.

extreme points and was shown to outperform all other methods that employ cues for segmentation (including GrabCut (GC) [9]). In our experiments, we initialized GC by setting area outside bounding box extended by extreme points to background, and extreme points to foreground, however GC did not produce any meaningful segmentation to warrant further exploration. We also evaluated combination of the confidence map and extreme points (gaussians) as two separate input channels. The mean Dice score results for all experiments are summarized in Table 1, organized by testing on each organ.

4.2 Weakly Supervised Segmentation

In order to evaluate the efficacy of our model in producing accurate segmentation for fully supervised training, we fine-tuned our model on the segmentation data of a new-to-the-model organ (liver, CHAOS data set [11]). Using a patient-level 25/10/65 split of the data (Fig. 2d), we produced segmentation on data collected from 65% of the patients for which ground truth segmentation was also available. Next, we trained 2 versions of U-Net [8] in a fully-supervised manner using a

Table 1. Mean Dice (mDice) score (%) on SegTHOR data organized by organ type. CM–Confidence Map, EP–Extreme Points. CM achieves higher mDice compared to EP. CM+EP inputs CM and EP (gaussians) as separate input channels. Results in the last column are the best achieved by a fully-supervised model without using any cue.

Organ	CM (**Ours**)	EP	CM+EP (**Ours**)	Best (No Cues)
Aorta	94.00 ± 2.02	92.80 ± 1.89	$\mathbf{94.41 \pm 1.87}$	86 ± 5
Esophagus	$\mathbf{89.87 \pm 4.36}$	88.14 ± 4.50	$89.83 \pm \mathbf{4.16}$	67 ± 4
Heart	95.97 ± 2.09	95.41 ± 2.05	$\mathbf{96.53 \pm 1.94}$	90 ± 1
Trachea	$\mathbf{91.87 \pm 4.07}$	$90.05 \pm \mathbf{3.90}$	91.24 ± 4.27	83 ± 6

patient-level 65/15/20 split of the data, as shown in Fig. 2. Both versions of the U-Net were identical in experimental settings (hyper-parameters, training, starting model) and training images used, and differed by using either ground-truth segmentation (U-Net GT) or the ones generated by our model (U-Net) for training. The U-Net GT model achieved mean Dice score (%) of 91.70 ± 13.00, compared to 90.35 ± 9.89 by U-Net trained on generated segmentation.

5   Discussion and Conclusion

We evaluated a new approach to incorporate cues from extreme points into neural network by computing a confidence map that is used during training. This was enabled by our algorithm for quickly computing distance of points from line segment. Our approach, when compared with the state-of-the-art baseline under identical and unbiased conditions resulted in improved mean Dice score across all four organs in the test set, with closely-matching variance in the Dice scores across samples. Interestingly, a combination of our confidence map and extreme points (gaussians) further improved the mean Dice for 2 out 4 organs while reducing variance. This strongly suggests that confidence map provide superior guidance to neural networks for segmentation, compared to extreme points alone.

On qualitative evaluation, the segmentation results were found to be consistent. We probed the samples which resulted in lower Dice score compared to the group mean and observed that these were slices where the organ occupied a small area within the image. Resizing such instances for input to the network is associated with two factors: (i) lack of texture in resized image, and (ii) rescaling binary segmentation can introduce non-trivial noise in the loss function. We posit these factors reduce the quantitative measures of segmentation performance. We further evaluated our model's ability to produce segmentation for fully-supervised learning. We observed that U-Net trained using segmentation produced by our model achieves slightly lower mean Dice score than the gold standard (U-Net GT), but achieves lower variance compared to U-Net GT.

Our findings suggest that to quickly annotate large data sets, it may suffice to: (1) Fine-tune a pre-trained model using a fully annotated small proportion of the data, (2) Use pre-trained model along with extreme points as cue to predict segmentation on the rest of the unlabeled data, (3) Use the generated labels to train a fully-supervised algorithm. Such an approach would help reduce the annotation time and expense drastically and allow more data to be labeled.

References

1. Cai, J., et al.: Accurate weakly-supervised deep lesion segmentation using large-scale clinical annotations: slice-propagated 3D mask generation from 2D RECIST. In: Medical Image Computing and Computer Assisted Interventions (MICCAI) (2018)
2. Chen, L.C., Papandreou, G., Kokkinos, I., Murphy, K., Yuille, A.L.: DeepLab: semantic image segmentation with deep convolutional nets, atrous convolution, and fully connected crfs. IEEE Trans. Pattern Anal. Mach. Intell. (TPAMI) **40**(4), 834–848 (2018)
3. He, K., Zhang, X., Ren, S., Sun, J.: Deep residual learning for image recognition. In: IEEE Conference on Computer Vision and Pattern Recognition (CVPR) (2016)
4. Kingma, D.P., Ba, J.: Adam: a method for stochastic optimization. In: International Conference on Learning Representation (ICLR) (2015)
5. Maninis, K., Caelles, S., Pont-Tuset, J., Van Gool, L.: Deep extreme cut: from extreme points to object segmentation. In: IEEE Conference on Computer Vision and Pattern Recognition (CVPR) (2018)
6. Papadopoulos, D.P., Uijlings, J.R., Keller, F., Ferrari, V.: Extreme clicking for efficient object annotation. In: IEEE International Conference on Computer Vision (ICCV) (2017)
7. Rajchl, M., et al.: DeepCut: object segmentation from bounding box annotations using convolutional neural networks. IEEE Trans. Med. Imaging (TMI) **36**(2), 674–683 (2017)
8. Ronneberger, O., Fischer, P., Brox, T.: U-Net: convolutional networks for biomedical image segmentation. In: Navab, N., Hornegger, J., Wells, W.M., Frangi, A.F. (eds.) MICCAI 2015. LNCS, vol. 9351, pp. 234–241. Springer, Cham (2015). https://doi.org/10.1007/978-3-319-24574-4_28
9. Rother, C., Kolmogorov, V., Blake, A.: GrabCut: interactive foreground extraction using iterated graph cuts. In: ACM Transaction on Graphics (2004)
10. Schlegl, T., Waldstein, S.M., Vogl, W.-D., Schmidt-Erfurth, U., Langs, G.: Predicting semantic descriptions from medical images with convolutional neural networks. In: Ourselin, S., Alexander, D.C., Westin, C.-F., Cardoso, M.J. (eds.) IPMI 2015. LNCS, vol. 9123, pp. 437–448. Springer, Cham (2015). https://doi.org/10.1007/978-3-319-19992-4_34
11. Selver, M.A., et al.: CHAOS - Combined (CT-MR) Healthy Abdominal Organ Segmentation (2018). chaos.grand-challenge.org
12. Trullo, R., Petitjean, C., Ruan, S., Dubray, B., Nie, D., Shen, D.: Segmentation of organs at risk in thoracic CT images using a SharpMask architecture and conditional random fields. In: International Symposium on Biomedical Imaging (ISBI) (2017)
13. Zhao, H., Shi, J., Qi, X., Wang, X., Jia, J.: Pyramid scene parsing network. In: IEEE Conference on Computer Vision and Pattern Recognition (CVPR) (2017)

Hetero-Modal Variational Encoder-Decoder for Joint Modality Completion and Segmentation

Reuben Dorent[(✉)], Samuel Joutard, Marc Modat, Sébastien Ourselin,
and Tom Vercauteren

School of Biomedical Engineering and Imaging Sciences,
King's College London, London, UK
reuben.dorent@kcl.ac.uk

Abstract. We propose a new deep learning method for tumour segmentation when dealing with missing imaging modalities. Instead of producing one network for each possible subset of observed modalities or using arithmetic operations to combine feature maps, our hetero-modal variational 3D encoder-decoder independently embeds all observed modalities into a shared latent representation. Missing data and tumour segmentation can be then generated from this embedding. In our scenario, the input is a random subset of modalities. We demonstrate that the optimisation problem can be seen as a mixture sampling. In addition to this, we introduce a new network architecture building upon both the 3D U-Net and the Multi-Modal Variational Auto-Encoder (MVAE). Finally, we evaluate our method on BraTS2018 using subsets of the imaging modalities as input. Our model outperforms the current state-of-the-art method for dealing with missing modalities and achieves similar performance to the subset-specific equivalent networks.

1 Introduction

Tumour segmentation and associated volume quantification plays an essential role during the diagnosis, follow-up and surgical planning stages of primary brain tumours. Multiple imaging sequences are usually employed to distinguish and assess the key tumour components such as the whole tumour, the peritumoral edema and the enhancing region. The common sequences are T1-weighted (T1), contrast enhanced T1-weighted (T1c), T2-weighted (T2) and Fluid Attenuation Inversion Recovery (FLAIR) images. These modalities reveal different characteristics of brain tissues. In practice, the set of acquired modalities may vary during the clinical assessment. For this reason, we aim to automatically segment these key components given an arbitrary set of modalities.

Methods based on deep learning currently achieve the best performance in brain tumour segmentation. Most of them require the full set of n modalities as input [4,9], while a scenario of missing modalities is common in practice. Segmentation with missing data can be achieved by: 1/ Training a model for each

© Springer Nature Switzerland AG 2019
D. Shen et al. (Eds.): MICCAI 2019, LNCS 11765, pp. 74–82, 2019.
https://doi.org/10.1007/978-3-030-32245-8_9

possible subset of modalities; 2/ Synthesising missing modalities [6] in order to then perform full modality segmentation; 3/ Creating a common feature space which encodes the shared information from which the segmentation is created [3,12]. The two first options involve training and handling a different network for each of the $2^n - 1$ combinations. These two solutions are cumbersome and computationally sub-optimal since duplicate information is extracted $2^n - 1$ times. In contrast, encoding the modalities into a common feature space produces a single model that shares feature extraction.

The current state-of-the-art network architecture which allows for missing modalities is HeMIS [3] and related extensions [12]. Feature maps are first extracted independently for each modality, then their first and second moments are computed across the modalities and used for predicting the final segmentation. However, using these arithmetic operations does not force the network to learn a shared latent representation. In contrast, Multi-modal Variational Auto-Encoders (MVAE) [13] provide a principled formulation to create a common representation: the n modalities and the segmentation map are considered conditionally independent given the common latent variable z.

While our goal to segment the tumour with missing modalities, auto-encoding and modality completion promote informativeness of the latent space and can be seen as regularizers, similarly to [9]. Ideally, all the modality-specific information should be encoded in the common latent space, meaning that the model should be able to reconstruct all the observed modalities. Additionally, the information loss related to any missing modality should be minimal (modality completion).

In this paper, we introduce a hetero-modal variational encoder-decoder for tumour segmentation and missing modalities completion. The contribution of this work is four-fold. First, we extend the MVAE for 3D tumour segmentation from multimodal datasets with missing modalities. Secondly, we propose a principled formulation of the optimisation process based on a mixture sampling procedure. Thirdly, we adapt the 3D U-Net in a variational framework for this task. Finally, we show that our model outperforms HeMIS in terms of tumour segmentation while comparing favourably with equivalent subset-specific models.

2   Method

2.1   Multi-modal Variational Auto-Encoders (MVAE)

The MVAE [13] aims at identifying a model in which n modalities $\mathbf{x} = (x_1, .., x_n)$ are conditionally independent given a hidden latent variable z. We consider the directed latent-variable model parameterised by θ (typically the weights of a decoding network $f_\theta(\cdot)$ going from the latent space to the image space):

$$p_\theta(z, x_1, ..., x_n) = p(z) \prod_{i=1}^{n} p_\theta(x_i|z) \qquad (1)$$

where $p(z)$ is a prior on the latent space, which we classically choose as a standard normal distribution $z \sim \mathcal{N}(0, I)$. The goal is then to maximise the marginal log-likelihood $\mathcal{L}(\mathbf{x}; \theta) = \log(p_\theta(x_1, ..., x_n))$ with respect to θ. However, the integral

$p_\theta(x_1, ..., x_n) = \int p_\theta(\mathbf{x}|z)p(z)$ is computationally intractable. [5] proposed to optimise, with respect to (ϕ, θ), the evidence lower-bound (ELBO):

$$\mathcal{L}(\mathbf{x}; \theta) \geq \text{ELBO}(\mathbf{x}; \theta, \phi) \triangleq E_{q_\phi(z|\mathbf{x})}[\log(p_\theta(\mathbf{x}|z))] - \text{KL}[q_\phi(z|\mathbf{x})||p(z)] \qquad (2)$$

where $q_\phi(z|\mathbf{x})$ is a tractable variational posterior that aims to approximate the intractable true posterior $p_\theta(z|\mathbf{x})$. For this purpose, $q_\phi(z|\mathbf{x})$ is typically modelled as a Gaussian after an encoding of $\mathbf{x}$ into a mean and diagonal covariance by a neural network, $h_\phi(\mathbf{x}) = (\mu_\phi(\mathbf{x}), \Sigma_\phi(\mathbf{x}))$, such that:

$$q_\phi(z|\mathbf{x}) = \mathcal{N}(z; \mu_\phi(\mathbf{x}), \Sigma_\phi(\mathbf{x})) \qquad (3)$$

The KL divergence between the two Gaussians $q_\phi(z|\mathbf{x})$ and $p(z)$ can be computed in closed form given by their means and covariances. In contrast, estimating $E_{q_\phi(z|\mathbf{x})}[\log(p_\theta(\mathbf{x}|z))]$ is done by sampling the hidden variable z according to the Gaussian $q_\phi(\cdot|\mathbf{x})$ and then decoding it as $f_\theta(z)$ in image space to evaluate $p_\theta(\mathbf{x}|z)$. To make sampling from $z|\mathbf{x}$ amenable to back-propagation, reparametrisation is used [5]: $\mu_\phi(\mathbf{x}) + \Sigma_\phi(\mathbf{x}) \times \epsilon$ where $\epsilon \sim \mathcal{N}(0, I)$.

Wu et al. [13] extended this variational formulation to a multi-modal setting. The authors remarked that $p_\theta(z|\mathbf{x}) \propto p(z) \prod_{i=1}^n \frac{p_\theta(z|x_i)}{p(z)}$. This expression shows that $p_\theta(z|\mathbf{x})$ can be decomposed into n modality-specific terms. For this reason, the authors approximate each $\frac{p_\theta(z|x_i)}{p(z)}$ with a modality-specific variational posterior $q_{\phi_i}(z|x_i)$. Similarly to (3), $q_{\phi_i}(z|x_i)$ is modelled as a Gaussian distribution after an encoding of x_i into a mean and a diagonal covariance by a neural network, $h_{\phi_i}(x_i) = (\mu_{\phi_i}(x_i), \Sigma_{\phi_i}(x_i))$, such that $q_i(z|x_i) = \mathcal{N}(z; \mu_{\phi_i}(x_i), \Sigma_{\phi_i}(x_i))$. Finally, [1] demonstrates that $q_\phi(z|\mathbf{x}) \propto p(z) \prod_{i=1}^n q_{\phi_i}(z|x_i)$ is Gaussian with mean μ_ϕ and covariance Σ_ϕ defined by:

$$\Sigma_\phi = (I + \sum_i \Sigma_{\phi_i}^{-1})^{-1} \text{ and } \mu_\phi = \Sigma_\phi^{-1}(\sum_i \Sigma_{\phi_i}^{-1} \mu_{\phi_i}) \qquad (4)$$

This formulation allows for encoding each modality independently and fusing their encoding using a closed-form formula.

However, from this well-posed multimodal extension of the ELBO, [13] resort to a ad hoc training sampling procedure. At each training iteration, the extremes cases (one modality and all the modalities) and random modality subsets are used concurrently. This option is highly memory consuming, not suitable for 3D images and not adapted to the clinical scenarios where some imaging subsets are clinically more frequent than others. The next section proposes to include this prior information in our principled training procedure via ancestral sampling.

2.2   Mixture Sampling for Modality Completion and Segmentation

In our scenario, the clinician provides a subset of $n = 4$ imaging modalities with some subsets of input modalities being more likely to be provided than others. We use an encoder-decoder to produce the missing modalities as well as the

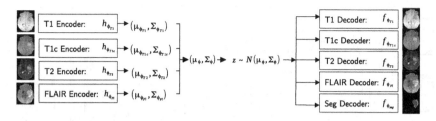

Fig. 1. MVAE architecture. Each imaging modality is encoded independently, the mean and covariance of each $q(z|x_i)$ are fused using the closed-form formula (4). A sample z is randomly drawn and is decoded into imaging modalities and the segmentation map

tumour segmentation. Although segmentation could be considered as a missing modality, we chose not to encode it as it is not observed in practice. Consequently, our model is composed of 4 encoders and 5 decoders (see Fig. 1).

Without loss of generality, we consider a training set providing the complete n modalities per subject. Consequently, during training, we can artificially remove some modalities as input yet evaluate the reconstruction error on all the modalities. When the training set is incomplete, the reconstruction error is only evaluated on the available data.

Let $\mathcal{P}$ denote the set of all possible non-empty combinations of the n modalities. Our goal is to maximise (2) when z has been encoded via a random subset $\pi \in \mathcal{P}$ drawn with probability α_π. This is exactly the ancestral sampling of a mixture model: we first draw the class label (here the subset) and then we draw a sample from the distribution associated to this class. For this reason, we model $q_\phi(z|\mathbf{x})$ as a mixture where the probabilities α_π are chosen to be representative of the clinical scenario:

$$q_\phi(z|\mathbf{x}) = \sum_{\pi \in \mathcal{P}} \alpha_\pi q_\phi^\pi(z|\mathbf{x}_\pi)$$

We choose $q_\phi^\pi(z|\mathbf{x}_\pi)$ as Gaussian. Given the convexity of the KL divergence and the fact that $\sum_{\pi \in \mathcal{P}} \alpha_\pi = 1$, we obtain:

$$\mathrm{KL}[q_\phi(z|\mathbf{x})||p(z)] \leq \sum_\pi \alpha_\pi \, \mathrm{KL}[q_\phi^\pi(z|\mathbf{x}_\pi)||p(z)]$$

Finally, our lower-bound is a weighted sum of the subset-specific lower-bound:

$$\mathcal{L}(\mathbf{x}; \theta) \geq \sum_{\pi \in \mathcal{P}} \alpha_\pi \underbrace{(E_{q_\phi^\pi(z|\mathbf{x}_\pi)}[\log(p_\theta(\mathbf{x}|z))] - \mathrm{KL}[q_\phi^\pi(z|\mathbf{x}_\pi)||p(z)])}_{\mathrm{ELBO}_\pi(\mathbf{x})} \qquad (5)$$

The single Gaussian prior model for $p(z)$ promotes consistency of the embedding z across the subsets of modalities π ($q_\phi^\pi(z|\mathbf{x}_\pi)$) and in turn across the full set of modalities ($q_\phi(z|\mathbf{x})$). In our optimisation procedure, at each iteration, we propose to randomly draw a subset π with a probability α_π as the model input and optimise $\mathrm{ELBO}_\pi(\mathbf{x})$. Classical modelling of $p_\theta(.|z)$ includes Gaussian distribution for image reconstruction and Bernoulli distribution for classification.

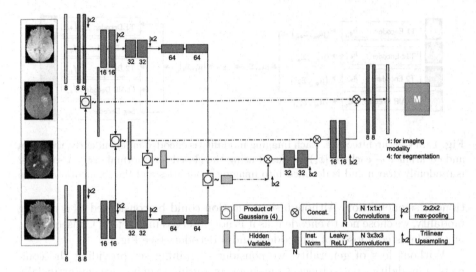

Fig. 2. Our 3D variational encoder-decoder (*U-HVED*). Only two encoders and one decoders are shown. Product of Gaussian is defined in (4)

2.3   Network Architecture: 3D Variational Encoder-Decoder

To exploit our framework we propose a novel network architecture: a 3D encoder-decoder with variational skip-connections. Our model is a mix between a 3D U-Net [10] and the MVAE [13].

In the U-net architecture, context information is extracted via the contracting path (encoder) and precise localisation is produced by the expanding part (decoder). In addition, information is captured at different levels via the skip-connections. To avoid a trivial identity function, existing auto-encoder architectures do not use skip-connections. In our case, the encoding of the latent variable is multi-modal and the imposed consistency of the latent representation creates a bottleneck. Skip-connections therefore do not allow for trivial identity mapping and can be included in our architecture.

We propose to use a multi-level latent variable to generate them. Figure 2 shows our network architecture. Unlike the existing hierarchical VAE models [11,14], we propose a fully convolutional network. Each modality i is independently encoded which produces 4 multi-scale means and variances $(\mu_i^k, \Sigma_i^k)_{k \in [1,..,4]}$. At each level, the means and the variances of the modalities present in the input subset x_π are combined via the product of Gaussian defined in (4). We then decode the multi-scale latent variable for each of the modalities and the segmentation. Consequently, we have n encoders and $n+1$ decoders. We assert that it is the first deep network which allows for missing modalities and performs 3D imaging reconstruction and segmentation in a variational manner.

3   Data and Implementation Details

Data. We evaluate our method on the training set of BRATS18 [7]. The training set contains the scans of 285 patients, 210 with high grade glioma and 75 with low grade glioma. Each patient was scanned with four sequences (T1, T1c, T2 and FLAIR) and pre-processed by the organisers: scans have been skull-striped and re-sampled to an isotropic 1 mm resolution, and the four sequences of the each patient have been co-registered. The ground truth was obtained by manual segmentation results given by experts. The segmentation classes include the following tumour tissue labels: (1) necrotic core and non-enhancing tumour, (2) oedema, (3) enhancing core.

Implementation Details. As pre-processing step, we used histogram-based scale standardisation method [8] followed by a zero mean and unit-variance normalisation. As a data augmentation, we randomly flip the axes and include a rotation with a random angle in $[-10°, 10°]$. The networks were implemented in Tensorflow using NiftyNet [2]. We used Adam as optimiser with initial learning rate 10^{-3} divided by 4 every 10^4 iterations, batch size 1 and maximal iteration 60k. Early stopping is performed if a plateau of performance is reached on the validation data set. At each iteration, a $112 \times 112 \times 112$ random patch is fed to the network. We did a 3-fold validation by random split of the data set a training (70%), validation (10%) and testing (20%) sets. We regularize with a $L2$ weight decay of 10^{-5}. During training, we uniformly draw a number of modalities i between 1 and 4 and uniformly draw a subset π of size i. During inference, given a subset of modalities, we randomly draw 10 hidden variable z from $q(.|\mathbf{x}_\pi)$ and decode them and average the outputs. Implementation is publicly available[1].

Choices of the Losses. The reconstruction loss follows from $p_\theta(x_i|z)$. For the segmentation we use the sum of the cross-entropy L_{cross} and the dice loss function L_{dice} [4]. For the imaging reconstruction loss, we used the classic L_2 loss. Additionally, given a drawn subset π, our loss includes the closed-form KL divergence between the Gaussians $q_\phi(z|\mathbf{x}_\pi)$ and $p(z)$. For weighting the regularization losses (KL divergence and reconstruction loss), we did a grid search over weights in $[0, 0.1, 1]$. Finally, the loss associated to maximising the ELBO (5) is:

$$L = L_{dice} + L_{cross} + 0.1 * L_2 + 0.1 * \text{KL}$$

4   Experiments and Results

Model Comparison. To evaluate the performance of our model (*U-HVED*), we compare it to three different approaches: The first, *HeMIS* is the model described in [3] and is the current state-of-the-art for segmentation with missing modalities. The second, *U-HeMIS*, is a particular case of our method where

---

[1] https://github.com/ReubenDo/U-HVED.

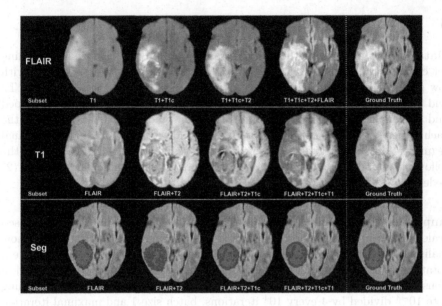

Fig. 3. Example of FLAIR and T1 completion and tumour segmentation given a subset of modalities as input. Green: edema; Red: non-enhancing core; Blue: enhancing core. (Color figure online)

the modalities are encoded as *U-HVED* and the skip-connection are the first and second moments of the modality-specific feature maps such as in *HeMIS*. *U-HeMIS* has only one decoder for tumour segmentation. The third approach, *Single*, is the "brute-force" method in which for each possible subset of modalities, we train a U-Net network where the observed modalities are concatenated as input. The encoder and decoder are those of our model. Given the 3-fold validation, we consequently trained 45 *Single* networks.

Missing Modalities Completion. Unlike these three approaches, *U-HVED* (*Ours*) generates missing modalities. Since image completion is a means rather than an end, we only provided a qualitative evaluation (Fig. 3) of T1 and FLAIR reconstruction examples. We find the reconstruction to be good quality, given that VAEs classically suffer of blurriness. Interestingly, our model tries to reconstruct the tumour information even when the tumour information is missing or not clear, such as in T1 scans. Moreover, comparable reconstructions are performed using 3 modalities and 4 modalities. This suggests that our network can effectively learn a common representation of the imaging modalities.

Tumour Segmentation. In order to evaluate the robustness of our model, we present qualitative results in Fig. 3 and comparative results with other methods in Table 1 for all the possible input subsets. We used the Dice Similarity as

Table 1. Comparison of the different models (Dice %) for the different combinations of available modalities. Modalities present are denoted by ●, the missing ones by ○. * denotes significant improvement provided by a Wilcoxon test ($p < 0.05$)

Modalities				Complete				Core				Enhancing			
F	T_1	T_1c	T_2	HeMIS	U-HeMIS	U-HVED	Sing	HeMIS	U-HeMIS	U-HVED	Sing	HeMIS	U-HeMIS	U-HVED	Sing
○	○	○	●	38.6	79.2	**80.9***	82.6	19.5	50.0	**54.1***	54.9	0.0	23.3	**30.8***	34.2
○	○	●	○	2.6	58.5	**62.4***	70.4	6.5	58.5	**66.7***	71.5	11.1	60.8	**65.5***	70.4
○	●	○	○	0.0	**54.3***	52.4	72.7	0.0	**37.9**	37.2	59.2	0.0	12.4	**13.7***	32.2
●	○	○	○	55.2	79.9	**82.1***	81.5	16.2	49.8	**50.4**	55.5	6.6	**24.9**	24.8	26.3
○	○	●	●	48.2	81.0	**82.7***	83.2	45.8	69.1	**73.7***	73.3	55.8	68.6	**70.2***	70.1
○	●	●	○	15.4	63.8	**66.8***	70.6	30.4	64.0	**69.7***	73.9	42.6	65.3	**67.0***	71.9
●	●	○	○	71.1	83.9	**84.3**	83.3	11.9	**56.7***	55.3	54.3	1.2	**29.0***	24.2	30.7
○	●	○	●	47.3	80.8	**82.2***	83.1	17.2	53.4	**57.2***	59.7	0.6	28.3	**30.7***	33.4
●	○	○	●	74.8	86.0	**87.5***	86.3	17.7	58.7	**59.7**	57.7	0.8	28.0	**34.6***	31.0
●	○	●	○	68.4	83.3	**85.5***	85.3	41.4	67.6	**72.9***	72.0	53.8	68.0	**70.3***	69.9
●	●	●	○	70.2	85.1	**86.2***	85.1	48.8	70.7	**74.2***	74.9	60.9	69.9	**71.1**	70.1
●	●	○	●	75.2	87.0	**88.0***	85.7	18.7	61.0	**61.5**	57.9	1.0	33.4	**34.1**	34.1
●	○	●	●	75.6	87.0	**88.6***	85.8	54.9	72.2	**75.6***	75.2	60.5	69.7	**71.2***	72.2
○	●	●	●	44.2	82.1	**83.3***	81.5	46.6	70.7	**75.3***	74.7	55.1	69.7	**71.1***	71.1
●	●	●	●	73.8	87.6	**88.8***	87.5	55.3	73.4	**76.4***	78.4	61.1	70.8	**71.7***	72.7
Means				50.7	78.6	**80.1***	81.6	28.7	59.7	**64.0***	66.2	27.4	48.1	**50.0***	52.7

metric. First, the U-Net architecture in *U-HeMIS* always achieves better performance than the original 2D fully-convolutionnal *HeMIS*. This highlights the efficiency of the 3D U-net architecture. Secondly, *U-HVED (Ours)* outperforms significantly *U-HeMIS* in most of the cases: 13 out of 15 cases for the complete tumour, 10 out of 15 cases for the core tumour; 11 out 15 cases for the enhancing tumour. This demonstrates that auto-encoding and modality completion improves the segmentation performance. Finally, *U-HVED* achieves similar performance to the 15 subset-specific models (*Single*). Again, this suggests that the imaging modalities are efficiently embedded in the latent space.

5   Discussion and Conclusion

In this work, we demonstrate the efficacy of a multi-modal variational approach for segmentation with missing modalities. Our model outperforms the state-of-the-art approach HeMIS [3]. In fact, HeMIS could be seen as the non-variational version of our method where: 1/one does not sample but uses the mean of the latent variable instead; 2/the modality-specific covariances are set up to the identity, $\Sigma_i = I$; 3/only the segmentation is reconstructed from the hidden variable. In this case, each modality are independently encoded and averaged such as HeMIS. Finally, our method (*U-HVED*) offers promising insight for leveraging large but incomplete data sets. For future work, we want to provide an analysis of the the learned embedding. This task is particularly challenging due to the multi-scale representation of the hidden variable.

Acknowledgement. We thank C. Sudre, W. Li, B. Murray, Z. Eaton-Rosen, F. Bragman, L. Fidon and T. Varsavsky for their useful comments. This work was supported by the Wellcome Trust [203148/Z/16/Z] and EPSRC [NS/A000049/1]. TV is supported by a Medtronic/RAEng Research Chair [RCSRF1819/7/34].

References

1. Cao, Y., Fleet, D.J.: Generalized product of experts for automatic and principled fusion of Gaussian Process Predictions. CoRR arXiv:1410.7827 (2014)
2. Gibson, E., Li, W., et al.: NiftyNet: a deep-learning platform for medical imaging. Comput. Meth. Progr. Biomed. **158**, 113–122 (2018)
3. Havaei, M., Guizard, N., Chapados, N., Bengio, Y.: HeMIS: hetero-modal image segmentation. In: Ourselin, S., Joskowicz, L., Sabuncu, M.R., Unal, G., Wells, W. (eds.) MICCAI 2016. LNCS, vol. 9901, pp. 469–477. Springer, Cham (2016). https://doi.org/10.1007/978-3-319-46723-8_54
4. Isensee, F., Kickingereder, P., Wick, W., Bendszus, M., Maier-Hein, K.H.: No new-net. In: Crimi, A., Bakas, S., Kuijf, H., Keyvan, F., Reyes, M., van Walsum, T. (eds.) BrainLes 2018. LNCS, vol. 11384, pp. 234–244. Springer, Cham (2019). https://doi.org/10.1007/978-3-030-11726-9_21
5. Kingma, D.P., Welling, M.: Auto-encoding variational bayes. In: ICLR (2014)
6. Li, R., et al.: Deep learning based imaging data completion for improved brain disease diagnosis. In: Golland, P., Hata, N., Barillot, C., Hornegger, J., Howe, R. (eds.) MICCAI 2014. LNCS, vol. 8675, pp. 305–312. Springer, Cham (2014). https://doi.org/10.1007/978-3-319-10443-0_39
7. Menze, B.H., et al.: The multimodal brain tumor image segmentation benchmark BRATS. IEEE Trans. Med. Imaging **34**, 1993–2024 (2015)
8. Milletari, F., Navab, N., Ahmadi, S.: V-net: fully convolutional neural networks for volumetric medical image segmentation. In: International Conference on 3D Vision (3DV), pp. 565–571 (2016)
9. Myronenko, A.: 3D MRI brain tumor segmentation using autoencoder regularization. In: Crimi, A., Bakas, S., Kuijf, H., Keyvan, F., Reyes, M., van Walsum, T. (eds.) BrainLes 2018. LNCS, vol. 11384, pp. 311–320. Springer, Cham (2019). https://doi.org/10.1007/978-3-030-11726-9_28
10. Ronneberger, O., Fischer, P., Brox, T.: U-Net: convolutional networks for biomedical image segmentation. In: Navab, N., Hornegger, J., Wells, W.M., Frangi, A.F. (eds.) MICCAI 2015. LNCS, vol. 9351, pp. 234–241. Springer, Cham (2015). https://doi.org/10.1007/978-3-319-24574-4_28
11. Sønderby, C.K., Raiko, T., Maaløe, L., Sønderby, S.R.K., Winther, O.: Ladder variational autoencoders. In: NeurIPS, pp. 3738–3746 (2016)
12. Varsavsky, T., Eaton-Rosen, Z., Sudre, C.H., Nachev, P., Cardoso, M.J.: PIMMS: permutation invariant multi-modal segmentation. In: Stoyanov, D., et al. (eds.) DLMIA/ML-CDS -2018. LNCS, vol. 11045, pp. 201–209. Springer, Cham (2018). https://doi.org/10.1007/978-3-030-00889-5_23
13. Wu, M., Goodman, N.: Multimodal generative models for scalable weakly-supervised learning. In: NeurIPS, pp. 5580–5590 (2018)
14. Zhao, S., Song, J., Ermon, S.: Learning hierarchical features from deep generative models. In: ICML, pp. 4091–4099 (2017)

Instance Segmentation from Volumetric Biomedical Images Without Voxel-Wise Labeling

Meng Dong, Dong Liu[✉], Zhiwei Xiong, Xuejin Chen, Yueyi Zhang,
Zheng-Jun Zha, Guoqiang Bi, and Feng Wu

University of Science and Technology of China, Hefei, China
dongeliu@ustc.edu.cn

Abstract. Volumetric instance segmentation plays a significant role in biomedical morphological analyses. The improvement of segmentation accuracy has been accelerated by the progress of deep learning-based methods. However, such methods usually rely heavily on plenty of precise annotation, which is time-consuming and may need some expert knowledge to label manually. Although there are several studies focusing on weakly supervised methods in order to save the labeling cost, previous approaches still more or less require voxel-wise annotation. In this paper, we propose a weakly supervised instance segmentation method that needs no voxel-wise labeling. Our approach takes advantage of two advanced techniques: one is the popular proposal-based framework (Faster R-CNN in this paper) for instance detection, and the other is the peak response mapping (PRM) for finding visual cues of instances. Then a new thresholding method combines detected boxes and visual cues to generate final instance segmentation results. We conduct experiments on two biomedical datasets, one of which is a large-scale mouse brain dataset at single-neuron resolution collected by ourselves. Results on both datasets validate the effectiveness of our proposed method.

Keywords: Biomedical image analysis · Peak response mapping · Volumetric instance segmentation · Weak supervision

1 Introduction

Instance segmentation is a pixel-level visual analysis task, which seeks to not only label precise class-aware masks but also produce instance-aware tags to distinguish same-class individual regions. With accurately segmented instances (e.g. somas), the morphological analyses of biomedical images can be made meticulous and more informative. With the progress of exploring deep learning-based methods for computer vision tasks, the popular multi-task approach [4] achieves excellent performance for instance segmentation on natural images, which performs object detection first and then generates instance masks by the following

© Springer Nature Switzerland AG 2019
D. Shen et al. (Eds.): MICCAI 2019, LNCS 11765, pp. 83–91, 2019.
https://doi.org/10.1007/978-3-030-32245-8_10

mask branch. The approach has been extended and its superiority has been verified for biomedical images [13]. However, exploiting the advanced deep learning methods on biomedical images still faces challenges. One major problem is that these methods usually rely heavily on pixel/voxel-wise detailed labeling, which is laborious and time-consuming especially for volumetric images. Labeling biomedical images may also need some expert knowledge, leading to even higher cost.

Many attempts have been made on biomedical images [1,11,13] aiming at saving labeling cost with weakly- or semi-supervised learning methods. Yang et al. [11] present an active learning method for 2D biomedical image segmentation, which can improve segmentation accuracy through suggesting the most effective rather than all samples for labeling. In [1], a sparse annotation approach is proposed for semantic segmentation from volumetric images: only several slices have pixel-wise labeling because of the structural similarity between sequential 2D images. Zhao et al. [13] apply a modified Mask R-CNN [4] to volumetric data for instance segmentation, and they use bounding boxes for all instances and voxel-wise labels for a small proportion of instances. However, the above mentioned works still more or less demand pixel-wise or voxel-wise annotation.

In fact, there are several existing studies about instance segmentation for natural images without pixel-wise labeling, i.e. with only bounding boxes or image-level classes. A commonly used strategy is self-training: the model is trained in full supervision using labels generated by the model itself in an iterative manner [5], and the rough labels can be refined after several iterations. But these methods are usually sensitive to the initial approximate labels and the iterative procedure is a heavy computation burden. In [9], a visualization method for deep image classification CNN has been explored, which is a top-down attention way. The saliency maps can be extracted by a single back-propagation, and the maps are also used as visual cues for weakly supervised semantic segmentation. Similarly, Zhou et al. [14] come up with a new idea for instance segmentation with only image-level class tags. They use locally class-aware peak response mapping (PRM) results as instance representations, and combine them with a segment proposal retrieving operation to produce the instance segmentation results.

Inspired by the above works, in this paper, we address the problem of 3D instance segmentation from volumetric biomedical images with only bounding-box labeling. We split the task into detection and segmentation, detection can be fulfilled by a deep network-based detector, while segmentation utilizes visual cues from PRM results. But the PRM results are usually not complete to produce segmentation masks, hence we design an advanced thresholding method to employ PRM for segmentation. Our main contributions are as follows:

- To our best knowledge, we propose the first weakly supervised instance segmentation method for volumetric biomedical images that does not rely on any voxel-wise annotation. Instead, our model can be trained with only bounding box annotation.
- We extend the peak response mapping into detection network so as to generate high-quality visual cues to benefit the following thresholding phase.

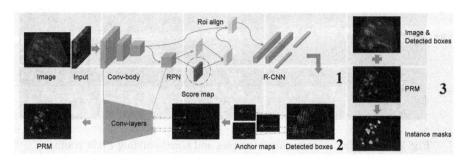

Fig. 1. The pipeline of our approach: Part 1 is the detection phase; Part 2 denotes the peak response mapping for extracting visual cues, which is fulfilled by the back-propagation of the anchor locations of the detected boxes through the Conv-layers; Part 3 shows the local thresholding phase. Best viewed in color.

- We design an advanced thresholding method that employs the visual cues extracted from deep learning-based model. And experiments verify that our thresholding method achieves more precise segmentation.
- We provide a mouse brain image dataset at single-neuron resolution, which is acquired by florescence staining and confocal microscopy imaging techniques. We label soma with bounding box for training set, but give voxel-wise mask annotation for testing set.

Our data and code have been published at https://braindata.bitahub.com/.

2   Method

The pipeline of our approach is shown in Fig. 1, the primary component is a proposal-based detector (denoted in pink background), which can be trained end-to-end with bounding boxes. Instance segmentation includes three steps: (1) the instances (e.g. cells) are detected as boxes; (2) the visual cues for each instance are obtained by PRM, i.e. the back-propagation from score-map layer to input layer; (3) the final instance masks will be segmented by a local thresholding method which utilizes the detected boxes, visual cues, and image intensity.

3D Faster R-CNN for Instance Detection. We extend Faster R-CNN [8] into 3D version for volumetric image task, including conv-body, region proposal networks (RPN) and region convolutional network (R-CNN). And the roi-align layer is also changed to 3D using trilinear interpolation among 8 neighbor voxels for aligning feature maps for each proposal box. Particularly, for the consideration of reducing computing burden for volumetric data, we select a small but still efficient network as the conv-body of detector for feature extraction, whose structure inherits the down-stream part of DSN [3]. And we may modify this network to adapt to different data. Since Faster R-CNN is a proposal-based

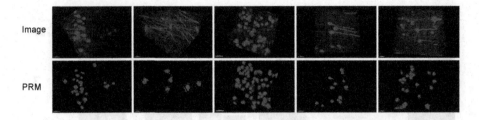

Image

PRM

Fig. 2. Mouse brain soma data examples and corresponding PRM results.

detector that depends on the default anchors, it is essential to carefully set sizes and aspect ratios for anchors to fit the size distribution of targets. Another important related factor is feature stride, which determines the granularity of sliding anchors. We decrease stride for smaller targets by adjusting conv-body, specifically, removing the last pooling layer and the following layers to reduce stride from 8 to 4. In this way, we can improve the cover rate of anchors and keep more detailed features for small targets. Note that we do not use more complex network structure for the sake of computation burden.

Peak Response Mapping for Visual Cues. PRM implemented in [14] depends on a class peak stimulation layer, which is learnt to predict the class probability corresponding to spatial locations. Inspired by this, we observe that due to the characteristics of detector structure, the score map of RPN is a typical class response map related to locations. Therefore, we assume that those high scores can also indicate the strongly informative voxels, and we propose a new PRM way based on object detection framework. RPN predicts the *score* and *location regression value* for each local anchor, which are used to produce proposal candidates. We call the anchor locations "anchor maps" as in Fig. 1. (The highlighted points actually locate at multiple channels of score maps and we only show one channel for visual simplicity.) Then proposals with high scores will be sent to R-CNN for further classification to filter out false positives and keep confident boxes as final detection results. During the procedure we record the source anchor location of each detected box and keep the specific location at anchor maps as peaks. Later the PRM phase will start from the peaks at score maps, which is interpreted as a random walker procedure from the peaks to the bottom layer in [14]. Assuming that U and V are the input and output feature map of a convolution layer in the forward process, whose filter size is $s \times h \times w$. The visiting probability of the random walker or the correlation between spatial locations U_{ijk} and V_{pqt} during PRM can be formulated by

$$P\left(U_{ijk}\right) = \sum_{p=i-\frac{s}{2}}^{i+\frac{s}{2}} \sum_{q=j-\frac{h}{2}}^{j+\frac{h}{2}} \sum_{t=k-\frac{w}{2}}^{k+\frac{w}{2}} P\left(U_{ijk}|V_{pqt}\right) \times P\left(V_{pqt}\right) \quad (1)$$

where the conditional probability is

$$P\left(U_{ijk}|V_{pqt}\right) = Z_{pqt} \times \widehat{U}_{ijk} W^{+}_{(i-p)(j-q)(k-t)} \quad (2)$$

$\widehat{U}_{ijk}$ denotes the activation value at location (i, j, k) of U during the forward process. W^+ means that we only reserve the positive weights of filter and Z_{pqt} is normalization factor to ensure $\sum_{i,j,k} P(U_{ijk}|V_{pqt}) = 1$. Note that the PRM can be realized using normal gradient back-propagation during inference and does not require any extra conditions or constraints for network training.

An Advanced 2D Otsu for Instance Segmentation. Figure 2 shows several examples of visual cues produced by PRM, from which we can tell the contour or boundaries of soma instance. But the PRM is not perfect enough as instance mask for two defects: (1) the regions highlighted as the most discriminative parts are usually not complete and may be broken; (2) other instances may also appear around targets in PRM, so only utilizing PRM can not remove such false regions. Hence, we propose a thresholding method for segmentation that utilizes the PRM results but in addition utilizes the grayscale information. Our method is an advanced 2D Otsu algorithm, but different from the traditional 2D Otsu where the second-dimension is using manually crafted features [12], we use the visual cues extracted from the deep learning-based detection network as the second dimension, which provides complementary information to the local intensity. In order to balance the weights between PRM and intensity, we rescale both into the same dynamic range, and we design a 2D oblique segmentation on the 2D histogram to leverage the complementary information. Specifically, assuming G and P are the intensity and PRM values of voxels inside one detected box, which constitute the two axes of the 2D histogram. Then the thresholding acts with an oblique decision boundary: $\text{sign}(G + k \times P - b)$ where k and b are the slope and bias. And k is set as 1 for the same sale of G and P, and b is searched in a recursion way aiming to maximize the between-class variance. Once the decision boundary is fixed, the segmentation can be accomplished by the thresholding.

3   Experiments and Results

We conduct experiments on two volumetric biomedical datasets, both are optical microscopy images: mouse brain soma dataset collected by ourselves and nuclei of HL60 cells [6,10]. Our method uses merely bounding box labels for training and evaluates instance segmentation performance on voxel-wise labeled test set. Considering that we aim to tackle both volumetric data and learning without voxel-wise annotation problems for instance segmentation task, so we select several competitive methods satisfying both conditions as comparison.

Mouse Brain Soma Data. Our mouse brain soma data is acquired by fluorescence staining and confocal microscopy imaging techniques, whose resolution is high enough to distinguish each neuron. For the training set, we label soma with inscribed sphere and get bounding box labels by extending the globules.

Table 1. Results of average precision with three volumetric mask IoU thresholds on our mouse brain soma dataset. All of these methods do not require voxel-wise labeling.

Method	Instance segmentation AP		
	IoU 0.3	IoU 0.4	IoU 0.5
NeuroGPS [7]	0.4965	0.3960	0.2705
DSN [2]	0.5459	0.4236	0.2512
Detection+1D Otsu	0.6563	0.5077	0.3904
Detection+2D Otsu (w/o PRM)	0.6741	0.5333	0.3992
Detection+2D Otsu (w/ PRM)	**0.7024**	**0.5864**	**0.4253**

Table 2. Results on the HL60 cells dataset in terms of F1 score (the box IoU threshold is 0.4). Det denotes detection.

Method	Voxel-wise labeling	Detection F1			Segmentation F1		
		Track1	Track2	Mean	Track1	Track2	Mean
Mask R-CNN [13]	20%	0.9967	**0.9599**	**0.9783**	0.9416	0.8437	0.8927
VoxResNet [13]	4/13	0.9965	0.9221	0.9593	0.9610	0.7873	0.8742
Det+1D Otsu	0	**0.9970**	0.9545	0.9758	0.7708	0.5668	0.6688
Det+2D Otsu (w/o PRM)	0				0.8792	0.6230	0.7511
Det+2D Otsu (w/ PRM)	0				**0.8902**	**0.7399**	**0.8151**

All images are processed into the same size of $128 \times 256 \times 256$ and saved as 16bit images whose physical resolution is $1\mu m^3$/voxel. Figure 2 shows several image examples. We have 3000 and 228 images for training and testing respectively. Considering the small soma targets and the memory limitation for CNN to handle volumetric data, we set feature stride as 4, input size as $64\times256\times256$ and batch size as 4 on two GeForce GTX 1080Ti's. Note that we can use such big input size thanks to the compact network structure. During inference, the detector firstly outputs boxes and corresponding scores. Afterwards the visual cues are produced by back-propagation for every box. Then the thresholding is completed off-line.

For there is no existing report on our soma data, we compare our method with two advanced methods including an optimization-based method NeuroGPS [7] and a learning-based semantic segmentation method DSN using course mask label [2], both of which do not need voxel-wise label. NeuroGPS is designed for neuron images like our soma data, which aims to find the most appropriate center coordinates and its radius for soma, so we regard the detected solid globules as instance masks. For DSN we find all the connected components as instance segmentation results. And for both baselines those too small masks are excluded to balance precision and recall. In addition, to verify the advantage of our 2D Otsu algorithm, we also check the results of simple but still powerful thresholding methods including 1D Otsu with grayscale only and 2D Otsu whose second dimension is Gaussian filtered grayscale. We evaluate the performance using

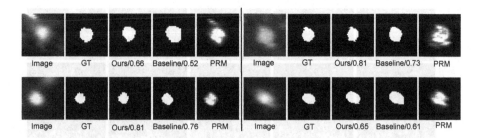

Fig. 3. Our proposed 2D Otsu with PRM produces segmentation results with more fine details, where IoU is calculated between segmentation result and ground-truth (GT).

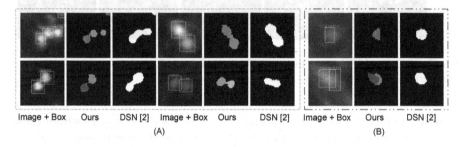

Fig. 4. (A) Detection helps identify instance individual in crowded-instance cases. (B) Failure cases. Best viewed in color.

Average Precision (AP) with three different IoU thresholds for volumetric masks, and results are shown in Table 1. Our approach achieves the best performance for all the metrics. And the ablation study shown in latter three rows indicates that with PRM as visual cues the segmentation AP can gain up to 5.3%.

Nuclei of HL60 Cells. We also apply our method to nuclei of HL60 cells [6,10], a synthetic dataset that contains two tracks and has full voxel-wise annotation for all instances. Note that this dataset is synthetic and the existing reported methods still more or less require voxel-wise labeling, thus the comparison is not fair. However, this is the only public dataset for our task and we conduct experiment on this dataset to verify the generality of our method. We follow the training/test split in [13]. Because the cells in this dataset are larger than those in our soma data, we use feature stride as 8. Also considering that this dataset has voxel-wise annotation and the related work from [13] is more competitive, we compare both detection and instance segmentation performance with the results in [13], using the same evaluation metric: F1 score with IoU threshold of 0.4. We also perform ablation study to verify our PRM-based 2D Otsu algorithm. Table 2 presents F1 scores of all methods. Our approach can achieve comparable detection performance with [13]. For instance segmentation, our method performs not as well as [13] because we use no voxel-wise label in

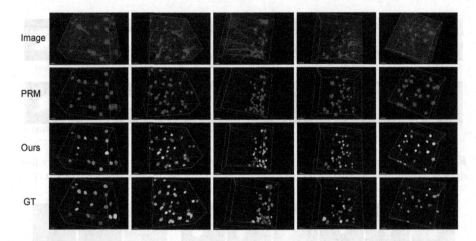

Fig. 5. Visualized PRM and instance segmentation results, where different instances are marked with random colors. Best viewed in color.

training, and for fairness the F1 scores in bold shows the best ones without any voxel-wise label. However, as this dataset is synthetic, it may not reveal the real-world cases.

Visualization Results. To better understand the effect of PRM and detection and visually evaluate our method, here we illustrate three groups of soma images in both 2D and 3D views. Figure 3 shows how PRM benefits thresholding. These results suggest that with PRM as a guidance the segmented mask has a closer appearance to the ground truth, especially in fine details. Although the visual cues from PRM might be not complete, the discriminative regions serve as complementary information to intensity and improve the mask contour. Examples in Fig. 4 reflect the influence of detection on instance segmentation. Group A shows that detected boxes help identify soma instances in dense-soma case even when they touch each other. While in some low-contrast or cropped regions, the segmentation may be not good enough for the boxes not precisely detected. Figure 5 illustrates some results in 3D view. We can see that our method can detect and segment soma in diverse intensity, density, shapes as well as from complex background, and the appearance is quite close to the ground truth.

4   Conclusion

In this paper, we propose a weakly supervised instance segmentation method for volumetric biomedical images not requiring any voxel-wise label. The network can be trained as a simple detector with bounding boxes only. And instance segmentation can be accomplished by PRM combined with an advanced thresholding algorithm. We design experiments on two datasets and results demonstrate the efficiency of the proposed method. Our approach can save considerable labeling efforts and has potential to be applied to other related segmentation tasks.

Acknowledgements. This work was supported by the Natural Science Foundation of China under Grant 91732304, and by the Fundamental Research Funds for the Central Universities under Grant WK2380000002.

References

1. Çiçek, Ö., et al.: 3D U-Net: Learning dense volumetric segmentation from sparse annotation. In: MICCAI. pp. 424–432 (2016)
2. Dong, M., et al.: 3D CNN-based soma segmentation from brain images at single-neuron resolution. In: ICIP. pp. 126–130 (2018)
3. Dou, Q., et al.: 3D deeply supervised network for automatic liver segmentation from CT volumes. In: MICCAI. pp. 149–157 (2016)
4. He, K., et al.: Mask R-CNN. In: ICCV. pp. 2961–2969 (2017)
5. Khoreva, A., et al.: Simple does it: Weakly supervised instance and semantic segmentation. In: CVPR. pp. 876–885 (2017)
6. Maška, M., et al.: A benchmark for comparison of cell tracking algorithms. Bioinformatics **30**(11), 1609–1617 (2014)
7. Quan, T., et al.: NeuroGPS: Automated localization of neurons for brain circuits using L1 minimization model. Scientific Reports 3, Article No. 1414 (2013)
8. Ren, S., et al.: Faster R-CNN: Towards real-time object detection with region proposal networks. In: NIPS. pp. 91–99 (2015)
9. Simonyan, K., et al.: Deep inside convolutional networks: Visualising image classification models and saliency maps. arXiv preprint arXiv:1312.6034 (2013)
10. Ulman, V., et al.: An objective comparison of cell-tracking algorithms. Nature Methods 14(12), Article No. 1141 (2017)
11. Yang, L., et al.: Suggestive annotation: A deep active learning framework for biomedical image segmentation. In: MICCAI. pp. 399–407 (2017)
12. Zhang, J., et al.: Image segmentation based on 2D Otsu method with histogram analysis. CASCON. **6**, 105–108 (2008)
13. Zhao, Z., et al.: Deep learning based instance segmentation in 3D biomedical images using weak annotation. In: MICCAI. pp. 352–360 (2018)
14. Zhou, Y., et al.: Weakly supervised instance segmentation using class peak response. In: CVPR. pp. 3791–3800 (2018)

Optimizing the Dice Score and Jaccard Index for Medical Image Segmentation: Theory and Practice

Jeroen Bertels[1], Tom Eelbode[1(✉)], Maxim Berman[1], Dirk Vandermeulen[1], Frederik Maes[1], Raf Bisschops[2], and Matthew B. Blaschko[1]

[1] ESAT, Center for Processing Speech and Images, KU Leuven, Leuven, Belgium
tom.eelbode@kuleuven.be
[2] Gastroenterology and hepatology, UZ Leuven, Leuven, Belgium

Abstract. The Dice score and Jaccard index are commonly used metrics for the evaluation of segmentation tasks in medical imaging. Convolutional neural networks trained for image segmentation tasks are usually optimized for (weighted) cross-entropy. This introduces an adverse discrepancy between the learning optimization objective (the loss) and the end target metric. Recent works in computer vision have proposed soft surrogates to alleviate this discrepancy and directly optimize the desired metric, either through relaxations (soft-Dice, soft-Jaccard) or submodular optimization (Lovász-softmax). The aim of this study is two-fold. First, we investigate the theoretical differences in a risk minimization framework and question the existence of a weighted cross-entropy loss with weights theoretically optimized to surrogate Dice or Jaccard. Second, we empirically investigate the behavior of the aforementioned loss functions w.r.t. evaluation with Dice score and Jaccard index on five medical segmentation tasks. Through the application of relative approximation bounds, we show that all surrogates are equivalent up to a multiplicative factor, and that no optimal weighting of cross-entropy exists to approximate Dice or Jaccard measures. We validate these findings empirically and show that, while it is important to opt for one of the target metric surrogates rather than a cross-entropy-based loss, the choice of the surrogate does not make a statistical difference on a wide range of medical segmentation tasks.

Keywords: Dice · Jaccard · Risk minimization · Cross-entropy

1 Introduction

The Dice score and Jaccard index have become some of the most popular performance metrics in medical image segmentation [1–3, 11, 18]. Zijdenbos et al. were among the first to suggest the Dice score for medical image analysis by

---

J. Bertels and T. Eelbode have contributed equally to this work.

© Springer Nature Switzerland AG 2019
D. Shen et al. (Eds.): MICCAI 2019, LNCS 11765, pp. 92–100, 2019.
https://doi.org/10.1007/978-3-030-32245-8_11

evaluating the quality of automated white matter lesion segmentations [22]. In scenarios with large class imbalance, with an excessive number of (correctly classified) background voxels, they show that the Dice score is a special case of the kappa index, a chance-corrected measure of agreement. They further note that the Dice score reflects both size and localization agreement, more in line with perceptual quality compared to pixel-wise accuracy.

Risk minimization principle says we should minimize during training time the loss that we will be using to evaluate the performance at test time [21]. This has motivated the introduction of differentiable approximations for Dice score (e.g. soft Dice [19]) and Jaccard index (e.g. soft Jaccard [16,20] or its more recent convex extension Lovász-softmax [5]) in order to incorporate it into gradient-based training schemes, such as stochastic gradient descent (SGD). These can be used for training segmentation models, including convolutional neural networks (CNNs) [19]. Nevertheless, training with the pixel-wise cross-entropy loss, or its weighted variant, remains highly popular, even when the evaluation is performed using the Dice score or Jaccard index [6,11]. In the MICCAI 2018 proceedings, 47 out of 77 learning-based segmentation papers used such a per-pixel loss even though the evaluation was performed with Dice score.

This raises the question to what extent a loss function has impact on the prediction quality, and whether there are principled reasons for choosing one set of loss functions over another. In this work, we consider from a theoretical perspective the relationship between Dice score and Jaccard index, and work out that one approximates the other under risk minimization. We further question the existence of a well-weighted cross-entropy loss as a surrogate for Dice or Jaccard. We find an approximation bound between Dice and Jaccard losses, but no such approximation exists for cross-entropy. We are able to validate our findings empirically on five medical tasks, finding that all of the metric-sensitive losses are favourable over (weighted) cross-entropy, but that generally no mutual statistical difference can be observed among the former.

2 Risk Minimization with Dice and Related Similarities

When performing discriminative training of machine learning methods, such as SGD for a CNN [9], we are performing risk minimization. To learn a mapping f from an observed input x to a hidden variable y, empirical risk minimization optimizes the expectation of a loss function over a finite training set:

$$\arg\min_{f\in\mathcal{F}} \underbrace{\frac{1}{n}\sum_{i=1}^{n}\ell(f(x_i),y_i)}_{=:\hat{\mathcal{R}}(f)}, \tag{1}$$

where ℓ is a loss function and $\mathcal{F}$ is a function class of interest, e.g. the set of functions that can be represented by a neural network with a given topology. We will denote the bootstrap distribution arising from a sample $\mathcal{S} := \{(x_i,y_i)\}_{1\leq i\leq n}$ of size n as P_n, and we may equivalently denote $\hat{\mathcal{R}}(f) = \mathbb{E}_{(x,y)\sim P_n}[\ell(x,y)]$.

In binary medical image segmentation, y can be thought of as a set of pixels labeled as foreground. It is therefore well defined to consider set theoretic notions such as $y \cap \tilde{y}$ for two different segmentations. This motivates the use of multiple set theoretic similarity measures between two segmentations y and $\tilde{y}$ including the Dice score D, the Jaccard index J, the Hamming similarity H, and what we will call the weighted Hamming similarity H_γ:

$$D(y, \tilde{y}) := \frac{2|y \cap \tilde{y}|}{|y| + |\tilde{y}|}, \quad J(y, \tilde{y}) := \frac{|y \cap \tilde{y}|}{|y \cup \tilde{y}|}, \quad H(y, \tilde{y}) := 1 - \frac{|y \setminus \tilde{y}| + |\tilde{y} \setminus y|}{d}, \quad (2)$$

$$H_\gamma(y, \tilde{y}) := 1 - \gamma \frac{|y \setminus \tilde{y}|}{|y|} - (1 - \gamma) \frac{|\tilde{y} \setminus y|}{d - |y|}, \quad (3)$$

where d denotes the number of pixels and $0 \leq \gamma \leq 1$. We note that all these similarities are between 0 and 1, and that H_γ generalizes H with equality when $\gamma = \frac{|y|}{d}$. A further important relationship is that between the Jaccard index and the Dice coefficient. It is well known that

$$J(y, \tilde{y}) = \frac{D(y, \tilde{y})}{2 - D(y, \tilde{y})} \text{ and } D(y, \tilde{y}) = \frac{2J(y, \tilde{y})}{1 + J(y, \tilde{y})}. \quad (4)$$

Indeed, in the risk minimization framework for medical image segmentation, there are numerous examples where each of these measures are optimized [8,15, 19].

In risk minimization, we replace a similarity $S : \mathcal{Y} \times \mathcal{Y} \to [0, 1]$ with its corresponding loss $1 - S$, and aim at minimizing this loss in expectation. To train a neural network by backpropagation [9] it is necessary to replace this value with a differentiable surrogate. For the Hamming similarity, cross-entropy loss and other convex surrogates are statistically consistent [4,13]. To optimize the weighted Hamming similarity, one may employ weighted loss functions [14] such as weighted cross entropy. Similarly, differentiable surrogates have been proposed both for the Dice score (e.g. soft Dice [19]) and Jaccard index (e.g. soft Jaccard [17] and Lovász-softmax [5]). Next, we hereby discuss the absolute and relative approximations between Dice and Jaccard and inspect the existence of an approximation through a weighted Hamming similarity.

Definition 1 (Absolute approximation). *A similarity S is absolutely approximated by $\tilde{S}$ with error $\varepsilon \geq 0$ if the following holds for all y and $\tilde{y}$:*

$$|S(y, \tilde{y}) - \tilde{S}(y, \tilde{y})| \leq \varepsilon. \quad (5)$$

Definition 2 (Relative approximation). *A similarity S is relatively approximated by $\tilde{S}$ with error $\varepsilon \geq 0$ if the following holds for all y and $\tilde{y}$:*

$$\frac{\tilde{S}(y, \tilde{y})}{1 + \varepsilon} \leq S(y, \tilde{y}) \leq \tilde{S}(y, \tilde{y})(1 + \varepsilon). \quad (6)$$

We note that both notions of approximation are symmetric in S and $\tilde{S}$.

Proposition 1. *J and D approximate each other with relative error of* 1 *and absolute error of* $3 - 2\sqrt{2} = 0.17157\ldots$.

Proof. The relative error between J and D is given by (cf. Eq. (4))

$$\min_{\varepsilon \geq 0} \varepsilon, \text{ s.t. } x \leq \frac{x}{2 - x}(1 + \varepsilon), \ \forall \ 0 \leq x \leq 1. \tag{7}$$

$$x \leq \frac{x}{2 - x}(1 + \varepsilon) \implies 1 - x \leq \varepsilon \implies \varepsilon = 1. \tag{8}$$

The absolute error between J and D is given by

$$\varepsilon = \sup_{0 \leq x \leq 1} \left| x - \frac{x}{2 - x} \right| = 3 - 2\sqrt{2}, \tag{9}$$

which can be verified straightforwardly by first order conditions:

$$\frac{\partial}{\partial x}\left(x - \frac{x}{2 - x} \right) = 0 \implies (2 - x)^2 - 2 = 0 \implies x = 2 - \sqrt{2}. \ \Box \ (10)$$

$\Box$

Proposition 2. *D and H_γ (where γ is chosen to minimize the approximation factor between D and H_γ) do not relatively approximate each other, and absolutely approximate each other with an error of* 1. *We note that the absolute error bound is trivial as D and H_γ are both similarities in the range* $[0, 1]$.

Proof. For relative error, consider the case that $|y \setminus \tilde{y}| = 0$, $|\tilde{y} \setminus y| = \alpha d$, and $|y \cap \tilde{y}| = \alpha^2 d$ for some $0 \leq \alpha < \frac{\sqrt{5}-1}{2}$:

$$\inf_{\gamma} \sup_{y, \tilde{y}} 1 - \gamma \frac{|y \setminus \tilde{y}|}{|y|} - (1 - \gamma)\frac{|\tilde{y} \setminus y|}{d - |y|} - \frac{2|y \cap \tilde{y}|}{|y \triangle \tilde{y}| + 2|y \cap \tilde{y}|}(1 + \varepsilon) \leq 0 \tag{11}$$

$$\implies \sup_{0 \leq \alpha < \frac{\sqrt{5}-1}{2}} 1 - \frac{\alpha}{1 - \alpha^2} - \frac{2\alpha^2}{\alpha + 2\alpha^2}(1 + \varepsilon) \leq 0 \tag{12}$$

If we let $\alpha \to 0$, it must be the case that $\varepsilon \to \infty$. To show that the absolute approximation error is 1, we similarly take

$$\lim_{\alpha \to 0} 1 - \frac{\alpha}{1 - \alpha^2} - \frac{2\alpha}{1 + 2\alpha} = 1. \tag{13}$$

$\Box$

Corollary 1. *D and H do not relatively approximate each other, and absolutely approximate each other with an error of* 1.

From these bounds, we see that a (weighted) binary loss can be an arbitrarily bad approximation for Dice when segmenting small objects, while the Jaccard loss gives multiplicative and additive approximation guarantees. Furthermore,

Eq. (4) implies that $1 - D(y, \tilde{y}) \leq 1 - J(y, \tilde{y}) \implies \mathbb{E}_{(x,y) \sim P_n}[1 - D(y, f(x))] \leq \mathbb{E}_{(x,y) \sim P_n}[1 - J(y, f(x))]$ and optimization with risk computed with the Jaccard loss minimizes an upper bound on risk computed with the Dice loss. Similarly setting $\varphi(x) = 2x/(1 + x)$, by application of Jensen's inequality we arrive at $\mathbb{E}_{(x,y) \sim P_n}[1 - J(y, f(x))] = \mathbb{E}_{(x,y) \sim P_n}[\varphi(1 - D(y, f(x)))] \leq \varphi(\mathbb{E}_{(x,y) \sim P_n}[1 - D(y, f(x))])$ and optimizing the Dice loss minimizes an upper bound on the Jaccard loss as φ is a monotonic function over $[0, 1]$.

3 Empirical Setup

To test the aforementioned properties empirically, we investigate the performance of segmentation networks trained with different loss functions: cross-entropy (CE), weighted cross-entropy (wCE), soft Dice (sDice), soft Jaccard (sJaccard), and Lovász-sigmoid. We validate by cross-validation on five medical binary segmentation tasks. Three tasks are publicly available 3D datasets: BRATS 2018 (limited to whole tumor segmentation [2]; BR18, 285 images), ISLES 2017 (follow-up stroke lesion segmentation [1]; IS17, 43 images) and ISLES 2018 (acute stroke lesion segmentation [3]; IS18, 94 images). Furthermore, we expand the empirical setup with two in-house 2D datasets: lower-left third molar segmentation from panoramic dental radiographs (MO17, 400 images) and segmentation of colorectal polyps from colonoscopy images (PO18, 1166 images).

Network Architectures and Preprocessing. For BR18, IS17 and IS18 we implement a U-Net-like [18] architecture with 3D convolutions, starting from a top-ranked implementation during last year's BRATS challenge [10] with less filters and an encoder depth of 7 layers. For MO17 the same architecture with 2D convolutions is used. For PO18 a VGG16 backbone architecture with atrous convolutions and pretrained on ImageNet [7] is used. We use all image modalities available in each dataset as input, excluding perfusion data for IS17 and IS18. In order to fit memory, these inputs are resized and cropped. Data augmentation consisted of Gaussian noise, translations, flips, and in-plane rotations.

Training Procedure. We perform an initial training of the CNNs with cross-entropy loss. We use Adam [12] with an initial learning rate of 10^{-3} for the randomly initialized networks, and 10^{-4} for the ImageNet-initialized network. This learning rate is decreased when the validation loss stagnates. We stop the training when the validation loss starts increasing. Batch sizes are 40 for MO17, 16 for PO18, and 4 for all public datasets. After initial convergence with cross-entropy, we continue training using one of the five different loss functions: CE, wCE, sDice, sJaccard and Lovász. For wCE, theory suggests that no optimal approximation w.r.t. Dice or Jaccard can be derived before training (see Sect. 2). To set the weights, we therefore resort to the common heuristic of balancing foreground and background equally [19]. Thus, the weight applied to the foreground class is $1/(2p)$ and the weight applied to the background class is $1/(2 - 2p)$, with p the foreground prior. We use the same optimization procedure as described for the initial training, with an initial learning rate of 10^{-3} for MO17 and 10^{-4} for all other datasets, which lead to appropriate convergence.

4 Results and Discussion

In the following discussion, we distinguish between two groups of losses. First, CE and wCE losses, which are surrogates for the (weighted) Hamming loss. Second, sDice, sJaccard and Lovász losses, which are surrogates either for the Dice score or Jaccard index, and which we group as *metric-sensitive losses*. Table 1 lists the average Dice scores and Jaccard indexes obtained after five-fold cross-validation for each dataset and loss under study. For each fold, we choose the best performing model w.r.t. the validation loss. We perform a pairwise non-parametric significance test (bootstrapping) with a p-value of 0.05 to assess inferiority or superiority between pairs of optimization methods.

Table 1. Dice scores and Jaccard indexes obtained for each dataset with the different losses. Values in italic point to a significant lower result compared to each of the metric-sensitive losses. Underlined values point to a significant lower result within the two groups of losses considered: the group of CE and wCE losses, and the group of metric-sensitive losses. Values in bold point to a significant better result compared to all other losses. Values in parentheses are dataset sizes.

	Dataset	$loss \rightarrow$	CE	wCE	sDice	sJaccard	Lovász
Dice score	BR18		*0.768*	*0.735*	0.823	0.823	**0.827**
	IS17		*0.260*	0.311	0.331	0.321	0.305
	IS18		*0.463*	*0.474*	**0.538**	0.528	0.508
	MO17		0.930	*0.860*	0.932	0.931	0.932
	PO18		*0.635*	*0.602*	0.656	0.651	0.649
Jaccard index	BR18		*0.654*	*0.602*	0.717	0.720	0.722
	IS17		*0.177*	0.212	0.227	0.217	0.204
	IS18		*0.345*	*0.344*	**0.407**	0.399	0.382
	MO17		0.873	*0.769*	0.877	0.875	0.877
	PO18		*0.541*	*0.488*	0.559	0.554	0.553

Equivalence of J and D. The theory suggests an equivalence between Dice and Jaccard metrics (Proposition 1). This equivalence appears in our results: in particular, we found the rankings of the performance of the different losses to be the same in terms of Dice score and in terms of Jaccard index.

Performance of the Surrogates. It is clear that CE and wCE lead to lower Dice scores and Jaccard indexes than the metric-sensitive losses (highlighted in italic). Only for MO17 does CE lead to similar performance compared to the metric-sensitive losses, likely due to a more uniform distribution of foreground and background pixels for this dataset. This trend was expected due to the theoretical divergence between cross-entropy losses and the metric-sensitive losses and holds with current works optimizing Dice or Jaccard measures directly via

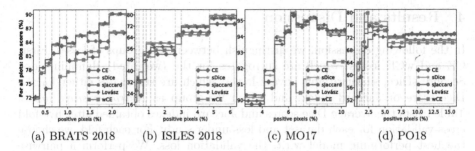

(a) BRATS 2018　　　(b) ISLES 2018　　　(c) MO17　　　(d) PO18

Fig. 1. Dice score as a function of the relative ratio of foreground pixels for four datasets. The scores are averaged within the 10 regions bordered by the dashed lines; each region contains 1/10 of the dataset. Metric-sensitive losses perform as well or better than cross-entropy over most of the relative area ranges. ISLES 2017 omitted for lack of statistical relevance given its lower number of samples.

their surrogates. Moreover, we found in general no statistically significant difference within the group of metric-sensitive losses w.r.t. Dice or Jaccard. This further confirms our theoretical findings and leaves the researcher a free choice.

Weighting of Cross-Entropy. We note that wCE is generally performing poorly compared to CE (inferior performances are underlined). A better choice of weights might lead to a better performance of wCE. However, it is clear from our results that the weighting is highly task-dependent. Finding a better weighting is therefore non-trivial, compared to using one of the metric-sensitive losses. Moreover, as highlighted in our subsequent scale-specific study, wCE does yield a better performance within some restricted ranges of object scales. In accordance with theory, it is likely that no single weighting would yield appropriate surrogates to the target metrics across all datasets and scales.

Scale-Specific Study. In general, a segmentation dataset contains objects of variable size. It is generally assumed that Dice or Jaccard-sensitive losses have most impact for refining the segmentations of samples of small size, thanks to their invariance to scale, which cross-entropy does not have [5]. The dependence of the approximation bound on the Hamming loss in Eq. (3) on the number of positive pixels in the ground truth $|y|$ also points towards a loss of segmentation accuracy in terms of Dice score in the small-sample regime when optimizing with Hamming loss or cross-entropy. We study this dependence in Fig. 1, showing the average Dice scores as a function of the ground truth object size for the different optimization methods. We found that the applicability of metric-sensitive losses goes beyond the small-size regime, and that it is possible for CE to perform poorly across almost all scales. This is most evident in BR18 and IS18; even in the other datasets, the cross-entropy curve is dominated by other optimization methods. Furthermore, while wCE improves on CE on some datasets and area ranges, it can also vastly underperform the metric-sensitive losses as in BR18 and MO17, further indicating that a simple re-weighting of cross-entropy is not sufficient to capture the target metric across all object scales and datasets.

5   Conclusion

We compared optimization with five different loss functions from both theoretical and empirical perspectives. We find Jaccard and Dice approximate each other relatively and absolutely, while no approximation by a weighted Hamming similarity (i.e. a set theoretical equivalent for weighted cross-entropy) can be found. We confirm these findings empirically by evaluation on five medical segmentation tasks. We can show that there is generally no significant difference between the use of either of the metric-sensitive loss functions. Cross-entropy and its weighted version are however inferior to the latter when evaluated on Dice and Jaccard. This is in line with theory, which predicts that Jaccard controls the Dice loss. Nevertheless, the use of per-pixel losses remains highly popular. Of the 77 learning-based segmentation papers in the MICCAI 2018 proceedings that perform evaluation with Dice, 47 trained using a per-pixel loss. The theory and empirical results presented here suggest that wider adoption of metric-sensitive losses like Dice and Jaccard is warranted.

Acknowledgements. This work is funded in part by Internal Funds KU Leuven (grant # C24/18/047). The computational resources were partly provided by the Flemish Supercomputer Center (VSC). J.B. is part of NEXIS, a project that has received funding from the European Union's Horizon 2020 Research and Innovations Programme (grant # 780026). R.B. is supported by FWO and Fujifilm. M.B. and M.B.B. acknowledge support from FWO (grant # G0A2716N), an Amazon Research Award, an NVIDIA GPU grant, and the Facebook AI Research Partnership. The authors thank H. Willekens, C. Camps, C. Hassan, E. Coron, P. Bhandari, H. Neumann, O. Pech and A. Repici for their effort and collaboration.

References

1. ISLES challenge (2017). http://www.isles-challenge.org/ISLES2017/
2. BRATS challenge (2018). https://www.med.upenn.edu/sbia/brats2018.html
3. ISLES challenge (2018). http://www.isles-challenge.org/ISLES2018/
4. Bartlett, P.L., Jordan, M.I., McAuliffe, J.D.: Convexity, classification, and risk bounds. J. Am. Stat. Assoc. **101**(473), 138–156 (2006)
5. Berman, M., Rannen Triki, A., Blaschko, M.B.: The Lovász-Softmax loss: a tractable surrogate for the optimization of the intersection-over-union measure in neural networks (2018)
6. Chen, L., Bentley, P., Rueckert, D.: Fully automatic acute ischemic lesion segmentation in DWI using convolutional neural networks. NeuroImage Clin. **15**, 633–643 (2017)
7. Chen, L., Papandreou, G., Kokkinos, I., Murphy, K., Yuille, A.L.: DeepLab: semantic image segmentation with deep convolutional nets, atrous convolution, and fully connected CRFs. IEEE-TPAMI **40**(4), 834–848 (2018)
8. England, J.R., Cheng, P.M.: Artificial intelligence for medical image analysis: a guide for authors and reviewers. AJR Am. J. Roentgenol. **212**(3), 513–519 (2019)
9. Goodfellow, I., Bengio, Y., Courville, A.: Deep Learning. MIT Press, Cambridge (2016)

10. Isensee, F., Kickingereder, P., Wick, W., Bendszus, M., Maier-Hein, K.H.: No New-Net (2018)
11. Kamnitsas, K., et al.: Efficient multi-scale 3D CNN with fully connected CRF for accurate brain lesion segmentation. MIA **36**, 61–78 (2017)
12. Kingma, D.P., Ba, J.: Adam: a method for stochastic optimization. arXiv:1412.6980 (2014)
13. Lapin, M., Hein, M., Schiele, B.: Loss functions for top-k error (2016)
14. Ling, C.X., Sheng, V.S.: Cost-sensitive learning. In: Sammut, C., Webb, G.I. (eds.) Encyclopedia of Machine Learning, pp. 231–235. Springer, Boston (2010). https://doi.org/10.1007/978-0-387-30164-8
15. Salehi, S.S.M., Erdogmus, D., Gholipour, A.: Tversky loss function for image segmentation using 3D fully convolutional deep networks. In: Wang, Q., Shi, Y., Suk, H.-I., Suzuki, K. (eds.) MLMI 2017. LNCS, vol. 10541, pp. 379–387. Springer, Cham (2017). https://doi.org/10.1007/978-3-319-67389-9_44
16. Nowozin, S.: Optimal decisions from probabilistic models: the intersection-over-union case, pp. 548–555 (2014)
17. Rahman, M.A., Wang, Y.: Optimizing intersection-over-union in deep neural networks for image segmentation. In: Bebis, G., et al. (eds.) ISVC 2016. LNCS, vol. 10072, pp. 234–244. Springer, Cham (2016). https://doi.org/10.1007/978-3-319-50835-1_22
18. Ronneberger, O., Fischer, P., Brox, T.: U-Net: convolutional networks for biomedical image segmentation. In: Navab, N., Hornegger, J., Wells, W.M., Frangi, A.F. (eds.) MICCAI 2015. LNCS, vol. 9351, pp. 234–241. Springer, Cham (2015). https://doi.org/10.1007/978-3-319-24574-4_28
19. Sudre, C.H., Li, W., Vercauteren, T., Ourselin, S., Jorge Cardoso, M.: Generalised dice overlap as a deep learning loss function for highly unbalanced segmentations. In: Cardoso, M.J., et al. (eds.) DLMIA/ML-CDS 2017. LNCS, vol. 10553, pp. 240–248. Springer, Cham (2017). https://doi.org/10.1007/978-3-319-67558-9_28
20. Tarlow, D., Adams, R.P.: Revisiting uncertainty in graph cut solutions (2012)
21. Vapnik, V.N.: The Nature of Statistical Learning Theory. Springer, New York (1995). https://doi.org/10.1007/978-1-4757-2440-0
22. Zijdenbos, A.P., Dawant, B.M., Margolin, R.A., Palmer, A.C.: Morphometric analysis of white matter lesions in MR images: method and validation. IEEE Trans. Med. Imaging **13**(4), 716–724 (1994)

Dual Adaptive Pyramid Network for Cross-Stain Histopathology Image Segmentation

Xianxu Hou[1,2], Jingxin Liu[1,2,3(✉)], Bolei Xu[1,2], Bozhi Liu[1,2], Xin Chen[4], Mohammad Ilyas[5], Ian Ellis[5], Jon Garibaldi[4], and Guoping Qiu[1,2,4]

[1] College of Information Engineering, Shenzhen University, Shenzhen, China
jingxin.liu@outlook.com
[2] Guangdong Key Laboratory of Intelligent Information Processing,
Shenzhen University, Shenzhen, China
[3] Histo Pathology Diagnostic Center, Shanghai, China
[4] School of Computer Science, University of Nottingham, Nottingham, UK
[5] School of Medicine, University of Nottingham, Nottingham, UK

Abstract. Supervised semantic segmentation normally assumes the test data being in a similar data domain as the training data. However, in practice, the domain mismatch between the training and unseen data could lead to a significant performance drop. Obtaining accurate pixelwise label for images in different domains is tedious and labor intensive, especially for histopathology images. In this paper, we propose a dual adaptive pyramid network (DAPNet) for histopathological gland segmentation adapting from one stain domain to another. We tackle the domain adaptation problem on two levels: (1) the image-level considers the differences of image color and style; (2) the feature-level addresses the spatial inconsistency between two domains. The two components are implemented as domain classifiers with adversarial training. We evaluate our new approach using two gland segmentation datasets with H&E and DAB-H stains respectively. The extensive experiments and ablation study demonstrate the effectiveness of our approach on the domain adaptive segmentation task. We show that the proposed approach performs favorably against other state-of-the-art methods.

Keywords: Gland segmentation · Histopathology · Domain adaptation

1 Introduction

Deep convolutional neural networks (DCNNs) have achieved remarkable success in the field of medical image segmentation [5], which aims to identify and segment specific regions, such as organs or lesions in MR images, and cellular

---

X. Hou and J. Liu—Equal contribution.

© Springer Nature Switzerland AG 2019
D. Shen et al. (Eds.): MICCAI 2019, LNCS 11765, pp. 101–109, 2019.
https://doi.org/10.1007/978-3-030-32245-8_12

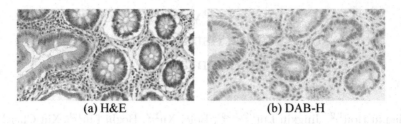

(a) H&E   (b) DAB-H

Fig. 1. Image examples of different histopathological stains. (a) Hematoxylin and Eosin; (b) Diaminobenzidene and Hematoxylin.

structures or tumor regions in pathological images. Although excellent performance has been achieved on benchmark dataset, deep segmentation models have poor generalization capability to unseen datasets [10] due to the domain shift between the training and test data.

Such domain shift is commonly observed especially in histopathology image analysis. For instance, the Hematoxylin and Eosin (H&E) stained colon image has significantly different visual appearances from that stained by Diaminobenzidene and Hematoxylin (DAB-H) (Fig. 1). Thus, the model trained on one (source) dataset would not generalize well when applied to the other (target) dataset. Although fine-tuning the model with labelled target data could possibly alleviate the impact of domain shift, manually annotating is a time-consuming, expensive and subjective process in medical area. Therefore, it is of great interest to develop algorithms to adapt segmentation models from a source domain to a visually different target domain without requiring additional labels in the target domain.

Domain adaptation algorithms have been developed to address the domain-shift problem. The main insight behind these methods is trying to align visual appearance or feature distribution between the source and target domains. Zhang *et al.* [11] render the source image with the target domain "style", and then learn domain-invariant representations in an adversarial manner. AdapSeg [9] is developed to align the two domain images in the structured output space. CyCADA [3] unifies adversarial adaptation methods together with cycle-consistent image translation techniques.

In this paper, we propose a DCNN-based domain adaptation algorithm for histopathology image segmentation, referred to as Dual Adaptive Pyramid Network (DAPNet). The proposed DAPNet is designed to reduce the discrepancy between two domains by incorporating two domain adaptation components on image level and feature level. The image-level adaptation considers the overall difference between source and target domain like image color and style, while feature-level adaptation addresses the spatial inconsistency of the two domains. In particular, each component is implemented as a domain classifier with an adversarial training strategy to learn domain-invariant features.

The contribution of this work can be summarized as follows. First, we develop a deep unsupervised domain adaptation algorithm for histopathology image seg-

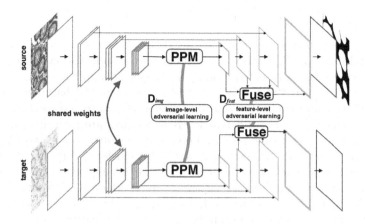

Fig. 2. Overview of our DAPNet. Both source and target domain images are fed to the segmentation network. The training procedure optimizes the segmentation loss based on the source ground truth, and two domain classification losses of image-level and feature-level adversarial learning modules to make the segmentation output close to the image labels of the source domain.

mentation. Second, we propose two domain adaptation components to alleviate the domain discrepancy at the image and feature levels based on pyramid features. Third, we conduct extensive experiments and our proposed DAPNet outperforms other state-of-the-art methods.

2   Method

In this work, we aim to learn gland segmentation model from images with a certain stain type and apply the learned model to a different stain scenario. The training data is used as the source domain S while the test data with a different stain type is regarded as the target domain T. In the S domain, we have access to the stained images X_S as well as the corresponding ground-truth labels Y_S. In the target domain T, we only have the unlabelled stained images X_T.

2.1   Model Overview

The overview of the proposed DAPNet is illustrated in Fig. 2. It contains a semantic segmentation network G and two adversarial learning modules D_{img} and D_{feat}. During training, both the source images x_s and target images x_t are fed into the network G as inputs. The source images and the corresponding labels are used to optimize G for the segmentation task, while both source and target images are used for optimizing domain adaptation losses by adversarial learning with D_{img} and D_{feat}.

2.2   Segmentation Network

As shown in Fig. 2, our segmentation network consists of 3 components. First a dilated ResNet-18 [2] is used as backbone to encode the input images. In order to achieve larger receptive field of our model, we apply a Pyramid Pooling Module (PPM) from PSPNet [12] on the last layer of the backbone network. The PPM separates the feature map into different pooled representations with varied pyramid levels. The different levels of features are then upsampled and concatenated as the pyramid pooling global feature. Furthermore, we adopt skip connections from U-Net [7] and a pyramid feature fusion architecture to achieve final segmentation. The decoded feature maps are upsampled to the same spatial resolution and merged by concatenation in a pyramidal way. The output feature maps undergo a 1×1 convolutional layer to reduce the dimension of channel to 512. Our method involves downsampling pyramid feature extraction and upsampling pyramid feature fusion. However, the CyCADA needs to first map source training data into the target domain in pixel level.

The segmentation task is learned by minimizing both standard cross-entropy loss and Dice coefficient for images from the source domain:

$$\mathcal{L}_{seg} = \mathbb{E}_{x_s \sim X_S}[-y_s log(\widetilde{y}_s)] + \alpha \mathbb{E}_{x_s \sim X_S}[-\frac{2y_s\widetilde{y}_s}{y_s + \widetilde{y}_s}] \tag{1}$$

where y_s stands for ground-truth labels, $\widetilde{y}_s$ stands for predicted labels and α is the trade-off parameter.

2.3   Domain Adaptation

Image-Level Adaptation. In this work, image-level representation refers to the PPM outputs of the segmentation network G. Image-level adaptation helps to reduce the shift by the global image difference such as image color and image style between the source and target domains. To eliminate the domain distribution mismatch, we employ a discriminator D_{img} to distinguish PPM features between source images and target images. At the same time, D_{img} also guides the training of segmentation network in an adversarial manner. In particular, we employ PatchGAN [4], a fully convolutional neural operating on image patches, from which we can get a two-dimensional feature map as the discriminator outputs. The loss for training D_{img} is formulated as follows:

$$\mathcal{L}_{img} = \mathbb{E}_{x_t \sim X_T}[logD_{img}(p_t)] + \mathbb{E}_{x_s \sim X_S}[log(1 - D_{img}(p_s))] \tag{2}$$

where p_s and p_t denote the PPM outputs of the segmentation network G for source domain and target domain.

Feature-Level Adaptation. The feature-level representation refers to the fused feature maps before feeding into the final segmentation classifier. Aligning the feature-level representations helps to reduce the segmentation differences in both global layout and local context. Similar to image-level adaptation, we also train a domain classifier D_{feat} formulated as a PatchGAN to align the feature-level distribution. Let us denote the final fused feature representation as f_s and

f_t for source domain and target domain respectively. The loss for D_{feat} is written as follows:

$$\mathcal{L}_{feat} = \mathbb{E}_{x_t \sim X_T}[logD_{feat}(f_t)] + \mathbb{E}_{x_s \sim X_S}[log(1 - D_{feat}(f_s))] \tag{3}$$

2.4 Overall Training Objective

We integrate the segmentation module for source images and the two domain adaptation modules to train all the networks G, D_{img} and D_{feat} jointly. The overall objective function can be formulated as follows:

$$\min_{G} \max_{D_{img}, D_{feat}} \mathcal{L}_{seg}(x_s, y_s) + \lambda_1 \mathcal{L}_{img}(x_s, x_t) + \lambda_2 \mathcal{L}_{feat}(x_s, x_t) \tag{4}$$

where λ_1 and λ_2 are two trade-off parameters. The min-max game is optimized by adversarial training and G is used to achieve segmentation for images in target domain during test.

3 Experiments and Results

3.1 Datasets

Two colorectal cancer gland segmentation datasets with different stains are used to evaluate our model. **Warwick-QU** dataset [8], introduced in gland segmentation challenge in MICCAI 2015, consists of 165 H&E stained images cropped from whole slide images (WSIs). The WSIs are acquired in 20× optical magnification. In our experiments, the dataset is separated into training and test sets with 85 and 80 images respectively. **GlandVision** dataset [1] contains 20 DAB-H stained colon images with size of 1280 × 1024, which were captured with 10× optical magnification. We randomly select 14 images for training and the rest for test. It is noted that those two datasets are labelled with different strategies. The masks in Warwick-QU cover the whole glandular structures, while GlandVision only considers the lumen regions.

3.2 Implementation Details

Our DAPNet employs 3 × 3 kernel for convolutional operations followed by a batch normalization layer. We train all the models using Adam optimization with a batch size of 4 for 300 epochs. We randomly crop image patches of size 256 × 256 for training. The initial learning rate is 10^{-3}, which is kept the same for the first 150 epochs and linearly decayed to zero over the next 150 epochs. The hyper-parameters α, λ_1 and λ_2 are set to 1, 0.002 and 0.005 respectively. Our method is based on LSGAN [6], which replaces the negative log likelihood objective by a least square loss. This loss achieves a more stable model training and generates higher quality results.

3.3   Results

We evaluate the performance of our DAPNet for gland segmentation in both adaptive directions. In particular, we denote Warwick-QU (source) to GlandVision (target) as Warwick-QU → GlandVision and vice versa, and the test images in the target domain are used for evaluation. Extensive experiments including comparisons to the state-of-the-art methods and ablation study are provided.

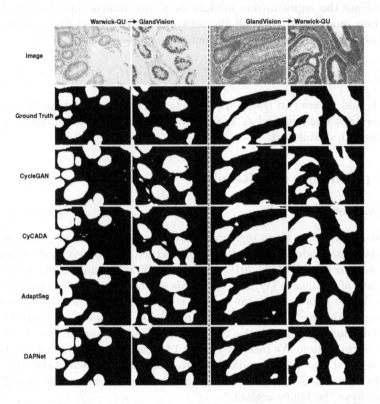

Fig. 3. Qualitative results of gland segmentation adapting from Warwick-QU to Gland-Vision dataset (left two columns) and vice versa (right two columns).

We compare our DAPNet with three state-of-the-art unsupervised domain adaptation methods: CycleGAN [13], CyCADA [3] and AdaptSeg [9]. The comparison with CycleGAN is achieved by two stages. We first use CycleGAN transforms the source domain images to target domain, and then use the transformed images along with the corresponding label in the source domain to train the segmentation network G. We report the segmentation results using Pixel Accuracy (Acc.) and the Intersection over Union (IoU) in Table 1. We can observe that our model DAPNet outperforms all the other methods for domain adaptation between WarwickQU and GlandVision in both directions. We have repeated the model training and testing for 3 times with random parameter initializations

Table 1. Comparison with state-of-the-art methods for semantic segmentation on GlandVision adapting from Warwick-QU and vice versa.

Method	Warwick-QU → GlandVision		Warwick-QU → GlandVision	
	Acc	IoU	Acc	IoU
CycleGAN [13]	0.84	0.60	0.74	0.54
CyCADA [3]	0.84	0.62	0.73	0.54
AdapSeg [9]	0.81	0.67	0.72	0.52
DAPNet-NA	0.80	0.58	0.73	0.50
DAPNet-IA	0.85	0.60	0.75	0.55
DAPNet-FA	0.83	0.63	0.74	0.53
DAPNet	**0.88**	**0.68**	**0.76**	**0.57**

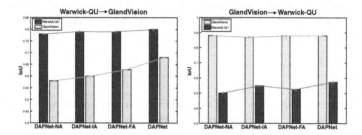

Fig. 4. Performance comparison of different variants of our proposed model in terms of IoU measurements. The trained models are applied to both the source and target domain images for test. The segmentation performance for the source domain maintains at a high level while the performance of the target domain is boosted.

and the same hyper-parameters. All tests have shown that our proposed method consistently outperforms other methods with statistical significance (paired t-test with p < 0.01). Specifically, when adapting from Warwick-QU to Gland-Vision, the averaged accuracy and IoU are 0.88 ± 0.0083 (Mean ± SD) and 0.68 ± 0.0021 respectively. On the other hand, the averaged accuracy and IoU are 0.76 ± 0.0105 and 0.57 ± 0.0108 respectively adapting from GlandVision to Warwick-QU. Moreover, Fig. 3 presents qualitative results of two example images for each of the domain adaptation case. Both CycleGAN and CyCADA can successfully detect the gland structures, but the predicted masks contain irregular spot noise. AdaptSeg with only image-level adaptation can hardly segment the gland boundaries clearly. Our proposed DAPNet produces significantly better predictions with accurate layout.

We further conduct ablation study to demonstrate the necessity of the two domain adaptation components of our model. In particular, we compare DAP-Net with its three variants, the model trained without domain adaptation modules (DAPNet-NA), only image-level adaptation module (DAPNet-IA) and only feature-level adaptation module (DAPNet-FA). As shown in Table 1, we observe that the performance of the DAPNet-NA drops significantly due to the domain shift and the best results are achieved with DAPNet. It is clear that the two adaptation components can effectively alleviate the discrepancy between two domains. We also show that domain adaptation modules can boosts the segmentation performance on target domain without affecting the results on source domain (see Fig. 4).

4   Conclusions

In this paper, we study the unsupervised domain adaptive segmentation task for histopathology images. We have proposed a dual adaptive pyramid network with two domain adaptation components by adversarial training on both image and feature levels. The model is trained without target domain labels and the test procedure works as normal segmentation networks. Experimental results show that the proposed DAPNet can effectively boost the performance on unlabelled target datasets, and outperform other state-of-the-art approaches.

References

1. Fu, H., Qiu, G., Ilyas, M., Shu, J.: GlandVision: a novel polar space random field model for glandular biological structure detection. In: Proceedings of the British Machine Vision Conference, pp. 42.1–42.12. BMVA Press (2012)
2. He, K., Zhang, X., Ren, S., Sun, J.: Deep residual learning for image recognition. In: Proceedings of the IEEE Conference on Computer Vision and Pattern Recognition, pp. 770–778 (2016)
3. Hoffman, J., et al.: CyCADA: cycle-consistent adversarial domain adaptation. In: International Conference on Machine Learning, pp. 1994–2003 (2018)
4. Isola, P., Zhu, J.Y., Zhou, T., Efros, A.A.: Image-to-image translation with conditional adversarial networks. In: Proceedings of the IEEE Conference on Computer Vision and Pattern Recognition, pp. 1125–1134 (2017)
5. Litjens, G., et al.: A survey on deep learning in medical image analysis. Med. Image Anal. **42**, 60–88 (2017)
6. Mao, X., Li, Q., Xie, H., Lau, R.Y., Wang, Z., Paul Smolley, S.: Least squares generative adversarial networks. In: Proceedings of the IEEE International Conference on Computer Vision, pp. 2794–2802 (2017)
7. Ronneberger, O., Fischer, P., Brox, T.: U-Net: convolutional networks for biomedical image segmentation. In: Navab, N., Hornegger, J., Wells, W.M., Frangi, A.F. (eds.) MICCAI 2015. LNCS, vol. 9351, pp. 234–241. Springer, Cham (2015). https://doi.org/10.1007/978-3-319-24574-4_28
8. Sirinukunwattana, K., et al.: Gland segmentation in colon histology images: the GlaS challenge contest. Med. Image Anal. **35**, 489–502 (2017)
9. Tsai, Y.H., Hung, W.C., Schulter, S., Sohn, K., Yang, M.H., Chandraker, M.: Learning to adapt structured output space for semantic segmentation. In: Proceedings of the IEEE Conference on Computer Vision and Pattern Recognition, pp. 7472–7481 (2018)
10. Tzeng, E., Hoffman, J., Saenko, K., Darrell, T.: Adversarial discriminative domain adaptation. In: Proceedings of the IEEE Conference on Computer Vision and Pattern Recognition, pp. 7167–7176 (2017)

11. Zhang, Y., Qiu, Z., Yao, T., Liu, D., Mei, T.: Fully convolutional adaptation networks for semantic segmentation. In: Proceedings of the IEEE Conference on Computer Vision and Pattern Recognition, pp. 6810–6818 (2018)
12. Zhao, H., Shi, J., Qi, X., Wang, X., Jia, J.: Pyramid scene parsing network. In: Proceedings of the IEEE Conference on Computer Vision and Pattern Recognition, pp. 2881–2890 (2017)
13. Zhu, J.Y., Park, T., Isola, P., Efros, A.A.: Unpaired image-to-image translation using cycle-consistent adversarial networks. In: Proceedings of the IEEE International Conference on Computer Vision, pp. 2223–2232 (2017)

HD-Net: Hybrid Discriminative Network for Prostate Segmentation in MR Images

Haozhe Jia[1], Yang Song[2], Heng Huang[3], Weidong Cai[4], and Yong Xia[1,5(✉)]

[1] National Engineering Laboratory for Integrated Aero-Space-Ground-Ocean Big Data Application Technology, School of Computer Science and Engineering, Northwestern Polytechnical University, Xi'an 710072, China
yxia@nwpu.edu.cn
[2] School of Computer Science and Engineering, University of New South Wales, Sydney, NSW 2052, Australia
[3] Department of Electrical and Computer Engineering, University of Pittsburgh, Pittsburgh, PA 15261, USA
[4] School of Computer Science, University of Sydney, Sydney, NSW 2006, Australia
[5] Research & Development Institute of Northwestern Polytechnical University in Shenzhen, Shenzhen 518057, China

Abstract. Efficient and accurate segmentation of prostate gland facilitates the prediction of the pathologic stage and treatment response. Recently, deep learning methods have been proposed to tackle this issue. However, the effectiveness of these methods is often limited by inadequate semantic discrimination and spatial context modeling. To address these issues, we propose the Hybrid Discriminative Network (HD-Net), which consists of a 3D segmentation decoder using channel attention block to generate semantically consistent volumetric features and an auxiliary 2D boundary decoder guiding the segmentation network to focus on the semantically discriminative intra-slice features. Meanwhile, we further design the pyramid convolution block and residual refinement block for HD-Net to fully exploit multi-scale spatial contextual information of the prostate gland. In addition, to reduce the information loss in propagation and fully fuse the multi-scale feature maps, we introduce inter-scale dense shortcuts for both decoders. We evaluated our model on the Prostate MR Image Segmentation 2012 (PROMISE12) challenge dataset and achieved a synthetic score of 90.34, setting a new state of the art.

1 Introduction

Accurate segmentation of the prostate gland using magnetic resonance (MR) imaging is critical to the diagnosis and treatment of prostate diseases. Due to the anatomical variation across subjects and the interference of adjacent structures with similar appearances, approaches based on the traditional machine learning algorithms [3,9] still suffer from low accuracy and poor generalization.

Recent works based on the 3D fully convolutional encoder-decoder [5] have shown convincing performance on this task. The design focus has been on effective ways of exploiting spatial context, which is an important cue for prostate

© Springer Nature Switzerland AG 2019
D. Shen et al. (Eds.): MICCAI 2019, LNCS 11765, pp. 110–118, 2019.
https://doi.org/10.1007/978-3-030-32245-8_13

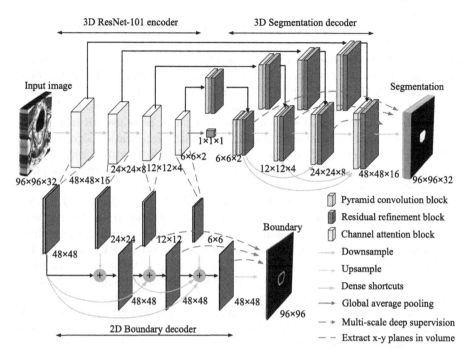

Fig. 1. An overview of the HD-Net, including: 3D ResNet-101 encoder, 3D up-bottom segmentation decoder, and 2D bottom-up boundary decoder.

segmentation. Milletari et al. [6] incorporated the Dice loss and unique data augmentation into a volumetric and fully convolutional network called V-Net to improve the segmentation result. Yu et al. [11] introduced both long and short residual connections to a 3D fully convolutional encoder-decoder to exploit the spatial contextual information, and achieved the top performance in the PROMISE 12 challenge [1] at that time. Zhu et al. [13] adopted dense connections and long connections to alleviate the vanishing gradient and overfitting issues encountered in the training process. Nie et al. [7] proposed an adversarial model ASDNet, which adopted region-attention based semi-supervised loss to address the insufficient data problem for training the complex networks. However, due to the large variability in the appearance of the gland capsule and its low contrast and high similarity to adjacent structures, these methods still reveal inadequate intra-class consistency and inter-class discrimination, which typically reflects in poor segmentation performance on the regions with the same semantic label but different appearances (usually inside the prostate gland) or the regions with similar appearances but different semantic labels (usually on the boundary of the prostate gland). Furthermore, prostate MR images normally have complex spatial contextual information due to the widely existed anisotropic voxel resolution. 3D isotropic convolutions [5,6] tend to be less-capable of segmenting the volumetric prostate gland accurately.

In this paper, we propose a Hybrid Discriminative Network (HD-Net) for automated prostate gland segmentation in MR images, as illustrated in Fig. 1. This HD-Net model has a 2D + 3D encoder-decoder structure, including a ResNet-101-based 3D encoder, a 3D segmentation decoder, and a 2D boundary decoder. In the training phase, the encoder and two decoders are trained in an end-to-end manner; whereas in the inference phase, the trained HD-Net without the boundary decoder is employed to segment prostate MR images. We evaluated our model against several state-of-the-art segmentation algorithms on the PROMISE 12 challenge dataset [1], and our HD-Net outperformed all the other methods. The further ablation experiment results demonstrate the effectiveness of each component of HD-Net.

The contributions of this work are three-fold: (1) we design a 3D ResNet encoder to characterize prostate MR images, a 3D segmentation decoder with channel attention to extract semantically consistent features, and an auxiliary 2D boundary decoder to guide the segmentation decoder with the intra-slice discriminative features on both sides of the prostate boundary; (2) we use a modified design of the pyramid convolution block and residual refinement block, and incorporate them into both decoders to fully exploit the multi-scale spatial contextual information of the prostate gland; and (3) we introduce inter-scale dense shortcuts to both decoders, aiming to reduce the information loss and to fuse multi-scale feature maps effectively.

2   Method

2.1   3D ResNet Encoder

In the proposed HD-Net, we use the ImageNet pre-trained ResNet-101 [4] as the backbone encoder model (Fig. 1). Here, considering the limited image size and uncontrollable computing complexity, we only utilize the first three res-blocks of ResNet-101, which means our encoder has four stages of feature map scale. Since the original ResNet-101 was constructed for 2D natural images, we need to extend it to 3D medical image segmentation. Specifically, we use $7 \times 7 \times 3$ 3D convolution to replace 7×7 2D convolution in the first convolutional layer of ResNet-101. For the other convolutional layers, we directly transform $x \times x$ 2D convolutions to $x \times x \times 1$ 3D convolutions. Such extension makes it feasible to use the pre-trained ResNet-101 to initialize our encoder to transfer the knowledge learned on the large-scale ImageNet images to characterize prostate MR images. In addition, similar to [10], we also add a global average pooling layer [12] on top of the segmentation network to get the strongest semantic consistency.

2.2   3D Segmentation Decoder

Channel Attention Block. For segmentation architecture with encoder-decoder style, it was observed that the features produced at the early stages of the network reveal fine spatial information but have weak semantic guidance,

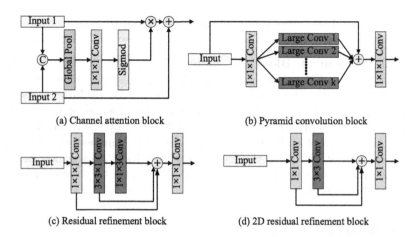

Fig. 2. Detailed structures of the channel attention block, pyramid convolution block, residual refinement block and 2D residual refinement block of boundary network. C, × and + represent concatenation, matrix multiplication and matrix summation, respectively. At each scale stage, the number of large convolutions and the corresponding kernel size are $(31 \times 31 \times 11, 23 \times 23 \times 9, 19 \times 19 \times 7, 15 \times 15 \times 5)$, $(19 \times 19 \times 7, 15 \times 15 \times 5, 9 \times 9 \times 3)$, $(9 \times 9 \times 3, 7 \times 7 \times 3)$ and $3 \times 3 \times 1$, respectively.

whereas the later-stage features have strong semantic consistency and discrimination but give coarse spatial prediction. Some studies [2,10] introduced channel-wise semantic attention to generate features with more discriminative capability. Based on these considerations, in the decoder of the segmentation network, we propose a channel attention block to provide up-bottom semantic discriminative guidance. As illustrated in Fig. 2(a), the channel attention block has two input feature maps from two adjacent stages. We first concatenate these two feature maps together and use global average pooling to generate the channel-wise attention. Then we multiply the obtained channel-wise attention vector with the early-stage feature map to enhance its semantic discrimination. Last, we combine the enhanced feature map with the later-stage feature map as the output feature map. With this design, the segmentation network not only integrate multi-scale context information, but also can pay more attention to the feature maps that are associated with more semantic information.

Pyramid Convolution Block. According to [8], in semantic segmentation task, large kernel convolution can promote voxel classification ability of deep network besides its inherent spatial localization capability. However, considering the variability in size and shape of the gland capsule, here we design the pyramid convolutional block to generate more discriminative features. Specifically, inside the pyramid convolution block, several 3D convolutions with different kernel sizes are constructed in parallel and the numbers of 3D convolutions are adaptive to the scale of feature map, as illustrated in Fig. 2(b). Pyramid kernels can fuse local and global image contents at multiple scales and reduce information loss.

In addition, to reduce computational complexity, we further apply convolution decomposition to reduce the parameters of the large kernel 3D convolution.

Residual Refinement Block. To address the anisotropic spatial context, within each stage of the decoder, we introduce the residual refinement block instead of the traditional isotropic block with $3 \times 3 \times 3$ convolutions. As illustrated in Fig. 2(c), the input to residual refinement block is passed to a $3 \times 3 \times 1$ and then a $1 \times 1 \times 3$ 3D convolutions in turn. Inspired by the residual connection [4], the outputs of both 3D convolutions are then summed with the input together as the output. With this design, the $3 \times 3 \times 1$ convolution helps to capture the 2D features inside the x-y planes, and the $1 \times 1 \times 3$ convolution can focus on between-slices features.

2.3   2D Boundary Decoder

Besides the intra-class consistency, the inter-class discrimination of adjacent region is also crucial for accurate semantic segmentation of the prostate. We suggest that a feasible solution to address this issue is to add the guidance of semantic boundary. To do this, we construct an auxiliary boundary network in a bottom-up fashion, so that the boundary network can use early-stage features to extract accurate prostate boundary and subsequently represent the extracted boundary with later-stage semantic information, as shown in Fig. 1. In addition, due to anisotropic spatial voxel resolution of prostate MR images, in each stage, we use 2D pyramid convolution blocks (of the same architecture as the 3D one but without the convolution kernel in z dimension) and 2D residual refinement block (shown in Fig. 2(d)) rather than 3D ones to obtain the prostate boundary on each x-y plane of the 3D feature maps. Since both decoders share one 3D encoder, the boundary decoder can guide the segmentation decoder to generate features on both sides of the prostate boundary with more semantic discrimination.

Note that we choose to model the 2D boundary information instead of 3D because compared to the whole image volume, the proportion of the boundary is low and the boundary of adjacent slices may have large variety in both shape and location, which all make it hard to model the 3D boundary information with deep network.

2.4   Further Refinements

To further reduce the potential information loss in the propagation and make full use of the inter-scale features, we introduce the inter-scale dense shortcuts in both decoders (Fig. 1). Since we construct segmentation decoder and boundary decoder in a up-bottom and bottom-up fashion, respectively. We apply different dense shortcuts strategies. Specifically, for segmentation network, the high stage input of the channel attention block is a combination of upsampled feature maps from all higher stages. In each stage of the boundary network, the input of the second refinement block further is the summation of the upsampled feature maps from all lower stages. With these specific inter-scale dense shortcuts, the HD-Net can fully fuse the features from different scales and directly propagates the forward and backward information from one scale stage to anther scale stage.

Throughout the whole HD-Net, we apply $1 \times 1 \times 1$ convolutions to adjust the channel number of feature maps. In addition, for explicit refinement and effective model optimization, instead of only using a final prediction supervision, we further add multi-scale side output supervisions to the segmentation decoder, which is accomplished by upsampling the multi-scale output feature maps of the residual refinement blocks of both decoders to the size of ground truths as segmentation results (Fig. 1). To reduce the influence of class imbalance in a dynamic way, we use mini-batch class weighted cross entropy loss for both sub-models:

$$L_{ce}(x, class) = \sum_{b=1}^{N} (r_b(-x[class] + \log(\sum_j \exp(x[j])))) \tag{1}$$

where x is the network prediction and the class weight r_b is the ratio of the numbers of voxels in the prostate and non-prostate regions in mini-batch b. The final loss of the HD-Net is $L = L_s + \lambda L_b$, a combination of the segmentation network loss L_s and boundary network loss L_b with the balance parameter λ.

3 Experiments and Results

Datasets: We used the PROMISE12 challenge database [1] to evaluate the proposed HD-Net. The dataset contains 50 training and 30 test T2-weighted MR images. The corresponding ground truths of the whole prostate annotated by the experts are available in the training set and that of the test set is withheld for online independent evaluation. We trained the proposed method on the training set and submitted the segmentation of the test set to the ongoing challenge for an evaluation score.

Implementation Details: We implemented the proposed method based on the Pytorch framework with two Nvidia Geforce GTX 1080Ti 11GB GPUs. We performed some simple image preprocessing, including bias field correction, voxel spacing unification to a fixed size of $0.625 \times 0.625 \times 1.5$ mm and intensity normalization into zero mean and unit variance. We employed several online data augmentations to reduce the potential overfitting caused by limited training images, including random flipping (up-down or left-right in x-y planes), random rotation (± 25, 90, 180, or 270° in x-y planes), random Gaussian noise addition (σ from 0.3 to 0.7) and random 3D scaling (± 0.2). We trained the network using the Adam optimizer with a batch size of 16 and betas of (0.9, 0.999). The initial learning rate was $1e^{-3}$ and decayed by multiplied with $(1 - \frac{iteration}{max_i teration})^{0.9}$. The loss combination weight λ was set to 0.5 after some comparisons. In the inference phase, for each MR image, we extracted the sub-volumes with a fixed stride of $24 \times 24 \times 8$ and averaged the predictions from the overlapping volumes to get the final segmentation.

Table 1. Quantitative results for segmentation obtained by the proposed HD-Net and top-ranking algorithms in the PROMISE 12 challenge leader board.

Method	DSC (%)	ABD (mm)	95HD (mm)	aRVD (%)	Score
HD-Net (ours)	91.35	1.36	**3.93**	5.10	**90.34**
whu_mlgroup	91.41	1.35	4.27	6.04	89.59
Revised_U-Net	91.30	1.31	3.97	**4.58**	89.56
kakatao	**91.76**	**1.29**	4.14	5.88	89.54
sakinis.tomas	91.33	1.34	4.15	6.03	89.44
pxl_cmg	91.23	1.40	4.28	5.67	89.39
Isensee (nnU-Net)	91.61	1.31	4.00	7.13	89.28
segsegseg	91.37	1.37	4.38	6.73	89.13
mls.dl.eecs	91.37	1.38	4.58	6.79	88.92
fly2019	90.12	1.62	5.09	6.98	88.73

Table 2. Quantitative results of the ablation experiments. RRB: residual refinement block, PB: pyramid convolution block, CAB: channel attention block, IDS: inter-scale dense shortcuts, DS: multi-scale deep supervision, BD: boundary decoder.

Method	Mean DSC (%)
ResNet-101+RRB	89.67
ResNet-101+RRB+PB	90.35
ResNet-101+RRB+PB+CAB	91.10
ResNet-101+RRB+PB+CAB+IDS	91.53
ResNet-101+RRB+PB+CAB+IDS+DS	91.66
ResNet-101+RRB+PB+CAB+IDS+DS+BD	91.81

Comparison with State-of-the-Art Methods: In Table 1, we compared our HD-Net with nine top-ranking methods listed on the PROMISE12 challenge leaderboard. Note that the dice similarity coefficient (DSC), average boundary distance (ABD), 95% Hausdorff distance (95HD) and absolute relative volume difference (aRVD) of the whole prostate gland, apex part (first 1/3 of the prostate volume), and base part (last 1/3 of the prostate volume) and a synthetic score were generated by the online validation system. At the writing of this paper, our proposed approach is ranked the first out of 291 entries. Due to the limitation of space, we can only list the results of all metrics on the whole prostate gland. From the results in Table 1, we can see that although some methods achieved better performance on a single metric, our HD-Net gained the overall best performance. Our HD-Net also has the best result on 95HD and second best result on aRVD, which indicates gland volumes segmented by our HD-Net have few outliers and globally match the ground truths, respectively.

Ablation Study: We also conducted an ablation study on the training set with a 5-fold cross validation to evaluate the contributions of the pyramid convolution block, channel attention block, inter-scale dense shortcuts, multi-scale deep supervision and boundary decoder to the overall performance of the proposed HD-Net. The results are given in Table 2. It shows that all components in the HD-Net are beneficial to the overall segmentation performance. In particular, it is clear to see that using pyramid convolution block and further incorporating channel attention block significantly increased DSC by 0.68% and 0.75%. Such results demonstrate that our HD-Net is highly effective in the fully exploitation of spatial image contextual information and of semantic discrimination between the prostate and surrounding tissues. Meanwhile, the results also show that adding inter-scale dense shortcuts can increase the DSC by more than 0.4%, which indicates its effectiveness in the reduction the information loss and the further fusion of the inter-scale features. In addition, we can observe the boundary decoder and multi-scale deep supervision can contribute to a further performance improvement by 0.15% and 0.13%, respectively.

4   Conclusions

In this paper, we propose the HD-Net, a novel fully convolutional encoder-decoder with a 3D segmentation decoder and an auxiliary 2D boundary decoder, for the segmentation of prostate gland in volumetric MR images. Specifically, we introduce the channel attention block to enhance semantic discrimination, use both pyramid convolution block and residual refinement block to fully exploit the spatial contextual information, and adopt the multi-scale deep supervision to further improve the performance. Moreover, we incorporate inter-scale dense shortcuts into both decoders to reduce the information loss and fuse the multi-scale features. Our experimental results suggest that the proposed HD-Net outperforms nine recent methods and sets the new state of the art on the PROMISE12 challenge dataset.

Acknowledgement. This work was supported in part by the National Natural Science Foundation of China under Grants 61771397, in part by the Science and Technology Innovation Committee of Shenzhen Municipality, China, under Grants JCYJ20180306171334997, in part by Synergy Innovation Foundation of the University and Enterprise for Graduate Students in Northwestern Polytechnical University under Grants XQ201911, in part by the Project for Graduate Innovation team of Northwestern Polytechnical University, and in part by the US NIH R01 AG049371 and the US NSF IIS 1836938, DBI 1836866, IIS 1845666, IIS 1852606, IIS 1838627, IIS 1837956.

References

1. MICCAI grand challenge: Prostate MR image segmentation 2012 (2012). https://promise12.grand-challenge.org/Home/
2. Chen, L., et al.: SCA-CNN: spatial and channel-wise attention in convolutional networks for image captioning. In: CVPR, pp. 5659–5667 (2017)

3. Guo, Y., Gao, Y., Shen, D.: Deformable MR prostate segmentation via deep feature learning and sparse patch matching. IEEE TMI **35**(4), 1077–1089 (2016)
4. He, K., Zhang, X., Ren, S., et al.: Deep residual learning for image recognition. In: CVPR, pp. 770–778 (2016)
5. Long, J., Shelhamer, E., Darrell, T.: Fully convolutional networks for semantic segmentation. In: CVPR, pp. 3431–3440 (2015)
6. Milletari, F., Navab, N., Ahmadi, S.A.: V-Net: fully convolutional neural networks for volumetric medical image segmentation. In: 3DV, pp. 565–571. IEEE (2016)
7. Nie, D., Gao, Y., Wang, L., Shen, D.: ASDNet: attention based semi-supervised deep networks for medical image segmentation. In: Frangi, A.F., Schnabel, J.A., Davatzikos, C., Alberola-López, C., Fichtinger, G. (eds.) MICCAI 2018. LNCS, vol. 11073, pp. 370–378. Springer, Cham (2018). https://doi.org/10.1007/978-3-030-00937-3_43
8. Peng, C., Zhang, X., Yu, G., Luo, G., Sun, J.: Large kernel matters-improve semantic segmentation by global convolutional network. In: CVPR, pp. 4353–4361 (2017)
9. Toth, R., Madabhushi, A.: Multifeature landmark-free active appearance models: application to prostate MRI segmentation. IEEE TMI **31**(8), 1638–1650 (2012)
10. Yu, C., Wang, J., Peng, C., Gao, C., Yu, G., Sang, N.: Learning a discriminative feature network for semantic segmentation. In: CVPR, pp. 1857–1866 (2018)
11. Yu, L., Yang, X., Chen, H., Qin, J., Heng, P.A.: Volumetric ConvNets with mixed residual connections for automated prostate segmentation from 3D MR images. In: AAAI, pp. 66–72 (2017)
12. Zhao, H., Shi, J., Qi, X., Wang, X., Jia, J.: Pyramid scene parsing network. In: CVPR, pp. 2881–2890 (2017)
13. Zhu, Q., Du, B., Wu, J., Yan, P.: A deep learning health data analysis approach: automatic 3D prostate MR segmentation with densely-connected volumetric ConvNets. In: IJCNN, pp. 1–6. IEEE (2018)

PHiSeg: Capturing Uncertainty
in Medical Image Segmentation

Christian F. Baumgartner[1]([✉]), Kerem C. Tezcan[1], Krishna Chaitanya[1],
Andreas M. Hötker[2], Urs J. Muehlematter[2], Khoschy Schawkat[2,4],
Anton S. Becker[2,3], Olivio Donati[2], and Ender Konukoglu[1]

[1] Computer Vision Lab, ETH Zürich, Zürich, Switzerland
baumgartner@vision.ee.ethz.ch
[2] University Hospital Zürich, Zürich, Switzerland
[3] Memorial Sloan Kettering Cancer Center, New York, USA
[4] Beth Israel Deaconess Medical Center, Harvard Medical School, Boston, USA

Abstract. Segmentation of anatomical structures and pathologies is
inherently ambiguous. For instance, structure borders may not be clearly
visible or different experts may have different styles of annotating. The
majority of current state-of-the-art methods do not account for such
ambiguities but rather learn a single mapping from image to segmentation. In this work, we propose a novel method to model the conditional
probability distribution of the segmentations given an input image. We
derive a hierarchical probabilistic model, in which separate latent variables are responsible for modelling the segmentation at different resolutions. Inference in this model can be efficiently performed using the
variational autoencoder framework. We show that our proposed method
can be used to generate significantly more realistic and diverse segmentation samples compared to recent related work, both, when trained with
annotations from a single or multiple annotators. The code for this paper
is freely available at https://github.com/baumgach/PHiSeg-code.

1   Introduction

Semantic segmentation of anatomical structures and pathologies is a crucial step
in clinical diagnosis and many downstream tasks. The majority of recent automated segmentation methods treat the problem as a one-to-one mapping from
image to output mask (e.g. [6]). However, medical segmentation problems are
often characterised by ambiguities and multiple hypotheses may be plausible [10].
This is in part due to inherent uncertainties such as poor contrast or other restrictions imposed by the image acquisition, but also due to variations in annotation
"styles" between different experts. To account for such ambiguities it is crucial

Electronic supplementary material The online version of this chapter (https://
doi.org/10.1007/978-3-030-32245-8_14) contains supplementary material, which is
available to authorized users.

© Springer Nature Switzerland AG 2019
D. Shen et al. (Eds.): MICCAI 2019, LNCS 11765, pp. 119–127, 2019.
https://doi.org/10.1007/978-3-030-32245-8_14

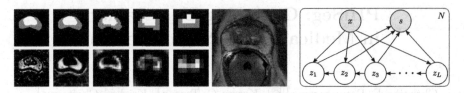

Fig. 1. (Left) Example of hierarchical segmentation generation with segmentation output at each level ($\hat{s}_\ell$) in the top row, right to left, and corresponding residual refinements to the prostate peripheral zone class in the bottom row. (Right) Corresponding graphical model (for N independent samples).

that prediction systems provide access to the full distribution of plausible outcomes without sacrificing accuracy. Predicting only the most likely hypothesis may lead to misdiagnosis and may negatively affect downstream tasks.

Recent work proposed to account for the uncertainty in the learned model parameters using an approximate Bayesian inference over the network weights [2]. However, it was shown that this method may produce samples that vary pixel by pixel and thus may not capture complex correlation structures in the distribution of segmentations [4]. A different line of work accounts for the possibility of different outcomes by training an ensemble of M networks [5] or by training a single network with M heads [7]. Both approaches, however, can only produce a fixed number of hypotheses. This problem is overcome by the conditional variational autoencoder (cVAE), an extension of [3] for modelling conditional segmentation masks given an input image [8]. Finally, the recently proposed probabilistic U-NET combines the cVAE framework with a U-NET architecture [4]. The authors showed that, given ground-truth annotations from multiple experts, the method can produce an unlimited number of realistic segmentation samples. Moreover, the method was shown to outperform various related methods including network ensembles, M-heads [7] and the Bayesian SegNet [2].

However, as we will show, the probabilistic U-NET produces samples with limited diversity. We believe this may be due to the fact that stochasticity is only introduced in the highest resolution level of the U-NET, and because the network can choose to ignore the random draws from the latent space since it is only concatenated to the channels. In this work, we propose a novel hierarchical probabilistic model which can produce segmentation samples closely matching the ground-truth distribution of a number of annotators. Inspired by Laplacian Pyramids, the model generates image-conditional segmentation samples by generating the output at a low resolution and then continuously refining the distribution of segmentations at increasingly higher resolutions. In contrast to prior work, the variations on *each resolution level* are governed by a separate latent variable, thereby avoiding the problems mentioned above. This process is illustrated in Fig. 1. We show that compared to recent work, our proposed Probabilistic Hierarchical Segmentation (PHiSeg) produces samples of significantly better quality for two challenging segmentation tasks, both, when trained with multiple annotations, and a single annotation per image. Furthermore, the mean prediction of our model performs on par with the standard U-NET in terms of segmentation accuracy.

2 Methods

We start by assuming that the segmentations s given an input image x are generated from L levels of latent variables z_ℓ according to the graphical model shown in Fig. 1. Thus, the conditional distribution $p(s|x)$ is given by the following expression for the general case of L latent levels:

$$p(\mathbf{s}|\mathbf{x}) = \int p(\mathbf{s}|\mathbf{z}_1, \ldots, \mathbf{z}_L) p(\mathbf{z}_1|\mathbf{z}_2, \mathbf{x}) \cdots p(\mathbf{z}_{L-1}|\mathbf{z}_L, \mathbf{x}) p(\mathbf{z}_L|\mathbf{x}) d\mathbf{z}_1 \cdots d\mathbf{z}_L. \quad (1)$$

We further assume that each latent variable z_ℓ is responsible for modelling the conditional target segmentations at $2^{-\ell+1}$ of the original image resolution (e.g. z_1 and z_3 model the segmentation at the original and at $1/4$ of the original resolution, respectively.). This does not result from the graphical model itself but is rather enforced by our implementation thereof as will become clear shortly.

We aim to approximate the posterior distribution of $p(\mathbf{z}|\mathbf{s}, \mathbf{x})$ using a variational approximation $q(\mathbf{z}|\mathbf{s}, \mathbf{x})$ where we used $\mathbf{z}$ to denote $\{\mathbf{z}_1, \ldots, \mathbf{z}_L\}$. It can be shown that $\log p(\mathbf{s}|\mathbf{x}) = \mathcal{L}(\mathbf{s}|\mathbf{x}) + \text{KL}(q(\mathbf{z}|\mathbf{s}, \mathbf{x})||p(\mathbf{z}|\mathbf{s}, \mathbf{x}))$, where $\mathcal{L}$ denotes the *evidence lower bound*, and $\text{KL}(\cdot, \cdot)$ the Kullback-Leibler divergence [3,4,8]. Since $\text{KL}(\cdot, \cdot) \geq 0$, $\mathcal{L}$ is a lower bound on the conditional log probability with equality when the approximation q matches the posterior exactly. Using the decomposition in Eq. 1 we find that for our model

$$\mathcal{L} = \mathbb{E}_{q(\mathbf{z}_1, \ldots, \mathbf{z}_L|\mathbf{x}, \mathbf{s})} \left[\log p(\mathbf{s}|\mathbf{z}_1, \ldots, \mathbf{z}_L) \right] - \alpha_L \, \text{KL} \left[q(\mathbf{z}_L|\mathbf{s}, \mathbf{x})||p(\mathbf{z}_L|\mathbf{x}) \right]$$
$$- \sum_{\ell=1}^{L-1} \alpha_\ell \, \mathbb{E}_{q(\mathbf{z}_{\ell+1}|\mathbf{s}, \mathbf{x})} \left[\text{KL} \left[q(\mathbf{z}_\ell|\mathbf{z}_{\ell+1}, \mathbf{s}, \mathbf{x})||p(\mathbf{z}_\ell|\mathbf{z}_{\ell+1}, \mathbf{x}) \right] \right], \quad (2)$$

with $\alpha_\ell = 1$. A complete derivation can be found in Appendix A. The α_ℓ are additional heuristic variables which we introduced to help account for dimensionality differences between the $\mathbf{z}_\ell$ (explained below). Following standard practice we parametrise the prior and posterior distributions as axis aligned normal distributions $\mathcal{N}(\mathbf{z}|\mu, \sigma)$. Specifically, we define

$$p(\mathbf{z}_\ell|\mathbf{z}_{\ell+1}, \mathbf{x}) = \mathcal{N} \left(\mathbf{z}|\phi_\ell^{(\mu)}(\mathbf{z}_{\ell+1}, \mathbf{x}), \phi_\ell^{(\sigma)}(\mathbf{z}_{\ell+1}, \mathbf{x}) \right) \quad (3)$$

$$q(\mathbf{z}_\ell|\mathbf{z}_{\ell+1}, \mathbf{x}, \mathbf{s}) = \mathcal{N} \left(\mathbf{z}|\theta_\ell^{(\mu)}(\mathbf{z}_{\ell+1}, \mathbf{s}, \mathbf{x}), \theta_\ell^{(\sigma)}(\mathbf{z}_{\ell+1}, \mathbf{s}, \mathbf{x}) \right), \quad (4)$$

where the ϕ, θ are functions parametrised by neural networks. Note that in contrast to the variational autoencoder [3], the $p(\mathbf{z}_\ell|\cdot, \mathbf{x})$ are also parametrised by neural networks similar to [4,8]. Lastly, we model $p(\mathbf{s}|\mathbf{z})$ as the usual categorical distribution with parameters (i.e. softmax probabilities) predicted by another neural network. By parametrising all distributions using neural networks, this can be seen as a hierarchical conditional variational autoencoder with the posteriors $q(\mathbf{z}_\ell | \cdot, \mathbf{s}, \mathbf{x})$ and priors $p(\mathbf{z}_\ell | \cdot, \mathbf{s})$ encoding $\mathbf{x}$ and $\mathbf{s}$ into latent representations $\mathbf{z}_\ell$, and the likelihood $p(\mathbf{s} | \mathbf{z})$ acting as the decoder. Our implementation of this model using a neural network for $L = 3$ is shown in Fig. 2. In that figure it can be seen that the total number of resolution levels of the network (i.e. number of downsampling steps plus one) can be larger than the number of latent levels. The example in Fig. 2 has a total of 4 resolution levels, of which only $L = 3$ are latent levels. We obtained the best results with 7 total resolution levels of which $L = 5$ are latent levels. The prior and posterior nets have identical structure but do not share any weights. Similar to previous work, all three subnetworks are used for training but testing is performed by using only the prior and the likelihood networks [3,4,8].

From Fig. 2 it can be seen that latent variables $\mathbf{z}_\ell$ will form the skip connections in a U-NET-like architecture. However, unlike [6] and [4], each skip connection corresponds to a latent variable $\mathbf{z}_\ell$ such that no information can flow from the image to the segmentation output without passing a sampling step. We do not map the latent variables to a 1-D vector but rather choose to keep the structured relationship between the variables. We found that this substantially improves segmentation accuracy. As a result, latent variable $\mathbf{z}_\ell$ has a dimensionality of $r_x 2^{-\ell+1} \times r_y 2^{-\ell+1} \times D$, where D is a hyper-parameter and $D = 2$ for all experiments, and r_x, r_y are the dimensions of the input images. The latent variable $\mathbf{z}_\ell$ is limited to modelling the data at $2^{-\ell+1}$ of the original resolution due to the downsampling operations before it. It then passes up the learned representation to the latent space embedding above ($\mathbf{z}_{\ell-1}$) to perform a refinement at double the resolution. This continues until the top level is reached. To further enforce this behaviour the likelihood network is designed to generate only *residual* changes of the segmentation masks for all $\mathbf{z}_\ell$ except the bottom one. This is achieved through the addition layers before the outputs (see Fig. 2). Our model bears some resemblance to the Ladder Network [9] which is also a hierarchical latent variable model where inference results in an autoencoder with skip connections. Our work differs substantially from that work in how inference is performed. Furthermore, to our knowledge, the Ladder Network was never applied to structured prediction problems.

Training and Predictions: We aim to find the neural network parameters which maximise the lower bound $\mathcal{L}$ in Eq. 2. The analytical form of the individual terms is prescribed by our model assumptions: since the posterior and prior both are modelled by normal distributions, the KL terms can be calculated analytically [3]. Our choice of likelihood results in a cross entropy term $\mathrm{CE}(\hat{\mathbf{s}}_1, \mathbf{s}_{gt})$, with $\hat{\mathbf{s}}_1$ the predicted segmentation and $\mathbf{s}_{gt}$ the corresponding ground-truth. Similar to previous work we found that it is sufficient to evaluate all of the expectations using a single sample [3]. Two deviations from the above theory were necessary for stable training. First, the magnitude of the KL terms depends on the dimensionality of $\mathbf{z}_\ell$. However, since the dimensionality of $\mathbf{z}_\ell$ in our model grows with $O(2^\ell)$, this led to optimisation problems. To counteract this, we heuristically set

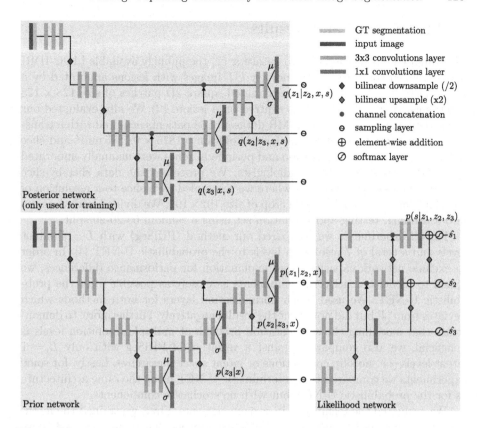

Fig. 2. Schematic network architecture of the proposed method for $L = 3$ latent levels and 4 resolution levels.

the weights $\alpha_\ell = 2^{\ell-1}$ in Eq. 2. Secondly, to enforce the desired behaviour that $\mathbf{z}_\ell$ should only model the data at its corresponding resolution, we added deep supervision to the output of each resolution level ($\hat{\mathbf{s}}_\ell$ in Fig. 2). The cost function used for this is again the cross entropy loss, $\mathrm{CE}(ups(\hat{\mathbf{s}}_\ell), \mathbf{s}_{gt})$ for $\ell > 1$, where $ups(\cdot)$ denotes a nearest neighbour upsampling to match the size of $\mathbf{s}_{gt}$. While $\mathbf{z}_\ell$ can only model the data at a certain resolution, it may ignore this responsibility and focus only on matching the prior and posterior. Deep supervision effectively prevents this behaviour.

We trained the model using the Adam optimiser with a learning rate of 10^{-3} and a batch-size of 12. We used batch-normalisation on all non-output layers. All models were trained for 48 h on a NVIDIA Titan Xp GPU and the model with the lowest total loss on a held-out validation set was selected.

After the model is trained, segmentation samples for an input image $\mathbf{x}$ can be generated by first obtaining samples $\mathbf{z}_\ell$ using the prior network and then decoding them using the likelihood network.

3   Experiments and Results

We evaluated our method on two datasets: (1) the publicly available LIDC-IDRI dataset which comprises 1018 thoracic CT images with lesions annotated by 4 radiologists [1]. Similar to [4] we extracted square 2D patches of size 128×128 pixels such that each patch was centred on a lesion. (2) We also evaluated our method on an in-house prostate MR dataset of 68 patients acquired with a transverse T2-weighted sequence (in-plane resolution $0.1875 \times 0.1875 \, \text{mm}^2$ and slice thickness $3.3 \, \text{mm}$). The transition and peripheral zones were manually annotated by 4 radiologists and 2 non-radiologists. We processed the data slice-by-slice (approx. 25 slices per volume), where we resampled each slice to a resolution of $0.6 \times 0.6 \, \text{mm}^2$ and took a central crop of size 192×192. We divided both datasets into a training, testing and validation set using a random 60-20-20 split.

For all experiments we compared our method (PHiSeg) with $L = 5$ latent levels and a total of 7 resolution levels to the probabilistic U-NET [4]. In order to exclude network capacity as an explanation for performance differences, we aimed to model our network components as closely as possible after the probabilistic U-NET. We used batch normalisation layers for both methods which deviates from [4] but did not affect the results negatively. Furthermore, to demonstrate that modelling the segmentation problem at multiple resolution levels is beneficial, we also compared against a variation of PHiSeg with only $L = 1$ latent levels (i.e. no skip connections or latent space hierarchy). Lastly, for some experiments we compared to a deterministic U-NET using the same architecture as for the probabilistic U-NET but with no stochastic components.

We evaluated the techniques in two experiments. First, we trained the methods using the masks from all available annotators, where in each batch we randomly sampled one annotation per image. We were interested in assessing how closely the distribution of generated samples matched the distribution of ground-truth annotations. To this end, we used the generalised energy distance $D^2_{\text{GED}}(p_{gt}, p_{\mathbf{s}}) = 2 \, \mathbb{E}[d(\mathbf{s}, \mathbf{y})] - \mathbb{E}[d(\mathbf{s}, \mathbf{s}')] - \mathbb{E}[d(\mathbf{y}, \mathbf{y}')]$, where d is 1 minus the intersection over union, i.e. $d(\cdot, \cdot) = 1 - \text{IoU}(\cdot, \cdot)$, and $\mathbf{s}, \mathbf{s}', \mathbf{y}, \mathbf{y}'$ are samples from the learned distribution $p_{\mathbf{s}}$, and ground-truth distribution p_{gt} [4]. The GED reduces the sample quality to a single, easy-to-understand number but, as a consequence, cannot be interpreted visually. Therefore, we additionally aimed to produce pixel-wise maps showing variability among the segmentation samples. We found the expected cross entropy between the mean segmentation mask and the samples to be a good measure, i.e. $\gamma(s_i) = \mathbb{E}[\text{CE}(\bar{s}_i, s_i)]$ with i the pixel position and $\bar{s}_i$ the mean prediction. γ is statistically similar to variance with the L2-distance replaced by CE. However, we believe it is more suitable for measuring segmentation variability. Examples of our γ-maps along with sample segmentations are shown in Fig. 3. We quantify how well the γ-maps for each method predict regions with large uncertainty using the average normalised cross correlation (NCC) between the γ-maps and the CE error maps obtained with respect to each annotator:

$$\mathcal{S}_{\text{NCC}}(p_{gt}, p_{\mathbf{s}}) = \mathbb{E}_{\mathbf{y} \sim p_{gt}} \left[\text{NCC}(\mathbb{E}_{\mathbf{s} \sim p_{\mathbf{s}}}[\text{CE}(\bar{\mathbf{s}}, \mathbf{s})], \mathbb{E}_{\mathbf{s} \sim p_{\mathbf{s}}}[\text{CE}(\mathbf{y}, \mathbf{s})]) \right]. \quad (5)$$

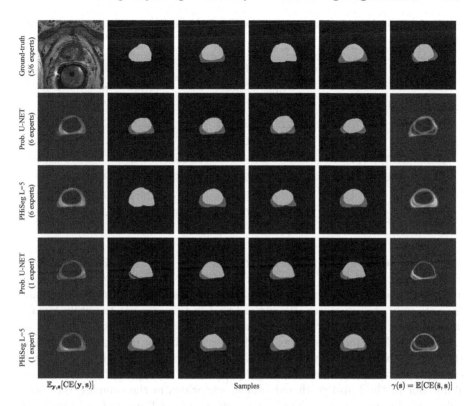

Fig. 3. Ground-truth annotations and samples for two of the evaluated methods trained with masks from 6 or 1 experts(s). Average error maps $\mathbb{E}_{\mathbf{y},\mathbf{s}}[\mathrm{CE}(\mathbf{y},\mathbf{s})]$ and γ-maps $(\mathbb{E}[\mathrm{CE}(\bar{\mathbf{s}},\mathbf{s})])$ for each model are shown in the left and right-most column, respectively.

Results for both D^2_{GED} and $\mathcal{S}_{\mathrm{NCC}}$ are shown in the top part of Table 1. All measures were evaluated with 100 samples drawn from the learned models.

Secondly, we set out to investigate the models' ability to infer the inherent uncertainties in the annotations from *just one* annotation per training image. To this end, we trained the above models by using only the annotations of a single expert. For the evaluation we then computed the D^2_{GED} and $\mathcal{S}_{\mathrm{NCC}}$ using all available annotators. Additionally, we evaluated the models in terms of conventional Dice score evaluated with masks from the single annotator as ground-truth. To get a single prediction from the probabilistic models we used $\bar{\mathbf{s}}$. This allowed us to obtain an indication of conventional segmentation accuracy. The results are shown in the bottom part of Table 1.

We observed that when using all annotators for training, PHiSeg ($L = 5$) produced significantly better D^2_{GED} and $\mathcal{S}_{\mathrm{NCC}}$ scores compared to all other methods. This can be observed qualitatively in Fig. 3 for a prostate slice with large inter-expert disagreements. Both, the prob. U-NET and PHiSeg ($L = 5$) produced realistic samples but PHiSeg ($L = 5$) was able to capture a wider vari-

Table 1. Quantitative results for all metric. Statistically significant improvements ($p < 0.01$ with paired student's t-test) over all other methods are indicated in bold.

	# experts	LIDC-IDRI			Prostate dataset		
		D^2_{GED}	$\mathcal{S}_{\mathrm{NCC}}$	Dice	D^2_{GED}	$\mathcal{S}_{\mathrm{NCC}}$	Dice
Prob. U-NET	All	0.2393	0.7749	–	0.1322	0.7763	–
PHiSeg ($L = 1$)	All	0.2934	0.7944	–	0.1608	0.7452	–
PHiSeg ($L = 5$)	All	**0.2248**	**0.8453**	–	**0.0864**	**0.8185**	–
Det. U-NET	1	–	–	0.5297	–	–	0.8364
Prob. U-NET	1	0.4452	0.5999	0.5238	0.2198	0.6022	0.8290
PHiSeg ($L = 1$)	1	0.4695	0.6013	0.5275	0.2462	0.6683	0.7942
PHiSeg ($L = 5$)	1	**0.3225**	**0.7337**	0.5408	0.2044	**0.6917**	0.8540

ability. Furthermore, as indicated by the high $\mathcal{S}_{\mathrm{NCC}}$ values, PHiSeg's ($L = 5$) γ-maps were found to be very predictive of where in the image the method's average prediction errors will occur. Similar results were obtained when training with only one annotator. We noticed that in this scenario the prob. U-NET may in some cases fail to learn variation in the data and revert back to an almost entirely deterministic behaviour (see fourth row in Fig. 3). We believe this can be explained by the prob. U-NET's architecture which, in contrast to our method, allows the encoder-decoder structure to bypass the stochasticity. While our method also predicted smaller variations in the samples, they were still markedly more diverse. The lower performance of PhiSeg ($L = 1$) indicates that using multiple resolution levels is crucial for our method. More samples for the prostate and LIDC-IDRI datasets can be found in Appendix B. From Table 1 it can be seen that no significant differences between the Dice scores were found for any of the methods (except PHiSeg's ($L = 1$)), including the det. U-NET. From this we conclude that neither PHiSeg ($L = 5$) nor the prob. U-NET suffer in segmentation performance due to their stochastic elements.

4   Discussion and Conclusion

We introduced a novel hierarchical probabilistic method for modelling the conditional distribution of segmentation masks given an input image. We have shown that our method substantially outperforms the state-of-the-art on a number of metrics. Furthermore, we demonstrated that PHiSeg was able to predict its own errors significantly better compared to previous work. We believe that proper modelling of uncertainty is indispensable for clinical acceptance of deep neural networks and that having access to the segmentation's probability distribution will have applications in numerous downstream tasks.

Acknowledgements. This work was partially supported by the Swiss Data Science Center. One of the Titan X Pascal used for this research was donated by the NVIDIA Corporation.

References

1. Armato, S.G., et al.: The lung image database consortium (LIDC) and image database resource initiative (IDRI): a completed reference database of lung nodules on CT scans. Med. Phys. **38**(2), 915–931 (2011)
2. Kendall, A., Badrinarayanan, V., Cipolla, R.: Bayesian SegNet: model uncertainty in deep convolutional encoder-decoder architectures for scene understanding. arXiv:1511.02680 (2015)
3. Kingma, D., Welling, M.: Auto-encoding variational bayes. arXiv:1312.6114 (2013)
4. Kohl, S., et al.: A probabilistic U-Net for segmentation of ambiguous images. In: Proceedings of NIPS, pp. 6965–6975 (2018)
5. Lakshminarayanan, B., Pritzel, A., Blundell, C.: Simple and scalable predictive uncertainty estimation using deep ensembles. In: Proceedings of NIPS, pp. 6402–6413 (2017)
6. Ronneberger, O., Fischer, P., Brox, T.: U-Net: convolutional networks for biomedical image segmentation. In: Navab, N., Hornegger, J., Wells, W.M., Frangi, A.F. (eds.) MICCAI 2015. LNCS, vol. 9351, pp. 234–241. Springer, Cham (2015). https://doi.org/10.1007/978-3-319-24574-4_28
7. Rupprecht, C., et al.: Learning in an uncertain world: Representing ambiguity through multiple hypotheses. In: Proceedings of CVPR, pp. 3591–3600 (2017)
8. Sohn, K., Lee, H., Yan, X.: Learning structured output representation using deep conditional generative models. In: Proceedings of NIPS, pp. 3483–3491 (2015)
9. Valpola, H.: From neural PCA to deep unsupervised learning. In: Perspectives of Neural Computing, pp. 143–171. Elsevier (2015)
10. Warfield, S.K., Zou, K.H., Wells, W.M.: Validation of image segmentation and expert quality with an expectation-maximization algorithm. In: Dohi, T., Kikinis, R. (eds.) MICCAI 2002. LNCS, vol. 2488, pp. 298–306. Springer, Heidelberg (2002). https://doi.org/10.1007/3-540-45786-0_37

Neural Style Transfer Improves 3D Cardiovascular MR Image Segmentation on Inconsistent Data

Chunwei Ma, Zhanghexuan Ji, and Mingchen Gao[(✉)]

Department of Computer Science and Engineering, University at Buffalo,
The State University of New York, Buffalo, USA
{chunweim,zhanghex,mgao8}@buffalo.edu

Abstract. Three-dimensional medical image segmentation is one of the most important problems in medical image analysis and plays a key role in downstream diagnosis and treatment. Recent years, deep neural networks have made groundbreaking success in medical image segmentation problem. However, due to the high variance in instrumental parameters, experimental protocols, and subject appearances, the generalization of deep learning models is often hindered by the inconsistency in medical images generated by different machines and hospitals. In this work, we present StyleSegor, an efficient and easy-to-use strategy to alleviate this inconsistency issue. Specifically, neural style transfer algorithm is applied to unlabeled data in order to minimize the differences in image properties including brightness, contrast, texture, etc. between the labeled and unlabeled data. We also apply probabilistic adjustment on the network output and integrate multiple predictions through ensemble learning. On a publicly available whole heart segmentation benchmarking dataset from MICCAI HVSMR 2016 challenge, we have demonstrated an elevated dice accuracy surpassing current state-of-the-art method and notably, an improvement of the total score by 29.91%. StyleSegor is thus corroborated to be an accurate tool for 3D whole heart segmentation especially on highly inconsistent data, and is available at https://github.com/horsepurve/StyleSegor.

Keywords: Whole heart segmentation · Atrous convolutional network · Neural style transfer

1 Introduction

The segmentation of 3D cardiac magnetic resonance (MR) images is the prerequisite for downstream diagnosis and treatment including heart disease identification and surgical planning. And there has been intensive research on the automatic algorithms for this segmentation problem, for purpose of alleviating the arduous manual labeling. Deep neural networks have made tremendous achievement on this task and many different architectures have been proposed,

© Springer Nature Switzerland AG 2019
D. Shen et al. (Eds.): MICCAI 2019, LNCS 11765, pp. 128–136, 2019.
https://doi.org/10.1007/978-3-030-32245-8_15

such as 3D U-Net [3], VoxResNet [1], 3D-DSN [5], DenseVosNet [11], VFN [10], and their ensemble meta-learner [13], which improved the segmentation performance to the dice score of myocardium at ~0.833 and that of blood pool at ~0.939.

However, the current accuracy of 3D cardiovascular MR image segmentation is still not well satisfactory for wider practice due to several issues. First, the morphological variation within the HVSMR data, originated from a variety of congenital heart defects, leads to difficulty in segmentation. Dong et al. [4] proposed an unsupervised domain adaptation network to enforce prediction masks to be similar across domains. However, the shapes of myocardium and blood pool are much more complex than lungs in 2D X-rays images. More important, we have observed non-negligible inter-subject variation within the training and testing images, including brightness, resolution, texture, and signal to noise ratio. In HVSMR data, the training samples are generally of high quality while the quality of the testing samples is relatively low. In a training image (Fig. 1A), the intensity distribution (gray line in Fig. 1D) exhibits three distinguishable peaks whereas the testing image (Fig. 1B and E) shows a substantial overlap of myocardium signal and background signal. This dataset shift phenomena [7] significantly hampered the generalization of deep neural network models. Zhao et al. [12] proposed using learned transforms to generate samples used in data augmentation aiming at one-shot segmentation. In our preliminary experiments, we found that augmenting the training set with images generated from the low-quality domain contributed little to the overall performance.

To address these challenges, we propose StyleSegor, a novel pipeline for 3D MR image segmentation of cardiac and vascular structures. StyleSegor has three main advantages. First, we adopted atrous convolution network with atrous spatial pyramid pooling module as an efficient way to retain as many details of feature maps as possible and achieve better segmentation on subtle structures. Second, we leverage neural style transfer to minimize the inter-subject variation. Every slice sample in the testing data is directly transferred to the same style of a target from the training set. Third, in order to fully utilize both the original and the transformed image data, an ensemble learning scheme is developed through voting of multiple predictions. On the HVSMR 2016 challenge dataset, StyleSegor has demonstrated superior performance compared with other methods, and notably, an improvement of the total score by 29.91%, showing the effectiveness of our strategy.

2   Methods

The complete pipeline of StyleSegor is shown in Fig. 2. The standard ResNet-101 and VGG-16 networks serve as the backbones for segmentation and style transfer, respectively. The network is pre-trained on the combination of images from three orthogonal planes and then fine-tuned separately on images from each plane. Each testing slice goes through style transfer network to generate its transferred counterpart, which is in turn segmented using the fine-tuned segmentation model.

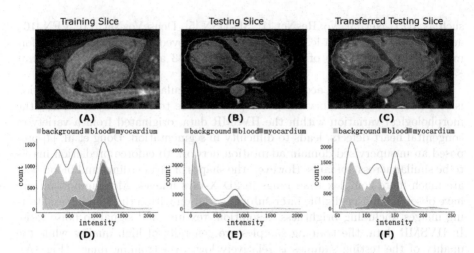

Fig. 1. Two representative slices from training (A) and testing set (B) and the transferred testing slice (C) are shown. Their intensity distributions are presented in D, E, and F, in which the intensity distributions of background, myocardium and blood pool are illustrated by gray, red, and green areas, respectively, and the gray lines show overall intensity distributions. (Color figure online)

2.1   Atrous Convolutional Neural Network for Dense Image Segmentation

For our baseline model, we modified DeepLabv3 [2], the state-of-the-art 2D semantic segmentation network, with ResNet-101 backbone. In order to fully utilize multi-scale information of feature maps elicited from ResNet, a pyramid of atrous convolution layer with various atrous rates $r = (6, 12, 18)$ is constructed on top of the last block of ResNet. Besides the three atrous convolution layers, the features from a 1×1 convolution and a bilinearly upsampled duplication of the input feature map are also considered. These 5 layers compose the atrous spatial pyramid pooling (ASPP) module whose feature maps are all concatenated. Finally, three 1×1 convolution layers are used to generate the final logits. Two batch normalization layers and two dropout layers (dropout rates being 0.5 and 0.1) are inserted between the final 3 convolution layers.

2.2   Neural Style Transfer on Inconsistent Data

Due to the large inconsistency between the training and testing data (Fig. 3 A), we apply a neural style transfer algorithm [6] on all 10 testing samples. Specifically, two types of loss, content loss and style loss are optimized, to change the style of a testing slice x to be similar to that of a target training slice y, while simultaneously impose constraint on the generated image $\hat{y}$ to maintain its content. Formally, given a feature extraction network ϕ that has J layers generating feature maps, the content loss is written as

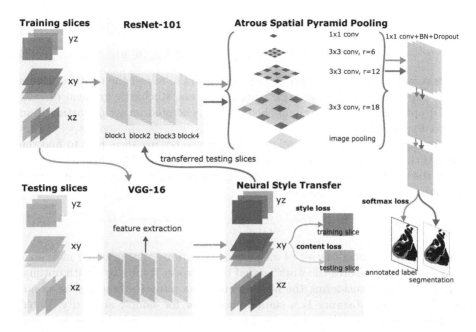

Fig. 2. Schematic illustration of StyleSegor workflow. A modified DeepLabv3 model with ResNet-101 backbone acts as our segmentation network and three models are trained in parallel for three planes $xy, yz, and\ zx$ (blue arrows). Meanwhile, testing slices are transferred to target styles guided by content loss and style loss, and then are fed into the segmentation network (red arrows). (Color figure online)

$$\ell^{\phi}_{content}(\hat{\boldsymbol{y}}, \boldsymbol{x}) = \sum_{j=1}^{J} \frac{1}{C_j H_j W_j} \parallel \phi_j(\hat{\boldsymbol{y}}) - \phi_j(\boldsymbol{x}) \parallel^2_2, \tag{1}$$

where C_j, H_j, W_j are the dimensions of the feature maps in the jth layer.

On the other hand, in order to measure the discrepancy between the generated slice $\hat{\boldsymbol{y}}$ and target slice $\boldsymbol{y}$, Gram matrix, originally designed to capture texture information, is to be computed. The jth Gram matrix for $\boldsymbol{y}$ is

$$G^{\phi}_j(\boldsymbol{y})_{i,k} = \frac{1}{C_j H_j W_j} \sum_{h=1}^{H_j} \sum_{w=1}^{W_j} \phi_j(\boldsymbol{y})_{h,w,i} \phi_j(\boldsymbol{y})_{h,w,k}, \tag{2}$$

that is, the i, k position at the jth Gram matrix measures the correlation (inner product) of the ith and the kth feature maps in the jth layer. Subsequently, the style loss is

$$\ell^{\phi}_{style}(\hat{\boldsymbol{y}}, \boldsymbol{y}) = \sum_{j=1}^{J} \parallel G^{\phi}_j(\hat{\boldsymbol{y}}) - G^{\phi}_j(\boldsymbol{y}) \parallel^2_2 . \tag{3}$$

The total loss is a weighted combination of content loss ans style loss

$$\ell^{\phi}_{total}(\hat{\boldsymbol{y}}, \boldsymbol{x}, \boldsymbol{y}) = \alpha \ell^{\phi}_{content}(\hat{\boldsymbol{y}}, \boldsymbol{x}) + \beta \ell^{\phi}_{style}(\hat{\boldsymbol{y}}, \boldsymbol{y}), \tag{4}$$

where α and β are user-specified hyper parameters to adjust the relative weights of the two losses. During the style transfer process, stochastic gradient descent (SGD) optimization is directly applied on the generated image $\hat{\boldsymbol{y}}$ starting from the content image $\boldsymbol{x}$.

Until now, a remaining question is, for a given testing slice, how to find the optimal training slice as its target slice. We address this problem in several steps. First, the pairwise similarities of all training and testing samples are measured through the 1st Wasserstein metric

$$W(r, g) = \inf_{\gamma \in \Gamma(r,g)} \mathbb{E}_{(x,y) \sim \gamma} \| x - y \|, \tag{5}$$

where $\Gamma(r, g)$ denotes the set of all joint distributions $\gamma(x, y)$ whose marginals are r, g, which measures the work needed to transport from x to y with optimal transport plan. Considering the high difference in intensity ranges across samples, Wasserstein distance is a suitable indicator for sample similarity. Based on these similarities, all samples are clustered using hierarchical clustering algorithm [8], and the training samples reside in one cluster serve as the style library (the first cluster in Fig. 3A). Using our baseline network, the percentages of the three labels within each testing slice are used to measure the distance between two slices, and the slice in the style library with the smallest Euclidean distance to the testing slice is chosen as the target style.

Because in StyleSegor, a full training process is required for every content-style pair, we use VGG-16, a lightweight network, as the feature extraction network ϕ and the feature maps after the $2^{nd}, 4^{th}, 7^{th}, 10^{th}$ convolution layers are used to compute the Gram matrices (see Fig. 2).

2.3   Probabilistic Adjustment and Ensemble Learning

Based on the observation that the signals of myocardium and blood pool tend to be overwhelmed by the background signal (Fig. 3E and H), we perform a probabilistic adjustment step and adjust the score for one label at position i by conditioning on the scores of other labels

$$c(p_k) = \arg\max_{k \in (1,2,3)} p_k \prod_{j \neq k} \left(1 - \frac{e^{p_j}}{\sum_{q \in (1,2,3)} e^{p_q}} \right), \tag{6}$$

where $p_k, k \in (1, 2, 3)$ is the logits output from the network for three labels. For example, the score of myocardium is multiplied by the probabilities of both non-blood pool and non-background (Fig. 3F and I).

In machine learning practice, model ensemble is oft-used to take advantage of multiple models and predictions. Here we adopt a voting scheme to integrate segmentations obtained from both original and transformed images. The final label at position i is the voting of $c(p_k^{(xy)}), c(p_k^{(yz)}), c(p_k^{(zx)})$ and $c(\sum_{xy,yz,zx} p_k)$ derived from the original images and $c(p_k^{'(xy)}), c(p_k^{'(yz)}), c(p_k^{'(zx)})$ and $c(\sum_{xy,yz,zx} p_k')$ derived from the transferred images (Fig. 3J).

3   Experimental Results

Dataset and Training Process. We evaluate the performance of StyleSegor on HVSMR, the dataset for MICCAI 2016 Challenge on Whole-Heart and Great Vessel Segmentation from 3D Cardiovascular MRI in Congenital Heart Disease. Imaging was done in an axial view on a 1.5T scanner. Ten 3D MR scans, as well as the manually labeled annotations for myocardium and great vessel, are provided for training, but the labels for 10 testing scans are not made publicly available for fair comparison. After carefully investigating the properties of testing images, we observed that the signal of myocardium in testing samples is especially lower than in training samples (see Fig. 1A, D and B, E). The clustering result of training and testing samples based on Wasserstein metric is shown in Fig. 3A, where training samples are marked from 0 to 9 and testing samples from 11 to 19. Clearly, all testing sample reside in the same cluster, which is significantly different from another cluster of training samples. In our style transfer network, the weights of style and content loss α and β are set at 10^6 and 1, respectively, and the optimization terminates after 50 epochs, which typically takes 3s for one content-style pair on a GTX 1080 Ti card. The VGG-16 network is trained on ImageNet dataset.

To fully make use of the slices from three orthogonal planes, all slices are collected for training for 20 epochs with learning rate starting at 0.01. Then the slices derived from xy, yz, and zx planes are used to fine-tune the model separately with learning rate starting from 0.002 for another 20 epochs each. A poly learning rate policy is employed where the starting learning rate is reduced by multiplying $(1 - \frac{epoch}{max\_epoch})$. To accelerate the training process, the segmentation network is pre-trained on COCO dataset. During the training of our baseline model, a series of data augmentation strategy is applied. Each original image is randomly scaled with the rates ranged from 0.5 to 2.0 and a 480×480 patch is cropped then goes through random left-right flipping and random Gaussian blurring. Because the training images are randomly scaled during training, in testing process, each testing image is scaled with scaling rate $= (0.5, 0.75, 1, 1.25, 1.5, 2.0)$ and the accumulated score map is used to produce final segmentation.

A representative testing slice and the transferred slice of it are shown in Fig. 1B and C, while the intensity distribution of background, blood pool, and myocardium are illustrated in Fig. 1E and F. Interestingly, after style transfer, not only the brightness, contrast, texture of the image but also the distribution of the three labels are transformed to be very similar to the training image, and the myocardium signal is smartly elevated.

Quantitative Comparisons. The comparison of StyleSegor and our baseline network, along with other segmentation methods are shown in Table 1, and the

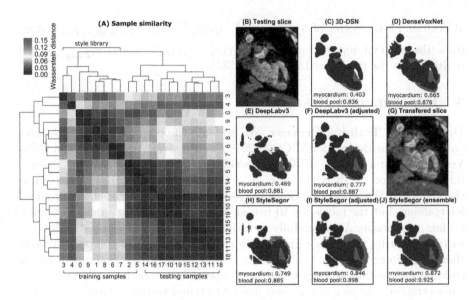

Fig. 3. Clustering result of the 20 samples (A) and segmentation results on a representative testing slice (B to J). The blue and red colors in B to J represent blood pool and myocardium, respectively. The dice scores of the two labels are also shown. The ground truth labels for testing data are not made publicly available. (Color figure online)

visualization of those segmentation results is provided in Fig. 3B to J. After probabilistic adjustment, although our baseline model only performs 2D convolution, it comes up with satisfactory segmentation with dice score of myocardium at 0.808 and that of blood pool at 0.919, and notably, by virtue of the large field of view, it produces the best Hausdorff distance at 3.105 mm compared with previous methods. After style transfer, the segmentation performance of myocardium is promoted to 0.825 and that of blood pool to 0.923, suggesting that with the promotion of myocardium signal, the myocardium structures are better recognized by the same model. However, we notice that after transfer, the Hausdorff distance of myocardium segmentation is enlarged to 4.633 mm, probably caused by false positive prediction of myocardium label brought by style transfer. And this false positive prediction is likely to be eliminated by the ensemble of multiple predictions. As shown in the last row of Table 1, the ensemble result is better than either StyleSegor or DeepLabv3, with dice score of myocardium at 0.839 and that of blood pool at 0.937. Notably, the Hausdorff distances are greatly minimized to 2.832 mm for myocardium and 4.023 mm for blood pool, and the overall score is boosted to 0.304, a 29.91% improvement compared with previously best result, demonstrating StyleSegor's strength to locate the region of interest.

Table 1. Comparison of different methods on HVSMR 2016 dataset. The weights of relative contributions of Dice, Average distance boundary (ADB), and Hausdorff distance to the Overall score are 0.5, −0.25, and −0.03, respectively.

Method	Myocardium			Blood pool			Overall score
	Dice	ADB [mm]	Hausdorff [mm]	Dice	ADB [mm]	Hausdorff [mm]	
3D U-Net [3]	0.694±0.076	1.461±0.397	10.221±4.339	0.926±0.016	0.940±0.192	8.628±3.390	-0.419
3D DSN [5]	0.739±0.072	1.035±0.240	5.248±1.332	0.928±0.014	1.017±0.181	7.704±2.892	-0.162
VoxResNet [1]	0.774±0.067	1.026±0.400	6.572±0.013	0.929±0.013	0.981±0.186	9.966±3.021	-0.202
DenseVoxNet [11]	0.821±0.041	0.964±0.292	7.294±3.340	0.931±0.011	0.938±0.224	9.533±4.194	-0.161
Wolterink et. al [9]	0.802±0.060	0.957±0.302	6.126±3.565	0.926±0.018	0.885±0.223	7.069±2.857	-0.036
VFN [10]	0.773±0.098	0.877±0.318	4.626±2.319	0.935±0.009	0.770±0.098	5.420±2.152	0.108
Zheng et. al [13]	0.833±0.054	**0.681±0.178**	3.285±1.370	**0.939±0.008**	0.733±0.143	5.670±2.808	0.234
DeepLabv3 (baseline)	0.648±0.156	1.234±0.531	5.960±3.921	0.920±0.025	0.983±0.309	7.343±2.999	-0.214
StyleSegor (baseline)	0.744±0.085	1.061±0.322	5.610±2.641	0.923±0.022	1.000±0.285	5.778±2.999	-0.061
DeepLabv3 (adjusted)	0.808±0.057	0.820±0.230	3.105±1.033	0.916±0.018	1.038±0.227	7.887±2.787	0.031
StyleSegor (adjusted)	0.825±0.031	0.934±0.237	4.633±2.241	0.923±0.014	1.073±0.191	7.435±2.649	-0.030
StyleSegor (ensemble)	**0.839±0.037**	0.689±0.140	**2.832±0.660**	0.937±0.014	**0.731±0.182**	4.023±1.299	**0.304**

4 Conclusion

In this paper, we present StyleSegor, a novel pipeline for 3D cardiac MR image segmentation. The neural style transfer algorithm automatically transfers the testing images towards the domain of training images, making them easier to be processed by the same model. Our StyleSegor pipeline is also easy to be used in other tasks such as disease detection and classification when data inconsistency is an inevitable issue, e.g., tasks involving datasets collected from different hospitals or institutions.

References

1. Chen, H., Dou, Q., Yu, L., Qin, J., Heng, P.A.: VoxResNet: deep voxelwise residual networks for brain segmentation from 3D MR images. NeuroImage **170**, 446–455 (2018)
2. Chen, L.C., Zhu, Y., Papandreou, G., Schroff, F., Adam, H.: Encoder-decoder with Atrous separable convolution for semantic image segmentation. In: ECCV, pp. 801–818 (2018)
3. Çiçek, Ö., Abdulkadir, A., Lienkamp, S.S., Brox, T., Ronneberger, O.: 3D U-Net: learning dense volumetric segmentation from sparse annotation. In: Ourselin, S., Joskowicz, L., Sabuncu, M.R., Unal, G., Wells, W. (eds.) MICCAI 2016. LNCS, vol. 9901, pp. 424–432. Springer, Cham (2016). https://doi.org/10.1007/978-3-319-46723-8_49
4. Dong, N., Kampffmeyer, M., Liang, X., Wang, Z., Dai, W., Xing, E.: Unsupervised domain adaptation for automatic estimation of cardiothoracic ratio. In: Frangi, A.F., Schnabel, J.A., Davatzikos, C., Alberola-López, C., Fichtinger, G. (eds.) MICCAI 2018. LNCS, vol. 11071, pp. 544–552. Springer, Cham (2018). https://doi.org/10.1007/978-3-030-00934-2_61
5. Dou, Q., et al.: 3D deeply supervised network for automated segmentation of volumetric medical images. Med. Image Anal. **41**, 40–54 (2017)
6. Gatys, L.A., Ecker, A.S., Bethge, M.: Image style transfer using convolutional neural networks. In: CVPR, pp. 2414–2423 (2016)

7. Gretton, A., Smola, A., Huang, J., Schmittfull, M., Borgwardt, K., Schölkopf, B.: Covariate Shift and Local Learning by Distribution Matching, pp. 131–160. MIT Press, Cambridge (2009)
8. Müllner, D.: Modern hierarchical, agglomerative clustering algorithms. arXiv preprint arXiv:1109.2378 (2011)
9. Wolterink, J.M., Leiner, T., Viergever, M.A., Išgum, I.: Dilated convolutional neural networks for cardiovascular MR segmentation in congenital heart disease. In: Zuluaga, M.A., Bhatia, K., Kainz, B., Moghari, M.H., Pace, D.F. (eds.) RAMBO/HVSMR -2016. LNCS, vol. 10129, pp. 95–102. Springer, Cham (2017). https://doi.org/10.1007/978-3-319-52280-7_9
10. Xia, Y., Xie, L., Liu, F., Zhu, Z., Fishman, E.K., Yuille, A.L.: Bridging the gap between 2D and 3D organ segmentation with volumetric fusion net. In: Frangi, A.F., Schnabel, J.A., Davatzikos, C., Alberola-López, C., Fichtinger, G. (eds.) MICCAI 2018. LNCS, vol. 11073, pp. 445–453. Springer, Cham (2018). https://doi.org/10.1007/978-3-030-00937-3_51
11. Yu, L., et al.: Automatic 3D cardiovascular MR segmentation with densely-connected volumetric convnets. In: Descoteaux, M., Maier-Hein, L., Franz, A., Jannin, P., Collins, D.L., Duchesne, S. (eds.) MICCAI 2017. LNCS, vol. 10434, pp. 287–295. Springer, Cham (2017). https://doi.org/10.1007/978-3-319-66185-8_33
12. Zhao, A., Balakrishnan, G., Durand, F., Guttag, J.V., Dalca, A.V.: Data augmentation using learned transformations for one-shot medical image segmentation. In: CVPR, pp. 8543–8553 (2019)
13. Zheng, H., et al.: A new ensemble learning framework for 3D biomedical image segmentation. In: AAAI (2019)

Supervised Uncertainty Quantification for Segmentation with Multiple Annotations

Shi Hu[1(✉)], Daniel Worrall[1], Stefan Knegt[1], Bas Veeling[1], Henkjan Huisman[2], and Max Welling[1]

[1] University of Amsterdam, Amsterdam, The Netherlands
s.hu@uva.nl
[2] Radboud University Medical Center, Nijmegen, The Netherlands

Abstract. The accurate estimation of predictive uncertainty carries importance in medical scenarios such as lung node segmentation. Unfortunately, most existing works on predictive uncertainty do not return *calibrated* uncertainty estimates, which could be used in practice. In this work we exploit multi-grader annotation variability as a source of 'groundtruth' aleatoric uncertainty, which can be treated as a target in a supervised learning problem. We combine this groundtruth uncertainty with a Probabilistic U-Net and test on the LIDC-IDRI lung nodule CT dataset and MICCAI2012 prostate MRI dataset. We find that we are able to improve predictive uncertainty estimates. We also find that we can improve sample accuracy and sample diversity. In real-world applications, our method could inform doctors about the confidence of the segmentation results.

Keywords: Uncertainty · Image segmentation · Deep learning

1 Introduction

In recent years, deep learning has propelled the state of the art in segmentation in medical imaging [6,10,11,16,22]. However, previous works tend to focus on maximizing accuracy, ignoring predictive uncertainty. Modeling uncertainty at the per-pixel level is as important as accuracy, especially in medical scenarios, since it informs clinicians about the trustworthiness of a model's outputs [13,21].

Typically, there are two main types of uncertainty one cares about, *aleatoric* and *epistemic* [15]. Aleatoric uncertainty is a measure of the intrinsic, irreducible noise found in data, usually associated with the data acquisition process. Epistemic uncertainty is our uncertainty over the true values of a model's parameters, which arises from the finite size of training sets. With increasing training set size, epistemic uncertainty tends asymptotically to zero [8]. In practice, these two sources of uncertainty are difficult to quantify. Typically epistemic uncertainty is very hard to evaluate since one would need access to the groundtruth model to measure it, but it is possible to form a meaningful estimate of aleatoric uncertainty since we do have access to groundtruth data. Consider a training

© Springer Nature Switzerland AG 2019
D. Shen et al. (Eds.): MICCAI 2019, LNCS 11765, pp. 137–145, 2019.
https://doi.org/10.1007/978-3-030-32245-8_16

set of N images $\{x_i\}_{i=1}^N$. If for the ith image we are able to acquire D grader segmentations $\{y_i^1, ..., y_i^D\}$, then we define aleatoric uncertainty to be the per-pixel variance among these segmentations $\mathbb{V}_{p(\mathcal{D})}[y_i] = \frac{1}{D}\sum_{j=1}^D (y_i^j - \bar{y}_i)^2$, where $\bar{y}_i = \frac{1}{D}\sum_{j=1}^D y_i^j$. Datasets containing multiple annotations exist in the literature, such as [1,2,7,18], and it is surprising that to date the authors cannot find examples of intergrader variability being exploited.

In this paper, we build a segmentation model based on the Probabilistic U-Net [16], exploiting intergrader variability as a target for aleatoric uncertainty. With this model one can draw diverse segmentations from its output and gain quantitative, calibrated aleatoric uncertainty estimates. We further add a source of epistemic uncertainty, which the model previously did not have. To view these two uncertainties we deploy an uncertainty decomposition in the output-space based on the law of total variance. We find improved predictive performance as well as better aleatoric uncertainty estimation over previous works, while also achieving higher sample diversity, which we did not explicitly design in.

2   Background and Related Works

Below we provide an overview of predictive uncertainty for deep learning.

Predictive Uncertainty. Consider a training set $\mathcal{D} = \{(x_i, y_i)\}_{i=1}^N$ with inputs x_i and target segmentations y_i, and a neural network with parameters/hidden variables θ. We can think of the neural network as a conditional distribution $p(y|x, \theta)$. Given test image x_*, the posterior predictive distribution [19] is $p(y_*|x_*, \mathcal{D}) = \int p(y_*|x_*, \theta)p(\theta|\mathcal{D})\,\mathrm{d}\theta$, where $p(\theta|\mathcal{D})$ is a posterior distribution over θ given the training data. This quantity is intractable to find [4], so it is typically approximated by some $q_\lambda(\theta)$ from a tractable family of distributions, where λ is called the *variational parameters*. Typically the approximation is fitted by minimizing the reverse KL-divergence $\mathrm{KL}[q_\lambda(\theta) \parallel p(\theta|\mathcal{D})]$. This is intractable, since it contains the intractable posterior term, but can be rearranged into the ELBO *evidence lower-bound* [4]:

$$\min_\lambda \mathrm{KL}[q_\lambda(\theta) \parallel p(\theta|\mathcal{D})] = \max_\lambda \mathbb{E}_{q_\lambda(\theta)}[\log p(\mathcal{D}|\theta)] + \mathrm{KL}[q_\lambda(\theta) \parallel p(\theta)] \quad (1)$$

where $p(\theta)$ is a prior on θ and $p(\mathcal{D}|\theta) = \prod_{i=1}^N p(y_i|x_i, \theta)$. The *predictive uncertainty* is the variance of the posterior predictive distribution.

Aleatoric and Epistemic Uncertainty. The predictive uncertainty can be decomposed into two parts. By the law of total variance, we can write predictive variances as a sum of these two independent components:

$$\underbrace{\mathbb{V}_{p(y|\theta,x)}[y]}_{\text{predictive uncertainty}} = \underbrace{\mathbb{E}_{q_\lambda(\theta)}[\mathbb{V}_{p(y|\theta,x)}[y]]}_{\text{aleatoric uncertainty}} + \underbrace{\mathbb{V}_{q_\lambda(\theta)}[\mathbb{E}_{p(y|\theta,x)}[y]]}_{\text{epistemic uncertainty}}, \quad (2)$$

where we have used the notation $\mathbb{E}$ and $\mathbb{V}$ for the expectation and variance operator. We have labeled the two right-hand terms as *aleatoric* and *epistemic* uncertainty. The aleatoric term measures the average of the output variance $\mathbb{V}_{p(y|\theta,x)}[y]$, under all settings of the variables θ. If $q_\lambda(\theta)$ were a delta peak, we would expect this term not to vanish and thus is it associated with aleatoric (data) uncertainty [21]. The epistemic term measures fluctuations in the mean prediction. These fluctuations exist because of uncertainty in the approximate posterior $q_\lambda(\theta)$. If $q_\lambda(\theta)$ were a delta peak, then this term would vanish to zero, and thus we associate it with epistemic (model) uncertainty [13,21].

Current techniques for estimating aleatoric and epistemic uncertainty follow similar line. In Tanno et $al.$ [21] the authors treat MRI superresolution as a regression problem. They build a CNN directly outputting $\mathbb{E}_{p(y|\theta,x)}[y]$ and $\mathbb{V}_{p(y|\theta,x)}[y]$. They model epistemic uncertainty using variational dropout [14]. Bragman et $al.$ [5] build on this technique, applying it to radiotherapy-treatment planning and multi-task learning. Concurrent to [21] Kendall and Gal proposed a similar method using Monte Carlo (MC) instead of variational dropout [9]. They also proposed a method which would work for classification, where they predict a mean and variance in the logit-space just before a sigmoid. Jungo et $al.$ [12] estimate epistemic uncertainty in the context of postoperative brain tumor cavity segmentation using MC dropout [9]. In [3] Ayhan and Berens treat the data augmentation process as part of the approximate posterior $q_\lambda(\theta)$. They claim this is aleatoric uncertainty, but from their method it appears they really compute epistemic uncertainty. None of these works quantitatively evaluates the quality of the epistemic and aleatoric uncertainties. In this work, we show that the aleatoric uncertainty can indeed be measured.

The Probabilistic U-Net. In the Probabilistic U-Net [16], the approximate posterior distribution is given the form $q_\lambda(z|x,y)$, where we have set $\theta = z$. The hidden variables are thus activations $z|x,y$ dependent on the training data. A (conditional) prior over z is given by a $prior$ $network$ $p_\lambda(z|x)$. To train this setup, the authors employ a variant of the ELBO with a β-weight on the KL-penalty

$$\max_\lambda -\frac{1}{N} \sum_{i=1}^{N} \left(\mathbb{E}_{q_\lambda(z|x_i,y_i)} [\log p_\lambda(y_i|x_i,z)] + \beta \cdot \mathrm{KL}[q_\lambda(z|x_i,y_i) \parallel p_\lambda(z|x_i)] \right). \quad (3)$$

Again, λ represents the variational parameters to be optimized. Since at test time we do not have access to y, we use the prior network and Monte Carlo sample in $p(y_*|x_*,\mathcal{D}) = \int p_\lambda(y_*|x_*,z)p_\lambda(z|x_*)\,\mathrm{d}z$. The specific form of the likelihood $p(y|x,z)$ can be found in the original paper [16]. This method is known to produce very diverse samples, from which we could estimate aleatoric uncertainty. In this paper, we endow the Probabilistic U-Net with a mechanism to estimate epistemic uncertainty and extend this method yet further, such that the aleatoric uncertainty estimates are automatically calibrated to the training set.

3   Method

We improve upon the Probabilistic U-Net model with two innovations. First, the original framework does not contain a mechanism to measure epistemic uncertainty. This can be included by adding variational dropout [14] after the last convolution layer in the U-Net. This corresponds to setting $\theta = (z, w)$ and $q_\lambda(\theta) = q_\lambda(w)q_\lambda(z|x, y)$, where w are CNN weights. The objective defined in Eq. 3 then changes to:

$$\mathcal{L}_{vd}(\lambda) = -\frac{1}{N}\sum_{i=1}^{N}\mathbb{E}_{q_\lambda(w)q_\lambda(z|x_i, y_i)}\left[\log p_\lambda(y_i|x_i, z, w)\right] +$$

$$\beta \cdot \frac{1}{N}\sum_{i=1}^{N}\mathrm{KL}[q_\lambda(z|x_i, y_i) \parallel p_\lambda(z|x_i)] + \frac{1}{N}\mathrm{KL}[q_\lambda(w) \parallel p(w)]. \quad (4)$$

Notice that as N becomes very large the relative weight of the last KL term reduces, so the prior on w is ignored [8]. The objective is maximized when $q_\lambda(w)$ is a delta peak on the maximum likelihood parameters, corresponding to zero model uncertainty. For our second innovation, we use intergrader variability $\mathbb{V}_{p(\mathcal{D})}[y]$ as a training target for the predicted aleatoric uncertainty $\mathbb{E}_{q_\lambda(\theta)}[\mathbb{V}_{p(y|\theta, x)}[y]]$. We found directly minimizing the L_1 or L_2 distance between the two does not work well. Instead, since for binary variables the mean and variance are tied, we match the means $p_g = \mathbb{E}_{p(\mathcal{D})}[y]$ and $p_m = \mathbb{E}_{q_\lambda(\theta)}[\mathbb{E}_{p(y|\theta, x)}[y]]$ using a cross-entropy loss. This term is not part of the ELBO, so we are free to sample from the prior network since this is used at test-time. Introducing scaling coefficient γ our final training objective becomes

$$\mathcal{L}(\lambda) = \mathcal{L}_{vd}(\lambda) - \gamma \cdot \frac{1}{N}\sum_{i=1}^{N}[p_g \log p_m + (1 - p_g)\log(1 - p_m)]. \quad (5)$$

4   Experiments

Datasets and Implementation Details. We use two datasets where images have different but plausible annotations. First, the LIDC-IDRI dataset with 4 lesion annotations per image [1,2,7]. This dataset contains 1,018 lung CT scans from 1,010 lung patients with manual lesion annotations. We use the LIDC Matlab Toolbox [17] to process the slices and annotations with dimension 512×512, then center the lesions and crop the patches of size 128×128. This results in 15,096 image patches in total. We do not change the in-plane resolution. Second, the MICCAI2012 dataset with 3 prostate peripheral zone annotations per image [18]. This dataset contains 48 prostate MRI images and each image has multiple slides. We discard images that have fewer than 3 annotations, which leaves 44 images in total. For each image, the original dimension of a slide is 320×320, and we crop the central patch of size 128×128. This results in 614 image patches in total. The patches are treated independently and we feed each 2D patch to a model. Since this is a very small dataset, we use elastic transformation [20] to augment the dataset to prevent overfitting.

For each dataset, we split the train/validation/test sets with ratio 70%/15%/15%. Different than [16], we put all annotations of an image in the same mini-batch. Table 1 shows some hyperparameters used for each dataset.

Table 1. Hyperparamters details.

Hyperparameters	LIDC	MICCAI2012
# epochs	800	1000
Mini-batch size	32	12
β	1	100
γ	100	100
Data augmentation?	None	Elastic transformation
Adam learning rate	1e-6	1e-4

Table 2. D^2_{GED} comparison (lower is better). Each result is computed over five random seeds.

Method	LIDC	MICCAI2012
Kohl et al. [16]	0.346 ± 0.038	0.382 ± 0.017
Kendall and Gal [13]	0.553 ± 0.010	0.571 ± 0.028
Ours	$\mathbf{0.267 \pm 0.012}$	$\mathbf{0.373 \pm 0.021}$

The ones not presented in this table are similar to [16]. For ease of comparison, all experiments on the same dataset use the same hyperparameters. Lastly, we run all experiments on NVIDIA TITAN Xp GPUs.

Sample Accuracy and Diversity. Figure 1 compares our generative results with Kendall and Gal model. In each plot, the first row is a patch in test and its true annotations. The second row is the samples generated by the Kendall and Gal model [13]. The third row is our samples. The annotations for most images exhibit some variability as they come from different graders. In general, we observe that the samples from our model are able to cover different modality in the annotations, whereas in Kendall and Gal there is limited diversity, and thus cannot cover all the variations in the true annotations.

Quantitatively, we evaluate the generative results using the generalized energy distance (or D^2_{GED}) metric [16]: $2\,\mathbb{E}[d(S,Y)] - \mathbb{E}[d(S,S')] - \mathbb{E}[d(Y,Y')]$, where d is the complement of the Intersection over Union (IoU): $d(a,b) = 1 - \mathrm{IoU}(a,b)$. S and S' are independent samples from a model, and Y and Y' are independent samples from the graders. Thus, the first term measures the expected difference between the samples and annotations, the second among the samples themselves and the third among the annotations themselves. In other words, this metric evaluates both the accuracy and diversity of the samples. Table 2 compares the D^2_{GED} scores on the LIDC and MICCAI2012 datasets. Since our model improves upon the Probabilistic U-Net model, we also present their numerical results for a reference[1]. Their generative results do not look very

---

[1] We use the PyTorch implementation for the Probabilistic U-Net model from https://github.com/stefanknegt/Probabilistic-Unet-Pytorch.

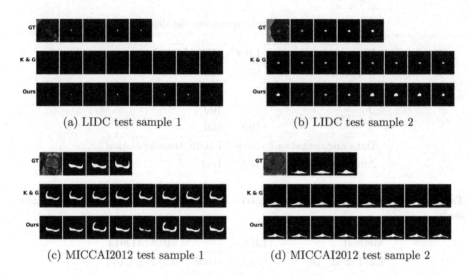

(a) LIDC test sample 1   (b) LIDC test sample 2

(c) MICCAI2012 test sample 1   (d) MICCAI2012 test sample 2

Fig. 1. Samples comparison (zoom in on detail).

differently from ours, so we omit them in Fig. 1. For each model in Table 2, we generate 50 samples for evaluation. The table shows our model achieves better D^2_{GED} on both datasets.

Uncertainty Decomposition. Figure 2 shows the aleatoric and epistemic uncertainty decomposition results. For each plot, the first row shows the results from Kendall and Gal [13] and the second row shows ours. To make the scales of these plots comparable, we set an upper threshold on the intensity values. Any value larger than the threshold will be treated as the threshold. For the true and predicted data uncertainty plots, we use the same threshold as we want to visually compare their similarity. In contrast, there is no label for the epistemic uncertainty, so we use a scale that fits well with most intensity pixels in a plot.

In general, we observe that Kendall and Gal makes plausible predictions on the shape of the data uncertainty, but tends to underestimate its scale, whereas we are relatively close to the ground truth in terms of both the shape and scale. Furthermore, the former tends to have high model uncertainty, especially at the image borders, whereas ours are usually around the point of interest. Although we do not know the true appearance of the model uncertainty, it should be high on the objects that do not occur often in the training set. In both test sets, the new objects usually appear around the center rather than at the borders. Therefore, we argue our epistemic uncertainty prediction is more sensible.

Quantitatively, Table 3 compares the data uncertainty prediction performance of the two models. As mentioned, the scale of the data uncertainty predictions from Kendall and Gal tends to be smaller than the ground truth. We want to establish a fair image similarity comparison that takes into account of this fact. Thus, for the true and predicted data uncertainty map a and b, we measure

Table 3. Data uncertainty prediction comparison using the normalized cross-correlation (higher is better). Each result is computed over three random seeds.

Method	LIDC	MICCAI2012
Kendall and Gal [13]	0.597 ± 0.006	0.299 ± 0.011
Ours	**0.669 ± 0.011**	**0.345 ± 0.005**

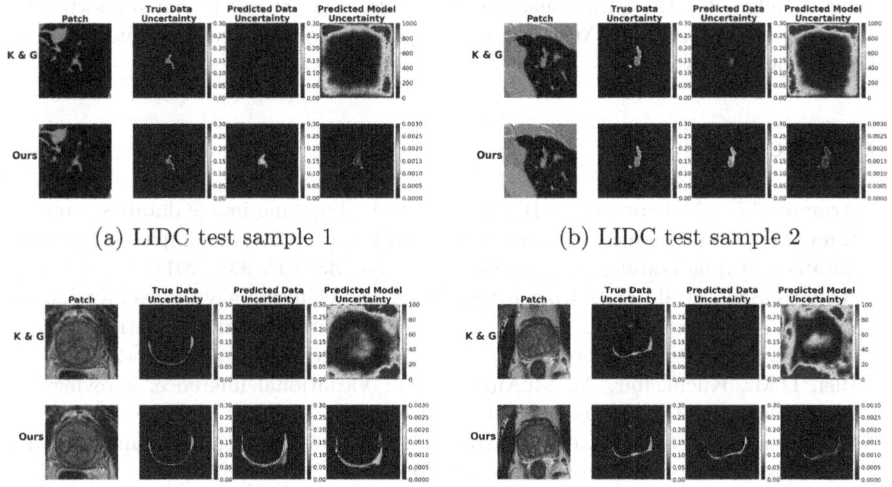

(a) LIDC test sample 1   (b) LIDC test sample 2

(c) MICCAI2012 test sample 1   (d) MICCAI2012 test sample 2

Fig. 2. Uncertainty quantification comparison.

their similarity using the normalized cross-correlation $\frac{1}{n\sigma_a\sigma_b}\sum_{x,y}(a_{x,y} - \mu_a) \cdot (b_{x,y} - \mu_b)$, where n is the total number of pixels in an uncertainty map, and μ and σ are the mean and the standard deviation of a uncertainty map. Since we normalize the scales of the uncertainty maps a and b, the output value represents their intrinsic similarity. In Table 3, we report the average normalized cross-correlation score over all test images for each dataset. Our model achieves higher data uncertainty correlations in both cases.

5   Conclusions

In this work we designed a model for segmentation based on the Probabilistic U-Net [16] which outputs two kinds of quantifiable uncertainty, aleatoric (data) uncertainty and epistemic (model) uncertainty. We leveraged intergrader variability as a target for calibrated aleatoric uncertainty, which, as far as we know, related works have surprisingly not used. We showcased our model on the LIDC-IDRI lung nodule CT dataset [1,2,7] and MICCAI2012 prostate MRI dataset [18], demonstrating that we could improve predictive uncertainty estimates.

We also found that we could improve sample accuracy and sample diversity. In real-world applications, our method could inform doctors if they can trust the segmentation results to decide in real-time whether to continue a treatment path or not. As future work, we would like to improve the quality of the epistemic uncertainty.

Acknowledgements. We thank Dimitrios Mavroeidis for helpful discussions and Arsenii Ashukha for the variational dropout code. This research was supported by NWO Perspective Grants DLMedIA and EDL, as well as the in-cash and in-kind contributions by Philips.

References

1. Armato, S.G., McLennan, G., Bidaut, L., et al.: The lung image database consortium (LIDC) and image database resource initiative (IDRI): a completed reference database of lung nodules on ct scans. Med Phys. **38**, 915–931 (2011)
2. Armato, S.G., et al.: Data from LIDC-IDRI. The Cancer Imaging Archive (2015)
3. Ayhan, M.S., Berens, P.: Test-time data augmentation for estimation of heteroscedastic aleatoric uncertainty in deep neural networks. In: MIDL (2018)
4. Blei, D.M., Kucukelbir, A., McAuliffe, J.D.: Variational inference: a review for statisticians. CoRR abs/1601.00670 (2016)
5. Bragman, F.J., et al.: Quality control in radiotherapy-treatment planning using multi-task learning and uncertainty estimation. In: MIDL (2018)
6. Causey, J., et al.: Highly accurate model for prediction of lung nodule malignancy with CT scans. CoRR abs/1802.01756 (2018)
7. Clark, K., et al.: The cancer imaging archive (TCIA): maintaining and operating a public information repository. J. Digit. Imaging **26**, 1045–1057 (2013)
8. Gal, Y.: Uncertainty in deep learning. Ph.D. thesis, University of Cambridge (2016)
9. Gal, Y., Ghahramani, Z.: Dropout as a Bayesian approximation: representing model uncertainty in deep learning. In: ICML (2016)
10. Gruetzemacher, R., Gupta, A., Paradice, D.B.: 3D deep learning for detecting pulmonary nodules in CT scans. JAMIA **25**, 1301–1310 (2018)
11. Gu, Y., et al.: Automatic lung nodule detection using A 3D deep convolutional neural network combined with a multi-scale prediction strategy in chest CTs. Comput. Biol. Med. **103**, 220–231 (2018)
12. Jungo, A., Meier, R., Ermis, E., Herrmann, E., Reyes, M.: Uncertainty-driven sanity check: application to postoperative brain tumor cavity segmentation. In: MIDL (2018)
13. Kendall, A., Gal, Y.: What uncertainties do we need in Bayesian deep learning for computer vision? In: NIPS (2017)
14. Kingma, D.P., Salimans, T., Welling, M.: Variational dropout and the local reparameterization trick. In: NIPS (2015)
15. Kiureghian, A.D., Ditlevsen, O.: Aleatory or epistemic? Does it matter? Struct. Saf. **31**, 105–112 (2009)
16. Kohl, S.A., et al.: A probabilistic u-net for segmentation of ambiguous images. In: NIPS (2018)
17. Lampert, T.A., Stumpf, A., Gancarski, P.: An empirical study of expert agreement and ground truth estimation. IEEE Trans. Image Process. **25**, 2557–2572 (2016)

18. Litjens, G., Debats, O., van de Ven, W., Karssemeijer, N., Huisman, H.: A pattern recognition approach to zonal segmentation of the prostate on MRI. In: Ayache, N., Delingette, H., Golland, P., Mori, K. (eds.) MICCAI 2012. LNCS, vol. 7511, pp. 413–420. Springer, Heidelberg (2012). https://doi.org/10.1007/978-3-642-33418-4_51

19. MacKay, D.J.C.: Bayesian interpolation. Neural Comput. **4**(3), 415–447 (1992)

20. Simard, P.Y., Steinkraus, D., Platt, J.C.: Best practices for convolutional neural networks applied to visual document analysis. In: International Conference on Document Analysis and Recognition (2003)

21. Tanno, R., et al.: Bayesian image quality transfer with CNNs: exploring uncertainty in dMRI super-resolution. In: Descoteaux, M., Maier-Hein, L., Franz, A., Jannin, P., Collins, D.L., Duchesne, S. (eds.) MICCAI 2017. LNCS, vol. 10433, pp. 611–619. Springer, Cham (2017). https://doi.org/10.1007/978-3-319-66182-7_70

22. Wang, S., et al.: Central focused convolutional neural networks: developing a data-driven model for lung nodule segmentation. Med. Image Anal. **40**, 172–183 (2017)

3D Tiled Convolution for Effective Segmentation of Volumetric Medical Images

Guodong Zeng[1,2,3] and Guoyan Zheng[1,2(✉)]

[1] School of Biomedical Engineering, Shanghai Jiao Tong University, Shanghai, China
guoyan.zheng@sjtu.edu.cn
[2] Institute of Medical Robotics, Shanghai Jiao Tong University, Shanghai, China
[3] ARTORG Center for Biomedical Engineering, University of Bern,
Bern, Switzerland

Abstract. Convolutional Neural Networks (CNNs) have achieved remarkable performance in many 2D computer vision and medical image analysis tasks. In clinical practice, however, a large part of the medical imaging data available are in 3D. This has motivated the development of 3D CNNs in order to benefit from more spatial context. Although weight sharing in CNNs significantly reduces the number of parameters that have to be learned, state-of-the-art 3D methods still depend on patch processing due to GPU memory restrictions caused by moving to fully 3D. The size of the input patch is usually small if no specialized hardware with large GPU memory is used, limiting the incorporation of larger context information for a better performance. In this paper, we propose a 3D Tiled Convolution (3D-TC) which learn a number of separate kernels within the same layer. 3D-TC has the advantage of significantly reducing the required GPU memory for 3D medical image processing task but with improved performance. Results obtained from comprehensive experiments conducted on both hip T1 MR images and pancreas CT images demonstrate the efficacy of the present method. Our implementation can be found at: https://github.com/guoyanzheng/LPNet.

Keywords: Segmentation · Deep learning · 3D tiled convolution · MRI · CT

1 Introduction

Convolutional Neural Networks (CNNs) have achieved state-of-the-art performance in many different 2D medical image analysis tasks. The common idea behind these solutions is to use deep convolutional networks with many hidden layers, aiming at learning discriminative feature embedding from raw data, rather than replying on handcrafted feature extraction. In clinical practice, however, a large part of the medical imaging data available are in 3D. This has motivated

© Springer Nature Switzerland AG 2019
D. Shen et al. (Eds.): MICCAI 2019, LNCS 11765, pp. 146–154, 2019.
https://doi.org/10.1007/978-3-030-32245-8_17

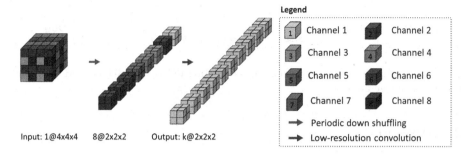

Fig. 1. A schematic view of 3D tiled convolutions which are implemented as a periodic down-shuffling operation with low-resolution convolutions. Here the down-shuffling factor is (2, 2, 2).

the development of 3D CNNs in order to benefit from more spatial context [1–6]. Due to GPU memory restrictions caused by moving to fully 3D, state-of-the-art methods [1–6] depend on subvolume/patch processing. The size of the input patch is usually small if no specialized hardware with large GPU memory is used, limiting the incorporation of larger context information for a better performance. In this paper, we present a novel and efficient approach for effective segmentation of volumetric images by leveraging context information in a large patch. Our contributions can be summarized as follows:

– First, inspired by [7], we propose a novel 3D Tiled Convolution (3D-TC) for volumetric image processing. 3D-TC is implemented with a periodic down-shuffling operation followed by conventional 3D convolutions. 3D-TC has the advantage of significantly reducing the size of the data for sub-sequential processing while using all the information available in the input irrespective of the down-shuffling factors. We apply 3D-TC directly to the input data, whose output will be used as the input for sub-sequential Fully Convolutional Networks (FCNs). A full-resolution dense prediction at the final output is then generated by using previously introduced Dense Upsampling Convolution (DUC) [8,9], which consists of low-resolution convolutions with a periodic up-shuffling operation to jointly learn the feature extraction and upsampling weights.
– Second, we extensively validate the proposed approach on two typical yet challenging volumetric image segmentation tasks, i.e., segmentation of hip bony structures from 3D T1 MR images of limited field of view and segmentation of pancreas from 3D CT images. We show that 3D-TC and DUC are network agnostic and can be combined with different FCNs for an improved performance.

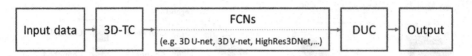

Fig. 2. A schematic view of how to augment existing FCNs with 3D-TC and DUC for volumetric image analysis.

2   Methods

2.1   3D Tiled Convolution

As shown in Fig. 1, 3D-TC consists of a periodic down-shuffling operator and low-resolution (LR) convolutions. 3D-TC is designed to be directly applicable to the input data with two goals in mind. First, different from conventional convolutions, where convolutional kernels are shared by all neurones in a particular layer, 3D-TC aims to learn $n_x \times n_y \times n_z$ separate kernels within the same layer, where n_x, n_y, n_z are the down-shuffling factors along the three spatial axes, respectively. Thus, irrespective of the down-shuffling facts, all data available in the input are used which is different from a simple down-sampling operation. Second, 3D-TC can significantly reduce the size of the data for sub-sequential processing. More specifically, let's assume that the size of input data (I^{HR}) is $(n_x \times d) \times (n_y \times h) \times (n_z \times w) \times C$ and the size of the output from 3D-TC is $d \times h \times w \times k$, where C is the number of channels in the input data; k is the number of feature maps in the output of 3D-TC. Instead of applying convolution to high resolution (HR) images, we first apply a periodic down-shuffling operator to the input data to get $C \times (n_x \times n_y \times n_z)$ channels of LR feature maps and then further apply convolutions with a kernel size of $3 \times 3 \times 3$ to get the k feature maps of size $(d \times h \times w)$. Mathematically, this can be described as:

$$TC(I^{LR}; W_1, b_1) = \phi(W_1 * PDS(I^{HR}) + b_1) \qquad (1)$$

where ϕ is an non-linear activation function that is applied element-wise; W_1, b_1 are trainable weights and bias, respectively; PDS is a periodic down-shuffling operator which aims to rearrange the tensor (T_{HR}) in the shape of $(n_x \times d) \times (n_y \times h) \times (n_z \times w) \times C$ to the tensor (T_{LR}) in the shape of $(d \times h \times w) \times (C \times (n_x \times n_y \times n_z))$. And the operation $T_{LR} = PDS(T_{HR})$ can be mathematically described as below:

$$\begin{aligned}
T_{LR}(x', y', z', c') = T_{HR}(&x' \times n_x + \lfloor mod(c', n_x \times C)/C \rfloor, \\
&y' \times n_y + \lfloor mod(c', n_x \times n_y \times C)/(n_x \times C) \rfloor, \\
&z' \times n_z + \lfloor c'/(n_x \times n_y \times C) \rfloor, \\
&mod(c', C))
\end{aligned} \qquad (2)$$

where x', y', z', c' are the coordinates of the voxels in the LR space, and $x' \in [0, d-1], y' \in [0, h-1], z' \in [0, w-1], c' \in [0, C \times n_x \times n_y \times n_z - 1]$.

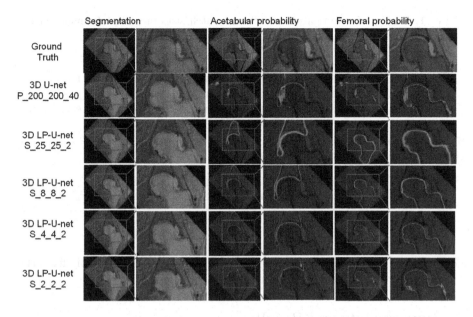

Fig. 3. Qualitative comparison of the segmentation results of 3D LP-U-Net with different shuffling factors and the 3D U-net with the largest patch size.

2.2 3D-TC and DUC Augmented FCNs for Image Segmentation

Both DUC and 3D-TC are network agnostic and can be combined with existing FCNs such as 3D U-net [1] for volumetric image analysis as shown in Fig. 2, as long as the dimensions of the output from 3D-TC satisfy the input requirement of the sub-sequential FCNs. The advantage of such a pipeline is apparent. When a 3D-TC with down-shuffling factors of (n_x, n_y, n_z) is applied to the input data, both the computational and the storage cost for the underlying networks will be reduced by a factor of $(n_x \times n_y \times n_z)$, allowing one to use large patch as the input but with reduced computational time. The full resolution result is then obtained at the final output by applying a DUC with up-shuffling factors of (n_x, n_y, n_z). To differentiate from the original 3D U-net, we call the 3D U-net augmented with 3D-TC and DUC as 3D large patch U-net (3D LP-U-net). Similarly we can derive 3D LP-V-net and LP-HighRes3DNet respectively by augmenting the original 3D V-net [2] and HighRes3DNet [5] with 3D-TC and DUC. In this study, we take the original 3D U-net, 3D V-net and HighRes3DNet as the base networks to evaluate the performance of the associated networks augmented with 3D-TC and DUC. For all the studies, a combination of cross entropy loss with Dice loss as introduced in [2] is used.

2.3 Implementation Details

All methods were implemented in Python using TensorFlow framework and were trained and tested on a desktop with a 3.6 GHz Intel(R) i7 CPU and a NVIDIA

Table 1. Results of investigation of different patch sizes on the performance of the original 3D U-net. Ace: the acetabulum; Femur: the proximal femur

Patch size	(50, 50, 40)		(96, 96, 96)		(200, 200, 40)	
Anatomy	Ace	Femur	Ace	Femur	Ace	Femur
DOC (%)	37.45 ± 5.73	30.62 ± 3.55	91.30 ± 5.84	95.89 ± 1.21	92.06 ± 5.37	96.84 ± 0.90
ASD (mm)	28.15 ± 5.04	29.27 ± 4.90	5.11 ± 7.57	1.41 ± 1.11	0.88 ± 0.76	0.63 ± 0.31

Table 2. Results when different shuffling factors were used for the 3D LP-U-net. The size of the input patch is fixed to $400 \times 400 \times 80$.

Shuffling factors	(2, 2, 2)		(4, 4, 2)		(8, 8, 2)		(16, 16, 2)		(25, 25, 2)	
Anatomy	Ace	Femur	Ace	Femur	Ace	Femur	Ace	Femur	Ace	Femur
DOC (%)	96.77 ± 1.27	97.41 ± 1.34	96.77 ± 1.26	97.95 ± 0.63	96.30 ± 0.97	97.25 ± 0.59	94.24 ± 1.73	95.75 ± 1.02	91.57 ± 2.03	93.82 ± 1.52
ASD (mm)	0.39 ± 0.28	0.43 ± 0.28	0.39 ± 0.28	0.33 ± 0.16	0.37 ± 0.11	0.41 ± 0.09	0.62 ± 0.23	0.64 ± 0.16	0.86 ± 0.25	0.96 ± 0.25

GTX 1080 Ti graphics card with 11 GB GPU memory. We empirically fixed the number of output feature maps from the 3D-TC as $k = 64$.

3 Experiments and Results

In this section, we present experimental results of the proposed pipeline for volumetric image analysis. Two datasets, i.e., an in-house dataset consisting of 25 T1 hip MR images with limited field of view and a publicly available dataset from National Institute of Health (NIH) containing 82 abdominal contrast enhanced 3D CT scans [10], were used in our study. For all the experiments described below, we used Dice Overlap Coefficients (DOC) and Average Surface Distance (ASD) as the evaluation metrics.

3.1 Ablation Study on Hip MR Images with Limited Field of View

Data and Augmentation. We used 25 3D T1 MR images, acquired from patients with hip pain. All images were resampled to have a uniform size of $480 \times 480 \times 160$ voxels with an average voxel spacing of 0.374 mm × 0.363 mm × 1.078 mm. Slice by slice manual segmentation was used to create the reference ground truth segmentation. In this study, we randomly distributed the 25 datasets into two groups with one group containing 20 datasets as the training data and the remaining 5 datasets as the testing data.

Ablation Study. We first investigated the influence of patch sizes on the performance of the original 3D U-net [1]. The results are presented in Table 1. It was observed that better performance was obtained when larger patch size was used. Due to the GPU memory constraint, $200 \times 200 \times 40$ is the maximum size that we can use.

We then examined the effect of different shuffling factors on the performance of 3D LP-U-net when a fixed patch size of $400 \times 400 \times 80$ was used. The results

Table 3. Results when different underlying FCNs were used.

Architectures	3D V-Net		3D LP-V-Net (2, 2, 2)		HighRes3DNet		LP-HighRes3DNet (4, 4, 1)	
Anatomy	Ace	Femur	Ace	Femur	Ace	Femur	Ace	Femur
DOC (%)	92.78 ± 0.50	96.67 ± 0.85	95.58 ± 1.43	97.11 ± 0.63	93.04 ± 4.31	93.58 ± 2.46	95.99 ± 1.18	97.38 ± 0.52
ASD (mm)	0.97 ± 0.97	0.59 ± 0.23	0.63 ± 0.58	0.49 ± 0.15	1.77 ± 2.34	1.50 ± 0.82	0.43 ± 0.18	0.44 ± 0.12

Table 4. Segmentation accuracy of 3D LP-U-net and three state-of-the-art methods.

Architectures (Used patch size)	3D U-net 200 × 200 × 40		3D V-net 200 × 200 × 40		HighRes3DNet 200 × 200 × 20		3D LP-U-Net (4, 4, 2) 400 × 400 × 80	
Anatomy	Ace	Femur	Ace	Femur	Ace	Femur	Ace	Femur
DOC (%)	94.01 ± 2.80	96.89 ± 0.85	93.35 ± 3.21	96.47 ± 1.54	90.51 ± 7.32	89.99 ± 4.91	**96.76 ± 0.92**	**98.14 ± 0.47**
ASD (mm)	0.96 ± 1.16	0.54 ± 0.20	0.91 ± 0.87	0.59 ± 0.36	3.74 ± 7.58	1.79 ± 0.83	**0.36 ± 0.20**	**0.27 ± 0.09**

are reported in Table 2. From this table, we can see that (1) the higher the shuffling factor, in general the less accurate the results but the best results were achieved when the shuffling factor was (4, 4, 2); (2) even with a shuffling factor as high as (25, 25, 2), we still get sub-millimeter segmentation accuracy for both structures; and (3) in comparison with the results reported in Table 1, 3D LP-U-net achieved better results than the original 3D U-net with the largest patch size when the shuffling factor was smaller than (16, 16, 2).

Figure 3 visually compares the segmentation results obtained by the 3D LP-U-net with a fixed patch size of 400 × 400 × 80 but different shuffling factors and the 3D U-net with the largest patch size. In this figure, we show both the overall segmentation and the probability of each structure as well as the results around the hip joint. From this figure, we observe that (1) less false positive segmentation was observed when comparing the results obtained by the 3D LP-U-net with those by the 3D U-net; and (2) for the 3D LP-U-net, the larger the shuffling factors, the higher the uncertainty around the boundary but the best results are obtained when the shuffling factors are (4, 4, 2).

Finally, we show that 3D-TC and DUC are agnostic to the base networks. To demonstrate such a capability, we compared the performance of the original 3D V-Net and HighRes3DNet when the maximally allowed patch sizes were used with that of 3D LP-V-Net with a shuffling factor (2, 2, 2) and LP-HighRes3DNet with a shuffling factor (4, 4, 1) when a fixed patch size of 400 × 400 × 80 was used. Please note that caused by high spatial resolution, the maximally allowed patch size for HighRes3DNet is 200 × 200 × 20 while for 3D V-Net, it is 200 × 200 × 40. The results are presented in Table 3, where results achieved by the 3D LP-V-Net and the LP-HighRes3DNet are better than those achieved by the associated base networks.

3.2   Validation on Hip MR Images

Using the same 25 T1 hip MR images with limited field of view as we used in the ablation study, we conducted a standard 5-fold cross validation experiment. We also adopted the same data augmentation strategy and the same training strategy as in the ablation study. In this cross validation study, for the 3D LP-U-net, we chose a fixed patch size of $400 \times 400 \times 80$ and a fixed shuffling factor of (4, 4, 2). We compared the performance of the 3D LP-U-net with state-of-the-art methods such as 3D U-net [1], 3D V-net [2], and HighRes3dNet [5] and the results are shown in Table 4. An average DOC of $96.76 \pm 0.92\%$, $94.01 \pm 2.80\%$, $93.35 \pm 3.21\%$ and $90.51 \pm 7.32\%$ was found for the 3D LP-U-net, the 3D U-net, the 3D V-net and the HighRes3DNet, respectively. The 3D LP-U-net showed significantly higher accuracy than all other three methods ($p < 0.01$). For ASD, the same significance was also observed. For the proximal femur, an average DOC of $98.14 \pm 0.47\%$, $96.89 \pm 0.85\%$, $96.47 \pm 1.54\%$ and $89.99 \pm 4.91\%$ was found for the 3D LP-U-net, the 3D U-net, the 3D V-net and the HighRes3DNet, respectively. The 3D LP-U-net showed significantly higher accuracy than all other three methods ($p < 0.01$) when segmenting the proximal femur. An average ASD of 0.27 ± 0.09 mm, 0.96 ± 1.16 mm, 0.91 ± 0.87 mm and 1.79 ± 0.83 mm was found for the 3D LP-U-net, the 3D U-net, the 3D V-net and the HighRes3DNet, respectively.

3.3   Validation on NIH Pancreas CT Dataset

We verified our approach on the NIH pancreas CT dataset [10] as well, which contains 82 contrast-enhanced abdominal CT volumes provided by an experienced radiologist. Following the training protocol [10], we conducted a 4-fold cross validation in a random split from 82 patients for training and testing folds, where each testing fold had 22, 20, 20, and 20 cases, respectively. We implemented a two-stage pipeline consisting of a coarse stage and a fine stage. In the coarse stage, we first trained a deep segmentation network to locate the rough region of the pancreas from a whole CT volume. The goal of the fine stage is then to train another deep segmentation network to further refine the results. In both stages, we used the 3D LP-U-net as the segmentation networks. During the training phase of the coarse stage, we chose a fixed patch size of $480 \times 480 \times 64$ voxels and a fixed shuffling factor of (4, 4 1). During the training phase of the fine stage, all training images were cropped by the bounding box calculated from the associated ground truth segmentation plus a padding of 20 voxels along all three spatial axes. Then all cropped images were resampled to a fixed size of $196 \times 128 \times 128$ voxels. For the 3D LP-U-net in the fine stage, we chose a fixed patch size of $176 \times 112 \times 96$ voxels and a fixed shuffling factor of (2, 2, 1).

Table 5 shows the accuracy comparison between our approach and previous state-of-the-art methods when evaluated on the NIH pancreas CT dataset. Our approach achieved a comparable average DOC with the state-of-the-art methods. Although the average DOC and the maximum DOC achieved by our approach are slightly worse than those achieved by [6], which is based on a complicated recurrent saliency transformation network with careful parameter fine-tuning, our approach achieved much better result in the worst case (68.39% by our approach vs. 62.81% by previous state-of-the-art), which guaranteed the reliability of our approach in clinical application.

Table 5. Accuracy (DOC, %) comparison between 3D LP-U-net and the state-of-the-arts on the NIH pancreas segmentation dataset.

Approach	Average	Max	Min
Roth et al. [10]	71.42 ± 10.11	86.29	23.99
Zhou et al. [11]	82.37 ± 5.68	90.85	62.43
Cai et al. [12]	82.4 ± 6.7	90.1	60.0
Roth et al. [13]	81.27 ± 6.27	88.96	50.69
Yu et al. [6]	$\mathbf{84.50 \pm 4.97}$	**91.02**	62.81
Our approach	83.0 ± 5.85	90.31	**68.39**

4   Conclusion

We proposed a simple yet effective 3D tiled convolution for 3D medical image analysis tasks. The 3D-TC consists of a periodic down-shuffling operation followed by low-resolution 3D convolutions. It can be directly applied to the input data and has the advantage of significantly reducing the size of the data for sub-sequential processing while using all the information available in the input irrespective of the down-shuffling factors. To achieve volumetric dense prediction at the output, we used a previously introduced dense upsampling convolution. We showed that 3D-TC and DUC were network agnostic and could be combined with different FCNs for an improved performance. Experimental results demonstrated the effectiveness of our framework on different semantic segmentation tasks. Our future work is to apply 3D-TC to other volumetric image processing tasks such as image synthesis and image super-resolution.

Acknowledgements. This study was partially supported by a start-up funding from Shanghai Jiao Tong University, China with Grant No. WF220882002 and the Swiss National Science Foundation via project 205321_163224/1.

References

1. Çiçek, Ö., Abdulkadir, A., Lienkamp, S.S., Brox, T., Ronneberger, O.: 3D U-Net: learning dense volumetric segmentation from sparse annotation. In: Ourselin, S., Joskowicz, L., Sabuncu, M.R., Unal, G., Wells, W. (eds.) MICCAI 2016. LNCS, vol. 9901, pp. 424–432. Springer, Cham (2016). https://doi.org/10.1007/978-3-319-46723-8_49
2. Milletari, F., Navab, N., Ahmadi, S.A.: V-Net: fully convolutional neural networks for volumetric medical image segmentation. In: Proceedings of 2016 International Conference on 3D Vision (3DV), pp. 565–571. IEEE (2016)
3. Dou, Q., et al.: 3D deeply supervised network for automated segmentation of volumetric medical images. Med. Image Anal. **41**, 40–54 (2017)
4. Kamnitsas, K., et al.: Efficient multi-scale 3D CNN with fully connected CRF for accurate brain lesion segmentation. Med. Image Anal. **36**, 61–78 (2017)

5. Li, W., Wang, G., Fidon, L., Ourselin, S., Cardoso, M.J., Vercauteren, T.: On the compactness, efficiency, and representation of 3D convolutional networks: brain parcellation as a pretext task. In: Niethammer, M., et al. (eds.) IPMI 2017. LNCS, vol. 10265, pp. 348–360. Springer, Cham (2017). https://doi.org/10.1007/978-3-319-59050-9_28

6. Yu, Q., Xie, L., Wang, Y., Zhou, Y., Fishman, E.K., Yuille, A.L.: Recurrent saliency transformation network: incorporating multi-stage visual cues for small organ segmentation. In: CVPR, pp. 8280–8289, June 2018

7. Ngiam, J., Chen, Z., Chia, D., Koh, P.W., Le, Q.V., Ng, A.Y.: Tiled convolutional neural networks. In: Advances in Neural Information Processing Systems, pp. 1279–1287 (2010)

8. Shi, W., et al.: Real-time single image and video super-resolution using an efficient sub-pixel convolutional neural network. In: CVPR, pp. 1874–1883 (2016)

9. Wang, P., et al.: Understanding convolution for semantic segmentation. In: 2018 IEEE Winter Conference on Applications of Computer Vision (WACV), pp. 1451–1460. IEEE (2018)

10. Roth, H.R., et al.: DeepOrgan: multi-level deep convolutional networks for automated pancreas segmentation. In: Navab, N., Hornegger, J., Wells, W.M., Frangi, A.F. (eds.) MICCAI 2015. LNCS, vol. 9349, pp. 556–564. Springer, Cham (2015). https://doi.org/10.1007/978-3-319-24553-9_68

11. Zhou, Y., Xie, L., Shen, W., Wang, Y., Fishman, E.K., Yuille, A.L.: A fixed-point model for pancreas segmentation in abdominal CT scans. In: Descoteaux, M., Maier-Hein, L., Franz, A., Jannin, P., Collins, D.L., Duchesne, S. (eds.) MICCAI 2017. LNCS, vol. 10433, pp. 693–701. Springer, Cham (2017). https://doi.org/10.1007/978-3-319-66182-7_79

12. Cai, J., Lu, L., Xie, Y., Xing, F., Yang, L.: Pancreas segmentation in MRI using graph-based decision fusion on convolutional neural networks. In: Descoteaux, M., Maier-Hein, L., Franz, A., Jannin, P., Collins, D.L., Duchesne, S. (eds.) MICCAI 2017. LNCS, vol. 10435, pp. 674–682. Springer, Cham (2017). https://doi.org/10.1007/978-3-319-66179-7_77

13. Roth, H.R., et al.: Spatial aggregation of holistically-nested convolutional neural networks for automated pancreas localization and segmentation. Med. Image Anal. **45**, 94–107 (2018)

Hyper-Pairing Network for Multi-phase Pancreatic Ductal Adenocarcinoma Segmentation

Yuyin Zhou[1(✉)], Yingwei Li[1], Zhishuai Zhang[1], Yan Wang[1], Angtian Wang[2], Elliot K. Fishman[3], Alan L. Yuille[1], and Seyoun Park[3]

[1] The Johns Hopkins University, Baltimore, MD 21218, USA
zhouyuyiner@gmail.com
[2] Huazhong University of Science and Technology, Wuhan 430074, China
[3] The Johns Hopkins University School of Medicine, Baltimore, MD 21287, USA

Abstract. Pancreatic ductal adenocarcinoma (PDAC) is one of the most lethal cancers with an overall five-year survival rate of 8%. Due to subtle texture changes of PDAC, pancreatic dual-phase imaging is recommended for better diagnosis of pancreatic disease. In this study, we aim at enhancing PDAC automatic segmentation by integrating multi-phase information (*i.e.*, arterial phase and venous phase). To this end, we present Hyper-Pairing Network (HPN), a 3D fully convolution neural network which effectively integrates information from different phases. The proposed approach consists of a dual path network where the two parallel streams are interconnected with hyper-connections for intensive information exchange. Additionally, a pairing loss is added to encourage the commonality between high-level feature representations of different phases. Compared to prior arts which use single phase data, HPN reports a significant improvement up to 7.73% (from 56.21% to 63.94%) in terms of DSC.

1 Introduction

Pancreatic ductal adenocarcinoma (PDAC) is the 4th most common cancer of death with an overall five-year survival rate of 8%. Currently, detection or segmentation at localized disease stage followed by complete resection can offer the best chance of survival, *i.e.*, with a 5-year survival rate of 32%. The accurate segmentation of PDAC mass is also important for further quantitative analysis, *e.g.*, survival prediction [1]. Computed tomography (CT) is the most commonly used imaging modality for the initial evaluation of PDAC. However, textures of PDAC on CT are very subtle (Fig. 1) and therefore can be easily neglected by even experienced radiologists. To our best knowledge, the state-of-the-art on this matter is [17], which only reports an average Dice of 56.46%. For better detection of PDAC mass, dual-phase pancreas protocol using contrast-enhanced CT imaging, which is comprised of arterial and venous phases with intravenous contrast delay, are recommended.

© Springer Nature Switzerland AG 2019
D. Shen et al. (Eds.): MICCAI 2019, LNCS 11765, pp. 155–163, 2019.
https://doi.org/10.1007/978-3-030-32245-8_18

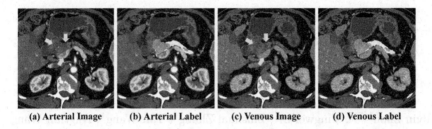

(a) Arterial Image   (b) Arterial Label   (c) Venous Image   (d) Venous Label

Fig. 1. Visual comparison of arterial and venous images (after alignment) as well as the manual segmentation of normal pancreas tissues (yellow), pancreatic duct (purple) and PDAC mass (green). Orange arrows indicate the ambiguous boundaries and differences of the abnormal appearances between the two phases. Best viewed in color. (Color figure online)

In recent years, deep learning has largely advanced the field of computer-aided diagnosis (CAD), especially in the field of biomedical image segmentation [4,10,11,16]. However, there are several challenges for applying existing segmentation algorithms to dual-phase images. Firstly, these algorithms are optimized for segmenting only one type of input, and therefore cannot be directly applied to handle multi-phase data. More importantly, how to properly handle the variations between different views requires a smart information exchange strategy between different phases. While how to efficiently integrate information from multi-modalities has been widely studied [3,6,15], the direction on learning multi-phase information has been rarely explored, especially for tumor detection and segmentation purposes.

To address these challenges, we propose a multi-phase segmentation algorithm, Hyper-Pairing Network (HPN), to enhance the segmentation performance especially for pancreatic abnormality. Following HyperDenseNet [3] which is effective on multi-modal image segmentation, we construct a dual-path network for handling multi-phase data, where each path is intended for one phase. To enable information exchange between different phases, we apply skip connections across different paths of the network [3], referred as *hyper-connections*. Moreover, by noticing that a standard segmentation loss (cross-entropy loss, Dice loss [8]) only aims at minimizing the differences between the final prediction and the groundtruth thus cannot well handle the variance between different views, we introduce an additional *pairing loss term* to encourage the commonality between high-level features across both phases for better incorporation of multi-phase information. We exploit three structures together in HPN including PDAC mass, normal pancreatic tissues, and pancreatic duct, which serves as an important clue for localizing PDAC. Extensive experiments demonstrate that the proposed HPN significantly outperforms prior arts by a large margin on all 3 targets.

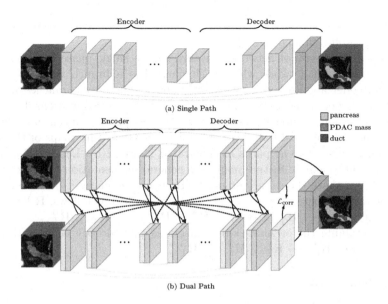

Fig. 2. (a) The single path network where only one phase is used. The dash arrows denote skip connections between low-level features and high-level features. (b) HPN structure where multiple phases are used. The black arrows between the two single path networks indicate hyper-connections between the two streams. An additional pairing loss is employed to regularize view variations, therefore can benefit the integration between different phases. Blue and pink stand for arterial and venous phase, respectively. (Color figure online)

2   Methodology

We hereby focus on dual-phase inputs while our approach can be generalized to multi-phase scans. With phase A and aligned phase B by the deformable registration, we have the set $\mathcal{S} = \{(\mathbf{X}_i^A, \mathbf{X}_i^B, \mathbf{Y}_i) | i = 1, ..., M\}$, where $\mathbf{X}_i^A \in \mathbb{R}^{W_i \times H_i \times L_i}$ is the i-th 3D volumetric CT images of phase A with the dimension $(W_i \times H_i \times L_i) = \mathcal{D}_i$ and $\mathbf{X}_i^B \in \mathbb{R}^{\mathcal{D}_i}$ is the corresponding aligned volume of phase B. $\mathbf{Y}_i = \{y_{ij} | j = 1, ..., \mathcal{D}_i\}$ denotes the corresponding voxel-wise label map of the i-th volume, where $y_{ij} \in \mathcal{L}$ is the label of the j-th voxel in the i-th image, and $\mathcal{L}$ denotes the label of the target structures. In this study, $\mathcal{L} = \{$normal pancreatic tissues, PDAC mass, pancreatic duct$\}$. The goal is to learn a model to predict label of each voxel $\hat{\mathbf{Y}} = f(\mathbf{X}^A, \mathbf{X}^B)$ by utilizing multi-phase information.

2.1   Hyper-connections

Segmentation networks (*e.g.*, UNet [2,10], FCN [7]) usually contain a contracting encoder part and a successive expanding decoder part to produce a full-resolution segmentation result as illustrated in Fig. 2(a). As the layer goes deeper, the output features evolve from low-level detailed representations to high-level abstract semantic representations. The encoder part and the decoder part share an equal number of resolution steps [2,10].

However, this type of network can only handle single-phase data. We construct a dual path network where each phase has a branch with a U-shape encoder-decoder architecture as mentioned above. These two branches are connected via hyper-connections which enrich feature representations by learning more complex combinations between the two phases. Specifically, hyper-connections are applied between layers which output feature maps of the same resolution across different paths as illustrated in Fig. 2(b). Let $\mathbf{R}_1, \mathbf{R}_2, ..., \mathbf{R}_T$ denote the intermediate feature maps of a general segmentation network, where $\mathbf{R}_t$ and $\mathbf{R}_{T-t}$ share the same resolution ($\mathbf{R}_t$ is on the encoder path and $\mathbf{R}_{T-t}$ is on the decoder path). Hyper-connections are applied as follows: $\mathbf{R}_t^A \longrightarrow \mathbf{R}_t^B$, $\mathbf{R}_t^B \longrightarrow \mathbf{R}_t^A$, $\mathbf{R}_t^A \longrightarrow \mathbf{R}_{T-t}^B$, $\mathbf{R}_t^B \longrightarrow \mathbf{R}_{T-t}^A$, $\mathbf{R}_{T-t}^A \longrightarrow \mathbf{R}_{T-t}^B$, $\mathbf{R}_{T-t}^B \longrightarrow \mathbf{R}_{T-t}^A$, while maintaining the original skip connections that already occur within the same path, i.e., $\mathbf{R}_t^A \longrightarrow \mathbf{R}_{T-t}^A$, $\mathbf{R}_t^B \longrightarrow \mathbf{R}_{T-t}^B$.

2.2   Pairing Loss

The standard loss for segmentation networks only aims at minimizing the difference between the groundtruth and the final estimation, which cannot well handle the variance between different views. Applying this loss alone is inferior in our situation since the training process involves heavy integration of both arterial information and venous information. To this end, we propose to apply an additional pairing loss, which encourages the commonality between the two sets of high-level semantic representations, to reduce view divergence.

We instantiate this additional objective as a correlation loss [13]. Mathematically, for any pair of aligned images (X_i^A, X_i^B) passing through the corresponding view sub-network, the two sets of high-level semantic representations (feature responses in later layers) corresponding to the two phases are denoted as $f_1(X_i^A; \mathbf{\Theta}_1)$ and $f_2(X_i^B; \mathbf{\Theta}_2)$, where the two sub-networks are parameterized by $\mathbf{\Theta}_1$ and $\mathbf{\Theta}_2$ respectively. The outputs of two branches will be simultaneously fed to the final classification layer. In order to better integrate the outcomes from the two branches, we propose to use a pairing loss which exploits the consensus of $f_1(X_i^A; \mathbf{\Theta}_1)$ and $f_2(X_i^B; \mathbf{\Theta}_2)$ during training. The loss is formulated as following:

$$\mathcal{L}_{corr}(X_i^A, X_i^B; \mathbf{\Theta}) = -\frac{\sum_{j=1}^N \left(f_1(X_{ij}^A) - \overline{f_1(X_i^A)} \right) \left(f_2(X_{ij}^B) - \overline{f_2(X_i^B)} \right)}{\sqrt{\sum_{j=1}^N \left(f_1(X_{ij}^A) - \overline{f_1(X_i^A)} \right)^2 \sum_{j=1}^N \left(f_2(X_{ij}^B) - \overline{f_2(X_i^B)} \right)^2}}, \quad (1)$$

where N denotes the total number of voxels in the i-th sample and $\mathbf{\Theta}$ denotes the parameters of the entire network. During the training stage, we impose this additional loss to further encourage the commonality between the two intermediate outputs. The overall loss is the weighted sum of this additional penalty term and the standard voxel-wise cross-entropy loss:

$$\mathcal{L}_{total} = -\frac{1}{N} \left[\sum_{j=1}^N \sum_{k=0}^K \mathbb{1}(y_{ij} = k) \log p_{ij}^k \right] + \lambda \mathcal{L}_{corr}(X_i^A, X_i^B; \mathbf{\Theta}), \quad (2)$$

where p_{ij}^k denotes the probability of the j-th voxel be classified as label k on the i-th sample and $\mathbb{1}(\cdot)$ is the indicator function. K is the total number of classes. The overall objective function is optimized via stochastic gradient descent.

3 Experiments

3.1 Experiment Setup

Data Acquisition. This is an institutional review board approved HIPAA compliant retrospective case control study. 239 patients with pathologically proven PDAC were retrospectively identified from the radiology and pathology databases from 2012 to 2017 and the cases with ≤ 4 cm tumor (PDAC mass) diameter were selected for the experiment. PDAC patients were scanned on a 64-slice multidetector CT scanner (Sensation 64, Siemens Healthineers) or a dual-source multidetector CT scanner (FLASH, Siemens Healthineers). PDAC patients were injected with 100–120 mL of iohexol (Omnipaque, GE Healthcare) at an injection rate of 4–5 mL/sec. Scan protocols were customized for each patient to minimize dose. Arterial phase imaging was performed with bolus triggering, usually 30 s post-injection, and venous phase imaging was performed 60 s.

Evaluation. Denote $\mathcal{Y}$ and $\mathcal{Z}$ as the set of foreground voxels in the ground-truth and prediction, *i.e.*, $\mathcal{Y} = \{i \mid y_i = 1\}$ and $\mathcal{Z} = \{i \mid z_i = 1\}$. The accuracy of segmentation is evaluated by the Dice-Sørensen coefficient (DSC): DSC $(\mathcal{Y}, \mathcal{Z}) = \frac{2 \times |\mathcal{Y} \cap \mathcal{Z}|}{|\mathcal{Y}| + |\mathcal{Z}|}$. We evaluate DSCs of all three targets, *i.e.*, abnormal pancreas, PDAC mass and pancreatic duct. All experiments are conducted by three-fold cross-validation, *i.e.*, training the models on two folds and testing them on the remaining one. Through our experiment, abnormal pancreas stands for the union of normal pancreatic tissues, PDAC mass and pancreatic duct. The average DSC of all cases as well as the standard deviations are reported.

3.2 Implementation Details

Our experiments were performed on the whole CT scan and the implementations are based on PyTorch. We adopt a variation of diffeomorphic demons with direction-dependent regularizations [9,12] for accurate and efficient deformable registration between the two phases. For data pre-processing, we truncated the raw intensity values within the range [−100, 240] HU and normalized each raw CT case to have zero mean and unit variance. The input sizes of all networks are set as $64 \times 64 \times 64$. The coefficient of the correlation loss λ is set as 0.5. No further post-processing strategies were applied.

We also used data augmentation during training. Different from single-phase segmentation which commonly uses rotation and scaling [5,17], virtual sets [14] are also utilized in this work. Even though arterial and venous phase scanning are customized for each patient, the level of enhancement can be different from patients by variation of blood circulation, which causes inter-subject

Table 1. DSC (%) comparison of abnormal pancreas, PDAC mass and pancreatic duct. We report results in the format of mean ± standard deviation.

Method	Abnormal pancreas	PDAC mass	pancreatic duct
3D-UNet-single-phase (Arterial)	78.35 ± 11.89	52.40 ± 27.53	38.35 ± 28.98
3D-UNet-single-phase (Venous)	79.61 ± 10.47	53.08 ± 27.06	40.25 ± 27.89
3D-UNet-multi-phase (fusion)	80.05 ± 10.56	52.88 ± 26.97	39.06 ± 27.33
3D-UNet-multi-phase-HyperNet	82.45 ± 9.98	54.36 ± 26.34	43.27 ± 26.33
3D-UNet-multi-phase-HyperNet-aug	83.67 ± 8.92	55.72 ± 26.01	43.53 ± 25.94
3D-UNet-multi-phase-HPN (Ours)	**84.32 ± 8.59**	**57.10 ± 24.76**	**44.93 ± 24.88**
3D-ResDSN-single-phase (Arterial)	83.85 ± 9.43	56.21 ± 26.33	47.04 ± 26.42
3D-ResDSN-single-phase (Venous)	84.92 ± 7.70	56.86 ± 26.67	49.81 ± 26.23
3D-ResDSN-multi-phase (fusion)	85.52 ± 7.84	57.59 ± 26.63	48.49 ± 26.37
3D-ResDSN-multi-phase-HyperNet	85.79 ± 8.86	60.87 ± 24.95	54.18 ± 24.74
3D-ResDSN-multi-phase-HyperNet-aug	85.87 ± 7.91	61.69 ± 23.24	54.07 ± 24.06
3D-ResDSN-multi-HPN (Ours)	**86.65 ± 7.46**	**63.94 ± 22.74**	**56.77 ± 23.33**

enhancement variations on each phase. Therefore we construct virtual examples by interpolating between venous and arterial data, similar to [14]. The i-th augmented training sample pair can be written as: $\tilde{X}_i^A = \lambda X_i^A + (1 - \lambda)X_i^B$, $\tilde{X}_i^B = \lambda X_i^B + (1 - \lambda)X_i^A$, where $\lambda \sim \text{Beta}(\alpha, \alpha) \in [0, 1]$. The final outcome of HPN is obtained by taking the union of predicted regions from models trained with the original paired sets and the virtual paired sets. We set the hyper-parameter $\alpha = 0.4$ following [14].

3.3 Results and Discussions

All results are summarized in Table 1. We compare the proposed HPN with the following algorithms: (1) single-phase algorithms which are trained exclusively on one phase (denoted as "single-phase"); (2) multi-phase algorithm where both arterial and venous data are trained using a dual path network bridged with hyper connections (denoted as "HyperNet"). In general, compared with single-phase algorithms, multi-phase algorithms (*i.e.*, HyperNet, HPN) observe significant improvements for all target structures. It is no surprise to observe such a phenomenon as more useful information is distilled for multi-phase algorithms.

Efficacy of Hyper-connections. To show the effectiveness of hyper-connections, output from different phases (using single-phase algorithms) are fused by taking at each position the average probability (denoted as "fusion"). However, we observe that simply fusing the outcomes from the different phases usually yield either similar or slightly better performances compared with single-phase algorithms. This indicates that simply fusing the estimations during the inference stage cannot effectively integrate multi-phase information. By contrast, hyper-connections enable the training process to be communicative between the

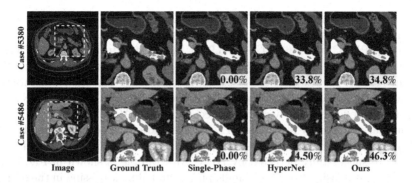

Fig. 3. Qualitative comparison of different methods, where HPN enhances PDAC mass segmentation (green) significantly compared with other methods. (Best viewed in color) (Color figure online)

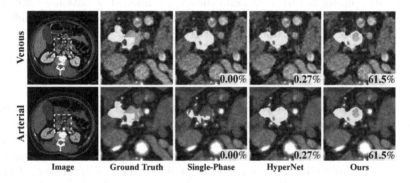

Fig. 4. Qualitative example where HPN detects the PDAC mass (green) while single-phase methods for both phases fail. From left to right: venous and arterial images (aligned), groundtruth, predictions of single-phase algorithms, HyperNet prediction, HPN prediction (overlayed with venous and arterial images). (Best viewed in color) (Color figure online)

two phase branches and thus can efficiently elevate the performance. Note that directly applying [3] yield unsatisfactory results. Our hyper-connections are not densely connected but are carefully designed based on previous state-of-the-art on PDAC segmentation [17] for better segmentation of PDAC. Meanwhile, we show much better performance of 63.94% compared to 56.46% reported in [17].

Efficacy of Data Augmentation. From Table 1, compared with HyperNet, HyperNet-aug witnesses performance gain especially for PDAC mass (*i.e.*, from 60.87% to 61.69% for 3D-ResDSN; from 54.36% to 55.72% for 3D-UNet), which validates the usefulness of using virtual paired sets as data augmentation.

Efficacy of HPN. We can observe additional benefit of our HPN over hyperNet-aug (*e.g.*, abnormal pancreas: 85.87% to 86.65%, PDAC mass: 61.69% to 63.94%, pancreatic duct: 54.07% to 56.77%, 3D-ResDSN). Overall, HPN observes an evident improvement compared with HyperNet, *i.e.*, abnormal pancreas: 85.79% to 86.65%, PDAC mass: 61.69% to 63.94%, pancreatic duct: 54.07% to 56.77% (3D-ResDSN). The *p-values* for testing significant difference between hyperNet and our HPN of all 3 targets are $p < 0.0001$, which suggests a general statistical improvement. We also show two qualitative examples in Fig. 3, where HPN shows much better segmentation accuracy especially for PDAC mass.

Another noteworthy fact is that 11/239 cases are false negatives which failed to detect any PDAC mass using either phase (Dice = 0%). Out of these 11 cases, 7 cases are successfully detected by HPN. An example is shown in Fig. 4—the PDAC mass is missing from both single phases and almost missing in the original HyperNet (DSC = 0.27%), but our HPN can detect a reasonable portion of the PDAC mass (DSC = 61.5%).

The deformable registration error by computing pancreas surface distances between two phases is 1.01 ± 0.52 mm (mean $\pm$ standard deviations) which can be considered as acceptable for this study. However, the effects between different alignments can be described as a further study.

4   Conclusions

Motivated by the fact that radiologists usually rely on analyzing multi-phase data for better image interpretations, we develop an end-to-end framework, HPN, for multi-phase image segmentation. Specifically, HPN consists of a dual path network where different paths are connected for multi-phase information exchange, and an additional loss is added for removing view divergence. Extensive experiment results demonstrate that the proposed HPN can substantially and significantly improve the segmentation performance, *i.e.*, HPN reports an improvement up to 7.73% in terms of DSC compared to prior arts which use single phase data. In the future, we plan to examine the behaviour of HPN when using different alignment strategies and try to extend the current approach to other multi-phase learning problems.

Acknowledgements. This work was supported by the Lustgarten Foundation for Pancreatic Cancer Research.

References

1. Attiyeh, M.A., Chakraborty, J., Doussot, A., Langdon-Embry, L., Mainarich, S., et al.: Survival prediction in pancreatic ductal adenocarcinoma by quantitative computed tomography image analysis. Ann. Surg. Oncol. **25**, 1034–1042 (2018)
2. Çiçek, Ö., Abdulkadir, A., Lienkamp, S.S., Brox, T., Ronneberger, O.: 3D U-Net: learning dense volumetric segmentation from sparse annotation. In: Ourselin, S., Joskowicz, L., Sabuncu, M.R., Unal, G., Wells, W. (eds.) MICCAI 2016. LNCS, vol. 9901, pp. 424–432. Springer, Cham (2016). https://doi.org/10.1007/978-3-319-46723-8_49

3. Dolz, J., Gopinath, K., Yuan, J., Lombaert, H., Desrosiers, C., Ayed, I.B.: HyperDense-Net: a hyper-densely connected CNN for multi-modal image segmentation. TMI **38**, 1116–1126 (2018)
4. Dou, Q., et al.: Automatic detection of cerebral microbleeds from MR images via 3D convolutional neural networks. TMI **35**(5), 1182–1195 (2016)
5. Kamnitsas, K., et al.: Efficient multi-scale 3D CNN with fully connected CRF for accurate brain lesion segmentation. arXiv
6. Li, Y., et al.: Multimodal hyper-connectivity of functional networks using functionally-weighted LASSO for MCI classification. Med. Image Anal. **52**, 80–96 (2019)
7. Long, J., Shelhamer, E., Darrell, T.: Fully convolutional networks for semantic segmentation. In: CVPR (2015)
8. Milletari, F., Navab, N., Ahmadi, S.: V-Net: fully convolutional neural networks for volumetric medical image segmentation. In: 3DV (2016)
9. Reaungamornrat, S., et al.: MIND demons: symmetric diffeomorphic deformable registration of MR and CT for image-guided spine surgery. TMI **35**(11), 2413–2424 (2016)
10. Ronneberger, O., Fischer, P., Brox, T.: U-Net: convolutional networks for biomedical image segmentation. In: Navab, N., Hornegger, J., Wells, W.M., Frangi, A.F. (eds.) MICCAI 2015. LNCS, vol. 9351, pp. 234–241. Springer, Cham (2015). https://doi.org/10.1007/978-3-319-24574-4_28
11. Roth, H.R., Lu, L., Farag, A., Sohn, A., Summers, R.M.: Spatial aggregation of holistically-nested networks for automated pancreas segmentation. In: Ourselin, S., Joskowicz, L., Sabuncu, M.R., Unal, G., Wells, W. (eds.) MICCAI 2016. LNCS, vol. 9901, pp. 451–459. Springer, Cham (2016). https://doi.org/10.1007/978-3-319-46723-8_52
12. Vercauteren, T., Pennec, X., Perchange, A., Ayache, N.: Diffeomorphic demons: efficient non-parametric image registration. NeuroImage **45**(1), S61–S82 (2009)
13. Yao, J., Zhu, X., Zhu, F., Huang, J.: Deep correlational learning for survival prediction from multi-modality data. In: Descoteaux, M., Maier-Hein, L., Franz, A., Jannin, P., Collins, D.L., Duchesne, S. (eds.) MICCAI 2017. LNCS, vol. 10434, pp. 406–414. Springer, Cham (2017). https://doi.org/10.1007/978-3-319-66185-8_46
14. Zhang, H., Cisse, M., Dauphin, Y.N., Lopez-Paz, D.: mixup: beyond empirical risk minimization. In: ICLR (2018)
15. Zhang, W., et al.: Deep convolutional neural networks for multi-modality isointense infant brain image segmentation. NeuroImage **108**, 214–224 (2015)
16. Zhu, W., et al.: AnatomyNet: deep learning for fast and fully automated whole-volume segmentation of head and neck anatomy. Med. Phys. **46**(2), 576–589 (2019)
17. Zhu, Z., Xia, Y., Xie, L., Fishman, E.K., Yuille, A.L.: Multi-scale coarse-to-fine segmentation for screening pancreatic ductal adenocarcinoma. arXiv (2018)

Statistical Intensity- and Shape-Modeling to Automate Cerebrovascular Segmentation from TOF-MRA Data

Shoujun Zhou[1], Na Li[1], Baochang Zhang[1], Cheng Wang[1],
Zonghan Wu[1], Jun Yang[2], and Aichi Chien[3](✉)

[1] Shenzhen Institutes of Advanced Technology, Chinese Academy of Sciences,
Beijing, China
[2] Guangzhou Special Service Recuperation Center of Rocket Force, PLA,
Beijing, China
[3] Department of Radiological Sciences,
David Geffen School of Medicine at UCLA, Los Angeles, USA
aichi@ucla.edu

Abstract. Complete, automatic, and fast segmentation of cerebrovascular Time-of-flight (TOF) Magnetic Resonance Angiography (MRA) is significant for the clinical application study, where vascular network coverage and accuracy are the focused issues. In our work, a novel statistical modeling method is proposed to efficiently improve the framework of Maximum a Posterior (MAP) and Markov Random Field (MRF), where the low-level process uses Gaussian mixture model to distinguish intensity information within the skull-stripped TOF-MRA data, and the high-level process embeds a new potential function of pair-wise sites into Markov neighborhood system (NBS). To explore vascular shape information in complex local context, the potential function employs vascular feature map and direction field. The Markov regularization parameter estimation is automated by using the machine-learning algorithm, which avoid the disadvantage of repeated trial-error-test to different data. This novel statistical model greatly improves segmentation accuracy and avoids vascular missing in the region of low contrast or low signal-to-noise ratio. Our experiments employ 109 public datasets from MIDAS data platform, in which 10 datasets is used to produce ground trues for quantitative validation. Existing statistical models are divided into 24 composite modes for cross comparisons, where the proposed strategy wins the best out of these modes on the evaluations.

Keywords: TOF-MRA · Cerebrovascular segmentation · Statistical modeling · MAP-MRF · Markov high-level model · Markov regularization parameter

This work was funded by the national NSFC (No. 81827805), and supported by the Key Laboratory of Health Informatics in Chinese Academy of Sciences, and also by Shenzhen Engineering Laboratory for Key Technology on Intervention Diagnosis and Treatment Integration.

D. Shen et al. (Eds.): MICCAI 2019, LNCS 11765, pp. 164–172, 2019.
https://doi.org/10.1007/978-3-030-32245-8_19

1 Introduction

Vascular disease diagnosis involves some medical imaging technologies. TOF-MRA is a non-invasive approach and widely used for clinical diagnosis of arteries and lesions [1]. For the cerebrovascular segmentation from TOF-MRA data, the model- and data-driven methods have been reviewed in [2, 3], which generally focused on scale analysis, deformation model, regional growth, statistical model, as well as the state-of-the-art deep-learning methods. These methods are generally affected by initial position deviation, artifacts and noise, and are high dependent on seed points or model parameters. The statistical models have received special attention so far, the popular ones [4–7] are still affected by exploring the finite mixture model (FMM) and its parameters, and cannot well cope with the variability of different imaging environments. In addition, their energy constraints are not sufficient to detect small-sized vessels or the main vascularity in low signal-to-noise ratio (SNR). Deep-learning methods [8, 9] realized the optimal segmentation on accuracy and completeness, while they are very hard to obtain vascular ground-truths (GT) by densely labeling on complex image context. Thus, a high-efficient statistical modeling is our main research motivation.

Related Works: The MAP-MRF framework [5–7] used FMM and neighborhood constraint as the low- and high-level models respectively. Given the observed data Y and Markov label field X, the framework realizes cerebrovascular segmentation with $p(X|Y) \propto p(Y|X)P(X)$, while the terms $p(Y|X)$ and $P(X)$ are modeled respectively as the Markov low- and high-level processes for data likelihood and data prior of the contextual information. Specifically, it is expressed as follows in a discrete mathematical way. The observed data on the lattice space $\Omega = \{s_n | n = 1, \ldots, N\}$ is modeled by FMM on $Y = \{y_s | s \in \Omega, y_s \in \mathcal{R}\}$, where y_s represents the intensity of voxel site s; while the high-level process models label field on the set $X = \{x_s | s \in \Omega, x_s \in \{L_V, L_B\}\}$ with L_V and L_B being the vessel and background classes. Based on MAP estimation [10], class label can be estimated by $x_s = argmax(p(x_s|y_s)) \propto argmax(p(y_s|x_s)p(x_s))$, and the class prior $P(x_s)$ is denoted as the Gibbs distribution with Hammersley-Clifford Theorem [10], i.e., $e^{-U(x_s)} / \sum_{x_s \in \{L_V, L_B\}} e^{-U(x_s)}$. The energy function $U(x_s)$ consists of low- and high-level energy forms, i.e., $U(x_s) = U_1(x_s) + U_2(x_s, x_{s'})$, and $s' \in \eta_s$ is the size of a neighborhood system (NBS). Existing low-level process used Rayleigh and Gaussian functions to construct the FMM [6, 7], where the model parameters were estimated by using the expectation maximization (EM) algorithm. Without loss of generality, there exists a negative correlation in between low-level energy and the likelihood probability for background and vessel class-labels, i.e.,

$$e^{-U_1(L_B)} \propto \frac{\sum_l w_l p_l(y_s; \theta_l)}{\sum_l w_l} \text{ with } l = 1, 2, 3, \text{ and } e^{-U_1(L_V)} \propto p_l(y_s; \theta_l) \text{ with } l = 4, \text{ where } \theta_l \text{ is}$$

the distribution parameter and the class proportions satisfy $\sum_l w_l = 1$. The high-level energy is the weighted sum of the potentials on pair-wise sites (PWS), i.e., $U_2(x_s, x_{s'}) = \sum_{s' \in \eta_s} \beta_c E(x_s, x_{s'})$ with regularization parameter β_c [7]. Traditional PWS-potential used the delta function [5–7] to calculate the PWS-potentials, i.e.,

$$E(x_s, x_{s'}) = 1 - \delta(x_s - x_{s'}), s' \in \eta_s \tag{1}$$

Unfortunately, that lead the existing high-level process only to remove the label-noise and keep the continuity of neighboring labels. With the cube size of $3 \times 3 \times 3$ voxels, the multi-pattern-NBS (MP-NBS) [7] generalized NBS energy by summing PWS-potentials on all of the patterns in clique-classes $c_{m,j}$ and minimizing the energy by

$$U_2(x_s, x_{s'}) = \min_m \left[\min_j \sum_{c_{m,j}} \beta_c E_{c_{m,j}}(x_s, x_{s'}) \right], j = 1, \cdots, N_{c_m}, m = 1, \cdots, M \tag{2}$$

where the traditional 6- and 26-NBSs are the particular cases of these patterns. Given f_{L_B} and f_{L_V} respectively the above two likelihood probabilities, Zhou et al. [7] expressed their posterior probabilities by using $p(L|y_s) \propto f_L \exp(-U_2(L, x_{s'}))$, $L = L_V$ or L_B. The site s is inferred as a vessel site when $p(L_V|y_s) - p(L_B|y_s) > 0$.

So far, the state-of-the-art statistical methods still face following limitations. The low-level process inevitably suffers from large fitting error of intensity-distribution in background region that occupies about 98% of original volume, thus may be impacted at the region of low contrast and/or low SNR. Another, their high-level process overly depends on the low-level one for initialization and iteration updating, and merely uses the summation of the delta functions based second order energy, like Eqs. (1)–(2), to denoise the label field. As a comparison, great difference on the results from between the traditional modeling strategies and ours is demonstrated in Fig. 1.

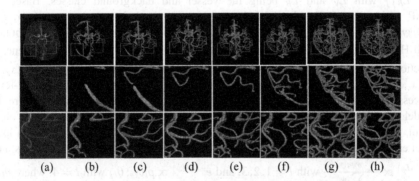

(a)   (b)   (c)   (d)   (e)   (f)   (g)   (h)

Fig. 1. Cerebrovascular segmentation results from TOF-MRA data by the existing statistical models and the proposed one. The 2nd and 3rd rows correspond to the yellow and blue boxes of the first row. (a) The maximum intensity projections (MIPs) of the raw data; (b)–(e) results by Lu et al.'s [5], Wen et al.'s [4], Hassouna et al.'s [6], and Zhou et al.'s [7]; (f) results by our low-level model, (g) results by our low- and high-level model. (h) the GTs.

2 Method

Our method steps contribute as: (1) preprocessing with skull-stripping and multi-scale filtering; (2) exerting a Gaussian mixture model (GMM) on the low-level process to generate intensity-based energy; (3) modeling the high-level process by using the vascular shape-prior PWS-potentials and NBS energy; (4) automating the regularization parameter estimation (RPE) by machine-learning algorithm.

2.1 Vascular Shape-Priors

The multiscale filtering [11] of the original data produces vessel Hessian characteristics. Given the original image intensity $I(s)$ at a site $s(x_1, x_2, x_3)$, the Hessian matrix is denoted by $H_\sigma(s) = \sigma^2 \partial^2 I_\sigma(s)/\partial x_i \partial x_j$ with dimensions $i, j = 1, 2, 3$; $I_\sigma(s)$ is the filtered result with Gaussian kernel at scale σ. The eigen-decomposed Hessian matrix has three eigenvalues $(\lambda_{1,\sigma}, \lambda_{2,\sigma}, \lambda_{3,\sigma}$ with $|\lambda_{1,\sigma}| \leq |\lambda_{2,\sigma}| \leq |\lambda_{3,\sigma}|)$ and the corresponding eigenvectors $(\vec{v}_{1,\sigma}, \vec{v}_{2,\sigma}, \vec{v}_{3,\sigma})$, where direction of $\vec{v}_{1,\sigma}$ indicates the direction locally parallel to the vascular ridge with minimum intensity variation. This filter responses to vascular ridges at different scales σ_k (with $k = 1, 2, \ldots$). The maximized response of each voxel is considered as the filter output and denoted by $\mathcal{V}(s)$ and the corresponding eigenvectors $\vec{v}_1(s)$ are obtained as the vascular feature map (VFM) and vascular direction field (VDF), as shown in Fig. 2 (right). Furthermore, the above vascular shape-prior features will be integrated with intensity distributions by our statistical modeling.

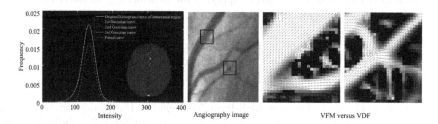

Fig. 2. (Left): Gaussian functions fit the intensity of skull-stripped TOF-MRA data. (Right): corresponding to the boxed regions in 2D original image, the VFMs are overlapped with VDFs.

2.2 Statistical Modeling with MAP-MRF

Without loss of generality, modeling cerebrovascular intensity distribution is greatly impacted by the fitting error in medium- and low-intensity range and also produces computational redundancy, while the skull-stripped intracranial area can stabilize the histogram fitting with Gaussian mixture model (GMM).

Low-Level Model. With skull-stripping algorithm [12], the resultant intensity distribution facilitates to divide the voxels of skull-stripping data into one vessel class (cerebral vasculature) and two background classes (brain tissues and cerebrospinal fluid). We use two Gaussian distributions to model the background classes, and another one for the vessel class, as shown in Fig. 2 (left). At each site s, the GMM of intensity value y_s is expressed as: $f_{GMM}(y_s) = \sum_{l=1}^{3} \frac{w_l}{\sqrt{2\pi}\sigma_l} exp\left(\frac{-(y_s-\mu_l)}{2\sigma_l^2}\right)$, where the parameters μ_l, σ_l, w_l ($l = 1, 2, 3$) are automatically estimated by K-means based pre-classification and parameter initialization and are followed by EM algorithm [7]. Note, the GMM does not involve shape-priors, while has the relation of $e^{-U_I(x_s)} \propto f_{GMM}(y_s)$ on the low-level energy $U_I(x_s)$ of vessel or background class.

High-Level Model. To segment vessels especially regain the latent vessels from low-contrast region, the VFM and VDF (as the shape-priors feature) are employed to construct the Markov high-level model. Unlike traditional PWS-potential in Eq. (1), a new one is pre-analyzed as follows. For the VDF, we denote PWS's direction vectors by $\vec{v}_1(s)$ and $\vec{v}_1(s')$ with $s' \in \eta_s$, the cosine of the angle between the two vectors is $\frac{\vec{v}_1(s)\cdot\vec{v}_1(s')}{|\vec{v}_1(s)||\vec{v}_1(s')|}$. Then, we get the first measure, namely, the normalized phase continuity of the two sites, which is denoted by $S_{s,s'} = 1 - \frac{|\vec{v}_1(s)\cdot\vec{v}_1(s')|}{|\vec{v}_1(s)||\vec{v}_1(s')|}$. For the VFM, we denote numerical difference of PWS-intensity by $\nabla V_{s,s'}$, and ∇V_{max} is the maximum value within the NBS, i.e., η_s. Then, we get the second measure, namely, normalized intensity smoothness of the PWS, which is expressed as $\nabla \mathcal{I}_{s,s'} = \frac{|\nabla V_{s,s'}|}{|\nabla V_{max}|}$. Combining the two measures, a compound measure of pair-wise sites is formed by using $\mathcal{E}_{s,s'} = \epsilon_1 \nabla \mathcal{I}_{s,s'} + \epsilon_2 S_{s,s'}$ with $\epsilon_1 + \epsilon_2 = 1$, where an average assignment will balance the two measures. Traditional minimum of the NBS energy with the PWS-potential of Eq. (1) only to regulate the label values at $x_s \neq x_{s'}$ that mainly situates in the edges of the vessels or the block-shaped structures. Applying the measure $\mathcal{E}_{s,r}$ to either edge (with $x_s \neq x_{s'}$) or background (with $x_s = x_{s'} = L_B$), a new PWS-potential is derived as

$$
\mathcal{P}(x_s, x_{s'}) = \begin{cases} 0 & x_s = x_{s'} = L_V \\ 1 - \mathcal{E}_{s,s'} & x_s = x_{s'} = L_B \\ \mathcal{E}_{s,s'} & x_s \neq x_{s'} \end{cases} \tag{3}
$$

where $x_s, x_{s'} \in \{L_V, L_B\}$. The new high-level NBS energy $U_{II}(x_s, x_{s'})$ can be derived from Eq. (2), when applying the potential $\mathcal{P}(x_s, x_{s'})$ to the MP-NBS. Different from Eqs. (1), (3) uses $\mathcal{E}_{s,s'}$ and $1 - \mathcal{E}_{s,s'}$ respectively at discontinuous edges and background to facilitate rerating the label field, thus improves vessel edges and regain the dim or slender vessels from low-contrast and/or low-SNR region.

Posterior Probability. Combining the above low- and high-level models with the MP-NBS, the new posterior probability is derived as

$$
x_s :\to f_{GMM}(y_s) \cdot exp(-U_{II}(x_s, x_{s'})) \tag{4}
$$

which combines the intensity information with vascular shape-priors, while the likelihood and prior probabilities is determined by the low- and high-level energy models $f_{GMM}(y_s)$ and $U_{II}(x_s, x_{s'})$ respectively. For Eq. (4), the iteration conditional mode [6, 10] and Bayesian rule [6, 7] can be used to iteratively solve a random field, namely, we infer that a site is the vessel site, if it meets $p(y_s|L_V)p(L_V) > p(y_s|L_B)p(L_B)$. The MRF process facilitates a global convergence within few iterations.

Regularization Parameter. Given a changeless constant β_c balancing the actions in between low- and high-level processes, Eq. (4) may produce uneven segmentation effects for individual data acquisitions. Thus, we estimate the parameter by using the maximum pseudo likelihood [10] with machine-learning, assuming that the spatial voxels meet homogeneous distribution. From an arbitrary initial label field (e.g., matrix zero), optimizing $\widehat{\beta}_c$ is to minimize the negative logarithm of the pseudo likelihood by

$$-ln\mathrm{PL}(x|\beta) = \sum_{s\in\Omega, s'\in\eta_s} \left[U_I(x_s) + U_{II}(x_s, x_{s'}) + \ln \sum_{x_s} \exp(-U_I(x_s) - U_{II}(x_s, x_{s'})) \right] \tag{5}$$

According to [7], a classical machine-learning process iteratively find the optimal $\widehat{\beta}_c$ through the gradient descent equation, i.e., $\beta_t = \beta_{t-1} + \gamma\nabla(ln\mathrm{PL}(x|\beta_{t-1}))$, with the step-size of γ and the negative gradient $-\nabla(ln\mathrm{PL}(x|\beta))$ derived as

$$\frac{\partial(ln\mathrm{PL}(x|\beta))}{\partial\beta} = \sum_{s\in\Omega} \left(\frac{f_{L_V}N_{L_V}e^{-\beta N_{L_V}} + f_{L_B}N_{L_B}e^{-\beta N_{L_B}}}{f_{L_V}e^{-\beta N_{L_V}} + f_{L_B}e^{-\beta N_{L_B}}} - \delta_{x_s-L_V}N_{L_V} - \delta_{x_s-L_B}N_{L_B} \right) \tag{6}$$

where the delta function $\delta_{x_s-L_V}$ produce 1 at $x_s = L_V$, the Gaussian functions f_{L_V} and f_{L_B} produce the conditional probability $p(y_s|L_V)$ and $p(y_s|L_B)$ for vessel- and background-class voxels respectively; the likelihood energies N_{L_V} and N_{L_B} are the derivatives of $U_2(x_s, x_{s'})$. Given an initial $\beta_0 = 0$, Eq. (6) is iteratively updated until β_t and $\nabla(-\ln PL(x|\beta_t))$ no longer change, then the obtained $\widehat{\beta}_c$ serves as a global parameter.

3 Experimental Results

To validate our algorithms of cerebrovascular segmentation, 109 sets of the public data (http://www.insight-journal.org/midas/community/view/21) of brain TOF-MRA were employed in the experiments. These datasets were acquired on a 3T MR unit, and the size of each volume was 128 slices of 448×448 voxels with voxel size of $0.5 \times 0.5 \times 0.8$ mm^3. We randomly selected 10 public datasets as training ones to produce their GTs, the remaining ones were for testing. The GTs were obtained by three neurosurgeons using MIMICS (i.e., the medical image processing software). The following experiments were carried out on a PC Inter(R) Core (TM) i7-4790 CPU @ 3.60 GHz, 24 GB-RAM; the main algorithms were coded by MATLAB 2018a; maximum connected regions of segmentation results were used for evaluations.

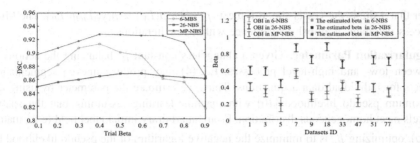

Fig. 3. Trial-error-test based PML-RPE verification on the training data. The left: for Normal001, three sets of DSCs on 6-, 26-, and MP-NBS are calculated with the candidate beta-values. The right: for 10 training datasets, i.e., Normal-001, -003, -005, -007, -009, -018, -033, -047, -051, -077, the estimated beta-values (colored points) all fall into the OBIs (colored line-segments). (Color figure online)

For the validation of RPE with different PWS-potentials, the gradient descent equation was applied to the training datasets. By using the trial-error-test, we took out 9 candidate beta-values uniformly from the interval [0, 1] to acquire segmentation results and the DSCs. Given β_T is the beta-value corresponding to the highest DSC, we can define the range $\beta_T \pm 0.05$ as the optimal beta-interval (OBI). Well, the results $\widehat{\beta}_c$ calculated by the PML on the training datasets were found all falling into the OBIs, as shown in Fig. 3, which facilitated to automate the RPE for testing datasets with individual statistical characteristics.

Our experiments consisted of cross validation of 24 composite modes with different low- and high-level models, as shown in Table 1. The cross-comparison was carried through in between their results and the corresponding GTs, where the Dice Similarity Coefficient (DSC) refers to $DSC = \frac{2TP}{2TP+FP+FN}$ with TP, FP and FN being the number of true positives, false positive, and false negative, respectively. Besides, clinical evaluation with the 99 testing datasets was proceeded through the observations of neurosurgeons. Their evaluation reports were divided into three-level cases, i.e. Good, general, and poor cases according to cerebrovascular network coverage, over-segmentation, and the percentage of pseudo-vascular structures. The visual effects of segmentation results from arbitrary 10 testing datasets were compared in Fig. 4.

Table 1. The DSCs and processing time (s) in cross validation of 24 composite modes.

Ref.	Low-level process without NBSs	Optimized high-level models with PWS-potential of Eq. (1) on the NBSs			Optimized high-level models with PWS-potential of Eq. (3) on the NBSs		
		6-NBS	26-NBS	MP-NBS	6-NBS	26-NBS	MP-NBS
[5]	.66 ± .06, 23	.51 ± .05, 35	.39 ± .06, 33	.52 ± .05, 49	.68 ± .06, 36	.68 ± .06, 46	.77 ± .08, 108
[4]	.49 ± .10, 19	.48 ± .09, 30	.48 ± .09, 31	.49 ± .09, 44	.50 ± .10, 33	.49 ± .10, 42	.50 ± .10, 105
[6, 7]	.77 ± .07, 22	.74 ± .07, 33	.70 ± .05, 34	.76 ± .07, 47	.77 ± .08, 36	.76 ± .08, 48	.77 ± .07, 107
Ours	.89 ± .03, 17	.84 ± .03, 28	.79 ± .03, 27	.85 ± .03, 41	.91 ± .02, 31	.91 ± .03, 40	.93 ± .02, 103

Note: each space in the table expresses the DSCs as mean value ± standard deviation and the average process times.

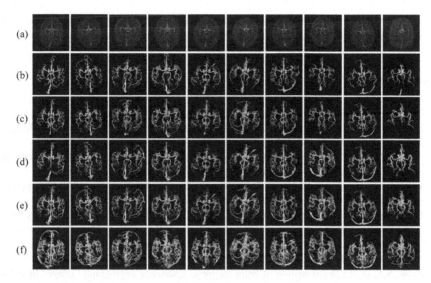

Fig. 4. Segmentation results from ten testing datasets (Normal-010, -017, -019, -021, -012, -013, -020, -022, -011, -029) by using five methods. The first row represents the MIPs of the raw datasets (a), while the segmentation results are shown in (b) by Lu's [5], (c) by Wen's [4], (d) by Hassouna's [6], (e) by Zhou's [7], and (f) by ours.

4   Discussion and Conclusions

Cerebrovascular segmentation and manual annotation from TOF-MRA dataset is a very hard and complicated work, which has to deal with a large number of personalized datasets and vast local environments with low-contrast or -SNR. Thus, we implemented cross-validation and numerical assessments on only 10 TOF-MRA datasets that have corresponding GTs by our manual annotation. In Table 1, the MP-NBS generates the highest DSC than other NBSs, while its computation time is longer, therefore, the statistical modeling with better calculation cost performance is to use GMM fitting skull-stripped data and use the shape-prior PWS-potential on the 6-NBS. Through qualitative comparison, Fig. 4 illustrates that all the methods show similar performance on the segmentation of the large size vessel or in high contrast region, while the proposed strategy greatly improves the segmentation effect of the small size vessel in low contrast region, e.g., Figure 4(f). According to the neurosurgeons, the proposed model performs well on most of the 99 testing datasets and is better than the other traditional models. For the RPE, we found that the estimated $\widehat{\beta}_c$ all fall into the OBIs corresponding to the maximum DSCs, see Fig. 3. For the model-driven methods, our statistical modeling has obtained the best effect among the existing ones that had been reported to win out the level set method in [5, 7].

Summarily, cerebrovascular segmentation from TOF-MRA data is of great significance, and also an open study so far. Our GMM and the optimized PWS-potential improves the traditional low- and high-level models on skull-tripped TOF-MRA data, and produces higher DSCs and better cerebrovascular network coverage. Such a novel statistical modeling strategy develops current MAP-MRF framework, and realizes the vascular segmentation with better accuracy, completeness, and computation speed.

References

1. Lin, A., et al.: Cerebrovascular imaging: which test is best? Neurosurgery **83**(1), 5–18 (2017)
2. Lesage, D., et al.: A review of 3D vessel lumen segmentation techniques: models, features and extraction schemes. Med. Image Anal. **13**(6), 819–845 (2009)
3. Moccia, S., et al.: Blood vessel segmentation algorithms — review of methods, datasets and evaluation metrics. Comput. Methods Programs Biomed. **158**, 71–91 (2018)
4. Wen, L., et al.: A novel statistical cerebrovascular segmentation algorithm with particle swarm optimization. Neurocomputing **148**, 569–577 (2015)
5. Lu, P., et al.: A vessel segmentation method for multi-modality angiographic images based on multi-scale filtering and statistical models. Biomed. Eng. Online **15**(1), 120 (2016)
6. Hassouna, M.S., et al.: Cerebrovascular segmentation from TOF using stochastic models. Med. Image Anal. **10**(1), 2–18 (2006)
7. Zhou, S.J., et al.: Segmentation of brain magnetic resonance angiography images based on MAP-MRF with multi-pattern neighborhood system and approximation of regularization coefficient. Med. Image Anal. **17**(8), 1220–1235 (2013)
8. Phellan, R., Peixinho, A., Falcão, A., Forkert, N.D.: Vascular segmentation in TOF MRA images of the brain using a deep convolutional neural network. In: Cardoso, M.J., et al. (eds.) LABELS/CVII/STENT -2017. LNCS, vol. 10552, pp. 39–46. Springer, Cham (2017). https://doi.org/10.1007/978-3-319-67534-3_5
9. Zhao, F.J., et al.: Semi-supervised cerebrovascular segmentation by hierarchical convolutional neural network. IEEE Access **6**, 67841–67852 (2018)
10. Li, S.Z.: Markov Random Field Modeling in Image Analysis. Springer, Tokyo (2001). https://doi.org/10.1007/978-4-431-67044-5
11. Jerman, T., et al.: Enhancement of vascular structures in 3D and 2D angiographic images. IEEE Trans. Med. Imaging **35**(9), 2107–2118 (2016)
12. Smith, S.M., et al.: Advances in functional and structural MR image analysis and implementation as FSL. Neuroimage **23**, S208–S219 (2004)

Segmentation of Vessels in Ultra High Frequency Ultrasound Sequences Using Contextual Memory

Tejas Sudharshan Mathai[1][(✉)], Vijay Gorantla[2], and John Galeotti[1]

[1] The Robotics Institute, Carnegie Mellon University, Pittsburgh, PA 15213, USA
tmathai@andrew.cmu.edu
[2] Department of Surgery, Wake Forest Institute for Regenerative Medicine,
Winston-Salem, NC 27101, USA

Abstract. High resolution images provided by Ultra High Frequency Ultrasound (UHFUS) scanners permit the vessel-based measurement of the Intimal-Media Thickness (IMT) in small vessels, such as those in the hand. However, it is challenging to precisely determine vessels in UHFUS sequences due to severe speckle noise obfuscating their boundaries. Current level set-based approaches are unable to identify poorly delineated boundaries and are not robust against varying speckle noise. While recent neural network-based methods, including recurrent neural networks, have shown promise at segmenting vessel contours, they are application specific and do not generalize to datasets acquired from different scanners, such as a traditional High Frequency Ultrasound (HFUS) machine, with different scan settings. Our goal for a segmentation approach was the accurate localization of vessel contours, and generalization to new data within and across biomedical imaging modalities. In this paper, we propose a novel ultrasound vessel segmentation network (USVS-Net) architecture that assimilates features extracted at different scales using Convolutional Long Short Term Memory (ConvLSTM) and segments vessel boundaries accurately. We show the results of our approach on UHFUS and HFUS sequences. To show broader applicability beyond US, we also trained and tested our approach on a Chest X-Ray dataset. To the best of our knowledge, this is the first learning-based approach to segment deforming vessel contours in both UHFUS and HFUS sequences.

Keywords: Ultrasound · Vasculature · Segmentation · Deep learning

1 Introduction

Intima-Media Thickness (IMT) is a parameter that quantifies risk in clinical applications, such as atherosclerotic plaque buildup [1]. In particular however,

Electronic supplementary material The online version of this chapter (https:// doi.org/10.1007/978-3-030-32245-8_20) contains supplementary material, which is available to authorized users.

© Springer Nature Switzerland AG 2019
D. Shen et al. (Eds.): MICCAI 2019, LNCS 11765, pp. 173–181, 2019.
https://doi.org/10.1007/978-3-030-32245-8_20

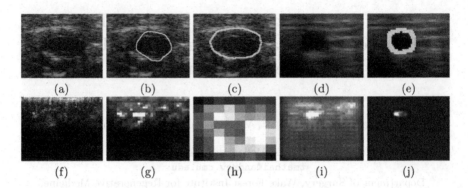

Fig. 1. (a) Still frame capturing a pulsating vessel acquired using UHFUS; (b) Segmentation (yellow contour) from a level set method [6] bleeds into the tissue region due to poor boundary contrast; (c) Final segmentation from the proposed USVS-Net; (d) Frame acquired using HFUS (zoomed), and (e) its associated final vessel segmentation; Activations of the network for the vessel imaged in (a) at different network depths: (f) downsampling level 1; (g) downsampling level 3; (h) downsampling level 5; (i) upsampling level 3; (j) upsampling level 1.

it can be used to track the functional progress of hand transplant recipients, where the gold standard for monitoring changes is currently histopathology [2]. Recently, Ultra-High Frequency Ultrasound (UHFUS) has been shown to quantitatively measure IMT through the resolution of vessel structures at 0.03 mm within a shallow tissue depth of ~1 cm [1]. However, this improved resolution is traded-off with an increase in speckle noise corrupting the vessel boundaries, which is in contrast to traditional ultrasound and high frequency ultrasound (HFUS) machines [1]. Furthermore, vessels at shallow depths contort themselves significantly (due to transducer pressure and motion) as opposed to vessels deeper in the body, such as the carotid artery [3,4]. Therefore, the key motivation of this work is the sub-mm localization of rapidly moving and pulsating vessel contours in UHFUS and HFUS sequences to compare changes in IMT over time.

Prior vessel-based segmentation approaches for ultrasound sequences fall into two categories: traditional and learning-based methods. Traditional approaches, such as state-of-the-art level set methods for HFUS and UHFUS [5,6], are quick to execute, but lack robustness needed in clinical use due to the fine-tuning of parameters. In contrast, learning-based approaches are resilient to changes in scan settings and variations in image quality. In particular, Convolutional Neural Networks (CNNs) [3,4] have made great strides in integrating features extracted at multiple scales through feature forwarding [7], residual learning [8], dilated convolutions [9] etc. However, these methods segment longitudinal vessels in ultrasound videos, and are task specific without adequately harnessing inter-frame vessel dynamics. Long Short Term Memory (LSTM) networks [10–15] intelligently combine multi-scale features to retain relevant features over video time steps, and only update the features when required. Some of these approaches have shown applicability to microscopy [10], X-Ray [11] etc. We tested the performance of these Convolutional LSTM (ConvLSTM) methods on the challenging task of segmenting highly deformable vessel contours in UHFUS and HFUS sequences. However, they did not accurately segment vessel cross-sections (see supplementary material). An ideal approach would accurately segment boundaries, while generalizing to data within and across biomedical imaging modalities.

In this paper, we propose a novel ConvLSTM-based ultrasound vessel segmentation network called USVS-Net to segment transverse vessel cross-sections in UHFUS and HFUS sequences. This network was influenced by methods designed for different anatomies (retina [16], cornea [17], microscopy [10], X-Ray [11]). Validation of our method was conducted on 38 UHFUS and 6 HFUS sequences respectively.

Contribution. (1) We propose a novel USVS-Net architecture that outperforms current ConvLSTM networks on vessel segmentation tasks. (2) To gauge the potential broader applicability of our work to other biomedical domains, we trained and tested our method on the Montgomery County Chest X-Ray dataset [18] with comparable results to the state-of-the-art [11].

2   Methods

As seen in Fig. 2, the proposed USVS-Net design is comprised of two sections: a downsampling encoder and a ConvLSTM-based decoder. Our network design is different from the traditional U-Net [7] based segmentation models, which treat each frame in a sequence independently. ConvLSTM-based models implement a memory mechanism [10–15] that considers the inter-relation between video frames to retain vessel appearance over multiple scales for dense pixel-wise predictions. By combining the ConvLSTM in the decoder with the spatial context gathered in the encoder, spatio-temporal vessel-related features are estimated for improved segmentation.

Encoder. The encoder structure is inspired by the approaches in [16,17], which have shown applicability to retina and cornea tissue interface segmentation. The blocks in the encoder pull out meaningful representations of the vessel appearance over multiple scales using dilated convolutions [9] and residual connections [8]. As shown in Fig. 1, the feature maps characterized at the first few layers of the encoder depict finely defined properties (edges, corners etc.), which are low-level attributes, and are limited due to their smaller receptive field. At the deeper layers of the network, coarse, but complex attributes are seen with poorly defined contours. At this level, more of the image is seen on a global scale due to the larger receptive field. Residual connections and dilated convolutions gather more spatial information, especially relating to faintly discernible boundaries [17], and inculcate this information from one block to the next to prevent holes in the final segmentation. Yet, this hierarchical representation is not enough on its own to model the dynamics of vessel movement in a video sequence. By forwarding the feature maps extracted at different scales to the ConvLSTM cells, which can retain relevant features of interest in memory, they can be integrated to produce segmentations of better quality and precision [10,11].

Decoder. Every encoder block forwards its output feature maps to a ConvLSTM unit in the decoder section. In this work, we incorporate the structured LSTM proposed in [12]. These LSTM cells consider the output of each encoder block as a single time step, and implement a memory mechanism wherein the features extracted at multiple scales are integrated in a coarse-to-fine manner. This is done by gating structures that carefully regulate the removal or addition of new information to the cell state. In this manner, global contextual information from the deepest encoder layer is observed by the LSTM unit first, and as the receptive fields are reduced, finer details about the vessel contour are added.

From Fig. 2, each LSTM unit uses three feature sets (input, hidden, and cell), and outputs information using three gates: forget, input, and output. The forget gate removes information from the cell state. The input gate determines the new information that will be incorporated into the cell state. Finally, the output of the LSTM unit is regulated by the output gate. Contrary to [12],

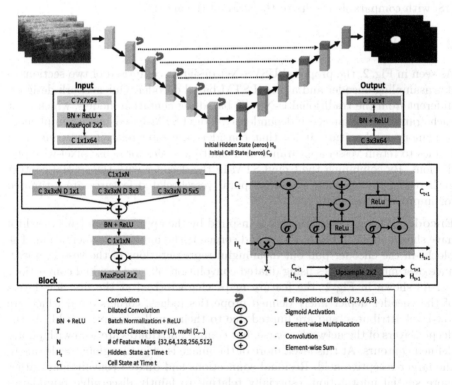

Fig. 2. The USVS-Net architecture contains encoding (purple) and decoding (green) sections. The encoder uses of residual connections and dilated convolutions to extract features, while the decoder uses structured ConvLSTM blocks to retain vessel shape attributes and segment the vessel. (Color figure online)

bi-directional LSTMs were not used in this work as our video sequences can be of arbitrary length with non-smooth vessel motion between consecutive frames, c.f. Fig. 3, making their implementation impractical. We employed convolution in the structured LSTM unit, and replaced the tanh operation with a ReLU as we empirically observed an improved segmentation accuracy. Similar to [11], the initial hidden and cell states were set to zero, and the hidden and cell states of the other LSTM units were upsampled from the LSTM unit below (see Fig. 2).

3   Experiments and Results

Data. Previously acquired (free-hand) deidentified video sequences from an existing research database [2, 6] were used in this work, and they came from two scanners: a Visualsonics Vevo 2100 UHFUS machine (Fujifilm, Canada), and a Diasus HFUS scanner (Dynamic Imaging, UK). The UHFUS scanner provided a 50 MHz transducer with physical resolution of 30 μm and a pixel spacing of 11.6 μm. 58 UHFUS sequences were used, each containing 100 2D B-scans with dimensions of 832×512 pixels. The HFUS scanner had a 10–22 MHz transducer with a pixel spacing of 92.5 μm. 26 HFUS sequences were used, each containing a variable number of 2D B-scans (50–250) with dimensions of 280×534 pixels. All the sequences contained arteries of the hand (eg. superficial palmar arch) with a wide range of adjustable gain settings (40–70 dB). Extensive probe motions were also acquired, such as longitudinal scanning, beating vessels, out-of-plane vessel deformation etc. An expert grader annotated all the 84 UHFUS and HFUS sequences. To show general applicability, we also retrained and tested our architecture on the Montgomery County Chest X-Ray dataset [18], which contained 138 annotated images with 58 abnormal and 80 normal cases.

Setup. Of the 58 UHFUS sequences, 20 were chosen for training and the remaining 38 were used for testing. Similarly, from the 26 HFUS sequences, 20 were chosen for training and the remaining 6 were used for testing. We ran a 3-fold cross-validation for the vessel segmentation task. To simulate a clinical application, an ensemble of the two best models with the lowest validation loss (from a single fold) were used for testing. Similar to [11], we also ran a 3-fold cross validation for the lung segmentation task in the CXR dataset.

Baseline Comparisons. For the vessel segmentation task, we compared our errors against those from a level set-based method [6], and two LSTM-based segmentation approaches: DecLSTM [10] and CFCM34 [11]. For the lung segmentation task, we compared against the state-of-the-art CFCM34 model [11].

Training. Our sequences contained variable image sizes and training a ConvLSTM with full-sized images is limited by GPU RAM. We trained our USVS-Net by scaling each B-scan to 256×256 pixels. Data augmentation (elastic deformation, blurring etc.) was done to increase the training set to ∼120,000 images. To compare against [11], we used the generalized dice coefficient [11] loss with the ADAM optimizer [19], and set the batch size to 16 with a learning rate of 0.00001 for 30 epochs. The final pixel level probabilities were classified using the

Table 1. Segmentation error comparison for the UHFUS (top) and HFUS (bottom) sequences. (* 33/38 sequences successful)

Method	DSC	HD (mm)	MAD (mm)	DFPD	DFND	Prec	Rec
Traditional* [6]	81.13 ± 3.72	0.21 ± 0.05	0.06 ± 0.02	**3.08 ± 1.68**	8.71 ± 0.55	**96.44 ± 2.56**	72.03 ± 4.9
DecLSTM [10]	88.83 ± 3.74	0.15 ± 0.06	0.04 ± 0.03	6.76 ± 1.05	**5.35 ± 1.4**	87.54 ± 4.45	92.46 ± 3.93
CFCM34 [11]	88.45 ± 3.97	0.15 ± 0.07	0.04 ± 0.04	6.41 ± 1.21	5.51 ± 1.39	88.07 ± 4.83	91.31 ± 3.87
USVS-Net	**92.15 ± 2.29**	**0.11 ± 0.03**	**0.03 ± 0.01**	6.83 ± 1.13	6.33 ± 1.36	**91.76 ± 3.78**	**93.2 ± 3.34**
Traditional [6]	83.6 ± 5.47	0.47 ± 0.13	0.08 ± 0.04	**2.08 ± 2.01**	6.02 ± 0.51	**95.13 ± 4.8**	75.42 ± 7.49
DecLSTM [10]	88.34 ± 5.21	0.39 ± 0.1	0.05 ± 0.3	4.23 ± 0.97	5.61 ± 0.78	87.21 ± 3.15	83.94 ± 7.61
CFCM34 [11]	89.44 ± 3.34	0.36 ± 0.09	0.05 ± 0.02	3.74 ± 1.04	5.23 ± 0.62	94.21 ± 3.48	85.74 ± 5.51
USVS-Net	**89.74 ± 3.05**	**0.36 ± 0.08**	**0.04 ± 0.02**	4.98 ± 0.86	**4.53 ± 1.03**	88.63 ± 0.05	**91.52 ± 0.05**

Table 2. Segmentation error comparison (pixels) for the Montgomery County Chest X-Ray dataset.

Method	DSC	HD	MAD	DFPD	DFND	Prec	Rec
CFCM34 [11]	**97.01 ± 1.82**	11.05 ± 10.78	0.13 ± 0.31	6.67 ± 0.97	**6.39 ± 0.98**	96.93 ± 2.42	**97.25 ± 2.67**
USVS-Net	96.89 ± 1.80	**10.29 ± 8.26**	**0.10 ± 0.19**	**6.64 ± 0.89**	6.73 ± 1.04	**97.15 ± 1.65**	96.57 ± 2.97

softmax function, and the connected component in the foreground class was considered the segmentation. For the DecLSTM [10], we used RMSProp optimizer [10], weighted cross-entropy loss [7], and a learning rate of 0.0001 for 30 epochs.

Metrics. We compared each baseline's results against the expert annotation. The following metrics were calculated to quantify errors: (1) Dice Similarity Coefficient (DSC) [6], (2) Hausdorff Distance (HD) in millimeters [6], (3) Mean Absolute Deviation (MAD) in millimeters [11], (4) Definite False Positive and Negative Distances (DFPD, DFND) [6], (5) Precision (Prec.) and (6) Recall (Rec.) [11]. Videos and additional visualizations are provided in the supplementary material that detail the results of vessel segmentation in UHFUS and HFUS sequences.

4   Discussion

UHFUS Results. Our primary assumption was that a vessel would be present in every frame of the video sequence. From Table 1 (top), the traditional level set approach only succeeded in segmenting vessels in 33 of 38 sequences, while the LSTM-based methods successfully segmented vessels in all sequences. The proposed USVS-Net matched the expert annotations with the highest DSC, and lowest HD and MAD errors among all baselines. We estimated the statistical significance of our results using paired t-tests for every baseline, and determined that our results were statistically significant ($p < 0.05$) for all metrics except DFPD. Our largest HD error of 0.14 mm was ~15× lower than the largest observed vessel diameter of 2.17 mm. Similarly, the average HD error was ~10× lower than the smallest observed vessel diameter of 1.1 mm. Although our method slightly over-segmented the boundaries (outer adventitia) as evidenced

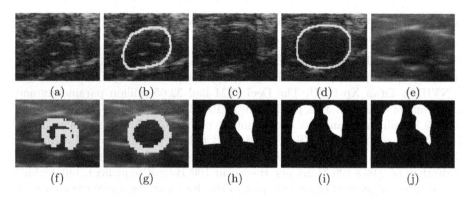

Fig. 3. (a) Frame 152 in a UHFUS sequence showing a completely contracted vessel, and (b) its associated segmentation; (c) Next frame 153 in the same sequence showing a patent vessel, and (d) its segmentation; (e) Zoomed view of a HFUS B-scan (gain set to maximum); (f) Segmentation by the CFCM34 [11] and (g) our segmentation result; (h) Ground truth lung segmentation from the CXR dataset; (i) Result from CFCM34, and (j) our result (note the improved segmentation due to better contextual information).

by the highest DFPD score, the low clinically relevant measures of HD and MAD were acceptable. Our primary intention for the USVS-Net was to segment vessels in UHFUS sequences, and through our results, we satisfactorily hit our target of sub-mm vessel localization in UHFUS sequences presenting with increased speckle, and large vessel motion.

HFUS Results. As seen in Table 1 (bottom), the performance of the CFCM34 and the USVS-Net is comparable. The USVS-Net edges out the CFCM34 with a higher DSC score, along with lower HD, MAD, and DFND errors, and a higher recall rate. We postulate that this is due to lower speckle and clearer contrast along the vessel boundaries. Again, we conducted paired t-tests to assess the statistical significance of our results, and report that the results were statistically significant ($p < 0.05$) for all metrics except DFPD and Precision. The largest HD error of 0.45 mm was ∼9.5× smaller than the largest observed vessel diameter of 4.35 mm, while the average HD error was ∼8× lower in contrast to the smallest vessel diameter of 2.9 mm. We note that the CFCM34 can be a useful alternative for clinical use in HFUS images, for which CFCM34 and USVS-Net could both be run (and results compared) for improved segmentation.

Chest X-Ray Results. To show the broader applicability of our approach to other biomedical imaging modalities, we took our network designed for UHFUS vessel segmentation, retrained, and validated it on CXR images. As seen in Table 2, the errors between the CFCM34 and the USVS-Net are comparable. CFCM34 has a higher DSC, lower DFND, and a higher recall rate, while we achieve slightly lower HD and MAD errors, lower DFPD and higher precision. As seen in Fig. 3, the dilated convolutions in the USVS-Net provide the utility of incorporating regions excluded by the CFCM34 in the final segmentation. The increased contextual information available at the deepest layers of the network allowed it to segment the lung regions better.

Performance. The network training and testing was performed using Tensorflow on a desktop using a 3.5 GHz Intel i7 processor, 16 GB DDR3 RAM, and a NVIDIA Titan Xp GPU. The DecLSTM had 32.65 million parameters and a runtime of 5.83 s (58.3 ms per B-scan in 100 B-scan sequence). The CFCM34 had 49.16 million parameters and a runtime of 8.45 s (84.5 ms per B-scan in 100 B-scan sequence). The USVS-Net had 64.34 million parameters and a runtime of 9.95 s (99.5 ms per B-scan in 100 B-scan sequence). The level set method had a runtime of 2.03 s (20.31 ms per B-scan in 100 B-scan sequence), but yielded less accurate segmentations in contrast to the deep learning approaches. Testing was done with an ensemble of two models with the lowest validation loss.

5   Conclusion and Future Work

In this paper, we proposed a novel architecture called the USVS-Net that segmented transverse vessel cross-sections in challenging UHFUS and HFUS sequences. The performance of the USVS-Net surpasses current state-of-the-art ConvLSTM-based architectures on UHFUS sequences presenting with highly deformable vessels, but the CFCM34 is also a viable clinical alternative to USVS-Net for HFUS video segmentation. We have also shown broader applicability of our approach to a Chest X-Ray dataset. To the best of our knowledge, this is the first work targeting the segmentation of rapidly deforming vessels in UHFUS and HFUS sequences. In the future, we plan to embed a level set-based framework in a ConvLSTM-based architecture.

Acknowledgements. These awards helped us in gathering data and designing initial algorithms: NIH 1R01EY021641, DOD awards W81XWH-14-1-0371 and W81XWH-14-1-0370, NVIDIA Corporation GPU donations, Carnegie Mellon Center for Machine Learning in Health (CMLH). Patent pending, US 62/860,392.

References

1. Mohler III, E.R., et al.: High frequency ultrasound for evaluation of intimal thickness. J. Am. Soc. Echocardiogr. **22**(10), 1129–1133 (2009)
2. Gorantla, V., et al.: Acute and chronic rejection in upper extremity transplantation: what have we learned? Hand Clin. **27**(4), 481–493 (2011)
3. Menchon-Lara, R.M., et al.: Fully automatic segmentation of ultrasound common carotid artery images based on machine learning. Neurocomputing **151**(1), 161–167 (2015)
4. Shin, J.Y., et al.: Automating carotid intima-media thickness video interpretation with convolutional neural networks. In: CVPR, pp. 2526–2535 (2016)
5. Chaniot, J., et al.: Vessel segmentation in high-frequency 2D/3D ultrasound images. In: IEEE International Ultrasonics Symposium, pp. 1–4 (2016)

6. Mathai, T.S., Jin, L., Gorantla, V., Galeotti, J.: Fast vessel segmentation and tracking in ultra high-frequency ultrasound images. In: Frangi, A.F., Schnabel, J.A., Davatzikos, C., Alberola-López, C., Fichtinger, G. (eds.) MICCAI 2018. LNCS, vol. 11073, pp. 746–754. Springer, Cham (2018). https://doi.org/10.1007/978-3-030-00937-3_85

7. Ronneberger, O., Fischer, P., Brox, T.: U-Net: convolutional networks for biomedical image segmentation. In: Navab, N., Hornegger, J., Wells, W.M., Frangi, A.F. (eds.) MICCAI 2015. LNCS, vol. 9351, pp. 234–241. Springer, Cham (2015). https://doi.org/10.1007/978-3-319-24574-4_28

8. He, K., et al.: Deep residual learning for image recognition. In: IEEE CVPR, pp. 770–778 (2016)

9. Koltun, V., et al.: Multi-scale context aggregation by dilated convolutions. In: ICLR (2016)

10. Arbelle, S., et al.: Microscopy cell segmentation via convolutional LSTM networks. In: IEEE ISBI, pp. 1008–1012 (2019)

11. Milletari, F., Rieke, N., Baust, M., Esposito, M., Navab, N.: CFCM: segmentation via coarse to fine context memory. In: Frangi, A.F., Schnabel, J.A., Davatzikos, C., Alberola-López, C., Fichtinger, G. (eds.) MICCAI 2018. LNCS, vol. 11073, pp. 667–674. Springer, Cham (2018). https://doi.org/10.1007/978-3-030-00937-3_76

12. Gao, Y., et al.: Fully convolutional structured LSTM networks for joint 4D medical image segmentation. In: IEEE ISBI, pp. 1104–1108 (2018)

13. Zhang, D., et al.: A multi-level convolutional LSTM model for the segmentation of left ventricle myocardium in infarcted porcine cine MR images. In: IEEE ISBI, pp. 470–473 (2018)

14. Zhao, C., et al.: Predicting tongue motion in unlabeled ultrasound videos using convolutional LSTM neural network. In: IEEE ICASSP, pp. 5926–5930 (2019)

15. Basty, N., Grau, V.: Super resolution of cardiac cine MRI sequences using deep learning. In: Stoyanov, D., et al. (eds.) RAMBO/BIA/TIA -2018. LNCS, vol. 11040, pp. 23–31. Springer, Cham (2018). https://doi.org/10.1007/978-3-030-00946-5_3

16. Apostolopoulos, S., De Zanet, S., Ciller, C., Wolf, S., Sznitman, R.: Pathological OCT retinal layer segmentation using branch residual U-shape networks. In: Descoteaux, M., Maier-Hein, L., Franz, A., Jannin, P., Collins, D.L., Duchesne, S. (eds.) MICCAI 2017. LNCS, vol. 10435, pp. 294–301. Springer, Cham (2017). https://doi.org/10.1007/978-3-319-66179-7_34

17. Mathai, T.S., et al.: Learning to segment corneal tissue interfaces in OCT images. In: IEEE ISBI, pp. 1432–1436 (2019)

18. Jaeger, S., et al.: Two public chest X-ray datasets for computer-aided screening of pulmonary diseases. Quant. Imaging Med. Surg. 4(6), 475–477 (2014)

19. Kingma, D., et al.: Adam: a method for stochastic optimization. In: ICLR (2015)

Accurate Esophageal Gross Tumor Volume Segmentation in PET/CT Using Two-Stream Chained 3D Deep Network Fusion

Dakai Jin[1($\boxtimes$)], Dazhou Guo[1], Tsung-Ying Ho[2($\boxtimes$)], Adam P. Harrison[1], Jing Xiao[3], Chen-kan Tseng[2], and Le Lu[1]

[1] PAII Inc., Bethesda, MD, USA
jindakai376@paii-labs.com
[2] Chang Gung Memorial Hospital, Linkou, Taiwan, ROC
tyho@cgmh.org.tw
[3] Ping An Technology, Shenzhen, China

Abstract. Gross tumor volume (GTV) segmentation is a critical step in esophageal cancer radiotherapy treatment planning. Inconsistencies across oncologists and prohibitive labor costs motivate automated approaches for this task. However, leading approaches are only applied to radiotherapy computed tomography (RTCT) images taken prior to treatment. This limits the performance as RTCT suffers from low contrast between the esophagus, tumor, and surrounding tissues. In this paper, we aim to exploit both RTCT and positron emission tomography (PET) imaging modalities to facilitate more accurate GTV segmentation. By utilizing PET, we emulate medical professionals who frequently delineate GTV boundaries through observation of the RTCT images obtained after prescribing radiotherapy and PET/CT images acquired earlier for cancer staging. To take advantage of both modalities, we present a two-stream chained segmentation approach that effectively fuses the CT and PET modalities via early and late 3D deep-network-based fusion. Furthermore, to effect the fusion and segmentation we propose a simple yet effective progressive semantically nested network (PSNN) model that outperforms more complicated models. Extensive 5-fold cross-validation on 110 esophageal cancer patients, the largest analysis to date, demonstrates that both the proposed two-stream chained segmentation pipeline and the PSNN model can significantly improve the quantitative performance over the previous state-of-the-art work by 11% in absolute Dice score (DSC) (from 0.654 ± 0.210 to 0.764 ± 0.134) and, at the same time, reducing the Hausdorff distance from 129 ± 73 mm to 47 ± 56 mm.

1 Introduction

Esophageal cancer ranks sixth in mortality amongst all cancers worldwide, accounting for 1 in 20 cancer deaths [1]. Because this disease is typically diagnosed at late stages, the primary treatment is a combination of chemotherapy

© Springer Nature Switzerland AG 2019
D. Shen et al. (Eds.): MICCAI 2019, LNCS 11765, pp. 182–191, 2019.
https://doi.org/10.1007/978-3-030-32245-8_21

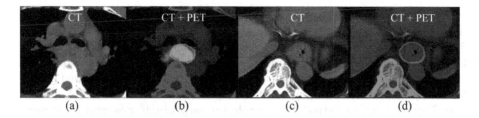

Fig. 1. Esophageal GTV examples in CT and PET images, where the green line indicates the GTV boundary. (a)–(b): although the GTV boundaries are hardly distinguishable in CT, it can be reasonably inferred with the help of the PET image, in spite of other false positive high-uptake regions. (c)–(d) here, no high uptake regions appear in PET; however, the esophagus wall enlargement evident in CT may indicate the GTV boundary [6].

and radiotherapy (RT). One of the most critical tasks in RT treatment planning is delineating the gross tumor volume (GTV), which serves as the basis for further contouring the clinical target volume [7]. Yet, manual segmentation consumes great amounts of time and effort from oncologists and is subject to inconsistencies [14]. Thus, there is great impetus to develop effective tools for automated GTV segmentation.

Deep convolutional neural networks (CNNs) have made remarkable progress in the field of medical image segmentation [2–4,8,9]. Yet, only a handful of studies have addressed automated esophageal GTV segmentation [15,16], all of which rely on only the radiotherapy computed tomography (RTCT) images. The assessment of GTV by CT has been shown to be error prone, due to the low contrast between the GTV and surrounding tissues [12]. Within the clinic these shortfalls are often addressed by correlating with the patient's positron emission tomography/computed tomography (PET/CT) scan, when available. These PET/CTs are taken on an earlier occasion to help stage the cancer and decide treatment protocols. Despite misalignments between the PET/CT and RTCT, PET still provide highly useful information to help manually delineate the GTV on the RTCT, due to its high contrast highlighting of malignant regions [11]. As shown in Fig. 1, CT and PET can each be crucial for accurate GTV delineation, due to their complementary strengths and weaknesses. While recent work has explored co-segmentation of tumors using PET and CT [17,18], these works only consider the PET/CT image. In contrast, leveraging the diagnostic PET to help perform GTV segmentation on an RTCT image requires contending with the unavoidable misalignments between the two scans acquired at different times.

To address this gap, we propose a new approach, depicted in Fig. 2, that uses a two-stream chained pipeline to incorporate the joint RTCT and PET information for accurate esophageal GTV segmentation. First, we manage the misalignment between the RTCT and PET/CT by registering them via an anatomy-based initialization. Next, we introduce a two-stream chained pipeline that combines and merges predictions from two independent sub-networks, one only trained using the RTCT and one trained using both RTCT and registered PET images. The former exploits the anatomical contextual information in CT, while the latter takes advantage of PET's sensitive, but sometimes spurious and overpoweringly strong contrast. The predictions of these two streams are then deeply fused together with the original RTCT to provide a final robust GTV prediction. Furthermore, we introduce a simple yet surprisingly powerful progressive semantically nested network (PSNN) model, which incorporates the strengths of both UNet [2] and P-HNN [3] by using deep supervision to progressively propagate high-level semantic features to lower-level, but higher resolution features. Using 5-fold cross-validation, we evaluate the proposed approach on 110 patients with RTCT and PET, which is more than two times larger than the previously largest reported dataset for esophageal GTV segmentation [15]. Experiments demonstrate that both our two-stream chained pipeline and the PSNN each provide significant performance improvements, resulting in an average Dice score (DSC) of $76.4\% \pm 13.4\%$, which is 11% higher over the previous state-of-the-art method using DenseUNet [15].

2   Methods

Figure 2 depicts an overview of our proposed two-stream chained esophageal GTV segmentation pipeline, which uses early and late 3D deep network fusions of CT and PET scans. Not shown is the registration step, which is detailed in Sect. 2.1.

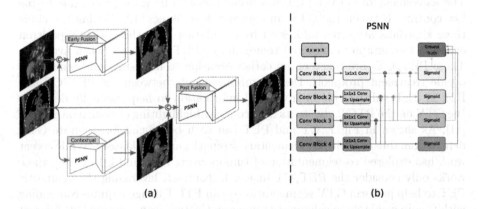

Fig. 2. (a) depicts our two-stream chained esophageal GTV segmentation method consisting of early fusion (EF) and late fusion (LF) networks, while (b) illustrates the PSNN model, which employs deep supervision at different scales within a parameterless high-to-low level image segmentation decoder. The first two and last two blocks are composed of two and three $3 \times 3 \times 3$ convolutional+BN+ReLU layers, respectively.

2.1   PET to RTCT Registration

To generate aligned PET/RTCT pairs, we register the former to the latter. This is made possible by the diagnostic CT accompanying the PET. To do this, we apply the cubic B-spline based deformable registration algorithm in a coarse to fine multi-scale deformation process [13]. We choose this option due to its good capacity for shape modeling and efficiency in capturing local non-rigid motions. However, to perform well, the registration algorithm must have a robust rigid initialization to manage patient pose and respiratory differences in the two CT scans. To accomplish this, we use the lung mass centers from the two CT scans as the initial matching positions. We compute mass centers from masks produced by the P-HNN model [3], which can robustly segment the lung field even in severely pathological cases. This leads to a reliable initial matching for the chest and upper abdominal regions, helping the success of the registration. The resulting deformation field is then applied to the diagnostic PET to align it to the RTCT at the planning stage. One registration example is illustrated in Fig. 3.

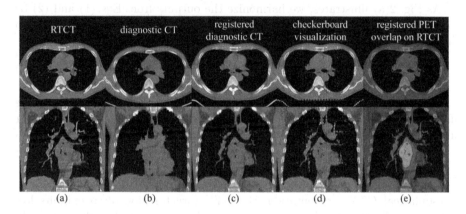

Fig. 3. Deformable registration results for a patient shown in axial and coronal views. (a) shows the RTCT image; (b, c) depicts the diagnostic CT image before and after the registration, respectively; (d) depicts a checkerboard visualization of the RTCT and registered diagnostic CT images; and (e) overlays the PET image, transformed using the diagnostic CT deformation field, on top of the RTCT.

2.2   Two-Stream Chained Deep Fusion

As mentioned, we aim to effectively exploit the complementary information within the PET and CT imaging spaces. To do this, we design a two-stream chained 3D deep network fusion pipeline. Assuming N data instances, we denote the training data as $S = \left\{ \left(X_n^{\text{CT}}, X_n^{\text{PET}}, Y_n \right) \right\}_{n=1}^{N}$, where X_n^{CT}, X_n^{PET}, and Y_n represent the input CT, registered PET, and binary ground truth GTV segmentation images, respectively. For simplicity and consistency, the same 3D segmentation backbone network (described in Sect. 2.3) is adopted. Dropping n for clarity, we first use two separate streams to generate segmentation maps using X^{CT} and $[X^{\text{CT}}, X^{\text{PET}}]$ as network input channels:

$$\hat{y}_j^{\text{CT}} = p_j^{\text{CT}} \left(y_j = 1 | X^{\text{CT}}; \mathbf{W}^{\text{CT}} \right), \tag{1}$$

$$\hat{y}_j^{\text{EF}} = p_j^{\text{EF}} \left(y_j = 1 | X^{\text{CT}}, X^{\text{PET}}; \mathbf{W}^{\text{EF}} \right), \tag{2}$$

where $p_j^{(\cdot)}(\cdot)$ and $\hat{y}_j^{(\cdot)}$ denote the CNN functions and output segmentation maps, respectively, $\mathbf{W}^{(\cdot)}$ represents the corresponding CNN parameters, and y_j indicates the ground truth GTV tumor mask values. We denote Eq. (2) as early fusion (EF), as the stream can be seen as an EF of CT and PET, enjoying the high spatial resolution and high tumor-intake contrast properties from the CT and PET, respectively. On the other hand, the stream in Eq. (1) provides predictions based on CT intensity alone, which can be particularly helpful in circumventing the biased influence from noisy non-malignant high uptake regions, which are not uncommon in PET.

As Fig. 2(a) illustrates, we harmonize the outputs from Eqs. (1) and (2) by concatenating them together with the original RTCT image as the inputs to a third network:

$$\hat{y}_j^{\text{LF}} = p_j^{\text{LF}} \left(y_j = 1 | X^{\text{CT}}, \hat{Y}^{\text{CT}}, \hat{Y}^{\text{EF}}; \mathbf{W}^{\text{CT}}, \mathbf{W}^{\text{EF}}, \mathbf{W}^{\text{LF}} \right). \tag{3}$$

In this way, the formulation of Eq. (3) can be seen as a late fusion (LF) of the aforementioned two streams of the CT and EF models. We use the DSC loss for all three sub-networks, training each in isolation.

2.3   PSNN Model

In esophageal GTV segmentation, the GTV target region often exhibits low contrast in CT, and the physician's manual delineation relies heavily upon high-level semantic information to disambiguate boundaries. In certain respects, this aligns with the intuition behind UNet, which decodes high-level features into lower-level space. Nonetheless, the decoding path in UNet consumes a great deal of parameters, adding to its complexity. On the other hand, models like P-HNN [3] use deep supervision to connect lower and higher-level features together using parameter-less pathways. However, unlike UNet, P-HNN propagates lower-level features <u>down</u> to high-level layers. Instead, a natural and simple means to combine the strengths of both P-HNN and UNet is to use essentially the same parameter blocks as P-HNN, but reverse the direction of the deeply-supervised pathways, to allow high-level information to propagate <u>up</u> to lower-level space. We denote such an approach as progressive semantically nested network (PSNN).

As shown in Fig. 2(b), a set of $1 \times 1 \times 1$ 3D convolutional layers are used to collapse the feature map after each convolutional block into a logit image, $i.e.,$ $\tilde{f}_j^{(\ell)}$, where j indexes the pixel locations. This is then combined with the previous

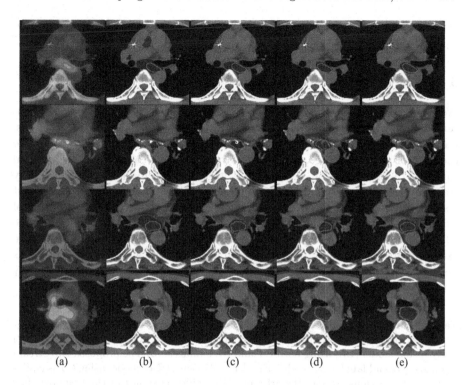

Fig. 4. Qualitative results of esophageal GTV segmentation. (a) RTCT overlayed with the registered PET channel; (b) GTV segmentation results using RTCT images with DenseUNet [15]; (c) Our results using Eq. (1), *i.e.*, RTCT-only stream using the proposed PSNN model; (d) Our results using Eq. (2) with PSNN, *i.e.*, EF of PET+RTCT images; (e) Our final GTV segmentation using Eq. (3) with PSNN, *i.e.*, EF and LF of PET+RTCT images. Red masks indicate automated segmentation results and green boundaries represent the ground truth. The first two rows demonstrate the importance of PET as using RTCT alone can cause under- or over-segmentation due to low contrast. The last two rows show cases where under- or over-segmentation can occur when the PET imaging channel is spuriously noisy. In all cases, the final EF+LF based GTV segmentation results achieve good accuracy and robustness. (Color figure online)

higher level segmentation logit image to create an aggregated segmentation map, *i.e.*, $f_j^{(\ell)}$, for the ℓth feature block by element-wise summation:

$$f_j^{(m)} = \tilde{f}_j^{(m)}, \tag{4}$$

$$f_j^{(\ell)} = \tilde{f}_j^{(\ell)} + g\left(f_j^{(\ell+1)}\right), \forall \ell \in \{m-1, \cdots, 1\}, \tag{5}$$

where m denotes the total number of predicted feature maps and $g(\cdot)$. denotes an upsampling, *i.e.*, bilinear upsampling. The PSNN model is trained using four deeply-supervised auxiliary losses at each convolutional block. As our experiments will demonstrate, PSNN can provide significant performance gains for

GTV segmentation over both a densely connected version of UNet [15] and P-HNN [3].

3 Experiments and Results

We extensively evaluate our approach using a dataset of 110 esophageal cancer patients, all diagnosed at stage II or later and undergoing RT treatments. Each patient has a diagnostic PET/CT pair and a treatment RTCT scan. To the best of our knowledge, this is the largest dataset collected for esophageal cancer GTV segmentation. All 3D GTV ground truth masks are delineated by two experienced radiation oncologists during routine clinical workflow. We first resample all imaging scans of registered PET and RTCT to a fixed resolution of $1.0 \times 1.0 \times 2.5$ mm. To generate positive training instances, we randomly sample $80 \times 80 \times 64$ sub-volumes centered inside the ground truth GTV mask. Negative examples are extracted by randomly sampling from the whole 3D volume. This results, on average, in 80 training sub-volumes per patient. We further apply random rotations in the x-y plane within $\pm 10°$ to augment the training data.

Table 1. Mean DSCs, HDs, and ASD_{GT}, and their standard deviations of GTV segmentation performance using: (1) Contextual model using only CT images (CT); (2) Early fusion model (EF) using both CT and PET images; (3) The proposed two-stream chained early and late fusion model (EF+LF). 3D DenseUNet model using CT is equivalent to the previous state-of-the-art work [15], which is shown in the first row. The best performance scores are shown in **bold**.

	CT	EF	EF+LF	DSC	HD (mm)	ASD_{GT} (mm)
3D DenseUNet	✓			0.654 ± 0.210	129.0 ± 73.0	5.2 ± 12.8
		✓		0.710 ± 0.189	116.0 ± 81.7	4.9 ± 10.3
			✓	0.745 ± 0.163	79.5 ± 70.9	4.7 ± 10.5
3D P-HNN	✓			0.710 ± 0.189	86.2 ± 67.4	4.3 ± 5.3
		✓		0.735 ± 0.158	57.9 ± 61.1	3.6 ± 3.7
			✓	0.755 ± 0.148	$\mathbf{47.2 \pm 52.3}$	3.8 ± 4.8
3D PSNN	✓			0.728 ± 0.158	66.9 ± 59.2	4.2 ± 5.4
		✓		0.758 ± 0.136	67.0 ± 59.1	$\mathbf{3.2 \pm 3.1}$
			✓	$\mathbf{0.764 \pm 0.134}$	$\mathbf{47.1 \pm 56.0}$	3.2 ± 3.3

Implementation Details: The Adam solver [10] is used to optimize all the 3D segmentation models with a momentum of 0.99 and a weight decay of 0.005 for 40 epochs. For testing, we use 3D sliding windows with sub-volumes of $80 \times 80 \times 64$ and strides of $48 \times 48 \times 32$ voxels. The probability maps of sub-volumes are aggregated to obtain the whole volume prediction.

We employ five-fold cross-validation protocol split at the patient level. Extensive comparisons of our PSNN model versus P-HNN [3] and DenseUNet [15] methods are reported, with the latter arguably representing the current state-of-the-art GTV segmentation approach using CT. Three quantitative metrics are utilized to evaluate the GTV segmentation performance: DSC, Hausdorff distance (HD) in "mm", and average surface distance with respect to the ground truth contour (ASD_{GT}) in "mm".

Results: Our quantitative results and comparisons are tabulated in Table 1. When all models are trained and evaluated using only RTCT, *i.e.*, Eq. (1), our proposed PSNN evidently outperforms the previous best esophageal GTV segmentation method, *i.e.*, DenseUNet [15], which straightforwardly combines DenseNet [5] and 3D UNet [2]. As can be seen, PSNN consistently improves upon [15] in all metrics: with an absolute increase of 7.4% in DSC (from 0.654 to 0.728) and significantly dropping in HD metric, despite being a simpler architecture. PSNN also outperforms the 3D version of P-HNN [3], which indicates that the semantically-nested high- to low-level information flow provides key performance increases.

Table 1 also outlines the performances of three deep models under different imaging configurations. Several conclusions can be drawn. First, all three networks trained using the EF of Eq. (2) consistently produce more accurate segmentation results than those trained with only RTCT, *i.e.*, Eq. (1). This validates the effectiveness of utilizing PET to complement RTCT for GTV segmentation. Second, the full two-stream chained fusion pipeline of Eq. (3) provides further performance improvements. Importantly, the performance boosts can be observed across all three deep CNNs, validating that the two-stream combination of EF and LF can universally improve upon different backbone segmentation models. Last, the best performing results are the PSNN model combined with chained EF+LF, demonstrating that each component of the system contributes to our final performance. When compared to the previous state-of-the-art work of GTV segmentation, which uses DenseUNet applied to RTCT images [15], our best performing model exceeds in all metrics of DSC, HD, and ASD_{GT} by 11%, 81.9 mm and 2.0 mm remarked margins (refer to Table 1), representing tangible and significant improvements. Figure 4 shows several qualitative examples visually underscoring the improvements that our two-stage PSNN approach provides.

4   Conclusion

This work has presented and validated a two-stream chained 3D deep network fusion pipeline to segment esophageal GTVs using both RTCT and PET+RTCT imaging channels. Diagnostic PET and RTCT are first longitudinally registered using semantically-based lung-mass center initialization to achieve robustness. We next employ the PSNN model as a new 3D segmentation architecture, which uses a simple, parameter-less, and deeply-supervised CNN decoding stream. The PSNN model is then used in a cascaded EF and LF scheme to segment the GTV. Extensive tests on the largest esophageal dataset to date demonstrate that our PSNN model can outperform the state-of-the-art P-HNN and DenseUNet networks with remarked margins. Additionally, we show that our 2-stream chained fusion pipeline produces further important improvements, providing an effective means to exploit the complementary information seen within PET and CT. Thus, our work represents a step forward toward accurate and automated esophageal GTV segmentation.

References

1. Bray, F., Ferlay, J., et al.: Global cancer statistics 2018: globocan estimates of incidence and mortality worldwide for 36 cancers in 185 countries. CA: A Cancer J. Clin. **68**(6), 394–424 (2018)
2. Çiçek, Ö., Abdulkadir, A., Lienkamp, S.S., Brox, T., Ronneberger, O.: 3D U-net: learning dense volumetric segmentation from sparse annotation. In: Ourselin, S., Joskowicz, L., Sabuncu, M.R., Unal, G., Wells, W. (eds.) MICCAI 2016. LNCS, vol. 9901, pp. 424–432. Springer, Cham (2016). https://doi.org/10.1007/978-3-319-46723-8_49
3. Harrison, A.P., Xu, Z., George, K., Lu, L., Summers, R.M., Mollura, D.J.: Progressive and multi-path holistically nested neural networks for pathological lung segmentation from CT images. In: Descoteaux, M., Maier-Hein, L., Franz, A., Jannin, P., Collins, D.L., Duchesne, S. (eds.) MICCAI 2017. LNCS, vol. 10435, pp. 621–629. Springer, Cham (2017). https://doi.org/10.1007/978-3-319-66179-7_71
4. Holger, R., Lu, L., Lay, N., et al.: Spatial aggregation of holistically-nested convolutional neural networks for automated pancreas localization and segmentation. Med. Image Anal. **45**, 94–107 (2018)
5. Huang, G., Liu, Z., van der Maaten, L., Weinberger, K.Q.: Densely connected convolutional networks. In: IEEE CVPR, pp. 2261–2269 (2017)
6. Iyer, R., Dubrow, R.: Imaging of esophageal cancer. Cancer Imaging **4**(2), 125 (2004)
7. Jin, D., Guo, D., Ho, T.Y., et al.: Deep esophageal clinical target volume delineation using encoded 3D spatial context of tumor, lymph nodes, and organs at risk. In: Shen, D., et al. (eds.) MICCAI 2019. LNCS, vol. 11765, pp. xx–yy. Springer, Heidelberg (2019)
8. Jin, D., Xu, Z., Harrison, A.P., George, K., Mollura, D.J.: 3D convolutional neural networks with graph refinement for airway segmentation using incomplete data labels. In: Wang, Q., Shi, Y., Suk, H.-I., Suzuki, K. (eds.) MLMI 2017. LNCS, vol. 10541, pp. 141–149. Springer, Cham (2017). https://doi.org/10.1007/978-3-319-67389-9_17
9. Jin, D., Xu, Z., Tang, Y., Harrison, A.P., Mollura, D.J.: CT-realistic lung nodule simulation from 3D conditional generative adversarial networks for robust lung segmentation. In: Frangi, A.F., Schnabel, J.A., Davatzikos, C., Alberola-López, C., Fichtinger, G. (eds.) MICCAI 2018. LNCS, vol. 11071, pp. 732–740. Springer, Cham (2018). https://doi.org/10.1007/978-3-030-00934-2_81
10. Kingma, D.P., Ba, J.: Adam: a method for stochastic optimization. arXiv:1412.6980 (2014)
11. Leong, T., Everitt, C., et al.: A prospective study to evaluate the impact of FDG-PET on CT-based radiotherapy treatment planning for oesophageal cancer. Radiother. Oncol. **78**(3), 254–261 (2006)
12. Muijs, C., Schreurs, L., et al.: Consequences of additional use of pet information for target volume delineation and radiotherapy dose distribution for esophageal cancer. Radiother. Oncol. **93**(3), 447–453 (2009)

13. Rueckert, D., Sonoda, L.I., Hayes, C.J., et al.: Nonrigid registration using free-form deformations: application to breast MR images. IEEE TMI **18**(8), 712–721 (1999)

14. Tai, P., Van Dyk, J., Yu, E., et al.: Variability of target volume delineation in cervical esophageal cancer. Int. J. Radiat. Oncol. Biol. Phys. **42**(2), 277–288 (1998)

15. Yousefi, S., et al.: Esophageal gross tumor volume segmentation using a 3D convolutional neural network. In: Frangi, A.F., Schnabel, J.A., Davatzikos, C., Alberola-López, C., Fichtinger, G. (eds.) MICCAI 2018. LNCS, vol. 11073, pp. 343–351. Springer, Cham (2018). https://doi.org/10.1007/978-3-030-00937-3_40

16. Hao, Z., Liu, J., Liu, J.: Esophagus tumor segmentation using fully convolutional neural network and graph cut. In: Jia, Y., Du, J., Zhang, W. (eds.) CISC 2017. LNEE, vol. 460, pp. 413–420. Springer, Singapore (2018). https://doi.org/10.1007/978-981-10-6499-9_39

17. Zhao, X., Li, L., et al.: Tumor co-segmentation in PET/CT using multi-modality fully convolutional neural network. Phys. Med. Biol. **64**(1), 015011 (2019)

18. Zhong, Z., Kim, Y., et al.: Simultaneous cosegmentation of tumors in PET-CT images using deep fully convolutional networks. Med. Phys. **46**(2), 619–633 (2019)

Mixed-Supervised Dual-Network for Medical Image Segmentation

Duo Wang[1,2], Ming Li[3], Nir Ben-Shlomo[4], C. Eduardo Corrales[4,5], Yu Cheng[6], Tao Zhang[1], and Jagadeesan Jayender[2,5(✉)]

[1] Department of Automation, Tsinghua University, Beijing, China
[2] Department of Radiology, Brigham and Women's Hospital, Boston, USA
[3] Department of Radiology and Radiation Oncology,
Huadong Hospital affiliated to Fudan University, Shanghai, China
[4] Department of Surgery, Brigham and Women's Hospital, Boston, USA
[5] Harvard Medical School, Boston, USA
jayender@bwh.harvard.edu
[6] Microsoft AI & Research, Redmond, WA, USA

Abstract. Deep learning based medical image segmentation models usually require large datasets with high-quality dense segmentations to train, which are very time-consuming and expensive to prepare. One way to tackle this difficulty is using the mixed-supervised learning framework, where only a part of data is densely annotated with segmentation label and the rest is weakly labeled with bounding boxes. The model is trained jointly in a multi-task learning setting. In this paper, we propose Mixed-Supervised Dual-Network (MSDN), a novel architecture which consists of two separate networks for the detection and segmentation tasks respectively, and a series of connection modules between the layers of the two networks. These connection modules are used to transfer useful information from the auxiliary detection task to help the segmentation task. We propose to use a recent technique called 'Squeeze and Excitation' in the connection module to boost the transfer. We conduct experiments on two medical image segmentation datasets. The proposed MSDN model outperforms multiple baselines.

Keywords: Mixed-supervised learning · Dual-network · Multi-task learning · Squeeze-and-Excitation · Medical image segmentation

1 Introduction

Image segmentation is an important application of medical image analysis. Recently, deep learning based methods [1–4] have achieved remarkable success in many medical image segmentation tasks, such as brain tumor and lung nodule segmentation. However, all these methods require a large amount of training data with high-quality dense annotations to train, which is very expensive and time-consuming to prepare.

© Springer Nature Switzerland AG 2019
D. Shen et al. (Eds.): MICCAI 2019, LNCS 11765, pp. 192–200, 2019.
https://doi.org/10.1007/978-3-030-32245-8_22

Therefore, weakly-supervised segmentation with insufficient labels, e.g. image tags [5] or bounding boxes [6] has attracted a lot of attention recently. Although great progress has been made, there still exists some gap in performance compared to the models trained with fully-supervised datasets. This makes it impractical for the medical image scenario, where accurate segmentation maps are required for disease diagnosis, surgical planning or pathological analysis. On the other hand, these weakly-supervised models are usually trained in multi-step iteration mode [5,6] or with prior medical knowledge [7], making it difficult to be scalable on real applications.

Another promising approach is the mixed-supervised segmentation, where only a part of data is densely annotated with segmentation map and the rest is labeled with weak form (such as with bounding boxes). Typical existing methods [8,14,15] consider training with such kind of data in a multi-task learning setting and exploit multi-stream network, where basic feature extractor is shared and different streams are used for data with different annotation forms. The work in [15] focuses on the optimal balance between the number of annotations needed for different supervision types and presents a budget-based cost-minimization framework in a mixed-supervision setting.

In this paper, we propose a novel architecture for mixed-supervised medical image segmentation. Considering the bounding boxes as weak annotation, our method takes the segmentation task as target task, which is augmented with object detection task (auxiliary task). Different from the multi-stream structure with shared backbone [8], our new architecture is made up of two separate networks for each task. The two networks are linked by a series of connection modules that lie between the corresponding layers. These connection modules take as input the convolution features of detection network and transfer useful information to the segmentation network to help the training of the segmentation task. We propose to use a recent feature attention technique called "Squeeze and Excitation" [9,10,13] in the connection module to boost the information transfer. The proposed model is named as Mixed-Supervised Dual-Network (MSDN). We perform evaluation on the lung nodule segmentation and the cochlea segmentation of CT images. Experimental results show that our model is able to outperform multiple baselines in both datasets.

2   Methods

2.1   Squeeze and Excitation

"Squeeze-and-Excitation" (SE) was first introduced in [9] and can be flexibly integrated in any CNN model. The SE module first squeezes the feature map by global average pooling and then passes the squeezed feature to the gating module to get the representation of channel-wise dependencies, which is used to recalibrate the feature map to emphasize on useful channels. The work in [10] refers to the SE module in [9] as Spatial Squeeze and Channel Excitation (cSE) and proposes a different version called Channel Squeeze and Spatial Excitation (sSE). The sSE module squeezes the feature map along channels to preserve more spatial information, thus is more suitable for image segmentation task. The two SE modules mentioned above are unary, as both the squeeze and excitation are operated on the same feature map. Roy *et al.* [13] builds a binary version of sSE and applies it to their two-armed architecture for few-shot segmentation. Since the sSE module is related to our method, we will give a more detailed introduction as follows (see Fig. 1).

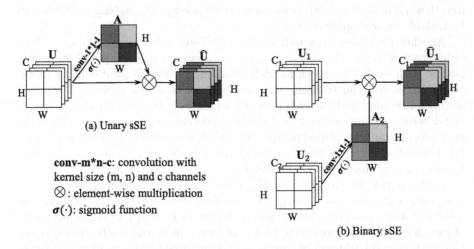

(a) Unary sSE

conv-m*n-c: convolution with kernel size (m, n) and c channels
⊗: element-wise multiplication
$\sigma(\cdot)$: sigmoid function

(b) Binary sSE

Fig. 1. Illustration of the Channel Squeeze and Spatial Excitation (sSE) architecture of Unary form (a) and Binary form (b).

We consider the feature map $\mathbf{U} = [\mathbf{u}^1, \mathbf{u}^2, ..., \mathbf{u}^C]$ from previous convolution layer as the input of the Unary sSE module and $\boldsymbol{u}^i \in \mathbb{R}^{W \times H}$ denotes its ith channel. The channel squeeze operation is achieved by 1×1 convolution with kernel weight $\mathbf{w}_{sq} \in \mathbb{R}^{1 \times C \times 1 \times 1}$. The squeezed feature is then passed through sigmoid function to derive the attention weight $\mathbf{A} \in \mathbb{R}^{W \times H}$. Then each feature channel of $\mathbf{U}$ is multiplied element-wise by $\mathbf{A}$ to get the spatially recalibrated feature $\widehat{\mathbf{U}}$ as output

$$\widehat{\mathbf{U}} = [\sigma(\mathbf{w}_{sq} * \mathbf{U}) \circ \mathbf{u}^1, \sigma(\mathbf{w}_{sq} * \mathbf{U}) \circ \mathbf{u}^2, ..., \sigma(\mathbf{w}_{sq} * \mathbf{U}) \circ \mathbf{u}^C] \tag{1}$$

Here ∘ denotes the Hadamard product, * denotes the convolution operation and σ denotes the sigmoid function.

Binary sSE extends the idea of Unary sSE, which takes two feature maps as inputs. One feature map is squeezed and used to recalibrate the other feature as output

$$\widehat{\mathbf{U}}_1 = [\sigma(\mathbf{w}_{sq} * \mathbf{U}_2) \circ \mathbf{u}_1^1, \sigma(\mathbf{w}_{sq} * \mathbf{U}_2) \circ \mathbf{u}_1^2, ..., \sigma(\mathbf{w}_{sq} * \mathbf{U}_2) \circ \mathbf{u}_1^C] \tag{2}$$

We propose to use the Binary sSE module as the connection between our dual-network architecture for information extraction and transfer.

2.2   Architectural Design

Our MSDN follows the setting of multi-task learning and is made up of two separate subnetworks for the segmentation and detection tasks respectively (as shown in Fig. 2). Both subnetworks are built from the U-Net and contain 9 feature stages, with 4 stages in the Encoder, 4 in the Decoder and 1 in the Bottleneck. Each feature stage consists of 2 dilated-convolution layers with 3 * 3 kernel, each followed by batch normalization [12] and rectified linear unit (ReLU). The output of each Encoder stage is skip-connected to the corresponding Decoder stage to recover spatial information lost during maxpooling. Dilation factors are set as [1, 2, 2, 2, 4, 2, 2, 2, 1] in the 9 feature stages respectively. The stride and padding are chosen accordingly to make the size of the output feature identical to that of the input. For the segmentation subnetwork, the sSE modules are added after each stage in its Encoder and Bottleneck, which take the segmentation and detection features from the same stage as input, squeeze the detection feature and recalibrate the segmentation feature. In this way, the segmentation subnetwork can extract useful information from the auxiliary detection subnetwork to facilitate its training.

The Segmentation Unit (**SU**) takes the extracted features into a 1 * 1 convolution layer followed by a channel-wise softmax to output a dense segmentation map with $C + 1$ channels, where C is the number of segmentation classes and we treat the background as another class. Dice loss [2] is used for the segmentation subnetwork training.

For the detection subnetwork, we build the Detection Unit (**DU**) under a single-stage object-detection paradigm, similarly to [8, 11]. The **DU** consists of a classifier block and a bounding box regressor block and takes as input the convolution feature from the detection subnetwork and produces class predictions for C target classes and object locations via bounding boxes. Note that all features from the Decoder stages are used for detection and the parameters of **DU** are shared. At each position of the feature, totally $A = 9$ reference bounding boxes of different shapes and sizes are built as anchors. The **DU** predicts the class label (C-length vector) of the object and the relative position (4-length vector) to the near ground-truth bounding boxes for each of the A anchors. Thus, the classifier (regressor) takes the feature from the Decoder of the detection subnetwork through 4 3 * 3 convolution layers with 256 channels and one 3 * 3 convolution layer with $C * A (4 * A)$ channels. A sigmoid function is used to scale the output of classifier to [0, 1]. The detection loss is the sum of the cross-entropy based focal loss for classification and the regularized-L1 loss for location [11].

During training, we mix the strongly- and weakly-annotated data and shuffle them. At each training iteration, we randomly select a batch of data as the input to our model. The strongly-annotated data I_s goes through the Encoder of the detection and segmentation subnetworks and its segmentation features are recalibrated by the detection features for the Decoder to derive the segmentation loss. The weakly-annotated data I_w only goes through the detection subnetwork to get the detection loss. The sum of the segmentation loss and detection loss is minimized to train the model.

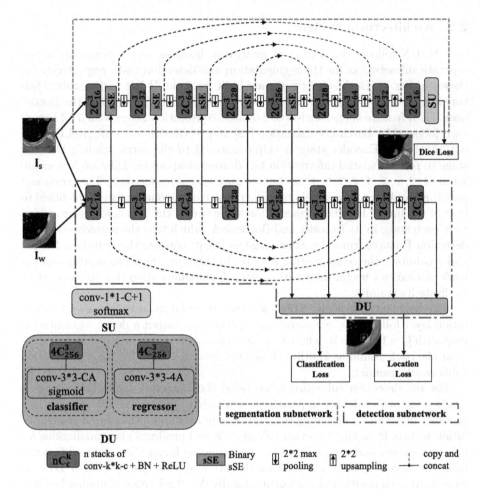

Fig. 2. Structure of Mixed-Supervised Dual-Network (MSDN).

The structure of our model is similar to that in [13], as we both build a dual architecture with two subnetworks and exploit sSE modules as connection. However, the work [13] focuses on the few-shot segmentation problem. The two subnetworks are used for the same segmentation task and trained jointly in the meta-learning mode. sSE modules exist in every feature stage of the base network. While, our model is designed for mixed-supervised segmentation problem, the two networks are used for different tasks and trained iteratively in multi-task learning mode. Because of that, the features of the two subnetworks in shallow layers may be relative to each other and those in deep layers may be task-specific. So we only use sSE in the shallow layers, specifically, in the Encoder and Bottleneck.

3   Experiments

We evaluate our model on two medical image segmentation datasets: lung nodule dataset and cochlea of inner ear dataset. The lung dataset consists of non-contrast CT of 320 nodules that was acquired on a 64-detector CT system (GE Light Speed VCT or GE Discovery CT750 HD, GE Healthcare, Milwaukee, WI, USA) using the scan parameters: section width, 1.25 mm; reconstruction interval, 1.25 mm; pitch, 0.984; 120 kV; and 35 mA; display field of view (DFOV) ranged from 28 cm to 36 cm; matrix size, 512 * 512, pixel size ranged from 0.55 mm to 0.7 mm. We randomly choose 160, 80 and 80 as training, validating and testing dataset. The inner ear dataset consisted of non-contrast temporal bone CT of 146 cochleas that was acquired on a Siemens Somatom scanner using the scan parameters: 120 kV; 167 mA, slice thickness, 1 mm; matrix size, 512 * 512, and pixel size, 0.40625. 66, 40 and 40 images are randomly split as training, validating and testing dataset. 5 different proportions of strongly-annotated data are tested. For both datasets, we measure the performance by the Dice score of target segmentation structure between the estimated and true label maps.

We use the Adam optimizer [17] to train all the models. The initial learning rate is set to 0.0001 and is reduced by a factor of 0.8 if the mean validation Dice score doesn't increase in 5 epochs. The training is stopped if the score doesn't increase by 20 epochs. Dropout [16] is used to the output of each convolution stage to avoid overfitting. During the training, we use a mini-batch of 4 images and if the validation Dice score goes up, we evaluate the model on the testing dataset. The best testing Dice score is reported as the final result. We perform data augmentation through random horizontal and vertical flipping, adding Gaussian noise and randomly cropping the image to a 128 * 128 patch centered around the target structure. All images are normalized by subtracting the mean and dividing by the standard deviation of the training data.

We compare **MSDN** with other 4 baselines, as shown in Table 1. All the models are trained following the same setting described aforementioned. A U-Net with the same number of convolution layers as the segmentation subnetwork of our model is used. For the **U-Net+Unary sSE**, Unary sSE module is added after every convolution stage. For the **Variant MS-Net**, we follow the thought of MS-Net [8] and build a multi-stream network based on U-Net, where all features from the Decoder are taken into the detection stream **DU**. We also compare to a reduced version of our model (**MSDN-**), where we remove the **DU** and only preserve the U-NET and the Binary sSE modules. Note that the **U-Net**, **U-Net+Unary sSE** and **MSDN-** are trained only with strongly-annotated data. We run each experiment repeatly for 3 times and the mean dice score with 95% confidence interval is listed in Table 1.

From the result, we can see that our model performs better than all the baselines in the same strong-weak data split. Compared with models trained in a fully-supervised manner, the performance is still comparable. When there are few strongly-annotated data for training, the performances of baselines decrease dramatically (see the last column). However, the performance of our model still remains good. The variation of MS-Net improves the results in some degree, but

Table 1. Mean of test Dice score (%).

Lung nodule segmentation					
Methods	Strong-weak data split (160 in total)				
	160-0	120-40	100-60	80-80	60-100
U-Net	84.04 ± 0.40	82.25 ± 0.39	81.85 ± 0.31	80.51 ± 0.59	80.18 ± 0.97
U-Net+Unary sSE	84.01 ± 0.11	82.15 ± 1.09	81.35 ± 1.39	82.08 ± 0.94	80.58 ± 0.01
Variant MS-Net[8]	-	82.75 ± 1.04	82.38 ± 0.53	81.72 ± 1.19	79.80 ± 1.26
MSDN-	**84.90 ± 0.60**	82.31 ± 1.14	82.17 ± 0.51	81.02 ± 1.10	80.50 ± 0.37
MSDN	-	**83.58 ± 1.20**	**83.56 ± 0.52**	**83.01 ± 0.69**	**82.37 ± 0.98**
Cochlea segmentation					
Methods	Strong-weak data split (66 in total)				
	66-0	44-22	33-33	22-44	11-55
U-Net	88.62 ± 0.08	87.41 ± 0.16	86.55 ± 0.81	85.01 ± 0.39	80.85 ± 0.42
U-Net+Unary sSE	**88.97 ± ± 0.12**	87.70 ± 0.49	85.30 ± 0.28	84.38 ± 0.03	82.23 ± 0.47
Variant MS-Net[8]	-	87.54 ± 0.36	86.03 ± 0.25	84.71 ± 0.53	82.60 ± 1.43
MSDN-	88.73 ± 0.33	86.73 ± 1.02	85.68 ± 0.35	85.10 ± 0.15	80.81 ± 0.47
MSDN	-	**87.91 ± 0.28**	**87.27 ± 1.08**	**87.11 ± 0.28**	**85.60 ± 1.76**

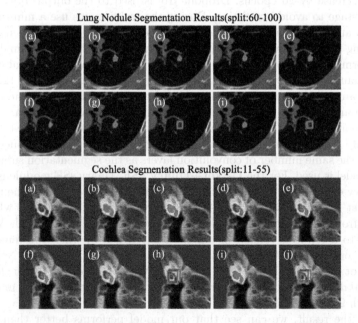

Fig. 3. (a) Original image. (b) Ground truth. (c) U-Net trained in full-supervised manner. (d) U-Net trained with only strongly-annotated data. (e) U-Net+Unary sSE. (f) MSDN-. (g),(h) Segmentation and detection results of Variant MS-Net. (i),(j) Segmentation and detection results of MSDN.

sometimes the performance is not stable. In contrast, our model works more stably. The use of sSE module, no matter Unary or Binary, could improve the training effect, but not as much as our model, which proves the effectiveness of our design. Some qualitative results are shown in Fig. 3.

4   Conclusion and Future Work

We propose Mixed-Supervised Dual-Network (MSDN), a novel multi-task learning architecture for mixed-supervised medical image segmentation. It is composed of two separate networks for the detection and segmentation tasks respectively, and a series of sSE modules as connection between the two networks so that the useful information of the detection task can be transferred to facilitate the segmentation task well. We perform experiments on two medical image datasets and our model outperforms multiple baselines. Currently, our model can only handle two-task problem. When there are more than two forms of annotations, our model can not directly be applied. In the future, we may consider to extend our method to fit for multi-task scenario [18,19].

Acknowledgement. This project was supported by the National Institute of Biomedical Imaging and Bioengineering of the National Institutes of Health through Grant Numbers P41EB015898 and R01EB025964, and China Scholarship Council (CSC). Unrelated to this publication, Jayender Jagadeesan owns equity in Navigation Sciences,Inc. He is a co-inventor of a navigation device to assist surgeons in tumor excision that is licensed to Navigation Sciences. Dr. Jagadeesan's interests were reviewed and are managed by BWH and Partners HealthCare in accordance with their conflict of interest policies.

References

1. Ronneberger, O., Fischer, P., Brox, T.: U-net: convolutional networks for biomedical image segmentation. In: Navab, N., Hornegger, J., Wells, W.M., Frangi, A.F. (eds.) MICCAI 2015. LNCS, vol. 9351, pp. 234–241. Springer, Cham (2015). https://doi.org/10.1007/978-3-319-24574-4_28
2. Milletari, F., Navab, N., Ahmadi, S.: V-net: fully convolutional neural networks for volumetric medical image segmentation. In: International Conference on 3D Vision, pp. 565–571 (2016)
3. Jiang, J., Hu, Y.C., Liu, C.J., et al.: Multiple resolution residually connected feature streams for automatic lung tumor segmentation from CT images. IEEE Trans. Med. Imaging **38**(1), 134–144 (2019)
4. Fan, G., Liu, H., Wu, Z., et al.: Deep learning-based automatic segmentation of lumbosacral nerves on CT for spinal intervention: a translational study. Am. J. Neuroradiol. **40**(6), 1074–1081 (2019)
5. Wang, X., You, S., Li, X., Ma, H.: Weakly-supervised semantic segmentation by iteratively mining common object features. CVPR **2018**, 1354–1362 (2018)
6. Rajchl, M., Lee, M.C., Oktay, O., et al.: DeepCut: object segmentation from bounding box annotations using convolutional neural networks. IEEE Trans. Med. Imaging **36**(2), 674–683 (2017)

7. Kervadec, H., Dolz, J., Tang, M., et al.: Constrained-CNN losses for weakly supervised segmentation. Med. Image Anal. **54**, 88–99 (2019)
8. Shah, M.P., Merchant, S.N., Awate, S.P.: MS-net: mixed-supervision fully-convolutional networks for full-resolution segmentation. In: Frangi, A.F., Schnabel, J.A., Davatzikos, C., Alberola-López, C., Fichtinger, G. (eds.) MICCAI 2018. LNCS, vol. 11073, pp. 379–387. Springer, Cham (2018). https://doi.org/10.1007/978-3-030-00937-3_44
9. Hu, J., Shen, L., Sun, G.: Squeeze-and-excitation networks. In: CVPR, vol. 2018, pp. 7132–7141 (2018)
10. Roy, A.G., Navab, N., Wachinger, C.: Concurrent spatial and channel 'squeeze & excitation' in fully convolutional networks. In: Frangi, A., Schnabel, J., Davatzikos, C., Alberola-López, C., Fichtinger, G. (eds.) MICCAI 2018. LNCS, vol. 11070, pp. 421–429. Springer, Cham (2018). https://doi.org/10.1007/978-3-030-00928-1_48
11. Lin, T.Y., Goyal, P., Girshick, R., He, K., Dollár, P.: Focal loss for dense object detection. In: ICCV 2017, pp. 2980–2988 (2017)
12. Ioffe, S., Szegedy, C.: Batch normalization: accelerating deep network training by reducing internal covariate shift. In: ICML 2015, pp. 448–456 (2015)
13. Roy, A.G., Siddiqui, S., Pölsterl, S., et al.: 'Squeeze and Excite' Guided Few-Shot Segmentation of Volumetric Images. arXiv preprint arXiv:1902.01314 (2019)
14. Mlynarski, P., Delingette, H., Criminisi, A., et al.: Deep Learning with Mixed Supervision for Brain Tumor Segmentation. arXiv preprint arXiv:1812.04571 (2018)
15. Bhalgat, Y., Shah, M., Awate, S.: Annotation-cost Minimization for Medical Image Segmentation using Suggestive Mixed Supervision Fully Convolutional Networks. arXiv preprint arXiv:1812.11302 (2018)
16. Srivastava, N., Hinton, G., Krizhevsky, A., et al.: Dropout: a simple way to prevent neural networks from overfitting. J. Mach. Learn. Res. **15**(1), 1929–1958 (2014)
17. Kingma, D.P., Ba, J.: Adam: a method for stochastic optimization. arXiv preprint arXiv:1412.6980 (2014)
18. Lu, Y., Kumar, A., Zhai, S., et al.: Fully-adaptive feature sharing in multi-task networks with applications in person attribute classification. In: CVPR 2017, pp. 5334–5343 (2017)
19. Wang, J., Cheng, Y., Schmidt Feris, R.: Walk and learn: facial attribute representation learning from egocentric video and contextual data. In: CVPR 2016, pp. 2295–2304 (2016)

Fully Automated Pancreas Segmentation with Two-Stage 3D Convolutional Neural Networks

Ningning Zhao[✉], Nuo Tong, Dan Ruan, and Ke Sheng

School of Medicine, University of California Los Angeles, Los Angeles, CA, USA
buaazhaonn@gmail.com

Abstract. Due to the fact that pancreas is an abdominal organ with very large variations in shape and size, automatic and accurate pancreas segmentation can be challenging for medical image analysis. In this work, we proposed a fully automated two stage framework for pancreas segmentation based on convolutional neural networks (CNN). In the first stage, a U-Net is trained for the down-sampled 3D volume segmentation. Then a candidate region covering the pancreas is extracted from the estimated labels. Motivated by the superior performance reported by renowned region based CNN, in the second stage, another 3D U-Net is trained on the candidate region generated in the first stage. We evaluated the performance of the proposed method on the NIH computed tomography (CT) dataset, and verified its superiority over other state-of-the-art 2D and 3D approaches for pancreas segmentation in terms of dice-sorensen coefficient (DSC) accuracy in testing. The mean DSC of the proposed method is 85.99%.

Keywords: Computed Tomography (CT) · Pancreas · Automate segmentation · Multi-stage · Deep convolutional neural network

1 Introduction

Automated and accurate organ segmentation is a fundamental step in medical image analysis, computer assisted diagnosis and radiation therapy plans. Recently, deep learning based methods such as convolutional neural networks (CNN) have demonstrated to be powerful tools for organ segmentation thanks to the availability of large annotated datasets and computational resources compared with traditional segmentation techniques.

One issue in organ segmentation is whether to deal with 2D slices or 3D volumes since training models on both 2D and 3D scans have their advantages and disadvantages. Specifically, training models on 3D volumes directly can leverage the inherent spatial and anatomical information in volumetric organs with the cost of significantly higher computational power and memory than training 2D models. On the contrary, there are usually more training samples for 2D network training by slicing volumes in three orthogonal planes (sagittal, coronal

© Springer Nature Switzerland AG 2019
D. Shen et al. (Eds.): MICCAI 2019, LNCS 11765, pp. 201–209, 2019.
https://doi.org/10.1007/978-3-030-32245-8_23

and transverse), which sacrifices the 3D geometric information. Moreover, the fusion of 2D segmentation results to construct 3D mask is necessary. Existing deep learning based techniques for pancreas segmentation include both cases. For example, 2D networks were explored in [8,9]. 3D network for pancreas segmentation were studied in [3,10]. In [2] and [7], the authors combined 2D and 3D networks for pancreas segmentation.

In addition, segmentation of the small, soft and flexible organs like pancreas automatically and accurately can be difficult due to its large variations in shape, size and the varying surrounding contents in comparison with the large organs (e.g., liver, kidney, stomach, etc.). Thus, much more accurate segmentation can be achieved by using smaller input region around the target. The coarse-to-fine multi-stage techniques have been explored widely to address this problem. The basic idea is to determine the regions of interest (ROIs)/candidate regions in a coarse step followed by refining the segmentation on the ROIs. However, the ROI generation through the bounding box estimation for pancreas can be difficult. Several methods to generate meaningful regions on 2D slices with recall of value 99% have been explored. For example, machine learning based techniques are implemented in [1,5] for candidate region generation through bounding box regression. A fixed-point algorithm during testing stage was studied in [9]. Recurrent neural networks were considered in [8] to keep the consistency between training and testing stages. [10] proposed to generate candidate regions using patch-based method.

In this work, we proposed a two-stage method for automated pancreas segmentation on 3D computed tomography (CT) scans, which contains two steps: (i) coarse segmentation on down-sampled 3D volumes for candidate region generation; (ii) to refine the pancreas segmentation on smaller regions-of-interest (ROIs) at the finest resolution scale. The performance of the proposed algorithm was demonstrated on the NIH dataset.

2   Method

We denote the 3D CT scans as X with size $W \times H \times D$. The down-sampled CT scans is X^R, where the superscript letter R is the decimation factor. The ground truth masks corresponding to the original and down-sampled CT scans are represented by Y and Y^R. $N = W \times H \times D$ is the total voxel number in the 3D scans. The vector version of the 3D volumes is denoted by their corresponding lower-case letters. For example, y is the vector version of ground truth mask Y. The two steps of the proposed method are detailed as follows.

2.1   Coarse Scale Segmentation

Due to the high dimensionality of the original 3D CT scans, training models on the original CT scans leads to high cost of the computational power and memory, which limits the depth and architecture of the networks. Thus, we first train a 3D U-Net on the down-sampled volume with a decimation factor $R = 4$. Based on the tight relationship between segmentation and localization, a candidate region of the pancreas can be extracted after obtaining the coarse scale segmentation mask. Note that the normalized bounding box of pancreas in down-sampled volume and original volume are the same since down-sampling operation cannot change the shape and location of the pancreas. Besides, the candidate region generation is conducted on 3D volumes instead of 2D slices since the location of pancreas on 3D volumes of different subjects are more consistent than that on 2D slices inter and/or intra subjects (Fig. 1).

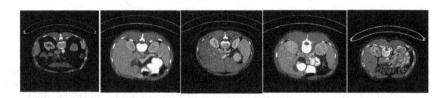

Fig. 1. CT slices from different subjects. The anatomical properties of pancreas (indicated by red mask) in different slices are quite different. (Color figure online)

2.2 Fine Scale Segmentation

In the second stage, another UNet of the same architecture is trained on the candidate regions generated in the first stage at the finest resolution scale. Since we cannot make sure that the ROIs generated in the first stage has both high precise and recall, the second stage during training and testing procedure are implemented in different ways.

In training, the bounding boxes are extracted from the ground-truth mask Y, and then enlarged by adding margins (10 pixels) along the three orthogonal axes. The candidate regions cropped with the enlarged ground truth bounding boxes (denoted as B_y) from the original 3D CT scans are the inputs of segmentation network in the second stage. Note that it is possible to train the networks of the two stages simultaneously since the ROIs used here are generated without the aid of the output in the first stage.

In testing, after obtaining the estimated label map $\hat{Y}^R$ from the down-sampled data X^R, we generated two bounding boxes in different ways: (i) We extracted a bounding box from $\hat{Y}^R$ directly and then enlarged it by adding margins of 2 pixels along different axes, denoted as $B_{\hat{y}}^R$. A bounding box covering the pancreas on the original CT scans was finally obtained by rescaling $B_{\hat{y}}^R$ through multiplying by R along different axes. (ii) After up-sampling $\hat{Y}^R$ with a factor R, one bounding box was extracted from it directly. The bounding box was then enlarged by adding 10 pixels of margin along different axes. Note that the differences between the

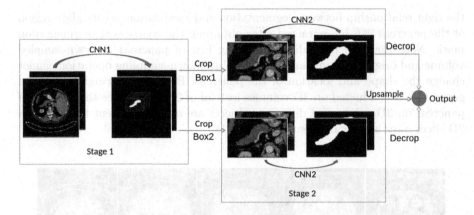

Fig. 2. Illustration of testing procedure. In Stage 2, three channels for pancreas segmentation are used. For the two channels represented by yellow arrows, two cropped regions are fed into the same network to produce two binary masks. In the channel represented by orange arrow, the estimated mask was up-sampled with a factor R = 4. The estimated mask in the three channels are finally combined through marginal voting. (Color figure online)

two bounding boxes come from the errors of sampling operation and different margins considered.

Since two bounding boxes are generated in the testing procedure, two estimated masks can be obtained by feeding the two cropped ROIs into the U-Net separately. Finally, the two estimated masks and the up-sampled pancreas mask estimated in the first stage were combined by marginal voting. Figure 2 explains the testing procedure of the proposed method.

2.3   Network Architecture and Loss Function

The architecture of the UNet employed in this work is shown in Fig. 3. Note that the architecture in stage 1 and stage 2 are the same. The parameters of the two networks in Stage 1 and Stage 2 can be trained simultaneously since they are independent during training.

The loss function is formulated as below. Note that the same loss function are used in both stages.

$$\mathcal{L} = \mathcal{L}_{\text{Dice}} + \gamma \mathcal{L}_{\text{Center}} \tag{1}$$

where γ is the penalty parameter. The dice loss and center loss are given by

$$\mathcal{L}_{\text{Dice}} = -\frac{\sum_i^N y_i \hat{y}_i}{\sum_i^N y_i + \hat{y}_i} - \frac{\sum_i^N (1 - y_i)(1 - \hat{y}_i)}{\sum_i^N 2 - y_i - \hat{y}_i} \tag{2}$$

$$\mathcal{L}_{\text{Center}} = \sum_{d=1}^{D} |f(Y_d) - f(\hat{Y}_d)| \tag{3}$$

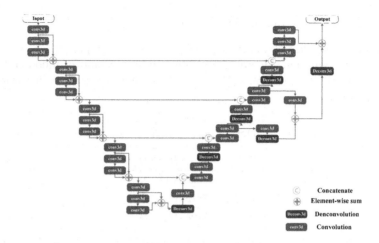

Fig. 3. The deep network architecture. The architecture of the U-Net used in the two stages are the same.

where

$$f(Y_d) = (c_{x,d}, c_{y,d}) = \frac{1}{\zeta} \sum_{v=1}^{H} \sum_{u=1}^{W} (u, v) \cdot Y_d(u, v) \tag{4}$$

where $f(Y_d)$ is the center point of dth slice of mask Y, which is denoted as the weighted sum of coordinates. $\zeta = \sum_{v=1}^{H} \sum_{u=1}^{W} (u, v) Y_d(u, v)$ is the spatial normalization factor. Note that both the dice loss and center loss are differentiable. In this work, the parameter γ is fixed as 10^{-3} for the initial 50 epochs and is decreased to 0 in the following epochs.

3   Experiments

3.1   Dataset

Our method is evaluated on the public NIH pancreatic segmentation dataset[1] [5]. There are 82 contrast-enhanced abdominal CT scans and corresponding annotated labels in this dataset. The CT scans have resolutions of 512×512 pixels with varying pixel sizes and slice thickness between $1.5 - 2.5$ mm. The pixel values for all the CT scans were clipped to $[-100, 240]$ HU, then rescaled to the range $[0, 1]$. Following previous work of pancreas segmentation, we used 4-fold cross-validation to assess the robustness of the model, i.e., 20 subjects are chosen for validation in each fold.

---

[1] https://wiki.cancerimagingarchive.net/display/Public/Pancreas-CT.

3.2   Quantitative Assessment Metrics

In both steps, the dice similarity coefficient (DSC) is employed for segmentation accuracy evaluation. Moreover, recall and intersection-over-union (IoU) are used to assess the localization performance. The metrics used in this work are expressed as below.

$$DSC = \frac{2\sum_i y_i \hat{y}_i}{\sum_i y_i + \sum_i \hat{y}_i} \tag{5}$$

$$Recall = \frac{Area(B_y \cap B_{\hat{y}})}{Area(B_y)} \tag{6}$$

$$IoU = \frac{Area(B_y \cap B_{\hat{y}})}{Area(B_y \cup B_{\hat{y}})} \tag{7}$$

where y and $\hat{y}$ are the ground truth and estimated masks. B_y and $B_{\hat{y}}$ are the bounding boxes extracted from the ground truth and estimated masks.

3.3   Results

Figure 4 shows the segmentation results from stage 1 and stage 2 respectively of three subjects in testing. For all the subjects, the overlaps between the estimated masks and ground truth masks in the second stage are larger compared to the overlaps in stage one. Quantitative results of the two-stage method are reported in Table 1. The mean DSC from stage 2 segmentation increases by at least 3%, compared to the stage 1 result.

The bounding box accuracy evaluated by recall and IoU is summarized in Table 2. The mean recalls of both bounding boxes are higher than 97%. The IoUs of the two bounding boxes from different subjects are all higher than 60% except for one subject whose IoU is lower than 40%. However, the segmentation performance of this subject also benefits from the two-stage method, i.e., DSC increased from 39.98% to 57.20%.

Table 1. Pancreas segmentation accuracy of the proposed method on the NIH dataset.

Fold	Stage 1			Stage 2		
	Mean DSC	Max DSC	Min DSC	Mean DSC	Max DSC	Min DSC
F0	82.18% ± 5.28%	89.31%	65.59%	85.82% ± 4.58%	91.20%	74.95%
F1	78.20% ± 10.60%	88.67%	39.98%	84.85% ± 6.75%	90.80%	57.20%
F2	83.23% ± 3.70%	89.61%	76.36%	86.52% ± 2.56%	91.14%	82.00%
F3	81.91% ± 6.84%	88.68%	78.69%	86.79% ± 2.43%	90.64%	82.13%

The comparison of pancreas segmentation using different methods are reported in Table 3. The proposed method outperforms the others in terms of the mean DSC.

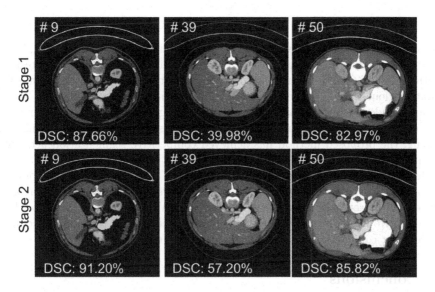

Fig. 4. Examples of segmentation results of the proposed method from subjects #9, #39 and #50. Red and yellow mask indicate the ground truth, prediction regions respectively. Best viewed in color. (Color figure online)

Table 2. Pancreas localization accuracy of the proposed method on the NIH dataset.

	Bounding box 1			Bounding box 2		
Fold	Mean Recall	Max Recall	Min Recall	Mean Recall	Max Recall	Min Recall
F0	98.44% ± 2.23%	100%	90.24%	99.41% ± 1.69%	100%	93.22%
F1	98.28% ± 2.24%	100%	90.74%	99.38% ± 1.39%	100%	93.89%
F2	97.67% ± 4.18%	100%	85.24%	98.71% ± 3.13%	100%	88.59%
F3	98.42% ± 1.95%	100%	93.42%	99.61% ± 0.73%	100%	97.78%
Fold	Mean IoU	Max IoU	Min IoU	Mean IoU	Max IoU	Min IoU
F0	81.04% ± 5.18%	88.23%	69.55%	69.52% ± 5.39%	77.68%	60.04%
F1	76.93% ± 13.37%	86.78%	20.80%	66.45% ± 11.60%	77.66%	18.35%
F2	77.74% ± 4.33%	84.85%	69.43%	66.78% ± 3.85%	72.61%	59.19%
F3	76.30% ± 12.69%	90.87%	42.42%	66.96% ± 10.15%	83.38%	40.51%

Table 3. Evaluation of different methods on the NIH dataset.

Method	Mean DSC	Max DSC	Min DSC
Roth et.al. MICCAI'2016 [6]	78.01% ± 8.20%	88.65%	34.11%
Holistically Nested 2D FCN [4]	81.27% ± 6.27%	88.96%	50.69%
Zhou et.al. MICCAI'2017 [9]	82.65% ± 5.47%	90.85%	63.02%
Attention-UNet [3]	83.10% ± 3.80%	-	-
ResDSN C2F [10]	84.59% ± 4.86%	**91.45%**	**69.62%**
Ours (Coarse)	81.91% ± 6.84%	89.61%	39.98%
Ours (Refine)	**85.99% ± 4.51%**	91.20%	57.20%

3.4 Discussion

According to the quantitative results about bounding box estimation in Table 2, it is difficult to achieve high IoUs for different subjects. Thus, a new testing method different from the training procedure is introduced. In testing, two candidate regions were extracted with the estimated mask in the first stage. Then, an up-sampled segmentation mask in the fist stage and two refined segmentation masks by majority voting. Although the inconsistency between training and testing, the proposed method has achieved competitive segmentation accuracy compared with state-of-the-art algorithms.

It is also interesting to note that more isolated false positive (FP) errors are introduced in the second stage segmentation for subject ♯39. The FP error is caused by the center loss term used for training. We noticed that the center loss term contribute to increase the convergence speed during training procedure. However, it can cause more isolated false positive errors.

4   Conclusions

A two-stage pancreas segmentation method was proposed in this work. Two deep networks of the same architecture were trained with down-sampled and original 3D CT scans for the purpose of coarse ROI definition and refined segmentation. We also proposed a novel testing framework, which can easily used for other small organ segmentation. The proposed method has achieved competitive segmentation accuracy compared with state-of-the-art algorithms.

References

1. Farag, A., Lu, L., Roth, H.R., Liu, J., Turkbey, E., Summers, R.M.: A bottom-up approach for pancreas segmentation using cascaded superpixels and (deep) image patch labeling. IEEE Trans. Med. Imaging **26**(1), 386–399 (2017)
2. Li, J., Lin, X., Che, H., Li, H., Qian, X.: Probability map guided bi-directional recurrent UNet for pancreas segmentation. Arxiv (2019), https://arxiv.org/abs/1903.00923
3. Oktay, O., et al.: Attention u-net: learning where to look for the pancreas. In: Medical Imaging with Deep Learning (MIDL) (2018)
4. Roth, H., et al.: Spatial aggregation of holistically-nested convolutional neural networks for automated pancreas localization and segmentation. Med. Image Anal. **45**, 94–107 (2017)
5. Roth, H.R., et al.: DeepOrgan: multi-level deep convolutional networks for automated pancreas segmentation. In: Navab, N., Hornegger, J., Wells, W.M., Frangi, A.F. (eds.) MICCAI 2015. LNCS, vol. 9349, pp. 556–564. Springer, Cham (2015). https://doi.org/10.1007/978-3-319-24553-9_68
6. Roth, H.R., Lu, L., Farag, A., Sohn, A., Summers, R.M.: Spatial aggregation of holistically-nested networks for automated pancreas segmentation. In: Ourselin, S., Joskowicz, L., Sabuncu, M.R., Unal, G., Wells, W. (eds.) MICCAI 2016. LNCS, vol. 9901, pp. 451–459. Springer, Cham (2016). https://doi.org/10.1007/978-3-319-46723-8_52

7. Xia, Y., Xie, L., Liu, F., Zhu, Z., Fishman, E.K., Yuille, A.L.: Bridging the gap between 2D and 3D organ segmentation with volumetric fusion net. In: Frangi, A.F., Schnabel, J.A., Davatzikos, C., Alberola-López, C., Fichtinger, G. (eds.) MICCAI 2018. LNCS, vol. 11073, pp. 445–453. Springer, Cham (2018). https://doi.org/10.1007/978-3-030-00937-3_51

8. Yu, Q., Xie, L., Wang, Y., Zhou, Y., Fishman, E.K., Yuille, A.L.: Recurrent saliency transformation network: incorporating multi-stage visual cues for small organ segmentation. In: IEEE Conference on Computer Vision and Pattern Recognition (CVPR) (2018)

9. Zhou, Y., Xie, L., Shen, W., Wang, Y., Fishman, E.K., Yuille, A.L.: A fixed-point model for pancreas segmentation in abdominal CT scans. In: International Conference on Medical Image Computing and Computer Assisted Intervention (MICCAI), vol. 1, pp. 693–701 (2017)

10. Zhu, Z., Xia, Y., Shen, W., Fishman, E., Yuille, A.: A 3D coarse-to-fine framework for volumetric medical image segmentation. In: International Conference on 3D Vision (2018)

Globally Guided Progressive Fusion Network for 3D Pancreas Segmentation

Chaowei Fang[1,2], Guanbin Li[3], Chengwei Pan[1], Yiming Li[1], and Yizhou Yu[1,2(✉)]

[1] Deepwise AI Lab, Beijing, China
yizhouy@acm.org
[2] The University of Hong Kong, Pokfulam, Hong Kong
[3] Sun Yat-sen University, Guangzhou, China

Abstract. Recently 3D volumetric organ segmentation attracts much research interest in medical image analysis due to its significance in computer aided diagnosis. This paper aims to address the pancreas segmentation task in 3D computed tomography volumes. We propose a novel end-to-end network, *Globally Guided Progressive Fusion Network*, as an effective and efficient solution to volumetric segmentation, which involves both global features and complicated 3D geometric information. A progressive fusion network is devised to extract 3D information from a moderate number of neighboring slices and predict a probability map for the segmentation of each slice. An independent branch for excavating global features from downsampled slices is further integrated into the network. Extensive experimental results demonstrate that our method achieves state-of-the-art performance on two pancreas datasets.

Keywords: Global guidance · Progressive fusion · End-to-end deep convolution network · Pancreas segmentation · Computed tomography

1 Introduction

Automatic organ segmentation, which is critical to computer aided diagnosis, is a fundamental topic in medical image analysis. This paper focuses on pancreas segmentation in 3D computed tomography (CT) volumes which is more difficult than segmentations of other organs such as liver, heart and kidneys [7].

Driven by the rapid development of deep learning techniques, significant progress has been achieved on 3D volumetric segmentation [8,10]. State-of-the-art methods primarily fall into two categories. The first category [13] is based on segmentation networks originally designed for 2D images, e.g. FCN [5]. However, only a small number of adjacent slices (usually 3) are stacked together

Electronic supplementary material The online version of this chapter (https://doi.org/10.1007/978-3-030-32245-8_24) contains supplementary material, which is available to authorized users.

© Springer Nature Switzerland AG 2019
D. Shen et al. (Eds.): MICCAI 2019, LNCS 11765, pp. 210–218, 2019.
https://doi.org/10.1007/978-3-030-32245-8_24

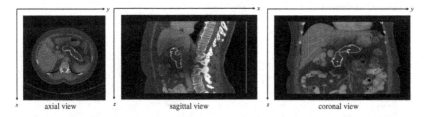

Fig. 1. An example of pancreas segmentation in the axial, sagittal and coronal views. The contour of the ground truth and our result is shown in red and green respectively. Blended regions indicate the probability map inferred from the global feature map. (Color figure online)

as the input to take advantage of network weights pretrained on natural image datasets such as Pascal VOC [3]. Although majority voting [12] can be used to incorporate pseudo 3D contextual information through 2D segmentation in slices along different views, powerful 3D features are still not exploited. Methods in the other category are based on 3D convolution layers, such as V-Net [6] and 3D U-Net [2,9]. Due to the huge memory overhead of 3D convolutions, the input is either decomposed into overlapping 3D patches [2], which ignores the global knowledge, or resized to a volume with a poor resolution [9], which likely gives rise to missed detections. Coarse-to-fine segmentation is a popular and effective choice for improving the accuracy [8,10,11]. However, it is severely dependent on the performance of its coarse segmentation model. Omission of regions of interest (ROIs) or inaccurate size of ROIs in the coarse segmentation often lead to irreparable loss. Most of these volumetric segmentation methods have been applied in pancreas segmentation such as [10,11,13].

In this paper, we focus on one fixed type of organs (pancreas) and the overall spatial arrangement of organs in any human body is more or less fixed as well. In such a specialized setting, both local and global contextual information is critical for achieving highly accurate segmentation results. To tackle the afore-mentioned challenges, we propose a novel end-to-end network, called *Globally Guided Progressive Fusion Network*. The backbone in our method is a progressive fusion network devised to extract 3D local contextual information from a moderate number of neighboring slices and predict a 2D probability map for the segmentation of each slice. However our progressive fusion network has limited complexity and receptive fields, which are inadequate for acquiring global contextual information. Thus a global guidance branch consisting of convolution layers is employed to excavate global features from a complete downsampled slice. We elegantly integrate this branch into the progressive fusion network through sub-pixel sampling. An example of the segmentation result of our method is presented in Fig. 1. In summary, the main contributions of our paper are as follows.

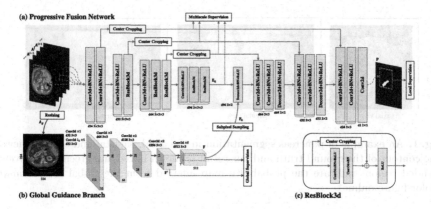

Fig. 2. The main pipeline of our method. More details are illustrated in supplemental material. (Best viewed in color) (Color figure online)

(1) A progressive fusion network is devised to extract 3D local contextual information from a 3D neighborhood. A unique aspect of this network is that the encoding part performs 3D convolutions while the decoding part performs 2D convolution and deconvolution operations.

(2) A global guidance branch is devised to replenish global contextual information to the progressive fusion network. The entire network, including the global branch, is trained in an end-to-end manner.

(3) Our method has been successfully validated on two pancreas segmentation datasets, achieving state-of-the-art performance.

2   Method

2.1   Overview

As discussed earlier, both local and global contextual information is critical for achieving highly accurate segmentation results. On the other hand, segmentation precision, especially around boundaries, is closely related to the spatial resolution of the input volume. However the huge memory consumption of 3D volumes prevents us from loading an entire high-resolution volume at once. Considering the above factors, we devise a novel end-to-end network, which segments every slice in a patchwise manner by predicting a probability map for each 2D image patch. This network consists of two modules: a progressive fusion network is devised to mine 3D local contextual features for a 2D image patch from its high-resolution 3D neighborhood; a global guidance branch is devised to replenish a complementary 2D global feature representation extracted from an entire downsampled slice. The overall architecture is presented in Fig. 2.

Given an $l \times h \times w$ input volume, where h and w represent the height and width of axial slices respectively and l is the number of axial slices, we define $\mathbf{A}^i$ ($h \times w$), $\mathbf{S}^i$ ($l \times h$) and $\mathbf{C}^i$ ($l \times w$) as the i-th slice in the axial, sagittal and coronal view, respectively. In the remainder of this section, we will use slices in the axial view to elaborate the aforementioned two modules. Suppose $\mathbf{A}^i$ is decomposed into N overlapping 2D patches $\{\mathbf{A}_k^i | k = 1, \cdots, N\}$.

2.2 Progressive Fusion Network

Local texture and shape features are valuable for organ segmentation, especially for accurate boundary localization. Hence we devise a progressive fusion network (Fig. 2(a)) based on the encoder-decoder architecture to extract 3D local contextual features for each 2D image patch $\mathbf{A}_k^i$ from its 3D neighborhood, which includes corresponding 2D patches from a moderate number (31) of adjacent slices, $\{\mathbf{A}_k^{i+t} | t = -T, \cdots, T\}$. The superscript i will be neglected by default for conciseness below.

The encoder, taking a 3D patch as the input, consists of 3D convolution layers and residual blocks [4], which are organized into 4 groups. Between every two consecutive groups, max pooling is used to reduce the spatial resolution of the feature map by half, giving rise to feature maps with 4 different scales. Inspired from [1], our network progressively fuses the slices in the input 3D patch by not performing the convolution operation in the 2 outmost slices in every 3D convolution layer because these two slices are of least relevance to the central slice. We choose T to be the number of 3D convolution layers so that there exists only one slice (the central slice) in the final group of feature maps, $\mathbf{E}_k$. The kernel size of each convolutional layer is set to $3 \times 3 \times 3$ and the overall receptive field of the encoder is 144×144, only covering part of the input patch. The decoder is set up with 2D convolution and deconvolution layers, producing the final segmentation result for the central slice. As in U-Net [2,9], there exist skip connections between corresponding encoder and decoder layers. Since our encoder and decoder as well as residual blocks deal with feature maps with different dimensionality, central cropping is performed to discard surplus features in skip connections.

2.3 Global Guidance Branch

Global contextual information is vital for providing absolute and relative positions with respect to distant objects. For example, the pancreas always lies in the upper center of the abdomen behind the stomach. To exploit global information, we devise a global guidance branch (Fig. 2(b)) to extract a global feature map from $\mathbf{A}_g$ with resolution $h_g \times w_g$, which is downsampled from the original slice $\mathbf{A}$. This branch consists of 13 convolution layers interleaved with 4 max pooling layers. The height and width of the global feature map $\mathbf{F}$ is $h_g/32$ and $w_g/32$ respectively. For every pixel in the local feature map $\mathbf{E}_k$, sub-pixel sampling is utilized to calculate a corresponding feature vector from $\mathbf{F}$, resulting a global feature map $\mathbf{F}_k$ for $\mathbf{A}_k$. $\mathbf{E}_k$ and $\mathbf{F}_k$ are concatenated and fed into the decoder in the progressive fusion network.

Algorithm 1. Inference procedure of our network.

Input: Slices: $\mathbf{A}^i$, $i = 1, \cdots, l$.
Output: Probability map: $\mathbf{P}^i$, $i = 1, \cdots, l$.
1: **for** each slice $\mathbf{A}$ in $\{\mathbf{A}^i\}$ **do**
2:      Downsample $\mathbf{A}$ to obtain $\mathbf{A}_g$;
3:      Compute $\mathbf{F}$ from $\mathbf{A}_g$ using the global guidance branch (Section 2.3);
4:      Decompose $\mathbf{A}$ into N overlapping patches $\{\mathbf{A}_k | k = 1, \cdots, N\}$;
5:      **for** $k = 1$ to N **do**
6:          Sample $\mathbf{F}$ to obtain a global feature map $\mathbf{F}_k$ for $\mathbf{A}_k$;
7:          Extract a local feature map $\mathbf{E}_k$ from a 3D neighborhood of $\mathbf{A}_k$ using the 3D encoder of our progressive fusion network (Section 2.2);
8:          Compute the probability map $\mathbf{P}_k$ for $\mathbf{A}_k$ by feeding concatenated $\mathbf{E}_k$ and $\mathbf{F}_k$ through the 2D decoder in our network;
9:      **end for**
10:     Merge $\{\mathbf{P}_k\}$ into $\mathbf{P}$ after disregarding peripheral overlapped pixels;
11: **end for**

2.4   Training Loss

Let $\mathbf{P}$ and $\mathbf{G}$ be the predicted and groundtruth segmentation of the slice $\mathbf{A}$ respectively. $p(x, y), g(x, y) \in \{0, 1\}$ indicates whether pixel (x, y) belongs to the predicted and groundtruth target region respectively. Binary cross entropy is used to measure the dissimilarity between $\mathbf{P}$ and $\mathbf{G}$,

$$C(\mathbf{P}, \mathbf{G}) = -\frac{1}{wh} \sum_{x=0}^{w-1} \sum_{y=0}^{h-1} g(x, y) \log p(x, y) + (1 - g(x, y)) \log(1 - p(x, y)). \quad (1)$$

We also use a fully connected layer to predict a probability map for each scale of the feature maps in the encoder. Let $\mathbf{P}_k^{(j)}$ be the probability map computed from the last feature map in the j-th scale. Multiscale supervision is imposed on these probability maps to enhance the training of the encoder. Likewise we also use $\mathbf{F}$ and the second last scale of feature $\mathbf{F}'$ to infer probability maps $\mathbf{P}^f$ and $\mathbf{P}^{f'}$ respectively, then impose additional supervision on the global guidance branch. The overall loss function can be summarized as follows,

$$L = \frac{1}{N} \sum_{k=1}^{N} [C(\mathbf{P}_k, \mathbf{G}_k) + \frac{1}{4} \sum_{j=1}^{4} C(\mathbf{P}_k^{(j)}, \mathbf{G}_k^{(j)})] + \alpha C(\mathbf{P}^f, \mathbf{G}^f) + \beta C(\mathbf{P}^{f'}, \mathbf{G}^{f'}), \quad (2)$$

where α and β are constants; $\mathbf{G}_k$, $\mathbf{G}_k^{(j)}$, $\mathbf{G}^f$ and $\mathbf{G}^{f'}$ are ground truths; $\mathbf{G}_k^{(j)}$ is downsampled from $\mathbf{G}_k$; $\mathbf{G}^f$ and $\mathbf{G}^{f'}$ are downsampled from the full resolution ground truth of $\mathbf{A}_g$.

The inference procedure is summarized in Algorithm 1. The same algorithm is applied to the segmentation of the slices from the sagittal and coronal views. The results for all three views are fused through weighted averaging [12] to produce the pseudo-3D segmentation result. Let the predictions for the axial, sagittal and coronal views are $\mathbf{V}_a$, $\mathbf{V}_s$ and $\mathbf{V}_c$ respectively. The final result is $\mathbf{V} = w_a \mathbf{V}_a + w_s \mathbf{V}_s + w_c \mathbf{V}_c$, where w_a, w_s and w_c are constants.

3   Experiments

3.1   Datasets

Two pancreas datasets are used to validate the performance of the proposed 3D volumetric segmentation algorithm in this paper.

(1) **MSD** (short for Medical Segmentation Decathlon challenge) provides 281 volumes of CT with labelled pancreas mask. The spatial resolution is 512×512 and the number of slices varies from 37 to 751. We randomly split them into 236 volumes for training, 5 for validation and 40 for testing.
(2) **NIHC** [7] contains 82 abdominal contrast enhanced 3D CT scans with the spatial resolution equal to 512×512 pixels and the number of slices falling between 181 and 466. We randomly split them into 48 volumes for training, 5 for validation and 29 for testing.

To measure the performance of segmentation algorithms, we first threshold the segmentation probability map by 0.5. Then Dice similarity coefficient (DSC) is used to calculate the similarity between the predicted segmentation mask and the ground truth.

3.2   Implementation

Because a patient's pancreas only occupies a small percentage of voxels in a CT volume, we use the following strategy to balance positive and negative training samples: two patches are cropped out from all slices of each volume; the central point of the first patch is randomly chosen from the whole volume while that of the second patch is randomly chosen from the box encompassing the pancreas. Random rotation and elastic deformation are applied to augment the training samples. The patch size is set to 256×256 for all views of NIHC and axial view of MSD. For the sagittal and coronal views of MSD, 128×256 patch size is utilized. The same patch size is used in validation and the number of overlapping pixels is set to 64. The global guidance branch is trained alone for 1000 epochs using a batch size of 32 and $\alpha = \beta = 0.5$. The progressive fusion network is also trained alone for 1000 epochs. Then the whole network is fine-tuned for another 800 epochs with $\alpha = 0.01$ and $\beta = 0$. We adopt a batch size of 4 in the latter two stages. The training process takes around 60 hours. Adam is adopted to optimize network parameters with learning rate of 10^{-4}. The model achieving the best performance on the validation set is chosen as the final version.

Parameters. In MSD, the difficulty of segmenting the sagittal and coronal slices is higher than segmenting axial slices as the resolution along the z axis varies much. We empirically set $w_a = 0.8$, $w_s = 0.1$ and $w_c = 0.1$ for MSD. w_a, w_s and w_c are set as $1/3$ for NIHC. h_g and w_g are set to 224 except for the sagittal and coronal views in MSD where 128 is used for h_g. N is set to 1 during testing.

Table 1. Comparisons with state-of-the-art segmentation algorithms.

Method	MSD			NIHC			#Params
	mean ± std	min	max	mean ± std	min	max	
3D Unet-Patch [8]	79.98 ± 7.71	61.14	93.73	78.36 ± 13.04	23.93	90.25	1.9×10^7
3D Unet-Full [9]	81.13 ± 8.20	61.84	93.49	81.43 ± 7.53	49.36	89.60	1.3×10^7
2D FCN8s-A [5]	82.24 ± 6.88	62.99	92.61	81.35 ± 5.87	60.57	88.16	1.3×10^8
2D RSTN-A [11]	83.29 ± 6.58	**66.23**	92.40	82.56 ± 5.18	63.36	89.82	2.7×10^8
2D GGPFN-A	84.56 ± 7.95	59.41	95.29	83.71 ± 5.83	66.33	90.13	1.4×10^7
P3D FCN8s [12]	82.52 ± 7.00	61.75	92.86	83.24 ± 5.63	61.53	90.13	4.0×10^8
P3D RSTN [11]	83.63 ± 6.65	64.21	93.02	84.45 ± 4.89	66.47	90.80	8.1×10^8
P3D GGPFN	**84.71 ± 7.13**	58.62	**95.54**	**85.46 ± 4.80**	**67.03**	**92.24**	4.2×10^7

Table 2. Ablation study on MSD.

Global guidance	3D fusion mode	T	mean ± std	min	max
✓	One-off	1	78.56 ± 8.63	58.76	93.62
✓	One-off	5	79.62 ± 7.65	**60.01**	93.63
✓	One-off	10	77.30 ± 8.38	59.21	92.69
✓	One-off	15	76.96 ± 9.38	57.67	94.26
✓	Progressive	5	80.30 ± 8.41	49.30	93.48
✓	Progressive	10	83.34 ± 7.90	54.38	94.70
×	Progressive	15	83.46 ± 8.15	56.94	94.28
✓	Progressive	15	**84.56 ± 7.95**	59.41	**95.29**

3.3 Experimental Results

Comparisons with State-of-the-Art Segmentation Algorithms. Comparisons against state-of-the-art volumetric segmentation algorithms are reported in Table 1. According to output type, we classify them into three categories: 3D models which predict 3D probability maps directly (such as UNet-Patch [8] and UNet-Full [9]), 2D models which produce 2D segmentation results over slices in the axial view (such as FCN8s [5]), Pseudo-3D (P3D) models which fuse 2D segmentation results for axial, sagittal and coronal views (such as RSTN [11]). Our globally guided progressive fusion network (GGPFN) can be easily integrated into the 2D and P3D segmentation frameworks. All models used for comparison here are retrained with the datasets adopted in this paper. Our method consistently performs better than FCN8s and RSTN in both 2D and P3D segmentation frameworks. For example, in the 2D framework, the mean DSC of our model is clearly higher than that of RSTN. With the help of the P3D segmentation framework, our algorithm achieves the best performance among all considered algorithms. Comparisons of precision-recall curves are presented in supplemental material.

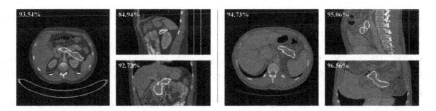

Fig. 3. Visualizations of segmentation results (green contours) produced by our method. The number on the top-left corner of each image indicate DSC metric. (Color figure online)

Ablation Study. To demonstrate the efficacy of our globally guided progressive fusion network, we conduct an ablation study (Table 2) on the testing set of the MSD dataset using slices along the axial view. We implement an one-off fusion mode, which directly fuses multiple adjacent slices into a single slice by using a single convolution layer and treating the multiple slices as channels of a single slice fed into this convolution layer. Our progressive fusion mode is able to make use of 3D information more effectively. As more slices are used, the advantages of our progressive fusion network become more prominent while the one-off mode fails to discover additional useful information when the number of slices exceeds 21. The feature map produced by the global guidance branch is also able to improve segmentation performance. The mean DSC is decreased by 0.011 when the global guidance branch is disabled.

Two examples of segmented pancreas organs using our method are visualized in Fig. 3. More results are shown in supplemental material.

4   Conclusions

In this paper, we have presented a novel end-to-end network for 3D pancreas segmentation. The proposed network consists of a progressive fusion network and a global guidance branch. Our new algorithm achieves state-of-the-art performance on two benchmark datasets. In our future work, we will extend the application of our algorithm to multi-organ segmentation scenes and improve its boundary locating capability.

References

1. Caballero, J., et al.: Real-time video super-resolution with spatio-temporal networks and motion compensation. In: 2017 IEEE Conference on Computer Vision and Pattern Recognition (CVPR), pp. 2848–2857 (2017)
2. Çiçek, Ö., Abdulkadir, A., Lienkamp, S.S., Brox, T., Ronneberger, O.: 3D U-Net: learning dense volumetric segmentation from sparse annotation. In: Ourselin, S., Joskowicz, L., Sabuncu, M.R., Unal, G., Wells, W. (eds.) MICCAI 2016. LNCS, vol. 9901, pp. 424–432. Springer, Cham (2016). https://doi.org/10.1007/978-3-319-46723-8_49

3. Everingham, M., Gool, L.J.V., Williams, C.K.I., Winn, J.M., Zisserman, A.: The PASCAL visual object classes (VOC) challenge. Int. J. Comput. Vis. **88**(2), 303–338 (2010)
4. He, K., Zhang, X., Ren, S., Sun, J.: Deep residual learning for image recognition. In: 2016 IEEE Conference on Computer Vision and Pattern Recognition (CVPR), pp. 770–778 (2016)
5. Long, J., Shelhamer, E., Darrell, T.: Fully convolutional networks for semantic segmentation. In: 2015 IEEE Conference on Computer Vision and Pattern Recognition (CVPR), pp. 3431–3440 (2015)
6. Milletari, F., Navab, N., Ahmadi, S.A.: V-Net: fully convolutional neural networks for volumetric medical image segmentation. In: 2016 Fourth International Conference on 3D Vision (3DV), pp. 565–571 (2016)
7. Roth, H.R., et al.: DeepOrgan: multi-level deep convolutional networks for automated pancreas segmentation. In: Navab, N., Hornegger, J., Wells, W.M., Frangi, A.F. (eds.) MICCAI 2015. LNCS, vol. 9349, pp. 556–564. Springer, Cham (2015). https://doi.org/10.1007/978-3-319-24553-9_68
8. Roth, H.R., et al.: An application of cascaded 3D fully convolutional networks for medical image segmentation. Comput. Med. Imaging Graph. **66**, 90–99 (2018)
9. Roth, H.R., et al.: Deep learning and its application to medical image segmentation. Med. Imaging Technol. **36**(2), 63–71 (2018)
10. Xia, Y., Xie, L., Liu, F., Zhu, Z., Fishman, E.K., Yuille, A.L.: Bridging the gap between 2D and 3D organ segmentation with volumetric fusion net. In: Frangi, A.F., Schnabel, J.A., Davatzikos, C., Alberola-López, C., Fichtinger, G. (eds.) MICCAI 2018. LNCS, vol. 11073, pp. 445–453. Springer, Cham (2018). https://doi.org/10.1007/978-3-030-00937-3_51
11. Yu, Q., Xie, L., Wang, Y., Zhou, Y., Fishman, E.K., Yuille, A.L.: Recurrent saliency transformation network: incorporating multi-stage visual cues for small organ segmentation. In: 2018 IEEE/CVF Conference on Computer Vision and Pattern Recognition, pp. 8280–8289 (2018)
12. Zhou, X., Ito, T., Takayama, R., Wang, S., Hara, T., Fujita, H.: Three-dimensional CT image segmentation by combining 2D fully convolutional network with 3D majority voting. In: Carneiro, G., et al. (eds.) LABELS/DLMIA -2016. LNCS, vol. 10008, pp. 111–120. Springer, Cham (2016). https://doi.org/10.1007/978-3-319-46976-8_12
13. Zhou, Y., Xie, L., Shen, W., Wang, Y., Fishman, E.K., Yuille, A.L.: A fixed-point model for pancreas segmentation in abdominal CT scans. In: Descoteaux, M., Maier-Hein, L., Franz, A., Jannin, P., Collins, D.L., Duchesne, S. (eds.) MICCAI 2017. LNCS, vol. 10433, pp. 693–701. Springer, Cham (2017). https://doi.org/10.1007/978-3-319-66182-7_79

Automatic Segmentation of Muscle Tissue and Inter-muscular Fat in Thigh and Calf MRI Images

Rula Amer[1]([⊠])(iD), Jannette Nassar[1](iD), David Bendahan[2], Hayit Greenspan[1](iD), and Noam Ben-Eliezer[1,3,4](iD)

[1] Department of Biomedical Engineering, Tel Aviv University, Tel Aviv, Israel
`rolaamer@mail.tau.ac.il`
[2] Aix Marseille Univ, CNRS, CRMBM, Marseille, France
[3] Center for Advanced Imaging Innovation and Research, New York University, New York, NY, USA
[4] Sagol School of Neuroscience, Tel Aviv University, Tel Aviv, Israel

Abstract. Magnetic resonance imaging (MRI) of thigh and calf muscles is one of the most effective techniques for estimating fat infiltration into muscular dystrophies. The infiltration of adipose tissue into the diseased muscle region varies in its severity across, and within, patients. In order to efficiently quantify the infiltration of fat, accurate segmentation of muscle and fat is needed. An estimation of the amount of infiltrated fat is typically done visually by experts. Several algorithmic solutions have been proposed for automatic segmentation. While these methods may work well in mild cases, they struggle in moderate and severe cases due to the high variability in the intensity of infiltration, and the tissue's heterogeneous nature. To address these challenges, we propose a deep-learning approach, producing robust results with high Dice Similarity Coefficient (DSC) of 0.964, 0.917 and 0.933 for muscle-region, healthy muscle and inter-muscular adipose tissue (IMAT) segmentation, respectively.

Keywords: MRI · Muscular dystrophy · Muscle and fat segmentation · Deep learning · Clustering

1 Introduction

Muscle dystrophies (MD) are an inherited class of disorders characterized by progressive muscle weakness that affects limb, axial, and facial muscles to a variable severity. Fat infiltration of the legs is a clinical manifestation of the disease, which is easily seen in MRI images. MD results in a loss of muscle mass causing a degradation of muscle strength [1].

Inter-muscular adipose tissue (IMAT) refers to infiltrated fat in the muscle region, and subcutaneous adipose tissue (SAT) refers to the outer fat surrounding

---

H. Greenspan and N. Ben-Eliezer—Equal contribution.

© Springer Nature Switzerland AG 2019
D. Shen et al. (Eds.): MICCAI 2019, LNCS 11765, pp. 219–227, 2019.
https://doi.org/10.1007/978-3-030-32245-8_25

the muscle. The two fat tissues are separated by a boundary called "fascia lata" which most of the studies try to detect.

It has been shown that the quantification of fat infiltration based on MRI techniques has a strong correlation with the disease progression and is therefore an accurate marker of disease state and severity [2]. In order to provide physicians with a precise disease bio-marker, an accurate segmentation of muscle tissue, subcutaneous fat and inter-muscular fat is needed. The "fascia lata" can be obscure and hard to find. The most common artifacts challenging the segmentation process are inconsistent pixel intensities and inhomogeneities across the MRI images.

Several works have been published for thigh and calf segmentation. Valentinitsch et al. [3] proposed a three-stage segmentation method using unsupervised multi-parametric k-means clustering to segment subcutaneous fat, intermuscular fat and muscle. Posetano et al. [4] introduced a fuzzy c-means approach, an active contour and Gaussian Mixture Model-Expectation Maximization (GMM-EM) algorithm for subcutaneous fat, muscle, inter-muscular fat and bone segmentation. The main problem facing those approaches is that segmentation using active contour based-methods gives unreliable results when the "fascia lata" is obscure. Chambers et al. [5] introduced muscle-region segmentation method refers to the live-wire approach for path search along the "fascia lata". Tan et al. [6] proposed a deformable model to reconstruct "fascia lata"'s surface. With the rapid development of deep-learning and its superior performance, automatic approaches based on Convolutional Neural Networks (CNNs) have been applied recently to the task of IMAT segmentation on thigh and calf MRI. Yao et al. [7] integrated deep-learning methods with traditional models, proposing a holistic neural networks and dual active contour model for "fascia lata" detection and muscle and IMAT classification.

In this work, we estimate an index that indicates the stage of the MD disease. This index is the ratio between the IMAT area and the whole region of muscle. Two stages are essential in order to calculate this index accurately. The first stage includes discarding the SAT, bone and bone marrow pixels, leaving us with the muscle-region. The next stage is to discriminate between the healthy muscle pixels and the IMAT pixels within the muscle-region. The "fascia lata" serves the experts a visual separation creating a reliable ground truth (GT) that enables supervised learning methods to accomplish this mission precisely. Thus, encouraged by it's high efficiency in semantic segmentation of small data sets, we employ the U-net architecture for the segmentation of the muscle-region. We show strong performance for a variety of cases, especially for severe fat infiltration, which is the hardest to segment. We also demonstrate the robustness of the network in the existence of MRI artifacts. Following segmentation, pixel-classification is performed to enable the distinction, on a pixel-level, of healthy muscle and IMAT. Pixels with fat infiltration are usually dispersed over the whole region of muscle. Moreover, the infiltration level varies across pixels. Consequently, the border between healthy muscle and IMAT pixels becomes blurry and a manual pixel-wise labeling becomes difficult and uncertain. Hence, a semi-

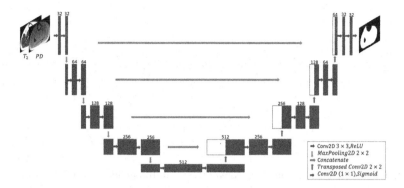

Fig. 1. The architecture of U-net used for muscle-region segmentation.

supervised method in this stage accounts for this limitation. Inspired by [8], we implement a patch based deep convolutional auto-encoder with a triplet-loss constraint to learn an interpretable latent feature representation and apply k-means in the embedded space to classify the pixels into two clusters. The integration of patches helps tackle the problem of small data, exploits the contextual information of the pixels and maintains the relationship to adjacent pixels. Results demonstrate the relevance of clustering to our task, and the ability of the overall system to predict the level of fat infiltration.

2   Methods

2.1   Data Set

Our data set includes 17 axial MR scans of patients' legs (thigh and calf) suffering from muscular disorders. A GT of the muscle regions for all the images was delineated by a domain expert.

The MR scans were scanned on a whole-body Siemens Prisma 3T scanner. A multi spin-echo sequence was used with relaxation time $(TR) = 1479$ ms, echo time $(TE) = 8.7$ ms, echo train length $(N_{echo}) = 17$, spatial resolution $= 1.5 \times 1.5$ mm^2 with a matrix size of 128×128. The regions were imaged acquiring 5 slices with slice thickness of 10 mm, the acquisition time for one scan is $5:07$ min.

To construct the T_2/PD maps, Bloch simulations were used to estimate the actual echo modulation curve (EMC). Simulations were repeated for a range of T_2, transmit field (B_1^+) and proton density (PD) values yielding a database of simulated EMCs, until the $[T_2, PD, B_1^+]$ set of values mostly matched the measured data at each voxel [9].

IMAT and healthy muscle ground truth is calculated on a pixel-by-pixel basis. The infiltration of subcutaneous fat into the diseased muscle region causes a mixture of two T_2 components to appear in each imaged voxel. An extension of the EMC algorithm was introduced [10] which is based on a two-T_2 component

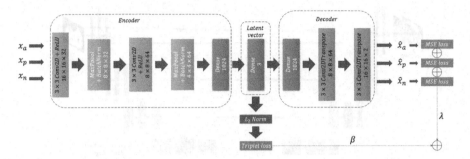

Fig. 2. The architecture of the deep convolutional auto-encoder and the losses used for muscle tissue classification.

decomposition of the signal in each imaged voxel, simultaneously estimating fat and water fractions within a single voxel. Voxels whose fat fraction was >50% were labelled as fat (i.e., diseased muscle), and the rest were labelled as muscle (i.e., healthy muscle). The fraction of IMAT area relative to the whole muscle region was calculated.

2.2 Muscle-Region Semantic Segmentation

In the first stage, we train a neural network to segment the region inside the "fascia lata". The subcutaneous adipose tissue (SAT), bone and bone marrow are masked out simultaneously by this method.

In the preprocessing stage, we separate the thighs\calf regions from the background by applying a canny edge detector in order to detect the outer edge. Then, we crop the image around the region of interest. The cropped image is then resized to (128×128). The intensity inhomogeneity that is inherent to the MRI images is corrected by using the N4ITK method [11]. After producing the T_2 and PD maps, we correct for extreme values in individual pixels within the T_2 images by taking the 98% percentile of the image intensity range and clipping the pixels above this value. We normalize each image to zero mean and unit variance before proceeding to the next step.

We employed a popular fully convolutional network (FCN)-based deep learning architecture, U-net [12], for the segmentation of muscle region. This U-net network has been demonstrated to work well on medical images with a very few learning samples and a strong use of data augmentation. The network architecture is illustrated in Fig. 1, The left part of the network is a contracting path and the right part is a symmetrical expanding path which decompresses the features back to its original size. The concatenating path consists of five levels with different resolution feature maps. Each level consists of two layers of 3×3 non-padded convolutions followed by a rectified linear unit (ReLU). Following the two convolution layers, we apply a 2×2 max pooling operation with stride 2 for down-sampling. After each down-sampling step we double the number of feature channels in the next two convolution layers. The expansive path consists of

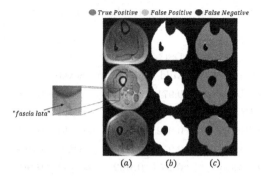

Fig. 3. Examples of muscle segmentation: (a) MRI images of three different patients: from top to bottom: mild, moderate and severe fat infiltration, (b) Delineated GT of muscle region used for training and testing, and (c) Overlap between GT and the output of the FCN.

five levels, where in each we halve the feature channels number. In each level we use a transposed convolution (a.k.a deconvolution) with a 2×2 kernel size and stride of 2. The transposed convolution optimally learns the up-sampling, which helps restore the image more precisely than using interpolation for up-sampling. Next, we concatenate those maps with the corresponding feature maps from the contracting path and apply two 3×3 convolutions, each followed by a ReLU. At the final layer a 1×1 convolution is used to map the feature vector to the desired number of classes.

Four types of inputs to the FCN were considered in this work: Two FCNs were fed by a concatenated T_2 and PD maps (2 channels). The difference between the two inputs lies in the preprocessing stage: one input was fed as it is without preprocessing, while the second input's inhomogeneous intensity was corrected and the T_2 maps were clipped. Two additional FCNs were used: in one network T_2 maps were the input (raw and preprocessed); in the other, PD maps were the input (raw and preprocessed). The purpose of these experiments was to explore the FCN's ability to reach excellent results in the existence of MRI artifacts and in the absence of inhomogeniety correction methods, as was used in previous works. The training set included 14 patients with the corresponding binary segmentation maps. The models were trained using Adam optimizer, with the default settings: $lr = 0.001$, $\beta_1 = 0.9$, $\beta_2 = 0.999$ and $\epsilon = 10^{-8}$. The loss that was optimized is soft Dice coefficient loss. The batch size was set to 8 and the models were trained for 100 epochs. We found it necessary to augment the original training images, increasing the number of images by 10, in order to improve the model's robustness in the presence of data variance. We randomly used shift (0.2 of image height and width), zoom (between 0.9 to 1.3 of image size), rotation ($0° - 30°$) and flip (vertical\horizontal).

Table 1. Quantitative comparison between the performance of the FCN on different input data types for muscle region segmentation (pp stands for preprocessing).

Input	DSC			
	Mild	Moderate	Severe	Combined
T_2+PD with pp	0.971	0.926	**0.964**	0.956
T_2+PD w/o pp	0.973	0.959	0.949	0.958
T_2 with pp	0.962	0.883	0.940	0.931
T_2 w/o pp	0.958	0.959	0.938	0.948
PD with pp	**0.974**	**0.962**	0.962	**0.964**
PD w/o pp	0.970	0.960	0.960	0.962

Table 2. Performance assessment of muscle tissue classification of our method compared to other clustering methods.

Method	Healthy muscle dice	IMAT Dice	ACC	NMI	ARI
k-means	0.877	0.906	0.906	0.565	0.654
DCAE + k-means	0.895	0.915	0.917	0.586	0.692
DCAE$_{TL}$ + k-means	**0.911**	**0.933**	**0.933**	**0.627**	**0.746**

2.3   Healthy Muscle and IMAT Classification

We further classified the region of muscle that we have segmented into two types of tissue: healthy muscle and IMAT pixels. We employed a patch-based deep convolutional auto-encoder (DCAE) to learn semantic feature representation incorporating deep metric learning. The learned embedding is utilized for tissue clustering with k-means algorithm. This method is motivated by our need to learn embedded feature representation of the two tissues with a constraint that imposes similarity across the patches of the same tissue and non-similarity between patches of different tissues.

Deep Convolutional Auto-Encoder and Triplet Loss (DCAE $_{TL}$). Since the clustering is performed for each pixel, we trained the DCAE on patches of size $16 \times 16 \times 2$ extracted around each pixel from the T_2 and PD images of the muscle region. The DCAE is composed of an encoder and a decoder. The encoder consists of two blocks with 32 and 64 feature maps. Each block is built of 3×3 convolutions followed by ReLU, 2×2 max pooling and batch-normalization. The output of the two fully convolution blocks is then flattened into 1024 units and followed by a dense layer that encodes the features in the embedded space. This is followed by L_2 normalization that constrains the embedding to live on a hypersphere. The decoder structure is composed of dense layer of 1024 reshaped to size $4 \times 4 \times 64$, followed by 3×3 transposed convolution layer with 32 filters and stride 2, and another 3×3 transposed convolution layer that reconstructs the input patch (see Fig. 2). The DCAE was trained with Adam optimizer with default settings, and batch size of 256 for 100 epochs. The loss consists of two parts: reconstruction loss and triplet loss. The reconstruction loss is the mean squared error (MSE). To train, we randomly select input patch triplet (x_a^i, x_p^i, x_n^i) from the training set. The distance of the anchor patch (x_a^i) from the positive patch (x_p^i), that roughly matches the anchor patch and the center pixel has same label as the anchor, is smaller than the distance from the negative patch (x_n^i). The auto-encoder is trained simultaneously on the three patches, transforms them to latent vectors $f(x_a^i)$, $f(x_p^i)$ and $f(x_n^i)$ and reconstructs each one to the original image $(\hat{x}_a^i, \hat{x}_p^i, \hat{x}_n^i)$. The latent vectors are used for the calculation of the triplet loss $(L_{triplet})$. The triplet loss over a batch N can be expressed as follows:

$$L_{triplet} = \sum_{i=1}^{N} \max \left\{ 0, \|f(x_a^i) - f(x_p^i)\|_2^2 - \|f(x_a^i) - f(x_n^i)\|_2^2 + \alpha \right\} \qquad (1)$$

where α is a margin that is enforced between positive and negative pairs and set to 1 in our experiments. The combined loss is defined in Eq. 2:

$$L_{total} = \beta L_{triplet} + \lambda (L_{MSE}(x_a^i, \hat{x}_a^i) + L_{MSE}(x_p^i, \hat{x}_p^i) + L_{MSE}(x_n^i, \hat{x}_n^i)) \quad (2)$$

Where β and λ are loss weights, experimentally set to $1/2$ and $1/6$, respectively. We compared this method with the classical k-means applied to the T_2 and PD values of each pixel and with deep convolutional auto-encoder followed by k-means (DCAE + k-means), where the DCAE is trained over patches with MSE loss and the k-means is applied to the embedded layer.

3   Results

The test set includes three patients with mild, moderate and severe fat infiltration. We evaluated the approach performance in terms of Dice Similarity Coefficient (DSC) of the predicted delineation to the GT annotation. The clustering performance of the evaluated clustering methods was evaluated with respect to the normalized mutual information (NMI), accuracy of clustering (ACC), and adjusted Rand index (ARI). NMI is a similarity measurement borrowed from information theory based on the mutual information of the ground-truth classes and the obtained clusters and normalized using the entropy of each. ARI is a variant Rand index that is adjusted for the chance grouping of elements. We also calculated the DSC for both healthy muscle and IMAT. The results for the muscle region segmentation are presented in Table 1 and show very high performance for the variety of inputs proving reliability and robustness of the method. Figure 3 shows results for muscle region segmentation. Our method succeeds to segment the muscle region with a small number of false positives and negatives around the "fascia lata" even when it becomes obscure and blurry in moderate and severe cases where the fat infiltration is high. Table 2 shows the results of clustering for the three clustering methods. The proposed method outperforms the competing methods in healthy muscle dice, IMAT dice, accuracy, NMI and ARI. Figure 4 shows the fraction of infiltrated fat area from the whole muscle region (healthy muscle + IMAT) which indicates the severity of fat infiltration. In addition to being agreeable with the corresponding GT, the fractions show a high correlation between our calculated index and the severity of the disease.

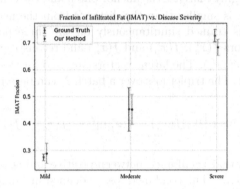

Fig. 4. Infiltrated fat (IMAT) as a fraction of the whole muscle in mild, moderate and severe cases compared to the GT.

4   Conclusions

This work presents a robust method to segment the muscle-region and classify the pixels within the region to healthy muscle pixels and IMAT pixels. We demonstrated the reliability of the proposed method when intensity inhomogeneity artifacts exist in MRI images. We tested the method on patients with mild, moderate and severe muscular dystrophies and proved that the method overcomes the issue of identifying the borders between tissues when the disease is in an advanced stage. We also calculated the fraction of the infiltrated fat and showed a high correlation between this index and the disease severity.

References

1. Mercuri, E., Muntoni, F.: Muscular dystrophies. Lancet **381**(9869), 845–860 (2013)
2. Wren, T.A., Bluml, S., Tseng-Ong, L., Gilsanz, V.: Three-point technique of fat quantification of muscle tissue as a marker of disease progression in duchenne muscular dystrophy: preliminary study. Am. J. Roentgenol. **190**(1), W8–W12 (2008)
3. Valentinitsch, A., et al.: Automated unsupervised multi-parametric classification of adipose tissue depots in skeletal muscle. J. Magn. Reson. Imaging **37**(4), 917–927 (2013)
4. Positano, V., Christiansen, T., Santarelli, M.F., Ringgaard, S., Landini, L., Gastaldelli, A.: Accurate segmentation of subcutaneous and intermuscular adipose tissue from mr images of the thigh. J. Magn. Reson. Imaging: Official J. Int. Soc. Magn. Reson. Med. **29**(3), 677–684 (2009)

5. Chambers, O., Milenkovic, J., Praznikar, A., Tasic, J.: Computer-based assessment for facioscapulohumeral dystrophy diagnosis. Comput. Methods Programs Biomed. **120**(1), 37–48 (2015)
6. Tan, C., et al.: Accurate thigh inter-muscular adipose quantification using a data-driven and sparsity-constrained deformable model. In: 2015 IEEE 12th International Symposium on Biomedical Imaging (ISBI), pp. 1130–1134. IEEE (2015)
7. Yao, J., Kovacs, W., Hsieh, N., Liu, C.-Y., Summers, R.M.: Holistic segmentation of intermuscular adipose tissues on thigh MRI. In: Descoteaux, M., Maier-Hein, L., Franz, A., Jannin, P., Collins, D.L., Duchesne, S. (eds.) MICCAI 2017. LNCS, vol. 10433, pp. 737–745. Springer, Cham (2017). https://doi.org/10.1007/978-3-319-66182-7_84
8. Karaletsos, T., Belongie, S., Ratsch, G.: Bayesian representation learning with oracle constraints. arXiv preprint arXiv:1506.05011 (2015)
9. Ben-Eliezer, N., Sodickson, D.K., Block, K.T.: Rapid and accurate T2 mapping from multi-spin-echo data using Bloch-simulation-based reconstruction. Magn. Reson. Med. **73**(2), 809–17 (2015)
10. Nassar, J., Le Fur, Y., Radunsky, D., Blumenfeld-Katzir, T., Bendahan, D., Ben-Eliezer, N.: Sub-voxel estimation of fat infiltration in degenerative muscle disorders using multi-T2 analysis - a quantitative disease biomarker. In: Montreal: 27th Proceedings of International Society for Magnetic Resonance in Medicine, p. 4011 (2019)
11. Tustison, N.J., et al.: N4ITK: improved N3 bias correction. IEEE Trans. Med. Imaging **29**(6), 1310 (2010)
12. Ronneberger, O., Fischer, P., Brox, T.: U-Net: convolutional networks for biomedical image segmentation. In: Navab, N., Hornegger, J., Wells, W.M., Frangi, A.F. (eds.) MICCAI 2015. LNCS, vol. 9351, pp. 234–241. Springer, Cham (2015). https://doi.org/10.1007/978-3-319-24574-4_28

Resource Optimized Neural Architecture Search for 3D Medical Image Segmentation

Woong Bae, Seungho Lee, Yeha Lee, Beomhee Park, Minki Chung, and Kyu-Hwan Jung[✉]

VUNO Inc., Seoul, South Korea
{iorism,bleaf.lee,yeha.lee,beomheep,brekkanegg,khwan.jung}@vuno.co

Abstract. Neural Architecture Search (NAS), a framework which automates the task of designing neural networks, has recently been actively studied in the field of deep learning. However, there are only a few NAS methods suitable for 3D medical image segmentation. Medical 3D images are generally very large; thus it is difficult to apply previous NAS methods due to their GPU computational burden and long training time. We propose the resource-optimized neural architecture search method which can be applied to 3D medical segmentation tasks in a short training time (1.39 days for 1 GB dataset) using a small amount of computation power (one RTX 2080Ti, 10.8 GB GPU memory). Excellent performance can also be achieved without retraining (fine-tuning) which is essential in most NAS methods. These advantages can be achieved by using a reinforcement learning-based controller with parameter sharing and focusing on the optimal search space configuration of macro search rather than micro search. Our experiments demonstrate that the proposed NAS method outperforms manually designed networks with state-of-the-art performance in 3D medical image segmentation.

Keywords: 3D medical image segmentation · AutoML · Neural Architecture Search (NAS) · Convolutional Neural Networks (CNN)

1 Introduction

Research using deep neural networks for 3D medical image segmentation has exploded over the last few years, producing excellent methods such as U-Net [9] and deep supervision [3]. However, the performance of these methods is highly influenced by manual tasks such as post-processing, hyperparameter tuning, and designing an optimal architecture. In particular, fine-tuning the hyperparameters and designing the best architecture require a great deal of time and computational power. To reduce these manual tasks, research in automated machine learning has been actively carried out for natural image processing tasks [1,6,8].

K.-H. Jung—contributed equally to this paper.

© Springer Nature Switzerland AG 2019
D. Shen et al. (Eds.): MICCAI 2019, LNCS 11765, pp. 228–236, 2019.
https://doi.org/10.1007/978-3-030-32245-8_26

Despite their success in natural image processing, these methods are difficult to apply to the segmentation of 3D medical image with high dimensions which requires enormous computational power. Automated methods developed for 3D medical image segmentation do not yet match state-of-the-art performances achieved by manually designed methods [7,10].

In this paper we propose a resource optimized neural architecture search for 3D medical image segmentation (RONASMIS) which takes a short training time (1.39 days for 1 GB dataset) and requires a small amount of GPU computational power (one RTX 2080Ti with 10.8 GB). The proposed framework differs from previous NAS frameworks by focusing on macro search rather than micro search, exploiting the characteristics of 3D medical images. We avoid retraining the network from scratch after finding the optimal architecture by continuously training the child network during the architecture search process without re-initializing the child network's weights. GPU memory is efficiently utilized by using addition-based skip connections and replacing depth-wise convolutions with normal convolutions. The search space only includes elements that significantly impact the final performance of 3D medical image segmentation, reducing the architecture complexity and GPU memory usage. To the best of our knowledge, our framework is the first to outperform state-of-the-art results in 3D medical image segmentation.

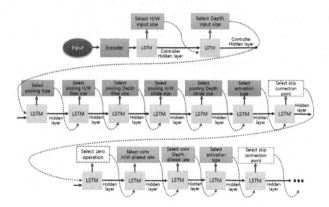

Fig. 1. The proposed RNN based controller and search space. The left figure shows the structure of the proposed controller with dotted boxes indicating that there is a point not applicable in certain sections. Table 1 shows the proposed search space.

2   Method

2.1   Resource-Optimized Search Space for Anisotropic 3D Medical Image and the Basic Architecture

Proposed Search Space: The search space we propose is shown in Table 1 of Fig. 1. Our search space is constructed differently from other NAS papers based on four main reasons:

Table 1. Proposed search space.

	Search space
Input patch size H/W	Equation 1
Input patch size depth	Equation 2
3D pooling type	Max, Avg
3D pooling H/W filter	1, 3, 5
3D pooling Depth filter	1, 3, 5
3D pooling H/W stride	1, 2
3D pooling Depth stride	1, 2
Activation type	ReLU, Leaky ReLU, ELU
Zero operation	0, 1
3D Conv H/W dilate rate	1, 2, 3, 4
3D Conv depth dilate rate	1, 2, 3, 4
Skip connection point	0–10

1. We include input patch sizes and the amount of down sampling in the search space taking into consideration the fact that most 3D medical images have anisotropic shapes. Images in our training data have shapes $4 \times 155 \times 240 \times 240$, $1 \times [90 \sim 130] \times 320 \times 320$, and $2 \times [11 \sim 24] \times [256 \sim 384] \times [256 \sim 384]$ in order of channel, depth, height, and width. The variation of input patch sizes and the number of down sampling operations were also considered by [5] which won the medical segmentation decathlon (MSD).
2. To effectively acquire the receptive field and preserve features' spatial resolution information as much as possible in the encoding process, we include the amount of pooling and dilation rate of 3D convolution in the search space.
3. One main goal of this paper is efficient utilization of GPU memory. A micro search space requires extensive GPU memory which is already burdensome for 3D medical image segmentation. We thus resort to focusing on a macro search space whereas other NAS methods consider either both micro and macro search space or just the prior [1,6,10].
4. Some studies show that connections between global features are pivotal [11]. Most NAS research considering micro search spaces receive inputs from one or two adjacent cells. We instead include skip connection points in our search space to maximize the effect of skip connections across the network.

Further, other NAS methods often apply skip connections to 1×1 convolution after concatenation with other inputs. This increases the number of parameters, resulting in more GPU memory usage than addition. As a remedy we use elementwise-sum based skip connection for macro search.

Most researchers manually determine the best 2D or 3D input patch size, type of down sampling operations along with their stride, and skip connection methods, taking into account available GPU memory and receptive field size

[3–5]. Cascaded learning methods are often used as an alternative; however, the training time takes longer and still requires hyper-parameter tuning [12]. Instead, we focus on constructing a resource optimized search space to reduce the time required to tune hyperparameters.

Three activation functions and two pooling operation types are included in our search space because they do not use additional GPU memory and may affect the segmentation performance depending on the task. To prevent overfitting of the child network, we also add a drop-path regularization (zero operation) which disables some operations or skip-connections at a specific node in the search space. This also helps the controller reliably construct the architecture [1,8].

We replace depth-wise convolution used in most NAS frameworks with normal convolution because the latter utilizes GPU memory more efficiently. It is commonly believed that depth-wise convolution saves more memory because it uses less parameters and requires fewer arithmetic operations. However, there are implementation issues in open source frameworks such as PyTorch which cause depth-wise convolution to inefficiently use up cache memory and more GPU memory when performing backpropagation.

Equations (1) and (2) show how to determine the input patch size in the search space given the the input training image dimensions.

$$\text{Search Space of Patch Size H/W} = \left\lfloor \frac{\max(H,W)}{S^4} \right\rfloor * S^4 - S^4 * \{0,1,2,3,4\} \quad (1)$$

$$\text{Search Space of Patch Size Depth} = \left\lfloor \frac{D}{S^4} \right\rfloor * S^4 - S^4 * \{0,1,2,3,4\} \quad (2)$$

where H, W, D are the median height, width, and depth sizes of training images respectively and S is the stride parameter for each stage. The height and width patch sizes are set equal and the depth is determined independently. The search space cardinality of each element is limited to 5 for any given input patch size.

When an image dimension in the intermediate stages becomes smaller than the largest pooling size, the search space for pooling stride is modified to smaller values. For example, the smallest depth size of prostate 3D images in the MSD challenge is 11. When using this particular image, the search space for pooling stride in the depth direction is set to $\{1\}$. This is necessary because the range of image sizes is unknown prior to training.

The Proposed Base Architecture: We use an architecture modified from U-Net [9] for our base architecture as shown in Fig. 2. The architecture combines the decoder $1 \times 1 \times 1$ convolution skip connections in DeepLabV3+ [2] and the deep supervision scheme proposed in [3]. Batch normalization is replaced with instance normalization to account for GPU memory.

Filled purple arrows indicate $1 \times 1 \times 1$ convolution skip connections that control the amount of information transfer between the encoder and decoder. The number of channels is halved, and the output is concatenated with the decoder's output. The unfilled purple and black arrows are a combination of 3D resize and element-wise-sum of outputs from stages 1, 2, and 3 which is a modified deep supervision method. The parameters considered in the search space are marked

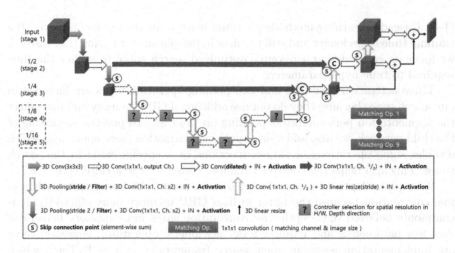

Fig. 2. The proposed base architecture.

bold in the box below the architecture diagram. Question marks denote positions in which feature sizes are determined by the pooling stride parameters in stages 3 and 4. The dotted green arrows indicate whether a zero operation should be used or not. Skip connections which send and receive features are marked with S circles.

When skip-connected features differ in channel sizes, most NAS frameworks concatenate all skip-connected features and apply $1 \times 1 \times 1$ convolution to each layer. On the other hand, we use a matching operation where $1 \times 1 \times 1$ convolutions are applied to all skip connected features with the corresponding channel size to decrease GPU memory usage and network parameters, and then perform an element-wise-sum. We expect this to transfer all import information contained in the features since features with various spatial resolutions are used during architecture search.

All 3D convolution kernels are $1 \times 1 \times 1$ or $3 \times 3 \times 3$ and the controller selects the convolution dilation rate. To stabilize training, the dilation rate of 3D convolution at stage 1 in the encoder part is fixed to 1, and the pooling strides at stage 1 and 2 are fixed to 2. The features in the inner-most stage can take resolutions ranging from 1/16 to 1/4 of the input image's resolution.

2.2   Training the Controller's Parameters for Architecture Selection

We use a parameter sharing based reinforcement learning proposed by ENAS [8] to train the controller. Parameter sharing is an excellent method which trains the controller by receiving a reward just from the newly constructed architecture without retraining the child network from scratch. This reduces the time necessary to reach the global optimum although performance may be affected by the initial architecture, number of episodes, number of training epochs for the child network, moving average baseline parameter, and the entropy's regularization coefficient. We assumed that the combination of sequential actions constitutes the optimal architecture. Thus, we distinguish distinct operations by adding unique values to the LSTM inputs. On the other hand, the reason we do not use the recently proposed differentiable NAS scheme is that the method uploads all operations on the GPU, requiring many expensive GPUs.

At each episode the controller creates 20 child networks and observes the corresponding validation dice scores of each network which are used as a reward to train the controller. The best performing child network is then selected to be trained using dice loss [4]. The dice score is calculated after thresholding pixel values lower than 0.5 to 0. The final architecture is determined by the sequence of actions taken by the controller.

3   Implementation Details and Experimental Results

3.1   Data and Implementation Details

Dataset: We conducted experiments on the brain, heart, and prostate 3D medical images used in the medical segmentation decathlon challenge(MSD, http://medicaldecathlon.com/). This dataset contains images with significantly varying 3D shape and channel sizes, making it appropriate for confirming our NAS method's performance. Because the labels for the test dataset are not publicly available, we evaluate performance with 5-fold cross validation as in [5,10], not on the test dataset.

Implementation Details: We preprocess the data by applying Z-score normalization to each channel independently. For the brain data, we cropped the images based on their non-zero minimum value of each dimension because many voxels contain zeros. The learning rate and weight decay of the child network were fixed as 0.001 and 0.00001 respectively without any learning rate decay methods. The controller also used a fixed learning rate and weight decay of 0.001 and 0.000001 respectively, with entropy regularization coefficient set as 0.0001. The ADAM optimizer was used for both the child and controller networks. Considering training time, the controller's training epochs were 150, 500, and 500 for brain, heart, and prostate tasks respectively. The child network was trained for 3 epochs per episode. To receive a more meaningful reward in the first epoch, the first child network arbitrarily used the architecture with the maximum input patch size including all skip connections and operations.

It is known that changes in batch normalization statistics hinder the training process early on when using drop-path regularization on NAS [1]. However, our training remains unaffected because batch normalization is replaced with instance normalization. The batch size was chosen based on available memory fixed as 2, 1, and 4 for brain, heart, and prostate tasks respectively. The code was implemented using PyTorch 1.0.0.

3.2   Experimental Results

Our comparison baselines include nnUnet [5] and SCNAS [10] as shown in Table 2. nnUnet achieves state-of-the-art performance and holds first place in the MSD competition. SCNAS is a gradient-based AutoML network with a micro search space developed for 3D medical image segmentation tasks. Our method achieves performance exceeding that obtained by SCNAS and nnUnet. Furthermore, this is achieved without using much memory, being small enough to be trained on just one RTX 2080Ti (10.8 GB GPU memory) and is computationally cheap, taking 3.1, 1.39, and 0.35 days to train on the brain, heart, prostate tasks respectively.

In the MSD challenge, most teams employ additional methods such as ensembling multiple neural networks, abundant data augmentation techniques, Test Time Augmentation (T.T.A), and post-processing methods. In contrast, we only use horizontal flip in the 2D axial dimension for data augmentation to evaluate the proposed NAS performance. We also did not use any pre-trained model weights, ensembling, T.T.A, nor post-processing methods. Furthermore, most teams use the 50% overlapped patch-wise inference method to improve performance [5,10]. This method increases the inference time and requires more computation. Instead, we use the one-shot inference method to process the whole image in a single forward pass for quick inference although this can degrade performance.

Figure 3 shows the entropy and reward sequence of each task and the resulting optimal architecture obtained for the heart task for a particular validation set. The uniformly decreasing entropy and steadily increasing rewards illustrate that the controller network was trained well and the result of the architecture is stable. In other words, the controller repeatedly suggests either the same or similar child networks producing consistent dice scores. In our experiments, the controller suggests the same network more than 80% of the time regardless of the validation set.

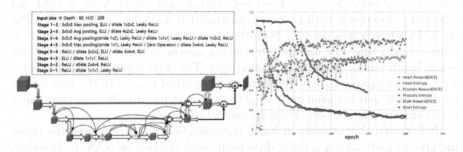

Fig. 3. Left: One of the optimal architectures chosen for the validation set of heart task. **Right:** The entropy of the controller and the reward of the selected architecture for each task.

Table 2. Mean Dice score for Brain tumor, Heart, and Prostate 3D segmentation tasks. V.D.A, Ensemble, T.T.A, and P.P indicate whether Various Data Augmentation, Ensembling, Test Time Augmentation, and Post-Processing were used to obtain the final result.

	3D U-ResNet [10]	SCNAS [10]	SCNAS (transfer)	nnUnet [5]	RONASMIS (non fine-tunning)
Brain Tumor	71.61	72.04	–	74.00	**74.14**
Heart	89.60	89.99	90.47	92.70	**92.72**
Prostate	63.77	65.30	67.92	74.54	**75.71**
V.D.A, Ensemble, T.T.A, P.P.	No	No	No	Yes	**No**
Training GPU	Tesla V100	Tesla V100	Tesla V100	-	**One RTX 2080Ti**
Inference of network	Overlapped patch-wise	Overlapped patch-wise	Overlapped patch-wise	Weighted overlapped patch-wise	**One-shot**

4   Conclusion

By configuring an efficient search space using macro search and utilizing parameter sharing for training a controller, we were able to apply NAS to 3D medical imaging segmentation tasks where previously developed NAS methods were difficult to apply. The proposed resource-optimized NAS framework outperforms state-of-the-art results obtained by manual design in the 3D medical image segmentation challenge. Furthermore, our proposed method is more meaningful in that it achieves excellent performance without using various data augmentation, ensembling, T.T.A, and post-processing.

Acknowledgement. This research was supported by a grant of the Korea Health Technology R&D Project(grant number: HI18C0673) through the Korea Health Industry Development Institute (KHIDI), funded by the Ministry of Health & Welfare, Republic of Korea and Industrial Strategic technology development program (grant number: 10072064) funded by the Ministry of Trade Industry and Energy, Republic of Korea.

References

1. Bender, G., Kindermans, P.J., Zoph, B., Vasudevan, V., Le, Q.: Understanding and simplifying one-shot architecture search. In: International Conference on Machine Learning, pp. 549–558 (2018)
2. Chen, L.-C., Zhu, Y., Papandreou, G., Schroff, F., Adam, H.: Encoder-decoder with atrous separable convolution for semantic image segmentation. In: Ferrari, V., Hebert, M., Sminchisescu, C., Weiss, Y. (eds.) ECCV 2018. LNCS, vol. 11211, pp. 833–851. Springer, Cham (2018). https://doi.org/10.1007/978-3-030-01234-2_49
3. Dou, Q., Chen, H., Jin, Y., Yu, L., Qin, J., Heng, P.-A.: 3D deeply supervised network for automatic liver segmentation from CT volumes. In: Ourselin, S., Joskowicz, L., Sabuncu, M.R., Unal, G., Wells, W. (eds.) MICCAI 2016. LNCS, vol. 9901, pp. 149–157. Springer, Cham (2016). https://doi.org/10.1007/978-3-319-46723-8_18

4. Drozdzal, M., Vorontsov, E., Chartrand, G., Kadoury, S., Pal, C.: The importance of skip connections in biomedical image segmentation. In: Carneiro, G., et al. (eds.) LABELS/DLMIA -2016. LNCS, vol. 10008, pp. 179–187. Springer, Cham (2016). https://doi.org/10.1007/978-3-319-46976-8_19

5. Isensee, F., et al.: nnU-Net: Self-adapting framework for u-net-based medical image segmentation. arXiv preprint arXiv:1809.10486 (2018)

6. Liu, H., Simonyan, K., Yang, Y.: DARTS: Differentiable architecture search. arXiv preprint arXiv:1806.09055 (2018)

7. Mortazi, A., Bagci, U.: Automatically designing CNN architectures for medical image segmentation. In: Shi, Y., Suk, H.-I., Liu, M. (eds.) MLMI 2018. LNCS, vol. 11046, pp. 98–106. Springer, Cham (2018). https://doi.org/10.1007/978-3-030-00919-9_12

8. Pham, H., Guan, M.Y., Zoph, B., Le, Q.V., Dean, J.: Efficient neural architecture search via parameter sharing. arXiv preprint arXiv:1802.03268 (2018)

9. Ronneberger, O., Fischer, P., Brox, T.: U-Net: convolutional networks for biomedical image segmentation. In: Navab, N., Hornegger, J., Wells, W.M., Frangi, A.F. (eds.) MICCAI 2015. LNCS, vol. 9351, pp. 234–241. Springer, Cham (2015). https://doi.org/10.1007/978-3-319-24574-4_28

10. Kim, S., et al.: Scalable neural architecture search for 3D medical image (2019). https://openreview.net/pdf?id=S1lhkdKkeV

11. Shah, M.P., Merchant, S.N., Awate, S.P.: MS-Net: mixed-supervision fully-convolutional networks for full-resolution segmentation. In: Frangi, A.F., Schnabel, J.A., Davatzikos, C., Alberola-López, C., Fichtinger, G. (eds.) MICCAI 2018. LNCS, vol. 11073, pp. 379–387. Springer, Cham (2018). https://doi.org/10.1007/978-3-030-00937-3_44

12. Wang, G., Li, W., Ourselin, S., Vercauteren, T.: Automatic brain tumor segmentation using cascaded anisotropic convolutional neural networks. In: Crimi, A., Bakas, S., Kuijf, H., Menze, B., Reyes, M. (eds.) BrainLes 2017. LNCS, vol. 10670, pp. 178–190. Springer, Cham (2018). https://doi.org/10.1007/978-3-319-75238-9_16

Radiomics-guided GAN for Segmentation of Liver Tumor Without Contrast Agents

Xiaojiao Xiao[1], Juanjuan Zhao[1(✉)], Yan Qiang[1], Jaron Chong[2],
XiaoTang Yang[3], Ntikurako Guy-Fernand Kazihise[1], Bo Chen[4,5,6],
and Shuo Li[4,5,6]

[1] College of Information and Computer, Taiyuan University of Technology,
Shanxi 030000, China
zhaojuanjuan@tyut.edu.cn
[2] Department of Radiology, Shanxi Province Cancer Hospital,
Shanxi Medical University, Taiyuan 030013, China
[3] Department of Radiology, McGill University, Montreal, QC, Canada
[4] Department of Medical Imaging, Western University, London, ON, Canada
[5] Department of Medical Biophysics, Western University, London, ON, Canada
[6] Digital Imaging Group of London, London, ON, Canada

Abstract. Segmentation of the liver tumor is critical for preoperative planning, surgical protocol guidance, and post-operative treatment. Because of using contrast agents (CA), current liver tumor imaging still suffers from high-risk, time-consumption and expensive issues. In this study, a new Radiomics-guided generative adversarial network (Radiomics-guided GAN) is proposed as a safe, short time-consumption and inexpensive clinical tool to segment liver tumor without CA. The innovative Radiomics-guided adversarial mechanism learns the mapping relationship between the contrast images and the non-contrast images, which leads to completing the segmentation. Radiomics-guided GAN contains a segmentor and a discriminator module: the discriminator innovatively uses the Radiomics-feature from the contrast images as prior knowledge to guide the segmentor's adversarial learning; the segmentor innovatively uses dense connection and skip connection to receive and share the guidance information, extracting the representing feature – Implicit Contract Radiomics (ICR) feature – in the non-contrast images. Our method yielded a pixel segmentation accuracy of 95.85%, and a Dice coefficient of 92.17 ± 0.79%, from 200 clinical subjects. The results illustrate that our method achieves the segmentation of liver tumor without CA and become the most potential useful tool for clinicians.

1 Introduction

Segmentation of liver tumor is critical for clinical treatment. It be used for preoperative planning, helping to improve the success rate of tumor resection [1]. Quantitative assessment of segmentation (such as tumor volume, diameter) be used to predict patient survival [2]. The segmentation results are combined with

© Springer Nature Switzerland AG 2019
D. Shen et al. (Eds.): MICCAI 2019, LNCS 11765, pp. 237–245, 2019.
https://doi.org/10.1007/978-3-030-32245-8_27

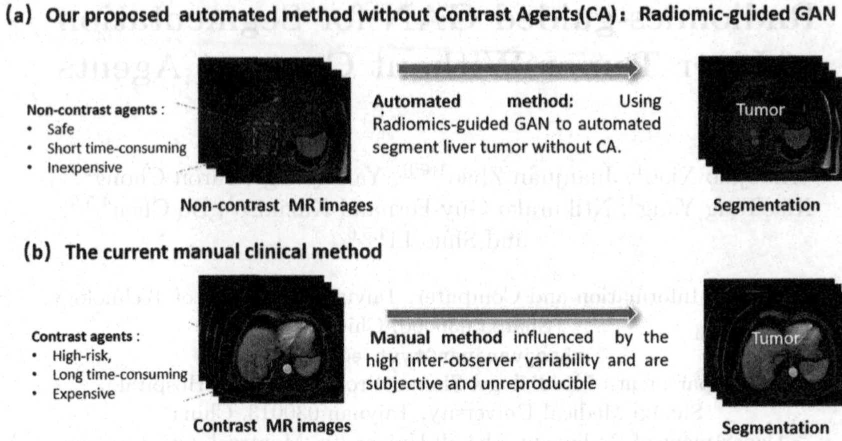

(a) Our proposed automated method without Contrast Agents(CA): Radiomic-guided GAN

Non-contrast agents :
• Safe
• Short time-consuming
• Inexpensive

Non-contrast MR images

Automated   method: Using
Radiomics-guided GAN to automated
segment liver tumor without CA.

Segmentation

(b) The current manual clinical method

Contrast agents :
• High-risk,
• Long time-consuming
• Expensive

Contrast MR images

Manual method influenced by the
high inter-observer variability and are
subjective and unreproducible

Segmentation

Fig. 1. (a) Our method utilizes the inherent Radiomics features of contrast images to guide GAN auto-segmented non-contrast images of liver tumors, which are safe, short-lived and inexpensive (b) The current manual clinical method is that the doctor manual segmentation by visual observation and experience, which is high risk, long time-consuming and expensive.

disease severity, patient age and comorbidities to select appropriate treatment options to prevent a further liver failure.

Most of the existing segmentation of the liver tumor methods is based on images of contrast agents (CA) [3]. Using CA could lead to high-risk, time-consuming and expensive issues. (1) High-risk is due to the potential toxicity of CA [4], after injecting the CA, very small amounts of at least some forms of gadolinium contrast (about 1% of the injected dose) are retained in the tissues. It may cause 10%–15% of the incidence of Contrast Induced Nephropathy (CIN), approximately 5% of patients have a completely normal renal function before the injection of CA. (2) The time-consuming comes from proper injection/administration of the CA costs additional patient time and the imaging process itself that requires multiple imaging techniques. (3) Expensive is due to higher cost of CA itself, and if not injected properly, results in wasted CA material, inefficient use of resources, and wasted MR scanner time. Therefore, segmentation without CA has become an urgent need in the clinic, particularly those with compromised kidney function.

Even in the manual segmentation of liver tumor without CA, there is no attempt. (1) In the non-contrast images, some tumors are almost invisible [5](as shown in Fig. 1), even if they be seen, the boundary of the tumor area are blurred. (2) The size, shape, and position of the tumor are complex and variable, and various in person, and have low contrast with surrounding tissues, uneven density inside the tumor, and various shapes.

The segmentation of non-contrast images has been success in cardiac fields, such as Xu [6] proposed method that simultaneous segmentation and quantification of myocardial infarction without contrast agents, but this method does not apply to liver segmentation. The heart images are dynamic, it takes advantage of the comprehensive spatio-temporal features, but spatio-temporal features do not exist on static images, so we propose to find out effective tumor features to replace it. Studies have proven that radiomics feature decodes tumor performance [7], which characterizes potential tumor microstructures and heterogeneity. Radiomics feature exists in non-contrast images but not immediately visible, however, it can be observed and extracted from the contrast images. Therefore, it is necessary to use visible Radiomics to guide the extraction of implicit contrast radiomics (ICR) feature in non-contrast images by adversarial learning and define this process as **Radiomics-guide adversarial mechanism**.

We propose a Radiomics-guided generation adversarial network (Radiomics-guided GAN) for segmentation of liver tumor from non-contrast images. With the strength of Radiomics-guide mechanism, the Radiomics feature extracted from the contrast images as prior guide knowledge input to the discriminator, which fused with semantic features by the Radiomics-guided Connection Layer (RgCL) lead to the pixel-level classification results. The results-guided are back-propagated to the Segmentor through the pixel-level guidance mixed loss function. Segmentor - Dilated Dense Block-UNet (DDB-UNet)- receives and maximizes the share information from back-propagated and guidance, learning the ICR features which could be applied to compare with the Radiomics features. Radiomics-guided GAN explores the mapping relationship between non-contrast and contrast images and provides an accuracy segmentation of liver tumor without CA.

Our contributions and advantages are three-fold. (1) For the first time, the segmentation of liver tumors without CA is enable. It produce safe, short time-consuming and inexpensive clinic tools. (2) Our DDB-UNet provides a join frame that maximum sharing of guidance information and extracting competitive features. (3) Our innovative Radiomics-guide adversarial mechanism integrates prior knowledge to guide the learning of the mapping relationship.

2   Radiomics-guided GAN

Radiomics-guided GAN segments tumor of non-contrast images (T2w sequence) in an innovative manner. Radiomics-guided GAN has two competing modules: the segmentor (Sect. 2.1) and discriminator (Sect. 2.2) (as shown in Fig. 2). The two modules interact with each other and consist of two seamlessly connected networks. The segmentor (as shown in Fig. 2(a)) establishes the Dilated Dense Block-UNet (DDB-UNet) framework for receiving the guidance information of the discriminator. Dilated convolution expands the receptive field and Dense connection maximizes the information flow and improve the shareability of features (as shown in Fig. 2(b)). UNet's skip connection architecture allows sharing of features and extracting the ICR feature of competition feedback information, thereby guiding the pixel-level accurately segment. The discriminator combines the Radiomics feature (as shown in Fig. 2(d)) with high-dimensional features by

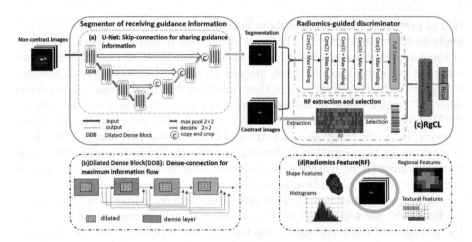

Fig. 2. (a) The architecture of Radiomics-guided GAN: segmentor of receiving guidance information and Radiomics-guided discriminator (b) DDB for extracting feature by expanding receptive fields and maximum information flow (c) Radiomics-guided Connection Layer (RgCL) (Sect. 2.2) (d) Radiomics feature extracted by PyRadiomics, which guide the adversarial learning by obtaining the characteristics of the contrast images.

RgCL (as shown in Fig. 2(c)) to guide segmentor by Radiomics-guide adversarial mechanism.

2.1   Segmentor of Receiving Guidance Information

Segmentor contains UNet of sharing guidance information and DDB of maximum information flow, UNet and DenseNet are both effective tools when using very few images for end-to-end training and are usually used separately. The two networks are reasonably integrated for sharing more information to extract competitive ICR features for a better deal with areas of low contrast caused without CA.

Skip-Connection for Sharing Guidance Information. In Fig. 2(a)), in order to more effectively receive the feedback information of the discriminator and the loss function, the architecture of the skip splicing connection allows the decoder to learn the relevant characteristics lost in the encoder pooling at each stage, sharing low-level information between the input and the output (e.g. boundary information, discriminator competition feedback information). The downsampling gradually reduces the spatial resolution and increases the semantic dimension to restore the abstract image representation, the upsampling process combines the downsampling layer information with the upsampling input information to restore the detail information and gradually restore the precision of images. Eventually extracted with Radiomics-guided competing ICR feature, and segmented images without CA.

Dense-Connection for Maximum Information Flow. In Fig. 2(b)), in order to further improve the information flow between layers, in dense block direct connections from any layers to all subsequent layers. Figure 1(b) illustrates the layout of the resulting Dilation Dense Block schematically. Consequently, the ℓth layer receives the feature-maps of all preceding layers, $x_0, ..., x_{\ell-1}$ as input:

$$x_\ell = H_\ell \left([x_0, x_1, ..., x_{\ell-1}] \right) \tag{1}$$

The above $H_\ell(.)$ represents a non-linear transformation, which is a combined operation, which may include a series of BN (Batch Normalization), ReLU, Pooling, and Conv operations. At the same time, in order to expand the receptive field while not reducing the resolution of the picture and introducing no additional parameters and calculations, a dilation rate is added for each dense block. The final design of each convolution block has a kernel size of 3×3 and each DDB has a dilation rate of $\{1, 2, 4, 8\}$.

2.2   Radiomics-guided Discriminator

The discriminator contains extracting semantic features network and inputting Radiomics feature as a priori knowledge layer, which are identified by Radiomics-guided connection layer (RgCL). These results are backpropagated to guide the segmentor in extracting IRC features.

Extracting Semantic Features Network. The input to the discriminator network is the probability of a T2 segmented image or a ground truth image in the form of a 64×64 patch, true and generated. Using the classic VGG16 [8], a convolutional layer of multiple smaller convolution kernels instead of a convolutional layer with a larger convolution kernel can reduce parameters on the one hand, and on the other hand, a more nonlinear mapping is performed, which increases the network. Fitting expression ability.

Radiomics-guided Connection Layer (RgCL). In Fig. 2(c), The Radiomics feature is used to connect with deep features extracted by VGG. We used a comprehensive opensource platform called PyRadiomics [9], which enables processing and extraction of radiomics features from medical images data using a large panel of engineered hard-coded feature algorithms. Radiomics can quantify a large panel of phenotypic characteristics, such as shape and texture, potentially reflecting biologic properties like inter tumor heterogeneities (as shown in Fig. 2(d)). In 200 patients, we analyze different tumor, and for each tumor, PyRadiomics automatically extracts 669 radiological features (14 shape features, 60 texture features, 395 regional features and 200 histograms features), and automatically selects the most important 15 features.

The discrimination result continuously optimizes VGG parameters through the back propagation of the discriminator loss function, and finally extracts more representative depth features under the guidance of Radiomics.

2.3   Pixel-Level-Guided Hybrid Loss Function

The loss function includes preliminary loss $loss_D$ and segment loss $loss_S$. Among them, input image x and its corresponding base fact y, and use x_i, y_i to represent the input and ground truth values at the pixel location, respectively. The loss function minimize $\log(1 - D(x, S(z))$ and adjust the parameters of D to maximize $\log D(X)$ by adjusting the parameters of S, which competing with each other, the two models are simultaneously enhanced to follow the minimum maximum game process. The traditional optimized loss function is defined as follows:

$$\min_{S} \max_{D} L_{GAN}(S, D) = E_{x,y \sim p_{data}(x,y)} \left[\log^{D(x,y)} \right]$$
$$+ E_{x \sim p_{data}(x)} \left[\log^{(1-D(x,S(x)))} \right] \tag{2}$$

During the training of network D, the loss gradient is propagated back to update the segmentation network. Work has shown that combining GAN losses with more traditional losses can effectively reduce ambiguity. In view of our segmentation task, in the loss method of G, we added an additional Dice loss function and a pixel classification cross entropy loss function. Therefore, the optimized objective function is defined as follows:

$$S^* = \arg\min\max L_{GAN}(S, D) + L_{dice}(S) + L_{Pix\_CE}(S) \tag{3}$$

among

$$L_{dice}(S) = 1 - 2 * \sum_i \frac{x_i y_i}{\sum_i x_i + \sum_i y_i} \tag{4}$$

$$L_{Pix\_CE}(S) = -\frac{1}{n \sum_x y \ln(a) + (1 - y) \ln(1 - a)} \tag{5}$$

3   Experimental Results

For the first time, Radiomics-guided GAN completed the segmentation of liver tumor directly from the non-contrast images with the dice coefficient of $92.17 \pm 0.79\%$, which is better than the current best method with 91.2%, even though it uses CA.

Dataset. An axial image dataset composed of 200 distinct subjects, each with a new untreated diagnosis of HCC, each underwent initial standard clinical liver MRI protocol examinations with corresponding pre-contrast (T2FS [5 mm], Diffusion Weighted Images [6 mm], T1-Pre Contrast [4 mm]) and post-contrast images (Arterial [4 mm], Portal-Venous [4 mm], Late [4 mm], 5-Min Delay [4 mm]) was collected. Gadolinium contrast used in these protocols was gadobutrol 0.1 mmol/kg on a 3T MRI scanner. A radiologist with 7 years of experience in MR Liver imaging analyzed the arterial and delayed enhancement images and verified manual segmentations of the dominant index HCC lesion in each scan as ground truth. The training phase uses 70% images in the dataset. All experiments were assessed with a 10-fold cross-validation test.

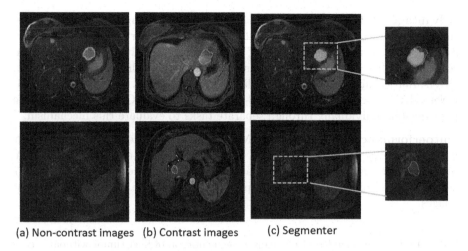

(a) Non-contrast images   (b) Contrast images   (c) Segmenter

Fig. 3. (a) The tumor boundary is blurred on the non-contrast images, and some are even invisible. (b) The CA can be made clear by the CA, and the doctor can complete the make. (c) Our method automatically segments the tumor areas (green plus red zone) on non-contrast images are consistent with the ground truth (yellow solid line) on contrast images. (Color figure online)

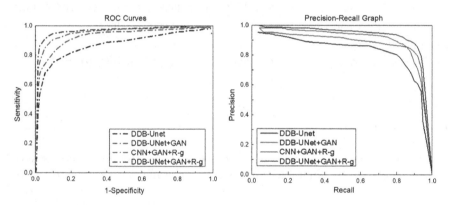

Fig. 4. ROCs and PRs figures proves that Radiomics-guide adversarial mechanism improves the efficiency of segmentation; The dense and skip connection of the segmenter (DDB-UNet) maximizes the sharing of the received feedback information than CNN; Radiomics feature be used as a priori knowledge to guide learning. It turns out that the method we proposed has a high accuracy.

Accurate Segmentation without Contrast Agents. In Fig. 3, our method directly segments the results from the non-contrast images Fig. 3(a) like the results of contrast images Fig. 3(b). It achieves an overall pixel accuracy of 95.85%, with a sensitivity of 90.37% and a specificity of 96.85%. In Fig. 4 displays the ROCs and PRs curves of our method, which has the highest results. The ground truth and result are binary images; each pixel is assessed for tumor or normality (0 or 1)

Advantage of Radiomics-guided GAN Mechanism. Figure 4 evidences that Radiomics-guided GAN has better segmentation performance in comparison to those frameworks because of Radiomics-guide adversarial mechanism: combined ability to share guide information from discriminator by DDB-UNet, adversarial learning (GAN) and Radiomics-guided (R-g). Our method (DDB-UNet+GAN+R-g),DDB-UNet, DDB-UNet+GAN, and CNN+GAN+R-g are implemented individually through separate tasks to evaluate this mechanism.

Outperformance than Existing Methods. Table 1 demonstrates that our method achieves direct segmentation of tumor from non-contrast images. The result achieves an overall pixel accuracy of 95.85%, the dice coefficient of 92.17 ± 0.79%, recall of 91.42%, which outperform than current methods on contrast images.

Table 1. Radiomics-guided GAN realized segmentation of liver tumor without a contrast agents and yielded higher performance than some existing methods [10–13]. Best results are bolded for each row.

Subject	Contrast or not	Accuracy	Dice	Recall
UNet as in [10]	Contrast	–	72.9%	–
Li et al. [11]	Contrast	82.67% ± 1.43%	80.06% ± 1.63%	84.34% ± 1.61%
Hoogi et al. [12]	Contrast	–	84.00% ± 0.03%	–
Jin et al. [13]	Contrast	–	91.2%	–
Our Method	Non-contrast	**95.85%**	**92.17 ± 0.79%**	**91.42%**

4 Conclusions

Radiomics-guided GAN have been proposed and, for the first time, achieved segmentation of liver tumor without CA. The experiment was conducted on 200 subjects and the results (a pixel classification accuracy of 95.85%, the dice of 92.17 ± 0.79%) demonstrate that Radiomics-guided GAN as a safe, short time-consumption and inexpensive clinical tool which aids in the clinical diagnosis of liver tumor assessments.

Acknowledgements. This work is partly supported by National Natural Science Foundation of China (Grant number 61872261), the open funding project of State Key Laboratory of Virtual Reality Technology and Systems, Beihang University (Grant No. 2018-VRLAB2018B07), Research Project Supported by Shanxi Scholarship Council of China (201801D121139).

References

1. Radtke, A., et al.: Computerassisted operative planning in adult living donor liver transplantation: a new way to resolve the dilemma of the middle hepatic vein. World J. Surg. **31**(1), 175 (2007)
2. Chapiro, J., et al.: Identifying staging markers for hepatocellular carcinoma before transarterial chemoembolization: comparison of three-dimensional quantitative versus nonthree-dimensional imaging markers. Radiology **275**(2), 438–447 (2014)
3. Sirlin, C.B., et al.: Consensus report from the 6th international forum for liver MRI using gadoxetic acid. J. Magn. Reson. Imaging **40**(32), 516–529 (2014)
4. Sadowski, E.A., et al.: Nephrogenic systemic fibrosis: risk factors and incidence estimation. Radiology **243**(1), 148–157 (2007)
5. Choi, J.Y., et al.: CT and MR imaging diagnosis and staging of hepatocellular carcinoma: part II. Extracellular agents, hepatobiliary agents, and ancillary imaging features. Radiology **273**(1), 30–50 (2014)
6. Xu, C., Xu, L., Brahm, G., Zhang, H., Li, S.: MuTGAN: simultaneous segmentation and quantification of myocardial infarction without contrast agents via joint adversarial learning. In: Frangi, A.F., Schnabel, J.A., Davatzikos, C., Alberola-López, C., Fichtinger, G. (eds.) MICCAI 2018. LNCS, vol. 11071, pp. 525–534. Springer, Cham (2018). https://doi.org/10.1007/978-3-030-00934-2_59
7. Aerts, H.J., et al.: Decoding tumour phenotype by noninvasive imaging using a quantitative radiomics approach. Nat. Commun. **5**, 4006 (2014)
8. Krizhevsky, A., et al.: ImageNet classification with deep convolutional neural networks. In: Advances in Neural Information Processing Systems, pp. 1097–1105 (2012)
9. Van Griethuysen, J.J., et al.: Computational radiomics system to decode the radiographic phenotype. Cancer Res. **77**(21), 104–107 (2017)
10. Ronneberger, O., Fischer, P., Brox, T.: U-Net: convolutional networks for biomedical image segmentation. In: Navab, N., Hornegger, J., Wells, W.M., Frangi, A.F. (eds.) MICCAI 2015. LNCS, vol. 9351, pp. 234–241. Springer, Cham (2015). https://doi.org/10.1007/978-3-319-24574-4_28
11. Li, W., et al.: Automatic segmentation of liver tumor in CT images with deep convolutional neural networks. J. Comput. Commun. **3**, 146–151 (2015)
12. Hoogi, A., et al.: Adaptive estimation of active contour parameters using convolutional neural networks and texture analysis. IEEE Trans. Med. Imaging **36**(3), 781–791 (2017)
13. Jin, Q., et al.: RA-UNet: a hybrid deep attention-aware network to extract liver and tumor in CT scans. arXiv preprint arXiv:1811.01328 (2018)

Liver Segmentation in Magnetic Resonance Imaging via Mean Shape Fitting with Fully Convolutional Neural Networks

Qi Zeng[1]([⊠]), Davood Karimi[1], Emily H. T. Pang[2], Shahed Mohammed[1],
Caitlin Schneider[1], Mohammad Honarvar[1], and Septimiu E. Salcudean[1]

[1] Department of Electrical and Computer Engineering,
University of British Columbia, Vancouver, BC, Canada
qizeng@ece.ubc.ca
[2] Vancouver General Hospital, Vancouver, BC, Canada

Abstract. In this work, we propose a novel learning-based segmentation technique for delineating liver volumes in magnetic resonance images. The method utilizes the shape prior of the liver for improved accuracy. Instead of labeling the tissue via binary classification, our method completes the segmentation by deforming a label template of the liver average shape based on the learned image features. The average shape of the liver we used is estimated from a large set of expert-labeled computed tomography images. A fully convolutional neural network (FCN) is trained to maximize the overlap between the deformed liver label template and the ground truth segmentation. The proposed method is validated with 51 T2-weighted liver image volumes and achieves an average Dice coefficient of 95.2% with a mean Hausdorff distance of 20.0 mm. Compared to the results obtained with a standard FCN-based method, a three-fold improvement of the Hausdorff distance is observed, indicating the substantial gains achieved by incorporating the shape prior.

1 Introduction

Over the last two decades, magnetic resonance imaging (MRI) has became a standard tool for the diagnosis of chronic liver diseases. Quantitative imaging techniques, such as magnetic resonance elastography (MRE) and proton density fat fraction (PDFF) have shown their potential to be the non-invasive gold standards for assessing hepatic fibrosis and steatosis [14]. Segmenting the liver in images with relatively high soft tissue contrast, such as T1 or T2-weighted MRI, is essential for analyzing the MRE and PDFF imaging data. The segmentation will be used to guide diagnosis in fused multi-parametric images. Figure 1 shows an example of patient data where the segmented T2-weighted image of the right liver lobe was used as background for MRE and PDFF overlays. In addition, automated liver segmentation has the potential to streamline pre-treatment

© Springer Nature Switzerland AG 2019
D. Shen et al. (Eds.): MICCAI 2019, LNCS 11765, pp. 246–254, 2019.
https://doi.org/10.1007/978-3-030-32245-8_28

planning for liver oncologic surgery or transplantation, to provide a more accurate means for diagnosing hepatomegaly or lobar redistribution, and to facilitate the follow-up of patients undergoing portal vein embolization.

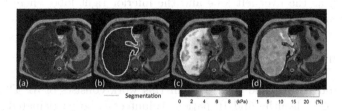

Fig. 1. Multi-parametric liver MRI example. (a) a T2-weighted slice, (b) liver tissue segmentation, (c) the MRE overlay presents liver tissue shear modulus E (unit is Kilopascal (kPa)), and (d) PDFF overlay presents liver tissue fat to water fraction (%).

Deep learning-based methods using fully convolutional neural networks (FCNs) represent the state of the art in medical image segmentation. These methods are effective in learning the complex mapping from the image domain to the segmentation domain using a cascade of convolutions, up-sampling, and down-sampling operations [9,16]. Existing FCN-based techniques commonly take the image intensity as the only source of information, ignoring other prior knowledge of the shape or size of the organ of interest. Recently, Milletari *et al.* proposed a FCN-based technique that utilizes such prior knowledge to segment 2D cardiac ultrasound images [10]. The idea was to predict the coefficients of a principal component analysis (PCA)-based shape model from the learned features to carry out the segmentation. Because this is a difficult task, the FCN architecture included a separate branch to refine the segmentation by focusing on patches around the predicted key-points. Al Arif *et al.* applied a similar shape-aware FCN technique to segment lateral cervical X-ray images and proposed to map the shape prior of cervical vertebra with signed distance functions [1]. Karimi *et al.* later developed a similar end-to-end shape model-based FCN technique to segment prostate in 3D MRI [6]. This study demonstrated the challenges of achieving FCN's convergence when predicting the coefficients of a 3D shape model and reported major difficulties in improving the segmentation performance. Moreover, the above studies focused mostly on segmenting relatively simple objects which have limited inter-subject variability. For 3D segmentation of large and complex organs, such as the liver, similar techniques might yield conservative results.

In this work, we propose a new way of incorporating shape prior in FCN based segmentation techniques, and we demonstrate the performance of our proposed method for liver segmentation in T2-weighted MRI images. The shape prior of the liver is extracted from a set of images with expert-provided liver segmentation as the estimated average liver shape. Our method produces the liver segmentation of a test image by deforming this average shape. A FCN is trained to estimate the deformation mapping between the average liver shape and the test image volume in the form of a dense deformation field (DDF). Opting for such a free-form deformation ensures that the model has sufficient flexibility to accommodate complex shapes and to better tackle the challenging regions such as the liver left lobe and the inferior right lobe where the image contrast is low and inter-subject variability is high.

2   Materials and Methods

Data Preparation. The data used in this work consists of 51 T2-weighted MRI scans of 15 healthy and 10 patient volunteers who participated in a liver MRI study approved by the University of British Columbia Clinical Research Ethics Board. Images were acquired with an Achieva 3T scanner (Philips Inc., Best, Netherlands) using a T2-weighted turbo spin echo (T2W-TSE) sequence with a SENSE Torso XL receiving coil. Details of the scan settings are as follows: $TR = 1400$ ms, $TE = 80$ ms, and flip angle $= 90°$. The reconstructed transverse slices were $432 \times 432 \times 25$ with a voxel size of $0.7 \times 0.7 \times 6$ mm^3. Preprocessing steps included: (1) N4 bias field correction [15], and (2) re-sampling to obtain isotropic voxels of size $1.4 \times 1.4 \times 1.4$ mm^3, resulting in an image size of $224 \times 224 \times 96$. For each volume, the liver was first manually segmented by an experienced research assistant. Then, a clinical radiologist edited this segmentation to obtain the ground truth. 40 out of the 51 image volumes (80%) were randomly selected for the training and cross-validation of the proposed method. The remaining 11 volumes (20%) were used as test data and remained unseen to the training and parameter tuning.

Segmentation with Mean Shape Fitting. Consider a training dataset consisting of N images $I = \{I_i\}_{i=1}^{N}$ and corresponding ground-truth segmentation masks $Y = \{Y_i\}_{i=1}^{N}$, where $I_i \in \mathbb{R}^3 \to \mathbb{R}$ and $Y_i \in \mathbb{R}^3 \to \{0, 1\}$, where 0 denotes the background and 1 denotes the foreground (liver). Our proposed segmentation method is based on deforming a "mean liver shape", in our case a binary label template, denoted with Z, to the desired segmentation of the image at hand.

The mean shape used in this work was created using the computed tomography (CT) liver images publicly available through the liver tumor segmentation challenge (LiTS) [2]. Liver surface meshes of the 131 volumes in this dataset were extracted as an atlas of the liver shape. We aligned the atlas and estimated the mean shape (Z) using a group-wise non-rigid point cloud registration algorithm [12]. The computed mean shape surface mesh was converted into a binary label mask as shown in Fig. 2 where the grid size and spacing were set to be the same as in our dataset described above.

In our proposed method, predicting the segmentation of an image amounts to estimating a "best fit" deformation field that deforms the liver mean shape to the liver tissue volume in the image. To achieve this, we train our FCN to estimate a 3D displacement vector for each voxel of the liver mean shape template, denoted by $u_i \in \mathbb{R}^3 \to \mathbb{R}^3$. The resulting free-form dense deformation field (DDF) gives the model complete flexibility in representing both local and global non-rigid deformations. To ensure efficient gradient back-propagation for FCN training, our DDF is implemented by linear operations such as grid warping and re-sampling as suggested in [4]. The estimated deformation vectors u_i are first added to the reference grid Cartesian coordinates of the mean shape template in $\mathbb{R}^3$. The deformed label mask is then computed via trilinear interpolation using the updated grid coordinates to produce the final segmentation mask.

Notice that our method does not use the commonly applied shape atlas representation, such as a statistical shape model (SSM). Instead, only the reg-istration between the mean shape and the input image volume was considered. The main challenge of incorporating additional shape modes in our method is

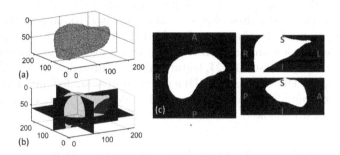

Fig. 2. Mean liver shape computed from the LiTS data: (a) the mean shape surface mesh (green) with the surface point cloud (blue), (b) the 3D orthogonal slices of the mean shape binary label template, and (c) the label template 2D views. (Color figure online)

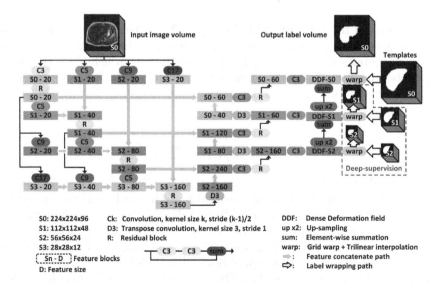

Fig. 3. Schematic representation of the FCN architecture used in this work. (Color figure online)

how to manage the convergence of the DDF for multiple modes in a consistent manner. Computing multiple DDFs for multiple shape modes is theoretically feasible, but hard to implement due to its high computational burden.

Network Design. Figure 3 shows the details of our FCN architecture. The overall design follows the V-net architecture [9] and consists of contracting and expanding paths of convolutional filters. In the contracting branch we compute features with different fields-of-view using 3D kernels of increasing sizes ($\{3^3, 5^3, 9^3, 17^3\}$) and strides ($\{1, 2, 4, 8\}$). This resulted in feature maps at four different scales $\{s0, s1, s2, s3\}$ with 20 features at each scale. Following the idea of feature reuse and dense connections proposed in [5], these feature maps are re-sized with additional convolution filters and forwarded to all coarser layers via concatenation paths. Residual blocks are also employed to improve the gradient back propagation [3]. In the expanding branch, feature maps are up-sampled via transpose-convolutions and concatenated with features from the contracting branch. At the scale of $\{s0, s1, s2\}$, feature maps go through a final convolutional layer to compute DDFs. Coarser DDFs are then up-sampled and added to the finer DDFs sequentially to improve the gradient flow. All convolution operations in this network are followed by a ReLU activation function [11].

Similarity Metric and Training Loss. The segmentation method performs the following loss function minimization:

$$\arg\min_{\theta} \frac{1}{N} \sum_{i=1}^{N} -J(T_\theta(Z, I_i), Y_i) + \gamma ||\nabla u_i||^2 \qquad (1)$$

where θ denotes the parameters of the FCN. The first term in the above loss function quantifies the similarity between the ground truth segmentation mask and the predicted segmentation mask, which is estimated by deforming the mean shape label template, Z. This deformation is denoted as $T_\theta(Z, I_i)$ because it is computed by the FCN as a function of the input image, I_i. For the similarity measure we use the Tversky metric [13]:

$$J = \frac{|TP|}{|TP| + \alpha |FP| + \beta |FN|} \qquad (2)$$

As an extension to the Dice similarity coefficient (DSC), the Tversky metric allows control over the trade-off between false positive (FP) and false negative (FN) by adjusting parameters α and β. For our data, we found that the setting of $\alpha = 0.6$ and $\beta = 0.4$ helps to reduce the number of false positives caused by over-segmentation into the surrounding tissue. The second term in our loss function is the L^2 norm of the DDF's first spatial derivative. This is a regularization term that is necessary to encourage the DDF to be locally smooth and thus avoid excessive local deformations [4]. Such deformations can occur due to spurious image features or image artifacts at the isolated small regions. The regularization parameter, γ, controls the trade-off between the two loss terms. Figure 4 shows how γ regularizes the DDF. The results reported in this paper were produced with $\gamma = 10^{-2}$, which we empirically found to lead to good results.

Training Strategy. We used 5-fold cross-validation to train an ensemble of 5 networks. The final segmentation mask is produced by averaging the results of the 5 networks. Each network was trained for 500 epochs using the Adam optimizer [7] with a batch size of 1. The initial learning rate was 10^{-5}, which was reduced by 5% after every 20 epochs. During training, three types of data augmentation were used: (1) B-spline local image deformation with an amplitude of 2 mm, (2) addition of Gaussian noise with a maximum amplitude of 10% of the average image intensity, (3) rigid image translation with a maximum of 5 mm in each of the x, y, z directions. As suggested by [8,16], deeply-supervised multi-scale training was introduced to our implementation as highlighted in Fig. 3 with red dashed lines. The lower-resolution ground-truth segmentation masks were generated by down-sampling the ground-truth at the original resolution.

3   Results and Discussion

We compare our method with the standard V-net [9] and report five results for our method: (1) Proposed-OneFCN: one FCN is trained without deep supervision to produce the DDF and the warped mean shape is considered as the final segmentation; (2) Proposed-OneFCN-DS: similar to (1), except that deep supervision at three different scales is used; (3) Proposed-Ensemble: five FCNs are

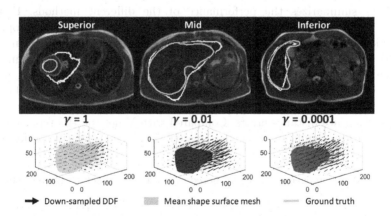

Fig. 4. An example of segmentations produced with $\gamma = \{1, 10^{-2}, 10^{-4}\}$. Top row: segmentation contours for the superior, mid, and inferior slices. Bottom row: 3D graphics to show how the label template is deformed. The DDF obtained with $\gamma = 1$ is too conservative causing the deformed template to fail to accurately delineate the liver boundary. The DDF with $\gamma = 10^{-4}$ is overly aggressive causing unexpected regions of over- and under-segmentation.

trained without deep supervision, the final segmentation is obtained by setting the threshold of the average label maps value produced by the five networks at 0.5; (4) Proposed-Ensemble-DS: similar to (3) except that networks are trained with deep supervision; and (5) Proposed-Baseline: we separately trained our FCN to generate the segmentation via the conventional binary labeling app-roach. The results presented show the performance of a classification approach with a more up-to-date FCN implementation than the V-net. Our evaluation cri-teria include Jaccard, Dice, false positive (FP), false negative (FN), Hausdorff Distance (HD), and mean surface distance (MSD).

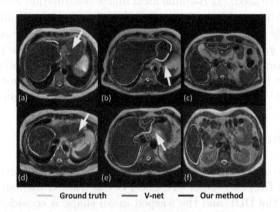

Ground truth   V-net   Our method

Fig. 5. Examples of results produced by our proposed method and V-net.

Table 1 summarizes the performance of the different methods. Figure 5 presents examples of image slices segmented by V-net and the Proposed-Ensemble technique. From the results, our method outperformed V-net in terms of all performance criteria. In terms of volume labeling accuracy, our method with network ensemble was able to achieved a mean Dice of 95.2%. A paired t-test showed a p-value of 0.003 when comparing the Dice scores achieved by our method with that of V-net. Our method also achieved improvements in terms of reduced surface distance errors. Compared with V-net the HD reported from our method was significantly smaller ($p = 0.04$). The conservative performance

Table 1. The comparison of the proposed method with V-net at different stages

Metrics	Jaccard (%)	DICE (%)	FN (%)	FP(%)	HD (mm)	MSD (mm)
V-net	86.9 ± 2.6	92.9 ± 1.5	3.7 ± 2.3	9.9 ± 2.6	60.3 ± 50.3	1.4 ± 0.3
Proposed-Baseline	88.4 ± 1.9	93.8 ± 1.0	3.2 ± 4.5	4.6 ± 2.7	63.8 ± 18.2	1.5 ± 0.3
Proposed-OneFCN	90.7 ± 1.0	95.1 ± 0.5	3.8 ± 2.8	5.6 ± 3.0	20.2 ± 9.8	1.0 ± 0.2
Proposed-OneFCN-DS	90.4 ± 2.1	94.9 ± 1.2	4.9 ± 4.2	4.9 ± 2.5	24.6 ± 10.2	1.1 ± 0.3
Proposed-ENS	90.9 ± 1.8	**95.2 ± 1.0**	3.3 ± 2.7	6.0 ± 3.0	**20.0 ± 12.1**	**0.9 ± 0.2**
Proposed-ENS-DS	90.9 ± 2.4	95.2 ± 1.3	5.5 ± 4.1	**3.8 ± 2.4**	23.8 ± 13.9	1.0 ± 0.3

of V-net in terms of a higher HD is due to its inconsistent results at the superior left lobe and the inferior right lobe as show on Fig. 5(a), (d) and (c). In comparison, our method was able to better avoid large segmentation errors, because the mean shape prior provided a good initial segmentation at these regions. When our proposed FCN structure was trained based on the conventional classification approach, it only achieved marginal improvements on the volume overlapping metrics, while no gain on surface distance metrics was observed. This demonstrates again the advantage of using the shape prior in further regulating the segmentation surface distance errors.

Although the use of Tversky metric allowed a higher penalty on the FP, a high FP rate (>5%) was still reported in all cases, indicating that accurately isolating the liver from surrounding tissue background is still a relatively challenging task for learning-based methods. It is also interesting to see that the overall performance of our method had no significant gain from introducing deep-supervision of the network training, except it might have helped to better regulate FP.

The purposed method was implemented using Tensorflow. With an NVIDIA TITAN RTX GPU, the training for 500 echos took approximately 24 h. For a test image volume, each FCN produces a segmentation in 0.8 s.

4 Conclusion

In the context of liver segmentation in 3D MRI T2-weighted image volumes, we proposed a new learning based method that utilizes prior shape information and non-rigid registration to improve the segmentation accuracy. Our method achieved significantly better results than the competing binary classification based method in terms of Dice and HD. Particularly, our method substantially reduced the maximum surface distance errors in the most challenging regions such as the superior left liver lobe and the inferior right lobe. Our technique can be easily extended to segment other more complicated organs when a good image atlas is available. A more detailed comparison study between the proposed method and some of the existing SSM-based techniques is warranted in a future study.

Acknowledgment. This project is funded by Natural Sciences and Engineering Research Council of Canada (NSERC). We deeply appreciate the support from the Charles A. Laszlo Chair in Biomedical Engineering held by Prof. Salcudean.

References

1. Al Arif, S.M.M.R., Knapp, K., Slabaugh, G.: SPNet: shape prediction using a fully convolutional neural network. In: Frangi, A.F., Schnabel, J.A., Davatzikos, C., Alberola-López, C., Fichtinger, G. (eds.) MICCAI 2018. LNCS, vol. 11070, pp. 430–439. Springer, Cham (2018). https://doi.org/10.1007/978-3-030-00928-1_49
2. Bilic, P., et al.: The liver tumor segmentation benchmark (LiTS). arXiv preprint arXiv:1901.04056 [cs.CV] (2019)

3. He, K., Zhang, X., Ren, S., Sun, J.: Deep residual learning for image recognition. In: IEEE CVPR, pp. 770–778 (2016)
4. Hu, Y., et al.: Adversarial deformation regularization for training image registration neural networks. In: Frangi, A.F., et al. (eds.) MICCAI 2018. LNCS, vol. 11070, pp. 774–782. Springer, Cham (2018). https://doi.org/10.1007/978-3-030-00928-1_87
5. Huang, G., Liu, Z., ven der Maaten, L., Weinberger, K.Q.: Densely connected convolutional networks. In: IEEE CVPR, pp. 2261–2269 (2017)
6. Karimi, D., et al.: Prostate segmentation in MRI using a convolutional neural network architecture and training strategy based on statistical shape models. Int. J. Comput. Assist. Radiol. Surg. 13(8), 1211–1219 (2018)
7. Kingma, D.P., Ba, J.: Adam: a method for stochastic optimization. arXiv preprint arXiv:1412.6980 [cs.LG] (2014)
8. Lee, C.Y., Xie, S., Gallagher, P., Zhang, Z., Tu, Z.: Deeply-supervised nets. In: PMLR, vol. 38, pp. 562–570 (2015)
9. Milletari, F., Navab, N., Ahmadi, S.: V-net: fully convolutional neural networks for volumetric medical image segmentation. In: 2016 Fourth International Conference on 3D Vision (3DV), pp. 565–571 (2016)
10. Milletari, F., et al.: Integrating statistical prior knowledge into convolutional neural networks. In: Descoteaux, M., et al. (eds.) MICCAI 2017. LNCS, vol. 10433, pp. 161–168. Springer, Cham (2017). https://doi.org/10.1007/978-3-319-66182-7_19
11. Nair, V., Hinton, G.E.: Rectified linear units improve restricted Boltzmann machines. In: ICML, pp. 807–814 (2010)
12. Rasoulian, A., Rohling, R., Abolmaesumi, P.: Group-wise registration of point sets for statistical shape models. IEEE Trans. Med. Imag. 31(11), 2025–2034 (2012)
13. Salehi, S.S.M., Erdogmus, D., Gholipour, A.: Tversky loss function for image segmentation using 3D fully convolutional deep networks. In: Wang, Q., et al. (eds.) MLMI 2017. LNCS, vol. 10541, pp. 379–387. Springer, Cham (2017). https://doi.org/10.1007/978-3-319-67389-9_44
14. Taouli, B., Ehman, R.L., Reeder, S.B.: Advanced MRI methods for assessment of chronic liver disease. AJR Am. J. Roentgenol. 193(1), 14–27 (2009)
15. Tustison, N.J., et al.: N4ITK: Improved N3 bias correction. IEEE Trans. Med. Imag. 29(6), 1310–1320 (2010)
16. Yang, D., et al.: Automatic liver segmentation using an adversarial image-to-image network. In: Descoteaux, M., et al. (eds.) MICCAI 2017. LNCS, vol. 10435, pp. 507–515. Springer, Cham (2017). https://doi.org/10.1007/978-3-319-66179-7_58

Unsupervised Domain Adaptation via Disentangled Representations: Application to Cross-Modality Liver Segmentation

Junlin Yang[1]($\boxtimes$), Nicha C. Dvornek[3], Fan Zhang[2], Julius Chapiro[3], MingDe Lin[3], and James S. Duncan[1,2,3,4]

[1] Department of Biomedical Engineering, Yale University, New Haven, CT, USA
junlin.yang@yale.edu
[2] Department of Electrical Engineering, Yale University, New Haven, CT, USA
[3] Department of Radiology and Biomedical Imaging, Yale School of Medicine, New Haven, CT, USA
[4] Department of Statistics and Data Science, Yale University, New Haven, CT, USA

Abstract. A deep learning model trained on some labeled data from a certain source domain generally performs poorly on data from different target domains due to domain shifts. Unsupervised domain adaptation methods address this problem by alleviating the domain shift between the labeled source data and the unlabeled target data. In this work, we achieve cross-modality domain adaptation, i.e. between CT and MRI images, via disentangled representations. Compared to learning a one-to-one mapping as the state-of-art CycleGAN, our model recovers a many-to-many mapping between domains to capture the complex cross-domain relations. It preserves semantic feature-level information by finding a shared content space instead of a direct pixelwise style transfer. Domain adaptation is achieved in two steps. First, images from each domain are embedded into two spaces, a shared domain-invariant content space and a domain-specific style space. Next, the representation in the content space is extracted to perform a task. We validated our method on a cross-modality liver segmentation task, to train a liver segmentation model on CT images that also performs well on MRI. Our method achieved Dice Similarity Coefficient (DSC) of 0.81, outperforming a CycleGAN-based method of 0.72. Moreover, our model achieved good generalization to joint-domain learning, in which unpaired data from different modalities are jointly learned to improve the segmentation performance on each individual modality. Lastly, under a multi-modal target domain with significant diversity, our approach exhibited the potential for diverse image generation and remained effective with DSC of 0.74 on multi-phasic MRI while the CycleGAN-based method performed poorly with a DSC of only 0.52.

This work was supported by NIH Grant 5R01 CA206180.

D. Shen et al. (Eds.): MICCAI 2019, LNCS 11765, pp. 255–263, 2019.
https://doi.org/10.1007/978-3-030-32245-8_29

1 Introduction

Deep neural networks have been very successful in a variety of computer vision tasks, including medical image analysis. The majority of neural networks conduct training and evaluation on images from the same distribution. However, real-world applications usually face varying visual domains. The distribution differences between training and test data, i.e. domain shifts, can lead to significant performance degradation. Data collection and manual annotation for every new task and domain are time-consuming and expensive, especially for medical imaging, where data are limited and are collected from different scanners, protocols, sites, and modalities. To solve this problem, domain adaptation algorithms look to build a model from a source data distribution that performs well on a different but related target data distribution [12]. In the context of medical image analysis, most prior studies on domain adaptation focus on aligning distributions of data from different scan protocols, scanners, and sites [4,9,11]. Related literature is relatively limited when it comes to different modalities.

In clinical practice, various imaging modalities may have valuable and complementary roles. For example, as a fast, less expensive, robust, and readily available modality, computed tomography (CT) plays a key role in the routine clinical examination of hepatocellular carcinoma (HCC), but has the disadvantages of radiation exposure and relatively low soft-tissue contrast. Magnetic resonance imaging (MRI) provides higher soft-tissue contrast for lesion detection and characterization but is more expensive, time-consuming, less robust, and more prone to artifacts. In practice, both multiphase contrast-enhanced MRI and CT may be used in the diagnosis and follow-up after treatment of HCC, and often require the same image analysis tasks, such as liver segmentation. While MRI acquisitions include more complex quantitative information than CT useful for liver segmentation, they are often less available clinically than CT images [8]. Thus, it would be helpful if we could learn a liver segmentation model from the more accessible CT data that also performs well on MRI images.

Given the significant domain shift, cross-modality domain adaptation is quite difficult (see Fig. 1). One promising approach utilizes CycleGAN, a pixel-wise style transfer model, for cross-modality domain adaptation in a segmentation task [3]. Compared to feature-based domain adaptation, it does not necessarily maintain the semantic feature-level information. More importantly, the cycle-consistency loss implies a one-to-one mapping between source domain and target domain and leads to lack of translated output diversity, generating very similar images. It thus fails to represent the complex real-world data distribution in the target domain and likely degrades the performance of segmentation or other follow-up analysis [5].

Our goal is to achieve domain adaptation between CT and MRI while maintaining the complex relationship between the two domains. Our model assumes the mapping to be many-to-many and learns it by disentangling the representation into content and style. A shared latent space is assumed to be found for both domains that preserves the semantic content information. Our main contributions are listed as follows. This is the first to achieve unsupervised domain adaptation for segmentation via disentangled representations in the field of medical imaging. Our model decomposes images across domains into a domain-invariant content space, which preserves the anatomical information, and a domain-specific style space, which represents modality information. We validated the superior performance of our model on a liver segmentation task with cross-modality domain adaptation and compared it to the state-of-art CycleGAN. We also demonstrated the generalizability of our model to joint-domain learning and robust adaptation to a multi-modal target domain with large variety.

2 Methodology

2.1 Assumptions

Let $x_1 \in \mathcal{X}_1$ and $x_2 \in \mathcal{X}_2$ be images from two domains, which differ in visual appearance but share common semantic content. We assume there exists a mapping, potentially many-to-many instead of deterministic one-to-one, between $\mathcal{X}_1$ and $\mathcal{X}_2$. Each image x_i from $\mathcal{X}_i$ can be embedded into and generated from a shared semantic content space $c \in \mathcal{C}$ that is domain-invariant and a style code $s_i \in \mathcal{S}_i$ that is domain-specific $(i = 1, 2)$ [2]. Specifically, MRI and CT of the abdomen from HCC patients can be considered as images from different domains $\mathcal{X}_1$ and $\mathcal{X}_2$, since they exhibit quite different visual appearance with the same anatomical structure shared behind them. Therefore, a shared domain-invariant space that preserves the anatomical information and a domain-specific style code for each modality can be found to recover the underlying mapping between MRI and CT. Due to the many-to-many assumption, the relatively complex underlying distribution of the target domain can be recovered.

2.2 Model

Our Domain Adaptation via Disentangled Representations (DADR) pipeline consists of two modules: Disentangled Representation Learning Module (DRLModule) and Segmentation Module (SegModule) (see Fig. 2). Of note, the DRL Module box in the DADR pipeline at the top is expanded in the left large box.

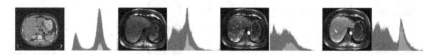

Fig. 1. Images and histograms of liver (yellow) and whole image (blue). From left to right: CT, multiphasic MRI sequence at three time points (pre-contrast, 20 s post-contrast i.e. arterial phase, 70 s post-contrast i.e. portal venous phase) (Color figure online)

DRLModule. The module consists of two main components, a variational autoencoder (VAE) for reconstruction and a generative adversarial network (GAN) for adversarial training. We train the VAE component for in-domain reconstruction, where reconstruction loss is minimized to encourage the encoders and generators to be inverses to each other. The GAN component for cross-domain translation is trained to encourage the disentanglement of the latent space, decomposing it into content and style subspaces [6,7]. Similar to Huang's work [2], the DRLModule consists of several jointly trained encoders E_{c_1}, E_{c_2}, E_{s_1}, E_{s_2}, generators G_1, G_2 and discriminators D_1, D_2, where $c_i = E_{c_i}(x_i) \sim p(c_i)$ and $s_i = E_{s_i}(x_i) \sim p(s_i)$ for $i = 1, 2$. Specifically, the generators are trying to fool the discriminators by successful cross-domain generation with swapped style code. Due to the disentangled style code $s_i \in \mathcal{S}_i$, the underlying mapping is assumed to be many-to-many. We have $p(c_1) = p(c_2)$ upon convergence, which is the shared content space that preserves anatomical information. The overall loss function is defined as the weighted sum of the three components:

$$L_{total} = \alpha L_{recon} + \beta L_{adv} + \gamma L_{latent} \tag{1}$$

(a) In-domain reconstruction, $L_{recon} = L_{recon}^1 + L_{recon}^2$

$$L_{recon}^i = \mathbb{E}_{x_i \sim X_i} \|G_i(E_{ci}(x_i), E_{si}(x_i)) - x_i\|_1 \tag{2}$$

(b) Cross-domain translation, $L_{adv} = L_{adv}^{1 \to 2} + L_{adv}^{2 \to 1}$

$$L_{adv}^{1 \to 2} = \mathbb{E}_{c_1 \sim p(c_1), s_2 \sim p(s_2)}[log(1 - D_2(x_{1 \to 2}))] + \mathbb{E}_{x_2 \sim X_2}[log(D_2(x_2))] \tag{3}$$

(c) Latent space reconstruction, $L_{latent} = L_{recon}^{c_1} + L_{recon}^{s_1} + L_{recon}^{c_2} + L_{recon}^{s_2}$

$$L_{recon}^{c_1} = \|E_{c_2}(x_{1 \to 2}) - c_1\|_1, L_{recon}^{s_2} = \|E_{s_2}(x_{1 \to 2}) - s_2\|_1 \tag{4}$$

Domain Adaptation with Content-Only Images. Once the disentangled representations are learned, content-only images can be reconstructed by using

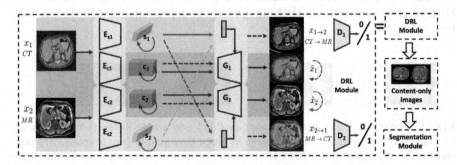

Fig. 2. Left: Framework for Disentangled Representation Learning Module. Solid line: in-domain reconstruction, Dotted line: cross-domain translation. Right: Pipeline of Domain Adaptation via Disentangled Representations (DADR)

the content code c_i without style code s_i. For both CT and MR, their content codes are embedded in a shared latent space that incorporates the anatomical structure information and excludes the modality appearance information. We train a segmentation model on content-only images from CT domain and apply it directly on content-only images from MR domain.

Joint-Domain Learning. Joint-domain learning aims to train a single model with data from both domains that works on both domains and outperforms models trained and tested separately on each domain. Our framework can easily generalize to joint-domain learning by including content-only images from both domains for the training segmentation module.

Implementation Details. The SegModule is a standard UNet [10]. Content encoders consist of convolutional layers and residual layers followed by batch normalization, while style encoders consist of convolutional layers, a global average pooling layer, and a fully-connected layer. Generators take the style code (vector of length 8) and content code (feature map of $64 \times 64 \times 256$) as inputs. A multilayer perceptron takes the style code and generates affine transformation parameters. Residual blocks in the generator are equipped with an Adaptive Instance Normalization (AdaIN) layer to take affine transformation parameters from the style code. Discriminators are convolutional neural networks for binary classification. For the loss function, $\alpha = 25, \beta = 10, \gamma = 0.1$ in our experiments. Experiments were conducted on two Nvidia 1080ti GPUs. The training time each fold is $\sim$5 h for DRLModule and $\sim$2 h for SegModule. Testing is very quick.

3 Experiments and Results

3.1 Datasets and Experimental Setup

We tested our methods on unpaired CT slices of 130 patients from LiTS challenge 2017 [1] and multi-phasic MRI slices of 20 local patients with HCC (see Fig. 1). CT and MR were divided into 5 folds for subject-wise cross-validation. A supervised UNet [10] trained and tested on pre-contrast MR serves as upper bound of domain adaptation, while a supervised UNet trained on CT and tested on pre-contrast MRI, without domain adaptation, provides the lower bound, which shows the relatively large domain shifts between CT and MRI (see Table 2).

For our DADR model, in experiment 1, 4 folds of CT and 4 folds of pre-contrast MR were used to train DRLModule, 4 folds of CT were used to train SegModule and 1 fold of pre-contrast MR were used to test SegModule. In experiment 2, it was the same as experiment 1, but 4 folds of pre-contrast MR were also used to train SegModule. In experiment 3, it was the same as experiment 1, except that pre-contrast MR were replaced with multi-phasic MR.

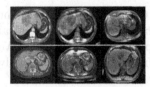

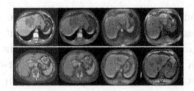

Fig. 3. Two examples of style transfer with CycleGAN, Left to right: CT, generated MR, MR

Fig. 4. Two examples of content-only images via disentangled representations, Left to right: CT, content-only CT, content-only MR, MR

3.2 Results

Experiment 1: Segmentation with Domain Adaptation. We evaluated Domain Adaptation with CycleGAN (DACGAN) and Domain Adaptation via Disentangled Representations (DADR) respectively and compared with UNet without Domain Adaptation (UNet w/o DA) (see Fig. 5 and Table 1).

Table 1. Comparison of Segmentation Results

Method	DICE	std
UNet w/o DA	0.26	0.07
DACGAN	0.72	0.05
DADR	**0.81**	**0.03**

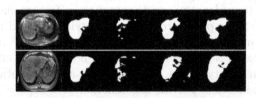

Fig. 5. Two examples of segmentation results. Left to right: pre-contrast MR, liver mask, predictions from UNet w/o DA, DACGAN, DADR

DACGAN. For comparison purposes, we trained a CycleGAN model with unpaired CT and pre-contrast MR images and performed style transfer on test CT images to generate synthetic MR images. A standard UNet was trained on synthetic MR images and validated on real precontrast MR images. It achieved a DSC score of 0.72 (see Table 1) with subject-wise 5-fold cross-validation. Figure 3 shows two examples of synthetic MR generated by CycleGAN.

DADR. Our DRLModule embeds cross-domain images into a shared content space and generates content-only images. Figure 4 shows two examples of content-only images via Disentanglement Representations. We trained the UNet model on content-only CT and validated on content-only MR with 5-fold cross-validation and achieved a DSC score of 0.81 (see Table 1).

Experiment 2: Joint-Domain Learning. Besides domain adaptation, our model can achieve joint-domain learning by feeding UNet with both content-only CT and content-only MR as training data. A single model that works on both CT and MR modality was obtained and outperformed two fully-supervised standard UNet models separately trained on each modality (see Table 2).

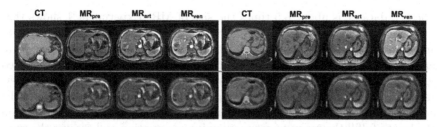

Fig. 6. Two examples of content-only images via disentangled representations for multi-phasic MR. first row: original images, second row: content-only images.

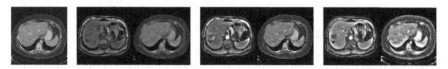

Fig. 7. Three examples of multi-modal style generation with reference, from left to right: CT, three pairs of reference MR and generated MR (pre-contrast, arterial, portal venous phase)

Experiment 3: Multi-modal Target Domain. We considered multi-phasic MR with three phases as multi-modal target domain with complex underlying distribution and conducted domain adaptation and style transfer on it.

A. Robust Domain Adaptation. A CycleGAN model was not able to handle such large variety in the multi-modal target domain e.g. multi-phasic MR. However, for our model, the shared content space provided a robust representation for anatomical information in multi-phasic MR; thus it remained effective even faced with the multi-modal target domain (see Fig. 6 and Table 3).

Table 2. Joint-domain Learning with DADR

Method	CT tested DSC	MR tested DSC
CT trained	0.901(0.020)	0.260(0.072)
MR trained	0.134(0.091)	0.869(0.044)
Joint CT & MR	**0.912(0.012)**	**0.891(0.040)**

Table 3. DA on Multi-modal Target Domain

Method	DICE	std
DACGAN	0.52	0.06
DADR	**0.74**	**0.04**

B. Diverse Style Transfer. Furthermore, our model can realize diverse style transfer by changing the style code while preserving the anatomical structure with the same content code. The style code can be randomly sampled in the style space or encoded from a reference image by style encoder E_{s_i} (see Fig. 7).

3.3 Analysis

We tested our model on unpaired CT and MRI data. It is noteworthy that it is a highly unbalanced cross-domain data, where CT is of better quality and the size of the CT dataset is about 6.5 times the size of MR. Experiment 1 shows that our model is superior to CycleGAN in terms of DSC score for cross-modality segmentation with domain adaptation. Experiment 2 shows a promising application of our model for joint-domain learning, which makes learning from unpaired medical images with different modalities a reality. Experiment 3 shows robustness of our model under multi-modal target domain with large diversity and the potential for diverse multi-modal style transfer. The disentangled representation is the key to fulfill the many-to-many mapping assumption and recover the complex relationship between two domains. It is also of vital importance to discover the shared latent space that preserves the semantic feature-level information.

4   Conclusions and Discussions

We proposed a cross-modality domain adaptation pipeline via disentangled representations, which may improve current clinical workflows and allow for robust intergration of multi-parametric MRI and CT data. Instead of one-to-one mapping, our model considers the complex mapping between CT and MR as many-to-many and preserves semantic feature-level information, thus ensuring robust cross-modality domain adaptation for a segmentation task. We validated and compared our model on CT and pre-phase MR from HCC patients with state-of-the-art methods. With multi-phasic MRI, our model demonstrated strong ability to handle multi-modal target domains with large variety. Furthermore, our model had good generalization towards joint-domain learning and showed the potential for multi-modal image generation, which can be further investigated in the future. In addition, we could focus on specific anatomical structures in the content space, such as liver and tumor, by including task-relevant loss to improve the results further.

References

1. Christ, P., Ettlinger, F., Grün, F., Lipkova, J., Kaissis, G.: LiTS-liver tumor segmentation challenge. ISBI and MICCAI (2017)
2. Huang, X., Liu, M.-Y., Belongie, S., Kautz, J.: Multimodal unsupervised image-to-image translation. In: Ferrari, V., Hebert, M., Sminchisescu, C., Weiss, Y. (eds.) ECCV 2018. LNCS, vol. 11207, pp. 179–196. Springer, Cham (2018). https://doi.org/10.1007/978-3-030-01219-9_11
3. Jiang, J., et al.: Tumor-aware, adversarial domain adaptation from CT to MRI for lung cancer segmentation. In: Frangi, A.F., Schnabel, J.A., Davatzikos, C., Alberola-López, C., Fichtinger, G. (eds.) MICCAI 2018. LNCS, vol. 11071, pp. 777–785. Springer, Cham (2018). https://doi.org/10.1007/978-3-030-00934-2_86
4. Kamnitsa, K., et al.: Unsupervised domain adaptation in brain lesion segmentation with adversarial networks. In: Niethammer, M., Niethammer, M., et al. (eds.) IPMI 2017. LNCS, vol. 10265, pp. 597–609. Springer, Cham (2017). https://doi.org/10.1007/978-3-319-59050-9_47

5. Lee, H.-Y., Tseng, H.-Y., Huang, J.-B., Singh, M., Yang, M.-H.: Diverse image-to-image translation via disentangled representations. In: Ferrari, V., Hebert, M., Sminchisescu, C., Weiss, Y. (eds.) ECCV 2018. LNCS, vol. 11205, pp. 36–52. Springer, Cham (2018). https://doi.org/10.1007/978-3-030-01246-5_3

6. Mathieu, M.F., Zhao, J.J., Zhao, J., Ramesh, A., Sprechmann, P., LeCun, Y.: Disentangling factors of variation in deep representation using adversarial training. In: Advances in Neural Information Processing Systems, pp. 5040–5048 (2016)

7. Narayanaswamy, S., et al.: Learning disentangled representations with semi-supervised deep generative models. In: Advances in Neural Information Processing Systems, pp. 5925–5935 (2017)

8. Oliva, M.R., Saini, S.: Liver cancer imaging: role of CT, MRI, US and PET. Cancer Imaging 4(Spec No A), S42 (2004)

9. Perone, C.S., Cohen-Adad, J.: Promises and limitations of deep learning for medical image segmentation. J. Med. Artif. Intell. 2 (2019)

10. Ronneberger, O., Fischer, P., Brox, T.: U-Net: convolutional networks for biomedical image segmentation. In: Navab, N., Hornegger, J., Wells, W.M., Frangi, A.F. (eds.) MICCAI 2015. LNCS, vol. 9351, pp. 234–241. Springer, Cham (2015). https://doi.org/10.1007/978-3-319-24574-4_28

11. Valindria, V.V., et al.: Domain adaptation for MRI organ segmentation using reverse classification accuracy. arXiv preprint arXiv:1806.00363 (2018)

12. Wang, M., Deng, W.: Deep visual domain adaptation: a survey. Neurocomputing **312**, 135–153 (2018)

Automatic Segmentation of Vestibular Schwannoma from T2-Weighted MRI by Deep Spatial Attention with Hardness-Weighted Loss

Guotai Wang[1,2,3]([✉]), Jonathan Shapey[3,2,7], Wenqi Li[4], Reuben Dorent[2], Alexis Dimitriadis[5], Sotirios Bisdas[6], Ian Paddick[5], Robert Bradford[5,7], Shaoting Zhang[8], Sébastien Ourselin[2], and Tom Vercauteren[2]

[1] School of Mechanical and Electrical Engineering,
University of Electronic Science and Technology of China, Chengdu, China
guotai.wang@uestc.edu.cn
[2] School of Biomedical Engineering and Imaging Sciences, King's College London, London, UK
[3] Wellcome/EPSRC Centre for Interventional and Surgical Sciences, University College London, London, UK
[4] NVIDIA, Cambridge, UK
[5] Queen Square Radiosurgery Centre (Gamma Knife), National Hospital for Neurology and Neurosurgery, London, UK
[6] Neuroimaging Analysis Centre, Queen Square, London, UK
[7] Department of Neurosurgery, National Hospital for Neurology and Neurosurgery, London, UK
[8] SenseTime Research, Shanghai, China

Abstract. Automatic segmentation of vestibular schwannoma (VS) tumors from magnetic resonance imaging (MRI) would facilitate efficient and accurate volume measurement to guide patient management and improve clinical workflow. The accuracy and robustness is challenged by low contrast, small target region and low through-plane resolution. We introduce a 2.5D convolutional neural network (CNN) able to exploit the different in-plane and through-plane resolutions encountered in standard of care imaging protocols. We propose an attention module with explicit supervision on the attention maps to enable the CNN to focus on the small target for more accurate segmentation. We also propose a hardness-weighted Dice loss function that gives higher weights to harder voxels to boost the training of CNNs. Experiments with ablation studies on the VS tumor segmentation task show that: (1) our 2.5D CNN outperforms its 2D and 3D counterparts, (2) our supervised attention mechanism outperforms unsupervised attention, (3) the voxel-level hardness-weighted Dice loss improves the segmentation accuracy. Our method achieved an average Dice score and ASSD of 0.87 and 0.43 mm respectively. This will facilitate patient management decisions in clinical practice.

The original version of this chapter was revised: an author's name has been corrected. The correction to this chapter is available at
https://doi.org/10.1007/978-3-030-32245-8_96

1   Introduction

Vestibular schwannoma (VS) is a benign tumor arising from one of the balance nerves connecting the brain and inner ear. The incidence of VS has risen significantly in recent years and is now estimated to be between 14 and 20 cases per million per year [4]. High-quality magnetic resonance imaging (MRI) is required for diagnosis and expectant management with serial imaging is usually advised for smaller tumors. Current MR protocols include contrast-enhanced T1-weighted (ceT1) and high-resolution T2-weighted (hrT2) images, but there is increasing concern about the potentially harmful cumulative side-effects of gadolinium contrast agents. Accurate measurement of VS tumor volume from MRI is desirable for growth detection and guiding management of the tumor. However, current clinical practice relies on labor-intensive manual segmentation.

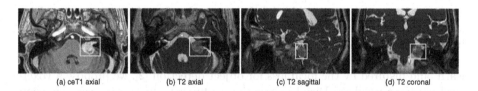

(a) ceT1 axial   (b) T2 axial   (c) T2 sagittal   (d) T2 coronal

Fig. 1. An example of VS tumor. (a) contrast-enhanced T1-weighted MRI. (b)-(d) T2-weighted MRI. Note the small target region, low contrast in T2, and low resolution in sagittal and coronal views.

This paper aims to automatically segment the VS tumor from T2-weighted MRI. This will improve clinical workflow and help to reduce the use of gadolinium contrast, thus improving patient safety. However, this task is challenging due to several reasons. First, T2 images have a relatively low contrast and the exact boundary of the tumor is hard to detect. Second, the VS tumor is a relatively small structure with large shape variations in the whole brain image. Besides, the image is often acquired with low through-plane resolution, as shown in Fig. 1.

In the literature, a Bayesian model was proposed for automatic VS tumor segmentation from ceT1 MRI [9], but it can hardly be applied to T2 images with much lower contrast. Semi-automated tools for this task suffer from inter-operator variations [8]. Recently, convolutional neural networks (CNNs) have achieved state-of-the-art performance for many segmentation tasks [1,3,6]. However, most of them are designed to segment images with isotropic resolution, and are not readily applicable to our VS images with high in-plane resolution and low through-plane resolution. To segment small structures, Yu et al. [12] used a coarse-to-fine approach with recurrent saliency transformation. Oktay et al. [5] learned an attention map to enable the CNN to focus on the target. However, the attention map was not explicitly supervised during training, and may not be well-aligned with the target region, which can limit the segmentation accuracy. Therefore, we hypothesise that end-to-end supervision on the

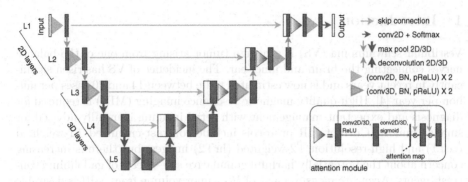

Fig. 2. The proposed 2.5D U-Net with spatial attention for VS tumor segmentation from anisotropic MRI. The attention module is depicted in the right bottom corner.

learning of attention map will lead to better results. Loss functions such as Dice loss [3] and generalized Dice loss [7] were also proposed to mitigate the class imbalance between foreground and background by image-level weighting during training. Considering the fact that some voxels are harder than the others to learn, and inspired by the focal loss for object detection [2], we propose a voxel-level hardness-weighted Dice loss function to further improve the segmentation accuracy.

The contribution of this paper is three-fold. First, to the best of our knowledge, this is the first work on automatic VS tumor segmentation using deep learning. We propose a 2.5D CNN combining 2D and 3D convolutions to deal with the low through-plane resolution. Second, we propose an attention module to enable the CNN to focus on the target region. Unlike previous works [5], we explicitly supervise the learning of attention maps so that they can highlight the target structure better. Finally, we propose a voxel-level hardness-weighted Dice loss function to boost the performance of CNNs. The proposed method was validated with T2-weighted MR images of 245 patients with VS tumor.

2   Methods

2.5D CNN for Segmentation of Images with Anisotropic Resolutions.
For our images with high in-plane resolution and low through-plane resolution, 2D CNNs applied slice-by-slice will ignore inter-slice correlation. Isotropic 3D CNNs may need to upsample the image to an isotropic 3D resolution to balance the physical receptive field (in terms of mm rather than voxels) along each axis, which requires more memory and may limit the depth or feature numbers of the CNNs. Therefore, it is desirable to design a 2.5D CNN that can not only use inter-slice features but also be more efficient than 3D CNNs. In addition, to make the receptive field isotropic in terms of physical dimensions, the number of convolution along each axis should be different when dealing with such images. In [10], a 2.5D CNN was proposed for brain tumor segmentation. However, it was designed for isotropically resampled 3D images and limited by a small physical receptive field along the through-plane axis.

The main structure of our proposed attention-based 2.5D CNN follows the typical encoder and decoder design of U-Net [6], as shown in Fig. 2. The encoder contains five levels of convolutions. The first two levels (L1–L2) and the other three levels (L3–L5) use 2D and 3D convolutions/max-poolings, respectively. This is motivated by the fact that the in-plane resolution of our VS tumor images is about 4 times that of the through-plane resolution. After the first two 2D in-plane max-pooling layers, the feature maps in L3 and the followings have a near-isotropic 3D resolution. At each level, we use a block of layers containing two convolution layers each followed by batch normalization (BN) and parametric rectified linear unit (pReLU). The number of output feature channels at level l is denoted as N_l. N_l is set as $16l$ in our experiments. The decoder contains similar blocks of 2D and 3D layers. Additionally, to deal with the small target region, we add a spatial attention module to each level of the decoder, which is depicted in Fig. 2 and detailed in the following.

Multi-scale Supervised Spatial Attention. Previous works have shown that spatial attention can enable the network to focus on the target region in a large image context [5] as it learns to give higher (lower) scores to voxels in the target region (background). Building upon these works, we further introduce an explicit supervision on the learning of attention to improve its accuracy. A spatial attention map is a single-channel image of attention coefficient $\alpha_i \in [0, 1]$ that is a score of relative importance for each spatial position i. The proposed attention module consists of two convolution layers. For an input feature map at level l with channel number N_l, the first convolution layer reduces the channel number to $N_l/2$ and is followed by ReLU. The second convolution layer further reduces the channel number to 1 and is followed by sigmoid to generate the spatial attention map $\mathcal{A}_l$ at level l. $\mathcal{A}_l$ is multiplied with the input feature map. We also use a residual connection in the attention module, as depicted in Fig. 2.

We propose an attention loss to supervise the learning of spatial attention explicitly during training. Let G denote the multi-channel one-hot ground truth segmentation of an image and G^f denote the single-channel binary foreground mask. For attention map $\mathcal{A}_l$ at level l, let G_l^f denote the average-pooled version of G^f so that it has the same resolution as $\mathcal{A}_l$. Our loss function for training is:

$$\mathcal{L} = \frac{1}{L} \sum_l \ell(\mathcal{A}_l, G_l^f) + \ell(P, G) \tag{1}$$

where L is the number of resolution levels ($L = 5$ in our case). $\ell(\mathcal{A}_l, G_l^f)$ measures the difference between $\mathcal{A}_l$ and G_l^f. This supervision drives the attention maps to be as close to the foreground mask as possible. P denotes the prediction output of CNN, i.e., the probability of belonging to each class for each voxel. $\ell(P, G)$ is the segmentation loss. The multi-scale supervision in Eq. (1) is similar to the holistic loss [11]. However, here we apply it to multi-scale attention maps rather than the network's final prediction output. The two terms in Eq. (1) share the same underlying loss function ℓ, as discussed in the following.

Voxel-Level Hardness-Weighted Dice Loss. A good choice of ℓ is the Dice loss [3] proposed to train CNNs for binary segmentation, and it has shown good performance in dealing with imbalanced foreground and background classes. For segmentation of small structures with low contrast, some voxels are harder than the others to learn. Treating all the voxels for a certain class equally as in [3] may limit the performance of CNNs on hard voxels. Therefore, we propose automatic hard voxel weighting in the loss function by defining a voxel-level weight:

$$w_{ci} = \lambda * abs(p_{ci} - g_{ci}) + (1.0 - \lambda) \tag{2}$$

where p_{ci} is the probability of being class c for voxel i predicted by a CNN, and g_{ci} is the corresponding ground truth value. $\lambda \in [0,1]$ controls the degree of hard voxel weighting. Our proposed hardness-weighted Dice loss (HDL) is defined as:

$$\ell_{HDL}(P,G) = 1.0 - \frac{1}{C}\sum_c \frac{2\sum_i w_{ci}p_{ci}g_{ci} + \epsilon}{\sum_i w_{ci}(p_{ci} + g_{ci}) + \epsilon} \tag{3}$$

where C is the channel number of P and G, and $\epsilon = 10^{-5}$ is a small number for numerical stability. Similarly to [3], the gradient of ℓ_{HDL} with respect to p_{ci} can be easily computed. Note that for the first term $\ell_{HDL}(\mathcal{A}_l, G_l^f)$ in Eq. (1) dealing with attention maps, the channel number C is one.

3   Experiments and Results

Data and Implementation. T2-weighted MRI of 245 patients with a single sporadic VS tumor were acquired in axial view before radiosurgery treatment, with high in-plane resolution around $0.4\,\mathrm{mm} \times 0.4\,\mathrm{mm}$, in-plane size 512×512, slice thickness and inter-slice spacing $1.5\,\mathrm{mm}$, and slice number 19 to 118. The ground truth was manually annotated by an experienced neurosurgeon and physicist using the Gamma Knife planning software (Leksell GammaPlan, Elekta, Sweden) that employs an in-plane semi-automated segmentation method. We randomly split the images into 178, 20 and 47 for training, validation and testing respectively. Each image was cropped with a cubic box of size $100\,\mathrm{mm} \times 50\,\mathrm{mm} \times 50\,\mathrm{mm}$ manually, and normalized by its intensity mean and standard deviation. The CNNs were implemented in Tensorflow and NiftyNet [1] on a Ubuntu desktop with an NVIDIA GTX 1080 Ti GPU[1]. For training, we used Adam optimizer with weight decay 10^{-7}, batch size 2. The learning rate was initialized to 10^{-4} and halved every 10k. The training was ended when performance on the validation set stopped to increase. For quantitative evaluation, we measured Dice, average symmetric surface distance (ASSD) and relative volume error (RVE) between segmentation results and the ground truth.

---

[1] Code available at: https://github.com/NifTK/VSSegmentation.

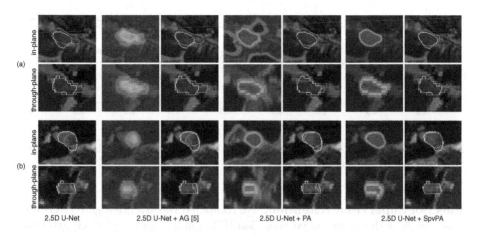

Fig. 3. Visual comparison of different attention mechanisms for VS tumor segmentation. Odd columns: segmentation results (green curves) and the ground truth (yellow curves). Even columns: attention maps at the highest resolution level (L1) of the decoder, where warmer color represents higher attention. (Color figure online)

Comparison of Different Networks. First, we evaluate the performance of our 2.5D network, and refer to our CNN without the attention module as 2.5D U-Net. Its 2D and 3D counterparts with the same configuration except the dimension of convolution/decovolution and max-pooling are referred to as 2D U-Net and 3D U-Net respectively. For 3D U-Net, the images were resampled to isotropic resolution of 0.4 mm × 0.4 mm × 0.4 mm. The performance of these networks trained with Dice loss is shown in Table 1. It can be observed that our 2.5D U-Net achieves higher accuracy than its 2D and 3D counterparts. In addition, it is more efficient than the other two. Its lower inference time than slice-by-slice 2D U-Net is due to the 3D down-sampled feature maps in L3-L5.

Table 1. Quantitative evaluation of different networks for VS tumor segmentation. Dice loss was used for training. AG: The attention gate proposed in [5]. PA: Our proposed attention module. SpvPA: The proposed attention with supervision. * denotes significant improvement from 2.5D U-Net based on a paired t-test ($p < 0.05$).

Network	Dice(%)	ASSD (mm)	RVE (%)	Time (s)
2D U-Net	80.38 ± 10.42	0.92 ± 0.68	18.01 ± 17.23	3.56 ± 0.36
3D U-Net	83.61 ± 13.69	0.84 ± 0.62	18.01 ± 17.48	3.90 ± 0.49
2.5D U-Net	85.69 ± 7.07	0.67 ± 0.45	16.02 ± 14.71	$\mathbf{3.49 \pm 0.39}$
2.5D U-Net + AG [5]	85.93 ± 6.96	$0.58 \pm 0.41^*$	15.45 ± 12.37	3.51 ± 0.34
2.5D U-Net + PA	86.09 ± 6.94	$0.55 \pm 0.32^*$	14.87 ± 12.19	3.52 ± 0.37
2.5D U-Net + SpvPA	$\mathbf{86.71 \pm 4.99^*}$	$\mathbf{0.53 \pm 0.29^*}$	$\mathbf{13.40 \pm 9.34^*}$	3.52 ± 0.37

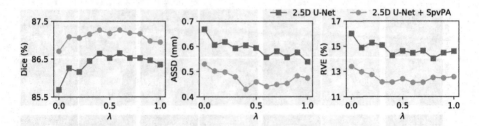

Fig. 4. Performance of 2.5D U-Net and 2.5D U-Net + SpvPA trained with the proposed voxel-level hardness-weighted Dice loss (HDL) with different values of λ.

Effect of Supervised Attention. We compared the attention gate (AG) proposed in [5] with our proposed attention (PA) module and supervised attention (SpvPA). These three variants were combined with our 2.5D U-Net respectively and trained with Dice loss. Quantitative evaluations in Table 1 show that both AG [5] and PA lead to an accuracy improvement from 2.5D U-Net without attention, and our proposed PA performs slightly better than AG [5]. By using our SpvPA, the segmentation accuracy can be further improved from that of PA.

Figure 3 shows a visual comparison of these three different attention methods. It can be observed that the attention map of AG [5] successfully suppresses most of the background region, but the magnitude for the target region is lower than that of PA and SpvPA. The attention map of PA highlights the target region, but also assigns high attention coefficients for strong edges in the input image. This is mainly because the input for the PA module is a concatenation of high-level and low-level features. Benefiting from our explicit supervision on the learning of attention, the attention map of SpvPA focuses more on the target region and is less blurry than that of AG [5].

Performance of Voxel-Level Hardness-Weighted Dice Loss. We additionally used HDL to train 2.5D U-Net and 2.5D U-Net + SpvPA respectively. The average Dice, ASSD and RVE of these two networks with different values of λ are shown in Fig. 4. Note that $\lambda = 0.0$ is the baseline without hard voxel weighting and a higher value of λ corresponds to assigning higher weights to harder voxels during training. The figure shows that our HDL with different values of λ leads to higher segmentation performance. An improvement of accuracy is observed when λ increases from 0.0 to 0.4. Interestingly, when λ is higher than 0.6, the segmentation accuracy decreases, as shown by the curves of Dice in Fig. 4. This indicates that giving too much emphasis to hard voxels may decrease the generalization ability of the CNNs. As a result, we suggest a proper range of λ as [0.4, 0.6]. Quantitative comparison between Dice loss [3] and our proposed HDL with $\lambda = 0.6$ is presented in Table 2. It shows that our proposed HDL outperforms Dice loss [3] for both 2.5D U-Net and 2.5D U-Net + SpvPA.

Table 2. Performance of two CNNs trained with different loss functions. * denotes significant improvement from Dice loss [3] based on a paired t-test ($p < 0.05$).

Network	Training loss	Dice(%)	ASSD (mm)	RVE (%)
2.5D U-Net	Dice loss [3]	85.69 ± 7.07	0.67 ± 0.45	16.02 ± 14.71
	HDL ($\lambda = 0.6$)	86.66 ± 6.01*	0.56 ± 0.37*	14.48 ± 12.30*
2.5D U-Net + SpvPA	Dice loss [3]	86.71 ± 4.99	0.53 ± 0.29	13.40 ± 9.34
	HDL ($\lambda = 0.6$)	$\mathbf{87.27 \pm 4.91}$	$\mathbf{0.43 \pm 0.31}$*	$\mathbf{12.14 \pm 8.94}$

4 Discussion and Conclusion

In this work, we propose a 2.5D CNN for automatic VS tumor segmentation from high-resolution T2-weighted MRI. Our network is a trade-off between standard 2D and 3D CNNs and specifically designed for images with high in-plane resolution and low through-plane resolution. Experiments show that it outperforms its 2D and 3D counterparts in terms of segmentation accuracy and efficiency. To deal with the small target region, we propose a multi-scale spatial attention mechanism with explicit supervision on the learning of attention maps. Experimental results demonstrate that the supervised attention can guide the network to focus more accurately on the target region, leading to higher accuracy of the final segmentation. We also combine automatic hard voxel weighting with existing Dice loss [3], and the proposed voxel-level hardness-weighted Dice loss can lead to further performance improvement. The weighting function only has one hyperparameter λ and experiments show that the performance was rather insensitive to the choice of λ when around 0.5. In the future, it would be of interest to apply our method to other datasets. Our segmentation method will facilitate the rapid adoption of these techniques into clinical practice, providing clinicians with the means for accurate automatically-generated segmentations that will be used to inform patient management decisions. Though our methods can also be applied to ceT1 images, this work on T2 image segmentation improves patient safety by enabling patients to undergo serial imaging without the need to use potentially harmful contrast agents.

Acknowledgements. This work was supported by Wellcome Trust [203145Z/16/Z; 203148/Z/16/Z; WT106882], and EPSRC [NS/A000050/1; NS/A000049/1] funding. TV is supported by a Medtronic/Royal Academy of Engineering Research Chair [RCSRF1819/7/34].

References

1. Gibson, E., et al.: NiftyNet: a deep-learning platform for medical imaging. Comput. Methods Programs Biomed. **158**, 113–122 (2018)
2. Lin, T.Y., Goyal, P., Girshick, R., He, K., Dollar, P.: Focal loss for dense object detection. In: ICCV, pp. 2999–3007 (2017)

3. Milletari, F., Navab, N., Ahmadi, S.A.: V-Net: fully convolutional neural networks for volumetric medical image segmentation. In: IC3DV, pp. 565–571 (2016)
4. Moffat, D.A., Hardy, D.G., Irving, R.M., Viani, L., Beynon, G.J., Baguley, D.M.: Referral patterns in vestibular schwannomas. Clin. Otolaryngol. Allied Sci. **20**(1), 80–83 (1995)
5. Oktay, O., et al.: Attention U-Net: learning where to look for the pancreas. arXiv Preprint arXiv:1804.03999 (2018)
6. Ronneberger, O., Fischer, P., Brox, T.: U-Net: convolutional networks for biomedical image segmentation. In: Navab, N., Hornegger, J., Wells, W.M., Frangi, A.F. (eds.) MICCAI 2015. LNCS, vol. 9351, pp. 234–241. Springer, Cham (2015). https://doi.org/10.1007/978-3-319-24574-4_28
7. Sudre, C.H., Li, W., Vercauteren, T., Ourselin, S., Jorge Cardoso, M.: Generalised dice overlap as a deep learning loss function for highly unbalanced segmentations. In: Cardoso, M.J., et al. (eds.) DLMIA/ML-CDS -2017. LNCS, vol. 10553, pp. 240–248. Springer, Cham (2017). https://doi.org/10.1007/978-3-319-67558-9_28
8. Tysome, J., et al.: A comparison of semi-automated volumetric vs linear measurement of small vestibular schwannomas. Eur. Arch. Oto-Rhino-Laryn. **275**(4), 867–874 (2018)
9. Vokurka, E.A., Herwadkar, A., Thacker, N.A., Ramsden, R.T., Jackson, A.: Using Bayesian tissue classification to improve the accuracy of vestibular schwannoma volume and growth measurement. Am. J. Neuroradiol. **23**(3), 459–467 (2002)
10. Wang, G., Li, W., Ourselin, S., Vercauteren, T.: Automatic brain tumor segmentation using cascaded anisotropic convolutional neural networks. In: Crimi, A., Bakas, S., Kuijf, H., Menze, B., Reyes, M. (eds.) BrainLes 2017. LNCS, vol. 10670, pp. 178–190. Springer, Cham (2018). https://doi.org/10.1007/978-3-319-75238-9_16
11. Xie, S., Diego, S., Jolla, L., Tu, Z., Diego, S., Jolla, L.: Holistically-nested edge detection. In: ICCV, pp. 1395–1403 (2015)
12. Yu, Q., Xie, L., Wang, Y., Zhou, Y., Fishman, E.K., Yuille, A.L.: Recurrent saliency transformation network: incorporating multi-stage visual cues for small organ segmentation. In: CVPR, pp. 8280–8289 (2018)

Learning Shape Representation on Sparse Point Clouds for Volumetric Image Segmentation

Fabian Balsiger[1]([✉])(iD), Yannick Soom[1], Olivier Scheidegger[2],
and Mauricio Reyes[1]

[1] Insel Data Science Center, Inselspital, Bern University Hospital,
University of Bern, Bern, Switzerland
fabian.balsiger@artorg.unibe.ch
[2] Support Center for Advanced Neuroimaging (SCAN),
Institute for Diagnostic and Interventional Neuroradiology, Inselspital,
Bern University Hospital, University of Bern, Bern, Switzerland

Abstract. Volumetric image segmentation with convolutional neural networks (CNNs) encounters several challenges, which are specific to medical images. Among these challenges are large volumes of interest, high class imbalances, and difficulties in learning shape representations. To tackle these challenges, we propose to improve over traditional CNN-based volumetric image segmentation through point-wise classification of point clouds. The sparsity of point clouds allows processing of entire image volumes, balancing highly imbalanced segmentation problems, and explicitly learning an anatomical shape. We build upon PointCNN, a neural network proposed to process point clouds, and propose here to jointly encode shape and volumetric information within the point cloud in a compact and computationally effective manner. We demonstrate how this approach can then be used to refine CNN-based segmentation, which yields significantly improved results in our experiments on the difficult task of peripheral nerve segmentation from magnetic resonance neurography images. By synthetic experiments, we further show the capability of our approach in learning an explicit anatomical shape representation.

Keywords: Shape representation · Point cloud · Segmentation · Magnetic resonance neurography · Peripheral nervous system

1 Introduction

Convolutional neural networks (CNNs) have enabled significant progress in medical image segmentation. Despite this progress, CNN-based segmentation still faces several challenges to process large volumes of interest. Among these challenges: difficulty to process target structures that span entire or large image volumes along with limited memory of graphics processing units (GPUs), limited image information between adjacent image slices due to highly anisotropic image

© Springer Nature Switzerland AG 2019
D. Shen et al. (Eds.): MICCAI 2019, LNCS 11765, pp. 273–281, 2019.
https://doi.org/10.1007/978-3-030-32245-8_31

resolutions (e.g., large image slice thicknesses and gaps), and highly imbalanced problems due to sparse target structures. Moreover, these challenges also hinder learning shape representations, which might be desirable for segmentation and especially for target structures with distinct anatomy [2,7,9].

These challenges have been addressed in a rather separate manner [6]. To tackle large volumes of interest and limited GPU memory, 2.5-D, dual-pathway, or patch-based processing has been proposed. Similarly, handling of anisotropic image resolution has been performed by only using a few image slices or entirely rely on slice-wise processing. Finally, dedicated loss functions were introduced to cope with highly imbalanced problems. An example with the aforementioned challenges existing is the segmentation of peripheral nerves from magnetic resonance neurography (MRN) images [1]. First, peripheral nerves span the entire image volume from the most proximal to most distal image slice. Second, they are hard to distinguish from muscular tissue, which hinders patch-based processing and calls for strategies incorporating global context information. Third, a large image slice thickness (4.4 mm) of the MRN images hinders 2.5-D and dual-pathway processing. Fourth, the problem is highly imbalanced with peripheral nerves on average only accounting for 0.14% of the voxels in the image volume. Lastly, peripheral nerves have a distinct tubular-like anatomical shape, which make them an excellent target for shape learning.

We propose to improve over traditional CNN-based volumetric image segmentation using the representation of a point cloud to tackle the aforementioned challenges. In particular, we refine a CNN-based segmentation by transforming the problem of volumetric image segmentation into a point cloud segmentation, wherein a voxel-wise classification becomes a point-wise classification (Fig. 1). This has several advantages: (i) point clouds are a more efficient way to represent sparse anatomical shapes than voxel-wise representations, (ii) the sparsity of point clouds allows processing entire image volumes at once and efficiently leveraging volumetric information, (iii) high class imbalances can be significantly reduced, and (iv) it allows learning anatomical shape explicitly. For instance, the right-most point cloud in Fig. 1 shows the compact representation of the entire structure with only 8930 points (0.12% of the voxels) and an almost balanced classification problem in the point cloud with 20211 points (i.e., from original 0.1/99.9 to 44/56 class ratio). We further propose to enrich point cloud information with image information extracted around each point, which enables us to maintain a compact model while jointly leveraging image information. As use case, we evaluated our approach to peripheral nerve segmentation from MRN images of the thigh, and show that the proposed approach can improve significantly over CNN-based segmentation. By synthetic experiments, we further show that our approach is capable of explicitly learning and exploiting the tubular-like shape of peripheral nerves for image segmentation.

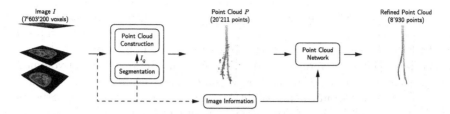

Fig. 1. Overview of the proposed approach. A volumetric image I is processed by a classifier to obtain a probability map I_Q. We then transform I_Q into the sparse representation of a point cloud P. The point cloud is processed by a point cloud network that classifies each point into foreground or background yielding a refined segmentation. The network incorporates not only Cartesian point coordinates but also image information around each point. In this work, we obtained image information from I_Q.

2 Methodology

2.1 Point Cloud Construction

In a first step, we transform a volumetric image I into a point cloud $P = [\mathbf{p}_1, \mathbf{p}_2, \ldots, \mathbf{p}_N]$ with N points $\mathbf{p}_i \in \mathbb{R}^3$ as follows: First, we obtain a probability map I_Q from a classifier trained to segment the target structure (CNN for peripheral nerves in our experiments). We threshold I_Q at θ to get the point cloud representation P, i.e., every voxel $\mathbf{v} \in I_Q$ with a probability $q \in [0,1]$ larger than θ is a point $\mathbf{p}_i = (x, y, z)$ with the Cartesian coordinates of $\mathbf{v}$. Therefore, a point cloud P consists of a different amount of points depending on the target structure's size as well as the classifier's segmentation confidence. We also remark, that no point correspondence is needed by the point cloud network.

2.2 Point Cloud Network

The point cloud network builds upon PointCNN introduced by Li et al. [5]. PointCNN follows the well-known encoding-decoding structure that gradually downsamples the point cloud to capture context followed by upsampling the point cloud and combining features through skip connections (Fig. 2a). The core of PointCNN is the $\mathcal{X}$-Conv operator, which is the counterpart of the convolution operator for unstructured data. At each encoding step, an input point cloud P_{in} is reduced to a set $P_{out} \subset P_{in}$ of $N = |P_{out}| \leq |P_{in}|$ representative points $\mathbf{p}$ using farthest point sampling. At each representative point $\mathbf{p}$, the $\mathcal{X}$-Conv operator extracts C features from the K nearest neighbor points of $\mathbf{p}$ in P_1 yielding a feature rich representative point $\mathbf{p}$. K can be seen as the receptive field of the network, which is increased towards the bottleneck by a dilation rate D, arriving ultimately at a receptive field of $D * K$. A decoding step works similarly, with the difference that P_{out} now has more points and fewer features compared to P_{in} ($|P_{out}| \geq |P_{in}|$). Further, the point clouds of the encoding path are concatenated following the principle of skip connections. After the last $\mathcal{X}$-Conv operator, two fully-connected (FC) layers reduce the features of each point to the number of classes. Finally, a softmax function assigns the class probabilities to each point.[1]

Despite the capability of PointCNN to reason on point clouds, it might be beneficial to jointly leverage the rich information contained in the volumetric images together with the Cartesian point coordinates. Inspired by [10], we extract image information from the probability map I_Q, which gives a strong indication of whether a point belongs to the target structure or not based on the raw image intensities. In particular, we define the image information for each point $\mathbf{p}$ to be features extracted from a volume of interest $I_{\mathbf{p}} \in \mathbb{R}^{X \times Y \times Z}$ centered at a point $\mathbf{p}$ (Fig. 2b). $I_{\mathbf{p}}$ is processed by a feature extraction module, which consists of a sequence of two 3-D convolutions (kernel size of 3 and stride of 1, 4 and 8 channels, respectively) with ReLU activation function, batch normalization, and max pooling operation. The features are then reshaped to a vector of size 64 and fed into the first $\mathcal{X}$-Conv operator together with the point's Cartesian coordinates. The feature extraction module and PointCNN can be trained end-to-end. We set $X = Y = Z = 5$ in our experiments. For reproducibility, the code is publicly available.[2]

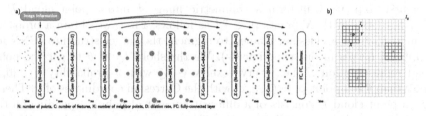

Fig. 2. (a) The proposed network architecture, which takes a point cloud and image information as input. The output is the probability of a point belonging to the target structure. The size of the dots • illustrates the number of features. (b) Illustration of the formation of the image information. We extract features from a volume of interest $I_{\mathbf{p}}$ (blue) from I_Q (light gray, probability values not shown for the sake of clarity) around each point $\mathbf{p}$ (•) in a point cloud, which yields the image information (Color figure online).

3   Experiments and Results

3.1   Data and Baselines

We used 52 MRN images of the thigh of healthy volunteers (n = 10) and patients (n = 42) to evaluate our method. The sciatic nerve has been manually segmented

---

[1] We remark that other point cloud architectures might also be feasible for the task at hand. Experiments with PointNet and PointNet++ [8], two popular architectures and pioneers in deep learning-based point cloud processing, showed slightly worse performance and are omitted here for clarity.

[2] https://github.com/fabianbalsiger/point-cloud-segmentation-miccai2019.

by three clinical raters and these manual segmentations have been merged using voxel-wise majority voting to obtain a consensus ground truth, to which all results were compared. In a four-fold cross-validation, a CNN was trained, as in [1], to segment the peripheral nerves using the consensus ground truth. This segmentation, termed CNN, served as baseline as well as for the construction of the point cloud P at threshold $\theta = 0.1$. As a second baseline CNN-P, we compared against a cascaded CNN [4] that uses I and the probability map I_Q of the baseline CNN as inputs, which simulates the use of the proposed image information originating from I_Q. We followed the same training procedure as for CNN. From the three rater segmentations, two human rater variabilities were additionally obtained for comparison: a rater-to-rater variability (R-R) and a rater-to-consensus ground truth variability (R-GT). We remark that R-R overestimates and R-GT tends to underestimate the true rater variability.

3.2 Network Training

We pre-processed the Cartesian coordinates of each P to lie in the unit cube $[-1, 1]^3$ and I_Q for extracting the image information to zero mean and unit variance on a subject level. We trained our network with $N = 2048$ input points. Therefore, during the training we randomly split a point cloud P into smaller point clouds with 2048 points. This extraction randomly permuted the point clouds during the training, and we added random 3-D rotations and jittering of the point clouds as additional data augmentation. A batch consisted of eight point clouds, and we trained the network for 40 epochs using Adam optimizer with a learning rate of 0.01 and cross-entropy loss. The training followed the same four-fold cross-validation as in Sect. 3.1 and hyperparameters were selected only on one fold. Note that during testing, we also randomly extract subsets of 2048 points until all points of a point cloud have been classified. We repeated this process ten times and did a majority voting to obtain the final point classification, which yielded slightly more robust classifications.

3.3 Ablation Study

To study the benefits of the proposed approach, we evaluated three variants: point cloud with Cartesian coordinates only (**Cartesian**, equivalent to

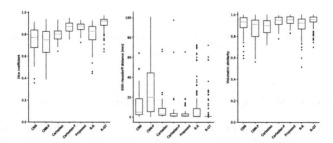

Fig. 3. Box-and-whisker plots for the metrics Dice coefficient, 95th Hausdorff distance, and volumetric similarity.

PointCNN only), point cloud with probability q (Cartesian-P), i.e., input is (x, y, z, q) similar to setting $X = Y = Z = 1$, and point cloud with image information from a $X = Y = Z = 5$ volume of interest (Proposed). Cartesian-P was added to show the benefit of neighborhood information around each point. Figure 3 shows box-and-whisker plots for the three metrics Dice coefficient (DICE), 95th Hausdorff distance (HD95), and volumetric similarity (VS). All point cloud-based variants outperform the CNN-based segmentations (CNN and CNN-P). With image information, our approach achieves statistically significant better results compared to the R-R variability for the DICE and the VS (both p ≤ 0.001) and on-par results for the HD95 (p = 0.100). Regarding R-GT variability, we achieve on-par performance for the VS (0.946 ± 0.041 vs. 0.944 ± 0.055, p = 0.600), and slightly decreased performances for the DICE (0.866 ± 0.044 vs. 0.899 ± 0.061, p ≤ 0.001) and the HD95 (4.5 ± 9.7 mm vs. 3.9 ± 11.1 mm, p ≤ 0.001). Compared to Cartesian-P, the Proposed image information performs slightly better, particularly for the HD95 with 4.5 ± 9.7 mm vs. 6.1 ± 16.1 mm (p = 0.57), although not statistically significant. Statistical tests with a Mann-Whitney U test and a significance level of 0.05.

The 3-D renderings in Fig. 4a illustrate the improvement of the final segmentation by the proposed method compared to CNN-based segmentation, Cartesian and Cartesian-P. The differences between Cartesian-P and Proposed are negligible in 3-D but accentuate in 2-D (Fig. 4b). In some few cases, a high HD95 was found mostly due to misclassification of points arranged in a tubular-like way in combination with image information of high probability, i.e. also misclassified by the CNN-based segmentation. We, therefore, investigated the sensitivity to shape and image information with a synthetic experiment, described below.

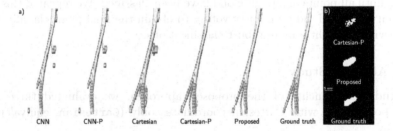

Fig. 4. Qualitative results: (a) 3-D renderings of segmentation results. (b) Worse in-plane segmentation results occurred with higher frequency for Cartesian-P than Proposed.

3.4 Sensitivity to Shape and Image Information

We conducted an experiment to confirm the hypothesis that our point cloud processing is capable of learning an explicit shape representation and is not only dependent on the probabilities of I_Q. We created two synthetic cases, one resembling a straight sciatic nerve and the other resembling a sciatic nerve with branching into tibial and fibular nerves. The nerves were manually drawn in ITK-SNAP[3] with a circular in-plane shape (diameter of ten voxels, based on the size of peripheral nerves in our data). For each case, we then assigned the probabilities $q = \{0.1, 0.3, 0.5, 0.7, 0.9\}$ to the synthetic nerves, which we additionally smoothed with a Gaussian filter ($\sigma = 1$) to simulate less confident boundaries arriving at a synthetic probability map I_Q. We then classified the cases using the proposed approach, which was trained on real data. Independent of the case or the probability, our approach consistently classified the point clouds correctly as peripheral nerves with Dice coefficients of 0.953 ± 0.015.

In a second experiment, we then investigated the influence of the shape and image information on false positive removal. Inspired by a case in our data, where a vein was misclassified, we manually draw a tubular-like false positive spanning from 1 up to 21 image slices (Fig. 5a shows a synthetic nerve with a false positive spanning 13 image slices). Intuitively, our approach should remove the false positive when it only spans a few image slices, independent of the image information's probability, because the shape does not resemble a peripheral nerve. Therefore, we varied the probability of the false positive ($q = \{0.1, 0.3, 0.5, 0.7, 0.9\}$) while fixing the probability of the synthetic nerve to be 0.5. The heat map in Fig. 5b shows that false positives spanning nine or fewer image slices get almost correctly removed independently of the image information's probability. Therefore, we concluded that the point cloud network learns a coarser anatomical shape resembling a peripheral nerve. It seems that shape is more important than the image information, which might only give an additional clue whether a certain point, e.g. at the boundary of the nerves, is classified as peripheral nerve or not.

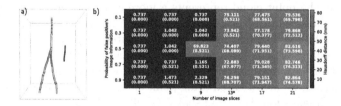

Fig. 5. Second synthetic experiment: (a) 3-D rendering of the synthetic sciatic nerve (in yellow) with a tubular-like false positive that spans 13 image slices (in red), (b) heat map of the Hausdorff distance (95th Hausdorff distance in parenthesis) after refinement depending on the image information's probability and size of the false positive. The asterisk indicates the false positive shown in (a) (Color figure online).

4   Discussion and Conclusion

We used point clouds combined with image information to improve volumetric image segmentation based on common challenges in CNN-based segmentation. Our approach comes with the benefit of processing entire image volumes by

---

[3] http://www.itksnap.org/.

leveraging the sparsity of a point cloud representation. Further, we showed that the point clouds allow us to explicitly learn the anatomical shape of the target anatomical structure. Jointly incorporating image information additionally improved the results on a coarse and local level (cf. Fig. 4). During the development, we also experimented with using the raw image intensities or Hessian matrix entries, inspired by [3], as image information. However, none of them improved the results compared to directly using I_Q. We hypothesize that this might be attributed to the rich information encoded in I_Q. But theoretically, any kind of image information can be incorporated into the network using the proposed scheme, which leaves room for tailoring the image information to specific applications. Finally, we remark that the quality of the point cloud depends on the quality of I_Q. This is a limitation of the presented approach. Selecting the threshold θ is a trade-off between including false positives and false negatives, and while our first results did not show high sensitivity to θ, a dedicated sensitivity analysis is subject to further work.

In regard to the presented application of peripheral nerve segmentation, we achieved promising results that even approach rater to consensus ground truth variability (R-GT). This variability is known to be difficult to achieve because every rater contributes itself to the consensus ground truth. For the Dice coefficient, it might be almost impossible to match R-GT due to the sensitivity of the Dice coefficient to small structures. As a next step, the results need to be confirmed on other anatomical regions than the thigh, which might give further insights into learning shape representations.

We think that the proposed transformation to point clouds might be applicable to other anatomical structures, where the conditions of sparse anatomical structure, i.e. the point cloud represents a more compact representation than a volumetric image, and distinct anatomical shape are present. Such anatomical structures could, for instance, be the vascular system (e.g., aorta segmentation) or the pulmonary system (e.g., airway tree segmentation). And as mentioned, the image information leaves room for tailoring to new applications.

In conclusion, we investigated using point clouds to improve volumetric medical image segmentation. By using sparse point clouds, combined with the proposed image information, our approach can reason over a coarser anatomical shape, which leads to significantly improved segmentation results.

Acknowledgement. This research was supported by the Swiss National Science Foundation (SNSF). The authors thank the NVIDIA Corporation for their GPU donation and Alain Jungo for fruitful discussions.

References

1. Balsiger, F., et al.: Segmentation of peripheral nerves from magnetic resonance neurography: a fully-automatic, deep learning-based approach. Front. Neurol. **9**, 777 (2018). https://doi.org/10.3389/fneur.2018.00777
2. Dalca, A.V., et al.: Anatomical priors in convolutional networks for unsupervised biomedical segmentation. In: CVPR, pp. 9290–9299 (2018)

3. Frangi, A.F., Niessen, W.J., Vincken, K.L., Viergever, M.A.: Multiscale vessel enhancement filtering. In: Wells, W.M., Colchester, A., Delp, S. (eds.) MICCAI 1998. LNCS, vol. 1496, pp. 130–137. Springer, Heidelberg (1998). https://doi.org/10.1007/BFb0056195

4. Havaei, M., et al.: Brain tumor segmentation with deep neural networks. Med. Image Anal. **35**, 18–31 (2017). https://doi.org/10.1016/j.media.2016.05.004

5. Li, Y., et al.: PointCNN: convolution on x-transformed points. In: NIPS 31, pp. 828–838. Curran Associates (2018)

6. Litjens, G., et al.: A survey on deep learning in medical image analysis. Med. Image Anal. **42**, 60–88 (2017). https://doi.org/10.1016/j.media.2017.07.005

7. Oktay, O., et al.: Anatomically constrained neural networks (ACNNs). IEEE Trans. Med. Imaging **37**(2), 384–395 (2018). https://doi.org/10.1109/TMI.2017.2743464

8. Qi, C.R., et al.: PointNet++: deep hierarchical feature learning on point sets in a metric space. In: NIPS 30, pp. 5099–5108. Curran Associates (2017)

9. Ravishankar, H., Venkataramani, R., Thiruvenkadam, S., Sudhakar, P., Vaidya, V.: Learning and incorporating shape models for semantic segmentation. In: Descoteaux, M., Maier-Hein, L., Franz, A., Jannin, P., Collins, D.L., Duchesne, S. (eds.) MICCAI 2017. LNCS, vol. 10433, pp. 203–211. Springer, Cham (2017). https://doi.org/10.1007/978-3-319-66182-7_24

10. Rempfler, M., et al.: Reconstructing cerebrovascular networks under local physiological constraints by integer programming. Med. Image Anal. **25**(1), 86–94 (2016). https://doi.org/10.1016/j.media.2015.03.008

Collaborative Multi-agent Learning for MR Knee Articular Cartilage Segmentation

Chaowei Tan[1], Zhennan Yan[2], Shaoting Zhang[2], Kang Li[1,3(✉)],
and Dimitris N. Metaxas[1]

[1] Department of Computer Science, Rutgers University, Piscataway, USA
Kang.li.research@gmail.com
[2] SenseTime Research, Princeton, USA
[3] Department of Orthopaedics, New Jersey Medical School,
Rutgers University, Newark, USA

Abstract. The 3D morphology and quantitative assessment of knee articular cartilages (i.e., femoral, tibial, and patellar cartilage) in magnetic resonance (MR) imaging is of great importance for knee radiographic osteoarthritis (OA) diagnostic decision making. However, effective and efficient delineation of all the knee articular cartilages in large-sized and high-resolution 3D MR knee data is still an open challenge. In this paper, we propose a novel framework to solve the MR knee cartilage segmentation task. The key contribution is the adversarial learning based collaborative multi-agent segmentation network. In the proposed network, we use three parallel segmentation agents to label cartilages in their respective region of interest (ROI), and then fuse the three cartilages by a novel ROI-fusion layer. The collaborative learning is driven by an adversarial sub-network. The ROI-fusion layer not only fuses the individual cartilages from multiple agents, but also backpropagates the training loss from the adversarial sub-network to each agent to enable joint learning of shape and spatial constraints. Extensive evaluations are conducted on a dataset including hundreds of MR knee volumes with diverse populations, and the proposed method shows superior performance.

Keywords: Collaborative multi-agent learning · Cartilage segmentation

1 Introduction

Osteoarthritis (OA) is the most common chronic health problem of human joints and the knee has the highest risk of developing OA in human lifetime. The knee articular cartilages (i.e., femoral, tibial, and patellar cartilage) are essential tissues for knee radiographic OA diagnosis. Eckstein et al. [2] indicated that the cartilage morphology outcomes (e.g., cartilage thickness and surface area) by

© Springer Nature Switzerland AG 2019
D. Shen et al. (Eds.): MICCAI 2019, LNCS 11765, pp. 282–290, 2019.
https://doi.org/10.1007/978-3-030-32245-8_32

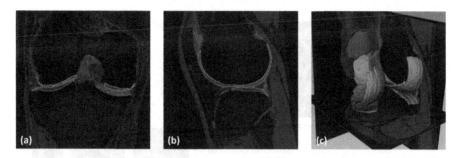

Fig. 1. (a) and (b) show the coronal and sagittal slices of a 3D MR knee data. The red, green and blue contours indicate the femoral cartilage (FC), tibial cartilage (TC) and patellar cartilage (PC), respectively. (c) demonstrates the cartilage labels in 3D (Color figure online).

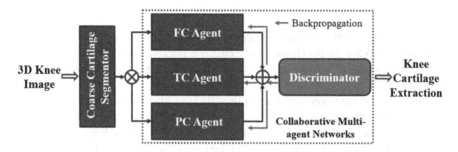

Fig. 2. Flowchart of the collaborative multi-agent learning for cartilage segmentation. (Color figure online)

measuring 3D magnetic resonance (MR) data in knee joint can help to identify the symptomatic and structural severity of knee OA. Hunter et al. [4] investigated the knee cartilage defects/losses by MR imaging as one important factor of knee OA. In order to capture the wide range and thin structure of cartilages in detail, MR data is usually in large size (millions of voxels) and high resolution. Figure 1 exhibits a 3D MR knee data from the Osteoarthritis Initiative (OAI) database[1], which has high resolution (0.365 mm × 0.365 mm × 0.7 mm) and large size (384 × 384 × 160). Effective and efficient segmentation of all articular cartilages in such high-resolution and large-sized data is challenging. Furthermore, the radiographic representations of cartilages may vary a lot in individuals with different age and pathology. Although the over-the-counter deep learning methods (e.g. VNet [6]) have shown superior performances in many segmentation tasks, simply applying VNet to the MR knee data may have low accuracy and result in crash of training due to huge GPU memory consumption. Besides, the task of multi-cartilage classification suffers from severe class imbalance problem. Xu et al. [10] showed a contextual additive network focusing on the boost of

---

[1] http://www.oai.ucsf.edu/.

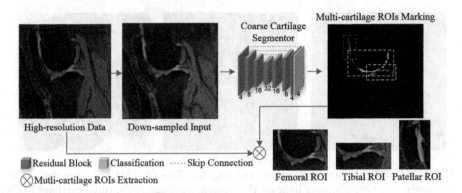

Fig. 3. Overview of the multiple cartilage ROIs extraction (only show the sagittal view). The number of feature maps in the network is displayed under each block.

memory efficiency for cartilage segmentation. The approach is based on small overlapping patches (a patch may only capture partial target) which may sacrifice certain accuracy. Some previous methods [3,7] present multi-task networks. They introduce the distinctive boundary features of organ to improve accuracy. But the tissue of cartilage has very thin structure and its topology may change in degenerative conditions. Xu et al. [9] segmented thin objects in 2D images through a myocardial infarction segmentation. Yet this 2D task-specific strategy may still suffer from the memory issue when applying for the 3D knee data.

In this paper, we propose a novel segmentation framework with collaborative multi-agent learning (shown in Fig. 2) for the task of knee cartilage labeling in large-sized and high-resolution 3D MR data. Through region of interest (ROI) extraction, three high-resolution cartilage ROIs are fed into different segmentation agents. The multiple agents collaborate by the help of discriminator and produce cartilage labels at the end. The ROI-fusion layer not only fuses the individual cartilages from multiple agents for discriminator, but also backpropagates the training errors from the adversarial sub-network to each agent to enable joint learning of shape and spatial constraints. Such collaborative multi-agent framework can obtain fine-grained segmentation in each ROI and ensure the spatial constraints between different cartilages. It satisfies the limits of GPU resources and enables smooth training on the challenging data. The experimental results show that the proposed method can extract all cartilages accurately.

2   Methods

The overview of the proposed framework is shown in Fig. 2. The coarse cartilage segmentor and ROI extraction (i.e., ⊗) steps aim to efficiently localize and extract three local regions of FC, TC and PC, and feed the ROIs to segmentation agents respectively. The blue dashed box shows the collaborative multi-agent cartilage segmentation module, which consists of three segmentation agents, one ROI-fusion layer (i.e., ⊕), and one joint-label discriminator.

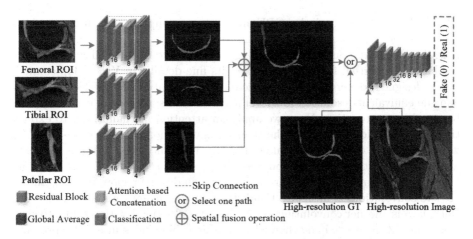

Fig. 4. Demonstration of the collaborative multi-agent learning framework for fine-grained cartilage segmentation. The agents yield binary labels and the spatial fusion operation outputs a 4-channel result (FC, TC, PC and background). (Color figure online)

ROI Extraction. In order to initialize the collaborative multi-agent learning, we first extract the ROIs of three cartilages. As shown in Fig. 3, by utilizing the location information of the multi-cartilage marks from the coarse segmentor, the image and label ROIs of FC, TC and PC are extracted from the original data. The segmentor's structure is like VNet [6], i.e., encoding-decoding. The encoding part contains 3 down-samplings (by convolutions of filter size 2 and stride 2) to obtain 3 different scales of feature maps. The decoding part has 3 up-samplings (by deconvolutions of filter size 2 and stride 2) to restore the scale of feature maps to reach the original input size. The blue block in this figure represents residual block followed by a down-sampling or up-sampling layer mentioned above when changing resolution. All the convolutional layers in the residual blocks have filter size 3, stride 1 and zero-padding 1. PReLU activation and batch normalization follow the convolutional and deconvolutional layers. The coarse cartilage segmentor is trained based on multi-class cross entropy loss ℓ_{mce} to obtain cartilage masks from the down-sampled MR data (e.g., $192 \times 192 \times 160$).

Collaborative Multi-agent Learning. In this learning stage (shown in Fig. 4), we construct one big network by three individual segmentation agents, one ROI-fusion layer, and one adversarial sub-network. The segmentation agent $A_{c=\{f,t,p\}}$ (f, t and p stand for FC, TC and PC, respectively) aims to generate fine cartilage binary mask $A_c(\mathbf{x}_{i,c})$ in the respective ROI $\mathbf{x}_{i,c}$ (its ground truth (GT) ROI is $\mathbf{y}_{i,c}$ and i is the data index). Each ROI is small enough to cover only one cartilage in it. Since the large portion of background and other cartilages are excluded, the class imbalance problem is relieved significantly. The small ROIs also reduce the requirement for the computational resources (i.e., GPU memories) and enable fine-grained segmentation in high-resolution data. All the segmentation agents have similar VNet-like pattern as the coarse segmentor. To balance the receptive field of neurons and the GPU memory consumption, we further reduce the down- and up-sampling operations to 2. Considering the thin characteristics and unclear boundary of cartilage, we need to better utilize the multi-resolution contextual features to capture its fine details. In VNet, skip connection is designed to merge the up-sampled high-level features I_h^{up} in decoding path and the equivalent-resolution low-level features I_l in symmetrical encoding path by simple concatenation. Here, we apply an attention mechanism [5] to extend the skip connections. Formally, the connecting operation becomes $o\,(\alpha \odot I_l, I_h^{up})$, where o denotes concatenation along the channel dimension, and $\odot$ is element-wise multiplication. The attention mask $\alpha = m\,(\sigma_r\,(c_l\,(I_l) + c_h\,(I_h^{up})))$ serves as a weight map that guides the learning to focus on desired region. Here, c_h and c_l are two convolutions of filter size 1 and stride 1; σ_r is an activation function (e.g., ReLU); m is another convolution of filter size 1 and stride 1 with sigmoid to contract the features to a single-channel mask. Light blue block in Fig. 4 represents the novel attention based concatenation.

Although individual agent can obtain fine segmentation in its ROI, the individual learning losses the mutual constraints between cartilages. In order to make the agents collaborate together to make use of the mutual position and shape priors of all the cartilages for better delineations, we propose a collaborative learning strategy. This strategy utilizes a ROI-fusion layer $\mathcal{F}$ to restore the single-cartilage output from each agent back to the original knee joint space where the mutual constraints and priors can be encoded. $\mathcal{F}(A_f, A_t, A_p)$ is implemented by using the location information of the three input ROIs to fuse the fine cartilage masks back to the original space. Then, the multi-cartilage priors are learned implicitly by adversarial learning strategy. We utilize a discriminator sub-network D to classify the fused multi-cartilage mask as "fake" and the whole GT label $\mathbf{y}_i$ as "real". In adversarial learning, the agents and the discriminator are trained alternatively. The parameters of agents are fixed when training the discriminator, and vice verse. In this way, discriminator sub-network can learn joint priors of multiple cartilages and guide the agents to produce better segmentation. It is important to note that the layer $\mathcal{F}$ not only fuses ROIs by their coordinates, but also passes the gradient updates from the discriminator to the agents during backpropagation, so that the two parts can be optimized in this alternating fashion. Since it is not intuitive to judge the labels without seeing the input in segmentation task, we borrow the idea of conditional generative adversarial nets, and treat the input MR knee image $\mathbf{x}_i$ as the conditioning variable. Figure 4 shows that the discriminator sub-network consists of 4 down-sampling convolutional layers, and the same residual block in the agents is also employed under each resolution level for contextual information learning. The input to the discriminator is a pair of MR knee image $\mathbf{x}_i$ and multi-label cartilage mask (either the GT label $\mathbf{y}_i$ or $\mathcal{F}(A_f, A_t, A_p)$). A global average layer is utilized at the end to generate a probability value for fake/real mask discrimination.

The loss functions of discriminator and agents are defined in Eqs. 1 and 2. Here, ℓ_b indicates the binary cross entropy loss. In Eq. 2, the first term $L_s = \ell_b\,[A_c\,(\mathbf{x}_{i,c}), \mathbf{y}_{i,c}]$ is to train each single segmentation agent. The second term $L_m = \ell_{mce}\,[\mathcal{F}(A_f, A_t, A_p), \mathbf{y}_i]$ and the third one are applied on the fused multi-cartilage mask for joint-label learning. The discriminator D and segmentation agents $A_{c=\{f,t,p\}}$ are alternatively trained by minimizing Eqs. 1 and 2.

$$\sum_i \{\ell_b [D(\mathbf{x}_i, \mathbf{y}_i), 1] + \ell_b [D(\mathbf{x}_i, \mathcal{F}(A_f, A_t, A_p)), 0]\} \tag{1}$$

$$\sum_i \left\{ \sum_{c=\{f,t,p\}} L_s(\mathbf{x}_{i,c}, \mathbf{y}_{i,c}) + L_m + \ell_b [D(\mathbf{x}_i, \mathcal{F}(A_f, A_t, A_p)), 1] \right\} \tag{2}$$

Table 1. Quantitative comparisons of approaches: mean and std of evaluation metrics.

	Femoral cartilage			Tibial cartilage			Patellar cartilage			All cartilages		
	DSC	VOE	ASD	DSC	VOE	ASD	DSC	VOE	ASD	DSC	VOE	ASD
D1	0.862	24.15	0.103	0.869	22.93	0.104	0.844	26.65	0.107	0.866	23.59	0.095
	0.024	3.621	0.042	0.034	5.184	0.061	0.052	7.429	0.049	0.023	3.475	0.026
D2	0.832	28.64	0.131	0.879	21.38	0.088	0.861	23.69	0.091	0.851	25.94	0.111
	0.025	3.618	0.059	0.038	5.972	0.055	0.040	6.027	0.051	0.023	3.393	0.036
C0	0.814	31.30	0.205	0.806	32.42	0.199	0.771	35.74	0.350	0.809	31.99	0.213
	0.029	4.155	0.095	0.033	4.577	0.055	0.132	14.56	0.129	0.031	4.350	0.095
P1	0.868	23.19	0.108	0.854	25.17	0.126	0.824	28.78	0.201	0.862	24.24	0.110
	0.023	3.514	0.067	0.029	4.173	0.059	0.104	12.45	0.439	0.023	3.457	0.048
P2	**0.900**	**18.82**	**0.074**	**0.889**	**19.81**	**0.082**	**0.880**	**21.19**	**0.075**	**0.893**	**19.19**	**0.073**
	0.037	6.006	0.041	0.038	6.072	0.051	0.043	6.594	0.038	0.034	5.434	0.034

3   Experiments

Experimental Settings. We validate our proposed method on the iMorphics dataset from the OAI database. This set includes 176 3D MR (sagittal DESS sequences) knee images. The set is splitted into training: 120, validation: 26, testing: 30. Patients are randomly and exclusively used in the three subsets. Fixed ROI size of each type of cartilage is pre-defined based on adequate evaluation on the training data. We compare the proposed method with the state-of-the-art dense atrous spatial pyramid pooling (DenseASPP) for semantic segmentation [11]. It integrates the ASPP architecture in a dense connection manner, which is able to generate large receptive field and multi-scale features for segmentation tasks. We also evaluate performances of the proposed coarse segmentor and individual agents to show the effectiveness of the collaborative learning. Dice similarity coefficient (DSC), volumetric overlap error (VOE) and average surface distance (ASD) between the GT labels and segmented results are reported. In the training (no pre-trained weights used), we set the batch size to 1 and multiply a factor of 0.95 every 10 epochs to reduce the learning rate (LR). The Adam (with initial LR 0.001) and stochastic gradient descent (SGD, with initial LR 0.0002) solvers are used for each agent and the discriminator. All the networks are trained and tested by a 12GB-RAM Titan X GPU.

Experimental Results. Quantitative comparisons are shown in Table 1. $C0$ represents the coarse cartilage extraction by the segmentor in Fig. 3. **P1** denotes

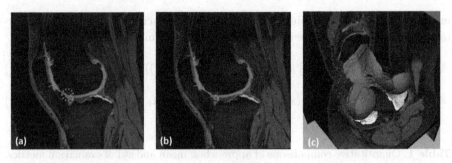

Fig. 5. Results of subject 1. (a) and (b) show the segmentation and GT labels for FC (red), TC (green), and PC (blue) in sagittal view. (c) is the segmented 3D cartilages (Color figure online).

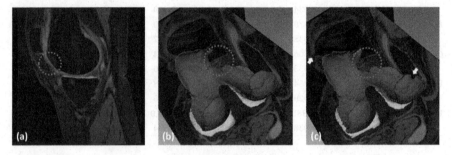

Fig. 6. Results of subject 2. (a) shows the segmented cartilages in sagittal view. (b) and (c) demonstrate the GT and segmentation results in 3D view. (Color figure online)

the fused results generated by the proposed segmentation agents, without the joint learning by the adversarial sub-network. **P2** represents results from the proposed method by employing the collaborative multi-agent learning framework as in Fig. 4. For comparison, we integrate two variants of DenseASPP into the collaborative multi-agent framework. In the first variant $D1$, the residual blocks and skip connections are replaced by DenseASPP blocks in the two down-sampled levels of the agent network. While in the second variant $D2$, only the deepest level is replaced with DenseASPP block.

From the table, we can see that the proposed segmentation **P2** achieves the best performance in all metrics. The mean results of $C0$ (i.e., a similar implementation of VNet) are relatively good and have no gross failure in our experiments. This shows that the coarse stage is reliable initialization. The proposed **P2** obviously outperforming **P1** shows that segmentation agents are improved with the help of the proposed collaborative learning strategy. The overall performances of the DenseASPP based variants $D1$ and $D2$ are close to that of **P1**. It indicates that the proposed agent network with the attention based concatenation is effective enough, compared to the DenseASPP blocks which have more complicated architecture. In addition, the results of the proposed method are comparable to those reported in some recent studies [1,10]. Xu et al. [10] reported a total DSC

(0.887 ± 0.024) value of FC and TC. Ambellan et al. [1] utilized both 2D and 3D deep learning based segmentations with statistical shape models as shape refinement postprocessing for femoral and tibial cartilages extraction. Using a similar set from OAI, they achieved[2] DSC (0.893 ± 0.024), VOE (19.4 ± 3.87) and ASD (0.19 ± 0.09) for FC, DSC (0.881 ± 0.038), VOE (21.05 ± 5.808) and ASD (0.223 ± 0.143) for TC. Without the sophisticated shape adjustment step, the proposed method acquires the comparable DSC and VOE scores, and much lower surface distance errors. Hence, the proposed framework can be used to automatically generate reliable assessments of all important articular cartilages in quantitative analysis for knee OA.

Visualization results (two examples) of the proposed method are showed in Figs. 5 and 6. The two patients have obvious shape variance of cartilages. In Fig. 5(a)–(c), the proposed method can accurately extract most of the cartilage regions and obtain smooth tissue boundaries. Furthermore, as indicated by green dashed circles in Fig. 5(a) and (c), our method can effectively capture a small cartilage defect. The green dashed circles in Fig. 6(a) and (c) indicate a possible cartilage damage/miss symptom well captured by our method. The 3D view exhibiting accurate 3D pattern of cartilage defects could be very useful in visual study of cartilage-related diseases. The yellow arrows in Fig. 6(c) show some minor errors occurred in some neighborhood areas due to unclear boundaries.

4   Conclusions

In this paper, we present a novel fully automatic method to segment three knee cartilages in 3D MR images based on a collaborative multi-agent learning archi-tecture. Each segmentation agent depicts the high-resolution cartilage mask in its coarsely (but efficiently) located ROI. A novel skip connection by multi-resolution attention mechanism is introduced to enhance the feature extraction of target, while suppressing confusing information in neighborhood areas. Then, the depicted multiple ROIs are spatially fused into the original space to form a multi-cartilage label image for collaborative learning. The collaboration of agents is implemented by the novel ROI-fusion layer followed by an adversarial discrim-inator to ensure the shape and position constraints. Learning of the agents and discriminator are conducted in an alternating fashion. In our experiments, the proposed method achieves robust and accurate segmentation for all important articular cartilages in high resolution and large 3D MR knee data. In future we will apply the method for quantifying cartilage biomarkers (e.g., volume, thick-ness, surface area) in large-scale studies and detecting cartilage defects for lesion estimation [2,4]. Besides the cartilages, the proposed framework could also be extended for other multi-organ segmentation tasks [8].

---

[2] [1] separately presents the results of FC, medial TC and lateral TC at two timepoints. For convenience, we average these results and get the approximate mean/std metrics.

References

1. Ambellan, F., Tack, A., Ehlke, M., Zachow, S.: Automated segmentation of knee bone and cartilage combining statistical shape knowledge and convolutional neural networks: data from the osteoarthritis initiative. Med. Image Anal. **52**, 109–118 (2018)
2. Eckstein, F., Wirth, W.: Quantitative cartilage imaging in knee osteoarthritis. Arthritis **2011** (2010)
3. He, K., Cao, X., Shi, Y., Nie, D., Gao, Y., Shen, D.: Pelvic organ segmentation using distinctive curve guided fully convolutional networks. IEEE Trans. Med. Imaging **38**(2), 585–595 (2019)
4. Hunter, D.J., et al.: Evolution of semi-quantitative whole joint assessment of knee OA: MOAKS (MRI Osteoarthritis Knee Score). Osteoarthr. Cartil. **19**(8), 990–1002 (2011)
5. Jetley, S., Lord, N.A., Lee, N., Torr, P.H.: Learn to pay attention. arXiv preprint. arXiv:1804.02391 (2018)
6. Milletari, F., Navab, N., Ahmadi, S.A.: V-net: fully convolutional neural networks for volumetric medical image segmentation. In: 2016 Fourth International Conference on 3D Vision (3DV), pp. 565–571. IEEE (2016)
7. Tan, C., Zhao, L., Yan, Z., Li, K., Metaxas, D., Zhan, Y.: Deep multi-task and task-specific feature learning network for robust shape preserved organ segmentation. In: ISBI, pp. 1221–1224. IEEE (2018)
8. Uzunbaş, M.G., Chen, C., Zhang, S., Pohl, K.M., Li, K., Metaxas, D.: Collaborative multi organ segmentation by integrating deformable and graphical models. In: Mori, K., Sakuma, I., Sato, Y., Barillot, C., Navab, N. (eds.) MICCAI 2013. LNCS, vol. 8150, pp. 157–164. Springer, Heidelberg (2013). https://doi.org/10.1007/978-3-642-40763-5_20
9. Xu, C., Xu, L., Brahm, G., Zhang, H., Li, S.: MuTGAN: simultaneous segmentation and quantification of myocardial infarction without contrast agents via joint adversarial learning. In: Frangi, A.F., Schnabel, J.A., Davatzikos, C., Alberola-López, C., Fichtinger, G. (eds.) MICCAI 2018. LNCS, vol. 11071, pp. 525–534. Springer, Cham (2018). https://doi.org/10.1007/978-3-030-00934-2_59
10. Xu, Z., Shen, Z., Niethammer, M.: Contextual additive networks to efficiently boost 3D image segmentations. In: Stoyanov, D., et al. (eds.) DLMIA/ML-CDS -2018. LNCS, vol. 11045, pp. 92–100. Springer, Cham (2018). https://doi.org/10.1007/978-3-030-00889-5_11
11. Yang, M., Yu, K., Zhang, C., Li, Z., Yang, K.: DenseASPP for semantic segmentation in street scenes. In: CVPR, pp. 3684–3692 (2018)

3D U²-Net: A 3D Universal U-Net for Multi-domain Medical Image Segmentation

Chao Huang[1,2], Hu Han[2,3], Qingsong Yao[2], Shankuan Zhu[1(✉)], and S. Kevin Zhou[2,3(✉)]

[1] Chronic Disease Research Institute and Department of Nutrition and Food Hygiene, School of Public Health, and Women's Hospital, School of Medicine, Zhejiang University, Hangzhou 310058, China
{huangchao09,zsk}@zju.edu.cn

[2] Medical Imaging, Robotics, Analytic Computing Laboratory/Engineering (MIRACLE), Key Lab of Intelligent Information Processing of Chinese Academy of Sciences (CAS), Institute of Computing Technology, CAS, Beijing 100190, China
{hanhu,zhoushaohua}@ict.ac.cn

[3] Peng Cheng Laboratory, Shenzhen, China

Abstract. Fully convolutional neural networks like U-Net have been the state-of-the-art methods in medical image segmentation. Practically, a network is highly specialized and trained separately for each segmentation task. Instead of a collection of multiple models, it is highly desirable to learn a universal data representation for different tasks, ideally a single model with the addition of a minimal number of parameters steered to each task. Inspired by the recent success of multi-domain learning in image classification, for the first time we explore a promising universal architecture that handles multiple medical segmentation tasks and is extendable for new tasks, regardless of different organs and imaging modalities. Our 3D Universal U-Net (3D U²-Net) is built upon separable convolution, assuming that *images from different domains have domain-specific spatial correlations which can be probed with channel-wise convolution while also share cross-channel correlations which can be modeled with pointwise convolution*. We evaluate the 3D U²-Net on five organ segmentation datasets. Experimental results show that this universal network is capable of competing with traditional models in terms of segmentation accuracy, while requiring only about 1% of the parameters. Additionally, we observe that the architecture can be easily and effectively adapted to a new domain without sacrificing performance in the domains used to learn the shared parameterization of the universal network. We put the code of 3D U²-Net into public domain (https://github.com/huangmozhilv/u2net_torch/).

C. Huang and S. Zhu were supported by Cyrus Tang Foundation & Zhejiang University Education Foundation. H. Han was supported by the Natural Science Foundation of China (61732004 and 61672496), External Cooperation Program of CAS (GJHZ1843), and Youth Innovation Promotion Association CAS (2018135). This work was done when C. Huang was an intern in MIRACLE.

© Springer Nature Switzerland AG 2019
D. Shen et al. (Eds.): MICCAI 2019, LNCS 11765, pp. 291–299, 2019.
https://doi.org/10.1007/978-3-030-32245-8_33

Keywords: Universal model · Multi-domain learning · Segmentation

1   Introduction

Image segmentation is crucial for clinical practice and health research. Fully convolutional neural networks (CNNs) like U-Net [15] have been the dominant approach in automatic medical imaging segmentation [4,11]. A practical segmentation model is learned by customizing a neural network architecture for a certain task or dataset and training it from scratch [11,16,18]. [7] learned a single segmentation CNN for brain datasets acquired with different scanners and/or protocols. Notwithstanding being powerful, these models are difficult to extend to new tasks with unseen contents because of the highly specialized design. [6] took one step further by presenting a self-adapting framework for various tasks, yielding mutually independent models for each task. On the contrary, human experts can easily learn to tackle multiple tasks and generalize to new tasks on the basis of acquired skills. Multiple previous works explored multi-task segmentation, wherein all organs of interest appear in the same image [9,17]. Here we consider a more realistic and challenging scenario: for a given dataset, only a local region of the human body is scanned and only one or several anatomical structures within the image are annotated. [12] focused on a similar topic and trained one single CNN on three tasks, however, the trained model was designed as such that it cannot be extended to other tasks. From this point of view, an effective and efficient method for image segmentation remains an open problem.

Bilen et al. [2,13,14] suggested that there might exist a universal data representation across different visual domains. Specifically, they introduced a new competition called Visual Decathlon Challenge[1], aiming to simultaneously model ten visual domains of different styles and contents, e.g., internet images, handwritten characters, sketches, planktons, etc. [13]. They referred to such a new topic as "multi-domain learning" and realized the universal representation by piggybacking parallel residual adapters on the model pre-trained with ImageNet. However, their work exclusively focuses on image classification. Naturally, one question occurs to us: *is it possible to build a single neural network that can deal with medical segmentation tasks from different domains?*

To achieve this goal, we draw inspiration from previous studies [3,5], particularly [5] which won the first place in the Visual Decathlon Challenge to date. [5] believed that [14] ignored the structural heterogeneity of various domains and attempted to address the issue by leveraging depthwise separable convolution. While standard convolution conducts the spatial and channel-wise computation at once, such convolution factors the computation into two sequential steps: first, depthwise convolution applies an independent convolutional filter per input channel, and then a pointwise convolution follows to linearly combine the output across all channels for every spatial location. The basic building block of their multi-domain network comprises a cohort of parallel channel-wise convolutions,

---

[1] https://www.robots.ox.ac.uk/~vgg/decathlon/.

one per domain, followed by one pointwise convolution shared by all domains. The insight is that the former is better to capture domain-specific spatial patterns while the latter probes the sharable cross-channel interdependencies. In this paper, we claim to note "depthwise separable convolution" as "separable convolution" and "depthwise convolution" as "channel-wise convolution" to avoid confusion with the depth dimension of the image volume.

Based on the separable convolution as introduced above, our work proposes a universal architecture for multi-domain medical image segmentation. The main idea behind is rather intuitive yet powerful: a basic network is first designed on the ground of 3D U-Net [4,15] (or V-Net [11]), and then any $3 \times 3 \times 3$ standard convolution with a stride of 1 is substituted by separable convolution similar to [5]. However, our approach substantially differ from [5] as following: (1) their work focuses on image classification which is fundamentally different from image segmentation here. (2) they obtain the ultimate multi-domain architecture in three steps: First, pre-training a ResNet-26 modified with separable convolution on ImageNet; Second, freezing and transferring the pointwise convolution weights to new network; Thirdly, training the new network on each domain separately and stacking the channel-wise convolutions together while sharing the pointwise convolution weights from the pre-trained model. Nevertheless, we manage to train across the domains together to obtain the final model. (3) we further adapt our universal network to a new domain by simply adding new channel-wise convolutions. To the best of our knowledge, this is the first time to learn an extendable universal network for multi-domain medical image segmentation.

2 Methods

2.1 Problem Definition

Let $\{D_1, D_2, \cdots, D_T\}$ be a set of T image domains, among which domain D_t consists of two paired image spaces of $\{X_t, Y_t\}$. $X_t \in \mathbb{R}^{C_t \times D \times H \times W}$ is the input image space and $Y_t \in \mathbb{R}^{C'_t \times D \times H \times W}$ is the output image space, i.e., segmentation masks. D, H and W are the spatial depth, height and width. C_t and C'_t are the numbers of imaging modalities and segmentation classes specific to each domain. To work well on all domains, our universal network contains domain-specific parameters as well as shared parameters. Let θ_t be the domain-specific parameters for domain D_t and θ_u be the universally shared parameters by all domains. Assuming $\{x_{t,i}, y_{t,i}\}$ as the ith training pair of domain D_t, then the output $\hat{Y}$ of the neural network $F(X)$ is

$$\hat{y}_{t,i} = F(x_{t,i}; \theta_u, \theta_t). \tag{1}$$

2.2 Domain Adapter

Domain adapter, the key component to ensure the success of our universal network, consists of both domain-specific parameters and shared parameters and is built upon separable convolution in place of standard convolution.

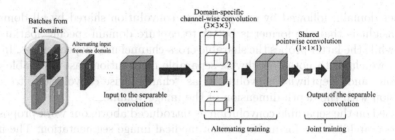

Fig. 1. Domain adapter based on separable convolution.

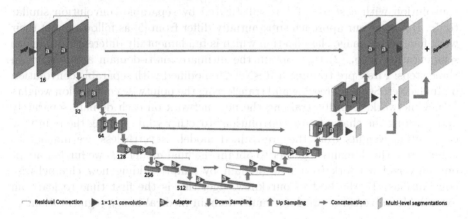

Fig. 2. The proposed 3D Universal U-Net (3D U²-Net).

In standard convolution with filter $W \in \mathbb{R}^{3\times3\times3\times C\times C'}$ applied to an input tensor $U \in \mathbb{R}^{C\times D\times H\times W}$, the output tensor $\hat{U} \in \mathbb{R}^{C'\times D\times H\times W}$ is obtained by applying C' filters $w \in \mathbb{R}^{3\times3\times3\times C}$ on the input in parallel and concatenating the C' output feature maps. A simple calculation tells that the total number of filter parameters in the above filters is $27 * C * C'$. Also, when training the models for the T domains separately, the number of parameters grows T times!

In separable convolution, the computation is factorized into two sequential steps. The first step applies C channel-wise filters $w \in \mathbb{R}^{3\times3\times3}$ to each channel of the input in parallel and concatenate the C output feature maps together. Here, *each domain has its own channel-wise filters*. The second step then applies C' pointwise filters $w \in \mathbb{R}^{1\times1\times1\times C}$ to output the final feature maps of C' channels. Here, *all domains share the same pointwise filters*. A simple calculation tells that the total number of weights in the above filters is $27 * C * T + C * C'$. How to assemble the domain-specific channel-wise convolutions and the shared pointwise convolution to form a domain adapter is illustrated in Fig. 1.

2.3 3D Universal U-Net (3D U²-Net)

As shown in Fig. 2, our universal network architecture is based on a basic network with six components: (1) input; (2) encoder path; (3) bottleneck block;

(4) decoder path; (5) deep supervision branch; and (6) output. Channels of the input and output could vary according to the number of imaging modalities and classes of different domains. In general, the input layer uses 16 filters. The encoder and decoder paths both contain five levels at different resolutions. Residual connection is applied within each level. Skip connection is employed to preserve more contextual information from the encoder counterpart for decoder path [15]. Inspired by [8], we incorporate a deep supervision branch alongside the end of decoder path via element-wise sum of multi-level segmentation maps to boost the final localization performance. To construct the universal network, domain adapters detailed above are inserted into basic network to replace any standard $3 \times 3 \times 3$ convolution with a stride of 1.

2.4 Loss Function

A hybrid loss function is employed by combining Lovász-Softmax loss [1], capable of improving intersection-over-union segmentation scores, and focal loss [10], aimed to alleviate class imbalance. During training the universal model, we sample a batch from each dataset in a round-robin fashion, allowing each domain to contribute to the shared parameters. Assuming that for the nth iteration the batch data pair $\{x_t, y_t\}$ is from domain D_t, the corresponding loss L_n is

$$L_n = L_L(x_t, y_t; \theta_u, \theta_t) + L_f(x_t, y_t; \theta_u, \theta_t), \tag{2}$$

where θ_t be the domain-specific parameters for domain D_t and θ_u be the universally shared parameters of the neural network. L_L is the Lovász-Softmax loss and L_f is the focal loss counterpart.

3   Experimental Results

In this section, we present extensive experiments to evaluate the proposed 3D U^2-Net in dealing with medical multi-organ segmentation: (1) independent models, aimed to reproduce the traditional methods, are obtained by training the basic network for each base domain separately; (2) shared model, which aims at investigating whether all parameters of a model can be shared by all domains and thus is gained by training the single basic network with all base domains together; and (3) universal model, which is our ultimate goal and is achieved by training the universal architecture with all base domains simultaneously. Notably, the first two represent two extreme multi-organ segmentation approaches and serve as baselines for the universal model. Additionally, we test the generalizability of both the shared model and universal model on one new domain.

Datasets: We use six public datasets from the Medical Segmentation Decathlon challenge[2] as introduced by [19]. The first five datasets are considered as base

---

[2] https://decathlon.grand-challenge.org/.

Table 1. Basic characteristics of the datasets.

Task	Modality	Data size	Image shape	Voxel spacing
Base01_Heart	MRI	20	$(90{\sim}130) \times 320 \times 320$	$1.37 \times 1.25 \times 1.25$
Base02_Liver	CT	131	$(74{\sim}987) \times 512 \times 512$	$(0.7{\sim}5) \times (0.557{\sim}1)$ $\times (0.557{\sim}1)$
Base03_Hippocampus	MRI	260	$(24{\sim}47) \times (40{\sim}59)$ $\times (31{\sim}43)$	$1 \times 1 \times 1$
Base04_Prostate	T2, ADC	32	$(11{\sim}24) \times (256{\sim}384)$ $\times (256{\sim}384)$	$(3{\sim}4) \times (0.6{\sim}0.75)$ $\times (0.6{\sim}0.75)$
Base05_Pancreas	CT	281	$(37{\sim}751) \times 512 \times 512$	$(0.7{\sim}7.5) \times (0.605{\sim}0.977)$ $\times (0.605{\sim}0.977)$
New_Spleen	CT	41	$(31{\sim}168) \times 512 \times 512$	$(1.25{\sim}7.5) \times (0.535{\sim}0.977)$ $\times (0.535{\sim}0.977)$

domains and are used to train the universal model. On the other hand, the last dataset is treated as the new domain and is used to test the adaptiveness of the universal model. Basic characteristics of the datasets are shown (Table 1). For each dataset, 80% of the samples are randomly extracted for training, while the remaining 20% are used as testing data.

Preprocessing: The datasets are highly diverse in terms of modality, image size and voxel spacing. Pre-processing procedures are conducted as below: (1) all images are cropped to the region of nonzero values, thereby reducing the image size to alleviate computation burden; (2) all images are resampled to the median voxel spacing of the corresponding dataset to retain spatial semantics; (3) for each patient, the image is clipped to the $[2.0, 98.0]$ percentiles of the intensity values of the entire image, followed by Z-score normalization with the mean and standard deviation of the image for each modality; and (4) the following data augmentation are applied: random elastic deformation, random rotation, random scaling and random mirroring. Data augmentation is done "on-the-fly" during training with batch generators[3], a python package maintained by the Division of Medical Image Computing at the German Cancer Research Center.

To accommodate the limited GPU memory, we train the network with patches randomly sampled from the whole images. While for inference, the patches are generated with a sliding window moving across the entire image with a stride of half patch size. As for the shared model and universal model, the input batch is of two patches with a size of $128 \times 128 \times 128$ and the number of down-sampling operations is set to 6. However, for the independent models, we adjust the input patch size and the resolution levels for each domain considering the image size in order to maximize the utilization of computation resources. If the median shape is smaller than $128 \times 128 \times 128$, we toggle between the input patch size and batch size to have the patch size of the same aspect ratio as the

---

[3] https://github.com/MIC-DKFZ/batchgenerators/.

Table 2. Quantitative results on base domains.

(Dice%)	Base01_ Heart	Base02_ Liver	Base03_ Hippocampus		Base04_ Prostate		Base05_ Pancreas	
	Left_atrium	Liver	Anterior	Posterior	PZ	TZ	Pancreas	Mean
Independent	93.26	95.02	89.62	87.74	58.39	87.18	78.78	84.28
Shared	92.73	93.40	89.25	87.30	68.38	89.30	57.57	82.56
Universal	91.98	93.54	89.34	87.05	68.50	89.21	62.08	83.10

median shape. The number of down-sampling operations per axis is set until the feature map size of the deepest layer reaches as small as 8. Specifically, to prepare the patches for shared model and universal model, we first extract a patch of size as in the independent model and then resize it to the above target patch size.

Implementation Details: The network is implemented in Pytorch 1.0.1 on an NVIDIA V100 GPU. The ADAM optimizer is applied with an initial learning rate of 3×10^{-4} and a weight decay of 10^{-5}. An epoch is defined as an iteration over 250 batches. Exponential moving average, l_{MA}^t, is monitored for training loss for every 30 epochs. The learning rate is reduced by a factor of 5 as long as l_{MA}^t does not decrease by 5×10^{-4}. We terminate the training once the learning rate is below 10^{-8}. During training the shared and universal models, we apply a round-robin fashion to feed the network sample batches from each domain in turn, so as to allow all the domains to contribute to the final model equally. The results are presented on the testing data.

Quantitative Results of Base Domains: Table 2 lists the mean Dice scores of the three models on each base domain. Comparing along the columns, we observe that the independent models obtain the highest scores on most domains and yield the highest overall mean score. However, strikingly both the shared model and the universal model achieve moderate performance for most domains comparable to the independent models, and gains significant increase regarding to peripheral zone (PZ) and transition zone (TZ) of Base04_Prostate. Compared to the shared model, we further observe that the universal model is better in the segmentation of pancreas for Base05_Pancreas. Besides, the universal model gets an overall higher mean score across all domains in comparison to the shared model. The increase in overall performance could be attributed to the use of domain-specific parameters that can agree with each domain well.

Model Complexity: When investigating the complexity of the models, we exclude the input layer, last layer and deep supervision branch as they are never shared across domains. The basic network used in the shared model is considered as reference. The number of parameters are computed and displayed in Table 3(a). Obviously the proposed 3D U^2-Net requires the least parameters, indicating that it can perform effectively across various domains. The overall

Table 3. (a) Model complexity. (b) Quantitative results on a new spleen domain.

	(a) #Par	(a) Ratio	(b) New_Spleen – Dice%	(b) #Added Par
Independent	126.7M	4.1×	92.37	30.7M
Shared	30.7M	1×	90.67	0
Universal	1.7M	0.06×	91.60	0.1M

number of parameters from the universal model is around **1%** of that of all independent models, while the two obtain comparable segmentation accuracy.

Quantitative Results of a New Domain: Furthermore, we conduct experiments to illustrate the effectiveness of adapting the trained shared model or universal model to a new task, which are implemented by freezing the corresponding shared pointwise convolutions or standard convolutions and adding and training all other domain-specific modules like input layer and channel-wise convolutions in parallel to the structures of the same kindred for this domain. Table 3(b) shows that the universal model performs better for the new domain 'New_Spleen' in comparison to the shared model, therefore indicating a superior generalization ability over the latter. This adds further evidence of the effectiveness of the domain-specific parameters. The universal model is adaptive to new domain with a few extra parameters, i.e., 0.3% compared to the traditional independent model, which is exactly what we anticipate in this paper.

4   Conclusions

In summary, we present a novel universal neural network named 3D U^2-Net for multi-organ segmentation problem, filling the gap of extendable multi-domain learning in image segmentation. Experimental results demonstrate that the proposed approach, with only a tiny portion of the parameters, obtains the segmentation performance comparable to the independent models trained in the traditional manner. As CT and MRI images are routine images on hand and the amount of human organs is constant, the universal model for multi-organ segmentation can be fully developed soon in the near future. Besides, the proposed framework could extend to many other multi-domain applications and thus facilitate the translation of neural networks to clinical practice.

References

1. Berman, M., Rannen Triki, A., Blaschko, M.B.: The lovász-softmax loss: a tractable surrogate for the optimization of the intersection-over-union measure in neural networks. In: Proceedings of CVPR, pp. 4413–4421 (2018)
2. Bilen, H., Vedaldi, A.: Universal representations: the missing link between faces, text, planktons, and cat breeds. arXiv:1701.07275 (2017)

3. Chollet, F.: Xception: deep learning with depthwise separable convolutions. In: Proceedings of CVPR, pp. 1251–1258 (2017)
4. Çiçek, Ö., Abdulkadir, A., Lienkamp, S.S., Brox, T., Ronneberger, O.: 3D U-Net: learning dense volumetric segmentation from sparse annotation. In: Ourselin, S., Joskowicz, L., Sabuncu, M.R., Unal, G., Wells, W. (eds.) MICCAI 2016. LNCS, vol. 9901, pp. 424–432. Springer, Cham (2016). https://doi.org/10.1007/978-3-319-46723-8_49
5. Guo, Y., Li, Y., Feris, R., Wang, L., Rosing, T.: Depthwise convolution is all you need for learning multiple visual domains. arXiv:1902.00927 (2019)
6. Isensee, F., et al.: nnU-Net: self-adapting framework for u-net-based medical image segmentation. arXiv:1809.10486 (2018)
7. Karani, N., Chaitanya, K., Baumgartner, C., Konukoglu, E.: A lifelong learning approach to brain MR segmentation across scanners and protocols. In: Frangi, A.F., Schnabel, J.A., Davatzikos, C., Alberola-López, C., Fichtinger, G. (eds.) MICCAI 2018. LNCS, vol. 11070, pp. 476–484. Springer, Cham (2018). https://doi.org/10.1007/978-3-030-00928-1_54
8. Kayalibay, B., Jensen, G., van der Smagt, P.: CNN-based segmentation of medical imaging data. arXiv:1701.03056 (2017)
9. Lay, N., Birkbeck, N., Zhang, J., Zhou, S.K.: Rapid multi-organ segmentation using context integration and discriminative models. In: Gee, J.C., Joshi, S., Pohl, K.M., Wells, W.M., Zöllei, L. (eds.) IPMI 2013. LNCS, vol. 7917, pp. 450–462. Springer, Heidelberg (2013). https://doi.org/10.1007/978-3-642-38868-2_38
10. Lin, T.Y., Goyal, P., Girshick, R., He, K., Dollár, P.: Focal loss for dense object detection. In: Proceedings of ICCV, pp. 2980–2988 (2017)
11. Milletari, F., Navab, N., Ahmadi, S.A.: V-Net: fully convolutional neural networks for volumetric medical image segmentation. In: Proceedings of 3DV, pp. 565–571 (2016)
12. Moeskops, P., et al.: Deep learning for multi-task medical image segmentation in multiple modalities. In: Ourselin, S., Joskowicz, L., Sabuncu, M.R., Unal, G., Wells, W. (eds.) MICCAI 2016. LNCS, vol. 9901, pp. 478–486. Springer, Cham (2016). https://doi.org/10.1007/978-3-319-46723-8_55
13. Rebuffi, S.A., Bilen, H., Vedaldi, A.: Learning multiple visual domains with residual adapters. In: Proceedings of NIPS, pp. 506–516 (2017)
14. Rebuffi, S.A., Bilen, H., Vedaldi, A.: Efficient parametrization of multi-domain deep neural networks. In: Proceedings of CVPR, pp. 8119–8127 (2018)
15. Ronneberger, O., Fischer, P., Brox, T.: U-Net: convolutional networks for biomedical image segmentation. In: Navab, N., Hornegger, J., Wells, W.M., Frangi, A.F. (eds.) MICCAI 2015. LNCS, vol. 9351, pp. 234–241. Springer, Cham (2015). https://doi.org/10.1007/978-3-319-24574-4_28
16. Roth, H.R., et al.: DeepOrgan: multi-level deep convolutional networks for automated pancreas segmentation. In: Navab, N., Hornegger, J., Wells, W.M., Frangi, A.F. (eds.) MICCAI 2015. LNCS, vol. 9349, pp. 556–564. Springer, Cham (2015). https://doi.org/10.1007/978-3-319-24553-9_68
17. Roth, H.R., et al.: Hierarchical 3D fully convolutional networks for multi-organ segmentation. arXiv:1704.06382 (2017)
18. Savioli, N., Montana, G., Lamata, P.: V-FCNN: volumetric fully convolution neural network for automatic atrial segmentation. arXiv:1808.01944 (2018)
19. Simpson, A.L., Antonelli, M., Bakas, S., et al.: A large annotated medical image dataset for the development and evaluation of segmentation algorithms. arXiv:1902.09063 (2019)

Impact of Adversarial Examples on Deep Learning Models for Biomedical Image Segmentation

Utku Ozbulak[1,3]([✉]), Arnout Van Messem[2,3], and Wesley De Neve[1,3]

[1] Department of Electronics and Information Systems,
Ghent University, Ghent, Belgium
[2] Department of Applied Mathematics, Computer Science and Statistics,
Ghent University, Ghent, Belgium
[3] Center for Biotech Data Science, Ghent University Global Campus,
Incheon, South Korea
{utku.ozbulak,arnout.vanmessem,wesley.deneve}@ugent.be

Abstract. Deep learning models, which are increasingly being used in the field of medical image analysis, come with a major security risk, namely, their vulnerability to adversarial examples. Adversarial examples are carefully crafted samples that force machine learning models to make mistakes during testing time. These malicious samples have been shown to be highly effective in misguiding classification tasks. However, research on the influence of adversarial examples on segmentation is significantly lacking. Given that a large portion of medical imaging problems are effectively segmentation problems, we analyze the impact of adversarial examples on deep learning-based image segmentation models. Specifically, we expose the vulnerability of these models to adversarial examples by proposing the Adaptive Segmentation Mask Attack (ASMA). This novel algorithm makes it possible to craft targeted adversarial examples that come with (1) high intersection-over-union rates between the target adversarial mask and the prediction and (2) with perturbation that is, for the most part, invisible to the bare eye. We lay out experimental and visual evidence by showing results obtained for the ISIC skin lesion segmentation challenge and the problem of glaucoma optic disc segmentation. An implementation of this algorithm and additional examples can be found at https://github.com/utkuozbulak/adaptive-segmentation-mask-attack.

1 Introduction

Recent studies adopt deep learning models at a quick pace to solve image-related problems for medical data sets. Provided that (1) labor expenses (i.e., salaries of nurses, doctors, and other relevant personnel) are a key driver of high costs in the medical field and that (2) increasingly super-human results are obtained by machine learning systems, an ongoing discussion is to replace or augment manual labor with automation for a number of medical diagnosis tasks [6]. However,

© Springer Nature Switzerland AG 2019
D. Shen et al. (Eds.): MICCAI 2019, LNCS 11765, pp. 300–308, 2019.
https://doi.org/10.1007/978-3-030-32245-8_34

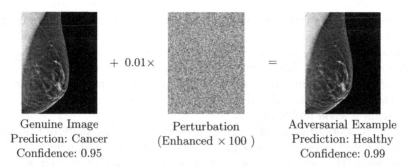

Genuine Image   Perturbation   Adversarial Example
Prediction: Cancer   (Enhanced × 100)   Prediction: Healthy
Confidence: 0.95   Confidence: 0.99

Fig. 1. A genuine image, initially classified as *cancer* with 0.95 confidence by a deep learning model, is perturbed to become an adversarial example. This adversarial example is then classified as *healthy* with 0.99 confidence by the same model.

a recent development called *adversarial examples* showed that deep learning models are vulnerable to gradient-based attacks [12]. These so-called adversarial examples are now considered a major security flaw, since they allow for the use of possible fraud schemes (e.g., for insurance claims) when deep learning models are deployed for clinical tasks [6].

The study of adversarial examples started with [12], in which the authors observed that small pixel modifications led to large changes in the prediction. Ever since, numerous attempts were made to mitigate the impact of adversarial examples and to fix this so-called security flaw, only to be found ineffective by subsequent studies [3]. Although the effects of adversarial examples are largely studied for non-medical datasets, it was also shown that classification problems in medical imaging datasets are of no exception to this exploit [6]. An adversarial example in the context of breast cancer classification is given in Fig. 1.

In the field of non-medical imaging, pixel by pixel detail is most of the time not task critical. As a result, segmentation problems are often expressed as detection or localization problems [5]. However, in medical imaging, precision is of utmost importance. Therefore, instead of detection or localization, segmentation covers a large portion of medical imaging problems [8].

Even though adversarial examples are studied extensively in the context of classification problems, it is only recently that studies started to investigate this phenomenon in the context of segmentation problems [1,13]. Thus far, in terms of segmentation, adversarial examples have been studied for the Pascal VOC [5] and Cityscapes [4] data sets, with a sole adversarial example generation method proposed in [13]. In particular, the Dense Adversary Generation (DAG) algorithm proposed in [13] aims to force deep learning models to segment all pixels wrong. Although the authors report that their algorithm is able to create adversarial examples in the context of segmentation, the resulting segmentation predictions, especially in the medical domain, are not realistic (i.e., the shape of the prediction immediately gives away that the input has been tampered with, since the prediction shape is not specified).

In this study, we focus on analyzing adversarial examples in the context of medical image segmentation problems. We demonstrate that adversarial examples indeed exist when dealing with medical image segmentation problems, discussing examples that have been obtained for glaucoma optic disc segmentation [10] and ISIC skin lesion segmentation [7]. Furthermore, we introduce a novel algorithm that is tailored to produce targeted adversarial examples for image segmentation problems.

To the best of our knowledge, this is the first study that analyzes the impact of adversarial examples, not only in the context of medical imaging but also in the case where the nature of the prediction is binary. Additionally, our algorithm is the first approach towards producing targeted adversarial examples for image segmentation that leads to a convincing prediction shape of choice, thus exposing a large security threat for image segmentation models. Our algorithm, while achieving targeted predictions with a high success rate, modifies the original image so subtly that the modifications on the original image are, for the most part, invisible to the bare eye.

2 Notation and Framework

In this section, we explain the datasets, the deep learning models, the notation, and the evaluation metrics used throughout the paper.

Framework—In order to show the effectiveness of the proposed approach, we evaluate our attack on two datasets: the first one is the glaucoma optic disc segmentation dataset [10] and the second one is the ISIC skin lesion segmentation dataset [7]. The results reported in Sect. 4 are obtained for two separate U-Net models which is one of the most used architectures in the field of medical segmentation [11]. These U-Net models have been trained on the two aforementioned datasets, achieving a segmentation effectiveness comparable to the state-of-the-art.

Neural Network Notation—We define the forward pass in a neural network as a function g with the weights and parameters of the same network detailed as θ. This function takes an input image $\mathbf{X}$ of size $C \times H \times W$, with C, H, and W representing the number of channels (i.e., 1 for grayscale images, 3 for colored images), the height, and the width of the input image, respectively. In this setting, $g(\theta, \mathbf{X})$ represents the prediction of this neural network for a given input image $\mathbf{X}$. The prediction is of size $M \times H \times W$, where M is the total number of classes (e.g., two in the case of binary segmentation). We define $\mathbf{Y} := \arg\max_M(g(\theta, \mathbf{X}))$ as the prediction of the neural network after discretization, containing prediction classes (i.e., values from 0 to $M - 1$) per pixel and having a size of $H \times W$.

Distance Metrics—When an adversarial example is generated, a distance metric is required in order to measure the difference between the original image and the generated image. Following previous studies [2], we use the Euclidean distance (L_2) and the max distance (L_∞), with the latter measuring the maximum change for a single pixel among all pixels.

Accuracy Metrics—In order to quantify the accuracy of the adversarial example generation, we calculate the intersection over union (IoU) and the pixel accuracy (PA) between the target mask and the predicted segmentation mask associated with the adversarial example produced. In our settings where the background label is selected as 0, IoU and PA are defined as follows:

$$\mathrm{IoU}(\mathbf{Y}^1, \mathbf{Y}^2) = \sum_{i,j} A_{i,j} \cap B_{i,j} \Big/ \sum_{i,j} B_{i,j}, \quad \mathrm{PA}(\mathbf{Y}^1, \mathbf{Y}^2) = \sum_{i,j} A_{i,j} \Big/ (H \times W),$$

for $(i,j) \in (\{1, \cdots, H\}, \{1, \cdots, W\})$ and where $A_{i,j} = \mathbb{1}_{\{\mathbf{Y}^2_{i,j} = \mathbf{Y}^1_{i,j}\}}$ and $B_{i,j} = \mathbb{1}_{\{\mathbf{Y}^2_{i,j} + \mathbf{Y}^1_{i,j} \neq 0\}}$, with $\mathbb{1}$ representing the indicator function.

3 Generating Adversarial Examples

To justify our design choices, we briefly highlight the differences between classification and segmentation in terms of adversarial example generation, before detailing our algorithm for generating adversarial examples for image segmentation.

Adversarial Target—In classification, the adversarial target is often a single class [9]. However, in segmentation, the target is a mask. Thus, the aim is to change the prediction of not just one but of a large number of labels.

Perturbation Multiplier—In the case of classification (when a single class is targeted), the optimization is influenced by only one source. However, in segmentation, as a consequence of the adversarial target being a mask, the optimization is influenced by a large number of sources (i.e., individual pixels). As a result, the perturbation multiplier (i.e., the learning rate) is harder to tune.

Keeping the aforementioned differences in mind and building upon the knowledge acquired from studying adversarial examples in classification problems, we propose the Adaptive Segmentation Mask Attack (ASMA), a novel algorithm for generating targeted adversarial examples for image segmentation models.

3.1 Adaptive Segmentation Mask Attack (ASMA)

As a starting point, we use the standard way of adversarial example generation, which is defined as follows:

$$\text{minimize } \| \mathbf{X} - (\mathbf{X} + \mathbf{P}) \|_2,$$
$$\text{such that } \arg\max\big(g(\theta, (\mathbf{X} + \mathbf{P}))\big) = \mathbf{Y}^A, \quad (\mathbf{X} + \mathbf{P}) \in [0,1]^{C \times H \times W}.$$

This equation iteratively aims at finding a small perturbation $\mathbf{P}$ that is sufficient to change the prediction of the model to $\mathbf{Y}^A$, which we will refer to as the target adversarial mask, while keeping the L_2 distance between the original image $\mathbf{X}$ and its adversarial counterpart $\mathbf{X}+\mathbf{P}$ minimal. In this setting, a perturbation is calculated in an iterative manner, multiplied with a constant, and then

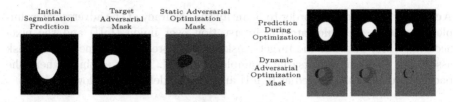

Fig. 2. An example adversarial optimization mask used by the static and the dynamic mask approaches, visualized in terms of the difference between the initial prediction and the targeted prediction (Color figure online).

added to the image: $\mathbf{X}_{n+1} = \mathbf{X}_n + \alpha\,\mathbf{P}_n$. We now detail how the perturbation $\mathbf{P}_n$ is calculated.

Static Segmentation Mask (SSM)—In the context of adversariality, a targeted segmentation attack must (i) increase the prediction likelihood of the selected foreground pixels in the target adversarial mask (i.e., blue areas in the static adversarial optimization mask in Fig. 2), while (ii) reducing the prediction likelihood of all other pixels that are not specified in the same mask (i.e., red areas in the static adversarial optimization mask in Fig. 2). To achieve this property, we write $\mathbf{P}_n$ as a sum of perturbations as follows:

$$\mathbf{P}_n = \sum_{c=0}^{M-1} \nabla_x\big(g(\theta, \mathbf{X}_n)_c \odot \mathbb{1}_{\{\mathbf{Y}^A = c\}}\big), \tag{1}$$

where $\odot$ denotes the Hadamard product and $\mathbf{Y}^A$, again, denotes the desired prediction mask for the adversarial example that contains class labels (as shown in Fig. 2). $g(\theta, \mathbf{X})_c$, on the other hand, denotes the channels of the prediction made by the neural network (i.e., in the case of binary prediction, $c = 0$ for background channel and $c = 1$ for foreground channel).

We will now describe how we improve this approach.

Adaptive Segmentation Mask (ASM)—When the static mask approach is used to generate adversarial examples, the gradient is sourced from the same number of target pixels in the target adversarial mask at each iteration. However, during the adversarial optimization, the prediction of certain pixels may already be correct (e.g., gray areas in the dynamic masks given in Fig. 2), and may thus not require any further optimization. In order to ensure that the optimization is only sourced from pixels whose predictions are not in line with the target adversarial mask, we introduce an approach that makes use of adaptive mask targeting. To achieve this property, we write $\mathbf{P}_n$ as follows:

$$\mathbf{P}_n = \sum_{c=0}^{M-1} \nabla_x\big(g(\theta, \mathbf{X}_n)_c \odot \mathbb{1}_{\{\mathbf{Y}^A = c\}} \odot \mathbb{1}_{\{\arg\max_M(g(\theta, \mathbf{X}_n)) \neq c\}}\big). \tag{2}$$

Writing $\mathbf{P}_n$ this way ensures that the gradient is only sourced from pixels whose labels are different from the target adversarial mask at each iteration.

Table 1. Experimental results in terms of image modification and prediction mask accuracy. We highlight the L_2 distances and IoU overlaps to emphasize the increase in the effectiveness of the optimization technique between the first and the last version. Note that numbers listed in this table are calculated for images whose pixel values are between 0 and 1.

Optimization	Glaucoma dataset				ISIC skin lesion dataset			
	Modification		Accuracy		Modification		Accuracy	
	L_2	L_∞	IoU	PA	L_2	L_∞	IoU	PA
SSM	**4.60**	0.22	**47%**	94%	**11.76**	0.24	**43%**	88%
	±1.76	±0.09	±18%	±2%	±4.11	0.05	±15%	±2%
ASM	2.82	0.17	94%	99%	4.11	0.16	89%	98%
	±1.29	±0.09	±7%	±1%	±2.23	±0.10	±9%	±1%
ASM + DPM (ASMA)	**2.47**	0.17	**97%**	99%	**3.88**	0.16	**89%**	98%
	±1.05	±0.09	±2%	±1%	±1.99	±0.09	±10%	±1%

Using the proposed adaptive segmentation mask approach, the number of pixels that source the optimization process starts high and as the prediction becomes in line with the target adversarial mask, lessens gradually.

Dynamic Perturbation Multiplier (DPM)—Since the usage of ASM progressively reduces the number of pixels the optimization sources from, setting the perturbation multiplier α to a fixed number either causes the optimization to halt when α is low or causes it to create large perturbations when α is high. Therefore, we employ a dynamic perturbation multiplier strategy in our adaptive mask approach, using $\alpha_n = \beta \times \text{IoU}(\mathbf{Y}^A, \mathbf{Y}_n) + \tau$, where β and τ are parameters used to calculate the final perturbation multiplier, also taking into account the IoU score of the prediction at the nth iteration. This method allows increasing the value of the multiplier dynamically as the number of pixels to be optimized decreases.

We name the adversarial example generation method that incorporates the aforementioned techniques (i.e., ASM and DPM) the **Adaptive Segmentation Mask Attack** (ASMA). Note our algorithm also works in the case where the prediction is not binary.

4   Experiments

Table 1 presents quantitative results on the viability of the proposed algorithm for adversarial example generation. Specifically, Table 1 shows the degree of perturbation in terms of L_2 and L_∞ distances, as well as the mask accuracy of the produced adversarial examples in terms of IoU and PA, hereby detailing the influence of the incremental updates (i.e., SSM, ASM, and DPM) that were discussed in Sect. 3.1. The values that can be found in Table 1 have been determined by calculating the mean and the standard deviation obtained from the

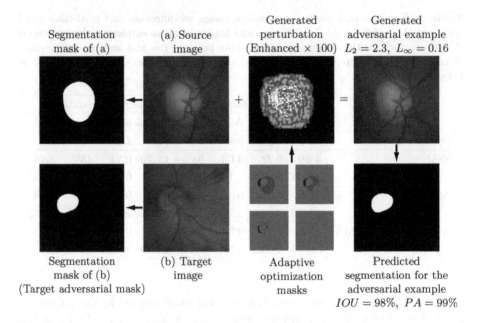

Fig. 3. An example optimization of an adversarial example for segmentation using ASMA. Best viewed in color.

optimization of 1000 adversarial examples. For each of those optimizations, the target adversarial mask is randomly selected among the masks of the other samples, so to have a realistic target in terms of medical image segmentation. To find an optimal perturbation multiplier when DPM is not incorporated, we used $\alpha \in \{1e-8, 1e-7, 1e-6, 1e-5\}$; when DPM is incorporated into the optimization, we use $\beta \in \{1e-6, 5e-6, 1e-5\}$ and $\tau = 1e-7$. Results are listed for the experiment that achieves the highest average IoU score throughout the 1000 generated adversarial examples for the selected set of parameters.

As can be observed from Table 1, the proposed method, when all enhancements introduced in Sect. 3.1 are incorporated, achieves 97% and 89% IoU overlap with the target mask that was used for initiating the optimization, with L_2 perturbations as low as 2.47 and 3.88 for the glaucoma optic disc and the ISIC skin lesion segmentation problems, respectively. For a more intuitive understanding, an L_2 perturbation of 3.88 corresponds to a modification of less than 1% of the images used in this study. Our experiments showed that, using ASMA, tuning the perturbation multiplier parameters β and τ is not a difficult task, as we were able to achieve high IOU overlap with low L_2 and L_∞ perturbations with only 3 possible combinations of β.

Apart from the quantitative results presented in Table 1, we also provide a qualitative overview of the approach used to generate adversarial examples in Fig. 3. Specifically, Fig. 3 shows the optimization procedure, a generated adversarial example, and the resulting predicted segmentation for a sample taken from the glaucoma optic disc dataset [10]. As can be seen, our algorithm is able to completely change the prediction to the desired output mask (taken from another sample in the dataset) with an IoU success rate of 98%.

5   Conclusions and Future Work

In this paper, we demonstrated that deep learning-based models for medical image segmentation are vulnerable to attacks using adversarial examples, hereby focusing on skin lesion and glaucoma optic disc segmentation. Specifically, we introduced the Adaptive Mask Segmentation Attack, a novel algorithm that is able to produce adversarial examples with realistic prediction masks that have been altered to be misclassified, using perturbations mostly invisible to the human eye. The source code of our adversarial attack, as well as additional examples, can be found at https://github.com/utkuozbulak/adaptive-segmentation-mask-attack.

Although we were able to observe similar results on different models, as well as transferability of our generated adversarial examples to other models, we leave it to future work to perform a more detailed analysis and to examine corresponding novel defense mechanisms against attacks that leverage realistic prediction masks.

Acknowledgements. The research activities described in this paper were funded by Ghent University Global Campus, Ghent University, imec, Flanders Innovation & Entrepreneurship (VLAIO), the Fund for Scientific Research-Flanders (FWO-Flanders), and the EU.

References

1. Arnab, A., Miksik, O., Torr, P.H.: On the robustness of semantic segmentation models to adversarial attacks. In: Proceedings of the IEEE Conference on Computer Vision and Pattern Recognition, pp. 888–897 (2018)
2. Carlini, N., Wagner, D.A.: Towards evaluating the robustness of neural networks. CoRR. arXiv:abs/1608.04644 (2016)
3. Carlini, N., Wagner, D.A.: Adversarial examples are not easily detected: bypassing ten detection methods. CoRR. arXiv:abs/1705.07263 (2017)
4. Cordts, M., et al.: The cityscapes dataset for semantic urban scene understanding. In: Proceedings of the IEEE Conference on Computer Vision and Pattern Recognition (CVPR) (2016)
5. Everingham, M., Eslami, S.M.A., Van Gool, L., Williams, C.K.I., Winn, J., Zisserman, A.: The pascal visual object classes challenge: a retrospective. Int. J. Comput. Vis. **111**(1), 98–136 (2015)
6. Finlayson, S.G., Kohane, I.S., Beam, A.L.: Adversarial attacks against medical deep learning systems. arXiv preprint. arXiv:1804.05296 (2018)
7. Gutman, D., et al.: Skin lesion analysis toward melanoma detection: a challenge at the international symposium on biomedical imaging (ISBI) 2016, hosted by the international skin imaging collaboration (ISIC). CoRR. abs/1605.01397 (2016)

8. Heimann, T., Meinzer, H.P.: Statistical shape models for 3d medical image segmentation: a review. Med. Image Anal. **13**(4), 543–563 (2009)
9. Kurakin, A., Goodfellow, I., Bengio, S.: Adversarial examples in the physical world. CoRR. arXiv:abs/1607.02533 (2016)
10. Pena-Betancor, C., et al.: Estimation of the relative amount of hemoglobin in the cup and neuroretinal rim using stereoscopic color fundus images. Invest. Ophthalmol. Vis. Sci. **56**(3), 1562–1568 (2015)
11. Ronneberger, O., Fischer, P., Brox, T.: U-Net: convolutional networks for biomedical image segmentation. In: Navab, N., Hornegger, J., Wells, W.M., Frangi, A.F. (eds.) MICCAI 2015. LNCS, vol. 9351, pp. 234–241. Springer, Cham (2015). https://doi.org/10.1007/978-3-319-24574-4_28
12. Szegedy, C., et al.: Intriguing properties of neural networks. CoRR. arXiv:abs/1312.6199 (2013)
13. Xie, C., Wang, J., Zhang, Z., Zhou, Y., Xie, L., Yuille, A.: Adversarial examples for semantic segmentation and object detection. In: Proceedings of the IEEE International Conference on Computer Vision, pp. 1369–1378 (2017)

Multi-resolution Path CNN with Deep Supervision for Intervertebral Disc Localization and Segmentation

Yunhe Gao, Chang Liu, and Liang Zhao[✉]

SenseTime Research, Shanghai, China
{gaoyunhe,liuchang,zhaoliang}@sensetime.com

Abstract. Automatic localization and segmentation of intervertebral discs (IVDs) from MR images plays a vital role in the diagnosis of pathological changes of IVDs. In this paper, we present a novel multi-resolution path network with deep supervision (MRP-DSN) to handle this challenging task. The MRP-DSN is based on a multi-scale backbone network, which is a DenseNet with densely connected atrous spatial pyramid pooling. More importantly, we introduce a multi-path network architecture that treats the segmentation of IVDs as a multi-task problem, i.e. segments IVDs into label maps at multiple resolutions, and then integrates them together for predicting the overall segmentation results. Each path is independently initialized and have a specific objective under deep supervision, which makes the training of each path more effective without interfering each other, thus results in more robust segmentation. We further design a training strategy that can eliminate the influence of unlabeled thoracic discs and make the training focus on the spine area. We evaluated our method on MICCAI 2018 IVDM3Seg Challenge dataset, the proposed MRP-DSN achieves superior performance.

1 Introduction

The intervertebral discs (IVDs) are fibrocartilage discs that connect adjacent vertebrae, they can provide flexibility to the spine, share the pressure between vertebrae, buffer impact and play vital roles of protecting the spinal cord and organs in the body. However, excessive activities or overload may lead to degeneration of the IVDs, causing lower back pain. Clinically, the MR image is the best non-invasive diagnostic method for IVDs. In order to obtain quantitative parameters and for the purpose of visualizing, doctors usually manually delineate the IVDs, which is tedious, time-consuming and lack of reproducibility, especially for 3D images. Therefore, a fully automatic localization and segmentation algorithm of the IVDs can greatly improve the speed as well as the quality of the diagnosis of IVD diseases.

In early studies, researchers typically used hand-crafted features [3,10] based on image intensity or texture features for IVD localization and segmentation. Graph-based methods are commonly used in the segmentation of vertebrae and

© Springer Nature Switzerland AG 2019
D. Shen et al. (Eds.): MICCAI 2019, LNCS 11765, pp. 309–317, 2019.
https://doi.org/10.1007/978-3-030-32245-8_35

discs. For example graph cut algorithm [1] were used for IVDs segmentation in spine MR images. As learning-based approaches gain more and more attention in the medical image analysis field, several marginal spacing learning [6] and regression-based methods [2] are proposed. However, those methods are limited by the representation capability of the hand-crafted features.

Recently, deep learning methods have revolutionized medical image analysis and computer vision field with its remarkable feature representation capability. For example, Ronneberger et al. [9] proposed U-net for cell segmentation from 2D images and Dou et al. [4] proposed 3D deeply-supervised convolutional neural network for 3D liver cancer segmentation. Deep learning methods also improve the performance of IVD localization and segmentation to a brand new level. For example, Zeng et al. [12] proposed a deeply supervise multi-scale FCN. Li et al. [8] proposed a 3D multi-scale FCN with random modality dropout scheme to better utilize multi-modality information and achieved decent accuracy for IVD localization and segmentation.

In this paper, we propose a novel multi-resolution path network with deep supervision (MRP-DSN), which treats the segmentation of IVDs as a multi-task problem, i.e. segment IVDs into label maps at multiple resolutions, and then integrates them together. This strategy can be easily extent to other network structures and other segmentation tasks. The MRP-DSN has a multi-scale back-bone network, which is based on DenseNet combined with densely connected atrous spatial pyramid pooling. Moreover, for the lumbar IVDs localization and segmentation tasks, we specially design a training strategy to avoid the influence of unlabeled thoracic IVDs, and make the network focus on the spine area without being affected by the external background. With the proposed multi-resolution path and deep supervision architecture and the specially designed training trategy, the proposed MRP-DSN achieves superior performance on the MICCAI 2018 IVDM3Seg challenge dataset.

2   Methodology

In this section, we will first introduce the structure of our backbone model, which is a DenseNet based network combined with atrous spatial pyramid pooling. Then we will elaborate the principle of multi-resolution path and deep supervision, then the proposed multi-resolution path network with deep supervision (MRP-DSN). Finally, we will introduce our specially designed training strategy for lumbar disc segmentation.

2.1   Multi-scale Backbone Network

Recent years, CNN based methods have made great progress on medical image segmentation. Inspired by U-Net [9], our backbone network has an encoder-decoder structure and short connections, but is not symmetric in down-sampling and up-sampling path, see in Fig. 1. Our backbone network is build upon dense blocks [5], where connections are linked among an layer to its all subsequent

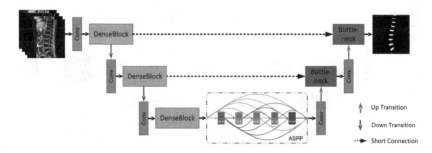

Fig. 1. Our multi-scale backbone network, it takes the 4-channel concatenated multi-modality image as input, and outputs the binary mask of IVDs.

layers. Specifically, each layer produces k feature maps and concatenate them to the its input feature maps, where k is the growth rate of the network and is set as 12 in our backbone network. Therefore, each layer can receive knowledge from all preceding layers, thus results in better information flow and feature reuse. However, redundant features may accumulate, so transition layers are used to reduce the number of channels to make the features more efficient. In our network the transition is performed combined with downsampling, and the reduction rate is set to 0.5.

Figure 3 shows the multi-modality MR images and the corresponding disc labels in the MICCAI 2018 IVDM3Seg challenge dataset. As can be seen that the size and interval of discs does not change much in scale, indicating that it is not a difficult problem for network to distinguish the IVDs from background, while the difficulty lies in how to make the segmentation result accurately fit to the edge of the discs. Since multiple times of downsamplings generates high-level but low-resolution feature maps, which cannot benefit the precise segmentation of edges, therefore, unlike U-Net, our backbone network performs two downsamplings. However, the receptive field of convolution kernel becomes smaller, which limits the network from capturing more global features. Therefore, we further use dilated convolution layers to build up densely connected atrous spatial pyramid pooling module (ASPP) [11] to solve this problem. In our model, we use the dilation rate of 3, 6, 12, 18 and 24.

2.2 Multi-resolution Path and Deep Supervision

Some literatures [4, 7] have studied the deep supervision training paradigm, and address that deep supervision can mitigate gradient vanishing during training and speed up convergence, moreover, it can also act as a feature regularization approach for early hidden layers. However, with the commonly using of residual connections, dense connections, batch normalization and etc in recent network structure, the gradient vanishing problem is greatly alleviated.

From another point of view, deep supervision can be seen as adding objectives at multiple resolutions to the network. Therefore, the segmentation of IVDs can

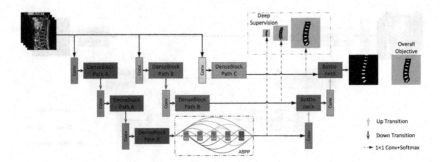

Fig. 2. The structure of proposed multi-resolution path CNN with deep supervision (MRP-DSN).

be seen as a multi-task problem, i.e. to segment IVDs into label maps in multiple resolutions, and then integrate them together to obtain the overall label map. Thus we propose a multi-resolution path CNN with deep supervision (MRP-DSN), see in Fig. 2. The encoder contains three separate paths, each path aims at encoding features into a specific resolution. Unlike [4], MRP-DSN adds supervision to the end of each path including the non-downsampled one. Specifically, 1×1 convolution layer following a softmax layer are used to obtain the dense prediction from feature maps at a certain resolution, the corresponding label is downsampled from the ground truth by bilinear interpolation. Finally, an overall loss is used to let the network learn to integrate multi-resolution segment label maps together into the final prediction. The parameters of each path are randomly initialized respectively and are not shared, moreover, each path has its own training objectives. Therefore, different paths can update individually without interfering each other, which makes the training more effective and are not likely to be stuck in the same local minima, and thus results in more robust segmentation.

When training segmentation network, cross entropy loss was used and the formula is as follow:

$$L(\mathcal{X}; \theta) = \sum_{x_i \in \mathcal{X}} -\log p(t_i | x_i; \theta), \tag{1}$$

where $\mathcal{X}$ denotes the images, $p(t_i | x_i; \theta)$ is the target class probability of pixel $x_i \in \mathcal{X}$ predicted with network parameters θ.

As MRP-DSN treats the segmentation of IVDs as a multi-task problem, each path should be equal, therefore, the weight of each loss is the same. Using d denotes the dth deep supervision, the total loss should be:

$$L_{total} = L_{overall} + \sum_{r \in D} L_d \tag{2}$$

2.3   Training Strategy

For the task of localization and segmentation of lumber IVDs, we specially designed a training strategy to further boost the performance. The multi-modality MR images and the corresponding ground truth labels are shown in Fig. 3. There are not only lumbar IVDs in most MR images, but also thoracic IVDs exist. Although those thoracic IVDs have similar appearance compared with the upper lumbar IVDs, they are marked as background. Obviously, opposite gradients will be given by two similar objects with different classes, and result in reducing the effectiveness of network training. Therefore, we ignore the loss of pixels above the uppermost lumbar IVDs with a certain distance when training.

To further improve the performance of the segmentation network, we made a natural assumption that only the spine part of the entire input image can provide valid training signals for IVD segmentation, while region outside the spine acts as a useless background.

We train a U-Net to coarsely predict the spine area, where the ground truth label of spine was generated by calculating the convex hull of the annotation of discs following with several dilation operations. When training the segmentation network, the predicted mask from the U-Net was used, loss from pixels outside the spine region and pixels that are above the uppermost lumbar IVDs with a certain distance will be ignored, i.e. ignore losses from the blue mask region in overall objective in Fig. 2. In the inference phase, the spine region is also predicted, for the prediction from the segmentation network, region outside the spine is set as background. Then the seven IVDs from bottom to up is retained, the others will be considered as thoracic IVDs and will be set as background.

3   Experiments

3.1   Dataset and Data Augmentation

We evaluated our proposed method on the MICCAI 2018 IVDM3Seg Challenge dataset, which consists of 16 sets of 3D multi-modality MR images from 8

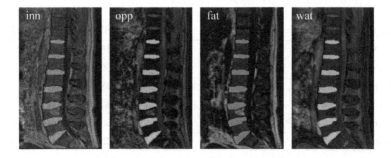

Fig. 3. Examples of multi-modality Dixon sequence, including in-phase, opposed-phase, fat and water from left to right. It should be noted that there are more than seven IVDs in the MR images, but only the lumber IVDs are our objective.

patients in two different stages. All images were scanned with a 1.5-Tesla MRI scanner of Siemens using Dixon protocol, which contains four self-aligned MRIs: in-phase, opposed-phase, fat and water, see in Fig. 3. The voxel spacing of each image is 2 mm × 1.25 mm × 1.25 mm. Seven lumber IVDs are annotated as ground truth labels.

Since each patient has two set of MR images, it may cause information leak if place images of one patient in both training set and validation set. Therefore, we divide the train/val dataset according to patient and perform 8-fold cross-validation. For the data augmentation, we use 3D deformation, random scale, random noise, and random crop. The evaluation metrics includes Dice similarity coefficient (DSC), average symmetric surface distance (ASSD), localization distance (LD), the localization distance is calculated with the morphological center of predict IVDs and the ground truth labels.

3.2 Result and Discussion

The quantitative evaluation result of 8-fold cross-validation are listed in Table 1, the values in the table are averaged among the 8 folds. The original U-Net can get fair segmentation results on IVDs, but is poor in term of ASSD, indicating that outliers exist in the segmentation results. After solving the contrary gradients of thoracic IVDs and making training focus on the spine region by add mask during training, the performance of U-Net is improved, especially the ASSD, which reveals the effectiveness of our training strategy. Compared with U-Net, our backbone network DenseNet is better in the aspects of DSC and ASSD, but slightly worse in LD. Although deep supervision can speed up convergence, the performance is only improved slightly, adding multi-resolution path is the same. By combining the multi-resolution path and deep supervision, our proposed MRP-DSN gives the best performance in all three metrics. The segmentation results of MRP-DSN are visualized in Fig. 4, the contours of MRP-DSN match with the ground truth very well.

Table 1. Quantitative evaluation results of cross-validation. M denotes mask, DS denotes deep supervision, MRP denotes multi-resolution path.

Method	DSC (%)	ASSD (mm)	LD (mm)
U-Net	91.26	0.616	0.512
U-Net+M	91.92	0.369	0.472
DenseNet+M	92.23	0.348	0.474
DenseNet+M+DS	92.27	0.344	0.476
DenseNet+M+MRP	92.28	0.333	0.484
DenseNet+M+MRP+DS (MRP-DSN)	**92.59**	**0.329**	**0.468**

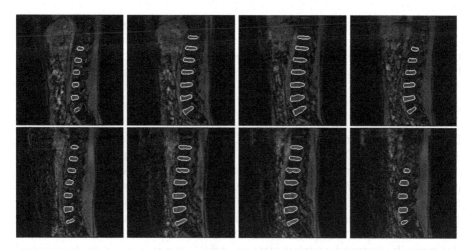

Fig. 4. Visualization of the prediction of MRP-DSN, the green line is the prediction of our approach, red line is ground truth and yellow line is the intersection (Color figure online).

Table 2. Comparison between MRP-DSN and DenseNet with deep supervision, where MP+DS is MRP-DSN, DS is DenseNet with deep supervision.

Resolution	DSC (%)		ASSD (mm)		LD (mm)	
	MP+DS	DS	MP+DS	DS	MP+DS	DS
1	**92.14**	91.95	**0.359**	0.369	**0.497**	0.503
1/2	**91.39**	90.95	**0.399**	0.427	**0.596**	0.663
1/4	**84.95**	84.58	**0.769**	0.776	**1.068**	1.120

We further exploit why MRP-DSN works better than DenseNet with deep supervision. Since the deep supervision we use is slightly different with that used by others, e.g. [4], it can output the results of three resolutions from encoder, therefore we can know what is encoded by network in different resolutions and calculate the metrics, results are shown in Table 2. The results from every resolution of both networks are worse than the overall prediction reported in Table 1, which indicates the integration of multiple relatively low-performance results from different resolutions can boost the overall performance. The results of MRP-DSN is better than DenseNet with deep supervision in every resolution, which shows that using separate paths to handle specific resolutions enables the network to encode more discriminative features, thus results in better performance. The result from 1/4 resolution is much poorer than the other two paths, shows that such low-resolution path contributes little to the overall performance gain. The low-resolution paths have larger receptive field, and can encode more high-level and global features. For the disc segmentation task, finding where the IVDs are is not a hard problem, the difficulty of the task lies in how to accurately delineate the contour of the discs. Therefore, such low-resolution high-level features are difficult to contribute to the segmentation of edges. This in turn proves that it is reasonable to reduce the number of downsampling when designing the backbone network.

4   Conclusion

In this paper, we present an effective 2D multi-resolution path CNN with deep supervision (MRP-DSN) for automatic localization and segmentation of intervertebral discs from multi-modal MR images. The MRP-DSN uses separate CNN paths to segment IVDs into different resolution label maps and then integrate them together. Since different paths are independently initialized and have their own objective function under deep supervision, they can learn more robust and more discriminative features without falling into the same local minima. With the specially designed training strategy, which ignores irrelevant background and unlabeled thoracic disc, and a multi-scale DenseNet-based backbone network, MRP-DSN achieved superior results on the IVDM3Seg challenge dataset. Extensive experiments demonstrate the effectiveness of MRP-DSN.

References

1. Ben Ayed, I., Punithakumar, K., Garvin, G., Romano, W., Li, S.: Graph cuts with invariant object-interaction priors: application to intervertebral disc segmentation. In: Székely, G., Hahn, H.K. (eds.) IPMI 2011. LNCS, vol. 6801, pp. 221–232. Springer, Heidelberg (2011). https://doi.org/10.1007/978-3-642-22092-0_19
2. Chen, C., et al.: Localization and segmentation of 3D intervertebral discs in MR images by data driven estimation. IEEE Trans. Med. Imaging **34**(8), 1719–1729 (2015)
3. Chevrefils, C., Cheriet, F., Aubin, C.É., Grimard, G.: Texture analysis for automatic segmentation of intervertebral disks of scoliotic spines from MR images. IEEE Trans. Inf. Technol. Biomed. **13**(4), 608–620 (2009)
4. Dou, Q., Chen, H., Jin, Y., Yu, L., Qin, J., Heng, P.-A.: 3D deeply supervised network for automatic liver segmentation from CT volumes. In: Ourselin, S., Joskowicz, L., Sabuncu, M.R., Unal, G., Wells, W. (eds.) MICCAI 2016. LNCS, vol. 9901, pp. 149–157. Springer, Cham (2016). https://doi.org/10.1007/978-3-319-46723-8_18
5. Huang, G., Liu, Z., Van Der Maaten, L., Weinberger, K.Q.: Densely connected convolutional networks. In: CVPR, vol. 1, p. 3 (2017)
6. Kelm, B.M., et al.: Spine detection in CT and MR using iterated marginal space learning. Med. Image Anal. **17**(8), 1283–1292 (2013)
7. Lee, C.Y., Xie, S., Gallagher, P., Zhang, Z., Tu, Z.: Deeply-supervised nets. In: Artificial Intelligence and Statistics, pp. 562–570 (2015)
8. Li, X., et al.: 3D multi-scale FCN with random modality voxel dropout learning for intervertebral disc localization and segmentation from multi-modality MR images. Med. Image Anal. **45**, 41–54 (2018)
9. Ronneberger, O., Fischer, P., Brox, T.: U-Net: convolutional networks for biomedical image segmentation. In: Navab, N., Hornegger, J., Wells, W.M., Frangi, A.F. (eds.) MICCAI 2015. LNCS, vol. 9351, pp. 234–241. Springer, Cham (2015). https://doi.org/10.1007/978-3-319-24574-4_28

10. Schmidt, S., et al.: Spine detection and labeling using a parts-based graphical model. In: Karssemeijer, N., Lelieveldt, B. (eds.) IPMI 2007. LNCS, vol. 4584, pp. 122–133. Springer, Heidelberg (2007). https://doi.org/10.1007/978-3-540-73273-0_11

11. Yang, M., Yu, K., Zhang, C., Li, Z., Yang, K.: DenseASPP for semantic segmentation in street scenes. In: Proceedings of the IEEE Conference on Computer Vision and Pattern Recognition, pp. 3684–3692 (2018)

12. Zeng, G., Zheng, G.: DSMS-FCN: a deeply supervised multi-scale fully convolutional network for automatic segmentation of intervertebral disc in 3D MR images. In: Glocker, B., Yao, J., Vrtovec, T., Frangi, A., Zheng, G. (eds.) MSKI 2017. LNCS, vol. 10734, pp. 148–159. Springer, Cham (2018). https://doi.org/10.1007/978-3-319-74113-0_13

Automatic Paraspinal Muscle Segmentation in Patients with Lumbar Pathology Using Deep Convolutional Neural Network

Wenyao Xia[1]([✉]), Maryse Fortin[2,3], Joshua Ahn[4], Hassan Rivaz[3,5], Michele C. Battié[6], Terry M. Peters[1], and Yiming Xiao[1]

[1] Robarts Research Institute, Western University, London, Canada
{wxia43,yxiao286}@uwo.ca
[2] Health, Kinesiology and Applied Physiology, Concordia University, Montreal, Canada
[3] PERFORM Centre, Concordia University, Montreal, Canada
[4] Department of Kinesiology, Western University, London, Canada
[5] Electrical and Computer Engineering, Concordia University, Montreal, Canada
[6] School of Physical Therapy and Western's Bone and Joint Institute, Western University, London, Canada

Abstract. Recent evidence suggests an association between low back pain (LBP) and changes in lumbar paraspinal muscle morphology and composition (i.e., fatty infiltration). Quantitative measurements of muscle cross-sectional areas (CSAs) from MRI scans are commonly used to examine the relationship between paraspinal muscle characters and different lumbar conditions. The current investigation primarily uses manual segmentation that is time-consuming, laborious, and can be inconsistent. However, no automatic MRI segmentation algorithms exist for pathological data, likely due to the complex paraspinal muscle anatomy and high variability in muscle composition among patients. We employed deep convolutional neural networks using U-Net+CRF-RNN with multidata training to automatically segment paraspinal muscles from T2-weighted MRI axial slices at the L4-L5 and L5-S1 spinal levels and achieved averaged Dice score of 93.9% and mean boundary distance of 1 mm. We also demonstrate the application using the segmentation results to reveal tissue characteristics of the muscles in relation to age and sex.

Keywords: Segmentation · Deep learning · Lumbar pathologies · MRI

1 Introduction

Low back pain (LBP) is the most common musculoskeletal disorder in adults, with a lifetime prevalence of up to 84% [1]. To better understand the underlying pathology and facilitate treatment and rehabilitation, there is an increasing

© Springer Nature Switzerland AG 2019
D. Shen et al. (Eds.): MICCAI 2019, LNCS 11765, pp. 318–325, 2019.
https://doi.org/10.1007/978-3-030-32245-8_36

interest to study the association between LBP and changes in morphology and composition (e.g., fat vs. muscle ratio) of lumbar paraspinal muscles. Most commonly, paraspinal muscle cross-sectional area (CSA) measurements are obtained from axial magnetic resonance imaging (MRI) scans, with published studies only relying on time-consuming and expertise-intensive manual segmentation for their analyses. So far, only a few methods [2–4] have been proposed for automatic paraspinal muscles segmentation, mostly based on computed tomography (CT) images and healthy subjects. However, much higher morphometric and composition variations exist in patients with LBP. In this paper, we use deep learning to automatically identify paraspinal muscles, including the multifidus and erector spinae muscles, as well as the intervertebral disc, spinal bone (i.e., spinous and transverse processes), and psoas muscles for computer-assisted analysis of LBP. More specifically, we leverage the strength of U-Net [5] and conditional random fields (CRF)-based probabilistic graphical modelling, which is reformulated as a Recurrent Neural Network (RNN) [6] to incorporate spatial information in tissue labeling. Furthermore, we also demonstrate the application of the proposed technique to help characterize muscle tissue properties in relation to the factors of sex and age, among a small cohort of patients with LBP.

2   Materials and Methods

2.1   Subjects, Imaging, and Preprocessing

Lumbosacral T2-weighted (T2w) MR images of 112 patients (59 male, age $= 30$–59y) were selected from the European research consortium project, Genodisc, on commonly diagnosed lumbar pathologies (physiol.ox.ac.uk/genodisc). For each sex, the subjects' ages are roughly uniformly distributed for the included range. Axial MRI slices of the L4-L5 and L5-S1 spinal levels at mid-disc were acquired for analysis. The multifidus (MF), erector spinae (ES) and psoas muscles, as well as the disc and spinal bone (9 labels) were manually segmented for all subjects at the L4-L5 and L5-S1 levels, using the software ITK-SNAP (itksnap.org). All cross-sectional MR images were first processed with N4 inhomogeneity correction [7] to remove field non-uniformity in the image (see Fig. 1). Then, the processed images were linearly transformed to the space of population-averaged paraspinal muscle atlases [8] at L4-L5 and L5-S1 spinal levels, and resampled to a standard image size of 256×256 with the resolution of $1 \times 1 \, mm^2$. This mitigates the large individual body size variation and images resolution differences for efficient feature learning. The manual segmentations were also transformed with the associated transformation and resampled to the same image size and resolution with nearest-neighborhood interpolation.

2.2   Deep Convolutional Neural Networks

With deep learning, many biomedical image segmentations can be performed with close-to-human accuracy. Instead of hand-crafting features to identify the

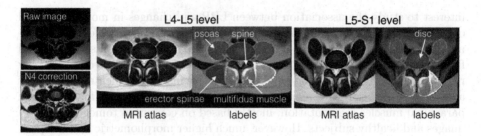

Fig. 1. Cross-sectional MRIs of paraspinal muscles at the L4-L5 and L5-S1 levels with different tissue classes using population-averaged MRI atlases.

target object, the discriminative image features can be learned automatically from examples via convolutional neural networks. In 2015, Ronneberger et al. [5], developed U-Net, which contains feature map concatenations and multiple de-convolution layers with learnable weight filters. In this study, we use U-Net to obtain the probability of each label given input MR image, $P(l_i|I)$ and we train a standard U-Net to directly predict all 9 labels from the input MRI image simultaneously. As described in [5], the standard U-Net consists of a contracting and expanding path, each with 4 resolution steps with a total of 23 convolution layers. We train our network using a combination of Dice coefficient and cross-entropy loss [9]: $L_{total} = L_{Dice} + L_{CE}$, where the Dice loss is computed for all samples individually and averaged over the batch.

2.3 Conditional Random Fields

Each muscle or bone component is highly localized and has smooth boundaries. However, due to image noise and local minima in training, the final label map tends to have small scattered mis-classifications. To resolve this problem, we combine conditional random fields [6] as recurrent neural networks with our U-Net to allow spatial constraints between labels. This can improve the delineation and integrity of our segmentations. We formulate our final labels as the inference from CRFs, given the probability map from U-Net and the input image. We model our CRFs to minimize the energy function:

$$E(x) = \sum_i \phi_u(l_i) + \sum_{i<j} \phi_p(l_i, l_j) \tag{1}$$

where $\phi_u(l_i) = -log(P(l_i|I))$ is the unary energy measuring the inverse likelihood of pixel i assigned as label l_i and $\phi_p(l_i, l_j)$ is the pairwise energy measuring likelihood of the neighboring pixel pair i and j assigned as label l_i and l_j, respectively. The pairwise energy term provides an image dependent smoothness cost, which encourages the neighboring pixels to share similar labels. The label l_i, which minimizes cost function (1), is chosen as our final label and we use the meanfield approximation algorithm [6] to efficiently minimize (1) with 6 iterations. The implementation workflow is shown in Fig. 2(b).

2.4   Multi-data Training with Gradient Magnitude Map

We also propose multi-data training to improve the efficiency of learning from examples with large morphological and intensity variations. Aside from the input training MRI, we compute the Laplacian gradient magnitude map of the training MRI and use them as additional samples to expand the training dataset. Instead of predicting labels based on input MRIs, the same network also has to learn how to identify the muscles & bones based on the gradient map, which contains no intensity information. The purpose of such augmentation training is to force the network to extract shared features between the MRI and its gradient magnitude for label classification. As a result, the network favors structural and spatial information from the MRI, and becomes less reliant on its intensity. The added gradient map is used solely for training and only the MRI is used for testing. The benefit of this approach is to increase the robustness of the trained model by reinforcing gradient feature learning (Fig. 2 (a)).

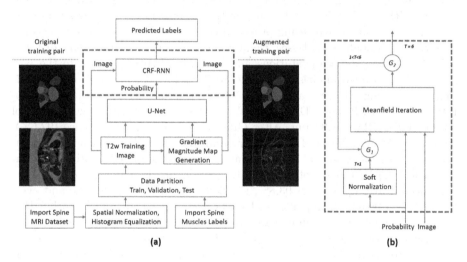

Fig. 2. (a) Overview of the proposed MRI segmentation pipeline. (b) Implementation of CRF-RNN, where G represents gating function and T represents iteration number.

2.5   Implementation and Training

Our neural networks were implemented in TensorFlow using the NiftyNet framework [10] and trained on a NVIDIA Titan XP GPU. We used Adam optimizer to train the network at a learning rate of 0.001. Of 112 patients, 75 were used for training, 10 for validation, and 27 for testing. Both training and testing datasets contained approximately equal splits in terms of gender and sex to fairly include muscle variations due to these factors. For training, the maximum iteration number was set at 15000 with a batch size of 20 and early stopping to prevent over-fitting.

2.6   Muscle-Fat Separation and Analysis

To demonstrate the application of the proposed segmentation method, we employed the segmentation results of the test dataset (27 patients) to obtain the CSAs of the multifidus and erector spinae muscles, as well as their fat percentages. We used k-means to separate the fat and muscle tissues while using the segmented muscle labels to constrain the region of interest. Spearman partial correlation between each of these metrics and the factor of sex or age was computed to reveal the physiological differences between different subgroups, as this relationship is being actively investigated in the LBP research.

3   Results

For segmentation, we first use Dice coefficient, sensitivity (recall), and positive predictive value (PPV) to quantitatively assess the performance of our trained neural networks. Experimental comparisons with standard U-Net and U-Net+CRF-RNN trained only with MRIs are also made to demonstrate the performance improvement using proposed training framework. Since Dice could be biased for imbalanced classes, we also compute the mean boundary distance (MBD) between the segmentations and the groundtruth to evaluate the performances of trained models. The Dice scores and MBDs are shown in Table 1. From our testing, we see that U-Net alone can produce highly accurate segmentation results with mean Dice of 92.4%, mean recall of 92.7%, mean PPV of 93.0%, and MBD of 1.93 mm. After CRF-RNN is incorporated, Dice (92.6%), PPV (93.4%), and MBD (1.48 mm) are improved, but there are no significant improvements for recall (92.7%). In comparison, the proposed multi-data training yields the best segmentation results for all muscle and bone components with overall average Dice of 93.8%, recall of 93.9%, PPV of 94.2%, and overall MBD of 1.00 mm. Comparing to U-Net+CRF-RNN trained only with MRIs, introducing multi-data training can improve the segmentation accuracies for all muscles and bones, especially for left & right psoas muscles with 3–4% improvements in terms of Dice and 1–2 mm improvements in terms of MBD. This is further reflected through the significant decrease in standard deviations for both Dice and MBD as shown in Table 1, indicating improvements in terms of robustness. We also performed paired-sample t-test using averaged Dice and MBD over all the labels. Our segmentations with multi-data training shows significant $(p < 0.05)$ and consistent improvement over U-Net+CRF-RNN with only MRI training both in terms of Dice $(p = 0.001)$ and MBD $(p = 0.043)$. As for U-Net vs. U-Net+CRF only trained with MRIs, there is no significant improvement in Dice $(p = 0.15)$, but there is significant improvement in terms of MBD $(p = 0.004)$.

To further illustrate the performance of our network, segmentation results for the two spine levels from our trained network using proposed framework are shown in Fig. 3. As seen from Fig. 3(c), U-Net+CRF-RNN reduces the small scattered false positives and smoothes the segmentation boundary. From Fig. 3(d), our network yields highly accurate segmentations for all muscle and bone components compared to the ground truth despite large muscle variations.

Table 1. Segmentation performance in different setups measured in Dice and mean boundary distance as mean ± standard deviation

Dice (%)	Spine	Disc	Left psoas	Right psoas	Left MF	Right MF	Left ES	Right ES	Overall
U-Net	91.8	96.9	90.5	91.5	94.4	93.9	89.7	90.5	92.4
	±2.9	±1.9	±15.1	±15.5	±2.6	±3.0	±6.5	±5.3	±3.9
U-Net+CRF	91.3	97.0	90.9	91.9	94.4	94.2	89.9	90.8	92.6
	±5.3	±2.4	±15.1	±15.5	±2.4	±2.3	±6.4	±5.1	±3.9
Multi-data training	92.7	97.4	94.6	94.8	95.0	94.5	90.6	91.3	93.9
	±2.9	±1.1	±4.3	±4.0	±2.3	±1.9	±5.8	±4.4	±0.2
Mean boundary distance (mm)	Spine	Disc	Left psoas	Right psoas	Left MF	Right MF	Left ES	Right ES	Overall
U-Net	1.26	1.09	2.99	4.04	1.10	1.30	1.89	1.80	1.93
	±1.4	±1.8	±4.6	±13.6	±0.7	±1.0	±1.1	±1.3	±1.9
U-Net+CRF	0.97	0.84	2.10	2.93	0.96	1.05	1.61	1.42	1.48
	±1.0	±0.8	±2.8	±13.5	±0.4	±0.5	±0.9	±0.8	±1.8
Multi-data training	0.68	0.57	1.18	0.93	0.87	0.94	1.46	1.34	1.00
	±0.2	±0.3	±1.0	±0.6	±0.4	±0.4	±0.8	±0.6	±0.3

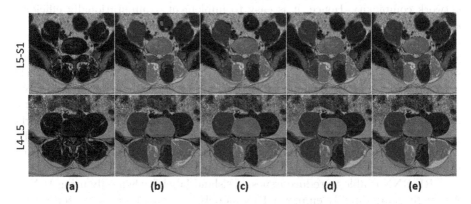

Fig. 3. Segmentation examples with MRIs at the L4-L5 and L5-S1 levels shown on the first and second rows, respectively. Columns: (a) Input T2w MRI (b) U-Net segmentation (c) U-Net+CRF-RNN segmentation (d) Our segmentation (e) Ground truth.

The results of the k-means algorithm to separate the muscle and fat tissue are demonstrated in Fig. 4. From the muscle morphometric analysis in the atlas reference space, at the L4-L5 level, the female group is significantly correlated ($p < 0.05$) with higher fat percentage within the multifidus muscles bilaterally ($r = 0.46$ for both sides) while controlling for age. At the same time, this metric within the left erector spinae muscles is positively correlated with increasing age ($r = 0.40$). At the L5-S1 level, the multifidus muscle fat content is correlated with sex (female) on both sides ($r = 0.53$ and 0.47 for the left and right). Our analysis with CSAs did not yield any significant correlations.

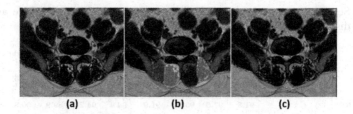

Fig. 4. Fat separation using k-means. (a) Input T2w MRI (b) Segmentations of multi-fidus and spinae muscles (c) Separated fat within the muscles (in orange color). (Color figure online)

4 Discussion and Future Work

Our results demonstrate that adding gradient magnitude images as additional training set can significantly improve the segmentation accuracy without increase network complexity. Hence, it is easy to implement, computationally efficient, and can be generalized to other MR or CT images. Although this technique is unconventional as we normally desire the network to learn the gradient features automatically, it can be very helpful to improve learning efficiency in applications with small datasets. Leveraging the automatic segmentation results, the muscle morphometric analysis demonstrates that female sex and aging is correlated with increased fatty infiltration in multifidus and erector spinae muscles among patients with lumbar pathologies. This trend is consistent with previous reports [11]. While the trend of fatty infiltration is similar on both sides of the body, only the left erector spinae muscle showed significant correlation with age. This is likely due to the side that is commonly affected by disease.

CRF-RNN is able to reduce issues of "island labels" when only using U-Net. Although many directly employ CRFs models as a post-processing step for U-Net, the RNN implementation allows end-to-end training. However, with high variations of muscle tissue properties, separation between muscles, especially between multifidus and erector spinae muscles, can be challenging. Future work will include improved definition of muscle groups with multi-contrast MRI, and we will also seek to incorporate models to enhance our network with the implied shape constraints to further improve the boundary smoothness of the segmentation. In the future, we will also include a wider age range of patients in the training set to further improve our network.

5 Conclusion

We have proposed the first technique with deep convolutional neural networks to automatically segment the paraspinal muscles from MRIs in patients with LBP, and further demonstrated its application to facilitate computer-assisted analysis of muscle characteristics. With CRF-RNN to help add spatial constraints to the tissue labeling, we proposed to incorporate additional gradient magnitude maps of the original images in training to enhance the performance without adding network complexity. We expect the resulting technique to greatly benefit the investigation of paraspinal muscle and common lumbar disorders.

Acknowledgment. This work was supported by CIHR, CFI, NSERC and BrainsCAN, as well as the Seventh Framework Programme (Health-2007-2013, grant agreement NO: 201626: GENODISC) and Canada Reearch Chairs program. We acknowledge the support of NVIDIA Corporation and thank Dr. Yingli Lu for his help.

References

1. Balagué, F., Mannion, A.F., Pellisé, F., Cedraschi, C.: Non-specific low back pain. Lancet **379**(9814), 482–491 (2012)
2. Kamiya, N., Li, J., Kume, M., et al.: Fully automatic segmentation of paraspinal muscles from 3D torso CT images via multi-scale iterative random forest classifications. Int. J. Comput. Assist. Radiol. Surg. **13**(11), 1697–1706 (2018)
3. Engstrom, C.M., Fripp, J., Jurcak, V., et al.: Segmentation of the quadratus lumborum muscle using statistical shape modeling. J. Magn. Reson. Imaging **33**(6), 1422–1429 (2011)
4. Wei, Y., Xu, B., Tao, X., Qu, J.: Paraspinal muscle segmentation in CT images using a single atlas. In: Proceedings of the PIC, pp. 211–215. IEEE (2015)
5. Ronneberger, O., Fischer, P., Brox, T.: U-Net: convolutional networks for biomedical image segmentation. In: Navab, N., Hornegger, J., Wells, W.M., Frangi, A.F. (eds.) MICCAI 2015. LNCS, vol. 9351, pp. 234–241. Springer, Cham (2015). https://doi.org/10.1007/978-3-319-24574-4_28
6. Zheng, S., Jayasumana, S., Romera-Paredes, B., et al.: Conditional random fields as recurrent neural networks. In: ICCV, pp. 1529–1537 (2015)
7. Tustison, N.J., Avants, B.B., Cook, P.A., et al.: N4ITK: improved N3 bias correction. IEEE Trans. Med. Imaging **29**(6), 1310 (2010)
8. Xiao, Y., Fortin, M., Battié, M.C., Rivaz, H.: Population-averaged MRI atlases for automated image processing and assessments of lumbar paraspinal muscles. Eur. Spine J. **27**(10), 2442–2448 (2018)
9. Isensee, F., Petersen, J., Klein, A., et al.: nnU-Net: self-adapting framework for u-Net-based medical image segmentation. arXiv preprint arXiv:1809.10486 (2018)
10. Gibson, E., Li, W., Sudre, C., et al.: NiftyNet: a deep-learning platform for medical imaging. Comput. Methods Programs Biomed. **158**, 113–122 (2018)
11. Urrutia, J., Besa, P., Lobos, D., et al.: Lumbar paraspinal muscle fat infiltration is independently associated with sex, age, and inter-vertebral disc degeneration in symptomatic patients. Skeletal Radiol. **47**(7), 955–961 (2018)

Constrained Domain Adaptation
for Segmentation

Mathilde Bateson$^{(\boxtimes)}$, Hoel Kervadec, Jose Dolz, Hervé Lombaert,
and Ismail Ben Ayed

ÉTS Montréal, Montreal, Canada
mathilde.bateson.1@ens.etsmtl.ca

Abstract. We propose to adapt segmentation networks with a constrained formulation, which embeds domain-invariant prior knowledge
about the segmentation regions. Such knowledge may take the form of
simple anatomical information, e.g., structure size or shape, estimated
from source samples or known *a priori*. Our method imposes domain-
invariant inequality constraints on a network output of unlabeled target samples. It implicitly matches prediction statistics between target
and source domains with permitted uncertainty of prior knowledge. We
address our constrained problem with a differentiable penalty, fully suited
for conventional gradient descent approaches, removing the need for computationally expensive Lagrangian optimization with dual projections.
Unlike current two-step adversarial training, our formulation is based on
a single loss in a single network, which simplifies adaptation by avoiding extra adversarial steps, while improving convergence and quality of
training. The comparison of our approach with state-of-the-art adversarial methods reveals substantially better performance on the challenging
task of adapting spine segmentation across different MRI modalities. Our
results also show a robustness to imprecision of size priors, approaching
the accuracy of a fully supervised model trained directly in a target
domain. Our method can be readily used for various constraints and
segmentation problems.

Keywords: Image segmentation · Domain adaptation ·
Constrained CNNs

1 Introduction

Convolutional neural networks (CNNs) are currently dominating segmentation
problems, yielding outstanding performances in a breadth of medical imaging
applications [14]. A major impediment of such supervised models is that they
require large amounts of training data built with scarce expert knowledge and
labor-intensive, pixel-level annotations. Typically, segmentation ground truth is
available for limited data, and supervised models are seriously challenged with

© Springer Nature Switzerland AG 2019
D. Shen et al. (Eds.): MICCAI 2019, LNCS 11765, pp. 326–334, 2019.
https://doi.org/10.1007/978-3-030-32245-8_37

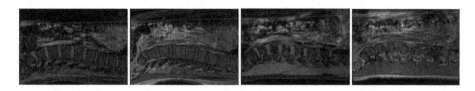

Fig. 1. Visualization of 2 aligned slice pairs in source (Wat) and target modality (IP).

new unlabeled samples (target data) that differ from the labeled training samples (source data) due, for instance, to variations in imaging modalities and protocols, vendors, machines and clinical sites; see Fig. 1. Unsupervised domain adaptation (UDA) tackles such substantial domain shifts between the distributions of the source and target data by learning domain-invariant representations, assuming labels are available only for the source. The subject is currently attracting substantial efforts, both in computer vision [7,20,21] and medical imaging [4,11,18,23]. While a large body of works focused on image classification [19,21], there is a rapidly growing interest into adapting segmentation networks [11,20], more so because building segmentation labels for each new domain is cumbersome.

In the recent literature, adversarial techniques have become the *de facto* choice in adapting segmentation networks, for medical [5,9,11,24] and color [3,7,8,20] images. These techniques match the feature distribution across domains by alternating the training of two networks, one learning a discriminator between source and target features and the other generating segmentations. While adversarial training achieved excellent performances in image classification [21], our experiments suggest that it may not be sufficient for segmentation, where learning a discriminator is much more complex than classification as it involves predictions in an exponentially large label space. This is in line with a few recent works in computer vision [22,25], which argue that adversarial formulations of classification may not be appropriate for segmentation, showing that better performances could be reached via other alternatives, e.g., self training [22] or curriculum learning [22,25]. Furthermore, a large label space might invalidate the assumption that the source and target share the same feature representation at all the abstraction levels of a deep network. In fact, recently, Tsai et al. [20] proposed adversarial training in the softmax-output space, outperforming feature-matching techniques in the context of color images. Such output space conveys domain-invariant information about segmentation structures, for instance, shape and spatial layout, even when the inputs across domains are substantially different. Finally, it is worth mentioning the recent classification study in [19], which argued that adversarial training is not sufficient for high-capacity models, as is the case for segmentation. For deep architectures, the authors of [19] showed experimentally that jointly minimizing source generalization error and feature divergence does not yield high accuracy on the target task.

We propose a general constrained domain adaptation formulation, which embeds domain-invariant prior knowledge about the segmentation regions. Such knowledge takes the form of simple anatomical information, e.g., region size or shape, which is either estimated from the source ground truth or known *a priori*. For instance, in the application we tackle in our experiments, we can use human-spine measurements that are well known in the literature [1] for constraining the sizes of the inter-vertebral discs in axial MRI slices. By imposing domain-invariant inequality constraints on the network outputs of unlabeled target samples, our method matches implicitly some prediction statistics of the target to the source, and allows uncertainty in the prior knowledge. We address our constrained problem with a differentiable penalty, which can be fully handled with SGD, removing the need for computationally expensive Lagrangian optimization with dual projections. Unlike two-step adversarial training, our method uses a single loss/network, which simplifies adaptation by avoiding extra adversarial steps, while improving training quality and efficiency. We juxtapose our approach to the state-of-art adversarial method in [20] on the challenging task of adapting spine segmentation across different MRI modalities. Our method achieves significantly better performances using simple and imprecise size priors, with a 16% improvement, approaching the performance of a supervised model. It can be readily used for various constraints and segmentation problems. Our code is publicly (and anonymously) available[1].

2   Formulation

Let $I_s : \Omega_s \subset \mathbb{R}^{2,3} \to \mathbb{R}$, $s = 1, \ldots, S$, denote the training images of the source domain. Assume that each of these has a ground-truth segmentation, which, for each pixel (or voxel) $i \in \Omega_s$, takes the form of binary simplex vector $\mathbf{y}_s(i) = (y_s^1(i), \ldots, y_s^K(i)) \in \{0, 1\}^K$, with K the number of classes (segmentation regions).

Given T unlabeled images of the target domain, $I_t : \Omega_t \subset \mathbb{R}^{2,3} \to \mathbb{R}$, $t = 1, \ldots, T$, we state unsupervised domain adaptation for segmentation as the following constrained optimization w.r.t parameters θ:

$$\min_{\theta} \sum_s \sum_{i \in \Omega_s} \mathcal{L}(\mathbf{y}_s(i), \mathbf{p}_s(i, \theta))$$

$$\text{s.t.} \quad f_c(\mathbf{P}_t(\theta)) \leq 0 \quad c = 1, \ldots, C; t = 1, \ldots, T \tag{1}$$

where $\mathbf{p}_x(i, \theta) = (p_x^1(i, \theta), \ldots, p_x^K(i, \theta)) \in [0, 1]^K$ is the softmax output of the network at pixel/voxel i in image $x \in \{t = 1, \ldots, T\} \cup \{t = 1, \ldots, S\}$, and $\mathbf{P}_x(\theta)$ is a $K \times |\Omega_x|$ matrix whose columns are the vectors of network outputs $\mathbf{p}_x(i, \theta), i \in \Omega_x$. In problem (1), $\mathcal{L}$ is a standard loss, e.g., the cross-entropy: $\mathcal{L}(\mathbf{y}_s(i), \mathbf{p}_s(i, \theta)) = -\sum_k y_s^k(i) \log p_s^k(i, \theta)$, computed on the source domain S. The inequality constraint can embed very useful prior knowledge that is invariant across domains and modalities, and is imposed on the network outputs for unlabeled target-domain data. Assume, for instance, that we have prior knowledge about the size (or cardinality) of the target segmentation region (or class) k.

---

[1] https://github.com/CDAMICCAI2019/CDA.

Such a knowledge is invariant w.r.t modalities, and does not have to be precise; it can be in the form of lower and upper bounds on region size. For instance, when we have an upper bound a on the size of region k, we can impose the following constraint: $\sum_{i \in \Omega_t} p_t^k(i, \theta) - a \leq 0$. In this case, the corresponding constraint c in the general-form constrained problem (1) uses particular function $f_c(\mathbf{P}_t(\theta)) = \sum_{i \in \Omega_t} p_t^k(i, \theta) - a$. In a similar way, one can impose a lower bound b on the size of region k using $f_c(\mathbf{P}_t(\theta)) = b - \sum_{i \in \Omega_t} p_t^k(i, \theta)$. Priors a and b can be learned from the ground-truth segmentations of the source domain (assuming such priors are invariant across domains). Also, depending on the application, such priors may correspond to anatomical knowledge. For instance, in the application we tackle in our experiments, we can use human spine measurements that are well known in the clinical literature [1] for constraining the sizes of the intervertebral discs in axial MRI slices. Our framework can be easily extended to more descriptive constraints, e.g., invariant shape moments [13], which do not change from one modality to another[2].

Even when the constraints are convex with respect to the network probability outputs, the problem in (1) is challenging for deep segmentation models that involve millions of parameters. In the general context of optimization, a standard technique to deal with hard inequality constraints is to solve the Lagrangian primal and dual problems in an alternating scheme [2]. For problem (1), this amounts to alternating the optimization of a CNN for the primal with stochastic optimization, e.g., SGD, and projected gradient-ascent iterates for the dual. However, despite the clear benefits of imposing hard constraints on CNNs, such a standard Lagrangian-dual optimization is avoided in the context of modern deep networks due, in part, to computational-tractability issues. As pointed out in [15, 17], there is a consensus within the community that imposing hard constraints on the outputs of deep CNNs that are common in modern image analysis problems is impractical: The use of Lagrangian-dual optimization for networks with millions of parameters requires training a whole CNN after each iterative dual step.

In the context of deep networks, equality or inequality constraints are typically handled in a "soft" manner by augmenting the loss with a *penalty* function [6,10,12]. The penalty-based approach is a simple alternative to Lagrangian optimization, and is well-known in the general context of constrained optimization; see [2], Sect. 4. In general, such penalty-based methods approximate a constrained minimization problem with an unconstrained one by adding a term, which increases when the constraints are violated. This is convenient for deep networks because it removes the requirement for explicit Lagrangian-dual optimization. The inequality constraints are fully handled within stochastic optimization, as in standard unconstrained losses, avoiding gradient ascent iterates/projections over the dual variables and reducing the computational load for training. For this work, we pursue a similar penalty approach, and replace constrained problem (1) by the following unconstrained problem:

---

[2] In fact, region size is the 0-order shape moment; one can use higher-order shape moments for richer descriptions of shape.

$$\min_{\theta} \sum_{s} \sum_{i \in \Omega_s} \mathcal{L}(\mathbf{y}_s(i), \mathbf{p}(i, \theta)) + \gamma \mathcal{F}(\theta) \qquad (2)$$

where γ is a positive constant and $\mathcal{F}$ a quadratic penalty, which takes the following form for the inequality constraints in (1):

$$\mathcal{F}(\theta) = \sum_{c=1}^{C} \sum_{t=1}^{T} [f_c(\mathbf{P}_t(\theta))]_+^2 \qquad (3)$$

with $[x]_+ = \max(0, x)$ denoting the rectifier linear unit function.

3   Experiments

3.1   Experimental Set-Up

Dataset. The proposed method was evaluated on the publicly available MIC-CAI 2018 IVDM3Seg Challenge[3] dataset. This dataset contains 16 3D multimodal magnetic resonance (MR) scans of the lower spine, with their corresponding manual segmentations, collected from 8 subjects at two different stages in a study investigating intervertebral discs (IVD) degeneration. In our experiments, we employed the water (Wat) modality as the labeled source domain S and the in-phase (IP) modality as the unlabeled target domain T, and the setting is binary classification ($K = 2$). While 13 scans were used for training, the remaining 3 scans were employed for validation.

Constrained versus Adversarial Domain Adaptation. We compared our constrained DA model to the adversarial approach proposed in [20], which encourages the output space to be invariant across domains. To do so, the penalty $\mathcal{F}$ in (2) is replaced by an adversarial loss, which enforces the alignment between the distributions of source and target image segmentations. During training, pairs of images from the source and target domain are fed into the segmentation network. Then, a discriminator uses the generated masks as inputs and attempts to identify the domain from which the masks come from (source, or target). In this setting, we focused on a single-level adversarial learning for simplicity (see [20] for more details).

Diverse Levels of Supervision. We used the penalty term in (3) on the size of the target region (the IVDs) bounded by two prior values, which were estimated from the ground truth. This setting is later on referred to as *Constraint*. We also experimented with three different levels of tightness of the bounds, $\pm 10\%$, $\pm 50\%$ and $\pm 70\%$ of variations with respect to the actual size, so as to evaluate the behaviour of our method in the case of imprecise prior knowledge. In addition, we employed a model trained on the source as the lower baseline –without any adaptation strategy– and a model trained on the target data, referred to as *Oracle*, which serves as an upper bound.

---

[3] https://ivdm3seg.weebly.com/.

Training and Implementation Details. As suggested in [20], we employ pairs of images from both domains, I_s and I_t, to train the deep models, which in our case correspond to the same 2D axial slice but from different modalities. For the segmentation network, we employ ENet [16], but any CNN segmentation network could be used. Regarding the DA adversarial approach, we employ the same segmentation network and include the discriminator proposed in [20]. Both the segmentation and the discrimination network were trained with Adam optimizer and a batch size of 1, for 100 epochs, and an initial learning rate of 5×10^{-4} and 10^{-4}, respectively. A baseline model trained on the source with full supervision was used as initialization. The γ parameter in (2) was set empirically to 2.5 in the proposed constrained adaptation model and to 0.1 in the adversarial approach.

Evaluation. In all our experiments, the Dice similarity coefficient (DSC) and the Hausdorff distance (HD) were employed as evaluation metrics to compare the different models.

3.2 Results

Quantitative metrics are reported in Table 1. First, we can observe that employing a model trained on source images to segment target images yields poor results, demonstrating the difficulty of CNNs to generalize well on a new domain. Adopting the adversarial strategy substantially improves the performance over the lower baseline, achieving a mean DSC of 65.3%. The proposed constrained DA models achieve a DSC value of 81.1%, 78.5% and 70.0% with tight ($Constraint_{10}$) and loose bounds ($Constraint_{50}$ and $Constraint_{70}$), respectively. This shows that, even with relaxed constraints, the proposed constrained DA model clearly outperforms the adversarial approach. Compared to the *Oracle*, the two best models –i.e., $Constraint_{10}$ and $Constraint_{50}$– reach 98% and 95% of its performance, demonstrating the efficiency of the proposed method and its robustness to the loosening of bounds. Regarding the HD values, we observe a similar pattern across the different models. Even though the adversarial approach reduces the HD to almost the half (1.67 pixels) compared to the lower baseline model (2.99 pixels), it is still far from the results obtained with our constrained models (1.10, 1.09 and 1.23 pixels). These findings are in line with the plots in Fig. 2, where the evolution of the training in terms of validation DSC is shown. In Fig. 2, *left* we can observe that the gap between the proposed and the adversarial approach holds during the whole training, with our constrained formulation yielding rapidly high validation Dice measures (first 20 epochs). This suggests that integrating the constraints help the learning process in domain adaptation.

Qualitative segmentations from the validation set are depicted in Fig. 3, from the easiest to the hardest subject. It can be observed that, if no adaptation is adopted, or even with the adversarial learning strategy, the network fails to successfully detect the 7 IVDs on all the subjects. While the adversarial approach segments 6 IVDs in the easiest subject (*top*), it is not able to correctly identify

Table 1. Quantitative comparisons of performance on the target domain for the different models.

	Source⟶Target					Target⟶Target
	No adaptation	Adversarial [20]	Constraint$_{10}$	Constraint$_{50}$	Constraint$_{70}$	Oracle
DSC	42.8 ± 5.29	65.3 ± 5.54	**81.1 ± 0.59**	78.5 ± 1.94	70.0 ± 4.11	82.9 ± 2.29
HD	2.99 ± 1.55	1.67 ± 1.64	1.10 ± 1.34	**1.09 ± 1.36**	1.23 ± 1.51	1.08 ± 1.35

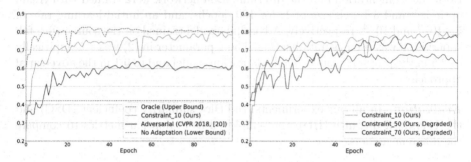

Fig. 2. Evolution of validation DSC over training for the different models. Comparison of the proposed model to the lower and upper bounds, as well as to the adversarial strategy is shown in the *left* figure, while an ablation study on the bounds is depicted in the *right*.

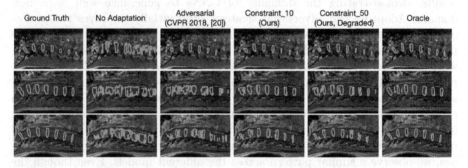

Fig. 3. Visual results in the validation set for several models. For better visibility results are depicted in the sagittal plane.

separate structures on harder cases. The segmentations achieved by the proposed constrained DA model present much better compactness and shape, where the 7 IVDs are distinguishable in all the subjects.

4   Conclusion

In this paper, we proposed a simple constrained formulation for domain adaptation in the context of semantic segmentation of medical images. Particularly, the proposed approach employs domain-invariant prior knowledge about the object of interest, in the form of target size, which is derived from the source ground truth. Unlike adversarial strategies, which are based on two-step training, our method tackles the UDA problem with a single constrained loss, simplifying the adaptation of the segmentation network. As demonstrated in our experiments, the performance is significantly improved with respect to a state-of-the art adversarial method, and is comparable to the upper baseline supervised on the target. The proposed learning framework is very flexible, being applicable to any architecture and capable of incorporating a wide variety of constraints.

References

1. Berry, J.L., Moran, J.M., Berg, W.S., Steffee, A.D.: A morphometric study of human lumbar and selected thoracic vertebrae. Spine **12**(4), 362–367 (1987)
2. Bertsekas, D.P.: Nonlinear Programming. Athena Scientific, Belmont (1995)
3. Chen, Y., Li, W., Van Gool, L.: Road: reality oriented adaptation for semantic segmentation of urban scenes. In: CVPR (2018)
4. Cheplygina, V., de Bruijne, M., Pluim, J.P.W.: Not-so-supervised: a survey of semi-supervised, multi-instance, and transfer learning in medical image analysis. MedIA **54**, 280–296 (2019)
5. Gholami, A., et al.: A novel domain adaptation framework for medical image segmentation. In: Crimi, A., Bakas, S., Kuijf, H., Keyvan, F., Reyes, M., van Walsum, T. (eds.) BrainLes 2018. LNCS, vol. 11384, pp. 289–298. Springer, Cham (2019). https://doi.org/10.1007/978-3-030-11726-9_26
6. He, F.S., Liu, Y., Schwing, A.G., Peng, J.: Learning to play in a day: faster deep reinforcement learning by optimality tightening. In: ICLR (2017)
7. Hoffman, J., et al.: CYCADA: cycle-consistent adversarial domain adaptation. In: ICML (2018)
8. Hong, W., Wang, Z., Yang, M., Yuan, J.: Conditional generative adversarial network for structured domain adaptation. In: CVPR (2018)
9. Javanmardi, M., Tasdizen, T.: Domain adaptation for biomedical image segmentation using adversarial training. In: ISBI (2018)
10. Jia, Z., Huang, X., Chang, E.I., Xu, Y.: Constrained deep weak supervision for histopathology image segmentation. IEEE TMI **36**(11), 2376–2388 (2017)
11. Kamnitsas, K., et al.: Unsupervised domain adaptation in brain lesion segmentation with adversarial networks. In: Niethammer, M., et al. (eds.) IPMI 2017. LNCS, vol. 10265, pp. 597–609. Springer, Cham (2017). https://doi.org/10.1007/978-3-319-59050-9_47
12. Kervadec, H., Dolz, J., Tang, M., Granger, E., Boykov, Y., Ayed, I.B.: Constrained-CNN losses for weakly supervised segmentation. MedIA **54**, 88–99 (2019)
13. Klodt, M., Cremers, D.: segmentation with moment constraints. In: ICCV (2011)
14. Litjens, G., et al.: A survey on deep learning in medical image analysis. MedIA **42**, 60–88 (2017)
15. Márquez-Neila, P., et al.: Imposing hard constraints on deep networks: promises and limitations. In: CVPR Workshop on Negative Results (2017)
16. Paszke, A., Chaurasia, A., Kim, S., Culurciello, E.: ENet: a deep neural network architecture for real-time semantic segmentation, arxiv preprint arXiv:1606.02147 (2016)
17. Pathak, D., Krähenbühl, P., Darrell, T.: Constrained convolutional neural networks for weakly supervised segmentation. In: ICCV (2015)

18. Ren, J., Hacihaliloglu, I., Singer, E.A., Foran, D.J., Qi, X.: Adversarial domain adaptation for classification of prostate histopathology whole-slide images. In: Frangi, A.F., Schnabel, J.A., Davatzikos, C., Alberola-López, C., Fichtinger, G. (eds.) MICCAI 2018. LNCS, vol. 11071, pp. 201–209. Springer, Cham (2018). https://doi.org/10.1007/978-3-030-00934-2_23
19. Shu, R., Bui, H.H., Narui, H., Ermon, S.: A DIRTT-T approach to unsupervised domain adaptation. In: ICLR (2018)
20. Tsai, Y., Hung, W., Schulter, S., Sohn, K., Yang, M., Chandraker, M.: Learning to adapt structured output space for semantic segmentation. In: CVPR (2018)
21. Tzeng, E., et al.: Adversarial discriminative domain adaptation. In: CVPR (2017)
22. Zhang, Y., David, P., Gong, B.: Curriculum domain adaptation for semantic segmentation of urban scenes. In: ICCV (2017)
23. Zhang, Y., Miao, S., Mansi, T., Liao, R.: Task driven generative modeling for unsupervised domain adaptation: application to X-ray image segmentation. In: Frangi, A.F., Schnabel, J.A., Davatzikos, C., Alberola-López, C., Fichtinger, G. (eds.) MICCAI 2018. LNCS, vol. 11071, pp. 599–607. Springer, Cham (2018). https://doi.org/10.1007/978-3-030-00934-2_67
24. Zhao, H., et al.: Supervised segmentation of un-annotated retinal fundus images by synthesis. IEEE TMI **38**(1), 46–56 (2019)
25. Zou, Y., Yu, Z., Kumar, B.V.K.V., Wang, J.: Unsupervised domain adaptation for semantic segmentation via class-balanced self-training. In: ECCV (2018)

Image Registration

Image-and-Spatial Transformer Networks for Structure-Guided Image Registration

Matthew C. H. Lee[1,2(✉)], Ozan Oktay[1,2], Andreas Schuh[1,2], Michiel Schaap[1,2], and Ben Glocker[1,2]

[1] HeartFlow, Redwood City, USA
[2] Biomedical Image Analysis Group, Imperial College London, London, UK
`matthew.lee13@imperial.ac.uk`

Abstract. Image registration with deep neural networks has become an active field of research and exciting avenue for a long standing problem in medical imaging. The goal is to learn a complex function that maps the appearance of input image pairs to parameters of a spatial transformation in order to align corresponding anatomical structures. We argue and show that the current direct, non-iterative approaches are sub-optimal, in particular if we seek accurate alignment of Structures-of-Interest (SoI). Information about SoI is often available at training time, for example, in form of segmentations or landmarks. We introduce a novel, generic framework, Image-and-Spatial Transformer Networks (ISTNs), to leverage SoI information allowing us to learn new image representations that are optimised for the downstream registration task. Thanks to these representations we can employ a test-specific, iterative refinement over the transformation parameters which yields highly accurate registration even with very limited training data. Performance is demonstrated on pairwise 3D brain registration and illustrative synthetic data.

1 Introduction

Image registration remains a fundamental problem in medical image computing, where the goal is to estimate a spatial transformation $T_\theta : \mathbb{R}^d \to \mathbb{R}^d$ mapping corresponding anatomical locations between d-dimensional images. The most widely used approach is intensity-based registration formalised as an optimisation problem seeking optimal transformation parameters θ that minimise a dissimilarity measure (or cost function) $\mathcal{L}(M \circ T_\theta, F)$, where M is the moving source image undergoing spatial transformation and F is the fixed target image. We refer the reader to [1] for a detailed overview of what we here call *traditional* methods, i.e., non-learning based approaches making use of iterative optimisation strategies to minimise the cost function for a given pair of images.

M. Schaap and B. Glocker—Shared senior authorship.

Electronic supplementary material The online version of this chapter (https://doi.org/10.1007/978-3-030-32245-8_38) contains supplementary material, which is available to authorized users.

ⓒ Springer Nature Switzerland AG 2019
D. Shen et al. (Eds.): MICCAI 2019, LNCS 11765, pp. 337–345, 2019.
https://doi.org/10.1007/978-3-030-32245-8_38

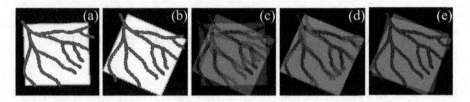

Fig. 1. A toy example (vessel trees on white box) illustrating the benefit of structure-guided image registration. The initial alignment of images (a, b) is shown in (c) and after intensity-based affine registration in (d). Registration focuses on aligning the white box ignoring Structures-of-Interest (SoI), i.e., the vessels. Our ISTNs learn to focus on the SoI yielding accurate alignment in (e).

Recently, the use of neural networks to learn the complex mapping from image appearance to spatial transformation has become an active field of research [2–7], providing a new perspective on tackling challenging registration problems. So called *supervised* approaches [2,3] have been used, which are similar in nature to methods used for image segmentation, where a convolutional neural network is trained to predict the transformation directly using examples of images and their ground truth transformation. Because actual ground truth for T_θ is not available, either random transformations are used to generate synthetic examples or a well established traditional registration method is employed to obtain reference transformations. Neither is optimal, as synthetic transformations might not be realistic and/or yield poor generalisation, while when employing a traditional method the prediction accuracy of the trained network is inherently limited by the accuracy of that method. One might argue that in this case the neural network is mostly learning to replicate the traditional method, although with a potentially remarkable computational speed up.

Due to the limitations of supervised methods, a number of works have then considered so called *unsupervised* approaches [6,7] where a neural network is trained based on the original cost function of traditional intensity-based methods minimising a dissimilarity measure such as mean squared intensity differences and others. While training over large number of examples might indeed be beneficial for optimising the cost function (it could have a regularisation effect or improve generalisation), these unsupervised approaches cannot be expected to perform fundamentally better compared to traditional methods as the exact same function is optimised. One might even argue that traditional methods are more flexible, as they can adapt to any new pair of test images, and are not limited to register images of similar appearance as the training data. For example, many of the traditional methods discussed in [1] can be equally used for brain MRI and lung CT with maybe only a few changes to some hyper-parameters. A recent hybrid approach [8] is combining an unsupervised and supervised cost function using a traditional method to generate training deformation fields.

Overall, one may argue that neural network based image registration, so far, has not taken full advantage of deep representation learning but mostly led

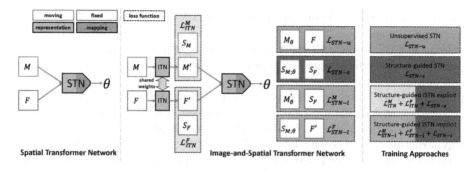

Fig. 2. Overview of image registration using Spatial Transformer Networks (STNs), with the classical model shown on the left mapping an image pair M, F *directly* to parameters θ of a spatial transformation (cf. [6,7]). Our Image-and-Spatial Transformer Networks (ISTNs) introduce a dedicated image transformer network (ITN) to learn to produce image representations M', F' optimised for the downstream registration task, as well as predicting θ. This gives raise to multiple ways of training ISTNs by combining different loss functions (see Sect. 2.2).

to a speed up in the time it takes to register two images. At the same time, one may argue that registration accuracy is of higher importance than speed in many clinical applications. We observe that neither the supervised nor the unsupervised methods exploit two key advantages of neural networks, which are (1) the ability to learn new representations that are optimised for a downstream task, and (2) the ability to incorporate and benefit from additional information during training that is unavailable (or very difficult to obtain) at test time.

Some exceptions to the second point are works that consider extra information such as segmentations or weak labels during training [4–6]. This additional supervision can help to guide the registration at test time in a different way than using image intensities alone. For example, the registration may focus on particular SoI (cf. Fig. 1). However, the current approaches do not retain or explicitly extract such extra information, so it cannot be used further at test time, for example, for refining the predicted, initial transformation parameters. In fact, most of the current works consider neural network based registration as a one-pass (non-iterative) process, which might be sub-optimal as we show in our results. The few works that discuss subsequent refinement either suggest to use a traditional (iterative) method [6], or to use the network in an auto-regressive way [7]. As both rely again on optimising the original intensity-based cost function the advantage over a traditional method remains unclear, and any extra information that was available during training is somewhat lost.

1.1 Contributions

To overcome these limitations, and to make best use of the key ability of neural networks to learn representations, we introduce Image-and-Spatial Transformer Networks (ISTNs) where a dedicated Image Transformer Network (ITN) is added to the head of a Spatial Transformer Network (STN) aiming to extract and retain information about SoIs, for which annotations are only required during training. While the STN predicts the parameters of the spatial transformation, the ITN produces a new image representation which is learned in an end-to-end fashion and optimised for the downstream registration task. This allows us to not only predict a good initial transformation at test time, but enables what we call *structure-guided* registration with an accurate test-specific, iterative refinement using the exact same model. An illustrative example of what ISTNs can do and why structure-guided registration can be useful is shown in Fig. 1. A schematic overview of our approach and how it relates to previous work that uses STNs only (such as [6,7]) is shown in Fig. 2.

2   Image-and-Spatial Transformer Networks

Spatial Transformer Networks [9] are the building block of most of the recent works on neural network based image registration. An STN is a neural network in itself commonly consisting of a few convolutional and fully connected layers that are able to learn a mapping from input images (M, F) to parameters θ of a spatial transformation T_θ. Taking advantage of the fact that image re-sampling is a differentiable operation, STNs can be trained end-to-end, and plugged as a module into larger networks (as originally used for improving image classification [9]). Revisiting the structure of an STN, we observe that there are two main components: a feature extraction part learning a new representation of the input using convolutional layers, and a second part that maps these representations to transformation parameters. We indicate this in Fig. 2 using different colours within the STN module. The representation that STNs may learn, however, is not exposed and remains hidden during inference. This is where our main contribution comes into play where we redesign the basic building block of the transformer module of neural network based image registration by introducing a dedicated Image Transformer Network.

2.1   Image Transformer Networks

We define ITNs to be convolutional neural networks that map an input image to an output image of the same size and dimension. In this paper we consider the case where the number of channels is the same for the input and output, although this does not have to be the case and other variants may be considered. The role of the ITN is to expose explicitly a learned image representation that is optimal for the downstream registration task solved by the STN. A shared ITN for inputs M and F learns to generate outputs M' and F' which are fed into a regular STN (cf. Fig. 2). This new architecture gives raise to a number of training approaches, in particular, when extra information about SoIs are available, such as image segmentations or landmarks.

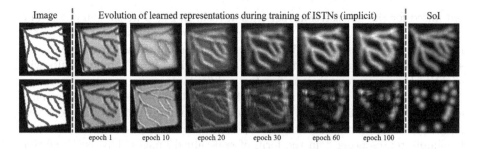

Fig. 3. For a toy example, we show the progress of the output of the ITN module in an ISTN model trained with the *implicit* loss function $\mathcal{L}_{ISTN-i}$ (cf. Eq. (2) in Sect. 2.2 and Fig. 2). The top row corresponds to a case where the SoI is a segmentation-like mask (shown on the most right). The bottom row shows training with landmark maps. The learned image representation allows accurate structure-guided registration with test-specific refinement at test time.

2.2 Explicit and Implicit Training of ISTNs

As indicated in Fig. 2, different loss functions can be considered for training ISTNs. Note that the unsupervised case using image intensities only, here corresponding to $\mathcal{L}_{STN-u}(M_\theta, F)$, is a special case of training an ISTN. We use M_θ as a short form of $M \circ T_\theta$. Similarly, we can incorporate auxiliary information in form of segmentations as in [6] or other structural or geometric information via a 'structure-guided' or 'supervised' loss $\mathcal{L}_{STN-s}(S_{M;\theta}, S_F)$. Here, S are images encoding SoIs (e.g., organ segmentations, anatomical landmarks, centerlines, etc.), and 'supervised' refers to the fact that such SoIs need annotations on the training data. Note, that neither $\mathcal{L}_{STN-u}$ nor $\mathcal{L}_{STN-s}$ will encourage the ITN to learn any directly useful representations. In order to facilitate this, we propose two different strategies for training ISTNs when auxiliary information about SoIs is available. The loss function for our *explicit* ISTN is defined as

$$\mathcal{L}_{ISTN-e} = \mathcal{L}_{ITN}^M + \mathcal{L}_{ITN}^F + \mathcal{L}_{STN-s} \qquad (1)$$

which combines the supervised STN with an ITN loss $\mathcal{L}_{ITN}(S_I, I')$ explicitly penalizing differences between the SoI encoding S_I and the ITN output I' for input image I. While the explicit loss has the desired effect of producing representations capturing the SoI information, the ITN and STN losses are somewhat decoupled where the ITN loss plays the role of deep supervison.

An intriguing alternative is the *implicit* ISTN with a loss function defined as

$$\mathcal{L}_{ISTN-i} = \mathcal{L}_{STN-i}^M + \mathcal{L}_{STN-i}^F + \mathcal{L}_{STN-s} \qquad (2)$$

Here, the two terms $\mathcal{L}_{STN-i}^M(M_\theta', S_F)$ and $\mathcal{L}_{STN-i}^F(S_{M;\theta}, F')$ intertwine the outputs of the ITN (M', F'), the SoI encodings (S_M, S_F) and the estimated transformation parameters θ from the STN. Combined with the supervised STN loss this gives raise to a fully end-to-end training of image representations that are optimised for the downstream registration task. In Fig. 3 we show how the ITN representations evolve over the course of training on an illustrative toy example both for the case of segmentations and landmark annotations. Due to space reasons, we omit the figure for the explicit ISTN which shows similar results with slightly sharper representations due to the ITN loss.

In this paper, for all above mentioned loss functions we use the mean squared error (MSE) loss. Other losses can be considered but we find MSE to work very well. It also allows us to flexibly incorporate different types of SoI information by simply representing it in the form of real-valued images. This is straightforward for binary segmentations, and anatomical landmarks can be, for example, encoded via distance maps or smoothed centroid maps (cf. bottom row of Fig. 3).

2.3   Test-Specific Iterative Refinement

The key of ISTNs is that they enable structure-guided, test-specific refinement based on the learned representations M' and F' that are exposed by the ITN. Though any registration technique can be used for refinement by using the inferred images M' and F' as inputs, we can also directly leverage the STN module itself to perform the refinement at inference time by iteratively updating the STN weights (keeping the ITN weights fixed) through minimization of a refinement loss denoted as $\mathcal{L}_{STN-r}(M'_\theta, F')$. Note, that no annotations are required for the test images to perform this iterative refinement, as the necessary representations M' and F' are generated by the trained ITN.

2.4   Transformation Models

STNs make no assumption about the employed spatial transformation model, and hence, our ISTN architecture remains generic allowing the integration of various linear and non-linear transformation models. In this paper, we consider two specific transformation models as a proof-of-concept. We employ a typical parameterisation for affine transformations decomposed into

$$T_\theta^{\text{affine}} = M_t R_\phi S_\psi^{-1} D_s S_\psi \qquad (3)$$

where M_t, R_ϕ, D_s and S_ψ are the translation, rotation, scaling and shearing matrices. This decomposition allows us to set intuitive bounds on the individual transformation parameters by using appropriately scaled tanh functions. For non-linear registration we employ a standard B-spline parameterisation using a regular grid of control points. Transformation parameters θ then correspond to control point displacements. Details on this, with emphasis on their applications and implementations within neural network architectures can be found in [7,10].

3   Experiments

We evaluate ISTNs on the task of pairwise registration of brain MRI (similar to [6,8]). In the first set of experiments, we use 420 individual subjects from the UK

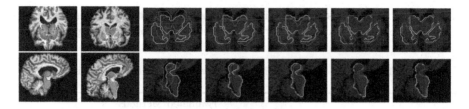

Fig. 4. Visual results for affine registration with SoI overlaid in red (moving), and green (fixed). On the left: the input images before registration. Close-ups from left to right: initial alignment, STN-u, STN-s, ISTN-e, ISTN-i. (Color figure online)

Biobank Imaging Study[1] to form 100 random pairs of moving and fixed images for training, 10 pairs for validation, and 100 pairs for testing. For each image, segmentations of sub-cortical structures are available. Images are skull-stripped and intensity normalised. Binarised segmentation label maps are used as the SoI information. Due to space reasons, we focus on the results while our publicly available code[2] contains details on architectural choices, hyper-parameters and training configurations.

We assess agreement of SoI after registration by calculating Dice scores and average surface distances (ASDs). We compare the explicit and implicit variants (ISTN-e and ISTN-i) with unsupervised and supervised models (STN-u and STN-s). These baselines are conceptually similar to the approaches in [6,7]. The baselines have been set up in a competitive way and we checked for proper convergence and best possible performance on the validation set.

Table 1 summarizes the quantitative results before and after iterative refinement using the four different approaches with affine and non-linear B-spline transformation models. For the B-splines we use a 30 mm control point spacing and start registration from rigidly pre-aligned images. For both affine and B-splines we provide numbers for the initial state (Id) and results when the SoI is used directly for registration as an upper bound "best-case" reference. We note that ISTN-e/i outperform STN-u/s for the one-pass predictions. Test-specific refinement boosts the accuracy significantly for all approaches. ISTNs achieve overall highest Dice scores and lowest ASDs, sometimes close to the best-case. STN-u/s after refinement converge to the same lower accuracy as no SoI information can be leveraged. Figure 4 shows qualitative results after refinement for affine registration, while Fig. 5 shows an example of learned SoI representations.

We repeat the experiments but with 1,000 pairs for training instead of 100. The one-pass predictions improve for all four methods with Dice scores of 0.75 (STN-u), 0.77 (STN-s), and 0.80 (ISTN-e/i) for affine, and 0.79, 0.83, and 0.86 (same order) for non-linear. Iterative refinement yields quasi identical results for STN-u/s as before when trained with 100 pairs, and slightly improves for ISTNs. Remarkably, ISTNs trained with only 100 pairs achieve much higher accuracy

---

[1] UK Biobank Resource under Application Number 12579.

[2] https://github.com/biomedia-mira/istn.

than STN-u and STN-s trained with 1,000 pairs, indicating excellent data efficiency and benefit of iterative, test-specific refinement for image registration.

Table 1. Summary of registration results when using 100 training images.

| T_θ | Metric | Refine | Id | Evaluated Methods | | | | SoI |
				STN-u	STN-s	ISTN-e	ISTN-i	
Affine	Dice	before	0.53	0.71	0.70	0.75	0.75	0.84
		after		0.79	0.79	0.83	0.82	
	ASD	before	2.41	1.11	1.10	0.93	0.89	0.50
		after		0.69	0.69	0.53	0.58	
B-Spline	Dice	before	0.70	0.74	0.77	0.80	0.81	0.91
		after		0.84	0.83	0.86	0.85	
	ASD	before	1.05	0.88	0.74	0.63	0.59	0.27
		after		0.51	0.52	0.45	0.46	

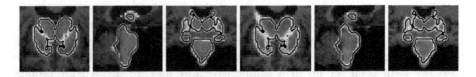

Fig. 5. Overlay of the learned representations of sub-cortical structures as heatmaps on top of a test input. The axial, sagittal and coronal slices on the left correspond to the ITN output of an *explicit* ISTN-e, the left shows the output for an *implicit* ISTN-i. Black contours show the ground truth segmentations.

4 Conclusion

ISTNs are a generic framework for neural network based structure-guided image registration with test-specific refinement using learned representations. In our experiments the explicit and implicit variants perform equally well and outperform unsupervised and supervised STNs both before and after refinement. Implicitly learned representations may be beneficial to prevent overfitting in cases where SoI information contains noise or corruption. This effect and other applications of ISTNs using different types of SoI will be explored in future work.

References

1. Sotiras, A., Davatzikos, C., Paragios, N.: Deformable medical image registration: a survey. IEEE Trans. Med. Imaging **32**(7), 1153 (2013)
2. Yang, X., Kwitt, R., Styner, M., Niethammer, M.: Quicksilver: fast predictive image registration-a deep learning approach. NeuroImage **158**, 378–396 (2017)

3. Sokooti, H., de Vos, B., Berendsen, F., Lelieveldt, B.P.F., Išgum, I., Staring, M.: Nonrigid image registration using multi-scale 3D convolutional neural networks. In: Descoteaux, M., Maier-Hein, L., Franz, A., Jannin, P., Collins, D.L., Duchesne, S. (eds.) MICCAI 2017. LNCS, vol. 10433, pp. 232–239. Springer, Cham (2017). https://doi.org/10.1007/978-3-319-66182-7_27

4. Rohé, M.-M., Datar, M., Heimann, T., Sermesant, M., Pennec, X.: SVF-Net: learning deformable image registration using shape matching. In: Descoteaux, M., Maier-Hein, L., Franz, A., Jannin, P., Collins, D.L., Duchesne, S. (eds.) MICCAI 2017. LNCS, vol. 10433, pp. 266–274. Springer, Cham (2017). https://doi.org/10.1007/978-3-319-66182-7_31

5. Hu, Y., et al.: Weakly-supervised convolutional neural networks for multimodal image registration. Med. Image Anal. **49**, 1–13 (2018)

6. Balakrishnan, G., Zhao, A., Sabuncu, M.R., Guttag, J., Dalca, A.V.: VoxelMorph: a learning framework for deformable medical image registration. IEEE Trans. Med. Imaging (2019)

7. de Vos, B.D., Berendsen, F.F., Viergever, M.A., Sokooti, H., Staring, M., Išgum, I.: A deep learning framework for unsupervised affine and deformable image registration. Med. Image Anal. **52**, 128–143 (2019)

8. Fan, J., Cao, X., Yap, P.T., Shen, D.: BIRNet: brain image registration using dual-supervised fully convolutional networks. Med. Image Anal. **54**, 193–206 (2019)

9. Jaderberg, M., Simonyan, K., Zisserman, A., Kavukcuoglu, K.: Spatial transformer networks. In: Advances in Neural Information Processing Systems (2015)

10. Sandkühler, R., Jud, C., Andermatt, S., Cattin, P.C.: AirLab: autograd image registration laboratory. arXiv preprint arXiv:1806.09907 (2018)

Probabilistic Multilayer Regularization Network for Unsupervised 3D Brain Image Registration

Lihao Liu, Xiaowei Hu, Lei Zhu$^{(\boxtimes)}$, and Pheng-Ann Heng

Department of Computer Science and Engineering,
The Chinese University of Hong Kong, Sha Tin, Hong Kong
lzhu@cse.cuhk.edu.hk

Abstract. Brain image registration transforms a pair of images into one system with the matched imaging contents, which is of essential importance for brain image analysis. This paper presents a novel framework for unsupervised 3D brain image registration by capturing the feature-level transformation relationships between the unaligned image and reference image. To achieve this, we develop a feature-level probabilistic model to provide the direct regularization to the hidden layers of two deep convolutional neural networks, which are constructed from two input images. This model design is developed into multiple layers of these two networks to capture the transformation relationships at different levels. We employ two common benchmark datasets for 3D brain image registration and perform various experiments to evaluate our method. Experimental results show that our method clearly outperforms state-of-the-art methods on both benchmark datasets by a large margin.

1 Introduction

Image registration aims to transform different images into one system with the matched imaging contents, which has significant applications in brain image analysis, including brain atlas creation [3], tumor growth monitoring [7] and multi-modality image fusion [5]. When we analyze a pair of brain images that were acquired from different sensors and viewpoints at different times, we need to transform one image (unaligned image) to another image (reference image) by establishing the anatomical correspondences [4,6,13]. The correspondence between the unaligned image x and the reference image y is usually formulated by a transformation function ϕ_z, which is parametrized by a latent variable z.

In order to capture the registration correspondence and estimate the latent registration variable, early works solved the optimization problems [1,2] in a high-dimensional deformation space, which is computationally expensive, thus limiting the practicability in clinical applications. Recently, methods based on the deep convolutional neural networks (CNNs) learned the latent variable in an end-to-end manner, which largely reduces the computational time and shows

© Springer Nature Switzerland AG 2019
D. Shen et al. (Eds.): MICCAI 2019, LNCS 11765, pp. 346–354, 2019.
https://doi.org/10.1007/978-3-030-32245-8_39

results outperforming previous approaches. For example, Sokooti *et al.* [16] developed a RegNet trained with the generated displacement vector fields to register CT images. Rohé *et al.* [14] learned to align the images by leveraging additional segmented shapes in a CNN. However, these methods leverage the manually-labeled ground truth to train the deep networks in a supervised manner, where the labeled real images are expensive and tedious to be obtained. Hence, training on the limited labeled data degrades the performance of image registration. Very recently, researchers explored the unsupervised learning strategies to learn the transformation function between the unaligned image and moving image without ground truth labels. Among them, Dalca *et al.* [4] developed a probabilistic generative model for image registration by using CNN to learn the latent spatial transformation variable. Krebs *et al.* [12] applied conditional variable autoencoder to regularize low-dimensional probabilistic latent variables for image registration. Kuang *et al.* [6] employed different regularization choices in the deep network to predict the latent variable for a better registration result. However, the existing deep-learning based methods take the unaligned and reference images as the input of a CNN and predict the latent variable directly, which *ignores the transformation relationships between these two images in the feature levels.* Thereby, the features learned at hidden layers of the CNN are not "transparent" to the latent variable, which reduces the discriminativeness of features for image registration.

In this paper, we present to *introduce direct regularizations to the hidden layers* of two deep convolutional neural networks (CNNs): one CNN to extract features from the unaligned image while another CNN from the reference image. We provide the regularizations by *adopting probabilistic models to capture the transformation relationship between each pair of hidden layers* in these two CNNs. These probabilistic models can be seen as the additional constraints to regularize the intermediate feature maps during the learning process. Furthermore, we embed the regularization terms into multiple layers of the CNNs and produce the feature-level latent variables in different layers. Finally, we combine the predicted feature-level latent variables of all layers and predict the final latent variable for 3D brain image registration. The whole network is trained end-to-end in an unsupervised manner. Experimental results on LPBA40 and MindBoggle101 dataset demonstrate that our method outperforms the current state-of-the-art methods by a large margin.

2   Methodology

2.1   Method Overview

Figure 1 presents the workflow of the overall architecture of our proposed network for the 3D brain image registration. To begin with, our method produces two sets of feature maps with different spatial resolutions by using two CNNs, which take the unaligned and reference 3D brain image (denoted as x and y) as the inputs. Then, we design a feature-level probabilistic inference model (see Sect. 2.2 and Fig. 1(b)) to estimate the feature-level latent variable, which represents the

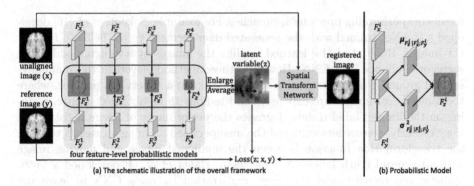

Fig. 1. (a) The schematic illustration of the overall framework. (b) The feature-level probabilistic model used in each pair of feature maps.

transformation relationship between the feature maps in the same layers of these two CNNs. We carry this estimation from the top layer (with the highest spatial resolution) to the bottom layer (with the lowest spatial resolution) in the CNNs. After that, we enlarge the obtained latent variable at all CNN layers to the same size of the input image using a linear interpolation, and then pixel-wisely average all the enlarged latent variables to produce the final latent variable z. Finally, we feed x and the final z into a spatial transform network (STN) [9] to generate an aligned image as the output of our network.

2.2 Feature-Level Probabilistic Model

Given a pair of feature maps (F_x^i, F_y^i) from the i-th layer of the two CNNs, our probabilistic model aims to estimate the i-th latent variable F_z^i, which parametrizes a spatial transformation function (denoted as $\psi_{F_z^i}$) for mapping F_x^i to F_y^i. According to the probabilistic model, we estimate F_z^i by maximizing the posterior registration probability $p(F_z^i|F_x^i; F_y^i)$ from the observed F_x^i and F_y^i. Similar to other works [4,12], we adopt a variational approach to compute $p(F_z^i|F_x^i; F_y^i)$ by first introducing an approximate posterior probability $q_\psi(F_z^i|F_x^i; F_y^i)$ and then minimizing a KL divergence between $p(F_z^i|F_x^i; F_y^i)$ and $q_\psi(F_z^i|F_x^i; F_y^i)$ to make these two distributions as similar as possible.

The minimization of KL divergence between $p(F_z^i|F_x^i; F_y^i)$ and $q_\psi(F_z^i|F_x^i; F_y^i)$ is defined as:

$$\min_{\psi} KL[q_\psi(F_z^i|F_x^i; F_y^i) \parallel p(F_z^i|F_x^i; F_y^i)]$$
$$= \min_{\psi} KL[q_\psi(F_z^i|F_x^i; F_y^i) \parallel p(F_z^i)] - E_q log\ p(F_y^i|F_z^i; F_x^i), \qquad (1)$$

where $q_\psi(F_z^i|F_x^i; F_y^i)$ comes from a multivariate normal distribution $\mathcal{N}$:

$$q_\psi(F_z^i|F_x^i; F_y^i) = \mathcal{N}(z; \mu_{F_z^i|F_x^i; F_y^i}, \sigma^2_{F_z^i|F_x^i; F_y^i}), \qquad (2)$$

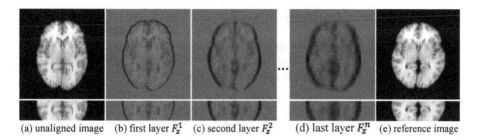

(a) unaligned image   (b) first layer F_z^1 (c) second layer F_z^2 (d) last layer F_z^n (e) reference image

Fig. 2. The visualization of (a) unaligned image; (b)–(d) the learned latent variables for different layers (from shallow layer to deep layer); (e) reference image.

where $\mu_{F_z^i|F_x^i;F_y^i}$ and $\sigma_{F_z^i|F_x^i;F_y^i}$ are the mean and standard variance of the distribution, and they are directly learned through the convolutional layers (see Fig. 1(b)) by using the combined feature maps of F_x^i and F_y^i. The $p(F_z^i)$ and $p(F_y^i|F_z^i;F_x^i)$ follow the multivariate normal distribution, which are modeled as:

$$p(F_z^i) = \mathcal{N}(F_z^i; 0, \sigma_{F_z^i}^2) , \tag{3}$$

$$p(F_y^i|F_z^i;F_x^i) = \mathcal{N}(F_y^i; F_x^i \circ \phi_{F_z^i}, \sigma_{F^i}^2) , \tag{4}$$

where σ_{F^i} is the variance (a diagonal matrix) of this distribution and $F_x^i \circ \phi_{F_z^i}$ is the noisy observed registered feature maps in which $\sigma_{F^i}^2$ is the variance of the noisy term; see [4] for detail definition.

2.3   Multilayer Fusion Network

As shown in Fig. 2, the feature maps at shallow CNN layers have high resolutions but with fruitful detail information, while the feature maps at deep layers have low resolutions but with high-level semantic information. The highly semantic features can help to register the global shape but neglecting many subtle details in the latent spatial variable; see Fig. 2(d). In contrast, as shown in Fig. 2(b), the fruitful details in the low-level latent variable capture the local detail registration deformation but fail to generate global shape registration correspondence. Motivated by this, we present to predict the final latent spatial transformation function between the two input images by leveraging features at multiple layers of the CNN to boost the registration performance. To achieve this, we leverage the feature-level probabilistic model to estimate the feature-level latent variable F_z^i by taking feature pairs from the shallowest layer to the deepest layer and fuse them together to compute the final latent variable z, which is then feed into the a spatial transform network (STN) [9] for generating the output registered image of our network.

2.4   Training and Testing Strategies

Loss Function. Our network predicts the latent registration transformation variable at each CNN layer and the output registered image. The total loss (denoted as $\mathcal{D}_{total}$) for each pair of images is defined as

$$\mathcal{D}_{total} = \mathcal{L}(z; x, y) + \sum_{i=1}^{n} w_i \mathcal{L}(F_z^i; F_x^i, F_y^i) , \qquad (5)$$

where $\mathcal{L}(z; x, y)$ denotes the KL divergence based loss of the prediction of the output registered image from the two input images (x and y); where $\mathcal{L}(F_z^i; F_x^i, F_y^i)$ is the KL divergence based loss generated of the registration transformation variable (F_z^i) prediction by taking two feature maps $(F_x^i$ and $(F_y^i))$ at the i-th layer of the CNNs as the input. n is the number of CNN layer and w_i is the loss weight of the i-th layer. We empirically set n and w_i as 4 and 1, respectively. According to [4], we start from the KL divergence in Eq. 1 and define the KL divergence-based loss in Eq. 5 as:

$$\mathcal{L}(Z; X, Y) = \frac{1}{2\sigma_{Z|X;Y}^2} ||Y - X \circ \phi_Z||^2 + \frac{1}{2} [tr(\sigma_{Z|X;Y}^2) + ||\mu_{Z|X;Y}|| - log\ det(\sigma_{Z|X;Y}^2)] ,$$
(6)

where $Z \in [z, F_z^i]$, $X \in [x, F_x^i]$ and $Y \in [y, F_y^i]$. The first term of Eq. 6 is a reconstruction loss for enforcing the registered image $X \circ \phi_Z$ to be similar to reference image Y. The second term is a closed form of first term of Eq. 1, and it encourages $q_\psi(Z|X; Y)$ and $p(Z)$ to be close. $\mu_{Z|X;Y}$ and $\sigma_{Z|X;Y}$ are the mean and standard variance of the distribution $q_\psi(Z|X; Y)$, and they are directly learned through convolutional layers; see Eq. 2.

Training Parameters. In our proposed model, we used the encoder architecture in [4] as the backbone for both CNNs. We adopted the initialization strategy of this work [8] to initialize the weights of all convolutional layers. Moreover, we set the initial learning rate as $1e^{-4}$, periodically reduced it by multiplying with 0.1, and stopped the learning process after 100 epochs. We employed the Adam optimizer [10] with the first momentum of 0.9, the second momentum of 0.999, and a weight decay of 0.0001 to minimize the loss (see Eq. 5) of the whole network. Our network was implemented using the Keras toolbox with a Tensorflow backend and we set the mini-batch size as one.

Inference. Given an unaligned image and a reference image, our network first estimates a latent variable from these two images and produces the registered image of the unaligned image by feeding the unaligned image and latent variable into the spatial transformation network (STN). Finally, we take the predicted registered image as the final output of our framework. Our method takes about 10 s to align a pair of images (size: $160 \times 192 \times 224$) on a single TITAN X GPU.

3 Experiments

3.1 Benchmark Datasets and Evaluation Metric

LPBA40. The LONI Probabilistic Brain Atlas (LPBA40) dataset [15] consists of 40 T1-weighted 3D brain MRI images from healthy subjects, and each volume has a brain mask and the corresponding segmentation mask (56 anatomical labels). We used the first 30 volumes as the training data and the remaining 10 volumes as the testing data. Note that we didn't use any segmentation mask during the training process.

MindBoggle101. MindBoggle101 dataset [11] contains 101 skull-stripped T1-weighted 3D brain MRI images from healthy subjects, and only 62 MRI images have their segmentation masks. For a fair comparison, we followed the recent work [13] and adopted 42 images for training and 20 images for testing.

Data Preprocessing and Evaluation Metric. We conducted the preprocessing steps for each 3D brain image, where these steps include brain extraction, voxel spacing re-sampling (1 mm), affine spatial normalization, "Whitening" operation, and intensity normalization; see [4] for detail. To evaluate the registration performance, we register each unaligned image as well as its segmentation mask, and measure the overlap between the registered segmentation mask and the segmentation mask of reference image using a widely-used Dice metric; see [4,6,13] for the details of the Dice definition. In general, a larger *Dice* indicates a better 3D brain registration result.

3.2 Experimental Results

Quantitative Comparison. We compared our method with three recent unsupervised brain image registration methods: UtilzReg [17], VoxelMorph [4], and FAIM [13]. Among them, UtilzReg adopted the hand-crafted features for image registration while the other two methods applied the CNN to predict the lantern variable for image registration. For a fair comparison, we obtained their results either by directly taking the results from their papers or by generating the results from the public codes provided by the authors using the recommended parameter setting. Moreover, we followed [13] and reported the Dice value on seven large regions of the human brain on LPBA40 dataset, where these regions are obtained by grouping all the tissues according to the regions of interests; see [13] for the details. For MindBoggle101 dataset, we followed [4,13] and compared the results on five large cortical regions, which are grouped from 25 cortical regions.

Tables 1 and 2 summary the quantitative results in terms of Dice on unsupervised 3D brain image registration in the two benchmark datasets. Apparently, Our method outperforms all the others for almost all the cases on these two benchmark datasets. It demonstrates that by introducing direct regularizations to multiple hidden layers in the deep convolutional neural networks, we can

Table 1. Comparison with the state-of-the-arts using Dice on the LPBA40 dataset.

	Frontal	Parietal	Occipital	Temporal	Cingulate	Putamen	Hippo
UtilzReg [17]	0.691	0.617	0.612	0.665	0.665	0.710	0.692
VoxelMorph [4]	0.669	0.610	0.605	0.652	0.663	0.700	0.689
FAIM [13]	0.676	0.617	0.608	0.658	0.675	0.710	0.696
Baseline-1	0.677	0.637	0.617	0.635	0.622	0.549	0.601
Baseline-2	0.702	0.661	0.648	0.664	0.665	0.602	0.682
Our method	**0.711**	**0.661**	**0.660**	**0.679**	**0.691**	**0.711**	**0.701**

Table 2. Comparison with the state-of-the-arts using Dice on the MindBoggle dataset.

	Frontal	Parietal	Occipital	Temporal	Cingulate
UtilzReg [17]	0.482	0.456	0.425	0.385	0.446
VoxelMorph [4]	0.534	0.527	0.510	0.433	0.483
FAIM [13]	0.572	0.551	**0.537**	0.469	0.508
Baseline-1	0.502	0.478	0.448	0.505	0.536
Baseline-2	0.560	0.545	0.433	0.523	0.546
Our method	**0.579**	**0.559**	0.430	**0.544**	**0.546**

obtain more discriminative features for latent variable prediction, thus producing more accurate registration results.

Visual Comparison. Figure 3 presents the visual comparison results produced by different registration methods. From the results, we can see that other methods tend to fail to the match the shape of the reference image or lose the structure details while our method is able to produce the result that is more consistent with the reference image and better preserves the internal structures.

Ablation Study. We performed an ablation study to evaluate the major components in our network design. Here, we considered two baselines. The first baseline (denoted as "Baseline-1") was a framework constructed by replacing the feature-level probabilistic model (see Sect. 2.2) in our network with an simple concatenation of F_x and F_y (shown in Fig. 1 for the latent variable estimation in each CNN layer, and also averaging the estimation result at all the CNN layers for computing the final latent variable, while the second baseline (denoted as "Baseline-2") only used the feature maps at the last CNN layers to compute the latent variable z. Tables 1 and 2 reported the comparison results, showing that the designed probabilistic model can effectively capture the transformation relationship between each pair of hidden layers in the two networks and adopting the probabilistic models to regularize multiple CNN layers leads to further improvement.

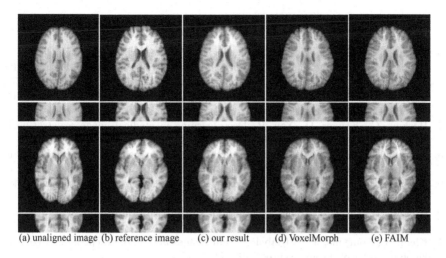

(a) unaligned image (b) reference image   (c) our result   (d) VoxelMorph   (e) FAIM

Fig. 3. Visual comparison of the results produced by our method and other methods.

4   Conclusion

This paper presents a deep neural network for boosting the 3D brain image registration. Our key idea is to develop feature-level probabilistic models to estimate the latent registration transformation variables from multiple layers of two convolutional neural networks (CNNs), which are constructed from two input images. Our network can provide the direct regularizations for hidden CNN layers and these direct regularizations introduce additional constraints for predicting the registration transformation variable, producing more discriminative features for image registration. Experimental results on two benchmark datasets demonstrate that our network clearly outperforms state-of-the-art methods.

Acknowledgment. The work described in this paper was supported by a grant from the Research Grants Council of Hong Kong Special Administrative Region, China (Project No. CUHK 14225616).

References

1. Avants, B.B., Epstein, C.L., Grossman, M., Gee, J.C.: Symmetric diffeomorphic image registration with cross-correlation: evaluating automated labeling of elderly and neurodegenerative brain. Med. Image Anal. **12**(1), 26–41 (2008)
2. Avants, B.B., Tustison, N.J., Song, G., Cook, P.A., Klein, A., Gee, J.C.: A reproducible evaluation of ANTs similarity metric performance in brain image registration. Neuroimage **54**(3), 2033–2044 (2011)
3. Chakravarty, M.M., Bertrand, G., Hodge, C.P., Sadikot, A.F., Collins, D.L.: The creation of a brain atlas for image guided neurosurgery using serial histological data. Neuroimage **30**(2), 359–376 (2006)
4. Dalca, A.V., Balakrishnan, G., Guttag, J., Sabuncu, M.R.: Unsupervised learning for fast probabilistic diffeomorphic registration. In: MICCAI, pp. 729–738 (2018)

5. Du, J., Li, W., Lu, K., Xiao, B.: An overview of multi-modal medical image fusion. Neurocomputing **215**, 3–20 (2016)
6. Fan, J., Cao, X., Xue, Z., Yap, P.-T., Shen, D.: Adversarial similarity network for evaluating image alignment in deep learning based registration. In: Frangi, A.F., Schnabel, J.A., Davatzikos, C., Alberola-López, C., Fichtinger, G. (eds.) MICCAI 2018. LNCS, vol. 11070, pp. 739–746. Springer, Cham (2018). https://doi.org/10.1007/978-3-030-00928-1_83
7. Haskins, G., Kruger, U., Yan, P.: Deep learning in medical image registration: a survey. arXiv preprint arXiv:1903.02026 (2019)
8. He, K., Zhang, X., Ren, S., Sun, J.: Delving deep into rectifiers: surpassing human-level performance on imagenet classification. In: CVPR, pp. 1026–1034 (2015)
9. Jaderberg, M., Simonyan, K., Zisserman, A., et al.: Spatial transformer networks. In: Advances in Neural Information Processing Systems, pp. 2017–2025 (2015)
10. Kingma, D.P., Ba, J.: Adam: a method for stochastic optimization. arXiv preprint arXiv:1412.6980 (2014)
11. Klein, A., Tourville, J.: 101 labeled brain images and a consistent human cortical labeling protocol. Front. Neurosci. **6**, 171 (2012)
12. Krebs, J., Mansi, T., Mailhé, B., Ayache, N., Delingette, H.: Unsupervised probabilistic deformation modeling for robust diffeomorphic registration. In: Stoyanov, D., et al. (eds.) DLMIA/ML-CDS -2018. LNCS, vol. 11045, pp. 101–109. Springer, Cham (2018). https://doi.org/10.1007/978-3-030-00889-5_12
13. Kuang, D., Schmah, T.: FAIM-a convnet method for unsupervised 3D medical image registration. arXiv preprint arXiv:1811.09243 (2018)
14. Rohé, M.-M., Datar, M., Heimann, T., Sermesant, M., Pennec, X.: SVF-Net: learning deformable image registration using shape matching. In: Descoteaux, M., Maier-Hein, L., Franz, A., Jannin, P., Collins, D.L., Duchesne, S. (eds.) MICCAI 2017. LNCS, vol. 10433, pp. 266–274. Springer, Cham (2017). https://doi.org/10.1007/978-3-319-66182-7_31
15. Shattuck, D.W., et al.: Construction of a 3D probabilistic atlas of human cortical structures. Neuroimage **39**(3), 1064–1080 (2008)
16. Sokooti, H., de Vos, B., Berendsen, F., Lelieveldt, B.P.F., Išgum, I., Staring, M.: Nonrigid image registration using multi-scale 3D convolutional neural networks. In: Descoteaux, M., Maier-Hein, L., Franz, A., Jannin, P., Collins, D.L., Duchesne, S. (eds.) MICCAI 2017. LNCS, vol. 10433, pp. 232–239. Springer, Cham (2017). https://doi.org/10.1007/978-3-319-66182-7_27
17. Vialard, F.X., Risser, L., Rueckert, D., Cotter, C.J.: Diffeomorphic 3D image registration via geodesic shooting using an efficient adjoint calculation. Int. J. Comput. Vis. **97**(2), 229–241 (2012)

A Deep Learning Approach to MR-less Spatial Normalization for Tau PET Images

Jennifer Alvén[1]([✉]), Kerstin Heurling[2], Ruben Smith[3], Olof Strandberg[3], Michael Schöll[2,3,4], Oskar Hansson[3], and Fredrik Kahl[1]

[1] Chalmers University of Technology, Gothenburg, Sweden
alven@chalmers.se
[2] Wallenberg Centre for Molecular and Translational Medicine and the Department of Psychiatry and Neurochemistry, University of Gothenburg, Gothenburg, Sweden
[3] Clinical Memory Research Unit, Lund University, Malmö, Sweden
[4] Dementia Research Centre, Institute of Neurology, University College London, London, UK

Abstract. The procedure of aligning a positron emission tomography (PET) image with a common coordinate system, *spatial normalization*, typically demands a corresponding structural magnetic resonance (MR) image. However, MR imaging is not always available or feasible for the subject, which calls for enabling spatial normalization without MR, *MR-less* spatial normalization. In this work, we propose a template-free approach to MR-less spatial normalization for [18F]flortaucipir tau PET images. We use a deep neural network that estimates an aligning transformation from the PET input image, and outputs the spatially normalized image as well as the parameterized transformation. In order to do so, the proposed network iteratively estimates a set of rigid and affine transformations by means of convolutional neural network regressors as well as spatial transformer layers. The network is trained and validated on 199 tau PET volumes with corresponding ground truth transformations, and tested on two different datasets. The proposed method shows competitive performance in terms of registration accuracy as well as speed, and compares favourably to previously published results.

1 Introduction

One of the necessary criteria for Alzheimer's disease (AD) diagnosis is the presence of abnormal tau protein in the brain. Normal tau protein is expressed ubiquitously in the central nervous system, but starts to aggregate and forms neurofibrillary tangles in AD. The positron emission tomography (PET) tracer [18F]flortaucipir binds to the aggregates of tau formed in AD, which makes it possible to visualize the distribution of tau pathology in the living human brain by means of tau PET [18].

In research settings, tau deposition is typically quantified in a common template space, e.g. defined by a magnetic resonance (MR) template brain image.

© Springer Nature Switzerland AG 2019
D. Shen et al. (Eds.): MICCAI 2019, LNCS 11765, pp. 355–363, 2019.
https://doi.org/10.1007/978-3-030-32245-8_40

This common template space provides anatomical information, which is insufficiently available in the PET scan alone, and enables region/voxel-wise analysis and comparisons. Consequently, this methodology requires spatial alignment of the acquired tau PET with this common coordinate system. This registration procedure, referred to as *spatial normalization*, is the focus of this paper.

Most approaches to spatial normalization utilize MR imaging, that is, the tau PET image is aligned with the template space via a MR image of the same subject. The alignment is typically carried out with image registration tools such as ANTs [1] or SPM [19]. One major disadvantage with this procedure is the need for the subject's MR; MR imaging is not necessarily available, and might be contraindicated or inconvenient for the subject. Enabling tau PET spatial normalization without MR, *MR-less spatial normalization*, would most definitely benefit large scale AD studies.

Common for all previous attempts on MR-less spatial normalization is the use of standard image registration techniques with an explicit PET template as target. The most simple approach uses one fix PET template, either computed as the mean over a set of training PET scans [6,15], or generated synthetically from MR template images [11]. More refined approaches use a learned PET template model to which the native PET scan is iteratively fitted and aligned. Variants of this approach are linear PET templates [3,16,17] and principal component analysis (PCA) models [7,8]. A deep learning based method for generating a synthetic PET template is proposed in [13], where a subject-specific template is predicted by a generative adversarial network (GAN) for each PET image. Note that a standard, non-learning, registration method is used when aligning the PET scan to the GAN-generated template.

None of the above-mentioned methods concern spatial normalization of PET scans using the tau tracer. These approaches are instead applied to β-amyloid PET or raclopride PET, i.e. PET scans using tracers that bind to other proteins than tau and showing less complex and more predictable uptake patterns. The only work on MR-less spatial normalization for tau PET that we are aware of is presented in [4], where the authors evaluate the three previously published template-based approaches [3,6,8] on tau PET scans. However, the paper notes that none of the compared template models (using a mean, linear and PCA template, respectively) capture the full variation of tau PETs. More specifically, a (linear) template model using the 1st PCA eigenvector only explained 28% of the variability within the tau PET dataset (consisting mainly of healthy subjects), while a PCA model, using the 1st and 2nd eigenvector, explained 42% of the total variance. For comparison, [7] reports a PCA model for β-amyloid PET where the 1st eigenvector accounts for 80% of the variability. This makes the template-based methods less robust and unreliable for general tau PET images.

In this work, we propose a template-free approach to MR-less spatial normalization for tau PET. In contrast to all previous attempts on MR-less spatial normalization, our method aligns the native PET scan directly without needing an explicit PET template. We use a deep neural network that takes a PET scan as input and outputs a parameterized transformation as well as the warped image. The implemented network includes convolutional neural network (CNN) regressors as well as spatial transformer layers, and is trainable end-to-end. Our solution is general, rather than being developed specifically for tau tracers, and can without alterations be applied to any application involving PET spatial normalization, e.g. PET scans of other body parts and/or with other PET tracers. We compare our method to a MR-dependent baseline, and to the template-based methods in [4]. Our approach outperforms the MR-dependent baseline in terms of registration accuracy as well as speed, and compares favourably to the template-based approaches.

2 A Deep Learning Approach to Spatial Normalization

Let $\mathcal{I}$ be the PET image in its original space and $\mathcal{I}_{\text{aligned}}$ be the same image aligned with the common template space via the coordinate transformation T, $\mathcal{I}_{\text{aligned}} = \mathcal{I} \circ T$. We restrict T to be a composition of a rigid transformation T_R and an affine transformation T_A, where T_R and T_A are parameterized as

$$T_R\left(\boldsymbol{r}, \boldsymbol{t}^{\text{rot}}\right) = \begin{bmatrix} R & \boldsymbol{t}^{\text{rot}} \\ \boldsymbol{0} & 1 \end{bmatrix}, \quad R = \exp \begin{bmatrix} 0 & -r_z & r_y \\ r_z & 0 & -r_x \\ -r_y & r_x & 0 \end{bmatrix}, \quad \boldsymbol{t}^{\text{rot}} = \begin{bmatrix} t_x^{\text{rot}} \\ t_y^{\text{rot}} \\ t_z^{\text{rot}} \end{bmatrix}, \quad (1)$$

$$T_A\left(\boldsymbol{a}, \boldsymbol{t}^{\text{aff}}\right) = \begin{bmatrix} A & \boldsymbol{t}^{\text{aff}} \\ \boldsymbol{0} & 1 \end{bmatrix}, \quad A = \begin{bmatrix} a_1 & a_2 & a_3 \\ a_4 & a_5 & a_6 \\ a_7 & a_8 & a_9 \end{bmatrix}, \quad \boldsymbol{t}^{\text{aff}} = \begin{bmatrix} t_x^{\text{aff}} \\ t_y^{\text{aff}} \\ t_z^{\text{aff}} \end{bmatrix}. \quad (2)$$

We describe the problem of spatially normalizing the input image $\mathcal{I}$ as the task of finding the estimates $\hat{T}_R$ and $\hat{T}_A$ that minimize a loss

$$\mathcal{L} = \mathcal{L}_{\text{MAE}}\left(\mathcal{I}_{\text{aligned}}, \mathcal{I} \circ (\hat{T}_A \cdot \hat{T}_R)\right) = \mathcal{L}_{\text{MAE}}\left(\mathcal{I} \circ (T_A \cdot T_R), \mathcal{I} \circ (\hat{T}_A \cdot \hat{T}_R)\right), \quad (3)$$

where $\mathcal{L}_{\text{MAE}}$ is the mean absolute intensity difference over all pixels.

We propose an inference method that uses a deep network consisting of CNN regressors and spatial transformer layers. We learn the network parameters in a supervised fashion, i.e. with access to the ground truth transformations T_R and T_A. Below, we describe the network in detail.

2.1 Network Design

We design two CNN regressors, $\mathcal{F}_R$ and $\mathcal{F}_A$, that each takes an image as input and outputs a rigid or an affine transformation respectively. Both networks include four consecutive convolutional layers followed by a global average pooling layer and dense layers. All convolutional layers use a $3 \times 3 \times 3$ kernel with a stride of two, ReLU activations and 20, 30, 40 and 50 filters respectively. The rigid regressor $\mathcal{F}_R$ is terminated with six parallel dense layers that each outputs one of the parameters in (1), while the affine regressor $\mathcal{F}_A$ is terminated with twelve parallel dense layers that each outputs one of the parameters in (2).

We pair each CNN with a spatial transformer that warps the input image according to the predicted transformation. Spatial transformer networks, introduced in [12], are designed to make the warping operation differentiable, and have successfully been used in previously published methods for deep medical image registration, e.g. [2,10,14,20].

We reason that small transformations are easier to predict than large ones, and we therefore let $\hat{T}_R$ and $\hat{T}_A$ be estimated in an iterative manner, more specifically as a composition of smaller transformations, i.e.

$$\hat{T}_R = \hat{T}_R^{(N)} \cdot \ldots \cdot \hat{T}_R^{(2)} \cdot \hat{T}_R^{(1)}, \quad \hat{T}_A = \hat{T}_A^{(M)} \cdot \ldots \cdot \hat{T}_A^{(2)} \cdot \hat{T}_A^{(1)}, \tag{4}$$

where N and M equal the number of rigid and affine transformations. Note that this scheme of estimating several consecutive transformations, instead of a single one, mirrors the scheme that is often present in standard registration methods.

The first rigid transformation $\hat{T}_R^{(1)}$ is estimated by feeding the original image $\mathcal{I}$ to the rigid regressor. Succeeding rigid transformations are computed with the warped image as input, i.e.

$$\hat{T}_R^{(i)} = \mathcal{F}_R \left[\mathcal{I} \circ \left(\hat{T}_R^{(i-1)} \cdot \ldots \cdot \hat{T}_R^{(1)} \right) \right]. \tag{5}$$

Similarly, the first affine transformation $\hat{T}_A^{(1)}$ is computed by feeding a rigidly warped image $\mathcal{I} \circ \hat{T}_R$ to the affine regressor. Succeeding affine transformations are computed with the warped image as input, i.e.

$$\hat{T}_A^{(i)} = \mathcal{F}_A \left[\mathcal{I} \circ \left(\hat{T}_A^{(i-1)} \cdot \ldots \cdot \hat{T}_A^{(1)} \cdot \hat{T}_R \right) \right]. \tag{6}$$

Note that the warped input image is always computed by feeding the spatial transformer with the original image $\mathcal{I}$ and a composition of all so far computed transformations. Thanks to the parametrization in (1) and (2), compositions of transformations can be implemented in a differentiable manner, and the network can be trained end-to-end.

To speed up learning, and to ensure that the rigid regressor outputs reasonable rigid transformations, we use an intermediate loss on the rigidly warped image. Thus, the full loss is given by

$$\mathcal{L} = \mathcal{L}_{\text{MAE}} \left(\mathcal{I} \circ T_R, \mathcal{I} \circ \hat{T}_R \right) + \mathcal{L}_{\text{MAE}} \left(\mathcal{I} \circ (T_A \cdot T_R), \mathcal{I} \circ (\hat{T}_A \cdot \hat{T}_R) \right). \tag{7}$$

In summary, the neural network takes the original PET image as input, computes rigid and affine transformations in an iterative manner and outputs the spatially normalized PET image. Since all the steps are designed to be differentiable, we learn the network parameters using stochastic gradient descent based methods on the loss (7). The framework is exemplified in Fig. 1.

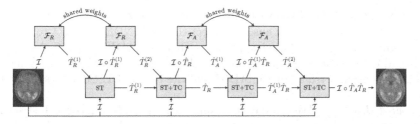

Fig. 1. Schematic illustration of the implemented network when $\hat{T}_R = \hat{T}_R^{(2)} \cdot \hat{T}_R^{(1)}$ and $\hat{T}_A = \hat{T}_A^{(2)} \cdot \hat{T}_A^{(1)}$. The network takes an image $\mathcal{I}$ as input and outputs a composed transformation $\hat{T}_A \cdot \hat{T}_R$ as well as the warped image. The network consists of two CNN regressors, $\mathcal{F}_R$ and $\mathcal{F}_A$, as well as spatial transformer (ST) layers and transformation composition (TC) layers.

3   Experimental Evaluation

Training and Validation Data. We use a dataset consisting of 199 subjects from the BioFINDER study, see http://biofinder.se/. This dataset contains subjects with a large variability in tau load and diagnosis [18]. The dataset is split into a training set (160 subjects) and a validation set (39 subjects). For each subject, there is a [18F]flortaucipir standardized uptake value (SUV) PET scan (non-smoothed), as well as ground truth transformations for spatial normalization pre-computed with a MR-dependent pipeline [9]. This pipeline includes preprocessing of the MR images (tailor-made for the BioFINDER data) as well as manual inspection, and when necessary, corrections.

Implementation Details. Each PET image is downsampled to a voxel size of $2 \times 2 \times 2$ mm and voxel intensities are standardized image-wise to the range $[-1, 1]$. We train and validate on full-size images, $91 \times 109 \times 91$ voxels, to learn large-scale translations, as well as on smaller patches, $33 \times 33 \times 33$ voxels, to learn rotations, scaling and shearing. Note that the network allows for different input sizes due to the global average pooling layer. The training patches are augmented by a random brightness shift. Training is done with the Nadam optimizer [5] and with l_2 weight regularization (regularization parameter is set to 10^{-3}). We use a batch size of 10 and 500 training steps per epoch. The validation loss monitors early stopping (training stops after 250 epochs without improvement) and learning rate decay (learning rate is decreased with a factor of 0.95 after 10 epochs without improvement).

Test Data. We use two different datasets for evaluation, (i) 37 additional subjects from the BioFINDER study and (ii) 111 subjects from the ADNI database, see http://adni.loni.usc.edu/. Compared to the BioFINDER data, the ADNI test set shows less variability in diagnosis, and contains subjects with a smaller average tau load. The difference in difficulty can be demonstrated by constructing a similar PCA model as in [4] for the both test sets. For the BioFINDER test set, such a model explains 36% of the variability, while the corresponding model explains 51% for the ADNI test set. Thus, we expect the BioFINDER test set to be more challenging for template-based approaches than the ADNI test set. Affine and non-rigid deformations computed by the MR-dependent methods in [4] and [9] are used as ground truth for the ADNI and the BioFINDER data respectively.

Compared Baselines. We evaluate our approach on the BioFINDER test set for three setups of rigid and affine transformations estimated in the iterative scheme:

$$\text{(a) } \hat{T}_R = \hat{T}_R^{(1)}, \ \hat{T}_A = \hat{T}_A^{(1)}, \ \text{ (b) } \hat{T}_R = \hat{T}_R^{(2)} \cdot \hat{T}_R^{(1)}, \ \hat{T}_A = \hat{T}_A^{(1)},$$
$$\text{(c) } \hat{T}_R = \hat{T}_R^{(2)} \cdot \hat{T}_R^{(1)}, \ \hat{T}_A = \hat{T}_A^{(2)} \cdot \hat{T}_A^{(1)}. \tag{8}$$

We also compare our results on the BioFINDER test set with a standard MR-dependent baseline: the PET image is aligned with the subject's skull-stripped T1 MR image via a rigid transformation, and thereafter, this MR image is aligned with the MR template space via a rigid, an affine and a deformable transformation. We use the ANTs software [1] with default parameters.

We evaluate the top-performing setup from (a)–(c) on the ADNI test set. We compare to the three template-based approaches in [4] (using mean, linear and PCA templates respectively), i.e. all MR-less methods previously evaluated on tau PET that we know of. Unfortunately, the code for these methods is not publicly available, but we have got access to paper's result on the ADNI test set.

Evaluation Metrics. To facilitate comparisons between subjects, we evaluate on SUV ratio (SUVR) images. The SUVR images are computed by normalizing the images with respect to the tau uptake in the cerebellum. As performance metrics, we use (i) the absolute percentage error over tau load in the *temporal meta-ROI*, defined in [18], which is a composite region including parts of the temporal cortex closely connected to tau deposition in AD subjects (entorhinal cortex, parahippocampal and fusiform gyrus, amygdala, inferior and middle temporal cortices), and (ii) the absolute percentage error over tau load in the whole brain. All ROIs are extracted from the population atlas used in [4]. Note that the same (atlas) ROIs are used when computing the SUVR tau load for the ground truth.

We use the mean residual error over the deformation fields (in mm) as an additional performance metric for the BioFINDER test set. We do not evaluate this metric on the ADNI test set since we do not have access to the competing method's deformation fields.

Experimental Results. See Tables 1 and 2 for the experimental results on the BioFINDER and the ADNI test set respectively. The proposed method clearly quantifies tau with less errors, and with more reliability, than the MR-dependent baseline and the compared MR-less approaches. The improvement in tau load quantification is statistically significant for both the temporal meta-ROI (the p-value equals 0.8% for a paired t-test of 'PCA templ.' vs. 'Ours, setup (c)' in Table 2) as well as for all ROIs. Figure 2 shows Bland-Altman plots of the tau deposition in the temporal meta-ROI for our top-performing approach (c)

Table 1. Absolute percentage error over (SUVR) tau load in the temporal meta-ROI ('SUVR-temp') and in the whole brain ('SUVR-all'), as well as the mean residual error over the deformation fields ("MRE"), for three different setups of our approach (a)–(c) and the MR-dependent baseline ("MR-baseline"), evaluated on the BioFINDER test set. The table reports the mean ± standard deviation for the BioFINDER test set.

	Ours, setup (a)	Ours, setup (b)	Ours, setup (c)	MR-baseline
SUVR-temp	2.30% ± 2.41%	2.14% ± 2.57%	**1.86% ± 1.95%**	2.04% ± 2.58%
SUVR-all	1.70% ± 1.55%	1.25% ± 2.01%	**1.21% ± 1.31%**	2.17% ± 2.52%
MRE	4.2 mm ± 5.3 mm	3.2 mm ± 3.7 mm	**2.9 mm ± 2.2 mm**	6.7 mm ± 4.6 mm

Table 2. Absolute percentage error over (SUVR) tau load in the temporal meta-ROI ('SUVR-temp') and in the whole brain ('SUVR-all') for the top-performing setup from Table 1, and for the methods in [4], evaluated on the ADNI test set. The table reports the mean ± standard deviation.

	[4], mean templ.	[4], linear templ.	[4], PCA templ.	Ours, setup (c)
SUVR-temp	1.72% ± 2.48%	1.77% ± 2.91%	1.57% ± 1.47%	**1.53% ± 1.38%**
SUVR-all	1.47% ± 2.21%	1.53% ± 2.67%	1.41% ± 1.34%	**1.16% ± 0.89%**

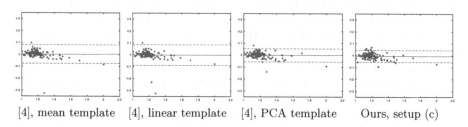

[4], mean template   [4], linear template   [4], PCA template   Ours, setup (c)

Fig. 2. Bland-Altman plot of the temporal meta-ROI SUVR for the compared methods. The figures show the difference in tau deposition between the MR-less and the MR-dependent method against the average of the two methods.

and the methods in [4] evaluated on the ADNI test set. The Bland-Altman plots confirm that the proposed method handles the most challenging cases, i.e. where the tau load error is larger than ±0.05, better than the template-based approaches. Our approach runs for 1.4 seconds per subject on a GeForce GTX 1080 Ti, significantly faster than the MR-dependent baseline, which runs for 30 min per subject on an Intel i7-8700 CPU. The run times for the compared methods in [4] are not reported.

4   Concluding Discussion

This work proposes a template-free approach to MR-less spatial normalization of [18F]flortaucipir PET scans, enabled by a deep neural network consisting of CNN regressors and spatial transformer layers. The network is trained and validated on 199 PET scans from the BioFINDER study.

We evaluate our method on 37 additional BioFINDER subjects, and outperform the standard, significantly slower, MR-dependent baseline. This shows that our method is robust and able to handle the high diversity among the subjects in the dataset without needing manual supervision. In addition, we compare the proposed method to the three methods in [4] evaluated on 111 test subjects from the ADNI database, which is a less challenging dataset. We perform better than the template-based approaches, despite that (i) our network is trained exclusively on BioFINDER data and run without fine-tuning on the ADNI test set and (ii) the compared approaches include non-rigid deformation while our does not.

Two possible extensions are (i) a more thorough evaluation of the optimal number of rigid and affine transformations used in the iterative scheme, and (ii) to implement and evaluate non-rigid deformation on top of these. A third extension could be to consider other loss functions, such as the difference between the estimated and the ground truth deformation fields.

It would be informative to evaluate our approach on other PET ligands than the tau tracer, such as a β-amyloid tracer. Further, the proposed approach could, with negligible modifications, be applied to tasks involving other modalities, e.g. as an alternative to multi-atlas based brain region parcellation on MR images. This would yield a larger selection of literature to compare with, as well as establish the applicability of our method. To allow for such future comparisons, we will make the code publicly available.

To enable a stand-alone tool for MR-less analysis of [18F]flortaucipir PET scans, we do not only need MR-less spatial normalization. Region-wise tau quantification demands region segmentations, which are most often derived from the MR image. It is questionable whether the anatomical information in a PET scan alone is sufficient for retrieving these regions, but a tool able to do so would surely challenge the MR-dependent gold standard in tau PET analysis.

References

1. Avants, B.B., et al.: A reproducible evaluation of ANTs similarity metric performance in brain image registration. NeuroImage **54**(3), 2033–2044 (2011)
2. Balakrishnan, G., et al.: An unsupervised learning model for deformable medical image registration. In: Proceedings of the CVPR, pp. 9252–9260 (2018)
3. Bourgeat, P., et al.: Comparison of MR-less PiB SUVR quantification methods. Neurobiol. Aging **36**, S159–S166 (2015)
4. Bourgeat, P., et al.: PET-only 18F-AV1451 tau quantification. In: Proceedings of the ISBI, pp. 1173–1176 (2017)
5. Dozat, T.: Incorporating nesterov momentum into adam (2016)
6. Edison, P., et al.: Comparison of MRI based and PET template based approaches in the quantitative analysis of amyloid imaging with PIB-PET. NeuroImage **70**, 423–433 (2013)
7. Fripp, J., et al.: Appearance modeling of 11C PiB PET images: characterizing amyloid deposition in Alzheimer's disease, mild cognitive impairment and healthy aging. NeuroImage **43**(3), 430–439 (2008)

8. Fripp, J., et al.: MR-less high dimensional spatial normalization of ^{11}C PiB PET images on a population of elderly, mild cognitive impaired and Alzheimer disease patients. In: Metaxas, D., Axel, L., Fichtinger, G., Székely, G. (eds.) MICCAI 2008. LNCS, vol. 5241, pp. 442–449. Springer, Heidelberg (2008). https://doi.org/10.1007/978-3-540-85988-8_53

9. Hansson, O., et al.: Tau pathology distribution in Alzheimer's disease corresponds differentially to cognition-relevant functional brain networks. Front. Neurosci. **11**, 167 (2017)

10. Hu, Y., et al.: Label-driven weakly-supervised learning for multimodal deformable image registration. In: Proceedings of the ISBI, pp. 1070–1074 (2018)

11. Hutton, C., et al.: Quantification of 18 F-florbetapir PET: comparison of two analysis methods. Eur. J. Nucl. Med. Mol. Imaging **42**(5), 725–732 (2015)

12. Jaderberg, M., et al.: Spatial transformer networks. In: Proceedings of the NIPS, pp. 2017–2025 (2015)

13. Kang, S.K., et al.: Adaptive template generation for amyloid PET using a deeplearning approach. Hum. Brain Mapp. **39**(9), 3769–3778 (2018)

14. Krebs, J., Mansi, T., Mailhé, B., Ayache, N., Delingette, H.: Unsupervised probabilistic deformation modeling for robust diffeomorphic registration. In: Stoyanov, D., et al. (eds.) DLMIA/ML-CDS-2018. LNCS, vol. 11045, pp. 101–109. Springer, Cham (2018). https://doi.org/10.1007/978-3-030-00889-5_12

15. Kuhn, F.P., et al.: Comparison of PET template-based and MRI-based image processing in the quantitative analysis of C 11-raclopride PET. Eur. J. Nucl. Med. Mol. Imaging **4**(1), 7 (2014)

16. Lilja, J., et al.: Spatial normalization of [18F] flutemetamol PET images utilizing an adaptive principal components template. J. Nucl. Med. **58**, 294 (2018)

17. Lundqvist, R., et al.: Implementation and validation of an adaptive template registration method for 18F-flutemetamol imaging data. J. Nucl. Med. **54**(8), 1472–1478 (2013)

18. Ossenkoppele, R., et al.: Discriminative accuracy of [18F]flortaucipir positron emission tomography for Alzheimer disease vs other neurodegenerative disorders. JAMA **320**(11), 1151–1162 (2018)

19. Penny, W.D., et al.: Statistical parametric mapping: the analysis of functional brain images. Elsevier (2011)

20. de Vos, B.D., Berendsen, F.F., Viergever, M.A., Staring, M., Išgum, I.: End-to-end unsupervised deformable image registration with a convolutional neural network. In: Cardoso, M.J., et al. (eds.) DLMIA/ML-CDS-2017. LNCS, vol. 10553, pp. 204–212. Springer, Cham (2017). https://doi.org/10.1007/978-3-319-67558-9_24

TopAwaRe: Topology-Aware Registration

Rune Kok Nielsen[1], Sune Darkner[1], and Aasa Feragen[1,2(✉)]

[1] Department of Computer Science, University of Copenhagen,
Universitetsparken 5, 2100 Copenhagen, Denmark
{darkner,aasa}@di.ku.dk
[2] DTU Compute, Technical University of Denmark,
Richard Petersens Plads 324, 2800 Kgs Lyngby, Denmark
afhar@dtu.dk

Abstract. Deformable registration, or nonlinear alignment of images, is a fundamental preprocessing tool in medical imaging. State-of-the-art algorithms restrict to diffeomorphisms to regularize an otherwise ill-posed problem. In particular, such models assume that a one-to-one matching exists between any pair of images. In a range of real-life-applications, however, one image may contain objects that another does not. In such cases, the one-to-one assumption is routinely accepted as unavoidable, leading to inaccurate preprocessing and, thus, inaccuracies in the subsequent analysis. We present a novel, piecewise-diffeomorphic deformation framework which models topological changes as explicitly encoded discontinuities in the deformation fields. We thus preserve the regularization properties of diffeomorphic models while locally avoiding their erroneous one-to-one assumption. The entire model is GPU-implemented, and validated on intersubject 3D registration of T1-weighted brain MRI. Qualitative and quantitative results show our ability to improve performance in pathological cases containing topological inconsistencies.

Keywords: Image registration · Diffeomorphisms · Topology-Aware

1 Introduction

Deformable image registration aims to align two images by non-linearly matching points between them, which is one of the most fundamental problems in medical imaging. Use cases include intra- and intersubject registration in e.g. longitudinal or population studies, respectively. To keep the optimization problem feasible, state-of-the-art registration frameworks limit themselves to *diffeomorphic* warps, which in particular assume a one-to-one mapping between the image domains. Real life is, however, rich with cases where one image contains matter that the other does not, thus violating the one-to-one assumption. Such pairs of images are *topologically different* in the sense that optimal alignment of the images requires tearing at least one of the image domains.

© Springer Nature Switzerland AG 2019
D. Shen et al. (Eds.): MICCAI 2019, LNCS 11765, pp. 364–372, 2019.
https://doi.org/10.1007/978-3-030-32245-8_41

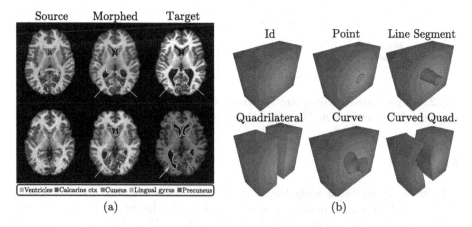

Fig. 1. (a): Diffeomorphic registration with ANTs [1] from sources with contracted ventricles to targets with expanded ventricles. The topological differences cause clear issues by the ventricles. (b) Toy example volume sliced in half following discontinuous deformation by various expansions using our deformation model.

We propose applying domain knowledge of the image topologies to handle topological changes during registration. We derive a novel framework for piecewise-diffeomorphic image registration, combining state-of-the-art diffeomorphic registration with a topology-altering model. The topology of the image domain is altered by expanding topological holes from predefined discontinuities in the form of points, curves or surfaces, as shown in Fig. 1(b). These *expansions* are simultaneously morphed into target shapes by a diffeomorphic model. We name this concept *Topology-Aware Registration* (TopAwaRe).

We validate the model on intersubject registration of T1-weighted brain MRI where some subjects have expanded ventricles in the back of the brain, which appears under pathological conditions including Alzheimer's disease. To motivate this challenge, consider the two examples in Fig. 1(a), where diffeomorphic registration locally fails due to the change of topology between source subjects with contracted ventricles and target subjects with expanded ventricles.

Related Work: Diffeomorphic registration methods [1,3] perform well when the diffeomorphic assumption is reasonable, but are in their nature unable to model discontinuities. The sliding motion between organs is a type of discontinuity that has received significant attention [5,9,10]. Other approaches to topological changes include individual parameterization of segmented organs [4] and supporting registration of pre-operative to post-recurrence scans of tumor patients by segmentation of pathological regions [6]. However, neither of these models support changing the topology within a connected region, nor modeling the interaction between an expanding hole and its surroundings. In recent years, deep learning models for registration have emerged [2]. However, these methods still optimize for global smoothness and do not account for topological changes.

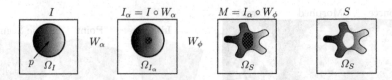

Fig. 2. Warp composition diagram: The source I is topologically altered by W_α expanding a spherical hole from p. The result I_α is morphed to match the target S.

2   Model

Deformable registration seeks the warp $W\colon \Omega_S \to \Omega_I$ aligning a source image $I\colon \Omega_I \to \mathbb{R}^d$ into the coordinate system of a target image $S\colon \Omega_S \to \mathbb{R}^d$. We denote the morphed image $M = I \circ W$, and W is then determined through an optimization process minimizing the combination $\mathcal{M}(S, I \circ W) + \mathcal{S}(W)$ of a matching term $\mathcal{M}$ and a regularization term $\mathcal{S}$ acting on the warp itself. The registration model controls a pull-back deformation vector field $u\colon \mathbb{R}^n \to \mathbb{R}^n$ such that $W = \mathrm{Id} - u$. In our proposed framework, the warp W is given by a composition $W = W_\alpha \circ W_\phi$ of respectively piecewise- and globally diffeomorphic warps W_α and W_ϕ (see Fig. 2). Here, W_α is controlled by a specialized topology-changing model and W_ϕ by a diffeomorphic registration model. The resulting W is piecewise-diffeomorphic with known discontinuities.

Topological differences are handled by inducing and expanding holes from predefined discontinuities, as illustrated in Fig. 2. The effects of an expansion are **(A)** discontinuous expansion in the deformation field and **(B)** changing intensity within the hole in the morphed image. This change of intensity is controlled through an alpha channel $\alpha\colon \Omega_S \to [0, 1]$ such that any $\boldsymbol{x} \in \Omega_S$ with $\alpha(\boldsymbol{x}) = 0$ is within a hole and $\alpha(\boldsymbol{x}) = 1$ is in the regular domain. We allow $0 < \alpha(\boldsymbol{x}) < 1$ to address partial volume effects near the boundaries. The morphed image then becomes a convex combination

$$M_\alpha(\boldsymbol{x}) = \alpha(\boldsymbol{x})M(\boldsymbol{x}) + (1 - \alpha(\boldsymbol{x}))\beta(\boldsymbol{x}), \tag{1}$$

where $\beta\colon \Omega_S \to \mathbb{R}^d$ decides within-hole intensity and thus affects optimization.

Expansions. We present the various types of expansions (illustrated in Fig. 1(b)) in order of increasing complexity following a common approach. We derive the case of single expansions as they are modeled individually and composed. As illustrated in Fig. 2, we introduce an intermediary domain Ω_{I_α} corresponding to the source image after being altered by the expansions, and specify $W_\alpha\colon \Omega_{I_\alpha} \to \Omega_I$ and $W_\phi\colon \Omega_S \to \Omega_{I_\alpha}$.

In radial expansion from a single point $p \in \Omega_I$, the radius of the resulting sphere in Ω_{I_α} is denoted by Π and optimized during registration. As the sphere constitutes a hole, any point $\boldsymbol{x} \in \Omega_{I_\alpha}$ within it is considered as background, i.e. $\alpha(\boldsymbol{x}) = 0$. The deformation caused by the growth is designed to be isotropic at p, decreasing in magnitude and have compact support. The pull-back displacement u_α caused by the expansion is given by the directional vector $\frac{\overrightarrow{px}}{||\overrightarrow{px}||}$ scaled by a radial basis function (RBF) $s\colon \Omega_{I_\alpha} \to \mathbb{R}^+$, such that

$$u_\alpha(x) = s(x)\frac{\overrightarrow{px}}{||\overrightarrow{px}||}. \tag{2}$$

The displacement magnitude s is affected by the radius Π and a smoothing parameter σ such that the reach of the displacement is exactly $(1+\sigma)\Pi$. In the pull-back mapping, any point within the sphere is sent to its center, giving

$$s(x) = ||\overrightarrow{px}|| \qquad \text{for } ||\overrightarrow{px}|| \le \Pi, \tag{3}$$

and any point outside is sent towards it based on a quadratic Wendland function

$$s(x) = \Pi\left(1 - \frac{\frac{||\overrightarrow{px}||}{\Pi} - 1}{\sigma}\right)_+^2 \qquad \text{for } ||\overrightarrow{px}|| > \Pi, \tag{4}$$

where $x \in \Omega_{I_\alpha}$ and $(\cdot)_+ = \max(\cdot, 0)$. The effects of Π and σ are illustrated in Fig. 3. It can be shown that s is invertible w.r.t. every $y \ne p$ by solving the quadratic equation

$$-\frac{1}{\sigma^2}\left(\frac{||\overrightarrow{px}||}{\Pi}\right)_x^2 + \left(1 + \frac{2}{\sigma} + \frac{2}{\sigma^2}\right)\frac{||\overrightarrow{px}||}{\Pi} + \left(-\frac{1}{\sigma^2} - \frac{2}{\sigma} - 1 - \frac{||\overrightarrow{py}||}{\Pi}\right) = 0, \tag{5}$$

for $||\overrightarrow{px}||$, such that $s^{-1}(y) = s(x)$ for $y = x - s(x)\frac{\overrightarrow{px}}{||\overrightarrow{px}||}$ thus resulting in $x = y + s^{-1}(y)\frac{\overrightarrow{py}}{||\overrightarrow{py}||}$.

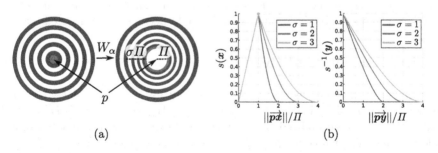

(a) (b)

Fig. 3. (a): Radial point expansion in a toy example with $\sigma = 2$. Note how the compression of the circles increases towards the center of expansion. (b) Scaling of displacement (left) and inverse displacement (right) w.r.t. distance to expansion center p for various σ after factoring out Π.

The line segment extends the model from a discrete point expanding radially to a straight line segment defined by two endpoints p_0 and p_1 expanding primarily along its normal directions and semi-radially at its endpoints. For a

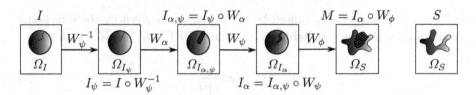

Fig. 4. The curved discontinuity is straightened from Ω_I to Ω_{I_ψ}, and its topology is then altered when moving to $\Omega_{I_{\psi,\alpha}}$. The curvature is then reintroduced going back to Ω_{I_α} where we apply W_ϕ as usual.

given $x \in \Omega_{I_\alpha}$, let p be the closest point on the segment $\overrightarrow{p_0 p_1}$, which is readily found by vector projection. The expansion is again modeled by a radius Π such that any x with $\|\overrightarrow{px}\| < \Pi$ is within the resulting hole, and the displacement is computed in the same way as for the sphere.

The quadrilateral extends the concept to expansion from a parallelogram in 3D. The discontinuity consists of all points contained in the parallelogram given by the corners p_0, p_1, p_2 and $p_0 + \overrightarrow{p_0 p_1} + \overrightarrow{p_0 p_2}$. Given a point x, we again find the closest point p in the discontinuity through vector projection, and determine the expansion as usual.

Curvature. The line segment and quadrilateral discontinuities assume the discontinuities in the source to be straight, which is seldom the case. However, any curved line segment or quadrilateral is diffeomorphic to its straight counterpart. Consider a curved discontinuity in Ω_I and let $W_\psi \colon \Omega_I \to \Omega_{I_\psi}$ be a diffeomorphism altering I to get a straight discontinuity in $I_\psi = I \circ W_\psi^{-1}$. We thus compute the change-of-topology in Ω_{I_ψ} with the usual model and return the result to Ω_{I_α} as shown in Fig. 4 (extending Fig. 2). As W_ψ only depends on the initial shape of the discontinuity in I it only needs to be computed once.

3   Experiments and Results

Our model is implemented for GPU processing using C++ and CUDA. The diffeomorphic model (TopAwaRe$_D$) controlling W_ϕ is based on LDDMM [3] and optimizes the normalized cross-correlation (as in [1]) over a time-dependent velocity field. The whole warp is optimized in a multi-scale scheme.

We validate our models via intersubject registration of T1-weighted MRI 3D brain volumes from the MICCAI2012 [7] database, which contains 32 subjects with 139 expert-labeled anatomical regions. From these, we identify 6 subjects of interest (SOI) with particularly expanded ventricles in the back, which cannot be registered correctly to a normal subject using diffeomorphic registration, as global continuity leads to an incorrect stretching of subcortical regions in order to map a normal ventricle to an expanded one (see Figs. 5 and 7). The results are thus divided into pairwise registrations between all 32 subjects ($N = 992$)

Source   TopAwaRe$_D$ TopAwaRe$_{PD}$ Target

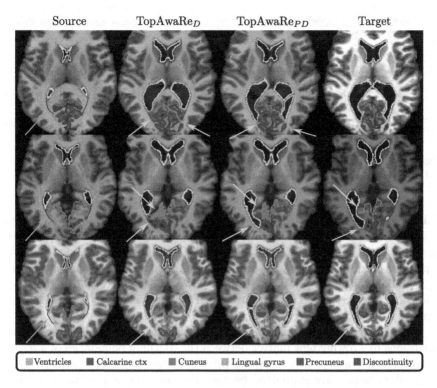

| Ventricles | Calcarine ctx | Cuneus | Lingual gyrus | Precuneus | Discontinuity |

Fig. 5. Registration from sources with contracted ventricles to expanded targets. The topological changes causes clear issues in their neighbourhoods. Blue arrows emphasize delineated discontinuities and yellow arrows point to subcortical regions incorrectly registered by the diffeomorphic model. (Color figure online)

and normal subjects to SOI ($N = 156$). All subjects are affinely preregistered to a common space of size $182 \times 218 \times 182$ voxels.

To facilitate TopAwaRe$_{PD}$, the two contracted ventricles of a single normal subject were manually delineated by 25 control points each. This subject was then registered to the rest and the control points coregistered accordingly to automatically obtain a discontinuity surface per source image (shown in Fig. 5). The background image β of Eq. (1) was set to a constant value of 0.2, corresponding roughly to the average intensity within the ventricles, such that points within the modeled holes are treated as ventricles when evaluating the results.

Validation of TopAwaRe$_D$: Over all samples, our base diffeomorphic implementation produces comparable results to those of the state-of-the-art ANTs framework [1] in terms of global Dice overlap of the 139 coregistered regions (Fig. 6). We thus conclude that our base model is on the level of the state-of-the-art and therefore a fair benchmark for the piecewise-diffeomorphic TopAwaRe$_{PD}$.

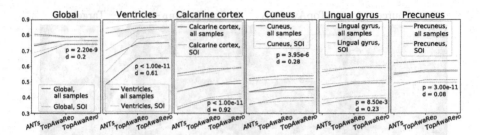

Fig. 6. Mean (solid) and standard deviations (dashed) of Dice overlaps over all samples and SOI. The p- and Cohen's d-values are for the paired t-tests (see below).

Validation of TopAwaRe$_{PD}$: To validate TopAwaRe$_{PD}$, we investigate the registration of the ventricles as well as four anatomical structures lying between them, both on all samples and the SOI. In Fig. 5 we illustrate a random selection of pairs of normal sources registered to targets with expanded ventricles. As in Fig. 1, the mistakes of the diffeomorphic registrations caused by the topological differences are evident. In particular, subcortical regions near the ventricles are clearly incorrectly registered as emphasized by the yellow arrows.

TopAwaRe$_{PD}$ captures the topological differences by modeling the ventricle expansions by growing new matter between the touching boundaries of a normal ventricle, and consequently prevents incorrect stretching of adjacent regions. These observations are supported by the Dice overlaps as presented in Fig. 6. Paired one-sided t-tests were performed on the SOI results for TopAwaRe$_{PD}$ versus TopAwaRe$_D$. To assess effect size, the p-values were supplemented by the corresponding Cohen's d (see p- and d-values in Fig. 6). With significance level 0.05 (Bonferroni corrected threshold 8.33e-3 for 6 tests) we obtain statistically significant improvement in all but the Lingual gyrus region which fails marginally. To further illustrate the differences, in Fig. 7 we show an example of a registration of a healthy control to an Alzheimer's patient from ADNI [8]. The

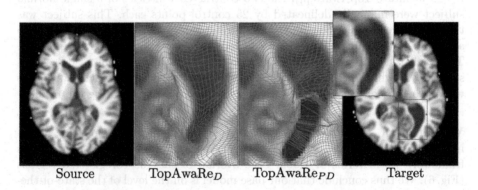

Fig. 7. Example registration from healthy subject to Alzheimer's patient shown with warp grids in selected region. Note: the grids are best viewed on a digital display.

diffeomorphic model stretches an open ventricle to match a large cavity while the piecewise-diffeomorphism opens a contracted ventricle. The warp grid shows how both the ventricle and surrounding tissue are affected by the diffeomorphic model's stretch similar to the effects on subcortical regions seen in Fig. 5.

4   Discussion and Conclusion

We have presented a novel framework for piecewise-diffeomorphic registration, preventing gross local misregistration caused by topological inconsistencies by applying knowledge of the underlying matter's topology. The model has been applied to a diverse dataset, showing that the piecewise-diffeomorphism can be used to prevent incorrect registration at and nearby certain topological differences. In particular, we show improvement in the face of expanded ventricles; a known side-effect of pathological conditions such as Alzheimer's disease.

The standard global Dice overlap is well suited to show that our diffeomorphic base model TopAwaRe$_D$ performs comparably to ANTs [1], but is less sensitive to improvements in the small subcortical regions shown in Fig. 5. Even the region-wise Dice overlap is insensitive to local changes if the majority of the region is not near the topological change. The improvements are, however, clear both from selected region-wise Dice coefficients and by visual inspection.

Our model depends on predefined discontinuities. Allowing discontinuities to occur anywhere may result in implausible warping but manual interaction may be costly. In our experiments it sufficed to manually delineate the collapsed ventricles of a single subject and coregister them to other subjects. This indicates some robustness towards the exact location and curvature of the discontinuities.

In its presented form, the framework is not symmetric. Specifically, the topology-altering model allows expansion from discontinuities in the source image but not vice-versa. This could be achieved by applying the model in both directions alongside a symmetric registration model [1].

One might expect the piecewise-diffeomorphic model to incur significant additional computational cost. However, as the size of an expansion is optimized by numerically estimating the gradient w.r.t. a single parameter, the increased cost is modest and the GPU implementation allows fast registration regardlessly.

The current practice in image registration is to accept the incorrect diffeomorphic assumption as unavoidable. We believe that, through additional specialization our model may provide a practical foundation for further improving registration of pathological tissue. We thus hope this might spark interest in the community to move beyond diffeomorphic image registration.

Acknowledgements. This research was supported by the Lundbeck Foundation and by the Centre for Stochastic Geometry and Advanced Bioimaging, funded by a grant from the Villum Foundation.

References

1. Avants, B.B., Epstein, C.L., Grossman, M., Gee, J.C.: Symmetric Diffeomorphic image registration with cross-correlation: evaluating automated labeling of elderly and neurodegenerative brain. Med. Image Anal. **12**(1), 26–41 (2008)
2. Balakrishnan, G., Zhao, A., Sabuncu, M.R., Guttag, J., Dalca, A.V.: An unsupervised learning model for deformable medical image registration. In: Conference on Computer Vision and Pattern Recognition (CVPR), pp. 9252–9260(2018)
3. Beg, M.F., Miller, M.I., Trouvé, A., Younes, L.: Computing large deformation metric mappings via geodesic flows of diffeomorphisms. Int. J. Comput. Vis. **61**(2), 139–157 (2005)
4. Berendsen, F.F., Kotte, A.N.T.J., Viergever, M.A., Pluim, J.P.W.: Registration of organs with sliding interfaces and changing topologies. In: SPIE, vol. 9034, pp. 90340E–90340E-7 (2014)
5. Delmon, V., Rit, S., Pinho, R., Sarrut, D.: Registration of sliding objects using direction dependent B-splines decomposition. Phys. Med. Biol. **58**(5), 1303 (2013)
6. Kwon, D., Niethammer, M., Akbari, H., Bilello, M., Davatzikos, C., Pohl, K.M.: PORTR: pre-operative and post-recurrence brain tumor registration. IEEE TMI (3), 651–667
7. Landman, B.A., et al.: MICCAI 2012 Workshop on Multi-Atlas Labeling. CreateSpace, Scotts Valley (2012)
8. Mueller, S.G., et al.: Ways toward an early diagnosis in Alzheimer's disease: the Alzheimer's disease neuroimaging initiative (ADNI). Alzheimer's Dement. **1**(1), 55–66 (2005)
9. Papież, B.W., Heinrich, M.P., Fehrenbach, J., Risser, L., Schnabel, J.A.: An implicit sliding-motion preserving regularisation via bilateral filtering for deformable image registration. Med. Image Anal. **18**(8), 1299–1311 (2014)
10. Risser, L., Baluwala, H.Y., Schnabel, J.A., Vialard, F.X.: Piecewise-diffeomorphic image registration: application to the motion estimation between 3D CT lung images with sliding conditions. Med. Image Anal. **17**(2), 182–193 (2012)

Multimodal Data Registration for Brain Structural Association Networks

David S. Lee[1(✉)], Ashish Sahib[1], Benjamin Wade[1], Katherine L. Narr[1,2],
Gerhard Hellemann[2], Roger P. Woods[1,2], and Shantanu H. Joshi[1]

[1] Ahmanson-Lovelace Brain Mapping Center, Department of Neurology,
University of California Los Angeles, Los Angeles, CA, USA
dalee@mednet.ucla.edu
[2] Department of Psychiatry and Biobehavioral Sciences,
University of California Los Angeles, Los Angeles, CA, USA

Abstract. We present a method for multimodal brain data registration that aligns shapes of nodal network configurations in an invertible manner. We use ideas from shape analysis to represent an individual subject data configuration as an element on a hypersphere, where geodesics have closed form solutions. The method not only performs inter-subject data registration, but also allows for the construction of a population data template to which all subject data configurations can be registered. Results show compression of data measures and significant reduction in variance after registration. We also observe increased predictive power of regions of interest (ROI) node identification, significant increases in pairwise network connectivity measures, as well as significant increases in canonical correlations with age after registration.

1 Introduction

Structural brain association networks are derived from correlations of cortical parcellated regions of interest (ROI) measures such as gray matter thickness, volume, surface area, etc., following voxel based or cortical based morphometry. Such networks, also termed as morphological networks yield complementary information to direct structural connectivity measures from diffusion weighted imaging (DWI) or connectivity measures from functional magnetic resonance imaging (fMRI) [8,9]. As opposed to explicit edge-based connections obtained from DWI, morphological networks are extracted by inferring covariance relationships between different nodal brain measures. Although the biological explanations of such inference-based networks are not yet fully developed, several studies have suggested that the structural covariance (i) encodes salient information about the large-scale brain organization, (ii) may be related to changes in brain development and may be perturbed by neurological and psychiatric diseases, (iii) may be modulated by biobehavioral factors, and (iv) may indicate maturational coupling (inter-subject correlations of longitudinal rates of change of cortical thickness) between brain regions [1]. Several methods have been proposed to analyze such inferred brain network associations. However there is still

© Springer Nature Switzerland AG 2019
D. Shen et al. (Eds.): MICCAI 2019, LNCS 11765, pp. 373–381, 2019.
https://doi.org/10.1007/978-3-030-32245-8_42

a need for improvement in the methodology for validation of statistical network models or even to conduct formal inference on network structural models. Such analyses are conducted in Euclidean spaces, where standard Pearson, or partial correlation coefficients are computed on the brain measures. Although the brains are preregistered to an atlas to account for spatial differences between subjects before computing such measures, we hypothesize that there may still remain other confounding factors (including biological demographic variables) that influence the underlying covariance structure. Generally network modeling methods perform multiple regression to factor out these nuisance variables. Such methods typically ignore the nonlinear geometry of the space of these measures. We thus suggest another level of data transformation or *alignment* to match the measures across ROIs and subjects. Our goal here is to perform statistical analysis of multivariate nodal network connectivity configurations in an invariant manner.

As an initial step, we propose representing multimodal brain data for each subject as a geometric configuration in an abstract multidimensional space and using statistical shape analysis methods for registering nodal data from brain measures across subjects [3, 10]. The data configuration can be identified and visualized in its native multidimensional variable space as well as transformed

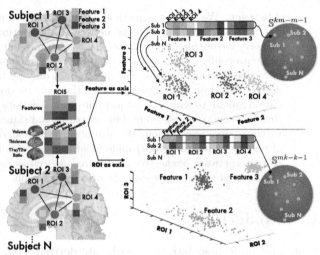

Fig. 1. Schematic for representation of subject data.

back to the population space using an invertible transform. The data configuration assumes a matrix form where rows denote observations and the columns denote features. For example, the rows can be ROIs and the columns can be vector valued measures for each ROI. In the variable space, these measures become axes of a coordinate system, and the ROIs become distinct nodes lying in this coordinate system, where a complete set of distinct ROIs in this coordinate system constitutes an individual subject. The subject space becomes a hypersphere, where shapes of data matrices, or nodal network configurations can be registered in a group-wise manner across a population. In this work, such registration is performed by Procrustes analysis, which includes scaling, translation, and exact rotations [3, 10]. A schematic overview of this representation is shown in Fig. 1. The novelty of this work lies in representing brain nodal data measures as configurations in a geometric space, and registering shapes of full data configurations formed from multiple ROIs and multidimensional measures for each ROI across subjects.

2   Multimodal Data Registration

Our data consists of averages of morphological features sampled from brain cortical surfaces for a population. However, we emphasize that the method is general, and can also be applied to functional measures from functional MRI or arterial spin labeling (ASL) measures. The morphological measures from surfaces are derived from atlas-based registrations of individual cortices from subjects using available methods such as Freesurfer [4], MSM [11], or BrainSuite [12]. Following registration, the cortex is parcellated into distinct regions of interest, and measures such as myelin (T1w/T2w fraction), cortical thickness, gray matter volume, or sulcal depths, are averaged over the ROIs. Thus for a single subject, one can have a vector of measures at each ROI.

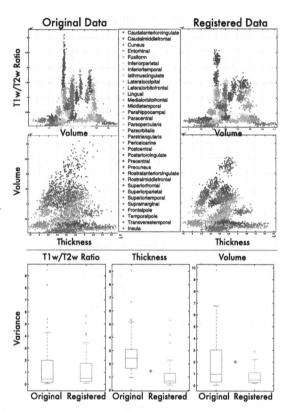

Fig. 2. Scatter plots of data (top) and variance (bottom) before and after registration. * denotes significant decreases (p < 0.05).

For a set of k ROIs and m measures per ROI, this multimodal dataset for a single subject is represented by a matrix configuration as $X = \{(x_1, \ldots, x_i, \ldots, x_k)\}$, where each $x_i = [w_1, w_2, \ldots, w_j, \ldots, w_m]^T$, $x_i \in \mathbb{R}^m$ is a multidimensional vector. Thus $X \in \mathbb{R}^{k \times m}$ is a matrix configuration. Since each of the values w_j represents different measurements such as thickness, volume, myelin (T1w/T2w fraction), their units are different, and thus should be standardized. Establishing the scale parameters in multimodal analyses generally remains a challenge, although several workarounds have been used previously. One could scale each of the measures as $[\alpha_1 w_1, \ldots, \alpha_j w_j, \ldots, \alpha_m w_m]^T$, where α_js are empirically chosen to bring the values of each feature to comparable units, or one could standardize the features using z-scores. In this paper, we empirically choose α_js based on prior observations of the data. Figure 1 shows the schematic of the data representation as well as the configuration of the data in the variable (ROI or feature) space.

2.1 Pairwise Subject Data Registration

Given such multimodal configurations for two subjects X_1 and X_2, our goal is to register them so that all the features are brought into a common space of configurations. Although each of the measures at each ROI have been scaled independently, there still remains a question of the global scale of the matrix, owing to inter-subject differences. Additionally, the two configurations may be shifted in space by a global translation. Thus before registering them, we perform global centering and scaling as follows. For a subject data matrix X_1, we compute a centered and a scaled matrix X_{1c}^s given by,

$$X_{1c} = (I_k - \frac{1}{k}\mathbf{1}_k\mathbf{1}_k^T)X_1 \tag{1}$$

$$X_{1c}^s = \frac{X_{1c}}{||X_{1c}||_F} = \frac{X_{1c}}{\sqrt{\sum_{i=1}^{k}||x_i - \bar{x}||^2}}, \tag{2}$$

where $|| \cdot ||_F$ denotes the Frobenius norm. Without loss of generality, we will denote the scaled and centered subject matrix X_{1c}^s as X_1 throughout this paper. We note that the scaling and centering operation maps the subject data matrix to a hypersphere $\mathbb{S}^{km-m-1}$. Finally, to register the two transformed subject configurations X_1 and X_2, we solve the problem of exact rotation $\hat{\Gamma}$ by minimizing the sum squared error as

$$\hat{\Gamma} = \underset{\Gamma}{\mathrm{argmin}}\,||X_1 - X_2\Gamma||^2, \tag{3}$$

where $\Gamma \in SO(n)$ is an element of the special orthogonal group. The solution to this problem can be estimated, even in noisy data [7]. We follow this method by first computing the singular value decomposition (SVD) of the product of X_1 and X_2^T as $X_1 X_2^T = UDV^T$, where $U, V \in SO(m)$. Then the exact rotation matrix is given by $\hat{\Gamma} = UV^T$.

2.2 Group-Wise Data Registration

While we can perform pairwise matching of subject data as shown above, the problem of groupwise registration can be solved in a variety of ways. We can assign a fixed subject as a template and register all data to it, in which case there is an introduction of bias due to the initial choice of the template. Alternatively, we can perform $\frac{N(N-1)}{2}$ pairwise registrations for all N subjects and average the resulting data. This can be done very fast, but the notion of averaging transforms for pairwise registrations is not straightforward and can potentially introduce errors. In our work, we estimate an average data template from the population by relying on the spherical geometry of the subject space. The geodesic between two data matrices X_1 and X_2 on the sphere is given by

$$\phi_t(X_1; f) = \cos\left(t \cos^{-1}\langle X_1, X_2\rangle_F\right) X_1 + \sin\left(t \cos^{-1}\langle X_1, X_2\rangle_F\right) f, \quad (4)$$

where $t \in [0, 1]$, $\langle \cdot, \cdot\rangle_F$ is the Frobenius inner product and $f = X_2 - \langle X_1, X_2\rangle_F X_1$. Then from Eq. 4, the geodesic distance is given by $\rho(X_1, X_2) = \int_0^1 \sqrt{\langle \dot{\phi}_t, \dot{\phi}_t\rangle_F} dt$. Next, we compute the average template using an iterative procedure that minimizes the sum squared geodesic distances to itself. Thus given a set of N subject data matrices $X_1, X_2, \ldots, X_N$, the average template is given as the local minimizer $\widehat{X_\mu} = \frac{1}{N} \text{argmin}_X \sum_{i=1}^{N} \rho(X_i, X)^2$. This iterative procedure is seeded with a Euclidean mean, projected on the sphere as the initial condition. Figure 2 shows an example of a group-wise registration of N subjects with $k = 33$ left hemisphere ROI measures of myelin, cortical thickness, and gray matter volume ($m = 3$).

2.3 Order of Data Representation

Thus far we represented the subject data matrix with ROIs as observations (rows), and measures such as thickness, myelin, volume as features (columns), as shown in the top scatter plot of Fig. 1. Another way to think about this is that from a given subject's brain, we sample (observe) k ROIs at once, and each ROI is described in terms of m features. In this case the method registers ROIs across subjects. Thus we expect a reduction in variance in the measures across all ROIs as well as an increased inter-subject correlation between ROIs for a given measure at a time. While this configuration seems easy to understand and will potentially find uses for subsequent group-wise statistical analyses, we could also flip the order of ROIs and measures. We note that this idea is similar to the $R-$ and $Q-$ analyses as introduced in Cattell et al. [2]. That is, each subject data matrix is now represented by a configuration $X \in \mathbb{R}^{k \times m}$, where rows ($m$) represent measures and columns (k) denote ROIs. Now, given a subject's brain, we sample (observe) m measures (thickness, volume, myelin etc.), and each measure is described in terms of k ROIs. While this data configuration doesn't seem an obvious choice to represent subjects, the method in this case will register measures across subjects. Thus we would expect an increase in pairwise ROI correlations for measures as well as potentially increased correlations of measures (thickness etc.) with external variables. This configuration may be potentially useful in harmonizing measures across subjects and in improving the sensitivity of group-wise network-based statistical analyses.

3   Results and Applications

3.1   Data

Our data consists of 93 subjects (44M/49F, ages from 20–64 years, mean age 36 ± 12 years) collected using the Human Connectome Project (HCP) MRI acquisition protocol. The structural scans consisted of a T1-weighted (T1w) multi-echo MPRAGE (voxel size (VS) = 0.8 mm isotropic; TR = 2.5 s; TE = 1.81:1.79:7.18 ms; TI = 1000 ms; flip angle (34) = 8.0 deg; acquisition time (TA) = 8:22 min) and a T2-weighted (T2w) acquisition (VS = 0.8 mm isotropic; TR = 3200 ms; TE = 564 ms; TA = 6:35 min). T1w and T2w imaging data were preprocessed using the HCP minimal processing pipeline [5]. After the automated Freesurfer (version 5.3) reconstruction implemented in the HCP pipeline, volume and thickness measures were extracted [4]. In addition, T1w/T2w ratio maps that indicate myelin contrast were also used as a measure for analysis [6]. We used 33 ROIs from the left hemisphere and all three measures were used for registration.

3.2   Data Registration Across ROI Nodes of Cortical Measures

Figure 2 shows results of data registration for a $k = 33, m = 3$ configuration. We display the results in two dimensions although all three measures were used for registration. It is observed that after registration, the individual data samples within each ROI are highly compressed compared to the original data. This compression observed in Fig. 2 is quantitatively compared by computing the variances of each cortical measure across ROIs in the original data before and after registration (bottom, Fig. 2). The variances of thickness and volume across all ROIs decreased significantly.

To assess whether the reduction in variance of ROIs translates to improvement in classifying ROI labels, we performed 10-fold cross validation of k-nearest-neighbor classification of ROI labels before and after alignment. The 10-fold mean prediction accuracy was

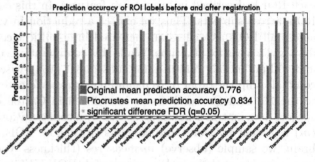

Fig. 3. Prediction accuracies of ROI labels.

higher after registration with 84% compared to 77% with p-value of 0.0036 (Fig. 3). The prediction accuracy was significantly higher after registration in the caudal middle frontal, fusiform, lateral orbitofrontal, lingual, pars opercularis, pars triangularis, rostral-middlefrontal, superior-frontal, and superior-temporal areas, and significantly lower in caudal anterior cingulate (FDR $q = 0.05$).

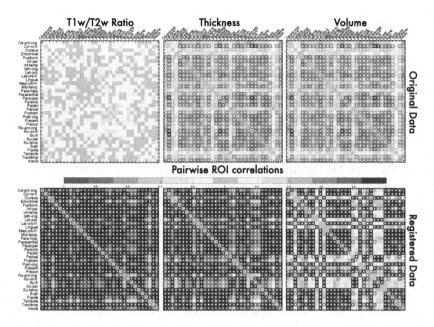

Fig. 4. ROI pairwise correlations before and after alignment. A white dot denotes significance (FDR corrected $q = 0.001$).

3.3 Registration Across Cortical Measures with ROIs as Features and Canonical Multivariate Correlations with Demographic Measures

Figure 4 shows pairwise ROI correlations between cortical measures. The correlations significantly improved (FDR corrected $q = 0.001$) across almost all areas after registration, demonstrating that the transposed representation is effective for aligning measures (with ROIs as features) across subjects.

Finally under this transposed configuration, we computed canonical correlations between all the 3 measures together with the population age following registration (Fig. 5). The correlations significantly increased (FDR corrected $q = 0.0001$) following registration, demonstrating that

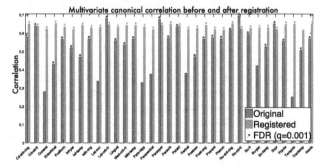

Fig. 5. Canonical correlations of cortical measures with age before and after registration.

registration of cortical measures across subjects may accentuate the relationship between the measures and a demographic variable such as age.

4   Discussion

We introduced an idea for shape matching of brain data configurations with applications to nodal network connectivity. The resulting data alignment has different applications depending upon the construction of the subject wise data matrix. We observed that formatting the data as a tall matrix (ROIs × measures) causes a reduction in overall variance in the ROI measures as well a decrease in the pairwise correlations between measures across ROIs (near diagonal covariance matrix). We conjecture that this property may be beneficial in partially reducing the influence of external confounding factors (not directly imaged in MRI). We propose to experimentally test this hypothesis in future work. On the other hand, formatting the data as a wide matrix (measures × ROIs) increases pairwise ROI correlations between measures as well as canonical correlations among demographic variables such as age. This characteristic is potentially useful in noisy observations where increased sensitivity in estimating the nodal correlations for network connectivity is desired. This may possibly lead to increased detection power under stringent multiple testing thresholds. Finally, in this paper, we only focused on global scaling, translation, and exact rotations, although in the future, other transformations of higher degree of freedom can be considered. We also plan to investigate the potential caveats of alignment decreasing or increasing useful information or/and noise, respectively.

Acknowledgments. This research was supported by the NIH/NIAAA award K25AA024192.

References

1. Alexander-Bloch, A., Giedd, J.N., Bullmore, E.: Imaging structural co-variance between human brain regions. Nat. Rev. Neurosci. **14**(5), 322 (2013)
2. Cattell, R.B.: The data box. In: Nesselroade, J.R., Cattell, R.B. (eds.) Handbook of Multivariate Experimental Psychology. Perspectives on Individual Differences, pp. 69–130. Springer, Boston (1988). https://doi.org/10.1007/978-1-4613-0893-5_3
3. Dryden, I.L., Mardia, K.: Statistical Shape Analysis. Wiley Series in Probability and Statistics: Probability and Statistics. Wiley, Hoboken (1998)
4. Fischl, B., van der Kouwe, A., Destrieux, C., et al.: Automatically parcellating the human cerebral cortex. Cereb. Cortex **14**(1), 11–22 (2004)
5. Glasser, M.F., Sotiropoulos, S.N., Wilson, J.A., Coalson, T.S., Fischl, B., et al.: The minimal preprocessing pipelines for the human connectome project. Neuroimage **80**, 105–124 (2013)
6. Glasser, M.F., Van Essen, D.C.: Mapping human cortical areas in vivo based on myelin content as revealed by T1-and T2-weighted MRI. J. Neurosci. **31**(32), 11597–11616 (2011)
7. Goryn, D., Hein, S.: On the estimation of rigid body rotation from noisy data. IEEE Trans. Pattern Anal. Mach. Intell. **17**(12), 1219–1220 (1995)
8. He, Y., Chen, Z.J., Evans, A.C.: Small-world anatomical networks in the human brain revealed by cortical thickness from MRI. Cereb. Cortex **17**(10), 2407–2419 (2007)

9. He, Y., Evans, A.: Graph theoretical modeling of brain connectivity. Curr. Opin. Neurol. **23**(4), 341–350 (2010)
10. Kendall, D.G.: Shape manifolds, procrustean metrics, and complex projective spaces. Bull. Lond. Math. Soc. **16**(2), 81–121 (1984)
11. Robinson, E.C., et al.: MSM: a new flexible framework for multimodal surface matching. Neuroimage **100**, 414–426 (2014)
12. Shattuck, D.W., Leahy, R.M.: BrainSuite: an automated cortical surface identification tool. Med. Image Anal. **6**(2), 129–142 (2002)

Dual-Stream Pyramid Registration Network

Xiaojun Hu[1,2], Miao Kang[1,2], Weilin Huang[1,2(✉)], Matthew R. Scott[1,2],
Roland Wiest[3], and Mauricio Reyes[4]

[1] Malong Technologies, Shenzhen, China
whuang@malong.com
[2] Shenzhen Malong Artificial Intelligence Research Center, Shenzhen, China
[3] Support Center for Advanced Neuroimaging,
University Institute for Diagnostic and Interventional Neuroradiology,
University Hospital, Bern, Switzerland
[4] Insel Data Science Center, Inselspital,
University Hospital, University of Bern, Bern, Switzerland

Abstract. We propose a Dual-Stream Pyramid Registration Network
(referred as Dual-PRNet) for unsupervised 3D medical image registration. Unlike recent CNN-based registration approaches, such as Voxel-
Morph, which explores a single-stream encoder-decoder network to compute a registration field from a pair of 3D volumes, we design a two-
stream architecture able to compute multi-scale registration fields from
convolutional feature pyramids. Our contributions are two-fold: (i) we
design a two-stream 3D encoder-decoder network which computes two
convolutional feature pyramids separately for a pair of input volumes,
resulting in strong deep representations that are meaningful for deformation estimation; (ii) we propose a pyramid registration module able to
predict multi-scale registration fields directly from the decoding feature
pyramids. This allows it to refine the registration fields gradually in a
coarse-to-fine manner *via* sequential warping, and enable the model with
the capability for handling significant deformations between two volumes, such as large displacements in spatial domain or slice space. The
proposed Dual-PRNet is evaluated on two standard benchmarks for brain
MRI registration, where it outperforms the state-of-the-art approaches
by a large margin, e.g., having improvements over recent VoxelMorph [2]
with 0.683 → 0.778 on the LPBA40, and 0.511 → 0.631 on the Mind-
boggle101, in term of average Dice score.

Keywords: Medical image registration · Encoder-decoder network ·
Deformable registration · Brain MRI

X. Hu and M. Kang—Contributed equally.

Electronic supplementary material The online version of this chapter (https://
doi.org/10.1007/978-3-030-32245-8_43) contains supplementary material, which is
available to authorized users.

1 Introduction

Deformable image registration has been widely used in image diagnostics, disease monitoring, and surgical navigation, with the goal of learning the anatomical correspondence between a moving image and a fixed image. A registration process mainly consists of three steps: establishing a deformation model, designing a similarity measurement function, and a parameter optimization step. Traditional deformable registration methods often cast it into a complex optimization problem that involves intensive computation by densely computing voxel-level similarities. Recent deep learning technologies have advanced this task significantly by developing learning-based approaches, which allow them to leverage strong feature learning capability of deep neural networks [2,3], resulting in fast training and inference, e.g., by just taking orders of magnitude less time [2].

Medical image registration often requires strong supervision information, such as ground-truth registration fields or anatomical landmarks. However, obtaining a large-scale medical dataset with such strong annotations is extremely expensive, which inevitably limits the applications of supervised approaches. Recently, unsupervised learning-based registration methods have been developed, by learning a registration function that maximizes the similarity between a moving image and a fixed image. For example, Balakrishnan *et al.* [2] proposed VoxelMorph which learns a parameterized registration function using a convolutional neural network (CNN). VoxelMorph estimates a deformation field by using an encoder-decoder CNN, and warps a moving image with a spatial transformation layer [1]. Kuang and Schmah [3] developed an unsupervised method, named as FAIM, which extends VoxelMorph by improving the network design with a new registration function. However, Lewis *et al.* [4] demonstrated that the performance of existing CNN-based approaches can be limited on challenging clinical applications where two medical images or volumes may have significant spatial displacements or large slice spaces. It is straightforward to handle such deformations by aligning them in a coarse-to-fine manner.

Contributions. Recent approaches on optical flow estimation [5] attempted to handle large displacements by gradually refining the estimated flows, which inspired the current work. They designed a cascaded architecture where multiple FlowNets were employed to gradually warp the images, while current paper describes a dual-stream single-model approach that implements sequential layer-wise refinements of registration fields, which in turn are used to warp the convolutional features rather than the images. This results in an end-to-end trainable model for 3D medical image registration.

Our work extends recent VoxelMorph [2] with two technical improvements, which are the key to boost the performance. (1) we develop a dual-stream encoder-decoder network able to compute two convolutional feature pyramids separately from a pair of input volumes, resulting in stronger deep representations for estimating multi-level deformations. (2) we propose a pyramid registration module which directly estimates registration fields from convolutional

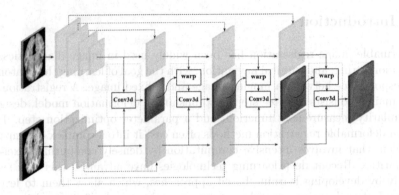

Fig. 1. Architecture of the proposed Dual-PRNet, which is a dual-stream encoder-decoder network, integrated with a new pyramid registration module.

features, resulting in a set of layer-wise registration fields that encode multi-level context information by sequentially warping the convolutional features. This enables the model with the ability to work on significant deformations. (3) we evaluate our model on the LPBA40 and the Mindboggle101, where our method improved the results of VoxelMorph [2] considerably, with $0.683 \rightarrow 0.778$ and $0.511 \rightarrow 0.631$ respectively, in term of average Dice score.

2   Dual-Stream Pyramid Registration Network

In this section, we describe the details of the proposed Dual-PRNet, including two main components: (i) a dual-stream encoder-decoder network for computing feature pyramids, and (ii) a pyramid registration module that estimates layer-wise registration fields in the decoding process.

2.1   Preliminaries

The goal of 3D medical image registration is to estimate a deformation field Φ which can warp a moving volume $M \subset R^3$ to a fixed volume $F \subset R^3$, so that the warped volume $W = M \circ \Phi \subset R^3$ can be accurately aligned to the fixed one F. We use $M \circ \Phi$ to denote the application of a deformation field Φ to the moving volume with a warping operation, and image registration can be formulated as an optimization problem:

$$\hat{\Phi} = \arg\min_{\Phi} \mathcal{L}(F, M, \Phi), \quad \mathcal{L}(F, M, \Phi) = \mathcal{L}_{sim}(F, M \circ \Phi) + \lambda\mathcal{L}_{smooth}(\Phi) \quad (1)$$

where $\mathcal{L}_{sim}$ is a function measuring image similarity between $M \circ \Phi$ and F, and $\mathcal{L}_{smooth}$ is a regularization constraint on Φ, which enforces spatial smoothness. Both $\mathcal{L}_{sim}$ and $\mathcal{L}_{smooth}$ can be defined in various forms. For example, Voxel-Morph [2] uses a CNN to compute a deformation field, $\Phi = f_\theta(F, M)$, where θ are learnable parameters of the CNN. The deformation warping is implemented by using a spatial transformer network [1], $M \circ \Phi = f_{stn}(M, \Phi)$. VoxelMorph uses a single-stream encoder-decoder architecture with skip connections, which are similar to U-Net [6]. A pair of volumes, M and F, are stacked as the input of VoxelMorph. More details of VoxelMorph are described in [2].

2.2 Dual-Stream Architecture

Our Dual-PRNet is built on the encoder-decoder architecture of VoxelMorph, but improves it by introducing a dual-stream design, as shown in Fig. 1. Specifically, the backbone of Dual-PRNet consists of a dual-stream encoder-decoder with shared parameters. We adopt the encoder as the same architecture of VoxRes-Net [7], which contains four down-sampling convolutional blocks. Each block has a 3D down-sampling convolutional layer with stride of 2. Thus the encoder reduces the spatial resolution of input volumes by a factor of 16 in total. Except for the first block, the down-sampling convolutional layer is followed by two ResBlocks, each of which contains two convolutional layers with a residual connection, similar to ResNet [8]. Batch normalization (BN) and ReLU operations are applied. More details of the network are presented in Fig. 1 of Supplementary Material (SM).

In the decoder stage, we apply skip connections on the corresponding convolutional maps in the encoding and decoding process. The features are fused using a Refine Unit, where the lower-resolution convolutional maps are up-sampled and added into the higher-resolution ones, by using a $1 \times 1 \times 1$ convolution layer. Finally, we obtain two feature pyramids with multi-resolution convolutional features computed from the moving volume and the fixed volume separately.

Dual-stream design allows us to first compute meaningful feature pyramids from two input volumes, and then predict deformable fields from the learned, stronger and more discriminative convolutional features, which is the key to boost the performance. This is different from existing single-stream networks, such as [2] and [3], which compute the convolutional features from two stacked volumes, and jointly estimate deformation fields using same convolutional filters. Furthermore, our dual-stream architecture can generate two paired feature pyramids where layer-wise deformation fields can be computed at multiple scales, allowing the model to generate more meaningful deformation fields by designing a new pyramid registration module, which is described next.

2.3 Pyramid Registration Module

VoxelMorph computes a single deformation field from the convolutional features at the last up-sampling layer in the decoding process, which limits its capability for handling large-scale deformations. Our pyramid registration module is able to predict multiple deformation fields with different resolutions, and generate pyramid deformation fields. As shown in Fig. 1, it computes a deformation field from a pair of convolutional features at each decoding layer. Each deformation field is computed by using a sequence of operations with feature warping, stacking, and convolution, except for the first deformation field where feature warping is not implemented. This results in a sequence of deformation fields with increasing resolutions, starting from the lowest-resolution decoding layer to the highest-resolution one. Our network includes four decoding layers, and thus generates four deformation fields sequentially.

Specifically, the first deformation field (Φ_1) is computed at the first decoding layer. We stack the convolutional features from two feature pyramids, and apply a 3D convolution with size of $3 \times 3 \times 3$ to estimate the deformation field, which is a 3D volume with the same shape of the corresponding convolutional maps. This deformation field is able to extract coarse-level context information, such as high-level anatomical structure of brain, which is then encoded into generating subsequent deformation field by feature warping: (i) the current deformation field is up-sampled by using bilinear interpolation with a factor of 2, denoted as $u(\Phi_1)$, and (ii) then is applied to warp the convolutional maps of the next layer from the moving volume, by using a grid sample operation, as shown in Fig. 1. Then the warped convolutional maps are stacked again with the corresponding convolutional features generated from the fixed volume, followed by a convolution operation to generate a new deformation field. This process is repeated at each decoding layer, and can be formulated as,

$$\Phi_i = C_i^{3\times3\times3}\left(P_i^M \circ u\left(\Phi_{i-1}\right),\ P_i^F\right) \tag{2}$$

where $i = 1, 2, ..., N$, and is empirically set to 4, indicating four decoding layers. $C_i^{3\times3\times3}$ denotes a 3D convolution at the i-th decoding layer. $\circ$ is the warping operation that maps the coordinates of P_i^M to P_i^F using $u(\Phi_{i-1})$, where P_i^M and P_i^F are the convolutional feature pyramids computed from the moving volume and the fixed volume at the i-th decoding layer.

Finally, the estimated deformation field is up-sampled by a factor of 2, and then is warped by the following deformation field estimated. Such up-sampling and warping operations are implemented sequentially and recurrently to generate a final deformation field, which encodes meaningful multi-level context information with multi-scale deformations. This allows the model to propagate strong context information over hierarchical decoding layers, where the estimated deformation fields are refined gradually in a coarse-to-fine manner, and thus aggregate both high-level context information and low-level detailed features. The high-level context information enables our model with the ability to work on large-scale deformations, while the fine-scale features allows it to preserve detailed anatomical structure. We integrate pyramid registration module into the dual-stream architecture, resulting in an end-to-end trainable model. We adopt a negative local cross correlation (NLCC) as loss function, which is coupled with a smooth regularization, by simply following VoxelMorph [2].

3 Experimental Results and Comparisons

The proposed Dual-PRNet is evaluated on 3D brain MRI registration on two public datasets, LPBA40 [9] and Mindboggle101 [10]. LPBA40 [9] contains 40 T1-weighted MR images, each of which was annotated with 56 subcortical ROIs.

Mindboggle101 [10] contains 101 T1-weighted MR images, which were annotated with 25 cortical regions, and can be used to evaluate registration results regarding fine brain structure.

Experimental Settings. Experiments were conducted by following [3]. On LPBA40, we train our model on 30 subjects, generating 30×29 volume pairs, and test on the remaining 10 subjects. We follow [3] to merge 56 labels into 7 regions on the LPBA40, and center-crop the volumes into a size of $160 \times 192 \times 160$. On Mindboggle101, the data was divided into 42 subjects (with 1722 pairs) for training, and 20 subjects with 380 pairs for testing. All volumes were cropped to $160 \times 192 \times 160$. For evaluation metrics, we adopted the Dice score, which measures the degree of overlap at the voxel level. The proposed Dual-PRNet was implemented in Pytorch and trained on 4 Titan Xp GPUs. Batch size was set to 4, due to the limitation of GPU memory. We adopt Adam optimization with a learning rate of 1e–4.

3.1   Performance on Large Displacements

Visualization. We first visualize the generated multi-resolution deformation fields in Fig. 2 (top). As can be found, the deformation field generated from a lower-resolution layer contains coarse and high-level context information, which is able to warp a volume at a larger scale. Conversely, the deformation field estimated from a higher-resolution layer can capture more detailed features. Figure 2 (bottom) shows the warped images by four deformation fields presented. The warped images are refined gradually toward the fixed image, by aggregating more detailed structural information. We investigate the capability of our Dual-PRNet for handling large displacements, and compare our registration results against that of VoxelMorph in Fig. 3. Our Dual-PRNet can align the image more accurately than VoxelMorph, especially on the regions containing large displacements, as indicated in green or red regions.

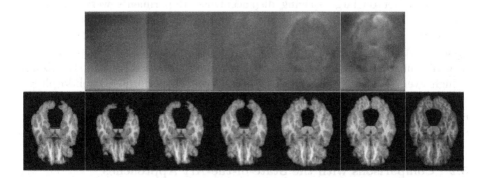

Fig. 2. Top: the generated deformation fields with increasing resolutions (left $\rightarrow$ right), and the last one is the final deformation field. Bottom: left $\rightarrow$ right: the moving image, the warped images by four deformation fields, and the fixed image.

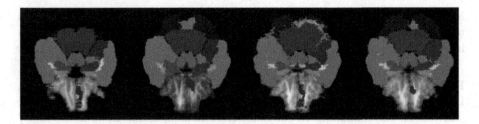

Fig. 3. Registration results on large displacements. From left to right: the moving image, the fixed image, results of VoxelMorph and Dual-PRNet. (Color figure online)

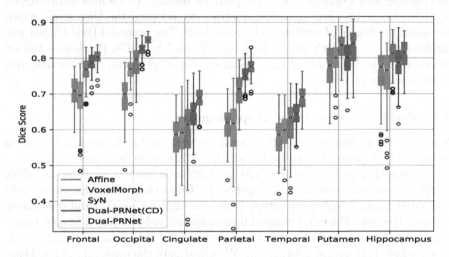

Fig. 4. Dice scores of different methods on LPBA40 (7 regions). Dual-PRNet (CD) indicates cross-dataset (CD) evaluation.

On Large Spacing Displacements. We further evaluate the performance of Dual-PRNet on large spacing displacements. Experiments were conducted on LPBA40, by reducing the slices of the moving volumes from $160 \times 192 \times 160$ to $160 \times 24 \times 160$. During testing, the estimated final deformation field is applied to the labels of the moving volume using zero-order interpolation. With a significant reduction of slices from 192 to 24, our Dual-PRNet can still obtain a high average Dice score of 0.711, which even outperforms VoxelMorph [2] using the original non-reduction volumes, with an average Dice score of 0.683 achieved. This demonstrates the strong robustness of our model against large spacing displacements.

3.2   Comparisons with the State-of-the-Art Approaches

We further compare our Dual-PRNet with a number of approaches: affine registration, SyN [9], and VoxelMorph [2], on LPBA40 and Mindboggle101 datasets.

Table 1. Dice scores of different methods on Mindboggle101. Dual-PRNet (CD) indicates cross-dataset (CD) evaluation.

Region	Frontal	Parietal	Occipital	Temporal	Cingulate	Average	Time(s)
Affine	0.455	0.406	0.354	0.469	0.450	0.427	–
SyN	0.558	0.496	0.446	0.578	0.549	0.525	–
VoxelMorph	0.532	0.459	0.480	0.585	0.499	0.511	**0.451**
Dual-PRNet	**0.602**	**0.690**	**0.550**	**0.695**	**0.618**	**0.631**	1.724
Dual-PRNet (CD)	0.558	0.640	0.504	0.633	0.570	0.581	–

We implemented affine registration method and SyN by using ANTs [11]. For VoxelMorph, we used the codes and models provided by the original authors.

Results and Comparisons. On LPBA40 database, as shown in Fig. 4, our method obtains an average Dice score of 0.778, and outperforms the others by a large margin, e.g., 0.731 of SyN and 0.683 of VoxelMorph. Our method achieves the best performance on all seven evaluated regions. The results on Mindboggle101 database are shown in Table 1, where our Dual-PRNet consistently outperforms the other three methods, and achieves best performance on all five regions. It reaches a high average Dice score of 0.631, compared to 0.525 of SyN and 0.511 of VoxelMorph. Furthermore, we evaluate the generalization capability of our Dual-PRNet by conducting external cross-dataset validation, e.g., training on LPBA40 and testing on Mindboggle101 and vice versa. We obtain an average Dice score of 0.747 on the LPBA40 and 0.581 on the Mindboggle101, which are compared favorably against that of VoxelMorph and SyN. Visualization results on the cross-dataset are compared in SM.

Discussions. We provide ablation studies to further verify the efficiency of each technical component: the dual-stream design and pyramid registration module. Our dual-stream architecture, by estimating a single deformation field as VoxelMorph, can achieve an average Dice score of 0.767 on the LPBA40, and 0.582 on the Mindboggle101, which improved the single-stream counterpart by +8.4% and +7.1% respectively. By integrating the pyramid registration module, the results are further increased, with +1.1% and +4.9% further improvements on the LPBA40 and Mindboggle101 respectively. Notice that the pyramid registration module has a larger improvement on the Mindboggle101, due to the more complicated anatomical structure provided in the Mindboggle101, which often require more accurate labels to identify subtle difference, and coarse-to-fine refinements of the deformation fields can naturally make more contribution.

4   Conclusion

We have presented a new Dual-Stream Pyramid Registration Network for unsupervised 3D medical image registration. We designed a two-stream 3D encoder-decoder network to compute two convolutional feature pyramids, and then proposed a pyramid registration module which predicts multi-scale registration fields directly from the decoding feature pyramids, allowing for recurrently refining the registration fields and convolutional features. This results in a high-performance model that can better handle large deformations in both spatial and spacing domains. With these technical improvements, our method achieved impressive performance for brain MRI registration, and significantly outperformed recent approaches.

References

1. Jaderberg, M., Simonyan, K., Zisserman, A.: Spatial transformer networks. In: NIPS, pp. 2017–2025 (2015)
2. Balakrishnan, G., Zhao, A., Sabuncu, M.R., Guttag, J., Dalca, A.V.: An unsupervised learning model for deformable medical image registration. In: CVPR, pp. 9252–9260 (2018)
3. Kuang, D., Schmah, T.: FAIM-A ConvNet method for unsupervised 3D medical image registration. arXiv preprint arXiv:1811.09243 (2018)
4. Lewis, K.M., Balakrishnan, G., Rost, N.S., Guttag, J., Dalca, A.V.: Fast learning-based registration of sparse clinical images. arXiv:1812.06932 (2018)
5. Ranjan, A., Black, M.J.: Optical flow estimation using a spatial pyramid network. In: CVPR, pp. 4161–4170 (2017)
6. Ronneberger, O., Fischer, P., Brox, T.: U-Net: convolutional networks for biomedical image segmentation. In: Navab, N., Hornegger, J., Wells, W.M., Frangi, A.F. (eds.) MICCAI 2015. LNCS, vol. 9351, pp. 234–241. Springer, Cham (2015). https://doi.org/10.1007/978-3-319-24574-4_28
7. Chen, H., Dou, Q., Yu, L., Qin, J., Heng, P.A.: VoxResNet: deep voxelwise residual networks for brain segmentation from 3D MR images. NeuroImage **170**, 446–455 (2018)
8. He, K., Zhang, X., Ren, S., Sun, J.: Deep residual learning for image recognition. In: CVPR, pp. 770–778 (2016)
9. Shattuck, D.W., et al.: Construction of a 3D probabilistic atlas of human cortical structures. Neuroimage **39**(3), 1064–1080 (2008)
10. Klein, A., Tourville, J.: 101 labeled brain images and a consistent human cortical labeling protocol. Front. Neurosci. **6**, 171 (2012)
11. Avants, B.B., Tustison, N.J., Song, G., Cook, P.A., Klein, A., Gee, J.C.: A reproducible evaluation of ants similarity metric performance in brain image registration. Neuroimage **54**(3), 2033–2044 (2011)

A Cooperative Autoencoder
for Population-Based Regularization
of CNN Image Registration

Riddhish Bhalodia[1,2]([✉]), Shireen Y. Elhabian[1,2], Ladislav Kavan[2],
and Ross T. Whitaker[1,2]

[1] Scientific Computing and Imaging Institute, University of Utah,
Salt Lake City, USA
[2] School of Computing, University of Utah, Salt Lake City, USA
riddhishb@sci.utah.edu

Abstract. Spatial transformations are enablers in a variety of medical image analysis applications that entail aligning images to a common coordinate systems. Population analysis of such transformations is expected to capture the underlying image and shape variations, and hence these transformations are required to produce *anatomically feasible* correspondences. This is usually enforced through some smoothness-based generic metric or regularization of the deformation field. Alternatively, population-based regularization has been shown to produce anatomically accurate correspondences in cases where anatomically unaware (i.e., data independent) regularization fail. Recently, deep networks have been used to generate spatial transformations in an unsupervised manner, and, once trained, these networks are computationally faster and as accurate as conventional, optimization-based registration methods. However, the deformation fields produced by these networks require smoothness penalties, just as the conventional registration methods, and ignores population-level statistics of the transformations. Here, we propose a novel neural network architecture that simultaneously learns and uses the population-level statistics of the spatial transformations to regularize the neural networks for unsupervised image registration. This regularization is in the form of a bottleneck autoencoder, which learns and adapts to the population of transformations required to align input images by encoding the transformations to a low dimensional manifold. The proposed architecture produces deformation fields that describe the population-level features and associated correspondences in an anatomically relevant manner and are statistically compact relative to the state-of-the-art approaches while maintaining computational efficiency. We demonstrate the efficacy of the proposed architecture on synthetic data sets, as well as 2D and 3D medical data.

Electronic supplementary material The online version of this chapter (https://doi.org/10.1007/978-3-030-32245-8_44) contains supplementary material, which is available to authorized users.

D. Shen et al. (Eds.): MICCAI 2019, LNCS 11765, pp. 391–400, 2019.
https://doi.org/10.1007/978-3-030-32245-8_44

1   Introduction

Spatial transformations between sets of images play an important role in medical image analysis and are usually used for bringing distinct subjects into *anatomical correspondence*. This has many uses, such as the alignment of a population into a common coordinate system to compare functional/structural properties of specific anatomy, alignment of a new subject to an atlas, and in the study of anatomical shapes, where the transformations among and between images describe the morphology. In all of these applications, there is an assumption, either explicit or implicit, that the ideal transformation should bring the images into an anatomical correspondence such that key parts of the anatomy are collocated in the transformed image(s). Some methods identify specific anatomical features and find transformations that ensure their alignment [1]. Others find transformations that align unidentified image intensities/features, but *regularize* the problem with a smoothness penalty on the class of transformations [2,3]. This approach has the advantage of potential generality, but it ignores known anatomical variability and correspondence. Thus, the *metric*, regularizations, or representations used to find these transformations do not incorporate any knowledge of transformations or class of transformations that best align members of a given population.

Existing body of literature suggests that anatomical correspondences can be better learned (even in the absence of semantic/functional knowledge) in the context of *populations* of images or shapes [4–6]. There is evidence that correct correspondence produces a population of transformations that is relatively easy to encode. This paper complements and extends these works by integrating population statistics (using non-linear models) into a deep neural network architecture for image registration, which we show is important for accurate characterization of anatomical correspondence.

Very recently, convolutional neural networks (CNNs) are utilized to regress coordinate transformations over the space of input images [7,8], in an *unsupervised* manner, by penalizing a metric of alignment between the input image pairs. These works are justified on the basis of computational speed or efficiency, as the feed-forward computation avoids non-linear, iterative optimization required for conventional image registration methods. However, CNNs for image registration offer other advantages, which are so far unexploited. In particular, CNNs do not rely on analytical representations of the coordinate transformation, the space of allowable transformations, or the optimization. This raises the possibility of incorporating empirical knowledge of the transformations, derived from a population of images, into the registration problem.

In this paper, we propose using population-based learning of regularizations or metrics for controlling the class of transformations that CNN learns. To achieve this, we introduce a novel neural network architecture that includes two subnetworks, namely *primary* and *secondary* networks, that work *cooperatively*. The primary network learns the transformations between pairs of images. The secondary network is a bottleneck autoencoder, that learns a low-dimensional description of the population of transformations, and *cooperates* with the primary network to enforce that the transformations adhere to a latent low-dimensional manifold.

2 Related Work

Deformable image registration has been explored extensively, however, challenges in generality, robustness, and efficiency remain. For brevity, we only focus below on the most closely related research.

Deformable registration is generally an ill-posed problem, and hence *regularization* is required to achieve plausible transformations, avoid non-smooth transformations, and provide anatomically consistent results. Deformation fields are a classical way to represent transformations, typically regularized through smoothness penalty, usually in the form of Dirichlet/elastic penalty on the deformation [9]. For relatively low-dimensional representations, such as b-splines [10], the basis introduces a degree of smoothness, although some methods apply penalties on the b-spline coefficients. Diffeomorphic registration uses static or dynamic (with time-dependent velocity), smooth flow fields to represent the deformation while guaranteeing invertibility, and has been applied to image alignment and shape analysis [2]. The smoothness in the diffeomorphic setting is typically introduced as part of the metric on the flow field.

Recently, CNNs have been used for image registration to boost the computational efficiency by avoiding the non-linear, iterative optimization routines of conventional methods. Supervised methods for CNN training showed promising results [11], but this requires large amounts of labeled training data (i.e., registration examples solved with other techniques). More recent work performs CNN-based registration in an unsupervised fashion [7,8]. The work of Balakrishnan et al. [8] shows promising results on learning 3D brain registration displacement fields, improving the computational cost (after training) over the state-of-the-art traditional registration methods, such as ANTs [12], while maintaining registration accuracy. Like most registration methods, this approach also uses smoothness on the deformation fields as a regularizer.

Early works by [4] considered anatomical landmarks on a set of anatomical shapes, and suggested that anatomical variability is relatively low-dimensional. Later work used information-theoretic criteria to parameterize correspondences on populations of shapes [5]. Deformable transformations between images have also been confined to a low-dimensional representation that captures population characteristics [13]. Statistical deformation models [13,14] learn the probability distribution (subspace or manifold) of the deformation fields for a given population to reduce the dimensionality of the solution space and constrain the registration process. Low-rank representations and spatially varying metrics have also been proposed for diffeomorphic registration [6,15]. All these methods use linear models (e.g. PCA or low-rank correlations) to feed population statistics back into the registration process. In this paper, we introduce nonlinear models of the population and integrate these into a network architecture for registration.

This paper proposes a neural network architecture where one network influences another. Few proposed systems of interacting neural networks include *generative adversarial networks* (GAN) [16] and its variants, and domain adaptation (DA) [17]. In these works, the primary network is *competing* with the secondary network as an adversary, and the steady states of these systems (in training) is a saddle point for the competing energies. In the proposed work, the primary network is minimizing both its loss as well as the reconstruction loss of the secondary network, in an unsupervised setting—and thus we call these architectures *cooperative networks*.

3   Methods

The proposed cooperative network architecture is depicted in Fig. 1. It consists of two interacting subnetworks, the *primary* network aims at solving the primary registration task, and the *secondary* network regularizes the solution space of the primary task. The architecture of the primary network is based on U-Net architecture (Fig. 2), in line with other registration approaches [8]. Given a source (I_S) and a target (I_T) image pair (2D/3D), the network produces a displacement field ϕ, corresponding to the warp that ideally should match I_S to I_T. This displacement field, with the source image, is passed through a spatial transform unit [18] to produce a registered image (I_R). The primary network uses an image matching term between I_R and I_T as the loss function (e.g., $\mathbb{L}_2$ norm or normalized cross-correlation). To re-iterate, the displacement fields ϕ are not required for training, and hence, this is an unsupervised image registration architecture.

The secondary network is a bottleneck autoencoder, which we call a *cooperative autoencoder* (CAE), that attempts to reconstruct the displacement field. The CAE's output is denoted as $\hat{\phi}$. The CAE is a CNN (Fig. 2) with an h-degrees-of-freedom bottleneck layer (i.e. the latent space) represents the low dimensional nonlinear manifold on which the displacement fields should lie (approximately). We add the CAE's reconstruction loss ($\mathbb{L}_2$ loss given as $||\phi - \hat{\phi}||^2$) to the primary registration loss. CAE acts as a regularizer and pushes the network objective function so that it prefers, among many possible solutions, displacement fields that are accurately represented by the CAE.

The final objective function constitutes three terms (Eq. 1). The first term represents the registration loss, the second term (weighted by $\alpha \geq 0$) is smoothness term [8], and, the third term (weighted by $\beta \geq 0$) is the CAE based regularization term.

$$Q = Loss(I_T, I_R) + \alpha ||\nabla \phi||^2 + \beta ||\phi - \hat{\phi}||^2 \qquad (1)$$

CAE training requires an initial set of transformation for a preliminary representation, hence, we start training with $\beta = 0$ (no CAE input), and a small smoothness with weight α. We found that this length of initialization phase does

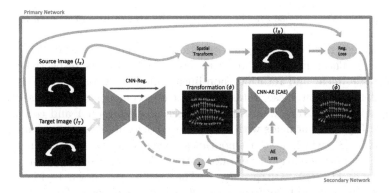

Fig. 1. Cooperative network architecture, with the *primary* unsupervised registration network depicted in the blue box, and the *secondary* autoencoder based regularizer network in the red box. (Color figure online)

not significantly affect the results of the system, and we always set it at 5% of total iterations. After the initialization phase, we turn on the CAE and set β to a non-zero value and $\alpha = 0$ (no smoothness), and train the primary and secondary network jointly (*cooperatively*).

4   Results

In this paper, we use the proposed method to register shapes, represented as binary images and/or distance transforms. The same method applies directly to medical images. For each dataset, we train each network on *all pairs* of images from the data, with random 25% of the pairs set aside for testing. To clarify, this testing set is of completely held out pairs of images and the remaining 75% of pairs is broken into training and validation set, Training on all pairs ensures that the CAE captures the inherent low-dimensional structure of the displacement fields while avoiding bias. However, the concept of cooperative networks is applicable to other training strategies (e.g. training with a given atlas image) or representations (e.g. momentum fields).

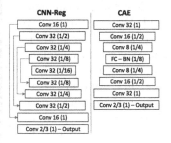

Fig. 2. Left: primary network architecture (input: pair of images, output: displacement field between the images), which is then fed into the Spatial Transform (Fig. 1). Right: architecture of the cooperative autoencoder.

Linear and Rotating Box-Bump

Our first didactic dataset is a set of 2D *box-bump* (as in [19]) images, where a protrusion on the surface of a rectangular shape is parameterized by its position along the side. We also use another synthetic dataset representative of rotational (non-linear) shape variations. Specifically, a protrusion is set atop of a circular base (parameterized by its angular position, between $[-50, +50]$ degrees from the center). These linear and rotating box-bump datasets respectively represent a single linear and rotating (non-linear) mode of variation. We apply the proposed method on these datasets with the secondary network as cooperative autoencoder (CAE) with the bottleneck of dimension 1 and compare the resulting displacement fields with unsupervised deformable registration (UnDR) proposed in [8], which uses a smoothness penalty on the displacement fields and encodes no population-level information. We use $\mathbb{L}_2$ difference as primary loss, i.e. $Loss(I_R, I_T) = ||I_T - I_R||^2$. The results are shown in Fig. 3, along with displacement fields and corresponding Dice coefficients, for a test pair of images. We see that the registration accuracy measured using the Dice coefficient is comparable for UnDR and the proposed method (UnDR-CAE), but produces vastly different displacement fields. Cooperating networks capture a single transverse/rotating component for linear/rotating box bump, respectively, each derived from population statistics. In comparison, UnDR (for both datasets) compresses the protrusion for the source and expands it for the target, which correctly aligns the source and target shapes, but it does not discover the shape variation of the population. This is an important distinction: unlike UnDR, CAE leverages information about the population statistics of the data.

The core idea of cooperative networks is to restrict displacement fields to a low dimensional manifold. For comparison, we also study some alternative strategies exploiting the same principle. The first option is to reduce the latent space of the primary network architecture (UnDR) to a single dimension bottleneck, which we call "UnDR-BN", this represents a conventional alternative to the CAE. The results for this approach are shown in Fig. 3 (UnDR-BN). These results show that UnDR-BN is similar to UnDR, which

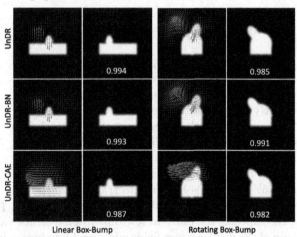

Fig. 3. Linear & rotating box-bump results with different methods, left figure shows the source with the field as produced by the network, and the right shows the false color difference image between the target and the registration output (white: correct overlap, green and magenta: mismatched pixels). (Color figure online)

can be explained, in part, by the *skip-connections* (Fig. 2) in the U-Net architecture used in UnDR. An alternative to UnDR-BN architecture can be to introduce a $\mathbb{L}_1$ penalty on this layer to encourage sparsity. In our experiments, this leads to similar results as UnDR-BN, and for brevity, we do not present those results in this paper. We also provide additional results (in supplementary material) with UnDR-BN, but with skip-connections of the U-Net architecture removed.

We hypothesize that cooperative networks can discover meaningful correspondences of shape, to validate we define landmarks (analytically) on the family of box-bump shapes (in correspondence with the bump movement) and we evaluate how well each method aligns these ground truth correspondences (*Landmark error* in Table 1), along with Dice coefficients measuring registration accuracy. The computational cost of discovering displacement fields for a given image pair (testing step), are similar for both UnDR and the proposed method, i.e. CAE does not lose any of its speed over UnDR (speed is the main advantage of UnDR [8]). UnDR-CAE registers with similar accuracy as UnDR (measured by Dice coefficient), but consistently achieves lower landmark errors due to the secondary network which learns population statistics. It is also interesting to see the latent space variations as discovered by the single dimension of CAE and the additional results for this is provided in supplementary material.

For the CAE, we report the reconstruction error ($\frac{\|\phi - \hat{\phi}\|_{L_2}}{\|\phi\|_{L_2}}$) in Table 1. For comparison, we train a separate autoencoder on the displacement fields produced by UnDR (Table 1). These results are in agreement with the key idea that the CAE helps the primary network to produce results closer to a low-dimensional manifold, as represented by the ability of the bottle-neck AE to accurately reconstruct its output.

Table 1. Results obtained with Cooperative AutoEncoder networks (CAE, bottleneck size, β coefficient) compared with Unsupervised Deformable Registration (UnDR) by [8]. Landmark errors for box-bump datasets are reported as the percentage of bump width. The AE error for UnDR refers to a separate autoencoder with bottleneck size same as CAE bottleneck (trained after UnDR). [†] The AE error is 63.3% for bottleneck size 1, 54.1% for 2, 49.4% for 4, 38.8% for 8, and 33.5% for 16. We also report the average test runtime to compute the displacement fields.

Dataset	Method	AE error	Dice coeff.	Landmark error	Test runtime
Linear Box-Bump	CAE (1, $\beta = 8$)	6.8%	0.98	26%	0.0185 s
Linear Box-Bump	UnDR	66.4%	0.97	124%	0.0184 s
Linear Box-Bump	UnDR-BN	65.8%	0.96	122%	0.0190 s
Rotate Box-Bump	CAE (1, $\beta = 8$)	12.3%	0.98	24%	0.0195 s
Rotate Box-Bump	UnDR	63.5%	0.99	101%	0.0193 s
Rotate Box-Bump	UnDR-BN	54.9%	0.99	102%	0.0196 s
Corpus Callosum	CAE (2, $\beta = 10$)	33.2%	0.89	5.7 mm	0.0237 s
Corpus Callosum	CAE (4, $\beta = 10$)	19.2%	0.93	5.1 mm	0.0237 s
Corpus Callosum	CAE (8, $\beta = 10$)	18.5%	0.95	4.5 mm	0.0237 s
Corpus Callosum	CAE (16, $\beta = 10$)	16.3%	0.96	5.2 mm	0.0237 s
Corpus Callosum	UnDR	33–63%[†]	0.93	6.5 mm	0.0234 s
Left Atrium (3D)	CAE (5, $\beta = 0.2$)	29.8%	0.76	9.9 mm	0.784 s
Left Atrium (3D)	UnDR	46.3%	0.75	10.1 mm	0.772 s

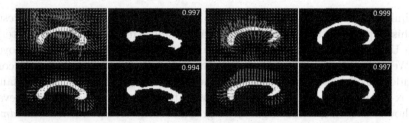

Fig. 4. Two corpus callosum source-target pairs, again one image showing the fields and the other a falsecolor between target and the registered output; top-row: UnDR, bottom-row: CAE.

Corpus Callosum (CC)

In this example, we use a dataset of 324 mid-saggital 2D slices of Corpus Callosum (CC) from the OASIS Brains dataset [20]. Unlike synthetic experiments discussed above, we do not know, apriori, the intrinsic dimensionality of the CC shapes. Therefore, we train the proposed architecture across a range of CAE bottleneck dimensions (2, 4, 8 and 16) and compare resulting Dice coefficients, autoencoder reconstructions, and landmark errors, as in Table 1. Networks are again trained using $\mathbb{L}_2$ difference as the primary loss. Landmarks were identified using features from the literature [21], and we had multiple raters identify the posterior and anterior points of the CC, the inferior tip of the splenium, the posterior tip of the genu, the posterior angle of the genu, and the interior notch of the splenium. Interrater RMS error is 1.4 mm, and the pixel/voxel size is 1 mm for these images. We see that the optimal bottleneck size for cooperative networks is 8 – increasing the bottleneck to 16 improves the Dice coefficient and AE error, but leads to worse landmark error, which suggests the CAE starts to overfit. The UnDR approach leads to comparable Dice scores, but worse autoencoder and landmark errors (Table 1). As in the synthetic experiments, to report the AE error for UnDR, we trained the autoencoder separately after UnDR training. CAE helps the primary network produce displacement fields that are close to a low-dimensional manifold—a result that is not achieved with the conventional smoothness penalty.

Left Atrium Appendage (LAA)

We apply the cooperative network on a 3D dataset of left atrium appendages (LAA). These images are represented as signed distance transforms, and hence we use the normalized cross-correlation loss as in [8], instead of a $\mathbb{L}_2$ image loss. The Dice scores, AE reconstruction

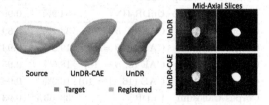

Fig. 5. The results of the 3D LAA registration produced by cooperative networks and UnDR.

accuracy and compute times are reported in Table 1. We also show the registration of a pair of LAA images in Fig. 5, and landmark (manually obtained clinically validated Ostia landmarks on LAA) reconstruction errors in Table 1.

5 Conclusions

This paper proposes a novel architecture proposed for CNN-based unsupervised image registration that uses a cooperative autoencoder (CAE) and enforces the displacement fields to lie in the vicinity of a low-dimensional manifold. CAE reconstruction loss acts as a regularizer term for unsupervised registration. Cooperative networks have comparable registration run times (Table 1) with UnDR, but much faster as compared to the conventional state-of-the-art registration methods (as analyzed in [8]). Cooperative networks produce meaningful correspondence representation between shapes as compared to other methods (evident by landmark reconstruction errors in Table 1), while maintaining the registration accuracy, making it a viable tool for obtaining fast alignment with anatomically feasible correspondence.

Acknowledgements. This work was supported by NIH [grant numbers R01-AR-076120-01, R01-HL135568-02, and P41-GM103545-19] and also supported by the National Institute of General Medical Sciences of the National Institutes of Health under grant number P41 GM103545-18.

References

1. Joshi, S.H., et al.: Diffeomorphic sulcal shape analysis on the cortex. IEEE Trans. Med. Imaging **31**(6), 1195–1212 (2012)
2. Beg, M.F., Miller, M.I., Trouvé, A., Younes, L.: Computing large deformation metric mappings via geodesic flows of diffeomorphisms. Int. J. Comput. Vis. **61**(2), 139–157 (2005)
3. Joshi, S.C., Miller, M.I.: Landmark matching via large deformation diffeomorphisms. IEEE Trans. Image Process. **9**(8), 1357–1370 (2000)
4. Grenander, U., Chow, Y., Keenan, D.M.: Hands: A Pattern Theoretic Study of Biological Shapes, vol. 2. Springer, Heidelberg (1991). https://doi.org/10.1007/978-1-4612-3046-5
5. Cates, J., Fletcher, P.T., Styner, M., Shenton, M., Whitaker, R.: Shape modeling and analysis with entropy-based particle systems. In: Karssemeijer, N., Lelieveldt, B. (eds.) IPMI 2007. LNCS, vol. 4584, pp. 333–345. Springer, Heidelberg (2007). https://doi.org/10.1007/978-3-540-73273-0_28
6. Vialard, F.-X., Risser, L.: Spatially-varying metric learning for diffeomorphic image registration: a variational framework. In: Golland, P., Hata, N., Barillot, C., Hornegger, J., Howe, R. (eds.) MICCAI 2014. LNCS, vol. 8673, pp. 227–234. Springer, Cham (2014). https://doi.org/10.1007/978-3-319-10404-1_29
7. de Vos, B.D., Berendsen, F.F., Viergever, M.A., Staring, M., Išgum, I.: End-to-end unsupervised deformable image registration with a convolutional neural network. In: Cardoso, M.J., et al. (eds.) DLMIA/ML-CDS -2017. LNCS, vol. 10553, pp. 204–212. Springer, Cham (2017). https://doi.org/10.1007/978-3-319-67558-9_24

8. Balakrishnan, G., Zhao, A., Sabuncu, M.R., Guttag, J., Dalca, A.V.: An unsupervised learning model for deformable medical image registration. In: CVPR, pp. 9252–9260 (2018)
9. Bajcsy, R., Kovačič, S.: Multiresolution elastic matching. Comput. Vis. Graph. Image Process. **46**(1), 1–21 (1989)
10. Rueckert, D., Sonoda, L.I., Hayes, C., Hill, D.L.G., Leach, M.O., Hawkes, D.J.: Nonrigid registration using free-form deformations: application to breast MR images. IEEE Trans. Med. Imaging **18**(8), 712–721 (1999)
11. Krebs, J., et al.: Robust non-rigid registration through agent-based action learning. In: Descoteaux, M., Maier-Hein, L., Franz, A., Jannin, P., Collins, D.L., Duchesne, S. (eds.) MICCAI 2017. LNCS, vol. 10433, pp. 344–352. Springer, Cham (2017). https://doi.org/10.1007/978-3-319-66182-7_40
12. Avants, B.B., Tustison, N.J., Song, G., Cook, P.A., Klein, A., Gee, J.C.: A reproducible evaluation of ants similarity metric performance in brain image registration. NeuroImage **54**(3), 2033–2044 (2011)
13. Rueckert, D., Frangi, A.F., Schnabel, J.A.: Automatic construction of 3-D statistical deformation models of the brain using nonrigid registration. IEEE Trans. Med. Imaging **22**(8), 1014–1025 (2003)
14. Joshi, S.C., Miller, M.I., Grenander, U.: On the geometry and shape of brain submanifolds. IJPRAI **11**(8), 1317–1343 (1997)
15. Schmah, T., Risser, L., Vialard, F.-X.: Left-invariant metrics for diffeomorphic image registration with spatially-varying regularisation. In: Mori, K., Sakuma, I., Sato, Y., Barillot, C., Navab, N. (eds.) MICCAI 2013. LNCS, vol. 8149, pp. 203–210. Springer, Heidelberg (2013). https://doi.org/10.1007/978-3-642-40811-3_26
16. Goodfellow, I., et al.: Generative adversarial nets. In: Advances in Neural Information Processing Systems 27, pp. 2672–2680. Curran Associates, Inc. (2014)
17. Ganin, Y., et al.: Domain-adversarial training of neural networks. J. Mach. Learn. Res. **17**(1), 2030–2096 (2016)
18. Jaderberg, M., Simonyan, K., Zisserman, A., Kavukcuoglu, K.: Spatial transformer networks. In: Advances in Neural Information Processing Systems 28, pp. 2017–2025. Curran Associates, Inc. (2015)
19. Thodberg, H.H.: Minimum description length shape and appearance models. In: Taylor, C., Noble, J.A. (eds.) IPMI 2003. LNCS, vol. 2732, pp. 51–62. Springer, Heidelberg (2003). https://doi.org/10.1007/978-3-540-45087-0_5
20. Marcus, D.S., Fotenos, A.F., Csernansky, J.G., Morris, J.C., Buckner, R.L.: Open access series of imaging studies: longitudinal MRI data in nondemented and demented older adults. J. Cogn. Neurosci. **22**, 2677–2684 (2010)
21. Sigirli, D., Ercan, I., Ozdemir, S.T., Taskapilioglu, O., Hakyemez, B., Turan, O.F.: Shape analysis of the corpus callosum and cerebellum in female MS patients with different clinical phenotypes. Anat. Rec.: Adv. Integr. Anat. Evol. Biol. **295**(7), 1202–1211 (2012)

Conditional Segmentation in Lieu of Image Registration

Yipeng Hu[1,2(✉)], Eli Gibson[3], Dean C. Barratt[1], Mark Emberton[4],
J. Alison Noble[2], and Tom Vercauteren[5]

[1] Centre for Medical Image Computing and Wellcome/EPSRC Centre
for Interventional and Surgical Sciences, University College London,
London, UK
yipeng.hu@ucl.ac.uk
[2] Institute of Biomedical Engineering, University of Oxford, Oxford, UK
[3] Digital Services, Digital Technology and Innovation,
Siemens Healthineers, Princeton, NJ, USA
[4] Division of Surgery and Interventional Science, University College London,
London, UK
[5] School of Biomedical Engineering and Imaging Sciences,
King's College London, London, UK

Abstract. Classical pairwise image registration methods search for a spatial transformation that optimises a numerical measure that indicates how well a pair of moving and fixed images are aligned. Current learning-based registration methods have adopted the same paradigm and typically predict, for any new input image pair, dense correspondences in the form of a dense displacement field or parameters of a spatial transformation model. However, in many applications of registration, the spatial transformation itself is only required to propagate points or regions of interest (ROIs). In such cases, detailed pixel- or voxel-level correspondence within or outside of these ROIs often have little clinical value. In this paper, we propose an alternative paradigm in which the location of corresponding image-specific ROIs, defined in one image, within another image is learnt. This results in replacing image registration by a *conditional segmentation* algorithm, which can build on typical image segmentation networks and their widely-adopted training strategies. Using the registration of 3D MRI and ultrasound images of the prostate as an example to demonstrate this new approach, we report a median target registration error (TRE) of 2.1 mm between the ground-truth ROIs defined on intraoperative ultrasound images and those propagated from the preoperative MR images. Significantly lower (>34%) TREs were obtained using the proposed conditional segmentation compared with those obtained from a previously-proposed spatial-transformation-predicting registration network trained with the same multiple ROI labels for individual image pairs. We conclude this work by using a quantitative bias-variance analysis to provide one explanation of the observed improvement in registration accuracy.

© Springer Nature Switzerland AG 2019
D. Shen et al. (Eds.): MICCAI 2019, LNCS 11765, pp. 401–409, 2019.
https://doi.org/10.1007/978-3-030-32245-8_45

1 Introduction

Recent medical image registration methods based on convolutional neural networks have adopted an end-to-end learning framework, in which a *moving* and *fixed* image pair is the input of the network that directly predicts a dense displacement field (DDF) or parameters of a parametric spatial transformation model [1]. These capture pixel- or voxel-level *dense correspondences*. Such networks have been trained by minimising unsupervised losses [2], adapted from classical or learned dissimilarity measures within pairs of images, or supervised losses measuring the difference to ground-truth transformations [3, 4]. Label similarity between anatomical segmentations has also been proposed to measure image alignment as a form of weak supervision [5] and has been combined with other losses [6, 7].

Predicting spatial transformations, as in the above-mentioned methods, enables physically-motivated prior knowledge on the deformation fields to be incorporated in the network training. Examples include parameterising the spatial transformation using rigid, spline-based models [1–3] or velocity fields [4], penalising implausible transformation through a regularisation term such as L^2-norm of DDF and bending energy [5–7], and minimising divergence between the predicted and the unpaired ground-truth deformations [8]. Figure 1 illustrates the training and prediction stages of these typical spatial-transformation-predicting registration networks.

Spatial-Transformation-Predicting Registration Networks

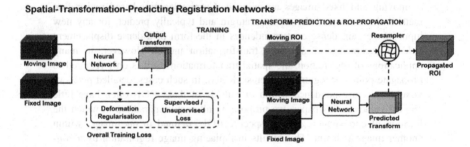

Fig. 1. Left: illustration of the training of spatial-transformation-predicting registration networks; Right: the ROIs are propagated from moving image to fixed image by the spatial transformation (predicted transform), predicted by the trained neural network.

A common purpose of image registration in medical applications is region-of-interest (ROI) propagation, also illustrated in Fig. 1. In multimodal image guided interventions, for instance, the registration-generated spatial transformation is used to warp one or more clinically useful ROIs, defined by inseparable pixel/voxel locations in the preoperative moving images, to intraoperative fixed images. These ROIs, such as patient-specific biopsy or pathology locations in a preoperative-image-derived procedure plan, are not necessarily anatomically-defined landmarks or identifiable in both images, and therefore are not consistently available for all cases *a priori*. Different to segmentation, a registration network predicts spatial transformation that defines dense correspondence, which can propagate any given ROI from a moving image to a fixed image.

However, clinically useful ROIs are often sparse for individual patients (e.g. a single target tumour), therefore propagating ROIs (equivalent to searching for a region-level correspondence) and searching for dense correspondence present very different challenges. This is partly because the regularised dense correspondence prediction encourages spatial smoothness and topology preservation, which may over-constrain localising ROIs in the fixed images that is of much greater clinical value. We postulate that, with the increasing availability in training data, predicting spatial transformation may limit the *clinically relevant registration accuracy* in such applications.

In this work, we propose to use a machine learning approach for *any* given ROI on a moving image to predict the image-specific ROI on a fixed image directly. This approach does not predict a spatial transformation and does not require deformation regularisation. Replacing the task of finding a spatial transformation with ROI propagation leads to a *conditional segmentation* approach, which is described in Sect. 2.

We report experimental results from a multimodal image registration application, in which MR and ultrasound images are aligned to guide targeted biopsy [9] and focal therapy [10] for prostate cancer patients. The contributions of this work include: (1) a novel conditional segmentation paradigm for ROI propagation tasks, which replaces commonly-adopted image registration methods; (2) the demonstration using clinical data that significantly improved registration accuracy can be achieved using the proposed conditional segmentation approach compared with a spatial-transformation-predicting registration network for a real-world application; and (3) a bias-variance analysis to further investigate the source of improvement shown for this application.

2   Method

2.1   Conditional Image Segmentation Paradigm for ROI Propagation

With clinically relevant ROIs having varying quantities, shapes, sizes and locations for each image pair, we formulate the ROI propagation task as a joint binary classification problem where each voxel on the fixed image is to be classified as either "belonging to" $(C_{k=1})$ or "not belonging to" $(C_{k=2})$ the ROI propagated from the moving image. Using a convolutional neural network with parameters θ, the posterior class probabilities, modelled by the network output, are given by $p_\theta(C_k|\mathbf{I}^{fix}, \mathbf{I}^{mov}, \mathbf{R}^{mov})$, where random vectors $\mathbf{I}^{fix}$, $\mathbf{I}^{mov}$ and $\mathbf{R}^{mov}$ represent the fixed image, the moving image and the ROI in the moving image (hereafter referred to as the "moving ROI"), respectively. Predicting $p_\theta(C_k|\mathbf{I}^{fix}, \mathbf{I}^{mov}, \mathbf{R}^{mov})$, in turn, represents a conditional segmentation problem, conditioned on a given moving image $\mathbf{I}^{mov}$ and a given moving ROI $\mathbf{R}^{mov}$.

As illustrated in Fig. 2, the conditional segmentation can be implemented with minimal adaptation to a standard image segmentation network by, for instance, concatenating the image pair $(\mathbf{I}^{fix}, \mathbf{I}^{mov})$ and moving ROI $\mathbf{R}^{mov}$ in the input layer. Unlike conventional spatial-transformation-predicting registration or multi-ROI segmentation methods, this network predicts any one single propagated ROI $\mathbf{R}^{fix}$ (potentially with a single foreground voxel) at a time during inference stage and can be trained with multiple training ROIs labelled from each of the training image pairs.

Proposed Conditional Segmentation Networks

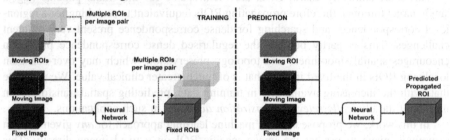

Fig. 2. Left: illustration of the training of the proposed conditional segmentation network; Right: individually propagated ROIs are directly predicted by the trained neural network.

2.2   A Supervised Training Approach

In this work, we implement a supervised conditional segmentation training approach, suitable for the multimodality 3D image registration application described in Sect. 3.

In training, N pairs of moving images $\{\mathbf{i}_n^{mov}\}$ and fixed images $\{\mathbf{i}_n^{fix}\}$ are available, $n = 1, \ldots, N$. For every image pair, M_n pairs of corresponding ROI labels $\{\mathbf{r}_{mn}^{mov}\}$ and $\{\mathbf{r}_{mn}^{fix}\}$, $m = 1, \ldots, M_n$, are delineated in the moving - and fixed images, respectively. $\{\mathbf{r}_{mn}^{fix}\}$ denotes the ground-truth for the propagated "fixed ROI" $\mathbf{R}^{fix}$. These ROIs need not to be labelled consistently across image pairs, individual images pairs may have different types anatomical structures or regions as training ROI labels and may have different numbers of ROI pairs, i.e. in general, $M_1 \neq M_2 \ldots \neq M_n$.

The fixed ROIs in this work are represented by binary masks, indicating ground-truth class probabilities at each voxel $p(C_k|\mathbf{r}_{mn}^{fix})$, for a foreground $C_{k=1}$ and a background class $C_{k=0}$. Without loss of generality, the moving ROIs are also represented by binary masks, each as an input of the neural network that predicts the conditional class probabilities $p_\theta(C_k|\mathbf{i}_n^{fix}, \mathbf{i}_n^{mov}, \mathbf{r}_{mn}^{mov})$. Given n^{th} image pair and M_n associated ROI pairs, the negative log-likelihood leads to a weighted cross-entropy loss function: $J_n(\theta) = -\sum_{m=1}^{M_n} \sum_{k=1}^{2} p(C_k|\mathbf{r}_{mn}^{fix}) \log p_\theta(C_k|\mathbf{i}_n^{fix}, \mathbf{i}_n^{mov}, \mathbf{r}_{mn}^{mov}) w_k$, where the weighting parameter w_k is the sample ratio between foreground and background voxels [11].

A typical image segmentation network, such as a 3D U-Net [12], can be adapted to take the input of an image pair and one of the moving ROI labels $(\mathbf{i}_n^{fix}, \mathbf{i}_n^{mov}, \mathbf{r}_{mn}^{mov})$. The previously-proposed two-stage sampling is adopted in a stochastic minibatch gradient descent optimisation, in which, image pairs are sampled first before sampling image-specific ROI labels. Thus, each minibatch has the same number of first-stage-sampled image pairs $(\mathbf{i}_n^{fix}, \mathbf{i}_n^{mov})$ and second-stage-sampled ROI pairs $(\mathbf{r}_{mn}^{mov}, \mathbf{r}_{mn}^{mov})$ and, collectively, they contribute to an unbiased estimator of the batch gradient [5]. During inference, given a new pair of images and a moving ROI, the trained network can predict where this ROI is propagated (or warped) to in the fixed image space.

2.3   Comparison to a DDF-Predicting Registration Network

We compared the proposed conditional segmentation network with a previously-proposed weakly-supervised registration network [5], because (1) it uses the same types of image and ROI data in training; and (2) it was proposed with a clinical aim for predicting ROIs, including the prostate gland, one or more image-visible lesions (potentially tumours) and surrounding organs, so these can be identified during ultrasound-guided interventional procedures [5, 8–10]. Once trained, the registration network does not need the moving ROI as input to predict a DDF for each image pair. Instead, it warps the ROI using the predicted DDF. The conditional segmentation network predicts a moved ROI directly, given the additional moving ROI. This difference is illustrated in Figs. 1 and 2. The details of both networks are summarised in Sect. 3.

Registration Accuracy: Two accuracy measures were computed in this study: Target registration error (TRE), defined as root-mean-square centroid distance, between the propagated moving ROIs and the ground-truth fixed ROIs, calculated over all ROI pairs for each test patient, and the Dice similarity coefficient (DSC) calculated between the pairs of ROIs representing the entire prostate. The training-independent TREs and DSCs are clinically informative in targeting the regions of surgical interest, such as prostate lesions, and in identifying vulnerable structures, such as rectum [9, 10]. They are reported based on the cross-validation experiments described in Sect. 3.

Physically Plausible Correspondence Prediction for Out-of-Sample ROIs: Predicting a new ROI at the inference stage could fail if this ROI is not within the ROI distribution represented by the training labels. However, it is reasonable to expect that a physically plausible mapping can be predicted on these novel landmarks using conditional segmentation without explicit deformation regularisation. This generalisability across different types of ROIs may be a result of potential anatomical, spatial and intensity correlations between these novel test ROIs and the training ROIs.

To test this generalisability, a set of *ad hoc* ROIs were selected if they do not have apparent representatives in the training data. For example, several patient-specific calcification clusters were found on unusual locations such as anterior regions of the prostate gland. The TREs on these ROIs are reported in addition to the overall results.

Bias-Variance versus Training Data Size: One of the potential advantages of avoiding deformation regularisation is to reduce the bias from the smoothness assumptions, such that more complicated correspondence can be learned from data, such as one-to-many or many-to-one mapping at voxel-level. Examples in this application include topological changes (presence of catheter in urethra and swelling during ablation) and high nonlinearity (between glandular zones and other structures).

To quantitatively investigate the bias for the two networks, we ran repeated experiments with bootstrap-sampled training/testing sets to decompose the variance due to random training data sampling and stochastic model training from the bias observed consistently across experiments. We propose two hypotheses, *Hypothesis A:* compared to the DDF-predicting network constrained by deformation regularisation (here, bending energy), the conditional segmentation would reduce the prediction bias, which is a component of the TRE; *Hypothesis B:* potential high-bias can limit generalisability in registration performance, represented by larger TREs on testing data, as training data increase. The Hypothesis B has an important practical value in informing the choice between these two types of networks, when training data size changes.

To test these hypotheses, we adopted a patient-level repeated cross-validation procedure [13] for both networks, by which, a set of training data sizes of interest is tested. The square of the bias and the variance on each ROI are then represented by the squared-distance d_{bias}^2 from the centre of the predicted centroids to the ground-truth and the average squared-distance d_{var}^2 to the centre from the centroids, respectively, over all samples estimated from the repeated cross-validation. This experiment does not take into account inter-training-data variability that will change as the training data size changes in cross-validation experiments, but it has been shown to be effective in estimating bias and variance of altering training data size [14], which was the concern in this study. The experiment details are described in Sect. 3.

3 Experiments

Without any initial alignment, a total of 115 pairs of T2-weighted MR and 3D transrectal ultrasound (TRUS) images from 80 prostate cancer patients who underwent TRUS-guided biopsy or therapy procedures were randomly sampled from clinical trial data (SmartTarget, NCT02341677, NCT02290561) for this study. Each patient may have multiple MR-TRUS image pairs according to the trial protocols. 3D TRUS volumes were reconstructed by rotational sagittal frames acquired by a bi-plane transrectal probe (Hitachi HI-VISION Preirus). All image volumes were normalised to zero-mean with unit-variance intensities after being resampled to $0.8 \times 0.8 \times 0.8$ mm^3 isotropic voxels. From these patients, a total of 910 pairs of corresponding anatomical ROIs were labelled and verified by second observers including consultant radiologists and senior imaging research fellows. Besides full gland segmentations for all cases, the ROIs defined landmarks including the apex and base of the prostate, the urethra, image-visible lesions, gland zonal separations, the vas deference and the seminal vesicles, and other patient-specific landmarks such as calcifications and fluid-filled cysts, with similar spatial and size distributions to those reported in the previous work [5].

Compared to the registration network architecture, only two changes were made to the original input and output layers to implement the conditional segmentation network: First, the additional single moving ROI label for each image pair, after being linearly-resampled to the fixed image size, is concatenated to the input layer with the image pair; second, instead of three displacement components, in x-, y- and z-channels, the conditional segmentation network outputs a single-channel logits layer, with a sigmoid function, to represent the foreground class probabilities in the fixed image space.

Compared to the registration network training, the conditional segmentation network training was found to be less sensitive to initialisation and learning rate as a result of not-predicting spatial transformations, required less memory without the 3D intensity resampler and did not need to tune the weighted deformation regularisation. Both networks had 32 initial channels and were trained with the same data using the Adam optimiser starting at a learning rate of 10^{-5}. For brevity, readers are referred to the referenced publication and the published demonstration code [5] for additional details, which were kept unchanged in this work to enable comparison. The networks were implemented in TensorFlow™ with open-source code from NiftyNet [15]. Each of the conditional segmentation networks and registration networks was trained for 48 and 72 h, respectively, both with a minibatch size of 2 using GeForce® GTX 1080Ti GPU cards with 11 GB memory on a high-performance computing cluster.

As part of the patient-level repeated k-fold cross-validation procedure, the TREs of individual patients were calculated. The cross-validation was repeated ten times, for each of the four tested training patient sizes 40, 60, 70, and 75 with k = 2, 4, 8, and 16, respectively, with increasing yet varying numbers of image pairs (ranging from 40 to 110). This resulted in 600 networks trained in total ($\sim 36{,}000$ GPU-hours) to compare the two types of networks. For each tested training size, the errors d_{bias}^2 and d_{var}^2 (described in Sect. 2.3), which represent the bias and variance in estimating ROI centroids, were estimated for individual ROIs from these ten samples.

4   Results

From the 16-fold cross-validation, the median (25th–75th percentiles) TRE and DSC are 2.1 (1.4–3.5) mm and 0.92 (0.90–0.94), respectively, for the proposed conditional segmentation networks, and 3.2 (2.3–6.4) mm and 0.90 (0.87–0.92) for the DDF-predicting registration networks. A statistically significant ($p < 0.001$) improvement of 34% in TREs was observed based on a paired Wilcoxon signed-rank test at a significance level $\alpha = 0.05$. TREs from the 70 manually selected *ad hoc* landmarks were also found to yield a lower median TRE of 2.8 (2.3–4.9) mm from the conditional segmentation, compared with 4.2 (3.0–7.8) mm using the registration network ($p < 0.001$).

As training set sizes increase, the TREs were found to decrease for both networks with lower mean TREs being obtained from the conditional segmentation for all different training set sizes, as shown in Fig. 3. Furthermore, the estimated variance decreased with more training data, although detecting differences in variance between the two networks was difficult due to the small sample sizes (10 from the repeated cross-validation). The estimated bias from the conditional segmentation is considerably lower for all training set sizes as shown in the median (25th–75th percentiles) d_{bias}^2 in Fig. 3. This suggests that (1) the prediction of spatial transformation may not be optimised for this task (here, a regularised DDF); (2) due to the high-and-non-decreasing bias observed from the registration network, the accuracy may not be improved by further increasing the training data; and (3) the lower TREs reported in this case can be attributed largely to the low-bias from the conditional segmentation network.

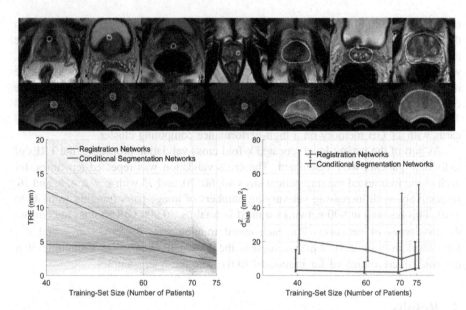

Fig. 3. Upper: example MR slices (1st row) with moving ROIs in blue contours, which are propagated to TRUS slices (2nd row) with the ground-truth ROIs in red areas; Lower: plots of mean TREs (left) and median d^2_{bias} (right) versus training-set sizes. See the text for details. (Color figure online)

5　Conclusion

While prior knowledge, such as deformation regularisation, has proven useful for improving the generalisation ability of registration networks with limited training data [8], the bias-variance analysis presented in this paper revealed that this approach can also produce a high prediction bias, which may not be reduced by increasing the training data size. Thus, we have proposed a conditional segmentation paradigm for ROI propagation applications that avoids estimating a spatial transformation to overcome this issue. Using a supervised neural network, we have demonstrated significantly improved TREs in a real-world surgical application where clinically meaningful ROIs corresponding to those defined in MR images are predicted in prostate ultrasound images.

Acknowledgement. This work is supported by the Wellcome/EPSRC Centre for Interventional and Surgical Sciences (203145Z/16/Z) and the Medical Image Analysis Network (EP/N026993/1). TV is supported by a Medtronic/RAEng Research Chair (RCSRF1819/7/34). Additional supports are from CRUK (C28070/A19985), the Wellcome (203145Z/16/Z; 203148/Z/16/Z) and the EPSRC (NS/A000050/1; NS/A000049/1).

References

1. DeTone, D., Malisiewicz, T., Rabinovich, A.: Deep image homography estimation. arXiv preprint arXiv:1606.03798 (2016)
2. de Vos, B.D., et al.: A deep learning framework for unsupervised affine and deformable image registration. Med. Image Anal. **52**, 128–143 (2019)
3. Eppenhof, K.A., et al.: Deformable image registration using convolutional neural networks. In: Medical Imaging 2018: Image Processing, vol. 10574, p. 105740S (2018)
4. Rohé, M.-M., Datar, M., Heimann, T., Sermesant, M., Pennec, X.: SVF-Net: learning deformable image registration using shape matching. In: Descoteaux, M., Maier-Hein, L., Franz, A., Jannin, P., Collins, D.Louis, Duchesne, S. (eds.) MICCAI 2017. LNCS, vol. 10433, pp. 266–274. Springer, Cham (2017). https://doi.org/10.1007/978-3-319-66182-7_31
5. Hu, Y., et al.: Weakly-supervised convolutional neural networks for multimodal image registration. Med. Image Anal. **49**, 1–13 (2018)
6. Balakrishnan, G., et al.: VoxelMorph: a learning framework for deformable medical image registration. IEEE Trans. Med. Imaging **38**, 1788–1800 (2019)
7. Hering, A., Kuckertz, S., Heldmann, S., Heinrich, M.P.: Enhancing label-driven deep deformable image registration with local distance metrics for state-of-the-art cardiac motion tracking. In: Handels, H., Deserno, T., Maier, A., Maier-Hein, K., Palm, C., Tolxdorff, T. (eds.) Bildverarbeitung für die Medizin 2019. I, pp. 309–314. Springer, Wiesbaden (2019). https://doi.org/10.1007/978-3-658-25326-4_69
8. Hu, Y., et al.: Adversarial deformation regularization for training image registration neural networks. In: Frangi, A.F., Schnabel, J.A., Davatzikos, C., Alberola-López, C., Fichtinger, G. (eds.) MICCAI 2018. LNCS, vol. 11070, pp. 774–782. Springer, Cham (2018). https://doi.org/10.1007/978-3-030-00928-1_87
9. Siddiqui, M.M., et al.: Comparison of MR/ultrasound fusion–guided biopsy with ultrasound-guided biopsy for the diagnosis of prostate cancer. JAMA **313**(4), 390–397 (2015)
10. Valerio, M., et al.: New and established technology in focal ablation of the prostate: a systematic review. Eur. Urol. **71**(1), 17–34 (2017)
11. Lawrence, S., et al.: Neural network classification and prior class probabilities. In: Neural Networks: Tricks of the Trade, pp. 299–313 (1998)
12. Çiçek, Ö., Abdulkadir, A., Lienkamp, S.S., Brox, T., Ronneberger, O.: 3D U-Net: learning dense volumetric segmentation from sparse annotation. In: Ourselin, S., Joskowicz, L., Sabuncu, M.R., Unal, G., Wells, W. (eds.) MICCAI 2016. LNCS, vol. 9901, pp. 424–432. Springer, Cham (2016). https://doi.org/10.1007/978-3-319-46723-8_49
13. Webb, G.I.: Multiboosting: a technique for combining boosting and wagging. Mach. Learn. **40**(2), 159–196 (2000)
14. Webb, G.I., Conilione, P.: Estimating bias and variance from data. Pre-publication manuscript (2005). http://users.monash.edu/~webb/Files/WebbConilione06.pdf
15. Gibson, E., et al.: NiftyNet: a deep-learning platform for medical imaging. Comput. Methods Programs Biomed. **158**, 113–122 (2018)

On the Applicability of Registration Uncertainty

Jie Luo[1,2(✉)], Alireza Sedghi[3], Karteek Popuri[4], Dana Cobzas[5],
Miaomiao Zhang[6], Frank Preiswerk[1], Matthew Toews[7], Alexandra Golby[1],
Masashi Sugiyama[2,8], William M. Wells III[1], and Sarah Frisken[1]

[1] Brigham and Women's Hospital, Harvard Medical School, Boston, USA
jluo5@bwh.harvard.edu
[2] Graduate School of Frontier Sciences, The University of Tokyo, Tokyo, Japan
[3] School of Computing, Queen's University, Kingston, Canada
[4] School of Engineering Science, Simon Fraser University, Burnaby, Canada
[5] Computing Science Department, University of Alberta, Edmonton, Canada
[6] McKelvey School of Engineering, Washington University in St. Louis,
St. Louis, USA
[7] Ecole de Technologie Superieure, Montreal, Canada
[8] Center for Advanced Intelligence Project, RIKEN, Tokyo, Japan

Abstract. Estimating the uncertainty in (probabilistic) image registration enables, e.g., surgeons to assess the operative risk based on the trustworthiness of the registered image data. If surgeons receive inaccurately calculated registration uncertainty and misplace unwarranted confidence in the alignment solutions, severe consequences may result. For probabilistic image registration (PIR), the predominant way to quantify the registration uncertainty is using summary statistics of the distribution of transformation parameters. The majority of existing research focuses on trying out different summary statistics as well as means to exploit them. Distinctively, in this paper, we study two rarely examined topics: (1) whether those summary statistics of the transformation distribution most informatively represent the registration uncertainty; (2) Does utilizing the registration uncertainty always be beneficial. We show that there are two types of uncertainties: the transformation uncertainty, U_t, and label uncertainty U_l. The conventional way of using U_t to quantify U_l is inappropriate and can be misleading. By a real data experiment, we also share a potentially critical finding that making use of the registration uncertainty may not always be an improvement.

Keywords: Image registration · Registration uncertainty

1 Introduction

Non-rigid image registration is the foundation for many image-guided medical tasks [1,2]. However, given the current state of the registration technology and the difficulty of the problem, an uncertainty measure that highlights locations

© Springer Nature Switzerland AG 2019
D. Shen et al. (Eds.): MICCAI 2019, LNCS 11765, pp. 410–419, 2019.
https://doi.org/10.1007/978-3-030-32245-8_46

where the algorithm had difficulty finding a proper alignment can be very helpful. Among the approaches that characterize the uncertainty of non-rigid image registration, the most popular, or perhaps the most successful framework is the probabilistic image registration (PIR) [3–17].

In contrast to traditional "point-estimate" image registration approaches that report a unique set of transformation parameters that best align two images, PIR models transformation parameters as random variables and estimates distributions over them. The mode of the distribution is then chosen as the most likely value of that transformation parameter. PIR has the advantage that the registration uncertainty can be naturally obtained from the distribution of transformation parameters. PIR methods can be broadly categorized into discrete probabilistic registration (DPR) [3,7,8,13] and continuous probabilistic registration (CPR) [4–6,9–12,14–18].

Related Work. Registration uncertainty is a measure of confidence in image alignment solutions. In the PIR literature, the predominant way to quantify the registration uncertainty is using summary statistics of the transformation distribution. Applications of various summary statistics have been proposed in previous research: the Shannon entropy and its variants of the categorical transformation distribution were used to measure the registration uncertainty of DPR [7]; the variance [4,12,14], standard deviation [11], inter-quartile range [6,20] and the covariance Frobenius norm [10] of the transformation distribution were used to quantify the registration uncertainty of CPR. In order to visually assess the registration uncertainty, each of these summary statistics was either mapped to a color scheme, or an object overlaid on the registered image. By inspecting the color of voxels or the geometry of that object, end users can infer the registration uncertainty, which suggests the confidence they can place in the registration result. Utilizing the registration uncertainty is presumably an advantage of PIR [19–21], to date, the majority of existing research focuses on trying out different summary statistics and means to exploit the registration uncertainty.

Clinical Motivation. In image-guided neurosurgery, surgeons need to correctly understand the registration uncertainty so as to make better informed decisions, e.g., If the surgeon observes a large registration error at location A and small error at location B, without knowledge of registration uncertainty, s/he would most likely assume a large error everywhere and thus entirely ignore the registration. With an accurate knowledge of uncertainty, once the surgeon knows that A lies in an area of high uncertainty while B lies in an area of low uncertainty, s/he would have greater confidence in the registration at B and other locations of low uncertainty. If surgeons are influenced by inaccurate amount of registration uncertainty and place unwarranted confidence in the alignment solutions, severe consequences may result [6,19,20].

The majority of research takes the registration uncertainty for granted. In this paper, we investigate two rarely examined topics: (1) whether summary statistics of the transformation distribution most informatively reflect the registration uncertainty; (2) Does utilizing the registration uncertainty always be beneficial. In Sect. 2, we identify and discuss two types of uncertainties: the transformation uncertainty U_t and label uncertainty U_l. By concrete examples, we show that the conventional way of using U_t to quantify U_l is inappropriate and can be misleading. In Sect. 3, by a real data example, we share a potentially critical finding that making use of the registration uncertainty may not always be an improvement. Finally, we summarize in Sect. 4. It should be noted that registration uncertainty is not equal to registration accuracy. There are excellent works which study standards of registration evaluation [22–24]. However, here we focus on the relation among different types of registration uncertainty.

2   The Ambiguity of Registration Uncertainty

For illustration purpose, we use DPR in all examples.

2.1   The DPR Set up

In the DPR setting, let I_t and I_s respectively be the target and source images $I_t, I_s : \Omega_I \to \mathbb{R}, \Omega_I \subset \mathbb{R}^d, d = 2$ or 3. The algorithm discretizes the transformation space into a set of K displacement vectors, $\mathcal{D} = \{\mathbf{d}_k\}_{k=1}^K, \mathbf{d}_k \in \mathbb{R}^d$. These displacement vectors radiate from voxels on I_t and point to their candidate transformation locations on I_s [2]. For every voxel v_i, the algorithm computes a unity-sum probabilistic vector $\mathcal{P}(v_i) = \{P_k(v_i)\}_{k=1}^K$ as the transformation distribution. $P_k(v_i)$ is the probability of displacement vector $\mathbf{d}_k$. In a standard DPR, the algorithm takes a displacement vector that has the highest probability in $\mathcal{P}(v_i)$ as the most likely transformation $\mathbf{d}_m$.

Conventionally, the uncertainty of registered v_i is quantified by the Shannon entropy of $\mathcal{P}(v_i)$ [7]. Since the algorithm takes $\mathbf{d}_m$ as its "point-estimate", the entropy provides a measure of the extent of dispersion from $\mathbf{d}_m$ of the rest of displacement vectors in $\mathcal{D}$. If other displacement vectors are all as equally likely to occur as $\mathbf{d}_m$, then the entropy is maximal, which indicates that it is completely uncertain which displacement vector should be chosen as the most likely transformation. When the probability of $\mathbf{d}_m$ is much higher than that of other displacement vectors, the entropy decreases, and there is greater certainty that $\mathbf{d}_m$ is the correct choice.

For example, $\mathcal{P}(v_l) = [0.25, 0.25, 0.25, 0.25]$ and $\mathcal{P}(v_r) = [0.1, 0.7, 0.1, 0.1]$ are two discrete transformation distributions. $\mathcal{P}(v_l)$ is uniformly distributed, and its entropy is $E(\mathcal{P}(v_l)) = 2$. $\mathcal{P}(v_r)$ has an obvious peak, and its entropy is $E(\mathcal{P}(v_r)) \approx 1.36$, which is lower than $E(\mathcal{P}(v_l))$. For a registered voxel, the entropy of its transformation distribution is usually mapped to a color scheme, clinicians can infer the level of confidence of the registration result by the color of the voxel.

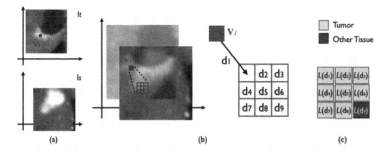

Fig. 1. (a) The target image I_t and souce image I_s; (b) The discretized transformation space $\mathcal{D}$; (c) The corresponding tissue label $L(\mathbf{d}_k)$ for $\mathcal{D}$.

2.2 Transformation Uncertainty and Label Uncertainty

In the context of neurosurgery, the goal of image registration is frequently to map the pre-operatively labeled tumor, and/or other tissue, onto the intra-operative patient space for resection. Since registration uncertainty is strongly linked to the goal of registration, here it should also reflect the confidence in the registered labels. However, does the conventional uncertainty measure of DPR, which is the entropy of transformation distribution, truly give insight into the trustworthiness of registered labels?

In a hypothetical DIR example, I_t and I_s in Fig. 1(a) are the intra-operative target and pre-operative source images, respectively. Voxel v_1 on I_t is the voxel we want to register. In Fig. 1(b), we can see that the discretized transformation space $\mathcal{D} = \{\mathbf{d}_k\}_{k=1}^9$ is a set of nine displacement vectors. Each displacement vector is linked to a candidate corresponding voxel of v_1. The labels $L(\mathbf{d}_k)$ are for voxels associated with $\mathbf{d}_k$. In this example, there are labels for the tumor and other tissue, as shown in Fig. 1(c).

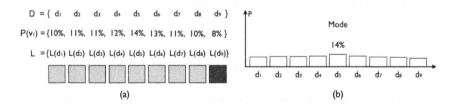

Fig. 2. (a) $\mathcal{P}(v_1)$ and corresponding labels; (b) The bar chart of $\mathcal{P}(v_1)$.

Figure 2 shows a transformation distribution $\mathcal{P}(v_1) = \{P_k(v_1)\}_{k=1}^9$ and its bar chart. We observe that $P_5(v_1)$ has the highest probability in $\mathcal{P}(v_1)$; therefore, $\mathbf{d}_5$'s corresponding label, $L(\mathbf{d}_5) = $ Tumor, will be assigned to the registered v_1.

Although $\mathcal{P}(v_1)$ has its mode at $P_5(v_1)$, the entire distribution is more or less uniformly distributed. The entropy of $\mathcal{P}(v_1)$, $E(\mathcal{P}(v_1)) \approx 3.15$, is close to the

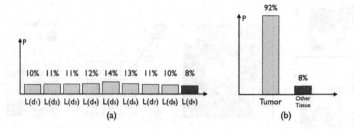

Fig. 3. (a) Bar chart of the transformation distribution $\mathcal{P}(v_1)$ taking into account $L(\mathbf{d_k})$; (b) The label distribution of the registered v_1.

maximum. Therefore, the conventional uncertainty measure will suggest that the registration uncertainty of v_1 is very high and highlight it with a bright color. Upon noticing the high degree of uncertainty in registered v_1, surgeons would place less confidence in its tumor label and make surgical plans accordingly.

On the other hand, let us take into account the label $L(\mathbf{d_k})$ associated with each $\mathbf{d_k}$ and form a label distribution. As shown in Fig. 3(a), even if $\mathbf{d_1}, \dots, \mathbf{d_8}$ are different displacement vectors, they correspond to the same label as the most likely displacement vector $\mathbf{d_5}$. If we accumulate the probability for all labels in $\mathcal{L}$, it is clear that "tumor" is the dominant one. Interestingly, despite being suggestive of having high registration uncertainty using the conventional uncertainty measure, the label distribution in Fig. 3(b) indicates that it is quite trustworthy to assign a tumor label to the registered v_1. In addition, the entropy of the label distribution is as low as 0.4, which also differs from the high entropy value computed from the transformation distribution.

In the example above, there appear to be two kinds of uncertainty. We name the uncertainty computed from the transformation distribution as the transformation uncertainty U_t, and the uncertainty relating to the goal of registration as label uncertainty U_l. Examples of U_l can be uncertainty in a categorical classification, or uncertainty in the intensity value of registered voxels.

In the PIR literature, the definition of registration uncertainty is ambiguous, because researchers do not differentiate U_t from U_l, and perhaps subconsciously use U_t to quantify U_l. The previous counter-intuitive example demonstrates that high U_t does not guarantee high U_l. In fact, the value of U_t can barely guarantee any useful information at all about the U_l.

More precisely, for point-estimate image registration, let Ω_T be the set of all estimated transformation, and Ω_L be the set of all possible corresponding labels (categorical labels or intensity values). The algorithm assigns a transformation $t \in \Omega_T$ to a voxel. By a non-linear function $f_{point}: \Omega_T \to \Omega_L$, the voxel will have its label $l \in \Omega_L$ as:

$$l = f_{point}(t). \tag{1}$$

In this case, the function f_{point} is surjective, and t always has a unique corresponding l. However, in the PIR setting, the voxel transformation becomes a random variable T. The corresponding label L is a function of T:

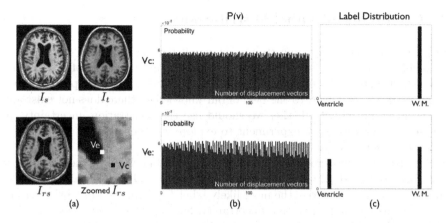

Fig. 4. (a) Input and result of the CUMC12 data example, v_c and v_e are two voxels of interest on the registered source image; (b) The transformation distribution of v_c and v_e in the DIR; (c) Label distributions of registered v_c and v_e.

$$L = f_{prob}(T). \tag{2}$$

therefore, it is also a random variable. Even if T and L are intuitively correlated, given different image context, there is no guaranteed analytical way to compute the uncertainty propagation from T to L. Thus it's inappropriate to measure the uncertainty of L, by the summary statistics of T.

In the registration community, researchers routinely distinguish between intensity match and e.g. DICE scores. It also makes sense to distinguish the transformation uncertainty and label uncertainty. In practice, U_t and U_l around certain areas, i.e., the tumor boundary, is quite dissimilar. Propagating U_t to the surgeon, as if it is the U_l can mislead them to place unwarranted confidence in the alignment solution and result in severe consequences.

Real Data Examples. As shown in Fig. 4, I_t and I_s are two brain MRI images arbitrarily chosen from the CUMC12 dataset. Subsequent to performing a DIR, we obtained the registered source image I_{rs}. The goal of this registration was to determine the categorical label, whether it is a ventricle or a white matter, for registered voxels of interest v_c and v_e. The transformation distribution of v_c is more uniformly distributed than that of v_e. Therefore, conventional entropy-based methods will report v_c as having higher registration uncertainty than v_e. However, as we form a label distribution in Fig. 4(c), it is clear that v_e, despite having a lower U_t, is assigned a label that is more uncertain. Examples that demonstrate the dissimilarity between U_t and U_l can be frequently found in the registration of various kind of images.

3   Credibility of Label Distribution

Utilizing the registration uncertainty, in particular the full label distribution, to benefit registration-based tasks is presumably an advantage of PIR. Many research of registration uncertainty reported positively over its impact in applications [19–21]. However, to the best of our knowledge, there does not exist any validation study about whether we should use the registration uncertainty. In this section, we design an experiment to explore whether utilizing the registration uncertainty always results in an improvement.

In PIR, the registered voxel has the corresponding label of the most likely transformation $L(\mathbf{d}_m)$, upon which the registration evaluation is also based [3–16]. Likewise, we can derive the most likely label L_m from the full label distribution. If utilizing the registration uncertainty, like reported in previous research, always be beneficial, then L_m should be always better than $L(\mathbf{d}_m)$.

In the following pilot experiment: an MRI image is arbitrarily chosen from the BRATS dataset [25] and synthetically deformed. Then we registered the original data with the deformed data using DIR. By doing so, we know the ground truth intensity for every registered voxel so that we can compare whether it is $L(\mathbf{d}_m)$ or L_m closer to the ground truth.

Here we are interested in the intensity label distributions of four registered voxels v_b, v_c, v_d and v_e, shown in Fig. 5(b), (c), (d), and (e) respectively. In Fig. 5, the red circle indicates the most likely intensity label L_m given by the full transformation distribution, the orange circle indicates the corresponding intensity label of the transformation mode $L(\mathbf{d}_m)$, and the green circle is the Ground Truth (GT). We observe that for v_b, L_m and $L(\mathbf{d}_m)$ are both equal to the GT. On the other hand, L_m and $I(\mathbf{d_m})$ for v_c, v_d and v_e, are not the same. As seen in Fig. 5(c), the L_m of the registered v_c is equal to the GT intensity, and is more accurate than $I(\mathbf{d_m})$. Yet, unexpectedly, for v_d and v_e, their $I(\mathbf{d_m})$ is closer to the GT than their L_m. Voxels such as v_d and v_e were found frequently in our experiments using other real data. This surprising result indicates that utilizing the full transformation distribution can actually give a poorer/less accurate estimation than using the transformation mode alone.

Researchers have attempted to present the visualized full label distribution of functional areas in fMRI to neurosurgeons [20]. However, based on the above finding, if L_m can give poorer estimation, the full label distribution might also have questionable credibility. Conveying such false information to surgeons would certainly be detrimental to the outcome of surgery.

It is noteworthy that in PIR, the estimation of T and L is influenced by the choice of hyper parameters, priors, and image context. Other PIR approaches can yield different findings. Nevertheless, studying the credibility of the label distribution before using it in practice warrants increased investigation.

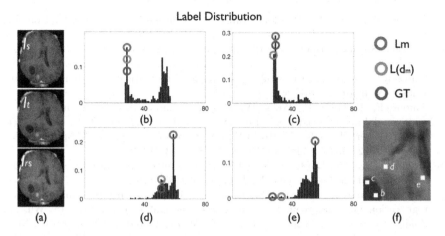

Fig. 5. (a) Input and result of the registration example; (b, c, d, e) Intensity label distributions of voxels v_b, v_c, v_d and v_e; (f) Approximate locations of tested voxels. (Color figure online)

4 Discussion

The majority of research takes the registration uncertainty for granted. We summarize current approaches of quantifying registration uncertainty and point out some fundamental problems which would make researchers rethink, or even rework approaches for quantifying and applying registration uncertainty.

At this stage, even the uncertainty is a useful addition to the registration result, we recommend treating it with caution: (1) It is advised to distinguish U_t and U_l in applications. Instead of using the unified term "registration uncertainty", i.e., we can use U_t to indicate the confidence for a predicted instrument location in neurosurgery; (2) Since the credibility of label distribution is unclear, we should avoid using U_l in clinical settings and put further effort in studying the implication of PIR results. We believe that this paper will serve as a foundation and draw more attention to this topic.

Acknowledgement. MS was supported by the International Research Center for Neurointelligence (WPI-IRCN) at The University of Tokyo Institutes for Advanced Study. This work was also supported by NIH grants P41EB015898, P41EB015902 and 5R01NS049251.

References

1. Maintz, J.B.A., Viergever, M.A.: A survey of medical image registration. Med. Image Anal. **2**(1), 1–36 (1998)
2. Sotiras, A., Davatzikos, C.: Deformable medical image registration: a survey. IEEE Trans. Med. Imaging **32**(7), 1153–1190 (2013)

3. Cobzas, D., Sen, A.: Random walks for deformable image registration. In: Fichtinger, G., Martel, A., Peters, T. (eds.) MICCAI 2011. LNCS, vol. 6892, pp. 557–565. Springer, Heidelberg (2011). https://doi.org/10.1007/978-3-642-23629-7_68

4. Simpson, I.J.A., et al.: Probabilistic inference of regularisation in non-rigid registration. NeuroImage. **59**, 2438–2451 (2012)

5. Janoos, F., Risholm, P., Wells, W.: Bayesian characterization of uncertainty in multi-modal image registration. In: Dawant, B.M., Christensen, G.E., Fitzpatrick, J.M., Rueckert, D. (eds.) WBIR 2012. LNCS, vol. 7359, pp. 50–59. Springer, Heidelberg (2012). https://doi.org/10.1007/978-3-642-31340-0_6

6. Risholm, P., et al.: Bayesian characterization of uncertainty in intra-subject non-rigid registration. Med. Image Anal. **17**(5), 538–555 (2013)

7. Lotfi, T., Tang, L., Andrews, S., Hamarneh, G.: Improving probabilistic image registration via reinforcement learning and uncertainty evaluation. In: Wu, G., Zhang, D., Shen, D., Yan, P., Suzuki, K., Wang, F. (eds.) MLMI 2013. LNCS, vol. 8184, pp. 187–194. Springer, Cham (2013). https://doi.org/10.1007/978-3-319-02267-3_24

8. Popuri, K., Cobzas, D., Jägersand, M.: A variational formulation for discrete registration. In: Mori, K., Sakuma, I., Sato, Y., Barillot, C., Navab, N. (eds.) MICCAI 2013. LNCS, vol. 8151, pp. 187–194. Springer, Heidelberg (2013). https://doi.org/10.1007/978-3-642-40760-4_24

9. Zhang, M., Singh, N., Fletcher, P.T.: Bayesian estimation of regularization and atlas building in diffeomorphic image registration. In: Gee, J.C., Joshi, S., Pohl, K.M., Wells, W.M., Zöllei, L. (eds.) IPMI 2013. LNCS, vol. 7917, pp. 37–48. Springer, Heidelberg (2013). https://doi.org/10.1007/978-3-642-38868-2_4

10. Wassermann, D., Toews, M., Niethammer, M., Wells, W.: Probabilistic diffeomorphic registration: representing uncertainty. In: Ourselin, S., Modat, M. (eds.) WBIR 2014. LNCS, vol. 8545, pp. 72–82. Springer, Cham (2014). https://doi.org/10.1007/978-3-319-08554-8_8

11. Simpson, I.J.A., et al.: Probabilistic non-linear registration with spatially adaptive regularisation. Med. Image Anal. **26**(1), 203–216 (2015)

12. Yang, X., Niethammer, M.: Uncertainty quantification for LDDMM using a low-rank Hessian approximation. In: Navab, N., Hornegger, J., Wells, W.M., Frangi, A.F. (eds.) MICCAI 2015. LNCS, vol. 9350, pp. 289–296. Springer, Cham (2015). https://doi.org/10.1007/978-3-319-24571-3_35

13. Heinrich, M.P., et al.: Deformable image registration by combining uncertainty estimates from supervoxel belief propagation. Med. Image Anal. **27**, 57–71 (2016)

14. Folgoc, L.L., et al.: Quantifying registration uncertainty with sparse Bayesian modelling. IEEE Trans. Image Process. **36**(2), 607–617 (2017)

15. Wang, J., Wells, W.M., Golland, P., Zhang, M.: Efficient Laplace approximation for Bayesian registration uncertainty quantification. In: Frangi, A.F., Schnabel, J.A., Davatzikos, C., Alberola-López, C., Fichtinger, G. (eds.) MICCAI 2018. LNCS, vol. 11070, pp. 880–888. Springer, Cham (2018). https://doi.org/10.1007/978-3-030-00928-1_99

16. Luo, J., et al.: A feature-driven active framework for ultrasound-based brain shift compensation. In: Frangi, A.F., Schnabel, J.A., Davatzikos, C., Alberola-López, C., Fichtinger, G. (eds.) MICCAI 2018. LNCS, vol. 11073, pp. 30–38. Springer, Cham (2018). https://doi.org/10.1007/978-3-030-00937-3_4

17. Dalca, A.V., Balakrishnan, G., Guttag, J., Sabuncu, M.R.: Unsupervised learning for fast probabilistic diffeomorphic registration. In: Frangi, A.F., Schnabel, J.A., Davatzikos, C., Alberola-López, C., Fichtinger, G. (eds.) MICCAI 2018. LNCS, vol. 11070, pp. 729–738. Springer, Cham (2018). https://doi.org/10.1007/978-3-030-00928-1_82

18. Sedghi, A., et al.: Semi-supervised image registration using deep learning. In: SPIE Medical Imaging, vol. 10951, p. 109511G (2019)

19. Risholm, P., Balter, J., Wells, W.M.: Estimation of delivered dose in radiotherapy: the influence of registration uncertainty. In: Fichtinger, G., Martel, A., Peters, T. (eds.) MICCAI 2011. LNCS, vol. 6891, pp. 548–555. Springer, Heidelberg (2011). https://doi.org/10.1007/978-3-642-23623-5_69

20. Risholm, P., Pieper, S., Samset, E., Wells, W.M.: Summarizing and visualizing uncertainty in non-rigid registration. In: Jiang, T., Navab, N., Pluim, J.P.W., Viergever, M.A. (eds.) MICCAI 2010. LNCS, vol. 6362, pp. 554–561. Springer, Heidelberg (2010). https://doi.org/10.1007/978-3-642-15745-5_68

21. Simpson, J.A., et al.: Ensemble learning incorporating uncertain registration. IEEE Trans. Med. Imaging $32(4)$, 748–756 (2013)

22. Rohlfing, T.: Image similarity and tissue overlaps as surrogates for image registration accuracy: widely used but unreliable. IEEE TMI $31(2)$, 153–163 (2012)

23. Fitzpatrick, J.M.: Fiducial registration error and target registration error are uncorrelated. In: Proceedings of SPIE, Medical Imaging 2009, vol. 7261 (2009) https://doi.org/10.1117/12.813601

24. Min, Z., et al.: Statistical model of total target registration error in image-guided surgery. IEEE Trans. Auto. Sci. Eng. $31(2)$, 1–15 (2019)

25. Menze, B.H., et al.: The multimodal brain tumor image segmentation benchmark (BRATS). IEEE Trans. Med. Imaging $34(10)$, 1993–2024 (2015)

DeepAtlas: Joint Semi-supervised Learning of Image Registration and Segmentation

Zhenlin Xu[✉] and Marc Niethammer

University of North Carolina, Chapel Hill, NC, USA
zhenlinx@cs.unc.edu

Abstract. Deep convolutional neural networks (CNNs) are state-of-the-art for semantic image segmentation, but typically require many labeled training samples. Obtaining 3D segmentations of medical images for supervised training is difficult and labor intensive. Motivated by classical approaches for joint segmentation and registration we therefore propose a deep learning framework that jointly learns networks for image registration and image segmentation. In contrast to previous work on deep unsupervised image registration, which showed the benefit of weak supervision via image segmentations, our approach can use existing segmentations when available and computes them via the segmentation network otherwise, thereby providing the same registration benefit. Conversely, segmentation network training benefits from the registration, which essentially provides a realistic form of data augmentation. Experiments on knee and brain 3D magnetic resonance (MR) images show that our approach achieves large simultaneous improvements of segmentation and registration accuracy (over independently trained networks) and allows training high-quality models with very limited training data. Specifically, in a one-shot-scenario (with only one manually labeled image) our approach increases Dice scores (%) over an unsupervised registration network by 2.7 and 1.8 on the knee and brain images respectively.

1 Introduction

Image segmentation and registration are two crucial tasks in medical image analysis. They are also highly related and can help each other. *E.g.*, labeled atlas images are used via image registration for segmentation. Segmentations can also provide extra supervision (in addition to image intensities) for image registration and are used to evaluate registration results. Consequentially, joint image registration and segmentation approaches have been proposed. *E.g.*, approaches based on active-contours [11] and Bayesian [7] or Markov random field formulations [6]. While these

---

Electronic supplementary material The online version of this chapter (https://doi.org/10.1007/978-3-030-32245-8_47) contains supplementary material, which is available to authorized users.

© Springer Nature Switzerland AG 2019
D. Shen et al. (Eds.): MICCAI 2019, LNCS 11765, pp. 420–429, 2019.
https://doi.org/10.1007/978-3-030-32245-8_47

methods jointly estimate registration and segmentation results, they operate on *individual* image pairs (instead of a population of images) and require the computationally costly minimization of an energy function.

Deep learning (DL) has been widely and successfully applied to medical image analysis. For supervised image segmentation, CNN-based approaches are faster and better than classical methods when many labeled training samples are available [5]. DL-based registration achieves similar performance to optimization-based approaches but is much faster. As true transformations are not available, training either uses estimates from optimization-based methods [10] or is unsupervised [2]. Recent work [3] shows that weak supervision via an additional image segmentation loss between registered images can improve results over unsupervised training, which relies on the images alone. In practice, obtaining segmentations for 3D medical images is difficult and labor intensive. Hence, manual segmentations will often not be available for a large fraction of image data.

We propose **DeepAtlas**, to jointly learn deep networks for weakly supervised registration and semi-supervised segmentation. Our contributions are:

- *We propose the first approach to jointly learn two deep neural networks for image registration and segmentation.* Previous joint approaches require joint optimizations for each image pair. Instead, we jointly learn from a population of images during training, but can independently use the resulting segmentation and registration networks at test time.
- *Our joint approach only requires few manual segmentations.* Our two networks mutually guide each other's training on unlabeled images via an anatomy similarity loss. This loss penalizes the dissimilarity of the warped segmentation of the moving image and the segmentation of the target image. When registering image pairs consisting of a manually labeled image and the estimate of a labeled image (via its network-predicted segmentation), this loss provides anatomy consistency supervision for registration and forces the predicted segmentation to match the manual segmentation after registration.
- *We evaluate our approach on large 3D brain and knee MRI datasets.* Using few manual segmentations, our method outperforms separately learned registration and segmentation networks. In the extreme case, where only one manually segmented image is available, our approach facilitates one-shot segmentation and boosts registration performance at the same time.

2   Method

Our goal is to improve registration and segmentation accuracy when few manual segmentations are available for a large set of images by jointly learning a segmentation and a registration network. Figure 1 illustrates our approach consisting of two parts: weakly-supervised registration learning (solid blue lines) and semi-supervised segmentation learning (dashed yellow lines). Our loss is the weighted sum of the registration regularization loss ($\mathcal{L}_r$), the image similarity loss ($\mathcal{L}_i$), the anatomy loss ($\mathcal{L}_a$) penalizing segmentation dissimilarity, and the supervised segmentation loss ($\mathcal{L}_{sp}$). The losses $\{\mathcal{L}_r, \mathcal{L}_i, \mathcal{L}_a\}$ drive the weakly supervised learning of registration (Sect. 2.1) and the losses $\{\mathcal{L}_a, \mathcal{L}_{sp}\}$ drive the semi-supervised learning of segmentation (Sect. 2.2). Section 2.3 details the implementation.

2.1   Weakly-Supervised Registration Learning

Given a pair of moving and target images I_m and I_t, a registration network $\mathcal{F}_R$ with parameters θ_r predicts a displacement field $\mathbf{u} = \mathcal{F}_R(I_m, I_t; \theta_r)$. This then allows warping the moving image to the target image space, $I_m^w = I_m \circ \Phi^{-1}$, where $\Phi^{-1} = \mathbf{u} + \mathrm{id}$ is the deformation map and id is the identity transform. A good map, Φ, maps related anatomical positions to each other. Unsupervised registration learning optimizes θ_r over an intensity similarity loss $\mathcal{L}_i$ (penalizing appearance differences between I_t and I_m^w) and a regularization loss $\mathcal{L}_r$ on $\mathbf{u}$ to encourage smooth transformations. Adding weak supervision by also matching segmentations between the target image (S_t) and the warped moving image $(S_m^w = S_m \circ \Phi^{-1})$ via an anatomy similarity loss $\mathcal{L}_a$ can improve registrations [3]. Weakly-supervised registration learning is then formulated as:

$$\theta_r^\star = \underset{\theta_r}{\mathrm{argmin}}\{\mathcal{L}_i(I_m \circ \Phi^{-1}, I_t) + \lambda_r \mathcal{L}_r(\Phi^{-1}) + \lambda_a \mathcal{L}_a(S_m \circ \Phi^{-1}, S_t)\}, \quad (1)$$

with weights $\lambda_r, \lambda_a \geq 0$. In practice, while a large set of images are often available, few of them have manual segmentations. In contrast to existing work, we estimate missing moving or target segmentations via our segmentation network (see Fig. 1). Hence, we provide weak supervision for *every* training image pair.

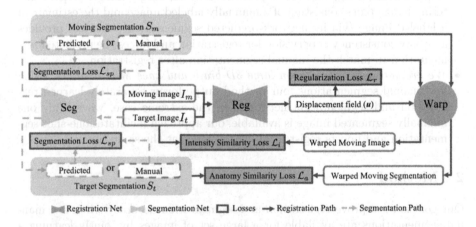

Fig. 1. *DeepAtlas* for joint learning of weakly supervised registration and semi-supervised segmentation. Unlabeled moving/target images are segmented by the segmentation network so that every training registration pair has weak supervision via the anatomy similarity loss which also guides segmentation learning on unlabeled images. (Color figure online)

2.2 Semi-supervised Segmentation Learning

The segmentation network $\mathcal{F}_S$ with parameters θ_s takes an image I as input and generates probabilistic segmentation maps for all semantic classes: $\hat{S} = \mathcal{F}_S(I; \theta_s)$. In addition to the typical supervised segmentation loss $\mathcal{L}_{sp}(\hat{S}, S)$ where S is a given manual segmentation, the anatomy similarity loss for registration $\mathcal{L}_a(S_m \circ \Phi^{-1}, S_t)$ also drives segmentation learning when S_m or S_t are predicted via $\mathcal{F}_S$ for unlabeled images. Specifically, we define these losses as:

$$\mathcal{L}_{seg} = \begin{cases} \lambda_a \mathcal{L}_a(S_m \circ \Phi^{-1}, \mathcal{F}_S(I_t)) + \lambda_{sp}\mathcal{L}_{sp}(\mathcal{F}_S(I_m), S_m), & \text{if } I_t \text{ is unlabeled;} \\ \lambda_a \mathcal{L}_a(\mathcal{F}_S(I_m) \circ \Phi^{-1}, S_t) + \lambda_{sp}\mathcal{L}_{sp}(\mathcal{F}_S(I_t), S_t), & \text{if } I_m \text{ is unlabeled;} \\ \lambda_a \mathcal{L}_a(S_m \circ \Phi^{-1}, S_t) + \lambda_{sp}\mathcal{L}_{sp}(\mathcal{F}_S(I_m), S_m), & \text{if } I_m \text{ and } I_t \text{ are labeled;} \\ 0, & \text{if both } I_t \text{ and } I_m \text{ are unlabeled.} \end{cases}$$

with weights $\lambda_a, \lambda_{sp} \geq 0$. $\mathcal{L}_a$ teaches $\mathcal{F}_S$ to segment an unlabeled image such that the predicted segmentation matches the manual segmentation of a labeled image via $\mathcal{F}_R$. In the case where the target image I_t is unlabeled, $\mathcal{L}_a$ is equivalent to a supervised segmentation loss on I_t, in which the single-atlas segmentation $S_m \circ \Phi^{-1}$ is the noisy true label. Note that we do not use two unlabeled images for training and $\mathcal{L}_a$ does not train the segmentation network when both images are labeled. We then train our segmentation network in a semi-supervised manner as follows:

$$\theta_s^\star = \underset{\theta_s}{\arg\min} \; \mathcal{L}_{seg}. \tag{2}$$

2.3 Implementation Details

Losses: Various choices are possible for the intensity/anatomy similarity, the segmentation, and the regularization losses. Our choices are as follows.

Anatomy Similarity and Supervised Segmentation Loss: A cross-entropy loss requires manually tuned class weights for imbalanced multi-class segmentations [8]. We use a soft multi-class Dice loss which addresses imbalances inherently:

$$\mathcal{L}_{dice}(S, S^\star) = 1 - \frac{1}{K} \sum_{k=1}^{K} \frac{\sum_x S_k(x) S_k^\star(x)}{\sum_x S_k(x) + \sum_x S_k^\star(x)}, \tag{3}$$

where k indicates a segmentation label (out of K) and x is voxel location. S and $S^\star$ are two segmentations to be compared.

Intensity Similarity Loss: We use normalized cross correlation (NCC) as:

$$\mathcal{L}_i(I_m^w, I_t) = 1 - NCC(I_m^w, I_t), \tag{4}$$

which will be in $[0, 2]$ and hence will encourage maximal correlation.

Regularization Loss: We use the bending energy [9]:

$$\mathcal{L}_r(\mathbf{u}) = \frac{1}{N} \sum_{\mathbf{x}} \sum_{i=1}^{d} \|H(u_i(\mathbf{x}))\|_F^2 \tag{5}$$

where $\| \cdot \|_F$ denotes the Frobenius norm, $H(u_i(\mathbf{x}))$ is the Hessian of the i-th component of $\mathbf{u}(\mathbf{x})$, and d denotes the spatial dimension ($d = 3$ in our case). N denotes the number of voxels. Note that this is a second-order generalization of diffusion regularization, where one penalizes $\|\nabla u_i(\mathbf{x})\|_2^2$ instead of $\|H(u_i(\mathbf{x}))\|_F^2$.

Alternating Training: It is in principle straightforward to optimize two networks according to Eqs. 1 and 2. However, as we work with the whole 3D images, not cropped patches, GPU memory is insufficient to simultaneously optimize the two networks in one forward pass. Hence, we alternately train one of the two networks while keeping the other fixed. We use a 1:20 ratio between training steps for the segmentation and registration networks, as the segmentation network converges faster. Since it is difficult to jointly train from scratch with unlabeled images, we independently pretrain both networks. When only few manual segmentations are available, *e.g.*, only one, separately training the segmentation network is challenging. In this case, we train the segmentation network from scratch using a fixed registration network trained unsupervisedly. We start alternating training when the segmentation network achieves reasonable performance.

Networks: DeepAtlas can use any CNN architecture for registration and segmentation. We use the network design of [2] for registration; and a customized light 3D U-Net design for segmentation with LeakyReLU instead of ReLU, and smaller feature size due to GPU memory limitations.

3   Experiments and Results

We show on a 3D knee and a 3D brain MRI dataset that our framework improves both registration and segmentation when many images with few manual segmentations are available: i.e. N of M images are labeled ($N \ll M$).

Mono-networks: We train single segmentation/registration models as baselines. For segmentation, fully supervised networks are trained with N labeled images; the registration networks are trained via Eq. 1 using all M training images with N images labeled; the anatomy similarity loss, $\mathcal{L}_a$, is only used for training pairs where both images have manual segmentations. Models trained with $N = M$ manual segmentations (*i.e.*, with manual segmentations for all images) provide our upper performance bound. All mono-networks are trained for a sufficient number of epochs until they over-fit. The best models based on validation performance are evaluated.

Moving   Target   Mono-0   Mono-5   DA-1   DA-5   Mono-200

Image   Manual Seg   DA-1   Mono-21   DA-21   Mono-65

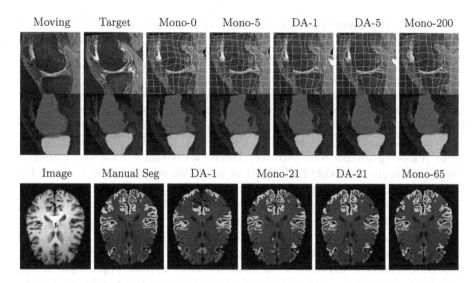

Fig. 2. Examples of knee MRI registration (top) and brain MRI segmentation (bottom) results. **Top:** The first two columns are the moving image/segmentation and the target image/segmentation followed by the warped moving images (with deformation grids)/segmentations by different models. **Bottom left to right:** original image, manual segmentation, and predictions of various models. Mono-i and DA-i represent the mono- and DA models with i manual segmentations respectively.

DeepAtlas (DA): We initialize the joint model with the trained mono-networks. In addition to the alternately trained DA models, we hold one network fixed all through training, termed **Semi-DeepAtlas (Semi-DA)**.

In one-shot learning (N = 1) experiments, training a supervised segmentation network based on a single labeled image is difficult; hence, we do not compute a segmentation mono-network in this case. For Semi-DA, we train a segmentation network from scratch with a fixed registration network that is trained unsupervised (N = 0). The DA model is initialized using the Semi-DA segmentation network and the unsupervised registration network.

Knee MRI Experiment: We test our method on 3D knee MRIs from the Osteoarthritis Initiative (OAI)[1] and corresponding segmentations of femur and tibia as well as femoral and tibial cartilage [1]. From a total of 507 labeled images, we use 200 for training, 53 for validation, and 254 for testing. To test registration performance we use 10,000 random image pairs from the test set. All images are affinely registered to an atlas built from the training images, resampled to isotropic spacing of 1 mm, cropped to $160 \times 160 \times 160$ and intensity normalized to $[0, 1]$. In addition, right knee images are flipped to be consistent with left knees. For training, the loss weights are $\lambda_r = 20{,}000$, $\lambda_a = 3$, and $\lambda_{sp} = 3$ based on

---

[1] https://nda.nih.gov/oai/.

approximate hyper-parameter tuning. Note that when computing $\mathcal{L}_r$ from the displacements, the image coordinates are scaled to $[-1, 1]$ for each dimension following the convention in the interpolation function of PyTorch.

Brain MRI Experiment: We also evaluate our method on the MindBoogle101 [4] brain MRIs with 32 cortical regions. We fuse corresponding segmentation labels of the left and right brain hemispheres. MindBoogle101 consists of images from multiple datasets, *e.g.*, OASIS-TRT-20, MMRR-21 and HLN-12. After removing images with incorrect labels, we obtain a total of 85 images. We use 5 images from OASIS-TRT-20 as validation set and 15 as test set. We use the remaining 65 images for training. Manual segmentations in the $N = 1$ and $N = 21$ experiments are only from the MMRR-21 subset; this simulates a common practical use case, where we only have few manual segmentations for one dataset and additional unlabeled images from other datasets, but desire to process a different, new dataset. All images are 1 mm isotropic, affinely-aligned, histogram-matched, and cropped to size $168 \times 200 \times 169$. We apply sagittal flipping for training data augmentation. We use the same loss weights as for the knee MRI experiment except for $\lambda_r = 5,000$, since cross-subject brain registrations require large deformations and hence less regularization.

Table 1. Segmentation and registration performance on 3D knee MRIs. Average (standard deviation) of Dice scores (%) for bones (femur and tibia) and cartilages (femoral and tibial). N of 200 training images are manually labeled.

N	Models	Segmentation Dice (%)			Registration Dice (%)		
		Bones	Cartilages	All	Bones	Cartilages	All
0	Mono	–	–	–	95.32(1.13)	65.71(5.86)	80.52(3.24)
1	Semi-DA	96.43(0.85)	76.67(3.24)	86.55(1.86)	–	–	–
	DA	**96.80(0.81)**	**77.63(3.22)**	**87.21(1.84)**	95.76(1.01)	70.77(5.68)	83.27(3.14)
5	Mono	96.51(1.69)	78.95(3.91)	87.73(2.37)	95.60(1.08)	68.13(5.98)	81.87(3.31)
	Semi-DA	96.97(1.26)	79.73(3.84)	88.35(2.22)	**96.38(0.81)**	73.48(5.26)	84.93(2.89)
	DA	**97.49(0.67)**	**80.35(3.64)**	**88.92(2.01)**	96.35(0.82)	**73.67(5.22)**	**85.01(2.86)**
10	Mono	97.29(1.03)	80.59(3.67)	88.94(2.07)	95.77(1.02)	69.45(5.93)	82.61(3.27)
	Semi-DA	97.60(0.76)	**81.21(3.58)**	89.40(1.99)	**96.66(0.72)**	74.67(5.01)	**85.66(2.73)**
	DA	**97.70(0.65)**	81.19(3.47)	**89.45(1.91)**	96.62(0.75)	**74.69(5.03)**	85.66(2.75)
200	Mono	98.24(0.34)	83.54(2.93)	90.89(1.56)	96.98(0.56)	77.33(4.34)	87.16(2.35)

Optimizer: We use Adam. The initial learning rates are 1e−3 for the mono-networks. Initial learning rates are 5e−4 for the registration network and 1e−4 for the segmentation network for Semi-DA and DA. Learning rates decay by 0.2 at various epochs across experiments. We use PyTorch and run on Nvidia V100 GPUs with 16 GB memory.

Results: All trained networks are evaluated using Dice overlap scores between predictions and the manual segmentations for the segmentation network, or between the warped moving segmentations and the target segmentations for the registration network. Tables 1 and 2 show results for the knee and brain MRI experiments respectively in Dice scores (%). Figure 2 shows examples of knee MRI registrations and brain MRI segmentations.

General Results: For both datasets across different numbers of manual segmentations, Semi-DA, which uses a fixed pre-trained network to help the training of the other network, boosts performance compared to separately trained mono-networks. DA, where both networks are alternately trained, achieves even better Dice scores in most cases. Based on a Mann-Whitney U-test with a significance level of 0.05 and a correction for multiple comparisons with a false discovery rate of 0.05, our models (DA/Semi-DA) result in significantly larger Dice scores than the mono-networks for all experiments. This demonstrates that segmentation and registration networks can indeed help each other by providing estimated supervision on unlabeled data.

Knee Results: On knee MRIs, our method improves segmentation scores over separately learned networks by about 1.2 and 0.5, and registration scores increase by about 3.1 and 3.0, when training with 5 and 10 manual segmentation respectively. Especially for the challenging cartilage structures, our joint learning boosts segmentation by 1.4 and 0.7, and registration by 5.5 and 5.2 for $N = 5$ and $N = 10$ respectively.

Brain Results: Dice scores for segmentation and registration increase by about 2.6 and 3.5 respectively for the cortical structures of the brain MRIs.

One-Shot Learning: In the one-shot experiments on both datasets, reasonable segmentation performance is achieved; moreover, DA increases the Dice score over unsupervised registration by about 2.7 and 1.8 on the knee and brain data respectively. This demonstrates the effectiveness of our framework for one-shot learning.

Qualitative Results: DA achieves more anatomically consistent registrations than the mono-networks on the knee (Fig. 2) and Brain MRI samples (see supplementary material).

4   Conclusion

We presented our DeepAtlas framework for joint learning of segmentation and registration networks using only few images with manual segmentations. By introducing

Table 2. Segmentation and registration performance on 3D brain MRIs. Average (Standard deviation) of Dice scores (%) for 31 cortical regions. N of 65 training images are manually labeled.

N	Models	Seg Dice (%)	Reg Dice (%)
0	Mono	–	54.75(2.37)
1	Semi-DA	61.19(1.49)	–
	DA	**61.22(1.40)**	56.54(2.32)
21	Mono	73.48(2.58)	59.47(2.34)
	Semi-DA	75.63(1.66)	62.92(2.14)
	DA	**76.06(1.50)**	**62.92(2.13)**
65	Mono	81.31(1.21)	63.25(2.07)

an anatomical similarity loss, the learned registrations are more anatomically consistent. Furthermore, the segmentation network is guided by a form of data augmentation provided via the registration network on unlabeled images. For both bone/cartilage structures in knee MRIs and cortical structures in brain MRIs, our approach shows large improvements over separately learned networks. When only given one manual segmentation, our method provides one-shot segmentation learning and greatly improves registration. This demonstrates that one network can benefit from imperfect supervision on unlabeled data provided by the other network. Our approach provides a general solution to the lack of manual segmentations when training segmentation and registration networks. For future work, introducing uncertainty measures for the segmentation and registration networks may help alleviate the effect of poor predictions of one network on the other. It would also be of interest to investigate multitask learning via layer sharing for the segmentation and registration networks. This may further improve performance and decrease model size.

Acknowledgements. Research reported in this publication was supported by the National Institutes of Health (NIH) and the National Science Foundation (NSF) under award numbers NSF EECS1711776 and NIH 1R01AR072013. The content is solely the responsibility of the authors and does not necessarily represent the official views of the NIH or the NSF.

References

1. Ambellan, F., Tack, A., Ehlke, M., Zachow, S.: Automated segmentation of knee bone and cartilage combining statistical shape knowledge and convolutional neural networks: data from the osteoarthritis initiative. MedIA **52**(2), 109–118 (2019). https://doi.org/10.1016/j.media.2018.11.009
2. Balakrishnan, G., Zhao, A., Sabuncu, M.R., Guttag, J., Dalca, A.V.: An unsupervised learning model for deformable medical image registration. In: CVPR, pp. 9252–9260 (2018)
3. Balakrishnan, G., Zhao, A., Sabuncu, M.R., Guttag, J., Dalca, A.V.: Voxelmorph: a learning framework for deformable medical image registration. IEEE TMI (2019)
4. Klein, A., Tourville, J.: 101 labeled brain images and a consistent human cortical labeling protocol. Front. Neurosci. **6**, 171 (2012). https://doi.org/10.3389/fnins.2012.00171
5. Litjens, G., et al.: A survey on deep learning in medical image analysis. MedIA **42**, 60–88 (2017)
6. Mahapatra, D., Sun, Y.: Joint registration and segmentation of dynamic cardiac perfusion images using MRFs. In: Jiang, T., Navab, N., Pluim, J.P.W., Viergever, M.A. (eds.) MICCAI 2010. LNCS, vol. 6361, pp. 493–501. Springer, Heidelberg (2010). https://doi.org/10.1007/978-3-642-15705-9_60
7. Pohl, K.M., Fisher, J., Grimson, W.E.L., Kikinis, R., Wells, W.M.: A Bayesian model for joint segmentation and registration. NeuroImage **31**(1), 228–239 (2006)
8. Ronneberger, O., Fischer, P., Brox, T.: U-Net: convolutional networks for biomedical image segmentation. In: Navab, N., Hornegger, J., Wells, W.M., Frangi, A.F. (eds.) MICCAI 2015. LNCS, vol. 9351, pp. 234–241. Springer, Cham (2015). https://doi.org/10.1007/978-3-319-24574-4_28

9. Rueckert, D., Sonoda, L.I., Hayes, C., Hill, D.L.G., Leach, M.O., Hawkes, D.J.: Nonrigid registration using free-form deformations: application to breast MR images. IEEE TMI **18**(8), 712–721 (1999). https://doi.org/10.1109/42.796284

10. Yang, X., Kwitt, R., Styner, M., Niethammer, M.: Quicksilver: fast predictive image registration - a deep learning approach. NeuroImage **158**, 378–396 (2017)

11. Yezzi, A., Zollei, L., Kapur, T.: A variational framework for joint segmentation and registration. In: MMBIA, pp. 44–51, December 2001. https://doi.org/10.1109/MMBIA.2001.991698

Linear Time Invariant Model Based Motion Correction (LiMo-MoCo) of Dynamic Radial Contrast Enhanced MRI

Jaume Coll-Font[1,2(✉)] ⓘ, Onur Afacan[1,2], Jeanne Chow[1,2], and Sila Kurugol[1,2]

[1] Boston Children's Hospital, Boston, MA, USA
[2] Harvard Medical School, Boston, MA, USA
jaume.coll-font@childrens.harvard.edu

Abstract. Early identification of kidney function deterioration is essential to determine which newborn patients with dilation of the renal pelvis (hydronephrosis) should undergo surgery. Kidney function can be measured by fitting a tracer kinetic (TK) model onto a series of Dynamic Contrast Enhanced (DCE) MR images and deriving the glomerular filtration rate (GFR) from the TK model. Unfortunately, heavy breathing and large bulk motion events create outliers and misalignments that introduce large errors in the TK estimates. Moreover, aligning the series of DCE images is not trivial due to the contrast differences between them and the undersampling artifacts due to fast imaging. We present a bulk motion detection and a linear time invariant (LTI) model-based motion correction approach for DCE-MRI alignment that leverages the temporal dynamics of the DCE data at each voxel. We evaluate our approach on 10 newborn patients that underwent DCE imaging without sedation. For each patient, we reconstructed the sequence of DCE images, detected and removed the volumes corrupted by motion using a self navigation approach, aligned the sequence using our approach and fitted the TK model to compute GFR. The results show that our approach correctly aligned all volumes and improved the TK model fit and, on average, reducing the normalized root-mean-squared error by 0.17.

1 Introduction

Congenital anomalies of the urinary tract, the most common being urinary tract dilation or hydronephrosis, is found in 2 to 7% of all maternal ultrasounds and can lead to chronic renal insufficiency (CRI). In these newborn patients, surgical intervention is indicated when there is clear evidence of renal function deterioration and delays in intervention can lead to potential lifelong complications and CRI. Hence, timely determination of which patients should undergo surgery is important to reduce the risk of developing CRI. The best measures of kidney function are glomerular filtration rate (GFR) and differential renal function. Dynamic Contrast Enhanced (DCE) MRI is a technology with great potential to simultaneously evaluate kidney function (GFR and DRF) and anatomy

D. Shen et al. (Eds.): MICCAI 2019, LNCS 11765, pp. 430–437, 2019.
https://doi.org/10.1007/978-3-030-32245-8_48

without ionizing radiation. DCE-MR imaging acquires a temporal sequence of volumes after injection of a contrast agent (CA) into the patient's bloodstream and kidney function is then measured by fitting a tracer kinetic (TK) model onto the series of DCE MR images. Unfortunately, current DCE methods are sensitive to motion and do not provide the high temporal resolution (3 s/volume) that is necessary to capture the rapidly changing dynamics of the arterial input function (AIF)—i.e. the input to the TK model that is necessary for accurate computation of kidney function.

Recent advances in MR imaging such as radial sampling and compressed-sensing (CS) reconstruction have allowed to attain sufficient spatio-temporal resolution to be able to reliably fit the TK model and estimate the GFR. However, there are still limitations that impede the accurate assessment of kidney function with DCE-MRI in clinical practice. One of them is motion due to breathing or changes of position of the subject, which cause miss-alignment of the voxels across time and introduces error in the TK model fit. These complications are particularly acute when imaging newborns, for whom sedation is avoided and who cannot hold their breath. Alignment of images in the DCE-MRI sequence acquired with radial sampling is especially challenging due to major contrast differences between volumes and low quality of the images due to presence of streaking artifacts from undersampling. Previous methods have attempted to register the sequence of volumes by reducing a PCA metric on the temporal covariance [5] or by registering onto templates generated using a TK model [1,8]. These methods, either implicitly or explicitly, model the temporal behavior of the DCE-MR signal to align the sequence of images. However, linear models like PCA are too simple to capture the behavior of DCE-MR data with presence of noise and TK models are too specific to the organs of interest to be fitted to the entire field of view (FOV) and the non-linear optimizations on which they depend are prone to converge to local minima, specially under the presence of noise.

Here, we introduce a new linear time invariant (LTI) model-based method to co-register a sequence of DCE volumes. Our method approximates the temporal behaviour of the CA in each patient as the response of an LTI system to an input—i.e. AIF. We iteratively fit the LTI model to the data, reconstruct template volumes from the LTI model and register each acquired volume to its corresponding template. Differently from other models, the LTI model is capable of accurately characterizing the organs of interest as well as the rest of the tissue. Moreover, it can be fitted with convex optimization that does not depend on an accurate initialization to converge to a global minimum.

2 Methods

Our registration approach is inspired by previous methods that use a TK model prior to register the sequence of volumes. These models characterize the signal intensity change due to CA in the tissue as the convolution of the AIF ($a(t)$) with a system response ($h(t)$). For example, Sourbron introduced the "seperable two-compartment" model, which characterizes the impulse response in the kidneys with Eq. (1).

$$h(t) = \frac{1}{T_P}e^{-t/T_P} + \frac{F_E}{T_P}e^{-t/T_P} * e^{-t/T_E}, \tag{1}$$

where T_P, T_E, F_E, F_P are the parameters of the model [9]. Unfortunately, estimating the parameters of such models requires solving a non-linear least-squares optimization, which can lead to convergence to local minima. Especially under the presence of streaking artifacts and large motion, this method is not robust and therefore results in inaccurate priors for registration.

2.1   LTI Model for Tissue Contrast Enhancement

Our approach overcomes this limitation with two modifications: an LTI model for $h(t)$ and a convex optimization to estimate its parameters without risk of converging into local minima. Hence, our model characterizes the DCE-MR data $s(t)$ as the convolution of the AIF with the impulse response of an LTI system ($s(t) = h(t) * a(t)$). Specifically, we approximate $h(t)$ as a sum of first-order, strictly proper transfer functions ($g_{p_k}(t)$) with poles (p_k) restricted to a low frequency section of the unit disk $\mathcal{D}_\rho$—with normalized frequency below $\rho = 0.014$. The resulting impulse response ($h(t) = \sum_{p_k \in \mathcal{D}_1} c_k g_{p_k}(t)$) decays over time and does not allow for large oscillations, matching the expected behavior of DCE-MR data.

To determine the exact form of $h(t)$, it is then necessary to find the minimum number of coefficients $c_k \in \mathcal{C}$ and transfer functions $g_{p_k}(t)$ that satisfy $s(t) = \sum_{p_k \in \mathcal{D}_\rho} c_k g_{p_k}(t) * a(t)$. To solve this problem, we use the system identification method by Yilmaz's et $al.$ [11]. This method solves a convex relaxation of the original l_0 norm minimization problem (Eq. 2) and uses a randomized version of the Frank-Wolfe algorithm [6] to optimize over all possible $p_k \in \mathcal{D}_\rho$.

$$\min_{\mathbf{c}} \sum_t \left[\sum_{p_k \in \mathcal{D}_\rho} c_k g_{p_k}(t) * a(t) - s(t) \right]^2 \qquad st. \sum_k |c_k| \leq \tau \tag{2}$$

In short, at every iteration k, the algorithm selects N random poles $p_n \in \mathcal{D}_\rho$, computes their corresponding impulse responses $\{g_{p_n}(t)\}_{n=0}^{N-1}$, and picks the one most aligned with the descent direction. Then, it updates the coefficients c_k such that $f(h^{k+1}) = \sum_t \left[h^{k+1}(t) * a(t) - s(t) \right]^2$ is minimized with $h^{k+1}(t) = h^k(t) + c_k g_{p_k}$.

The LTI model for DCE-MR data requires an AIF, $a(t)$, which is not typically known a priori and must be extracted from the data. In order to estimate it, we use the LTI model on the voxels that correspond to the aorta, now using a delta function as an input. First, we select the relevant voxels with a precomputed aorta mask, then we cluster them with K-means ($K = 10$) and, finally, we fit the LTI model to the mean signal from each cluster. This procedure provides denoised time intensity curves of the aorta, from which we select final AIF as the intensity curve with the highest peak to minimize the effect of inflow artifacts. Once the AIF is computed, we use it as an input function to the LTI model and fit the model to the rest of the tissue voxels. To reduce computational demands and noise, we also cluster the voxels within the tissue with K-means ($K = 1000$ clusters per slice) and fit the LTI model to each cluster mean.

2.2 LTI Model Based Groupwise Registration

The proposed registration algorithm, shown in Algorithm 1, consists of iteratively fitting the LTI model to the data and then registering each volume to its corresponding template generated with the LTI model. This iterative method is repeated until convergence of the registration parameters. However, we have observed that after 2 iterations, the diminishing returns in the quality of the registration are outweighted by the computational time required by the model fit and we terminate the optimization. To register each volume, our algorithm allows to choose any interpolation or optimization metric in the registration step—e.g. rigid or non-rigid registration, intensity or information based metrics and register the entire FOV or only the organs of interest. In this implementation, we choose to use a non-rigid registration using mutual information as an optimization metric. In particular, we used a 3rd order B-spline interpolation (spacing of 28 mm) with "AdvancedMattesMutualInformation" metric implemented in ELASTIX [7].

Algorithm 1. LiMo-MoCo

1: **procedure** LIMO($s(t)$)   ▷ DCE sequence s(t)
2:      $r(t) \leftarrow s(t)$ ▷ Initialize registered sequence
3:      **for** $i = 1, 2, \ldots I_{max}$ **do**
4:          estimate AIF
5:          **for** $sl = 1 \ldots S$ **do**   ▷ For each slice
6:              Cluster voxels in $r(t, sl)$ with K-means
7:              Fit LTI model to cluster means
8:              generate LTI template $m(t)$
9:              $r(t) \leftarrow reg(s(t), m(t))$ ▷ Register $s(t)$ to $m(t)$
10:      Interpolate bad volumes with $m(t)$
11:      **return** x_k

After registering the sequence of volumes, we correct those volumes that have been corrupted by rapid motion events. To that objective we use an outlier rejection algorithm that leverages the center of raw k-space data acquired with "stack-of-stars" [2] sampling scheme. This algorithm takes the signal acquired at the center of k-space with each spoke—i.e. the center of each line traversing k-space radially—and determines that a spoke is corrupted when its correlation with neighboring spokes decreases below a threshold. With this algorithm, we detected the volumes that included corrupted spokes and substituted them with the template volumes generated with the LTI model.

3   Experiments

We evaluated our algorithm on data from 10 infants with hydronephrosis (age 0–4 months) that underwent DCE-MRI of their kidneys. The data acquisition was done following IRB approval and with consent. The infants were fed, swaddled and rocked to sleep without sedation. We imaged each subject with a stack-of-stars sampling scheme and reconstructed the sequence of volumes with GRASP, a CS technique that uses total-variation regularization over time [4]. We used 34 k-space spokes per slice, leading to an average temporal resolution of 3.3 s. We then applied the proposed LiMo-MoCo Algorithm 1 for motion correction.

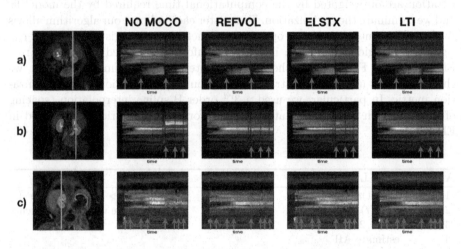

Fig. 1. Temporal evolution of the intensity of a line of voxels for three subjects. The first column shows a coronal image with the line of voxels marked in red as reference. The rest of the columns show the temporal evolution of the line of voxels for No-MoCo, REFVOL, gPCA and the proposed LiMo-MoCo, respectively. Green arrows indicate volumes corrupted by sudden motion. (Color figure online)

We evaluated the quality of the registration algorithm based on the TK model fit on the average time intensity curves throughout each kidney. Volume sequences with large outliers or changes in position will increase the TK fitting error, in contrast, proper detection of outliers and correction of motion will reduce it. Hence, we fitted the TK model (Eq. 1) to the data and computed the normalized root-mean-square error (nRMSE) of the fit. For each kidney we used wild bootstrap to estimate the variance of the nRMSE [3] and determined statistical significance of the results with the Wilcoxon statistical test [10].

We compared the results of the LiMo-MoCo against no motion compensation (No MoCo), registration to a fixed reference volume (REFVOL)[1] and a PCA-based groupwise registration for quantitative MRI (gPCA) [5]. For all cases, we used non-rigid registration with B-spline interpolation implemented in ELASTIX [7].

4   Results

Figure 1 shows the evolution in time of a line of voxels in a volume for three subjects. Without MoCo, all subjects showed different degrees of motion: (a) presented little motion in the form of oscillations, (b) motion events with corruption of volumes and large displacements and (c) small but continuous motion that corrupted several volumes.

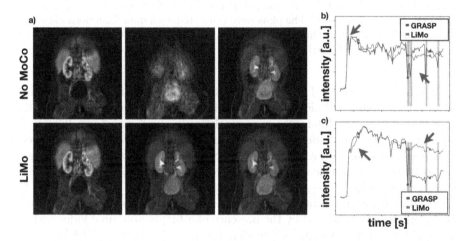

Fig. 2. (a) Coronal images at three different time instances of subject (b) for before alignment (top) and after aligning with LiMo-MoCo. Red and green marks indicate the voxels used to generate time intensity curves of the right panels. (b) and (c) show the time intensity curves of the areas marked in red (top) and green (bottom) in the coronal images for No MoCo and LiMo-MoCo. (Color figure online)

All MoCo algorithms recovered the continuity of the voxel intensities over time. However, the corrupted volumes—marked with green arrows—remained dark and some alignment errors prevailed. LiMo-MoCo corrects those displacements and impaints the outliers, hence correcting the time intensity curves in each voxel. These errors are more apparent in areas with small anatomical features, such as the aorta, where the signal shows large deviations after motion events. We illustrate this effect in Fig. 2 with the coronal plots over time and the time intensity curves of subject (b). The displacements and outliers observed in

---

[1] Determined as the volume with least motion detected by the center-of-k-space metric.

the coronal images create large deviations in intensity of the voxels near boundaries and eliminate the initial intensity peak in some voxels on the aorta.

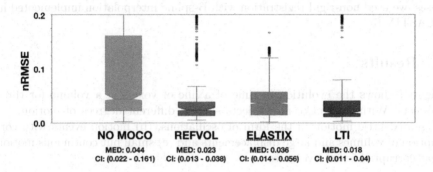

Fig. 3. Normalized Root Mean Squared Error for all four approaches (No MoCo, REFVOL, gPCA and LiMo). The plots were generated with data from both kidneys in 10 subjects and after applying wild bootstrap. Medians and 95% confidence intervals of each method are indicated below each box.

We show the numerical results in the nRMSE boxplots of Fig. 3. The median nRMSE for No MoCo, REFVOL, gPCA and LiMo are, respectively, 0.044, 0.023, 0.036 and 0.018. All differences were statistically significant ($p < 0.005$). As expected, there is a considerable decrease in nRMSE of all registration methods with respect to No MoCo. The median error of all MoCo methods was near the bottom 95% confidence interval of the No MoCo results. However, all MoCo algorithms exhibited heavy tails with considerable number of outliers: 300 for REFVOL, 107 for gPCA and 101 for LiMo. From those outliers, ~100 of them in each method were produced by the presence of a highly abnormal kidney whose signal did not match Sourbrone's model. The rest of outliers in REFVOL were caused by the failed alignment of a subject.

The results presented show that it is beneficial to apply alignment of any kind to the DCE-MR image sequences. However, including a model to enforce temporal consistency introduces robustness to the spurious bad registrations like the ones observed in the outliers of REFVOL. Moreover, including models tailored to DCE-MR data further improves the alignment and allows to interpolate volumes corrupted due to sudden motion. Future work should inform the LTI model fitting procedure about which volumes have been corrupted by sudden motion and make it robust to those.

5 Conclusions

We present a model-based approach to align temporal sequences of DCE volumes. Our approach characterizes the DCE data over time as the response of an LTI system to the contrast agent injected. It iteratively fits this model and registers the acquired volumes to the fitted model. We tested this approach on newborn patients that underwent DCE MRI for kidney function assessment and evaluated the improvement in TK model fit. The results suggest our approach provides better accuracy in TK model fitting and that correct alignment of the aorta is key to successful evaluation of GFR.

Acknowledgements. This work was supported partially by the Boston Children's Hospital Translational Research Program Pilot Grant 2018, Society of Pediatric Radiology Multi-center Research Grant 2019, Crohn's and Colitis Foundation of America's (CCFA) Career Development Award and AGA-Boston Scientific Technology and Innovation Award 2018 and by NIDDK of the National Institutes of Health under award number R01DK100404.

References

1. Buonaccorsi, G.A., et al.: Tracer kinetic model-driven registration for dynamic contrast-enhanced MRI time-series data. Magn. Reson. Med. **58**(5), 1010–1019 (2007). https://doi.org/10.1002/mrm.21405
2. Coll-Font, J., et al.: Self-navigated bulk motion detection for feed and wrap renal dynamic radial VIBE DCE-MRI. In: ISMRM (2019)
3. Davidson, R., Flachaire, E.: The wild bootstrap, tamed at last. J. Econom. **146**(1), 162–169 (2008). https://doi.org/10.1016/J.JECONOM.2008.08.003
4. Feng, L., et al.: Golden-angle radial sparse parallel MRI: combination of compressed sensing, parallel imaging, and golden-angle radial sampling for fast and flexible dynamic volumetric MRI. Magn. Reson. Med. **72**(3), 707–717 (2014). https://doi.org/10.1002/mrm.24980
5. Huizinga, W., et al.: PCA-based groupwise image registration for quantitative MRI. Med. Image Anal. **29**, 65–78 (2016). https://doi.org/10.1016/j.media.2015.12.004
6. Jaggi, M.: Revisiting Frank-Wolfe: projection-free sparse convex optimization. In: Proceedings of the 30th International Conference on Machine Learning, vol. 28, pp. 427–435 (2013)
7. Klein, S., et al.: Elastix: a toolbox for intensity-based medical image registration. IEEE Trans. Med. Imaging **29**(1), 196–205 (2010). https://doi.org/10.1109/TMI.2009.2035616
8. Kurugol, S., et al.: Motion-robust parameter estimation in abdominal diffusion-weighted MRI by simultaneous image registration and model estimation. Med. Image Anal. **39**, 124–132 (2017). https://doi.org/10.1016/J.MEDIA.2017.04.006
9. Sourbron, S.P., et al.: MRI-measurement of perfusion and glomerular filtration in the human kidney with a separable compartment model. Invest. Radiol. **43**(1), 40–48 (2008). https://doi.org/10.1097/RLI.0b013e31815597c5
10. Wilcoxon, F.: Individual comparisons by ranking methods. Biometrics Bull. **1**(6), 80 (1945)
11. Yilmaz, B., et al.: A randomized algorithm for parsimonious model identification. IEEE Trans. Autom. Control **63**(2), 532–539 (2018). https://doi.org/10.1109/TAC.2017.2723959

Incompressible Image Registration Using Divergence-Conforming B-Splines

Lucas Fidon[1]([✉]), Michael Ebner[1,2], Luis C. Garcia-Peraza-Herrera[1,2], Marc Modat[1], Sébastien Ourselin[1], and Tom Vercauteren[1]

[1] School of Biomedical Engineering and Imaging Sciences, King's College London, London, UK
lucas.fidon@kcl.ac.uk
[2] University College London, London, UK

Abstract. Anatomically plausible image registration often requires volumetric preservation. Previous approaches to incompressible image registration have exploited relaxed constraints, ad hoc optimisation methods or practically intractable computational schemes. Divergence-free velocity fields have been used to achieve incompressibility in the continuous domain, although, after discretisation, no guarantees have been provided. In this paper, we introduce stationary velocity fields (SVFs) parameterised by divergence-conforming B-splines in the context of image registration. We demonstrate that sparse linear constraints on the parameters of such divergence-conforming B-Splines SVFs lead to being exactly divergence-free at any point of the continuous spatial domain. In contrast to previous approaches, our framework can easily take advantage of modern solvers for constrained optimisation, symmetric registration approaches, arbitrary image similarity and additional regularisation terms. We study the numerical incompressibility error for the transformation in the case of an Euler integration, which gives theoretical insights on the improved accuracy error over previous methods. We evaluate the proposed framework using synthetically deformed multimodal brain images, and the STACOM'11 myocardial tracking challenge. Accuracy measurements demonstrate that our method compares favourably with state-of-the-art methods whilst achieving volume preservation.

1 Introduction

Medical image registration consists of finding a spatial transformation that aligns two or more images. The intrinsic ill-posedness of registration can lead to anatomically implausible transformations associated with unrealistic volumetric distortion of the anatomy. For certain anatomical regions, such as the myocardium, physiologically plausible image registration requires volumetric preservation which corresponds to so-called *incompressible* registration [2,7,10].

Electronic supplementary material The online version of this chapter (https://doi.org/10.1007/978-3-030-32245-8_49) contains supplementary material, which is available to authorized users.

© Springer Nature Switzerland AG 2019
D. Shen et al. (Eds.): MICCAI 2019, LNCS 11765, pp. 438–446, 2019.
https://doi.org/10.1007/978-3-030-32245-8_49

Incompressible medical image registration between a pair of images I_1, I_2 can be defined as a constrained optimisation problem:

$$\underset{\Phi \in \mathcal{D}(\Omega)}{\operatorname{argmin}}\ \mathcal{L}(I_1, I_2, \Phi) + R(\Phi) \quad \text{s.t.} \quad [\forall x \in \mathcal{M}, \quad \det(J_\Phi(x)) = 1] \tag{1}$$

where Ω is the image domain, $\mathcal{M} \subset \Omega$ is the incompressible region, $\mathcal{L}$ an image dissimilarity measure, R a regularisation term, $\mathcal{D}(\Omega)$ the group of diffeomorphic transformations from Ω onto itself, and J_Φ the Jacobian matrix of the transformation Φ.

In practice, to solve (1), the transformation must be parameterised by a finite number of parameters, and the constraint $\forall x \in \mathcal{M}$, $\det(J_\Phi(x)) = 1$ must be reduced to a finite number of equality constraints. There are two approaches to discretise the constraint: (1) relaxing the constraint into an additive soft constraint [1,3,5,9]. (2) using a specific parameterisation for the transformation [2,6,7]. Soft constraints introduce hyperparameters that are difficult to tune reliably and cannot guarantee an incompressible transformation. In [2], the transformation is parameterised by a divergence-free displacement. Yet, this approach only provides a first order approximation of an incompressible deformation, still requiring a soft constraint. Recently [6,7] proposed to parameterise the transformation by a divergence-free stationary velocity field (SVF). The transformation is obtained via the Lie exponential mapping $\exp: v \mapsto \Phi$ that maps any divergence-free SVF v into an incompressible transformation Φ [6,7]. This reduces the non-convex constraint in (1) to a linear constraint in the continuous domain. However, in [6,7] the SVF is parameterised as linear B-splines, and the linear constraint is discretised by imposing the constraint only on the points of the deformation grid. As a result, guarantees to obtain a continuous incompressible transformation do not hold anymore. To mitigate this issue, [6] proposed to work with images of higher resolution with a finer grid for the linear B-spline leading to the need for distributed super-computing. Moreover, [6,7] methods are limited to using sum of squared differences (SSD) as image similarity metric, which limits their applicability to images with similar intensity distributions.

In this paper, we propose a constrained optimisation framework for incompressible diffeomorphic registration that allows to use any smooth image similarity and regularisation penalty. As an efficient means of discrete SVF parameterisation for this problem, we introduce multivariate divergence-conforming B-splines that have recently raised interest in computational physics [4]. We demonstrate that their properties can be exploited to impose bounds on the divergence of the SVF over the entire continuous space using sparse linear constraints on its finite parameters. Our general problem formulation allows us to solve incompressible registration using any state-of-the-art optimiser for constrained non-convex optimisation (e.g. IPOPT [11]). For evaluation, we initially apply our method for multi-modal incompressible registration of synthetically deformed brains. We then compare our approach against the state-of-the-art results published for the STACOM'11 myocardial tracking challenge dataset [10] and achieve similar results while better retaining the incompressibility.

2   Method

Divergence-Conforming B-Splines. General B-splines are very popular to parameterise deformations and velocity fields over a continuous spatial domain Ω with a finite number of parameters $\phi_i \in \mathbb{R}^3$:

$$\forall (x,y,z) \in \Omega, \quad v(x,y,z) = \sum_i B_{i,X}^k(x) B_{i,Y}^k(y) B_{i,Z}^k(z) \phi_i, \tag{2}$$

where (x_i, y_i, z_i) are the knots of a regular grid of spacing $\delta x \times \delta y \times \delta z$ and $B_{i,U}^k$ are the 1D B-spline basis functions of order k in the direction $U \in \{X, Y, Z\}$ (see supplemental material for more details). Popular choices of the order are $k = 1$ (linear B-splines) [6,7] and $k = 3$ (cubic B-splines) [10]. A fundamental property of 1D B-spline basis functions of the variable u, on a regular grid of spacing δu with n knots is that:

$$\forall i, \quad \frac{dB_{i,U}^k}{du} = \frac{B_{i,U}^{k-1} - B_{i+1,U}^{k-1}}{\delta u} \tag{3}$$

This implies that the derivative of a 1D B-spline on a regular grid is also a 1D B-spline on the same grid, albeit of lower order. However, this property does not extend to 3D B-splines using definition (2). Especially, the divergence of those 3D B-splines are not B-splines, because of the mixed order appearing with first partial derivatives. This limitation makes it more difficult to relate properties of the velocity field v to the values of the parameters ϕ_i.

To overcome this limitation, we propose to use a 3D divergence-conforming B-splines [4] to parameterise v. The orders of the 3D B-splines basis of each component are chosen so that the divergence of v is, in a continuous sense, exactly a 1D B-spline of order k. Using the same notations as in (2), and using $\phi_i = (\phi_i^X, \phi_i^Y, \phi_i^Z)$, we have:

$$\forall (x,y,z) \in \Omega, \quad v(x,y,z) = \begin{pmatrix} \sum_i B_{i,X}^{k+1}(x) B_{i,Y}^k(y) B_{i,Z}^k(z) \phi_i^X \\ \sum_i B_{i,X}^k(x) B_{i,Y}^{k+1}(y) B_{i,Z}^k(z) \phi_i^Y \\ \sum_i B_{i,X}^k(x) B_{i,Y}^k(y) B_{i,Z}^{k+1}(z) \phi_i^Z \end{pmatrix} \tag{4}$$

Using (3), we obtain the continuous divergence $\nabla \cdot v$ for all $(x,y,z) \in \Omega$:

$$\nabla \cdot v(x,y,z) = \sum_i B_{i,X}^k(x) B_{i,Y}^k(y) B_{i,Z}^k(z) \psi_i$$

$$\text{s.t. } \forall i, \quad \psi_i = \frac{\phi_i^X - \phi_{i-1}^X}{\delta x} + \frac{\phi_i^Y - \phi_{i-1}^Y}{\delta y} + \frac{\phi_i^Z - \phi_{i-1}^Z}{\delta z} \tag{5}$$

As a consequence, the following lemma states that $\nabla \cdot v$ is uniformly bounded at any point of a continuous subregion $\mathcal{M} \subset \Omega$ provided that a finite number of linear constraints are satisfied by the coefficients $(\phi_i^X, \phi_i^Y, \phi_i^Z)$.

Lemma 1. *Let $k \geq 2$, and $\mathcal{M}$ be a non-empty subset of Ω. Let $\epsilon \geq 0$ and let $\mathbf{J}_{\mathcal{M}} = \{i \mid (\operatorname{supp} B_{i,X}^k \times \operatorname{supp} B_{i,Y}^k \times \operatorname{supp} B_{i,Z}^k) \cap \mathcal{M} \neq \emptyset\}$. If*

$$\forall i \in \mathbf{J}_{\mathcal{M}}, \quad -\epsilon \leq \frac{\phi_i^X - \phi_{i-1}^X}{\delta x} + \frac{\phi_i^Y - \phi_{i-1}^Y}{\delta y} + \frac{\phi_i^Z - \phi_{i-1}^Z}{\delta z} \leq \epsilon,$$

then at any point $m \in \mathcal{M}$, it holds that $|\nabla \cdot v(m)| \leq \epsilon$.

Proof. The proof follows from (5) and the fact that the value of a B-spline at any point m is bounded by the values of the B-spline coefficients associated to the knots that are close to m (see supplementary material for more details).

Optimisation Formulation and Implementation. In this section, we formulate the optimisation problem for diffeomorphic registration with the proposed incompressibility constraint on a subregion $\mathcal{M}$. Using Lemma 1 and previous notations, our (symmetric) optimisation formulation of (1) is:

$$\underset{\Theta = \{(\phi_i^X, \phi_i^Y, \phi_i^Z)\}_i}{\operatorname{argmin}} \quad \mathcal{L}(I_1 \circ \widetilde{\exp}(v(\Theta)), I_2) + \mathcal{L}(I_1, I_2 \circ \widetilde{\exp}(-v(\Theta))) + R(v(\Theta))$$

$$\text{s.t.} \quad \forall i \in \mathbf{J}_{\mathcal{M}}, \quad \frac{\phi_i^X - \phi_{i-1}^X}{\delta x} + \frac{\phi_i^Y - \phi_{i-1}^Y}{\delta y} + \frac{\phi_i^Z - \phi_{i-1}^Z}{\delta z} = 0 \tag{6}$$

where $\widetilde{\exp}$ is an approximation of the Lie exponential. Thus we obtain a constrained optimisation formulation that guarantees the SVF to be *exactly* divergence-free over the entire continuous subregion $\mathcal{M}$ and that can be solved with efficient state-of-the-art optimisers. Using state-of-the-art solvers like IPOPT, that uses a primal-dual interior-point filter line-search method, an approximated solution of (6) that satisfies the constraints up to machine precision can be obtained.

Lie Exponential Approximation and Incompressibility. As the Lie exponential has to be approximated in practice, having a divergence-free velocity field does not strictly guarantee that the resulting deformation will be incompressible. We now quantify this approximation in our framework with respect to the time step τ for the Euler method. Let v denote a (SVF) solution of (6) that fulfills the divergence-free constraint up to machine precision ϵ_{mach}. For any point $m \in \mathcal{M}$, the Jacobian of the first step of the Euler method, $I + \tau v$, fulfills:

$$\det(J_{I+\tau v}(m)) = 1 + \tau \nabla \cdot v(m) + \mathcal{O}(\tau^2) \quad \text{where} \quad |\nabla \cdot v(m)| \leq \epsilon_{mach}. \tag{7}$$

Then, by composing $1/\tau$ times, if the point m remains inside $\mathcal{M}$ during the Euler integration, the Jacobian of $\widetilde{\exp}(v)$ satisfies (see supplementary material):

$$\det(J_{\widetilde{\exp}(v)}(m)) = 1 + \mathcal{O}(\tau + \epsilon_{mach}) \tag{8}$$

This approximation is independent to the spatial spacing and only depends on the time integration step τ. This is, to the best of our knowledge, a new state-of-the-art approximation for an incompressible diffeomorphic deformation parameterised by an SVF. However, it is worth noting that (8) is only guaranteed if m

Table 1. Validation on incompressible multi-modal registration. RMSE values between predicted and ground-truth transformations are reported in mm. MAE ($|$Jacobian $- 1|$) stands for the Mean Absolute Error between the Jacobian map of the predicted transformation and a map uniformly equal to 1 (perfect incompressibility). For both metrics, we reported mean value (standard deviation) over 60 registrations.

Error measures	Affine	Cubic B-splines	Ours
RMSE (transformation)	2.28 (0.68)	0.96 (0.44)	**0.90 (0.45)**
MAE ($|$Jacobian $- 1|$)	0.0062 (0.005)	0.054 (0.02)	**0.00079 (0.0004)**

remains inside $\mathcal{M}$ during the Euler integration. Thus, when $\mathcal{M}$ is not equal to the entire spatial domain, this approximation may not hold for large deformations.

3   Evaluation on Synthetic Data for Incompressible Multi-modal Registration

We start by evaluating our method on synthetic incompressible registration in the context of multi-modal MRI data.

Data Generation Method. We used T1, T2 and PD brain images from the IXI dataset[1]. We generated realistic ground-truth incompressible transformations in two steps. First, we non-linearly registered a pair of T1 images coming from different patients using a classical cubic B-splines SVF v_0. Second, we generated a quasi-divergence-free SVF v by projecting v_0 on the space of quasi-divergence-free SVFs. This corresponds to solving:

$$\underset{\Theta = \{\phi_i\}_i}{\mathrm{argmin}} \frac{1}{2}\|v(\Theta) - v_0\|^2 \quad \text{s.t.} \quad \forall i, \quad \boldsymbol{\nabla} \cdot v(x_i, y_i, z_i) = 0 \tag{9}$$

where v and v_0 are parameterised with classical cubic B-splines as in (2). We note that any potential bias towards the space of divergence-conforming B-splines is avoided in this comparison. We used IPOPT [11] to solve (9).

Evaluation. We generated a ground-truth quasi-incompressible SVF for 10 patients using the previous generation procedure, taking as fixed images 10 other patients. Then for a given subject and for any pair of imaging modalities $M_1, M_2 \in \{T1, T2, PD\}$, we warped the first image $I(M_1)$ using the inverse of the ground-truth transformation. The task consists in estimating v_{GT} by registering $I(M_1) \circ \widetilde{\exp}(-v_{GT})$ to $I(M_2)$. We compared the proposed method with divergence-conforming B-splines SVF under incompressibility constraint to a classic registration approach based on cubic B-splines SVF similar to the one used to generate the ground-truth. We also performed an affine registration to illustrate that the ground-truth transformation is not just affine.

---

[1] https://brain-development.org/ixi-dataset/.

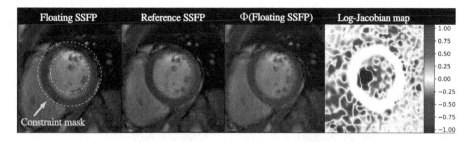

Fig. 1. We aim to register SSFP images at different times of the cardiac cycle. During the registration, the myocardium should not compress or expand. To impose this constraint we provide a mask of it to our algorithm (dashed in yellow). The floating image is warped into Φ(Floating SSFP) so that it matches the reference image, while keeping the deformation of the myocardium incompressible, as shown in the log-Jacobian map. Red and blue represent expansion and compression respectively. (Color figure online)

Implementation Details. We used `NiftyReg` [8] for the diffeomorphic registrations using cubic B-splines SVF. For both `NiftyReg` and our incompressible implementation we used the same hyperparameters (grid size 5 mm, 3 levels of pyramid) and objective function, consisting of Normalised Mutual Information (NMI) as a similarity measure (weight 0.95) and a bending energy regularisation term (weight 0.05). The optimiser differs, as we used `IPOPT` optimiser while a Conjugate Gradient approach is used in `NiftyReg`.

Results. `NiftyReg` and our approach recovered the ground-truth SVF up to a RMSE of the order of the images resolution, as shown in Table 1. In addition, our method recovered the incompressibility with a higher accuracy.

4   Evaluation for Myocardial Tracking

We evaluate the proposed method on the STACOM'11 myocardial tracking challenge [10]. In particular, this allows a direct comparison of our framework with iLogDemons [7] a state-of-the-art incompressible registration method.

Data. The STACOM'11 dataset[2] contains 4D cine Steady State Free Precession (SSFP) of a full cardiac cycle with 30 time points for 15 patients. Those SSFP come with 12 manually tracked landmarks. We used only 13 of the 15 patients available because we found a shift between the images and the landmarks for two of them which we reported to the organisers. The coordinates of the landmarks obtained by competitive methods of the challenge are available alongside the original data. This allows a direct comparison with our method.

---

[2] http://stacom.cardiacatlas.org/motion-tracking-challenge/.

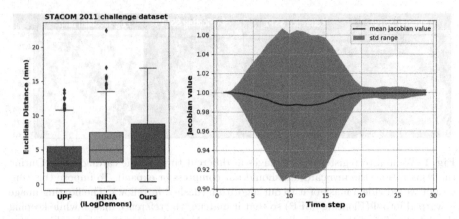

Fig. 2. (left) Distances to the landmarks after registering SSFP data. Our method achieves similar results to iLogDemons [7] for an incompressible registration. UPF [3] achieves the highest accuracy, but it does not guarantee incompressibility. (right) Evolution of the Jacobian values distribution in the incompressible region (myocardium) while registering the first frame to all other time frames. The Jacobian values are uniformly close to 1 for small and moderate deformations of the myocardium. For large deformations (frames at the opposite to the cardiac cycle) the mean Jacobian value is close to 1, but the dispersion of the Jacobian value distribution is large. This can be attributed to the use of a SVF.

Implementation Details. We used a similar implementation to the one of iLogDemons for this challenge, where we registered the first frame to all subsequent frames for each patient and used a manually delineated mask for the first frame. Yet, we used Local Normalised Cross Correlation as a similarity measure. We used a bending energy regularisation, and a grid size of 3 mm.

Results. The evaluation of the myocardial tracking is based on the manually annotated landmarks at End Diastole and End Systole. Using a Wilcoxon signed-rank test, we found that our results, shown in Fig. 2, are not statistically different from the results of iLogDemons [7] in terms of landmark tracking error. The log-Jacobian map of Fig. 1 illustrates our approximation results (8): for a small deformation, our registration framework can guarantee an incompressible deformation in a subregion with high accuracy. While Fig. 2 illustrates the degradation of this result for larger deformation, i.e. when registering frames at the opposite of the cardiac cycle.

5   Conclusion and Future Work

Limitations. Similar to [6,7], the divergence-free constraint is imposed on the stationary velocity field (SVF) in a subregion $\mathcal{M}$, rather than imposing incompressibility on $\mathcal{M}$. A voxel that is originally in $\mathcal{M}$ might exit $\mathcal{M}$ during the integration of the SVF and start being transported by velocity vectors that are not divergence-free (see supplemental material for a mathematical justification). In this case, the deformation of this voxel is no longer incompressible. As a result, using an SVF for incompressible registration applies only for deformations that are small enough or when the whole spatial domain is constrained to be divergence-free. Investigating other diffeomorphic parameterisations is left for future work.

Advantages Compared to Previous Methods. Our method for incompressible registration relies on the parameterisation of the velocity field by a divergence conforming B-splines [4]. In contrast to classical B-splines used in [6,7], it guarantees that the divergence of the velocity field is still a B-spline. This parameterisation along with constrained optimisation methods allows us to impose the velocity field to be divergence-free up to machine precision (10^{-16} in our experiments). This is irrespective of the grid resolution chosen for the velocity field. As a result, the proposed method is scalable to 3D images with high resolution. We also proved an error bound for the incompressibility of the deformation for the proposed method in the case an Euler integration of the velocity field is used (8). The study of the error bound for other integrators, that may require additional interpolations (e.g. scaling-and-squaring), is left for future works. Additionally, previous (quasi-)incompressible registration methods [6,7] have been limited to using SSD as image similarity metric. We are proposing the first incompressible non-linear registration method that supports any smooth image similarity measure and spatial regularization.

Acknowledgments. This project has received funding from the European Union's Horizon 2020 research and innovation programme under the Marie Skłodowska-Curie grant agreement TRABIT No 765148; Wellcome [203148/Z/16/Z; 203145Z/16/Z; WT101957], EPSRC [NS/A000049/1; NS/A000050/1; NS/A000027/1; EP/L016478/1]. TV is supported by a Medtronic/RAEng Research Chair [RCSRF1819\7\34].

References

1. Aganj, I., Reuter, M., Sabuncu, M.R., Fischl, B.: Avoiding symmetry-breaking spatial non-uniformity in deformable image registration via a quasi-volume-preserving constraint. NeuroImage **106**, 238–251 (2015)
2. Bistoquet, A., Oshinski, J., Škrinjar, O.: Myocardial deformation recovery from cine MRI using a nearly incompressible biventricular model. Med. Image Anal. **12**, 69–85 (2008)
3. De Craene, M., et al.: Temporal diffeomorphic free-form deformation: application to motion and strain estimation from 3D echocardiography. Med. Image Anal. **16**, 427–450 (2012)
4. Evans, J.A., Hughes, T.J.: Isogeometric divergence-conforming B-splines for the unsteady Navier-Stokes equations. J. Comput. Phys. **241**, 141–167 (2013)

5. Heyde, B., Alessandrini, M., Hermans, J., Barbosa, D., Claus, P., D'hooge, J.: Anatomical image registration using volume conservation to assess cardiac deformation from 3D ultrasound recordings. Trans. Med. Imaging **35**, 501–511 (2016)
6. Mang, A., Gholami, A., Davatzikos, C., Biros, G.: CLAIRE: a distributed-memory solver for constrained large deformation diffeomorphic image registration. arXiv preprint arXiv:1808.04487 (2018)
7. Mansi, T., Pennec, X., Sermesant, M., Delingette, H., Ayache, N.: ILogDemons: a demons-based registration algorithm for tracking incompressible elastic biological tissues. Int. J. Comput. Vis. **92**, 92–111 (2011)
8. Modat, M., et al.: Fast free-form deformation using graphics processing units. Comput. Methods Programs Biomed. **98**, 278–284 (2010)
9. Rohlfing, T., Maurer, C., Bluemke, D., Jacobs, M.: Volume-preserving nonrigid registration of MR breast images using free-form deformation with an incompressibility constraint. Trans. Med. Imaging **22**, 730–741 (2003)
10. Tobon-Gomez, C., et al.: Benchmarking framework for myocardial tracking and deformation algorithms: an open access database. Med. Image Anal. **17**, 632–648 (2013)
11. Wächter, A., Biegler, L.T.: On the implementation of an interior-point filter line-search algorithm for large-scale nonlinear programming. Math. Program. **106**, 25–57 (2006)

Cardiovascular Imaging

Direct Quantification for Coronary Artery Stenosis Using Multiview Learning

Dong Zhang[1,2], Guang Yang[3,4], Shu Zhao[1,2(✉)], Yanping Zhang[1,2], Heye Zhang[5], and Shuo Li[6]

[1] Key Laboratory of Intelligent Computing and Signal Processing, Ministry of Education, Anhui University, Hefei, China
zhaoshuzs2002@hotmail.com
[2] School of Computer Science and Technology, Anhui University, Hefei, China
[3] Cardiovascular Research Centre, Royal Brompton Hospital, London SW3 6NP, UK
[4] National Heart and Lung Institute, Imperial College London, London SW7 2AZ, UK
[5] School of Biomedical Engineering, Sun Yat-Sen University, Shenzhen, China
[6] Western University, London, ON, Canada

Abstract. The quantification of the coronary artery stenosis is of significant clinical importance in coronary artery diseases diagnosis and intervention treatment. It aims to quantify the morphological indices of the coronary artery lesions such as minimum lumen diameter, reference vessel diameter, lesion length and these indices are the reference of the interventional stent placement. In this study, we propose a direct multiview quantitative coronary angiography (DMQCA) model as an automatic clinical tool to quantify the coronary artery stenosis from X-ray coronary angiography images. The proposed DMQCA model consists of a multiview module with two attention mechanisms, a key-frame module and a regression module, to achieve direct accurate multiple-index estimation. The multi-view module comprehensively learns the spatiotemporal features of coronary arteries through a three-dimensional convolution. The attention mechanisms of each view focus on the subtle feature of the lesion region and capture the important context information. The key-frame module learns the subtle features of the stenosis through successive dilated residual blocks. The regression module finally generates the indice estimation from multiple features. We evaluate the proposed model over 2100 X-ray coronary angiography images collected from 105 subjects from two viewpoints. Compared to other direct quantification methods, our DMQCA model achieves more accurate quantification, enabling to provide a patient-specific assessment of coronary artery stenosis.

1 Introduction

The quantification of the coronary artery stenosis (e.g., multiple-index estimation of diameters and lengths for vessel) is of significant clinical importance [1]

© Springer Nature Switzerland AG 2019
D. Shen et al. (Eds.): MICCAI 2019, LNCS 11765, pp. 449–457, 2019.
https://doi.org/10.1007/978-3-030-32245-8_50

in coronary artery diseases (CAD) diagnosis and intervention treatment. In particular, the minimum lumen diameter (MLD), reference vessel diameter (RVD) and lesion length (LL) are the most valuable indices for the quantification of the coronary artery stenosis. The MLD and the RVD correlate with the severity of stenosis and the diameter stenosis have an important impact on the blood flow. The LL is crucial for the selection of appropriate stent size in coronary intervention. The accurate index estimation can increase the assessment capabilities for both diagnostic and interventional cardiology. However, current visual estimation or manual measurement from cardiologists exist differences and errors due to the subjective judgments [2]. Thus, the direct accurate quantification of the coronary artery stenosis from the X-ray coronary angiography is therefore highly in demand. It is more efficient, accurate, reliable and reproducible compared with visual estimation and manual measurement of the stenosis indices. Existing studies have only focused on the artery lesion grading [2], which only bring a rough description rather than an accurate quantification of the stenosis. Moreover, other studies have performed the quantitative coronary angiography (QCA) with a complex reconstruction [3] first, which can provide more vascular geometry information of the coronary arterial tree but is still not a direct quantification.

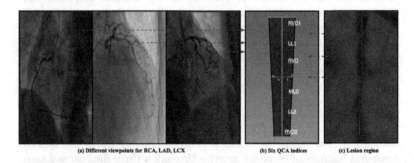

Fig. 1. The complex structures and variable locations of coronary arteries in X-ray coronary angiography images, and the lesion regions are relatively small. (a) A 46° left anterior oblique (LAO) viewpoint for the right coronary artery (RCA). A 44° right anterior oblique (RAO), 26° cranial (CRA) viewpoint for the left anterior descending artery (LAD). A 32° right anterior oblique, 20° caudal viewpoint (CAU) for the left circumflex coronary artery (LCX). The lesion regions are annotated in red-dashed box, the red coloured texts denote the locations and the red-dashed arrows denote modeling the lesion region as an ideal isosceles trapezoid. (b) The coronary artery is modeled as an ideal isosceles trapezoid and 6 quantitative indices are shown, including four vessel diameters (RVD1, RVD, MLD, RVD2) and two lesion lengths (LL1, LL2). Note that $RVD = (RVD2 \times LL1 + RVD1 \times LL2)/(LL1 + LL2)$. (c) A zoomed-in region of the coronary artery segment stenosis. (Color figure online)

Direct quantification of the coronary artery stenosis poses great challenges in feature representation learning. First, the complex structures and various locations of vessels in X-ray images (as shown in Fig. 1(a)). Coronary arteries have many extremely small branches and different shapes due to the individual differences. The severe occlusions always exist and coronary arteries lie in different locations of X-ray images due to the different viewpoints. Because of these, it is difficult to capture the expressive feature representation of different coronary arteries. Second, the artery stenosis is relatively small in the whole X-ray image (as shown in Fig. 1(a)). It is quite challenging to have a comprehensive observation when the angiogram images have high noise, poor contrast and nonuniform illumination. However, these lead to difficulties in capturing the discriminative features of the small lesion objects without segmentation. In this paper, a direct multiview [4,5] quantitative coronary angiography model (DMQCA) is proposed to quantify the artery stenosis in X-ray coronary angiography images. This quantification model includes a multiview (main-view, support-view) module with attention mechanisms, a key-frame module and a regression module. Our DMQCA model imitates viewing procedure of the reporting clinicians who make a comprehensive observation based on a main viewpoint, if necessary, a support viewpoint is also employed. As show in Fig. 2, the main-view module and the support-view module are comprised of successive 3D convolution (Conv) networks and integrate self-attention module and context attention module. In particular, the 3DConvs can extract the expressive spatio-temporal features of coronary artery over different time steps from 2D+T sequential X-ray images in each viewpoint. The self-attention [6] module models relationships between widely separated spatial regions in the feature maps. The context attention [7] can extract such regions that are important to the current image and such images that are important to the current view, respectively. Then it aggregates the representation of informative regions and images to form the ultimate representation of the image and view. The key-frame module consists of several dilated residual blocks, which are used to capture the subtle features for the stenosis. From the multiview modules and the key-frame module, the expressive spatio-temporal features and the subtle features are aggregated into the regression module, i.e., fully connected network, which is used to capture the relationship between the features and the multiple quantification indices.

The major contribution of this study lies in that we for the first time achieve a direct quantification of coronary artery stenosis from the X-ray coronary angiography images via deep learning. In DMQCA model, (1) we design a multiview learning model, which imitates viewing routines of the reporting clinicians to provide an expressive feature representation for quantitative measurement of the coronary artery stenosis, and (2) introduce two attention mechanisms, which are employed for the model to focus on the important features, especially for extracting the subtle features for artery stenosis.

2   Methods

The proposed DMQCA model is comprised of a multiview module with two attention mechanisms, a key-frame module and a regression module, to achieve direct multiple-index estimation. The workflow of our DMQCA model is summarized as Fig. 2.

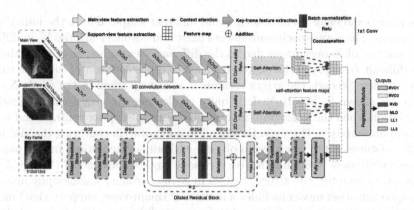

Fig. 2. The workflow of the DMQCA model. 3D convolution networks in each view are employed for extract multiview features of coronary artery. @# denotes the number of 3D convolution filters. The dilated residual block is employed for the feature in key frame. A self-attention and a context attention are employed for the subtle features of the stenosis and the important context information. A regression module is employed for the relationship between the quantitative indices and the expressive features.

2.1 DMQCA Formulation

Direct quantification for the coronary artery stenosis is described as a multi-output regression problem solved by our DMQCA model. Consider multiple quantitative indices $Y = \{y_1, y_2, y_3, \ldots, y_d\}$ and the objective of the DMQCA is to estimate Y from X-ray coronary angiography images X, which consist of two 2D+T image frames $X_m, X_s \in (x_1, x_2, \ldots, x_T, \mathbb{R}^{H \times W \times 3 \times T})$ of the main viewpoint and the support viewpoint, and a keyframe image $x_{key} \in \mathbb{R}^{H \times W \times 3}$, where H and W are the height and width of each frames respectively (H = W = 512), T is the temporal step (T = 10). Given a training dataset $D = \{X_{im}, X_{is}, x_{ikey}, Y_i\}_{i=1}^N$, we aim to learn the mapping $f: X \rightarrow Y \in \mathbb{R}^d$, and N is the number of training samples, d is the number of quantitative indices.

2.2 Comprehensive Observation for Quantification

The DMQCA model can mimic the reporting clinicians to make a comprehensive observation based on a main viewpoint, a support viewpoint and a key frame image. It can learn an expressive feature embedding of coronary arteries stenosis directly from X-ray coronary angiography images.

Multiview Feature Embedding Learning. A multiview learning module we design to learn an expressive feature for coronary arteries stenosis. It consists a main-view module and a support-view module, which use the same network architecture as shown in Fig. 2. 3DConvs networks are effective for learning the spatial and temporal features from 3D data. Interestingly, 2D+T image sequences can also be considered as 3D data. In our work, five successive 3DConv layers are designed for each view to extract the morphology (spatial) and kinematic (temporal) features from different temporal steps for coronary arteries. The input of 3DConvs is a set of T image frames. We set the different numbers and the different sizes of 3D convolutional filters (as shown in Fig. 2) with the same $1 \times 2 \times 2$ stride.

In order to capture the subtle features of the stenosis in each view, we apply the outputs of the Conv networks into a self-attention block, which models the relationships between the lesion region and the remote regions. In this block, the single image features $x \in R^{C \times M}$ of the frame sequences in current view from the previous layer are first transformed into two feature spaces f, g with different weights, where M is the number of spatial locations, C is the channel numbers, $f(x) = W_f x, g(x) = W_g x$. In addition, $\alpha_{j,i}$ indicates the contribution weight from the i_{th} location region when synthesizing the j_{th} location. The final output of the self-attention block is denoted as $o = (o_1, o_2, ..., o_i, ..., o_M) \in R^{C \times M}$, where,

$$S_{ij} = f(x_i)^\top g(x_i) \tag{1}$$

$$\alpha_{j,i} = \frac{exp(S_{ij})}{\sum_{i=1}^{M} exp(S_{ij})} \tag{2}$$

$$o_i = x_i + \gamma \sum_{i=1}^{M} \alpha_{j,i} h(x_i) \tag{3}$$

In the formulations above, $W_f, W_g \in R^{\frac{C}{8} \times C}$, $W_h \in R^{C \times C}$ are the weight matrices which are implemented as 1×1 convolutions, and the parameter γ is initialized as 0.

However, not all regions contribute equally to the representation of each frame meaning. Hence, we introduce the context attention to extract such regions that are important to the meaning of the frame image. Then we aggregate the representation of those regions to form an expressive feature vector of the frame. That is, we first feed the r_{th} region annotation x_{tr} through a one layer perception to get u_{tr} as the hidden feature of x_{tr}, then we measure the importance of the region with a region context vector u_r and get a importance weight β_{tr} through a softmax function. After that, we compute the t_{th} frame representation x_t as a weighted sum of the regions based on β_{tr}. Similarly, we again use the context attention mechanism to reward the frames that are important to the current view representation. A frame level context vector u_f is employed to measure the importance β_t of the t_{th} frame. Finally, the vector v denotes the view representation that summarizes the information of T frames in the current view. (Here we omit the equations of u_t, β_t, v for simplicity.)

$$u_{tr} = tanh(W_{tr} x_{tr} + b_{tr}) \tag{4}$$

$$\beta_{tr} = \frac{exp(u_{tr}^\top u_r)}{\sum_r exp(u_{tr}^\top u_r)} \tag{5}$$

$$x_t = \sum_r \beta_{tr} x_{tr} \tag{6}$$

Keyframe Feature Embedding Learning. A keyframe module we introduce to enhance the representation of the relatively small stenosis in different locations. The keyframe module consists of 6 successive dilated residual blocks, as shown in Fig. 2. Each dilated residual block employs two residual blocks [8] having two convolution layers with 3×3 filters, and a pooling layer. Then we use a fully connected layer to map the feature from dilated residual blocks to the same shape of the multiview modules.

Regression Module for the QCA Indices. A regression module we design to aggregate multiple features for direct index estimation. We denote V_m, V_s, K as the extracted features from the main view, the support view and the keyframe image, respectively. In order to regress the QCA indices according to the multiple features, V_m, V_s, K are concatenated and then we feed it into two fully connected layers with 512 and 6 units, each employing a LeakyReLU activation. The output of the regression module is $f(x_i) = W_o(V_m \oplus V_s \oplus K) + b_o$, where the $\oplus$ denotes the concatenation operator, W_o and b_o are the weight matrix and bias respectively. To minimize the difference between the outputs $f(x_i)$ and the ground truth, we employ the mean absolute error (MAE) as the loss function (Eq. 7), where the λ_{qca} is the l_2 norm regularization.

$$L_{qca} = \frac{1}{d \times N} \sum_{i=1}^{N} |f(x_i) - Y_i| + \lambda_{qca} \sum_i \|w_i\|_2^2 \tag{7}$$

3   Experiments and Results

3.1   Dataset and Configurations

A total of 105 patients of type A coronary artery lesions were retrospectively selected and they have completed coronary angiography using a clinical angiographic X-ray system (Philips Allura XPER). In particular, different severity of lesions locates main coronary artery branches, including 33 LADs, 26 LCXs and 46 RCAs. T $= 10$ frames X-ray images ($512 \times 512 \times 3$ pixels) are collected from two viewpoints for each patient. The keyframe images are extracted from main viewpoint, and the ground truth values are manually measured under the guidance of an experienced radiologist.

Our deep learning model was implemented using $TensorFlow$ 1.11.0 on a Ubuntu 16.04 machine, and was trained and tested on an NVIDIA Titan Xp 12 GB GPU. For the implementation, we used the Adam method to perform the optimization with decayed learning rate (the initial learning rate was 0.0002) and the l_2 norm regularization λ_{qca} was set to 10^{-6}. In our experiments, a 10-fold cross-validation is employed to provide an unbiased estimation of the MAE. It is of note that all the 2100 images are resized into $256 \times 256 \times 3$. For comparison studies, the Pearson correlation coefficient is used to evaluate the performance with two baseline methods CNNs, 3DCNNs and other direct quantification methods HOG+RF [9] (histogram of oriented gradients (HOG) feature we use), Indices-Net [10] and DMTRL [11].

Table 1. Our DMQCA model works best in comparison with two baseline methods, three direct quantification methods and different sub-frameworks including single view (Main, Sup) integrating keyframe (Key) information, main view, keyframe, main view without context attention (Main-ConAtt) and DMQCA without self-attention (**Ours-SelfAtt**).

Method	MAE	Pearson (%)	RVD1	RVD2	RVD	MLD	LL1	LL2
Sup+Key	1.3216 ± 0.7036	88.62 ± 12.73	0.8642	0.6902	0.7252	0.6642	2.4468	2.5389
Main+Key	1.3296 ± 0.6906	88.40 ± 11.93	0.7780	0.6735	0.8137	0.6275	2.4768	2.6079
Key	1.3188 ± 0.6724	88.72 ± 12.22	0.7864	0.7082	0.6895	**0.5648**	2.5605	2.6032
Main-ConAtt	1.3449 ± 0.7480	87.61 ± 14.87	0.8713	0.7538	0.7393	0.5936	2.4111	2.7000
Main	1.3352 ± 0.6916	87.89 ± 14.41	0.7998	0.6967	0.7162	0.6418	2.3867	2.7705
Ours-SelfAtt	1.3138 ± 0.6910	87.71 ± 12.77	0.7913	0.7409	0.6879	0.6258	2.5013	2.5353
† CNNs	1.3436 ± 0.6417	87.97 ± 13.75	0.7661	0.8067	0.7057	0.6510	2.5664	2.5659
$ 3DCNNs	1.3537 ± 0.7035	88.18 ± 11.53	0.7489	0.7342	0.7506	0.6014	2.5985	2.6887
‡ 3DCNNs	1.3291 ± 0.6778	87.86 ± 12.55	0.8143	0.6694	0.7881	0.6744	2.3800	2.6482
† HOG+RF [9]	1.4606 ± 0.6798	87.47 ± 14.04	0.7915	0.7114	0.7186	0.5943	2.9396	3.0086
† Indices-Net [10]	1.5105 ± 0.7475	85.45 ± 14.40	0.8402	0.7951	0.9090	0.7459	2.7612	3.0114
‡ DMTRL [11]	1.3117 ± 0.7403	88.44 ± 12.03	**0.7353**	**0.6591**	0.6984	0.5669	2.4350	2.7755
$ DMTRL [11]	1.3124 ± 0.7362	88.32 ± 14.31	0.7356	0.6823	0.6841	0.6140	2.4160	2.7422
Ours	**1.2737 ± 0.7115**	**89.14 ± 11.24**	0.7947	0.7486	**0.6669**	0.5669	**2.3330**	**2.5322**

† On Keyframe images. ‡ On Main view images. $ On Support view images

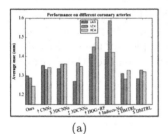
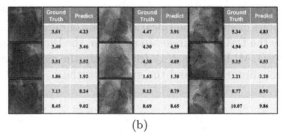

(a)   (b)

Fig. 3. (a) The experimental results of comparison methods on different coronary arteries. (b) The lesion regions are annotated in red-dashed box in main-view, support-view and keyframe (from top to bottom) images. The six indices RVD1, RVD2, RVD, MLD, LL1, LL2 (from top to bottom) of LAD, LCX, RCA (from left to right) quantified by our method are consistent with the ground truth. (Color figure online)

3.2   Results and Analysis

Quantitative Coronary Angiography. The experimental results show that our DMQCA model can accurately quantify the coronary artery stenosis. The obtained MAE and the Pearson correlation coefficient are 1.2737 ± 0.7115 mm and 89.14% ± 11.24%, respectively. For each quantitative indice, our method estimates the RVD, MLD, LL1 and LL2 with the superior average MAE of 0.6669 mm, 0.5669 mm, 2.3330 mm and 2.5322 mm.

Ablation Study I: Multiview Learning. We further demonstrate the value of our multiview model for capturing expressive representation. We design some sub-frameworks which just employ single view (main view or support view) with Keyframe (Sup+Key, Main+Key), single view (Main), Keyframe (Key), respectively. The quantitative results in Table 1 show that our multiview learning achieved better performance for quantitative coronary angiography in X-ray images.

Ablation Study II: Attention Mechanism. We employ a self-attention to force more attention to the lesion regions and apply a context attention to capture the important context information to enhance the representation of coronary arteries. To evaluate the performance of these two attention modules, we remove self-attention from DMQCA model and remove context attention from main-view framework, respectively. The superior experiment results in Table 1 prove the effectiveness of these two attention mechanisms.

Comparison with Some Existing Methods. In order to evaluate the performance of our DMQCA model, we make the comparison with two baseline methods and three direct quantification methods. As shown in Table 1, our proposed DMQCA model has also achieved better quantification performance in the QCA compared with these five methods. We further evaluate the performance of our DMQCA model on different coronary arteries (Fig. 3(a)). And Fig. 3(b) shows example quantification results of different coronary artery lesions obtained by the DMQCA model. In addition, the Bland-Altman plots of indices LL1, LL2, RVD, MLD in Fig. 4(a)–(d) indicate the agreement between the DMQCA quantification results and the ground truths.

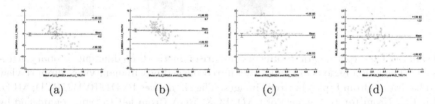

(a)   (b)   (c)   (d)

Fig. 4. Bland-Altman plots of the quantifications of LL1 (a), LL2 (b), RVD (c), MLD (d).

4   Conclusion

In this study, we have proposed a direct quantification model (namely DMQCA) for coronary artery stenosis by incorporating multiview learning and attention mechanisms. By aggregating the multiview features and keyframe feature for direct quantitative index estimation. The proposed method has been evaluated on 105 subjects and has yielded better quantitative results, by comparing with two baseline methods and three existing direct quantification methods. In addition, the experimental results show compelling evidence of our DMQCA method in quantitative coronary angiography.

Acknowledgments. This work was supported by the National Natural Science Foundation of China under Grants 61876001, 61602003 and 61673020, the Anhui Provincial Natural Science Foundation under Grant 1708085QF156.

References

1. Zhang, N., Yang, G., Gao, Z., et al.: Deep learning for diagnosis of chronic myocardial infarction on nonenhanced cardiac cine MRI. Radiology **291**(3), 606–617 (2019)
2. Wan, T., Feng, H., Tong, C., Li, D., Qin, Z.: Automated identification and grading of coronary artery stenoses with x-ray angiography. Comput. Methods Programs Biomed. **167**, 13–22 (2018)
3. Cong, W., Yang, J., Ai, D., Chen, Y., Liu, Y., Wang, Y.: Quantitative analysis of deformable model-based 3-d reconstruction of coronary artery from multiple angiograms. IEEE Trans. Biomed. Eng. **62**(8), 2079–2090 (2015)
4. Chen, J., et al.: Multiview two-task recursive attention model for left atrium and atrial scars segmentation. In: Frangi, A.F., Schnabel, J.A., Davatzikos, C., Alberola-López, C., Fichtinger, G. (eds.) MICCAI 2018. LNCS, vol. 11071, pp. 455–463. Springer, Cham (2018). https://doi.org/10.1007/978-3-030-00934-2_51
5. Yang, G., Chen, J., Gao, Z., et al.: Multiview sequential learning and dilated residual learning for a fully automatic delineation of the left atrium and pulmonary veins from late gadolinium-enhanced cardiac MRI images. In: 40th EMBC, pp. 1123–1127. IEEE (2018)
6. Zhang, H., Goodfellow, I., Metaxas, D., et al.: Self-attention generative adversarial networks. arXiv preprint arXiv:1805.08318 (2018)
7. Yang, Z., Yang, D., et al.: Hierarchical attention networks for document classification. In: Conference of the North American Chapter of the Association for Computational Linguistics: Human Language Technologies, pp. 1480–1489 (2017)
8. He, K., Zhang, X., Ren, S., Sun, J.: Deep residual learning for image recognition. In: IEEE Conference on Computer Vision and Pattern Recognition (CVPR) (2016)
9. Zhen, X., Wang, Z., Islam, A., Bhaduri, M., Chan, I., Li, S.: Direct estimation of cardiac bi-ventricular volumes with regression forests. In: Golland, P., Hata, N., Barillot, C., Hornegger, J., Howe, R. (eds.) MICCAI 2014. LNCS, vol. 8674, pp. 586–593. Springer, Cham (2014). https://doi.org/10.1007/978-3-319-10470-6_73
10. Xue, W., Islam, A., Bhaduri, M., Li, S.: Direct multitype cardiac indices estimation via joint representation and regression learning. IEEE Trans. Med. Imaging **36**(10), 2057–2067 (2017)
11. Xue, W., Brahm, G., Pandey, S., et al.: Full left ventricle quantification via deep multitask relationships learning. Med. Image Anal. **43**, 54–65 (2018)

Bayesian Optimization on Large Graphs via a Graph Convolutional Generative Model: Application in Cardiac Model Personalization

Jwala Dhamala[1(✉)], Sandesh Ghimire[1], John L. Sapp[2], B. Milan Horáček[2], and Linwei Wang[1]

[1] Rochester Institute of Technology, New York, USA
jd1336@rit.edu
[2] Dalhousie University, Halifax, Canada

Abstract. Personalization of cardiac models involves the optimization of organ tissue properties that vary spatially over the non-Euclidean geometry model of the heart. To represent the high-dimensional (HD) unknown of tissue properties, most existing works rely on a low-dimensional (LD) partitioning of the geometrical model. While this exploits the geometry of the heart, it is of limited expressiveness to allow partitioning that is small enough for effective optimization. Recently, a variational auto-encoder (VAE) was utilized as a more expressive generative model to embed the HD optimization into the LD latent space. Its Euclidean nature, however, neglects the rich geometrical information in the heart. In this paper, we present a novel graph convolutional VAE to allow generative modeling of non-Euclidean data, and utilize it to embed Bayesian optimization of large graphs into a small latent space. This approach bridges the gap of previous works by introducing an expressive generative model that is able to incorporate the knowledge of spatial proximity and hierarchical compositionality of the underlying geometry. It further allows transferring of the learned features across different geometries, which was not possible with a regular VAE. We demonstrate these benefits of the presented method in synthetic and real data experiments of estimating tissue excitability in a cardiac electrophysiological model.

Keywords: Graph convolution · Variational auto-encoder · Bayesian optimization · Model personalization

1 Introduction

Personalized computer models of the heart have shown promise in various clinical tasks such as risk stratification [2] and predicting treatment response [10]. With advances in medical imaging technologies, personalization of high-resolution anatomical models is now feasible. By contrast, organ tissue properties vary spatially over the three-dimensional anatomical domain but have to be estimated from indirect, sparse and noisy data, resulting in a difficult ill-posed optimization problem with a high-dimensional (HD) unknown.

© Springer Nature Switzerland AG 2019
D. Shen et al. (Eds.): MICCAI 2019, LNCS 11765, pp. 458–467, 2019.
https://doi.org/10.1007/978-3-030-32245-8_51

Most existing methods choose to represent spatially-varying tissue properties via a low-dimensional (LD) partitioning of the underlying geometrical model, either as pre-defined segments [11], or iteratively optimized in a coarse-to-fine fashion [5,10]. This LD-to-HD definition directly exploits the spatial proximity and hierarchical composition of the underlying geometry. However, it is of such limited expressiveness that the number of partitioning is either too low to faithfully represent high-resolution tissue properties, or too high to allow effective optimization. In contrast, recent work presented the use of a data-driven generative model of HD tissue properties, via a variational auto-encoder (VAE), to embed the optimization into a LD latent space [6]. Being more expressive, this VAE-based generative model is able to represent high-resolution tissue properties with a latent code sufficiently small for effective optimization. However, as the regular VAE is defined over Euclidean data, it does not take into account the valuable geometry information in the data, nor does it allow transferring among different geometry without first establishing point-by-point correspondence.

If we view organ tissue properties over a 3D geometrical model as an image, convolutional neural networks (CNNs) are a natural choice to incorporate knowledge of the spatial proximity and hierarchical composition of the image [4]. However, standard CNNs have been most successful on data with an underlying Euclidean structure (*i.e.*, image grids). Generalizing CNNs to non-Euclidean domains is an emerging area of research [4], where significant efforts have been presented on addressing the challenges of defining convolution [8], pooling, and up-sampling operations [12]. However, most developments to non-Euclidean CNNs are focused on supervised discriminative networks. To date, very limited work have been presented to enable generative modeling of non-Euclidean data.

In this paper, we present a novel VAE architecture that allows generative modeling of data over non-Euclidean domains, and utilize this generative model to embed Bayesian optimization of large graphs into a LD manifold. The presented approach bridges the gap of previous works by introducing an expressive generative model that is able to represent high-resolution tissue properties with a small latent code, while incorporating the geometrical knowledge in the data and being transferable across geometries. We evaluate the presented method in synthetic and real-data experiments of estimating tissue excitability in a cardiac electrophysiological model, where we compare the expressiveness of the generative model and the accuracy of the subsequent parameter optimization with those obtained by using a linear reconstruction model based on principal component analysis (PCA) and a regular fully-connected VAE [6]. We further demonstrate the feasibility of transferring the presented non-Euclidean VAE across patients. To our knowledge, this is the first introduction of a graph convolutional VAE and its use to enable Bayesian optimization over large graphs.

2 Background: Models of Cardiac Electrophysiology

Cardiac Electrophysiological Model: Among various computational models of cardiac electrophysiology, phenomenological models are widely used in parameter personalization as they are able to express key macroscopic properties of cardiac excitation with a small number of parameters [5,10]. We thus adopt the phenomenological two-variable Aliev-Panfilov (AP) model [1]:

$$\partial u/\partial t = \nabla(\mathbf{D}\nabla u) - cu(u - \theta)(u - 1) - uv,$$
$$\partial v/\partial t = \varepsilon(u, v)(-v - cu(u - \theta - 1)),$$

(1)

where u is the normalized transmembrane potential, and v is the recovery current. Parameter ε controls the coupling between u and v, $\mathbf{D}$ is the diffusion tensor, c controls the repolarization, and θ controls tissue excitability. As u is most sensitive to parameter θ in the AP model (1) [5], we focus on its estimation. Solving the AP model on a 3D discrete cardiac anatomy of meshfree nodes [5], we obtain a 3D electrophysiological model of the heart that describes the temporal evolution of 3D transmembrane potential $\mathbf{u}(t, \boldsymbol{\theta})$.

Measurement Model: $\mathbf{u}(t, \boldsymbol{\theta})$ is measured on the body surface following the quasi-static electromagnetic theory, solving which on a discrete subject-specific heart-thorax mesh gives a linear relationship between $\mathbf{u}(t, \boldsymbol{\theta})$ and its surface potential measurement $\mathbf{y}(t)$ as: $\mathbf{y}(t) = \mathbf{Hu}(t, \boldsymbol{\theta})$ [5].

3   Personalizing HD Parameters on Unstructured Meshes

We seek parameter $\boldsymbol{\theta}$ that minimizes the sum of squared errors between model output $M(\boldsymbol{\theta}) = \mathbf{Hu}(t, \boldsymbol{\theta})$ and patient's measurements $\mathbf{y}_d(t)$ as:

$$\hat{\boldsymbol{\theta}} = \arg\max_{\boldsymbol{\theta}}\{-\sum_t \|\mathbf{y}_d(t) - M(\boldsymbol{\theta})\|^2\}. \tag{2}$$

Directly solving (2) for the spatially-distributed $\boldsymbol{\theta}$ is difficult [5]. Below we describe how we learn a LD-to-HD generation of $\boldsymbol{\theta}$ that accounts for the underlying geometry, and embed the HD optimization into the expressive LD manifold.

3.1   Graph Convolutional VAE

We model the generation of spatially-distributed $\boldsymbol{\theta}$ with a VAE [9]. A VAE consists a probabilistic encoder network with parameters $\boldsymbol{\alpha}$ that approximates the intractable true posterior density as $q_{\boldsymbol{\alpha}}(\mathbf{z}|\boldsymbol{\theta})$; and a probabilistic decoder network with parameters $\boldsymbol{\beta}$ that represents the likelihood as $p_{\boldsymbol{\beta}}(\boldsymbol{\theta}|\mathbf{z})$. For data defined on a Euclidean grid, structural information is incorporated in VAE through CNNs. Here, we present a novel VAE architecture that enables convolution, pooling, and unpooling over non-Euclidean geometry of the heart.

Local Connectivity and Graph Convolution: We model the cardiac mesh as a graph: $\mathcal{G} = (\mathcal{V}, \mathcal{E}, \mathbf{U})$, where vertices $\mathcal{V}$ consist of all N meshfree nodes and edges $\mathcal{E}$ exist between each meshfree node and its k nearest neighbors. $\mathbf{U} \in [0, 1]^{N \times N \times 3}$ consists of edge attributes $\boldsymbol{v}(i, j)$, calculated as the normalized $(x_1 - x_2, y_1 - y_2, z_1 - z_2)$ if an edge $(i, j) \in \mathcal{E}$ exists between vertices at (x_1, y_1, z_1)

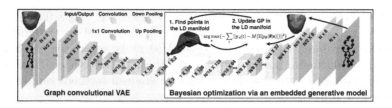

Fig. 1. Outline of the presented method, with dimensions labeled within the VAE.

and (x_2, y_2, z_2) and 0 otherwise. On this graph, we use a convolution operator based on spatial continuous convolution kernels because it was shown to allow better generalization to similar graphs [8]. In specific, given the graph $\mathcal{G}$ and M-dimensional input features $\{\mathbf{f}(i)|i \in \mathcal{V}\}$, the l-th convolution kernel is:

$$g_l(\boldsymbol{v}) = \sum_{\mathbf{p} \in \mathcal{P}} w_{\mathbf{p},l} \prod_{i=1}^{d} N_{i,p_i}^m(v_i), \tag{3}$$

where $((N_{1,i}^m)_{1 \leq i \leq k_1}, \ldots, (N_{d,i}^m)_{1 \leq i \leq k_d})$ denotes d open B-spline bases of degree m based on equidistant knot vectors with d-dimensional kernel size of $\mathbf{k} = (k_1, \ldots, k_d)$, $\mathcal{P}$ is the Cartesian product of the B-spline bases, and $w_{\mathbf{p},l}$ are the trainable parameters. Given kernel functions $\mathbf{g} = (g_1, \ldots, g_M)$ and input features $\mathbf{f} \in \mathcal{R}^M$, the spatial convolution operator for each vertex $i \in \mathcal{V}$ with a neighborhood $\mathcal{N}(i)$ based on its edge connectivity is then defined as:

$$(\mathbf{f} * \mathbf{g})(i) = \frac{1}{|\mathcal{N}(i)|} \sum_{l=1}^{M} \sum_{j \in \mathcal{N}(i)} f_l(j) g_l(\boldsymbol{v}(i,j)). \tag{4}$$

Hierarchical Composition and Pooling: To define pooling and unpooling operations necessary for the encoding-decoding architecture , a hierarchical representation of the graph is needed. We obtain this by an efficient multilevel graph clustering method based on minimizing the normalized cuts (Graclus) [7], which reduces the graph size by half the number of vertices at each coarsening.

We store hierarchical graph representation in matrices which reduces pooling/unpooling operations to efficient matrix multiplications. In specific, if $\mathcal{G}$ is a graph with N_1 vertices and $\mathcal{G}_c$ is its coarsened graph with $N_2 < N_1$ vertices, we populate a binary matrix $\mathbf{P}^{N_1 \times N_2}$, where $\mathbf{P}_{ij} = 1$ if the ith vertex in $\mathcal{G}$ was grouped to the jth vertex in $\mathcal{G}_c$ and $\mathbf{P}_{ij} = 0$ otherwise. Given M feature maps $\mathbf{F} \in \mathcal{R}^{N_1 \times M}$ over the vertices of graph $\mathcal{G}$ and $\mathbf{F}_c \in \mathcal{R}^{N_2 \times M}$ over graph $\mathcal{G}_c$, the average pooling in the encoder can be obtained by $\mathbf{F}_c = \mathbf{P}_n^{\mathrm{T}} \mathbf{F}$ and unpooling in the decoder by $\mathbf{F} = \mathbf{P}\mathbf{F}_c$, where $\mathbf{P}_n$ is column normalized from $\mathbf{P}$.

Graph Convolutional VAE: Using these building blocks we construct a VAE architecture as shown in Fig. 1. It is trained by optimizing the variational lower bound on the marginal likelihood of the training data

$\boldsymbol{\Theta} = \{\boldsymbol{\theta}^{(i)}\}_{i=1}^N$: $\mathcal{L}(\boldsymbol{\alpha}; \boldsymbol{\beta}; \boldsymbol{\theta}^{(i)}) = -D_{\mathrm{KL}}(q_{\boldsymbol{\alpha}}(\mathbf{z}|\boldsymbol{\theta}^{(i)})||p(\mathbf{z})) + E_{q_{\boldsymbol{\alpha}}(\mathbf{z}|\boldsymbol{\theta}^{(i)})}[\log p_{\boldsymbol{\beta}}(\boldsymbol{\theta}^{(i)}|\mathbf{z})]$. We set $q_{\boldsymbol{\alpha}}(\mathbf{z}|\boldsymbol{\theta})$ and $p_{\boldsymbol{\beta}}(\boldsymbol{\theta}|\mathbf{z})$ to be Gaussian parameterized by the graph convolutional networks. The prior $p(\mathbf{z}) \sim \mathcal{N}(0, 1)$ is set to be an isotropic Gaussian, producing an analytical form for the KL divergence. Using the reparameterization trick [9], standard stochastic gradient methods can be used to optimize $\mathcal{L}(\boldsymbol{\alpha}; \boldsymbol{\beta}; \boldsymbol{\theta}^{(i)})$.

3.2   Bayesian Optimization on Large Graphs

Bayesian optimization is a popular choice in optimizing complex objective functions such as (2) [3]. It begins by defining a surrogate over the objective function. The optimization then consists of two iterative steps: (1) actively find a point that optimizes a utility function based on the surrogate, and (2) update the surrogate with the newly-selected point. Direct Bayesian optimization over HD space is difficult and its use over large graphs has not been reported [3]. To enable this, we reformulate the original objective function in (2) as follows:

$$\hat{\mathbf{z}} = \arg\max_{\mathbf{z}}\{-\sum_t ||\mathbf{y}_d(t) - M(\mathrm{E}[p_{\boldsymbol{\beta}}(\boldsymbol{\theta}|\mathbf{z})])||^2\}. \tag{5}$$

This allows us to embed surrogate construction and active selection of training points in a LD manifold. We initialize the Gaussian process (GP) surrogate of (5) with a zero mean function and an anisotropic Matérn 5/2 kernel.

Active Selection of Training Points: To select a training point, we maximize the expected improvement (EI) utility function that favours a point with the highest expected improvement over the current optimum f^+ [3]:

$$\mathrm{EI}(\mathbf{z}) = (\mu(\mathbf{z}) - f^+)\Phi\left(\frac{\mu(\mathbf{z}) - f^+}{\sigma(\mathbf{z})}\right) + \sigma(\mathbf{z})\phi\left(\frac{\mu(\mathbf{z}) - f^+}{\sigma(\mathbf{z})}\right), \tag{6}$$

where $\mu(\mathbf{z})$ and $\sigma(\mathbf{z})$ are the predictive mean and standard deviation of the GP, Φ is the cumulative normal distribution, and ϕ is the normal density function. The first term promotes exploitation , while the second term promotes exploration.

GP Update: After picking a new point $\mathbf{z}^{(i)}$, the value of the optimization objective (5) is evaluated at $\mathbf{z}^{(i)}$ as $\mathcal{J}^{(i)}$. The GP is then updated by including the new input-output pair of $(\mathbf{z}^{(i)}, \mathcal{J}^{(i)})$ and maximizing the log marginal likelihood for kernel hyperparameters: length-scales and co-variance amplitude.

4   Synthetic Experiments

We evaluate the presented graph convolutional VAE (termed as gVAE) by: (1) its reconstruction accuracy , and (2) optimization accuracy of the gVAE-based Bayesian optimization, both in comparison to existing methods. Accuracy is evaluated by the sum of squared error (SSE) in θ, and the dice coefficient (DC) of the abnormal region obtained by thresholding θ with Otsu's method.

We synthetically generate data of heterogeneous tissue excitability via random region growing in each cardiac model. Beginning with a single meshfree node as abnormal, we randomly grow the abnormal region by adding one of the nearest neighbors of the abnormal nodes, until the abnormal region reaches a desired size (2% to 40% of the heart volume). On average, we generated $78,208 \pm 12,541$ data for training and $13,545 \pm 7654$ data each for validation and testing. The various layers and sizes of feature maps in each layer of the presented gVAE architecture are detailed in Fig. 1. We use B-spline basis degree of $m = 1$ with kernel size of $k_1 = k_2 = k_3 = 5$ in all graph convolution layers. All models are trained with a learning rate of 0.001 with Adam optimizer.

Table 1. Comparison of reconstruction accuracy with the presented gVAE, PCA, and fVAE with various depths [6] in five different geometries.

Anatomy	SSE					DC					Trainable parameters
	1	2	3	4	5	1	2	3	4	5	
PCA	12.73	14.18	12.35	23.85	23.26	39.80	39.87	41.31	49.17	54.42	NA
fVAE-3h [6]	8.03	8.45	8.44	13.07	13.70	61.77	66.20	60.45	70.30	70.72	2,087,822
fVAE-4h	7.97	8.29	8.33	12.47	13.99	61.76	64.60	61.58	71.51	69.84	2,613,134
fVAE-5h	7.42	8.01	8.19	13.96	12.41	64.59	65.72	62.21	68.04	74.50	3,138,446
gVAE	**6.66**	**6.89**	**6.79**	**11.28**	**11.43**	**68.43**	**70.92**	**70.70**	**75.10**	**76.86**	2,778,069

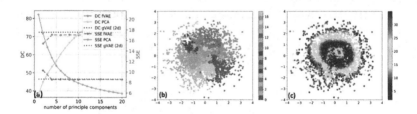

Fig. 2. (a) Comparison of reconstruction accuracy using gVAE with a 2d manifold *vs.* PCA and fVAE [6] with various-dimensional manifolds. (b)-(c): Plots of 2d latent codes from gVAE colored by infarct location (b) and infarct size (c).

gVAE as a Generative Model: On five different human heart models constructed from CT images, we first evaluate the ability of the presented gVAE model to reconstruct tissue excitability in comparison to: (1) PCA-based linear reconstruction, and (2) fully-connected VAE (termed as fVAE) [6] with three to five hidden layers (termed as fVAE-3h, -4h, and -5h, respectively). As summarized in Table 1, PCA being a linear model has the lowest accuracy. Compared to fVAE, the reconstruction accuracy of gVAE is consistently higher in both DC and SSE, even when its number of trainable parameters is similar to or lower than fVAE. However, gVAE is more expensive to train: 37.21 hrs *vs.* 7.51 mins for fVAE-3h in TITAN Xp GPU. Nevertheless, note that the number of trainable parameters for gVAE does not increase for larger meshes.

We further compare gVAE with two-dimensional (2d) latent codes *vs.* fVAE and PCA with various latent dimensions. As shown in Fig. 2(a), to achieve the reconstruction accuracy of gVAE with 2d latent codes, at least 13 principles components are required with PCA: this increase in dimension will make the subsequent optimization difficult. With fVAE, a similar SSE is attained with four latent dimensions, while a similar DC could not be attained with even 50 latent dimensions. This may be because fVAE does not consider the geometry underlying the spatial distribution of tissue excitability. Figure 2(b) and (c) show that the latent code learned with gVAE are clustered by the location of the abnormal tissue and its radial direction encodes the size of the abnormal tissue.

gVAE-Based Parameter Optimization: On 40 synthetic cases on two different heart geometries, we conduct experiments on estimating unknown tissue excitability. In each case, we set an abnormal region by using various combinations of AHA segments which are very different from the training set. Measurement data was simulated, sub-sampled and corrupted with 20 dB Gaussian noise. We compare the accuracy of gVAE-based Bayesian optimization with three previous approaches: (1) optimization on 17 fixed segments (termed as FS) [10,11], (2) coarse-to-fine optimization along a fixed multi-scale mesh hierarchy (termed as FH) [5], and (3) optimization on a LD manifold obtained with fVAE-3h [6]. Result in Fig. 3(a) shows that gVAE-based Bayesian optimization is more accurate than all other approaches in both DC and SSE (paired t-test, $p < 0.05$). Figure 3(c)–(f) shows visual comparison on a few examples. The computational cost of gVAE-based optimization is much lower than that of FH ($>$22x) and FS ($>$7.5x), and similar to that of fVAE-based optimization.

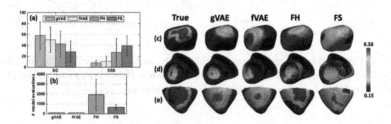

Fig. 3. (a) Accuracy and (b) computational cost of gVAE (green) versus fVAE [6] (yellow), FH [5] (purple), and FS [11] (red). (c)–(e): Examples of estimated parameters. (Color figure online)

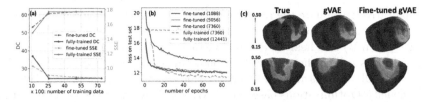

Fig. 4. (a) Reconstruction accuracy and (b) convergence of test losses from fine-tuned gVAE *vs.* gVAE trained from scratch (termed fully-trained) with varying training data size. (c) Examples of estimated parameters using gVAE fine-tuned with 7360 data.

Feature Sharing Across Geometries: To demonstrate the feasibility of transferring the presented gVAE across different geometries, we take a pre-trained gVAE, fix the learned features in the encoder's graph convolution layers, and fine-tune the remaining layers for a different anatomy. We compare this training strategy to training a gVAE from scratch. Results in Fig. 4(a) show that a pre-trained model can be fined-tuned with as small as 1088 new examples. In comparison, gVAE could not be trained from scratch with $\leq$ 7360 samples, shown both by the low reconstruction accuracy (Fig. 4(a): DC = 0.24; SSE = 17.68) and a flat test loss plot (Fig. 4(b)). Test loss plots in Fig. 4(b) also show that a pre-trained model starts with a lower loss and a larger size of training data leads to faster convergence. Parameter optimization via a gVAE fine-tuned with 7360 data on 20 cases achieved an average DC and SSE of 53.10 and 11.01 respectively. Figure 4(c) shows some examples of the estimated parameters.

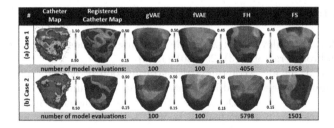

Fig. 5. Estimated parameters with gVAE, fVAE, FH, and FS on real-data studies. (Color figure online)

5   Real Data Experiments

We conduct real-data studies on two patients with chronic myocardial infarction. Patient-specific heart-thorax models are obtained from axial CT images. Using 120-lead ECG as measurements, we evaluate the presented gVAE in estimating tissue excitability in comparison to the fVAE [6], FH [5], and FS [11] methods. Training dataset and network architectures are as described in Sect. 4.

We qualitatively evaluate the results with *in-vivo* catheter mapping data which, as shown in Fig. 5, provides a reference for the location of the abnormal (red, voltage ≤0.5 mV) and healthy (purple, voltage >1.5 mV) regions.

Case 1 has a large heterogeneous abnormal region in the lateral LV region (Fig. 5(a)). All methods are able to localize this region, but with varying degree of heterogeneity. Optimizations based on gVAE and fVAE are much faster requiring only 100 model evaluations, in comparison to FH and FS that required 4056 and 1058 model evaluations, respectively. By contrast, case 2 has a smaller but dense abnormal region in the lateral LV (Fig. 5(b)). While all methods identify the general location of this abnormality, gVAE more accurately differentiates the region of dense core and border. In comparison, fVAE and FH estimate a larger border region; and the abnormal region revealed by FS is less accurate. Again, in this case, gVAE and fVAE required only 100 model evaluations, whereas FH and FS required 5798 and 1501 model evaluations, respectively.

Conclusion and Future Work: We presented a novel graph convolutional VAE and integrated it with Bayesian optimization to enable optimization on large graphs. In future, we will incorporate realistic data from high resolution 3D images and investigate transfer learning of models trained on these data for efficient model personalization.

Acknowledgements. This work is supported by the NSF under CAREER Award ACI-1350374 and the NHLBI of the NIH under Award R01HL145590.

References

1. Aliev, R.R., Panfilov, A.V.: A simple two-variable model of cardiac excitation. Chaos Solitons Fractals **7**(3), 293–301 (1996)
2. Arevalo, H.J., et al.: Arrhythmia risk stratification of patients after myocardial infarction using personalized heart models. Nat. Commun. **7**, 11437 (2016)
3. Brochu, E., Cora, V.M., De Freitas, N.: A tutorial on bayesian optimization of expensive cost functions, with application to active user modeling and hierarchical reinforcement learning. arXiv preprint arXiv:1012.2599 (2010)
4. Bronstein, M.M., Bruna, J., LeCun, Y., Szlam, A., Vandergheynst, P.: Geometric deep learning: going beyond euclidean data. IEEE Sign. Process. Mag. **34**(4), 18–42 (2017)
5. Dhamala, J., et al.: Spatially adaptive multi-scale optimization for local parameter estimation in cardiac electrophysiology. IEEE TMI **36**(9), 1966–1978 (2017)
6. Dhamala, J., Ghimire, S., Sapp, J.L., Horáček, B.M., Wang, L.: High-dimensional bayesian optimization of personalized cardiac model parameters via an embedded generative model. In: Frangi, A.F., Schnabel, J.A., Davatzikos, C., Alberola-López, C., Fichtinger, G. (eds.) MICCAI 2018. LNCS, vol. 11071, pp. 499–507. Springer, Cham (2018). https://doi.org/10.1007/978-3-030-00934-2_56
7. Dhillon, I.S., Guan, Y., Kulis, B.: Weighted graph cuts without eigenvectors a multilevel approach. IEEE TPAMI **29**(11), 1944–1957 (2007)

8. Fey, M., Eric Lenssen, J., Weichert, F., Müller, H.: Splinecnn: fast geometric deep learning with continuous b-spline kernels. In: CVPR, pp. 869–877 (2018)
9. Kingma, D.P., Welling, M.: Auto-encoding variational bayes. arXiv preprint arXiv:1312.6114 (2013)
10. Sermesant, M., Chabiniok, R., Chinchapatnam, P., et al.: Patient-specific electromechanical models of the heart for the prediction of pacing acute effects in crt: a preliminary clinical validation. Med. Image Anal. **16**(1), 201–215 (2012)
11. Wong, K.C.L., et al.: Strain-based regional nonlinear cardiac material properties estimation from medical images. In: Ayache, N., Delingette, H., Golland, P., Mori, K. (eds.) MICCAI 2012. LNCS, vol. 7510, pp. 617–624. Springer, Heidelberg (2012). https://doi.org/10.1007/978-3-642-33415-3_76
12. Ying, Z., You, J., Morris, C., Ren, X., Leskovec, J.: Hierarchical graph representation learning with differentiable pooling. In: NeurIPS, pp. 4805–4815 (2018)

Discriminative Coronary Artery Tracking via 3D CNN in Cardiac CT Angiography

Han Yang, Junxuan Chen, Ying Chi$^{(\boxtimes)}$, Xuansong Xie, and Xiansheng Hua

Alibaba Group, Hangzhou, China
xinyi.cy@alibaba-inc.com

Abstract. Extraction of the coronary artery centerline from cardiac CT angiography (CCTA) is a challenging yet prerequisite task for subsequent diagnosis in clinical practice. In this paper, a discriminative coronary artery tracking method (DCAT) is proposed to (semi) automatically extract coronary artery centerlines. It consists of two parts: a tracker and a discriminator. The tracker outputs orientation and radius of the vessel at each location, which is used to extract vessel-like objects. The discriminator provides a learning-based stop criterion during tracking, which can distinguish coronary artery from other vessel-like objects. We train the tracker and the discriminator simultaneously, which are proved to be helpful to each other. We evaluate the DCAT on the public dataset in CAT08 challenge and our method outperforms state-of-the-art methods. Furthermore, training of the discriminator only needs coarsely labeled centerline annotations, that enables training the DCAT model on a large set of data all of which have centerline annotations, but only a small fraction of which have accurate centerline and radius annotations. This reduces annotations effort greatly. Experimental results on a private collected clinical dataset demonstrate the effectiveness of this training schema.

Keywords: Coronary artery tracking · Discriminative · Convolutional neural network · Cardiac CT angiography

1 Introduction

Coronary artery disease is one of the leading cause of death in the world today [12]. To obtain the information of the coronary artery of a suspicious patient, cardiac CT angiography (CCTA) is widely used because of non-invasion and high sensitivity [7]. Typically it is difficult to observe a tubular structure such as coronary arteries in a 3D CCTA volume directly. So in the first step, coronary artery centerlines are extracted manually or (semi) automatically from the volume. Then doctors can examine a full coronary artery in an 2D curved planar reformation (CPR) image easily. To reduce the manual labor of the doctor, many (semi) automatic methods that extract coronary artery centerlines have been proposed.

© Springer Nature Switzerland AG 2019
D. Shen et al. (Eds.): MICCAI 2019, LNCS 11765, pp. 468–476, 2019.
https://doi.org/10.1007/978-3-030-32245-8_52

Most of the methods can be divided into three categories, i.e. shortest path based [6,10], segmentation based [9,14,16], and tracking based [1–3,11,13,15]. The first approach computes the shortest path in a vessel map between a start and an end point as the vessel centerline. Therefore, this method may need many interactions to extract the whole vessel tree. The second approach segments the vessels first and then extracts centerlines from the mask. It requires large amount of accurate labeled training data. For instance, [9] used over 100 synthetic and 40 real data with mask annotation to train a convolutional neural network (CNN). The third approach early used a tracker based on hand-crafted features to iteratively search tubular structures such as retinal vessel [15], ridge-based vessel [13] and liver vessel [3]. Recently, [11] proposed a CNNTracker to extract coronary artery centerlines and they obtained state-of-the-art (SOTA) performance. The CNNTracker can simultaneously predict the proper direction and step-size using a single CNN. However, it may fall into other vessel-like objects such as veins, because training samples are only extracted along the vessel centerlines and the stop criterion based on manual rules is inflexible. In addition, training scans used in [11] require accurate centerline and radius annotations, which is a time-consuming work.

In this paper, in order to solve the problems mentioned above, a discriminative coronary artery tracking method (DCAT) based on 3D CNN is proposed. The DCAT consists of a tracker and a discriminator. The tracker identifies proper orientation and radius of the artery at each location, which is used to extract vessel-like objects. The discriminator is a binary classifier which provides a learning-based stop criterion during tracking. Training samples for the discriminator come from everywhere in 3D CCTA, therefore, it has ability to distinguish coronary artery from other vessel-like objects. We simultaneously optimize these two tasks, which can promote each other. In addition, training of the discriminator only needs coarsely labeled centerline annotations, that enables training the DCAT model with small amount of precisely labeled data and large amount of coarsely labeled data simultaneously. This can reduce annotation effort greatly.

The main contributions of this paper include: (1) We propose DCAT, a discriminative coronary artery tracking method via 3D CNN. It has a tracker and a discriminator which can be jointly trained and promote each other. (2) Our DCAT can be trained with small amount of precisely labeled data and large amount of coarsely labeled data simultaneously. With this training schema, the model can be easily transferred to different domains with much less annotation workload. (3) We evaluate DCAT on the public dataset in CAT08 challenge and a private collected dataset. In both scenes, our method achieves SOTA performances.

2   Method

2.1   Discriminative Coronary Artery Tracking

The DCAT model contains a backbone and a functional head including a tracker and a discriminator shown in Fig. 1. The tracker is developed to identify the orientation of vessel-like objects. And then the discriminator is introduced to

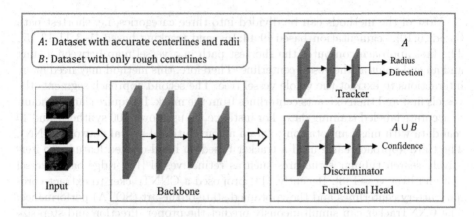

Fig. 1. Detailed illustration of our DCAT. The backbone is a 3D CNN combined with first 4 conv layers used in [11]. Dilation conv layer is used and dilation rate in layer 2 and 3 is 2 and 4 respectively. The tracker has three 3D conv layers and two outputs: radius r and direction probability distribution T. The discriminator has three 3D conv layers and a output confidence p.

distinguish the coronary artery from other vessel-like objects such as vein in 3D CCTA. It takes a 3D image patch of shape $w \times w \times w$ with isotropic voxel spacing v as input, and a direction probability distribution $T \in [0, 1]^N$ where N is the number of all possible directions in Fig. 2(a), a radius $r \in \mathbb{R}$ of the coronary artery and an identification confidence $p \in [0, 1]$ for being a part of coronary artery as outputs.

The tracker includes two task branches: a direction branch and a radius branch. As shown in Fig. 2(a), all possible directions $D \in \mathbb{R}^{N \times 3}$ are evenly distributed on a sphere [5]. The direction branch is a classifier to recognize the next proper direction $d \in D$ from current location. The radius branch is a regressor to predict the radius r of the coronary artery at current location.

Besides coronary artery, there are many other vessel-like objects like veins in CCTA. To prevent the tracker from falling into these objects which we are not interested in, we introduce a discriminator. It has three 3D convolutional layers and takes the same input features as the tracker. The first layer with kernel size $3 \times 3 \times 3$ outputs a feature map with 64 channels. The second layer is a $1 \times 1 \times 1$ convolutional layer with 64 output channels. At last, another $1 \times 1 \times 1$ convolutional layer outputs a probability scalar p.

The benefit of using the discriminator comes from three aspects. Firstly, we directly stop tracking according to the discriminator instead of the moving average normalized entropy of T used in [11]. As a result, our stop criterion is learning-based and more flexible while the one in [11] relies on manual designed rules. Secondly, our DCAT model has ability to distinguish coronary artery from background such as veins. At last, the discriminator is trained with various types of easily-labeled data so it can make the fundamental convolutional layers more robust.

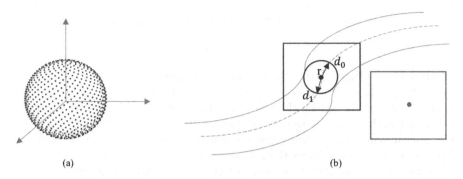

(a)   (b)

Fig. 2. (a) All possible directions distribute on the sphere. (b) A 2D simplified visualization of the coronary artery and training patches. The solid curves are lumen boundaries and the dash line is the centerline. A training sample for the tracker is represented by a box on the left. It has two reference directions d_0, d_1 and a reference radius r. The box on the left is also a positive sample for the discriminator while the box on the right is a negative sample.

2.2 Training and Testing Strategy

Training Procedure: The model can be fed with two kinds of dataset, we call them dataset A and B. Dataset A is labeled with point-wise centerlines and radii following the annotation standard [8]. Dataset B only has coarse centerlines where annotated points may be off-center in the coronary artery lumen. Training samples extracted along the centerlines in dataset A are used to train the tracker. And training samples extracted everywhere in the whole 3D CCTA volume from dataset $A \cup B$ are used to train the discriminator.

As shown in Fig. 2(b), training samples for the tracker are extracted along the centerlines. The corresponding direction label comprises two directions that from current location to the last and the next reference centerline points with a foot-step length of radius r, and the radius label is the reference radius r of the current location. The positive samples for the discriminator are extracted on the coronary artery. And the negative samples are extracted at the location outside the area defined by a certain minimum distance S to the centerlines.

During training, the Adam optimizer updates all trainable parameters in the backbone, the tracker and the discriminator to minimize the loss

$$\mathcal{L}_{DCAT} = \mathcal{L}_{dir} + \lambda \mathcal{L}_{reg} + \beta \mathcal{L}_{cls} \tag{1}$$

where $\mathcal{L}_{dir}$ is the categorical cross-entropy loss from direction task, $\mathcal{L}_{reg}$ is the squared error from radius regression task, and $\mathcal{L}_{cls}$ is the binary cross-entropy loss from discriminator task.

This joint training schema brings a practical benefit. When we need to transfer our model to a new data distribution, we can conveniently enlarge the amount of dataset B with coarsely labeled data in the new dataset. In this manner, we can significantly decrease the annotation workload. We will demonstrate this advantage in Sect. 3.2.

Testing Procedure: For a single coronary artery, when a start point x_0 in the coronary artery lumen is provided, two initial directions d_0, d_1 and radius r_0 are firstly determined by the tracker. Toward direction d_0, the tracker takes a step of length r_0 and arrives at location x_1 via operation: $x_1 = x_0 + r_0 * d_0$. The discriminator outputs a confidence that point x_1 is on the coronary artery. When the confidence is lower than a predefined threshold K, we stop tracking. Then we repeat this operation until termination. And the same processing is applied to direction d_1.

The two coronary ostium $O_0, O_1 \in \mathbb{R}^3$ and initial seed points $S \in \mathbb{R}^{M \times 3}$ in the coronary artery can be detected using two distance regression models described in [11]. Each seed point $s_i \in S$ is used as a start point to extract the relevant vessel v_i, and we push v_i into tree set V if one of its end covers O_0 or O_1. Seed points within a certain minimum distance to vessels in V are ignored because of being redundant. As a result, V is the complete coronary artery tree which is extracted automatically.

3   Experiments and Results

We conduct the experiments on the public CAT08 dataset and a private collected clinical dataset. In all experiments, we resample 3D CCTA scans to voxel spacing $v = 0.5$. The input shape w of the DCAT is 19 and the number of possible directions $N = 500$. In the objective loss function, we use 15 and 1 for the λ and β respectively. We set the threshold $K = 0.5$ for the discriminator. Considering the coronary artery radius is almost all less than 3 mm, we use 3 for S. And we apply random translation and rotation as data augmentation. The algorithm is implemented using Pytorch with an NVIDIA Tesla P100 GPU. In training stage, we train the DCAT model up to 100 epochs with a initial learning rate of 0.001.

We evaluate our DCAT based on the Rotterdam Coronary Artery Algorithm Evaluation Framework [8]. Extracted centerlines are evaluated by total overlap (OV), overlap until first error (OF), overlap of clinical relevant part (OT) and average inside accuracy (AI).

3.1   Experimental Results on CAT08 Dataset

The CAT08 dataset contains 8 CCTA scans with multi-expert collaborative annotations. Each annotation has four major coronary arteries and their accurate point-wise centerlines and corresponding radii. In this experiment we use a leave-one-out cross-validation strategy to evaluate 8 CCTA scans and compare our method with several SOTA methods i.e. HOTtractography [2], ModelDriven-Centerline [16], CNNTracker [11], and MHT [4] on the CAT08 leaderboard.

Table 1. Comparison of different approaches in the task of coronary artery centerline extraction. Upper corner mark of the method indicates corresponding challenge category. Challenge 1 is automatic. Challenge 2 provides one auxiliary point while challenge 3 provides more than one auxiliary points.

Method	OV(%)			OF(%)			OT(%)			AI(mm)		
	min.	max.	avg.	min.	max.	avg.	min.	max.	avg.	min.	max.	avg.
HOTtractography[2]	66.6	100.0	97.3	10.0	100.0	85.0	67.2	100.0	97.7	0.22	0.51	0.34
ModelDrivenCenterline[1]	68.7	99.9	92.4	17.1	100.0	80.6	69.7	100.0	93.4	**0.12**	0.47	0.21
CNNTracker[3]	61.3	100.0	95.7	12.9	100.0	87.1	62.2	100.0	97.1	0.14	0.43	0.23
MHT[3]	**94.5**	100.0	99.3	23.9	100.0	94.6	**94.5**	100.0	99.5	0.16	0.37	0.24
DCAT(Ours)[2]	83.1	**100.0**	**99.5**	**71.6**	**100.0**	**99.1**	83.1	**100.0**	**99.5**	0.15	**0.24**	**0.19**

As reported in Table 1, Our method surpasses other methods in average OV, OF, OT and AI. Some of them require more user interactions. For example, MHT even needs 2–5 points per vessel. In terms of computation time, MHT needs 6 min per CCTA image on average. ModelDrivenCenterline needs 1 min and HOTtractography needs less than 30 s. CNNTracker and Our DCAT take around 10 s due to the efficiency of the tracking based method.

In tracking-based methods, DCAT is obviously much better than the other one CNNTracker. In vessel 0 of dataset 0 (Fig. 4(a)), there is a long plaque with severe stenosis in proximal segment. CNNTracker could not pass through this area because of the inflexible stop criterion, which leads to an OF as low as 12.9%. Thanks to the discriminator, our DCAT can correctly extract complete vessel and the OV, OF, OT are 99.4%, 100.0%, 100.0% respectively.

We also conduct an experiment to show that the joint training of the discriminator and the tracker can promote the tracker. As illustrated in Fig. 3, when the tracker is trained with the discriminator, the direction loss and the radius loss both converge faster and better.

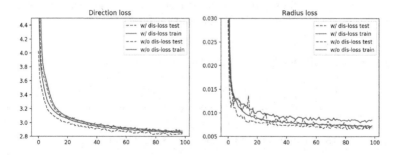

Fig. 3. Loss curves of direction classification and radius regression in the tracker. Solid lines denote training loss, and dash lines denote testing loss. The loss curves of the models that are trained with and without discriminator are represented in red and green respectively. (Color figure online)

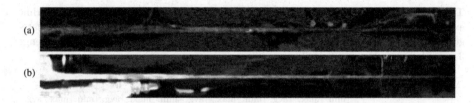

Fig. 4. Straightened CPR of extracted coronary artery in WL 300 and WW 800. (a) artery in the public CAT08 dataset. (b) artery in the private dataset.

3.2 Experimental Results on Private Dataset

The private dataset collected from clinic contains 18 training scans and 32 testing scans. Training data labeled on axis view has only coarse centerlines, while testing data contains accurate centerlines and radii following the annotation standard in [8]. As shown in Fig. 4, CCTA scans in the private dataset are much different from scans in the CAT08 dataset. We denote all of the 8 scans in public CAT08 dataset as A, and 18 training scans in our private dataset as B.

Low annotation cost and few interaction are two main requirements to widely utilize deep learning algorithms in clinic. To evaluate that our DCAT can reduce annotation cost, A is firstly used to train a model DCAT-A, and then we leverage the combination of A and B ($A \cup B$) to jointly train a model DCAT-A $\cup$ B following the framework illustrated in Fig. 1. In order to automatically extract coronary arteries, two distance regression models trained by $A \cup B$ are used to detect the ostium locations O_0, O_1 and initial start points S respectively. At last, we automatically test DCAT-A and DCAT-A$\cup$B on 32 precisely labeled testing scans in our private dataset.

As reported in Table 2, DCAT-A $\cup$ B surpasses DCAT-A in all metrics with a large margin especially OF. The only difference is that DCAT-A $\cup$ B uses additional easily labeled dataset B which has only coarse centerlines annotation. With this strategy, during training, we can increase the percentage of B in the combination of A $\cup$ B. It can reduce annotation effort greatly.

Table 2. Results for DCAT-A and DCAT-A $\cup$ B in the private dataset.

Method	OV(%)			OF(%)			OT(%)			AI(mm)		
	min.	max.	avg.	min.	max.	avg.	min.	max.	avg.	min.	max.	avg.
DCAT-A	45.3	100.0	85.6	34.9	100.0	82.1	79.6	100.0	87.8	0.23	0.51	0.35
DCAT-A $\cup$ B	**75.8**	**100.0**	**92.6**	**73.1**	**100.0**	**93.8**	**92.4**	**100.0**	**94.6**	**0.21**	**0.43**	**0.31**

4   Conclusion

In this paper, we propose a discriminative coronary artery tracking method (DCAT) via 3D CNN. The DCAT consists of a tracker and a discriminator which can be simultaneously trained. The discriminator provides a learning-based stop criterion which is more robust for tracking-based methods, and also, the discriminator and the tracker can promote each other. As a result, our DCAT achieves state-of-the-art performance in CAT08 challenge and a private clinical dataset. In addition, the DCAT can be jointly trained with a small subset of precisely labeled data and a large subset of easily labeled data. With this training schema, we can significantly decrease the annotation costs and make the method transfer to different domains easily, which is very helpful in practice.

References

1. Aylward, S.R., Bullitt, E.: Initialization, noise, singularities, and scale in height ridge traversal for tubular object centerline extraction. IEEE Trans. Med. Imaging **21**(2), 61–75 (2002)
2. Cetin, S., Unal, G.: A higher-order tensor vessel tractography for segmentation of vascular structures. IEEE Trans. Med. Imaging **34**(10), 2172–2185 (2015)
3. Friman, O., Hindennach, M., Kühnel, C., Peitgen, H.O.: Multiple hypothesis template tracking of small 3d vessel structures. Med. Image Anal. **14**(2), 160–171 (2010)
4. Friman, O., Kühnel, C., Peitgen, H.O.: Coronary centerline extraction using multiple hypothesis tracking and minimal paths. In: Proceedings of MICCAI, vol. 42 (2008)
5. González, Á.: Measurement of areas on a sphere using fibonacci and latitude-longitude lattices. Math. Geosci. **42**(1), 49 (2010)
6. Krissian, K., Bogunovic, H., Pozo, J., Villa-Uriol, M., Frangi, A.: Minimally interactive knowledge-based coronary tracking in cta using a minimal cost path. Insight J. (2008)
7. Leipsic, J., et al.: Scct guidelines for the interpretation and reporting of coronary ct angiography: a report of the society of cardiovascular computed tomography guidelines committee. J. Cardiovasc. Comput. Tomogr. **8**(5), 342–358 (2014)
8. Schaap, M., et al.: Standardized evaluation methodology and reference database for evaluating coronary artery centerline extraction algorithms. Med. Image Anal. **13**(5), 701–714 (2009)
9. Tetteh, G., et al.: Deepvesselnet: vessel segmentation, centerline prediction, and bifurcation detection in 3-d angiographic volumes. arXiv preprint arXiv:1803.09340 (2018)
10. Wink, O., Frangi, A.F., Verdonck, B., Viergever, M.A., Niessen, W.J.: 3D MRA coronary axis determination using a minimum cost path approach. Mag. Reson. Med. Official J. Int. Soc. Mag. Reson. Med. **47**(6), 1169–1175 (2002)
11. Wolterink, J.M., van Hamersvelt, R.W., Viergever, M.A., Leiner, T., Išgum, I.: Coronary artery centerline extraction in cardiac ct angiography using a cnn-based orientation classifier. Med. Image Anal. **51**, 46–60 (2019)
12. World Health Organization (WHO): The top ten causes of death - fact sheet n310 (2008)
13. Xiao, R., Yang, J., Li, T., Liu, Y.: Ridge-based automatic vascular centerline tracking in X-ray angiographic images. In: Yang, J., Fang, F., Sun, C. (eds.) IScIDE 2012. LNCS, vol. 7751, pp. 793–800. Springer, Heidelberg (2013). https://doi.org/10.1007/978-3-642-36669-7_96

14. Yang, G., et al.: Automatic centerline extraction of coronary arteries in coronary computed tomographic angiography. Int. J. Cardiovasc. Imaging **28**(4), 921–933 (2012)
15. Yin, Y., Adel, M., Bourennane, S.: Retinal vessel segmentation using a probabilistic tracking method. Pattern Recogn. **45**(4), 1235–1244 (2012)
16. Zheng, Y., Tek, H., Funka-Lea, G.: Robust and accurate coronary artery centerline extraction in CTA by combining model-driven and data-driven approaches. In: Mori, K., Sakuma, I., Sato, Y., Barillot, C., Navab, N. (eds.) MICCAI 2013. LNCS, vol. 8151, pp. 74–81. Springer, Heidelberg (2013). https://doi.org/10.1007/978-3-642-40760-4_10

Whole Heart and Great Vessel Segmentation in Congenital Heart Disease Using Deep Neural Networks and Graph Matching

Xiaowei Xu[1(✉)], Tianchen Wang[1], Yiyu Shi[1], Haiyun Yuan[2], Qianjun Jia[2], Meiping Huang[2], and Jian Zhuang[2]

[1] University of Notre Dame, Notre Dame, USA
{xxu8,twang9,yshi4}@nd.edu
[2] Guangdong General Hospital, Guangzhou, China
yhyyun@163.com, jiaqianjun@126.com, huangmeipng@126.com,
zhuangjian5413@tom.com

Abstract. Congenital heart disease (CHD) is the leading cause of mortality from birth defects, which occurs 1 in every 110 births in the United States. While various whole heart and great vessel segmentation frameworks have been developed in the literature, they are ineffective when applied to medical images in CHD, which have significant variations in heart structure and great vessel connections. To address the challenge, we leverage the power of deep learning in processing regular structures and that of graph algorithms in dealing with large variations, and propose a framework that combines both for whole heart and great vessel segmentation in CHD. Particularly, we first use deep learning to segment the four chambers and myocardium followed by blood pool, where variations are usually small. We then extract the connection information and apply graph matching to determine the categories of all the vessels. Experimental results using 68 3D CT images covering 14 types of CHD show that our method can increase Dice score by 12% on average compared with the state-of-the-art whole heart and great vessel segmentation method in normal anatomy. Our dataset is released to the public.

Keywords: Congenital heart disease · Segmentation · Deep neural networks · Graph matching

1 Introduction

Congenital heart disease (CHD) is the most common cause of infant death due to birth defects [3]. It usually comes with significant variations in heart structures and great vessel connections, which renders general whole heart and great vessel segmentation methods [9,11] in normal anatomy ineffective. Most existing segmentation methods dedicated to CHD target blood pool and myocardium only

© Springer Nature Switzerland AG 2019
D. Shen et al. (Eds.): MICCAI 2019, LNCS 11765, pp. 477–485, 2019.
https://doi.org/10.1007/978-3-030-32245-8_53

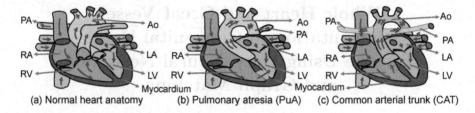

(a) Normal heart anatomy   (b) Pulmonary atresia (PuA)   (c) Common arterial trunk (CAT)

Fig. 1. Examples of large structure variations in CHD. In normal heart anatomy (a), PA is connected to RV. However, in pulmonary atresia (b), PA is rather small and connected to descending Ao. In common arterial trunk (c), Ao is connected to both RV and LV, and PA is connected to Ao.

[13,16]. Recently, semi-automated segmentation in CHD has also been explored [8], which requires users to locate an initial seed. However, fully automated segmentation of whole heart and great vessel segmentation in CHD still remains a missing piece in the literature.

Inspired by the success of graph matching in a number of applications with large variations [4], in this paper we propose to combine deep learning [6,7,12, 14,15] and graph matching for fully automated whole heart and great vessel segmentation in CHD. Particularly, we leverage deep learning to segment the four chambers and myocardium followed by blood pool, where variations are usually small and accuracy can be high. We then extract the vessel connection information and apply graph matching to determine the categories of all the vessels. Compared with the state-of-the-art method for whole heart and great vessel segmentation in normal anatomy, our method can achieve 12% higher Dice score. Our dataset including 68 3D CT images with 14 types of CHD is available at [1].

2   Background

Within normal heart anatomy as shown in Fig. 1(a), there are usually seven substructures: left ventricle (LV), right ventricle (RV), left atrium (LA), right atrium (RA), myocardium (Myo), faorta (Ao) and pulmonary artery (PA). Note that the area including RA, LA, LV, RV, PA, and Ao is defined as blood pool. However, CHD usually suffers from significant variations in heart structure and great vessel connections. Six common types of CHD [3] include: atrial septal defect (ASD), atrio-ventricular septal defect (AVSD), patent ductus arteriosus (PDA), pulmonary stenosis (PS), ventricular septal defect (VSD), co-arctation (CA). Figure 1(b) and (c) shows two less common types with larger variations, where we can notice that PA is connected to Ao rather than RV. As existing methods perform pixel-wise classification based on the surrounding pixels in the receptive field, the disappeared main trunk of PA renders them ineffective.

Table 1. The types of CHD in our dataset and the associated number of images. Note that some images may correspond to more than one type of CHD.

Common CHD						Less common CHD								Normal
ASD	AVSD	VSD	PDA	CA	PS	ToF	TGA	PAS	AD	CAT	AAA	SV	PuA	
17	4	26	7	4	4	7	4	3	20	4	8	2	7	2

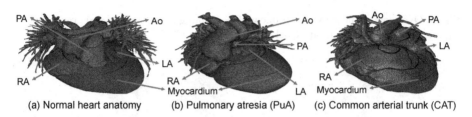

(a) Normal heart anatomy   (b) Pulmonary atresia (PuA)   (c) Common arterial trunk (CAT)

Fig. 2. Pulmonary atresia and common arterial trunk examples in our dataset, with large variations from normal heart anatomy.

3 Dataset

Our dataset consists of 68 3D CT images captured by a Simens biograph 64 machine. The ages of the associated patients range from 1 month to 21 years, with majority between 1 month and 2 years. The size of the images is $512 \times 512 \times (130 - 340)$, and the typical voxel size is $0.25 \times 0.25 \times 0.5 \,\mathrm{mm}^3$. The dataset covers 14 types of CHD, which include the six common types discussed in Sect. 2 plus eight less common ones (Tetrology of Fallot (ToF), transposition of great arteries (TGA), pulmonary artery sling (PAS), anomalous drainage (AD), common arterial trunk (CAT), aortic arch anomalies (AAA), single ventricle (SV), pulmonary atresia (PuA)). The number of images associated with each is summarized in Table 1. All labeling were performed by experienced radiologists, and the time for labeling each image is 1–1.5 h. The labels include seven substructures: LV, RV, LA, RA, Myo, Ao and PA. For easy processing, venae cavae (VC) and pulmonary vein (PV) are also labeled as part of RA and LA respectively, as they are connected and their boundaries are relatively hard to define. Anomalous vessels are also labeled as one of the above seven substructures based on their connections. Figure 2 shows 3D views of some examples in our dataset with significant structure variations.

4 Method

Overview: The overall framework is shown in Fig. 3. **Region of interest (RoI) cropping** extracts the area that includes the heart and its surrounding vessels. We resize the input image to a low resolution of $64 \times 64 \times 64$, and then adopt the same segmentation-based extraction as [9] to get the RoI. **Chambers and myocardium segmentation** resizes the extracted RoI to $64 \times 64 \times 64$ which

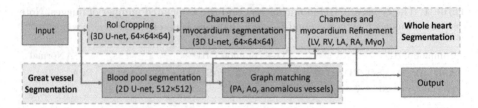

Fig. 3. Overview of the proposed framework combining deep learning and graph matching for whole heart and great vessel segmentation in CHD.

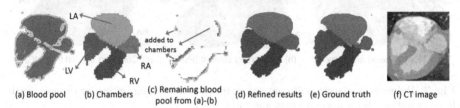

(a) Blood pool   (b) Chambers   (c) Remaining blood pool from (a)-(b)   (d) Refined results   (e) Ground truth   (f) CT image

Fig. 4. Illustration of chambers and myocardium refinement. (a) is obtained from blood pool segmentation (high resolution). (b) is from chambers and myocardium segmentation (low resolution). (c) is the remaining blood pool by subtracting chambers (b) from blood pool (a). It is added to the surrounding chambers to refine the boundaries (d). (e) and (f) are the ground truth and CT image, respectively.

is fed to a 3D U-net for segmentation. **Blood pool segmentation** is conducted on each 2D slice of the input using a 2D U-net [10] with an input size of 512×512. Note that in order to detect the blood pool boundary for easy graph extraction in graph matching later, we add another class blood pool boundary in the segmentation. **Chambers and myocardium refinement** refines the boundaries of chambers and myocardium based on the outputs of chambers and myocardium segmentation and blood pool segmentation. **Graph matching** identifies Ao, PA and anomalous vessels using the outputs of blood pool segmentation and chambers and myocardium segmentation. More details about chambers and myocardium refinement and graph matching are discussed as follows.

Chambers and Myocardium Refinement: To avoid excessive memory consumption and over-fitting [9], the input of 3D U-net is usually limited to low resolution or small size, and accordingly the chambers and myocardium segmentation results may lose boundary information. This is critical for CHD where significant variations exist. To address this issue, we refine the boundary of chambers and myocardium by reusing the blood pool segmentation results, which is in high resolution. Specifically, we remove the portion of blood pool that corresponds to the chambers from the results of blood pool segmentation, and the remaining blood pool is added to its surrounding chambers to refine the boundaries. With the refined boundary of chambers, the boundary of myocardium is also refined as the chambers and the myocardium share a large portion of boundaries as shown

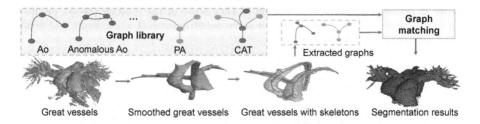

Fig. 5. Illustration of great vessel segmentation with graph matching. With smoothing, the skeleton of great vessels can be easily extracted, and then its corresponding graph is obtained for graph matching based classification of Ao, PA and anomalous vessels.

in Fig. 1. An illustration of the refinement process is shown in Fig. 4. Comparing (b) with (e), we can notice that part of the boundary information is lost, and the boundary is indeed refined after the process as shown in (d).

Graph Matching: Great vessels can be obtained by removing the chambers areas from the blood pool, which need to be segmented to identify Ao, PA as well as anomalous vessels. This is where significant variations can occur in CHD. To address this issue, we adopt a surface thinning algorithm [5] to obtain skeletons of blood vessels for graph matching, and the workflow is shown in Fig. 5. A graph library is built to represent all the possible connections of great vessels and anomalous vessels. We then extract the graphs corresponding to Ao, PA, and anomalous vessels or their mixtures. Note that these extracted graphs should be disconnected from each other to match with the ones in the library. However, due to inaccurate blood pool segmentation or small anomalous connections, the graphs are often fused together, making the matching difficult. To tackle this issue, we apply multiple smoothing in various scales to extract several candidate graphs. Then we match these graphs with the ones in the library to identify the most similar pairs. With graph matching, the categories of the extracted graphs as well as the categories of the corresponding vessels in these graphs can be determined (based on the labeled graphs in the library). The vessels that are left out in the smoothing process are finally classified by a simple region growing technique [2].

5   Experiments

Experiment Setup: All the experiments run on a Nvidia GTX 1080Ti GPU with 11 GB memory. We implement our 3D U-net using Pytorch based on [9]. For 2D U-net, most configurations remain the same with those of the 3D U-net except that 2D U-net adopts 5 levels and the number of filters in the initial level is 16. Both Dice loss and cross entropy loss are used, and the training epochs are 6 and 480 for 2D U-net and 3D U-net, respectively. Data augmentation is also adopted with the same configuration as in [9] for 3D U-net. Data normalization is the same as [9]. The learning rate is 0.0002 for the first 50% epochs, and

Table 2. Mean and standard deviation of Dice score of the state-of-the-art method Seg-CNN [9] and our method (in %) for seven substructures of whole heart and great vessel segmentation.

Method	LV	RV	LA	RA	Myo	Ao	PA	Average
Seg-CNN [9]	67.3	65.0	70.2	76.0	71.5	63.0	52.3	66.5
std	±13.9	±12.0	±7.8	±7.5	±8.3	±13.3	±12.3	±10.7
Our method	82.4	77.6	78.6	82.7	77.3	82.2	67.1	78.3
std	±10.5	±14.3	±7.4	±7.5	±8.3	±8.1	±19.8	±10.8

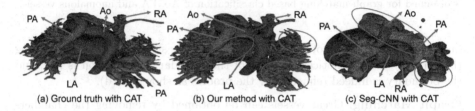

(a) Ground truth with CAT   (b) Our method with CAT   (c) Seg-CNN with CAT

Fig. 6. Visualized comparison between the state-of-the-art method Seg-CNN [9] and our method. The differences from the ground truth are highlighted by the red circles. (Color figure online)

Table 3. Mean and standard deviation of Dice score of the state-of-the-art method Seg-CNN [9] and our method (in %) in mild and severe CHDs.

Method	Mild CHD (VSD, ASD, AVSD, PDA)	Severe CHD (others)
Seg-CNN [9]	70.3 ± 8.3	62.7 ± 14.4
Our method	82.6 ± 6.2	74.1 ± 14.5

then 0.00002 afterward. We adopt Seg-CNN [9] that achieves the state-of-the-art performance in whole heart and great vessel segmentation within normal anatomy for comparison. The configuration is the same as that in [9].

For both methods, four-fold cross validation is performed (17 images for testing and 51 images for training). The split of our dataset considers the structures of CHD so that any structure in the testing dataset also has a similar presence in the training dataset, though they may be not of the same type of CHD. The Dice score is used for segmentation evaluation.

Results and Analysis: The comparison with Seg-CNN [9] is shown in Table 2. Our method can get 5.8%–19.2% higher mean Dice score across the seven substructures (12% higher on average). The highest improvement is achieved in Ao, which is due to its simple graph connection with successful graph matching. The least improvement is obtained in myocardium, which is due to the fact that myocardium is not well considered in the high-resolution blood pool segmentation. Visualization of CAT segmentation using our method and Seg-CNN is

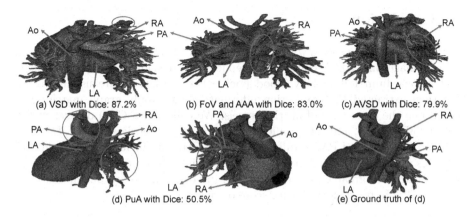

Fig. 7. Visualization of our segmentation results with (a) best, (b)(c) median, and (d) worst Dice scores among all the test images. The ground truth of (d) is shown in (e). Red circles indicate the segmentation error. (Color figure online)

shown in Fig. 6. Our method can clearly segment Ao and PA with some slight mis-segmentation between PA and LA. However, Seg-CNN segments the main part of Ao as PA, which is due to the fact that pixel-level segmentation by U-net is only based on the surrounding pixels, and the connection information is not well exploited.

The segmentation performance of our method and Seg-CNN [9] in different scenarios (mild and severe CHDs) [3] is shown in Table 3. Both methods achieve higher mean Dice with lower standard deviations in mild CHD than in severe CHD, as severe CHD has more complicated structure variations. Compared with Seg-CNN, our method can achieve about 12% higher mean Dice score on both mild and severe CHDs on average. Our method also achieves a 1.9% reduction on standard deviation of Dice score in mild CHD compared with Seg-CNN [9].

Finally, visualizations of segmentation results from our method with best, median and worst Dice score among all the test images are shown in Fig. 7. The segmentation result in Fig. 7(a) achieves the best accuracy, and most of the structures are segmented correctly, with some error in the tiny connections between RA and Ao as indicated by the red circle. The segmentation results in Fig. 7(b) and (c) have some more serious mis-segmentation: the one in Fig. 7(b) has an anomalous vein from RA which is segmented as part of Ao due to the boundary extraction error in blood pool segmentation, and the one in Fig. 7(c) suffers from the boundary extraction error between LA and PA. This type of error also leads to the result with the worst Dice score as shown in Fig. 7(d), with corresponding ground truth provided in (e). In the ground truth, a thick anomalous vein from RA crosses Ao, and PA has no trunk vessels and is of a very small volume. Compared with the ground truth, the thick anomalous vein from RA is mis-classified as PA, and the majority of PA is mis-classified as LA. In the future work, we will try to solve this problem to correctly extract all the critical boundaries.

6   Conclusion

In this paper we proposed a whole heart and great vessel segmentation framework for CT images in CHD. We first used deep learning to segment the four chambers and myocardium followed by blood pool, where variations are usually small. We then extracted the connection information and apply graph matching to determine the categories of all the vessels. We collected a CHD dataset in CT with 68 3D images, and the ground truth has seven categories: LV, RV, LA, RA, myocardium, Ao and PA. Totally 14 types of CHD are included in this dataset which is made publicly available. Compared with the state-of-the-art method for whole heart and great vessel segmentation in normal anatomy, our method can achieve 12% improvement in Dice score on average.

Acknowledgement. This work was approved by the Research Ethics Committee of Guangdong General Hospital, Gunagdong Academy of Medical Sciences with protocol No. 20140316. This work was supported by the National key Research and Development Program [2018YFC1002600], Science and Technology Planning Project of Guangdong Province, China [No. 2017A070701013, 2017B090904034, 2017030314 109, and 2019B020230003], and Guangdong peak project [DFJH201802].

References

1. Chd segmentation dataset. https://github.com/XiaoweiXu/Whole-heart-and-great-vessel-segmentation-of-chd_segmentation/tree/master
2. Adams, R., Bischof, L.: Seeded region growing. IEEE Trans. Pattern Anal. Mach. Intell. **16**(6), 641–647 (1994)
3. Bhat, V., BeLaVaL, V., Gadabanahalli, K., Raj, V., Shah, S.: Illustrated imaging essay on congenital heart diseases: multimodality approach part i: clinical perspective, anatomy and imaging techniques. J. Clin. Diagn. Res. JCDR **10**(5), TE01 (2016)
4. Lajevardi, S.M., Arakala, A., Davis, S.A., Horadam, K.J.: Retina verification system based on biometric graph matching. IEEE Trans. Image Process. **22**(9), 3625–3635 (2013)
5. Lee, T.C., Kashyap, R.L., Chu, C.N.: Building skeleton models via 3-d medial surface axis thinning algorithms. CVGIP Gr. Models Image Process. **56**(6), 462–478 (1994)
6. Li, B., Chenli, C., Xu, X., Jung, T., Shi, Y.: Exploiting computation power of blockchain for biomedical image segmentation. In: Proceedings of the IEEE Conference on Computer Vision and Pattern Recognition Workshops, pp. 0–0 (2019)
7. Liu, Z., et al.: Machine vision guided 3d medical image compression for efficient transmission and accurate segmentation in the clouds. arXiv preprint arXiv:1904.08487 (2019)
8. Pace, D.F., et al.: Iterative segmentation from limited training data: applications to congenital heart disease. In: Stoyanov, D., et al. (eds.) DLMIA/ML-CDS -2018. LNCS, vol. 11045, pp. 334–342. Springer, Cham (2018). https://doi.org/10.1007/978-3-030-00889-5_38

9. Payer, C., Štern, D., Bischof, H., Urschler, M.: Multi-label whole heart segmentation using0 CNNs and anatomical label configurations. In: Pop, M., et al. (eds.) STACOM 2017. LNCS, vol. 10663, pp. 190–198. Springer, Cham (2018). https:// doi.org/10.1007/978-3-319-75541-0_20

10. Ronneberger, O., Fischer, P., Brox, T.: U-Net: convolutional networks for biomedical image segmentation. In: Navab, N., Hornegger, J., Wells, W.M., Frangi, A.F. (eds.) MICCAI 2015. LNCS, vol. 9351, pp. 234–241. Springer, Cham (2015). https://doi.org/10.1007/978-3-319-24574-4_28

11. Wang, C., MacGillivray, T., Macnaught, G., Yang, G., Newby, D.: A two-stage 3d unet framework for multi-class segmentation on full resolution image. arXiv preprint arXiv:1804.04341 (2018)

12. Wang, T., Xiong, J., Xu, X., Shi, Y.: Scnn: A general distribution based statistical convolutional neural network with application to video object detection. arXiv preprint arXiv:1903.07663 (2019)

13. Wolterink, J.M., Leiner, T., Viergever, M.A., Išgum, I.: Dilated convolutional neural networks for cardiovascular MR segmentation in congenital heart disease. In: Zuluaga, M.A., Bhatia, K., Kainz, B., Moghari, M.H., Pace, D.F. (eds.) RAMBO/HVSMR -2016. LNCS, vol. 10129, pp. 95–102. Springer, Cham (2017). https://doi.org/10.1007/978-3-319-52280-7_9

14. Xu, X., et al.: Quantization of fully convolutional networks for accurate biomedical image segmentation. In: Proceedings of the IEEE Conference on Computer Vision and Pattern Recognition, pp. 8300–8308 (2018)

15. Xu, X., et al.: Dac-sdc low power object detection challenge for uav applications. arXiv preprint arXiv:1809.00110 (2018)

16. Yu, L., Yang, X., Qin, J., Heng, P.-A.: 3D FractalNet: dense volumetric segmentation for cardiovascular MRI volumes. In: Zuluaga, M.A., Bhatia, K., Kainz, B., Moghari, M.H., Pace, D.F. (eds.) RAMBO/HVSMR -2016. LNCS, vol. 10129, pp. 103–110. Springer, Cham (2017). https://doi.org/10.1007/978-3-319-52280-7_10

Harmonic Balance Techniques in Cardiovascular Fluid Mechanics

Taha Sabri Koltukluoğlu[1]([✉]) [iD], Gregor Cvijetić[2][iD], and Ralf Hiptmair[1][iD]

[1] Seminar for Applied Mathematics, ETH, Zurich, Switzerland
koltukluoglu@gmail.com
[2] Faculty of Mechanical Engineering and Naval Architecture, FSB, Zagreb, Croatia

Abstract. In cardiovascular fluid mechanics, the typical flow regime is unsteady and periodic in nature as dictated by cardiac dynamics. Most studies featuring computational simulations have approached the problem exploiting the traditional mathematical formulation in the time domain, an approach that incurs huge computational cost. This work explores the application of the harmonic balance method as an alternative numerical modeling tool to resolve the dynamic nature of blood flow. The method takes advantage of the pulsatile regime to transform the original problem into a family of equations in frequency space, while the combination of the corresponding solutions yields the periodic solution of the original problem. As a result of this study we conclude that only a few harmonics are required for resolving the presented fluid flow problem accurately and the method is worth of further investigation in this field.

1 Introduction

In cardiac dynamics, blood flow is heavily influenced by the dynamic nature of the heart beat, which results in an unsteady and periodic flow. When performing pulsatile flow simulations, the classical approach relies on the traditional time-stepping schemes, which require the definition of boundary conditions (BCs) at every time instant. In recent decades, phase-contrast magnetic resonance imaging (4D flow MRI) became relevant for data-based computational fluid dynamics (CFD) studies. Velocity components of blood flow can be measured in-vivo and non-invasively. In addition, three-directional flow can be resolved with the ability to measure the temporal evolution of blood flow within a 3D volume [7]. In CFD studies relying on 4D flow MRI data, sparsely measured velocity profiles are usually interpolated to generate velocity fields to be applied as dynamic BCs for each time instant. Such studies simply apply either linear or spline interpolation [8,11] for transient CFD simulations. Most of these studies have approached the transient problem exploiting the traditional mathematical formulation in the time domain, an approach that incurs huge computational cost.

In this work, an alternative and effective approach is proposed for temporal discretization. This method is known as the harmonic balance (HB) approach

© Springer Nature Switzerland AG 2019
D. Shen et al. (Eds.): MICCAI 2019, LNCS 11765, pp. 486–494, 2019.
https://doi.org/10.1007/978-3-030-32245-8_54

[6], so far mostly reported with preliminary results using mostly 2D or idealized cylindrical geometries [3,4,10]. To the best of authors' knowledge, the HB method is investigated in this work for the first time in the field of computational hemodynamics. The method is based on Fourier decomposition of the velocity field in time and enables the evaluation of its derivative with respect to time in frequency space. Furthermore, the HB discretization can easily be adapted to the sampling rate of measurements in time. This eliminates the necessity for completing the missing data for all time steps, as required in conventional methods. In 4D flow MRI, the velocity components are usually obtained by periodic averaging. The proposed method makes use of this information and proves to be accurate and remarkably effective in terms of computational time.

2   Mathematical Model

Let $\Omega \subset \mathbb{R}^3$ be an open set with boundary $\partial\Omega = \Gamma_i \cup \Gamma_o \cup \Gamma_w$. See Fig. 1a, where Γ_i, Γ_o and Γ_w represent the inlet, outlet and wall boundaries respectively. An incompressible Newtonian fluid is assumed to flow through Ω in the time interval $\mathbb{T} := [0; T]$, as the result of prescribed T-periodic inflow data at Γ_i. The velocity field prescribed at the inlet is characterized by the T-periodic function $g(t, x) = g(t + mT, x) : \mathbb{T} \times \Gamma_i \to \mathbb{R}^3$ with $m \in \mathbb{N}$. The density and dynamic viscosity of the fluid are denoted as ρ and μ respectively.

Considering the strain rate tensor $\nabla^s(\cdot) = [\nabla(\cdot) + (\nabla(\cdot))^T]/2$ and setting $\mathcal{U} = \{ v \in H^1(\Omega) \mid v|_{\Gamma_w} = 0 \}$, the Navier-Stokes equations read: for $t \in \mathbb{T}$, given the initial guess $u(0, x) = u(x)^{\{0\}}$, find $(u, p) \in \mathcal{U} \times L^2(\Omega)$, such that

$$\rho\left[\partial_t u + (\nabla u)u\right] - \mu\Delta u + \nabla p = 0 \qquad \text{in } \mathbb{T} \times \Omega \ , \tag{1}$$

$$\operatorname{div} u = 0 \qquad \text{in } \mathbb{T} \times \Omega \ , \tag{2}$$

$$u = g \qquad \text{on } \mathbb{T} \times \Gamma_i \ , \tag{3}$$

$$(-pI + 2\mu\nabla^s u)n = 0 \qquad \text{on } \mathbb{T} \times \Gamma_o \ . \tag{4}$$

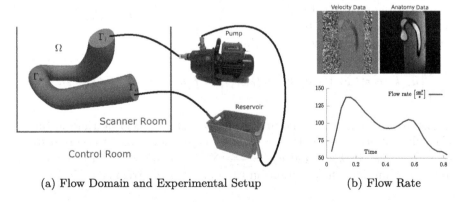

(a) Flow Domain and Experimental Setup   (b) Flow Rate

Fig. 1. Experimental setup (a) and flow rate waveform (b) obtained from 4D flow MRI acquisition in flow domain Ω with boundaries Γ_i : inlet, Γ_o : outlet and Γ_w : wall.

2.1 Harmonic Balance

In what follows, we will consider a time discretization of the momentum equation (1), which can be expressed in the following compact form

$$\partial_t u = f(u),$$ (5)

where $f(u) := -\left[(\nabla u)u - \nu \Delta u + \frac{\nabla p}{\rho} \right]$ (with $\nu := \frac{\mu}{\rho}$ being the kinematic viscosity), which encompasses the convective and diffusive terms along with the force term caused by the pressure. Equation (5) is an evolution equation. Further, $t \to u(t, x)$ is periodic in time with known period T. Therefore, we approximate $u \approx \tilde{u}(t, x) = \sum_{k=1}^{2n+1} c_k(x) \varphi_k(t)$ with the temporal expansion functions φ_k taken from the set

$$\mathcal{T} := \{ 1, \cos(\omega t), \sin(\omega t), \cos(2\omega t), \sin(2\omega t), \cdots, \cos(n\omega t), \sin(n\omega t) \},$$ (6)

where $\mathcal{T}$ represents a complete L^2-orthogonal system on $\mathbb{T}$ and $\omega = \frac{2\pi}{T}$ is the angular frequency. This gives rise to a Fourier spectral method [1] for approximation in time, which relies on the degree-n Fourier polynomial

$$\tilde{u}(t, x) = \frac{\widehat{u}_{c_0}(x)}{2} + \sum_{k=1}^{n} \left[\widehat{u}_{c_k}(x) \cos(k\omega t) + \widehat{u}_{s_k}(x) \sin(k\omega t) \right],$$ (7)

where $\widehat{u}_{c_k}$ for $k = 0 \cdots n$ and $\widehat{u}_{s_k}$ for $k = 1 \cdots n$ are the discrete spectrum of $\tilde{u}$.

In order to obtain a system of equations for the discrete spectrum, we demand that Eq. (5) be satisfied for $2n + 1$ time instants denoted as t_j. We employ a collocation approach and opt for equidistant collocation points

$$t_j := \frac{jT}{2n + 1}, \quad j = 1, 2, \cdots, 2n + 1.$$ (8)

The number of collocation points is equal to the number of terms in the Fourier polynomial (7). Finally, inserting (7) into (5), applying the derivative and demanding that (5) be satisfied at each t_j, the following $2n + 1$ equations are obtained in the frequency domain

$$\sum_{k=1}^{n} \left[\widehat{u}_{s_k} k\omega \cos(k\omega t_j) - \widehat{u}_{c_k} k\omega \sin(k\omega t_j) \right] = f(\tilde{u}(t_j, x)), \quad j = 1 \cdots 2n + 1.$$ (9)

Let $\tilde{u}^i := \tilde{u}(t_i, x)$ be the approximated velocity field at time instant t_i. The DFT of $\tilde{u}^i$ is given by the discrete cosine and sine transforms $\widehat{u}_{c_k} = \frac{2}{2n+1} \sum_{i=1}^{2n+1} \tilde{u}^i \cos(k\omega t_i)$ and $\widehat{u}_{s_k} = \frac{2}{2n+1} \sum_{i=1}^{2n+1} \tilde{u}^i \sin(k\omega t_i)$. Inserting the discrete spectrum into the equations in (9) and using the trigonometric identities,

$\sin(\alpha \pm \beta) = \sin(\alpha)\cos(\beta) \pm \cos(\alpha)\sin(\beta)$, results in the following approximation,

$$\sum_{k=1}^{n} \left[\frac{2k\omega}{2n+1} \sum_{i=1}^{2n+1} \tilde{u}^i \Big(\sin(k\omega t_i)\cos(k\omega t_j) - \cos(k\omega t_i)\sin(k\omega t_j) \Big) \right] = f(\tilde{u}^j)$$

$$\Rightarrow \frac{2\omega}{2n+1} \sum_{i=1}^{2n+1} \sum_{k=1}^{n} k\tilde{u}^i \sin(k\omega(t_i - t_j)) = f(\tilde{u}^j). \tag{10}$$

Setting $N = 2n+1$ and defining $c_{ij} = \frac{2\omega}{N}\sum_{k=1}^{n} k\sin(k\omega(t_i - t_j))$ for $i, j = 1 \cdots N$, we finally obtain from (10) the harmonically balanced momentum equations

$$\sum_{i=1}^{N} \tilde{u}^i c_{ij} + (\nabla \tilde{u}^j)\tilde{u}^j - \nu\Delta\tilde{u}^j + \frac{\nabla p^j}{\rho} = 0, \qquad j = 1, 2, \cdots, N. \tag{11}$$

Algorithm 1. SIMPLE & Block-Gauss-Seidel Algorithm for Harmonic Balance

Input : $(u^j)^{\{0\}}$, $(p^j)^{\{0\}}$, n ▷ Initial guesses $(\cdot)^{\{0\}}$ and harmonics

Output : $(u^j)^{\{k\}}, (p^j)^{\{k\}}$ ▷ Flow fields at last iteration k

1: **procedure** HARMONICBALANCELOOP($u^{\{0\}}, p^{\{0\}}, N = 2n + 1$)

2:      $g^j \leftarrow (u^j)^{\{0\}}$ on Γ_i for $j = 1 \cdots N$, $\quad m \leftarrow$ Number of HB iterations

3:      **for** $k \leftarrow 1, m$ **do**   ▷ HB iterations

4:          **for** $j \leftarrow 1, N$ **do**   ▷ Solve one SIMPLE iteration at each t_j

5:              $(u^j)^{\{k\}} \leftarrow$ Given $\sum_{i=1}^{N} \tilde{u}^i c_{ij}$, g^j, $(p^j)^{\{k-1\}}$ solve equation (11)

6:              $(p^j)^{\{k\}} \leftarrow$ Given $(u^j)^{\{k\}}$ solve for $(p^j)^{\{k\}}$

7:              Correct $(u^j)^{\{k\}}$ using $(p^j)^{\{k\}}$ and update HB coupling $\sum_{i=1}^{N} \tilde{u}^i c_{ij}$

8:          **if** each $|\mathscr{R}^j((u^j)^{\{k\}})| \ll 1$ **then**   ▷ Convergence criterion

9:              **return** $(u^j)^{\{m\}}, (p^j)^{\{m\}}$ for $j = 1 \cdots N$

The frequency domain equations are now expressed in terms of the time domain state variables $\tilde{u}^j$ at each time instant $t_j = \frac{jT}{2n+1}$. The original problem has been cast into the form of a set of coupled fluid flow problems, which yield the periodic solution of the original problem.

For the set of HB momentum equations (11), the SIMPLE algorithm [9] was employed to deal with the pressure-velocity coupling at each time instant t_j, separately. The temporal influence from neighbouring time instants is accounted for by the summation term $\sum_{i=1}^{N} \tilde{u}^i c_{ij}$. The numerical solution of the HB coupling is obtained using a block-Gauss-Seidel iterative algorithm. The spatial discretization of the corresponding equations was achieved using the finite volume method. Algorithm 1 describes the HB method in terms of a pseudo-code. The fields $(\cdot)^{\{k\}}$ will represent the fields $(\cdot)$ at k-th iteration of SIMPLE. Moreover, the equation residuals of the equations in (11) will be denoted by $\mathscr{R}^j((\boldsymbol{u}^j)^*)$ for each j, where $(\boldsymbol{u}^j)^*$ is the corresponding approximation of the solver. The calculation is considered converged when each of the N equation sets are converged.

3   Experimental Setup for 4D Flow MRI

A time-dependent experiment was performed using a glass replica of human aorta, which was placed in a 3T MRI scanner. The rigid geometry consists of aortic root, ascending aorta, aortic arch without branches and descending aorta as illustrated in Fig. 1a. Detailed explanation of the experimental setup is provided in [5] (Sect. 5.1). The acquired voxel size was 1.5 mm^3 isotropic, along with a time resolution of 33 ms. The period of one heart cycle was 0.825 s and 25 data were acquired per cardiac cycle. Controlling the flow rates, a Reynolds number of at most 1100 was achieved. The flow model in this work does not account for turbulence, which is a matter of current research. Finally, the obtained volumetric flow rate resulted in a wave containing two peaks of different magnitudes as shown in Fig. 1b. The observed flow rates are merely an approximation to the physiological flow rates and were dictated by limitations of the experimental setup.

The connection was made with a PVC tubing of total length 20 m with an inner diameter of 19 mm. The inlet and outlet of the pipe were connected to a reservoir in the control room creating an open circuit. A ball bearing valve was placed 1.5 m downstream the tube and was used to control the flow rate. Figure 1a illustrates the experimental setup.

Obtained raw measurements underwent a set of preprocessing tasks including denoising of the flow field, segmentation of the aorta, its smoothing and registration with the exact geometry and a divergence-free projection of the reconstructed flow field, which have all been comprehensively described in [5] (Sects. 3 and 5). Further, three computational meshes, denoted as $\mathbf{M_2}$, $\mathbf{M_4}$ and $\mathbf{M_7}$, were generated using the exact geometry of the aortic replica, with different numbers of cells, 215 000, 440 000 and 750 000 respectively.

In addition to the flow acquisition, reference flow solutions were numerically generated to serve as the ground truth for validation purposes. To achieve this, first an inflow boundary profile was reconstructed from a single steady-state flow MRI acquisition and the obtained flow field was smoothed using low-pass filtering (in order to reduce the measurement noise). Second, the acquired steady flow profile was dynamically adjusted over time and then applied as BC at the inlet for twenty periods to achieve a transient flow simulation with a periodic state of equilibrium. This was performed by multiplying each velocity component at the inlet with an appropriately chosen analytical periodic function of period 0.8 s and base frequency of 1.25 Hz. The function was chosen such that it contains two peaks of different magnitudes in one cycle, similar to the flow rates obtained from the dynamic experiments.

4   Numerical Experiments

Computed flow fields $\boldsymbol{u}_c$ and reference flow fields $\boldsymbol{u}_r$ were quantitatively compared using the following normalized root-mean square error integrated over time

$$\text{nRMSE}(\boldsymbol{u}_c, \boldsymbol{u}_r) = \left(\frac{100}{\underset{\text{T}, \Omega}{\text{avr}} |\boldsymbol{u}_r|} \right) \sqrt{ \frac{1}{V_\Omega \cdot T} \int_\text{T} \int_\Omega |\boldsymbol{u}_c - \boldsymbol{u}_r|^2 \, d\Omega \, dt}. \qquad (12)$$

Validation with a Single Mesh Geometry. As a first step, mesh $\mathbf{M_2}$ was employed to generate both the numerical reference solution, denoted by $\boldsymbol{u}_{\text{ext}}$, as well as the solutions based on the HB method, denoted by $\boldsymbol{u}_{\text{hb}}^n$ with $n = \{2, 5, 8, 10, 12\}$ number of harmonics. For this purpose, the reference flow solution was sparsely sampled multiple times at $2n + 1$ equidistantly placed time instants for each HB simulation, resulting in 5, 11, 17, 21 and 25 data points (samples) per cycle respectively. The samples were then used as the observational boundary data for the HB solver, which was run for 1 000 Gauss-Seidel iterations on mesh $\mathbf{M_2}$ using 48 processors. Quantitatively, the solutions $\boldsymbol{u}_{\text{hb}}^n$ were compared with the reference solution $\boldsymbol{u}_{\text{ext}}$ in terms of nRMSE($\boldsymbol{u}_{\text{hb}}^n$, $\boldsymbol{u}_{\text{ext}}$), resulting in 13.22%, 2.18%, 0.75%, 0.43% and 0.29% respectively. These results are summarized in Table 1 along with the corresponding wall clock times.

Table 1. Root mean square errors nRMSE($\boldsymbol{u}_{\text{hb}}^n$, $\boldsymbol{u}_{\text{ext}}$) evaluated against the ground truth $\boldsymbol{u}_{\text{ext}}$ and the corresponding wall clock times (WCT) in seconds.

$\boldsymbol{u}_c$	$\boldsymbol{u}_{\text{hb}}^2$	$\boldsymbol{u}_{\text{hb}}^5$	$\boldsymbol{u}_{\text{hb}}^8$	$\boldsymbol{u}_{\text{hb}}^{10}$	$\boldsymbol{u}_{\text{hb}}^{12}$
nRMSE($\boldsymbol{u}_c$, $\boldsymbol{u}_{\text{ext}}$)	13.22%	2.18%	0.75%	0.43%	0.29%
WCT in seconds	217 s	458 s	788 s	960 s	1 190 s

We observed that at least 8 harmonics are needed for the HB method to recover the velocity field with nRMSE below 1%. Considering the number of harmonics from 2 to 12, the errors dropped rapidly (from 13.22% to 0.29%), whereas further increase in the number of harmonics over 12 did not drastically improve the flow field. Finally, we conclude that the use of a moderate number of harmonics, e.g. between 8 and 12, is enough to reconstruct the flow field with an acceptable accuracy (errors below 1%). Hereafter, we make use of the HB method set with 12 harmonics. The corresponding HB solution is simply referred to as $\boldsymbol{u}_{\text{hb}}$ (instead of $\boldsymbol{u}_{\text{hb}}^{12}$).

Sensitivity to the Mesh Size Parameter. To further verify the processes, a much finer mesh, denoted by $\mathbf{M_7}$, was used to generate the numerical reference solution, denoted by $\boldsymbol{u}_{\text{ext}}$ and sampled at 25 time instants. The reference solution was then mapped to the meshes $\mathbf{M_2}$ and $\mathbf{M_4}$ using a cell volume weighted interpolation method [2] and resulting in reference flow fields denoted by $\boldsymbol{u}_{\text{ext}}^2$

and $\boldsymbol{u}_{\text{ext}}^4$ respectively. As such, there is now a source of error in terms of interpolation. In mesh $\mathbf{M_2}$, nRMSE($\boldsymbol{u}_{\text{hb}}$, $\boldsymbol{u}_{\text{ext}}^2$) was 2.93%, whereas, in mesh $\mathbf{M_4}$, the same metric evaluated against $\boldsymbol{u}_{\text{ext}}^4$ was 1.51%.

4.1   Comparison with a Classical Data-Based CFD Method

As additional validation of the HB method, we have considered a classical CFD approach based on traditional time-stepping schemes for comparison purposes. Instead of using a simple linear interpolation, we consider an inverse problem based on penalized regression spline (PRS) to reconstruct the inflow BCs at all time instants present in the traditional time discretization, for which the observations are not available. The regression model functions are of class C^2 and correspond to cubic splines with uniformly distributed nodes. For the PRS method, the momentum equation was discretized in time using backward differentiation, an implicit scheme of second order accuracy. The time steps were chosen such that the Courant number was below 0.3.

The simulations with the HB and PRS methods were run in computational meshes $\mathbf{M_2}$ and $\mathbf{M_4}$, using 48 and 96 processors respectively. The PRS simulation was run for 12 periods, where a periodic state of equilibrium was reached. The velocity fields $\boldsymbol{u}_{\text{hb}}$ and $\boldsymbol{u}_{\text{prs}}$, numerically obtained from HB and PRS methods respectively, were compared with the exact solution. The results are summarized in Table 2. Remarkably, the HB method yields almost the same accuracy as the PRS method, when compared with a reference solution. Furthermore, the error nRMSE($\boldsymbol{u}_{\text{hb}}$, $\boldsymbol{u}_{\text{prs}}$) between these solutions was 0.39% in $\mathbf{M_2}$ and 0.36% in $\mathbf{M_4}$. Finally, the WCT in $\mathbf{M_4}$ were 23 052 s for the PRS method and 1 512 s for the HB method, the latter being ≈15 times faster than the former. In total, the PRS method needed ≈ 6.4 h, whereas the HB method with $n = 12$ needed ≈25 min. This is a tremendous saving in terms of computational effort.

Table 2. Root mean square errors nRMSE($\boldsymbol{u}_{\text{hb}}, \boldsymbol{u}_{\text{ext}}^n$) and nRMSE($\boldsymbol{u}_{\text{prs}}, \boldsymbol{u}_{\text{ext}}^n$) for HB and PRS methods, evaluated against the reference solutions $\boldsymbol{u}_{\text{ext}}^2$ and $\boldsymbol{u}_{\text{ext}}^4$ mapped onto meshes $\mathbf{M_2}$ and $\mathbf{M_4}$ respectively. In addition, the corresponding wall clock times (WCT) in seconds is provided for each simulation (with 96 processors) on $\mathbf{M_4}$.

$\boldsymbol{u}_c$	nRMSE($\boldsymbol{u}_c$, $\boldsymbol{u}_{\text{ext}}^2$) on $\mathbf{M_2}$	nRMSE($\boldsymbol{u}_c$, $\boldsymbol{u}_{\text{ext}}^4$) on $\mathbf{M_4}$	WCT for $\boldsymbol{u}_c$ on $\mathbf{M_4}$
$\boldsymbol{u}_{\text{hb}}$	2.93%	1.51%	1 512 s
$\boldsymbol{u}_{\text{prs}}$	2.88%	1.47%	23 052 s

4.2   Simulations with Boundary Data from 4D Flow MRI

The performance and feasibility of both the HB and PRS methods was studied on $\mathbf{M_2}$ to reconstruct the velocity fields obtained from 4D flow MRI experiment. Computed flow patterns were first qualitatively compared by visual inspection.

The HB method proved to be able to reproduce the velocity field delivered by the PRS method without an appreciable difference. Finally, since no ground truth is available, the velocity fields obtained from HB and PRS methods were quantitatively compared, resulting in a metric nRMSE(u_{hb},u_{prs}) of 8.56%.

5   Conclusions

This work has investigated the harmonic balance method as a novel approach to perform pulsatile fluid flow simulations in computational hemodynamics, facilitating the combination of CFD with data obtained from 4D flow MRI. The method is being reported for the first time in a study combining CFD with 4D flow MRI and it shows a significant improvement regarding the trade-off between computational cost and accuracy.

Comparison has been performed against a classical CFD method based on a traditional time discretization scheme. The classical approach proves to be a time consuming process. In contrast, the harmonic balance method relies on a frequency-based temporal discretization scheme. Thereby, the velocity field is decomposed into its Fourier series and the method operates in the frequency domain. Based on our experiments, the harmonic balance method was about 15 times faster compared to the conventional transient simulations.

Our experience indicates that only a moderate number of harmonics is required to accurately resolve the periodic fluid flow problem. This makes the method extremely useful, for example, in data assimilation procedures based on 4D flow MRI acquisitions, where the fluid flow problem has to be solved many times. Regarding the number of time instants at which data is acquired per cardiac cycle, the method can be easily adjusted such that the discretized momentum equations are temporally registered with the measurements. In the case of 4D flow MRI, our experience indicates that it requires observational data at a number of time instants between 17 and 25. This corresponds to a number of harmonics of at least 8, which is a region in which the method has proved to be satisfactorily accurate.

This work does not include the mechanical models of the vessel walls but is a starting point for the adaptation of fluid-structure interaction studies. Hence, this investigation is the first of a series that will most likely address the deformation and dynamic response of the arterial walls.

Based on these results, we conclude that the HB numerical scheme reveals itself as a method with a tremendous potential in computational hemodynamics. The proposed approach enables pulsatile fluid flow simulations at a significantly smaller cost when compared with traditional methods, without exhibiting deterioration of the approximate solution.

References

1. Boyd, J.: Chebyshev and Fourier Spectral Methods, 2nd Revised edn. Dover Books on Mathematics. Dover Publications (2001)
2. Coetzee, R.V.: Volume weighted interpolation for unstructured meshes in the finite volume method. Ph.D. thesis, North-West University (2005)
3. Cvijetić, G., Jasak, H., Vukčević, V.: Finite volume implementation of the harmonic balance method for periodic non-linear flows. In: 4th AIAA Aerospace Sciences Meeting (2016). https://doi.org/10.2514/6.2016-0070
4. Hall, K.C., Ekici, K., Jeffrey, P.T., Earl, H.D.: Harmonic balance methods applied to computational fluid dynamics problems. Int. J. Comput. Fluid Dynam. **27**(2), 52–67 (2013). https://doi.org/10.1080/10618562.2012.742512
5. Koltukluoğlu, T.S., Blanco, P.J.: Boundary control in computational haemodynamics. J. Fluid Mech. **847**, 329–364 (2018). https://doi.org/10.1017/jfm.2018.329
6. Krack, M., Gross, J.: Harmonic Balance for Nonlinear Vibration Problems. Springer, Cham (2019). https://doi.org/10.1007/978-3-030-14023-6
7. Markl, M., Frydrychowicz, A., Kozerke, S., Hope, M., Wieben, O.: 4D flow MRI. Magn. Reson. Im. **36**(5), 1015–1036 (2012). https://doi.org/10.1002/jmri.23556
8. Miyazaki, S., et al.: Validation of numerical simulation methods in aortic arch using 4D flow MRI. Heart Vessels **32**(8), 1032–1044 (2017). https://doi.org/10.1007/s00380-017-0979-2
9. Patankar, S.V., Spalding, D.B.: A calculation procedure for heat, mass and momentum transfer in three-dimensional parabolic flows. J. Heat Mass Transf. **15**, 1787–1806 (1972). https://doi.org/10.1016/0017-9310(72)90054-3
10. Stokes, A.: On the approximation of nonlinear oscillations. J. Differ. Equ. **12**(3), 535–558 (1972). https://doi.org/10.1016/0022-0396(72)90024-1
11. Wake, A.K., Oshinski, J.N., Tannenbaum, A.R., Giddens, D.P.: Choice of in vivo versus idealized velocity boundary conditions influences physiologically relevant flow patterns in a subject-specific simulation of flow in the human carotid bifurcation. J. Biomech. Eng. **131**(2), 021013 (2009). https://doi.org/10.1115/1.3005157

Deep Learning Within *a Priori* Temporal Feature Spaces for Large-Scale Dynamic MR Image Reconstruction: Application to 5-D Cardiac MR Multitasking

Yuhua Chen[1,2](✉) , Jaime L. Shaw[2] , Yibin Xie[2] ,
Debiao Li[1,2] , and Anthony G. Christodoulou[2]

[1] Department of Bioengineering, University of California,
Los Angeles, CA 90095, USA
chyuhua@ucla.edu
[2] Biomedical Imaging Research Institute, Cedars-Sinai Medical Center,
Los Angeles, CA 90048, USA

Abstract. High spatiotemporal resolution dynamic magnetic resonance imaging (MRI) is a powerful clinical tool for imaging moving structures as well as to reveal and quantify other physical and physiological dynamics. The low speed of MRI necessitates acceleration methods such as deep learning reconstruction from under-sampled data. However, the massive size of many dynamic MRI problems prevents deep learning networks from directly exploiting global temporal relationships. In this work, we show that by applying deep neural networks inside *a priori* calculated temporal feature spaces, we enable deep learning reconstruction with global temporal modeling even for image sequences with >40,000 frames. One proposed variation of our approach using dilated multi-level Densely Connected Network (mDCN) speeds up feature space coordinate calculation by 3000x compared to conventional iterative methods, from 20 min to 0.39 s. Thus, the combination of low-rank tensor and deep learning models not only makes large-scale dynamic MRI feasible but also practical for routine clinical application (This work was supported by NIH 1R01EB028146).

Keywords: Image reconstruction · Low-Rank model · Deep learning

1 Introduction

Dynamic imaging plays an important role in many clinical MRI exams, assessing tissue health by visualizing and/or measuring any of several dynamic processes within the body: cardiac motion, respiration, T1 or T2 relaxation, contrast agent dynamics, and more. However, dynamic MRI is a relatively slow imaging modality, necessitating acceleration methods which can reconstruct images from "incomplete" image data. Thanks to the demonstrated ability of multilayer neural networks to learn highly efficient image representations and to rapidly decode imaging data, deep learning has become a popular approach for reconstructing static images (or individual frames of

© Springer Nature Switzerland AG 2019
D. Shen et al. (Eds.): MICCAI 2019, LNCS 11765, pp. 495–504, 2019.
https://doi.org/10.1007/978-3-030-32245-8_55

dynamic images) from snapshots of incomplete imaging data. This time-independent approach to image reconstruction ignores relationships between different frames of the image sequence; as a result, dynamic deep learning methods have recently been introduced, sharing data across sequences between 30 and 200 frames long [1–3].

A major unaddressed problem in dynamic deep learning MR image reconstruction is how to handle even longer image sequences—a challenge raised by two current trends in dynamic MRI. First, accelerated dynamic MRI techniques have pushed toward higher frame rates as a means of investigating dynamic processes with increased temporal resolution. Second, multi-dynamic/extra-dimensional MRI techniques [4–6] can now simultaneously image multiple dynamic processes at once by defining multiple "time dimensions" (i.e., time-varying independent variables), leading to exponential growth of frames per image sequence. These trends have led to massive problem sizes; for example, [6] reports image sequences between 20,000 frames and 140,000 frames long. Dynamic deep learning MR image reconstruction has not yet been demonstrated for image sequences of this size, largely due to GPU memory limitations and overfitting risks that stem from the increased numbers of weights required to exploit global temporal relationships by connecting all frames (even indirectly).

One memory-efficient approach for non–deep learning methods has been linear subspace modeling [7], a variant of low-rank imaging. There, rather than focusing on image sequences in the time-domain, images are modeled, reconstructed, and stored in a low-dimensional, subject-specific feature space. However, employing linear modeling alone is known to be less effective than combining this approach with sparse recovery inside the feature space [8, 9] (substantially slowing the reconstruction process) or replacing the linear subspace model with nonlinear manifold modeling [10] (discarding the memory benefits). These approaches all require slow iterative reconstruction, which compromises their practical application in the clinic, where reconstruction is expected to take seconds. This iterative reconstruction is especially slow for non-Cartesian acquisitions, which otherwise have excellent properties for dynamic imaging.

Here, we propose an approach combining the memory efficiency of linear subspace modeling with the quality of nonlinear manifold modeling. Our approach uses deep learning to recover image coordinates/feature maps within linear subspaces rather than directly recovering image sequences, allowing non-local temporal modeling across entire image sequences with many frames. Due to strong connections between deep learning and nonlinear manifold modeling [11], we interpret this approach as using deep learning to recover feature maps on a nonlinear manifold within a subject-specific linear subspace. Although the feature space changes with each subject and is determined from concurrent subject-specific auxiliary data, the transform learned by the network is generalized and can be applied in any linear subspace of the same dimensionality.

We evaluate this approach for 5-D cardiac MR Multitasking, a low-rank tensor approach with three time-dimensions (cardiac phase, respiratory phase, and inversion time) and >40,000 frames per image sequence, enabling non-ECG, free-breathing, myocardial T1 mapping [12]. For this evaluation, we compare mDCN [13] and the state-of-the-art DenseUnet [14] as example network architectures, training on 153 subjects. We further expanded the mDCN structure with dilated convolutional layers for a larger receptive field, which is proven to further improve the reconstruction performance. Our preliminary results show that our model can reduce image coordinate recovery time from 20 min for a single 2D slice into 0.39 s, an >3000x speed improvement which puts online clinical deployment within reach. Both networks were capable of fast image reconstruction, but mDCN was faster, smaller, more accurate, and more precise than the more widely-used DenseUnet.

1.1 Contributions

- We developed a new deep learning approach to dynamic MR imaging reconstruction
- Specifically, we show that applying deep neural networks inside low-dimensional data-driven temporal feature spaces allows time- and memory-efficient learning of global temporal relationships, even for image sequences with >40,000 frames.
- We modified a highly efficient neural network mDCN to produce high-quality images with less time and memory usage than the more-popular DenseUnet.

2 Method

2.1 Background

Dynamic MRI produces a spatiotemporal image sequence $I(\mathbf{x}, \mathbf{t})$, a function of spatial location (denoted by vector $\mathbf{x} = [x_1, x_2, x_3]^T$ containing up to three spatial directions x_i) and one or more time dimensions (denoted by vector $\mathbf{t} = [t_1, t_2, \cdots, t_R]^T$ containing R time-varying independent variables t_i). Here, we represent the discretized image sequence as a matrix $\mathbf{A} \in \mathbb{C}^{M \times N}$ with elements $A_{ij} = I(\mathbf{x}_i, \mathbf{t}_j)$, with M spatial locations (voxels), and N time points (frames). The matrix $\mathbf{A}$ is spatially encoded by the MR scanner, producing a vector of encoded data $\mathbf{d} = E(\mathbf{A})$, where $E(\cdot)$ typically comprises partial spatial Fourier encoding as well as additional spatial encoding from receiver sensitivity patterns.

The goal of image reconstruction is to recover the original image sequence $\mathbf{A}$ from the measured data $\mathbf{d}$, i.e., to find some operation f such that $\mathbf{A} = f(\mathbf{d})$. Typically, it is not possible to sample $\mathbf{d}$ at or above the spatiotemporal Nyquist rate, so the data are undersampled. This leads to an ill-posed inverse problem, such that a general $f(\cdot) = E^{-1}(\cdot)$ does not exist. However, due to strong relationships between different image frames of $\mathbf{A}$, dynamic MR images lie on low-dimensional manifolds [7, 10]; reconstruction methods can exploit these temporal relationships to find an f such that $f(E(\mathbf{A})) \approx \mathbf{A}$ for these images.

2.2   Subspace Formulation

When the image sequence contains many frames, $\mathbf{A}$ can be rather large, presenting substantial computational challenges for designing an f which produces $\mathbf{A}$ by exploiting global temporal relationships across all image frames. One memory-efficient approach to recover $\mathbf{A}$ while exploiting global temporal relationships has been to use linear subspace modeling: $I(\mathbf{x}, \mathbf{t}) = \sum_{l=1}^{L} u_\ell(\mathbf{x}) \varphi_\ell(\mathbf{t})$. This model implies that the matrix $\mathbf{A}$ has a low rank $L < \min(M, N)$ and can be efficiently factored as $\mathbf{A} = \mathbf{U}\boldsymbol{\Phi}$, where $\mathbf{U} \in \mathbb{C}^{M \times L}$ has elements $U_{i\ell} = u_\ell(\mathbf{x}_i)$ and $\boldsymbol{\Phi} \in \mathbb{C}^{L \times N}$ has elements $\Phi_{\ell j} = \varphi_\ell(\mathbf{t}_j)$. In this formulation, the columns of the spatial factor $\mathbf{U}$ are feature maps containing the coordinates for $I(\mathbf{x}, \mathbf{t})$ within a "temporal feature space" spanned by $\{\varphi_\ell(\mathbf{t}_j)\}_{\ell=1}^{L}$. Sampling can be designed to include high-speed auxiliary data as a subset of $\mathbf{d}$ (sometimes called subspace training data or navigator data), from which the temporal feature space can be directly extracted via principal component analysis (PCA). This predetermines $\boldsymbol{\Phi}$ and updates the problem formulation to

$$\mathbf{d} = E(\mathbf{U}\boldsymbol{\Phi}) = E_{\boldsymbol{\Phi}}(\mathbf{U}),$$

where the new goal of image reconstruction is to find an $f_{\boldsymbol{\Phi}}$ such that $f_{\boldsymbol{\Phi}}(\mathbf{d}) \approx \mathbf{U}$.

Linear subspace modeling alone is typically not enough to produce a high-quality $\mathbf{A}$ from a highly under-sampled $\mathbf{d}$, so this approach is often combined by sparse recovery methods such as compressed sensing to find a $\mathbf{U}$ which itself has a sparse representation $\Psi(\mathbf{U})$, e.g., by solving the nonlinear reconstruction problem

$$f_{\boldsymbol{\Phi}}(\mathbf{d}) = \arg \min_{\mathbf{U}} \| \mathbf{d} - E_{\boldsymbol{\Phi}}(\mathbf{U}) \|_2^2 + \lambda \| \Psi(\mathbf{U}) \|_1 . \tag{1}$$

In practice, (1) is solved $\mathbf{U}$ by "backprojecting" $\mathbf{d}$ onto the feature space as $E_{\boldsymbol{\Phi}}^*(\mathbf{d})$ (where * denotes the adjoint) or a pre-conditioned $E_{\boldsymbol{\Phi},\text{pc}}^*(\mathbf{d})$ and performing nonlinear iterative reconstruction such as the alternating direction method of multipliers (ADMM) upon the result entirely within the feature space [9]. This process is very slow, especially for non-Cartesian sampling patterns, for which $E_{\boldsymbol{\Phi}}(\cdot)$ comprises several non-invertible, non-separable multidimensional non-uniform fast Fourier transforms (NUFFTs) instead of invertible, separable FFTs.

2.3   Deep Learning Formulation

We aim to replace this slow, iterative process with a much faster deep learning network which exploits global temporal relationships while retaining the memory benefits of the linear subspace formulation. We constrain all processing of the network to occur within the L-dimensional temporal feature space (rather than the N-dimensional full temporal space), by: (1) backprojecting $\mathbf{d}$ onto the feature space as $\mathbf{U}_0 = E_{\boldsymbol{\Phi},\text{pc}}^*(\mathbf{d})$; then (2) passing $\mathbf{U}_0$ through a network to apply a learned reconstruction operator $g(\cdot)$:

$$\mathbf{U} = f_{\mathbf{\Phi}}(\mathbf{d})$$
$$= g(\mathbf{U}_0) = g\left(E_{\mathbf{\Phi},\mathrm{pc}}^*(\mathbf{d})\right).$$

This approach is compatible with a wide range of network architectures for a wide range of dynamic imaging applications. The specific network structure and application we used to evaluate our approach will be described in the next section.

3 Experiment

3.1 MR Multitasking Application, Training Data, and Preprocessing

To demonstrate and evaluate our reconstruction approach, we designed a series of experiments to replace the MR Multitasking spatial factor estimation process, i.e., iterative reconstruction by Eq. (1). Multitasking for non-ECG, free-breathing quantitative T1 mapping of the heart produces a 5-D image $I(\mathbf{x}, \mathbf{t})$ with two spatial dimensions and three time dimensions: $\mathbf{t} = [c, r, \tau]^T$, where c is cardiac phase, r is respiratory phase, and τ is inversion time. There is an image frame for each combination of 344 T1-recovery time-points (τ), 20 cardiac phases (c), and 6 respiratory phases (r), i.e., $344 \times 20 \times 6 = 41280$ frames (a data size equivalent to 23 min of video at 30 fps).

In our experiments, we used non-Cartesian multichannel MRI, such that $E_{\mathbf{\Phi}}(\mathbf{U}) = \Omega([\mathbf{SF}_{\mathrm{NU}}\mathbf{U}]\mathbf{\Phi})$, where $\mathbf{F}_{\mathrm{NU}}$ is the NUFFT, $\mathbf{S}$ applies coil sensitivity patterns, and Ω is the undersampling operator. We produced our network input according to $\mathbf{U}_0 = E_{\mathbf{\Phi},\mathrm{pc}}^*(\mathbf{d}) = \mathbf{S}^\dagger \mathbf{F}_{\mathrm{NU}}^H \mathbf{W} \Omega^*(\mathbf{d}) \mathbf{\Phi}^H$, where $\Omega^*(\cdot)\mathbf{\Phi}^H$ transforms the data into the temporal feature space, $\mathbf{F}_{\mathrm{NU}}^H \mathbf{W}$ regrids the non-Cartesian data by applying a density compensation function (the diagonal matrix $\mathbf{W}$) followed by the adjoint NUFFT $\mathbf{F}_{\mathrm{NU}}^H$ (a process similar to filtered backprojection), and where the pseudoinverse $\mathbf{S}^\dagger$ performs a complex coil combination.

A total of 191 subjects' worth of raw dynamic MRI data were collected via on-site Siemens 3T MRI scanners, and split into 8:1:1 ratio as training, validation, and testing set. We used a rank of $L = 32$ with image matrix size of 160×160, so the network was tasked with recovering a spatial factor $\mathbf{U}$ composed of 32 complex-valued 160×160 feature maps. In order to handle complex numbers, the real and imaginary parts of $\mathbf{U}$ were concatenated into a set of 64 real-valued 160×160 feature maps.

3.2 Training Parameters and Experiment Setting

The models were implemented in Tensorflow on a workstation with Nvidia GTX 1080TI GPU. Before feeding into the network, instance-wise normalization was done on both the input and label data by subtracting their mean and dividing by their standard deviation (std). We used Adam optimizer with a default learning rate of 1e-4 to minimize the L1 loss between the network output and the label data. Two network backbones were implemented and evaluated, one based on the mDCSRN [13] and the other based on the DenseUnet [14]. Both networks had the same densely-connected block setting (4 convolutional layers, 128 of growth rate, and ELU [15] nonlinear activation), whose details are shown in Fig. 1. To evaluate the effects of regularization, we applied different L1 and L2 regularization on the weights to avoid overfitting. We then further investigated how the dilation rate affects the reconstruction quality. For all the experiment, models were trained for 300 k steps, after which no further improvement was observed. The validation loss was monitored and the checkpoint with best validation loss was used to test the model performance.

To quantitatively analyze the results, we used three different measurements to compare results from the deep learning networks and the reference conventional iterative algorithm: (1) the normalized root mean square error (NRMSE) of the spatial factors; (2) three image similarity metrics, NRMSE, PSNR, and SSIM of the reconstructed image sequences for the whole cardiac cycle (20 frames) at the end-expiration (EE) respiratory phase, for inversion times corresponding to bright-blood and dark-blood contrast weighting (i.e., the two most clinically important qualitative image weightings); and (3) the accuracy and precision of T1 maps (i.e., the quantitative map produced by Multitasking). The timing of the network runtime was also recorded.

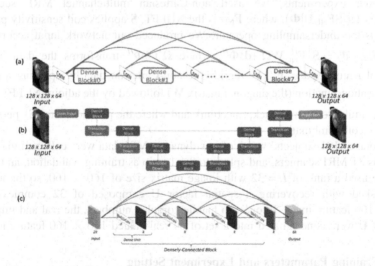

Fig. 1. Architecture of (a) the mDCN Network and (b) DenseUnet. Both have the same (c) DenseBlock (DB) with four 3 × 3 CONV layers. Dilation rate in CONV layers within a DB can vary and are notated as d1-4-8-1. DenseUnet has 4 resolution levels; the dilation rate of all layers is 1.

3.3 Results

The quantitative results of NRMSE on the spatial factor and image similarity metrics on cardiac cycles from different networks and configurations are shown in Table 1 and Table 2. Hyperparameter searching was only done on the *validation set* to avoid overfitting to the *test set*. mDCN with dilation 1-4-8-1 and regularization scale of 0.01 outperformed all other networks. In general, mDCN outperformed the more popular DenseUnet in both image quality and speed. An example case of reconstructed MR images showing multiple contrasts and time dimensions is also shown in Fig. 2.

Table 1. The similarity metrics compared to iterative reconstruction for different L1 & L2 regularization scale on the *validation set*. The 0.01 scale gave the best performance.

	mDCN *d1-4-8-1*			DenseUnet		
L1&L2 Reg. Scale	No-reg	1e-3	1e-2	No-reg	1e-3	1e-2
Image basis NRMSE	0.4460 (0.036)	0.4324 (0.036)	**0.4302 (0.038)**	0.4416 (0.035)	0.4440 (0.033)	*0.4415 (0.034)*
Cardiac cycle SSIM	0.8329 (0.069)	**0.8524 (0.069)**	0.8519 (0.070)	0.8450 (0.063)	0.8252 (0.059)	*0.8368 (0.062)*
	0.9164 (0.027)	0.9392 (0.026)	**0.9398 (0.037)**	0.9292 (0.025)	0.9033 (0.026)	*0.9128 (0.039)*
Cardiac cycle PSNR	29.44 (2.733)	30.51 (2.912)	**30.70 (2.850)**	29.97 (2.342)	29.16 (2.326)	*29.70 (2.024)*
	31.44 (3.052)	33.42 (3.081)	**33.74 (2.989)**	32.13 (2.243)	30.87 (2.385)	*31.97 (2.021)*
Cardiac cycle NRMSE	0.1754 (0.057)	0.1580 (0.056)	**0.1554 (0.061)**	0.1643 (0.052)	0.1773 (0.048)	*0.1673 (0.050)*
	0.1114 (0.044)	0.0894 (0.035)	**0.0863 (0.037)**	0.1007 (0.030)	0.1147 (0.028)	*0.1013 (0.025)*
Runtime per case	**0.39 s**			*0.46 s*		

Table 2. Comparison between different dilation rates of mDCN on validation set. mDCN d1-4-8-1 with the largest effective receptive field gave the best scores on both *validation & test* set.

	Validation set				Test set	
	mDCN			DenseUnet	mDCN	DenseUnet
Dilation	No dilation	d1241	d1481	No dilation	d1481	No dilation
Image basis NRMSE	*0.4402 (0.042)*	0.4350 (0.041)	**0.4302 (0.038)**	0.4415 (0.034)	**0.4450 (0.055)**	0.4493 (0.052)
Cardiac cycle SSIM	*0.8474 (0.065)*	0.8472 (0.071)	**0.8519 (0.070)**	0.8368 (0.062)	**0.8619 (0.070)**	0.8381 (0.079)
	0.9320 (0.024)	0.9351 (0.029)	**0.9398 (0.037)**	0.9128 (0.039)	**0.9382 (0.033)**	0.9068 (0.045)
Cardiac cycle PSNR	*29.54 (2.576)*	30.07 (3.126)	**30.70 (2.850)**	29.70 (2.024)	**30.07 (3.836)**	29.20 (3.374)
	31.20 (3.382)	32.49 (3.705)	**33.74 (2.989)**	31.97 (2.021)	**32.07 (4.300)**	31.27 (4.298)
Cardiac cycle NRMSE	*0.1723 (0.055)*	0.1680 (0.068)	**0.1554 (0.061)**	0.1673 (0.050)	**0.1556 (0.056)**	0.1687 (0.051)
	0.1161 (0.047)	0.1050 (0.057)	**0.0863 (0.037)**	0.1013 (0.025)	**0.1052 (0.053)**	0.1127 (0.043)

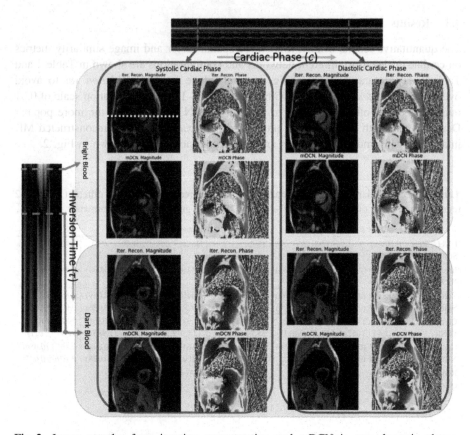

Fig. 2. Image samples from iterative reconstruction and mDCN in two dynamic phases: Inversion time (τ), showing T1 recovery, and cardiac phase (c), showing cardiac motion.

Bland-Altman plots of the T1 fitting results and sample T1 maps are given in Fig. 3. The mDCN maps were more accurate (smaller bias) and more precise (tighter limits of agreement) than DenseUnet. Neither network showed a statistically significant bias (mDCN: $p = 0.98$; DenseUnet: $p = 0.36$). The mDCN results were also more highly correlated to conventional results (mDCN: $R = 0.95$, DenseUnet $R = 0.90$).

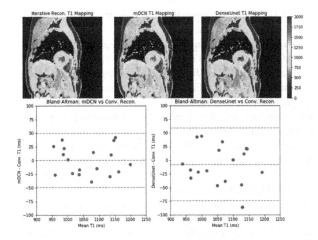

Fig. 3. T1 mapping results from conventional iterative reconstruction, mDCN, and DenseUnet. Bland-Altman analyses show that the mDCN is more accurate and precise than DenseUnet. In both cases, the limits of agreement are smaller than the ΔT1 of many diseases; e.g., median ΔT1 at 3 T between infarcted myocardium and remote myocardium in ST-segment elevation myocardial infarction (STEMI) patients was recently found to be 271 ms [16].

4 Conclusion

In this work, we have presented a fast, accurate approach to large-scale dynamic MRI reconstruction with global temporal modeling using a combination of low-rank modeling and deep learning. Our dilated mDCN provided similar-quality reconstructed images and T1 maps to conventional iterative methods, while reducing the time by >3000x. This reduction makes online reconstruction feasible for clinical application.

References

1. Schlemper, J., Caballero, J., Hajnal, J.V., Price, A.N., Rueckert, D.: A deep cascade of convolutional neural networks for dynamic MR image reconstruction. IEEE Trans. Med. Imaging **37**, 491–503 (2018)
2. Qin, C., Schlemper, J., Caballero, J., Price, A.N., Hajnal, J.V., Rueckert, D.: Convolutional recurrent neural networks for dynamic MR image reconstruction. IEEE Trans. Med. Imaging **38**, 280–290 (2019)
3. Biswas, S., Aggarwal, H.K., Jacob, M.: Dynamic MRI using model-based deep learning and SToRM priors: MoDL-SToRM. Mag. Reson. Med. **82**(1), 485–494 (2019)
4. Feng, L., Axel, L., Chandarana, H., Block, K.T., Sodickson, D.K., Otazo, R.: XD-GRASP: golden-angle radial MRI with reconstruction of extra motion-state dimensions using compressed sensing. Mag. Reson. Med. **75**, 775–788 (2016)
5. Cheng, J.Y., et al.: Comprehensive multi-dimensional MRI for the simultaneous assessment of cardiopulmonary anatomy and physiology. Sci. Rep. **7**, 5330 (2017)

6. Christodoulou, A.G.: Magnetic resonance multitasking for motion-resolved quantitative cardiovascular imaging. Nat. Biomed. Eng. **2**, 215–226 (2018)
7. Liang, Z.-P.: Spatiotemporal imaging with partially separable functions. In: Proceedings of the IEEE International Symposium Biomed Imaging, pp. 988–991 (2007)
8. Lingala, S.G., Hu, Y., DiBella, E., Jacob, M.: Accelerated dynamic MRI exploiting sparsity and low-rank structure: k-t SLR. IEEE Trans. Med. Imaging **30**, 1042–1054 (2011)
9. Zhao, B., Haldar, J.P., Christodoulou, A.G., Liang, Z.-P.: Image reconstruction from highly undersampled (k, t)-space data with joint partial separability and sparsity constraints. IEEE Trans. Med. Imaging **31**, 1809–1820 (2012)
10. Poddar, S., Jacob, M.: Dynamic MRI Using SmooThness Regularization on Manifolds (SToRM). IEEE Trans. Med. Imaging **35**, 1106–1115 (2016)
11. Bengio, Y., Courville, A., Vincent, P.: Representation learning: a review and new perspectives. IEEE Trans. Pattern Anal. Mach. Intell. **35**, 1798–1828 (2013)
12. Shaw, J.L.: Free-breathing, non-ECG, continuous myocardial T_1 mapping with cardiovascular magnetic resonance Multitasking. Mag. Reson. Med. **81**, 2450–2463 (2019)
13. Chen, Y., Shi, F., Christodoulou, A.G., Xie, Y., Zhou, Z., Li, D.: Efficient and accurate mri super-resolution using a generative adversarial network and 3D multi-level densely connected network. In: Frangi, A.F., Schnabel, J.A., Davatzikos, C., Alberola-López, C., Fichtinger, G. (eds.) MICCAI 2018. LNCS, vol. 11070, pp. 91–99. Springer, Cham (2018). https://doi.org/10.1007/978-3-030-00928-1_11
14. Jégou, S., Drozdzal, M., Vazquez, D., Romero, A., Bengio, Y.: The one hundred layers tiramisu: Fully convolutional densenets for semantic segmentation. In: Proceedings of the IEEE Conference on Computer Vision and Pattern Recognition Workshops, pp. 11–19 (2017)
15. Clevert, D.-A., Unterthiner, T., Hochreiter, S.: Fast and accurate deep network learning by exponential linear units (elus). arXiv preprint arXiv:1511.07289 (2015)
16. Kali, A., et al.: Native T1 mapping by 3-T CMR imaging for characterization of chronic myocardial infarctions. JACC Cardiovasc. Imaging **8**(9), 1019–1030 (2015)

k-t NEXT: Dynamic MR Image Reconstruction Exploiting Spatio-Temporal Correlations

Chen Qin[1]($\boxtimes$), Jo Schlemper[1], Jinming Duan[1,3], Gavin Seegoolam[1], Anthony Price[2], Joseph Hajnal[2], and Daniel Rueckert[1]

[1] Department of Computing, Imperial College London, London, UK
`c.qin15@imperial.ac.uk`
[2] Division of Imaging Sciences and Biomedical Engineering Department, King's College London, St. Thomas' Hospital, London, UK
[3] School of Computer Science, University of Birmingham, Birmingham, UK

Abstract. Dynamic magnetic resonance imaging (MRI) exhibits high correlations in *k*-space and time. In order to accelerate the dynamic MR imaging and to exploit *k-t* correlations from highly undersampled data, here we propose a novel deep learning based approach for dynamic MR image reconstruction, termed *k-t* NEXT (*k-t* NEtwork with X-*f* Transform). In particular, inspired by traditional methods such as *k-t* BLAST and *k-t* FOCUSS, we propose to reconstruct the true signals from aliased signals in *x-f* domain to exploit the spatio-temporal redundancies. Building on that, the proposed method then learns to recover the signals by alternating the reconstruction process between the *x-f* space and image space in an iterative fashion. This enables the network to effectively capture useful information and jointly exploit spatio-temporal correlations from both complementary domains. Experiments conducted on highly undersampled short-axis cardiac cine MRI scans demonstrate that our proposed method outperforms the current state-of-the-art dynamic MR reconstruction approaches both quantitatively and qualitatively.

1 Introduction

Dynamic Magnetic Resonance Imaging (MRI) is a non-invasive imaging technique to monitor dynamic processes such as cardiac motion by acquiring data in a *k-t* space that contains both temporal and spatial information. However, the acquisition speed is limited due to both physical and physiological constraints. It is well known that in dynamic MRI there exists significant correlations in *k*-space and time. In order to increase the acquisition rate, most strategies have

Electronic supplementary material The online version of this chapter (https://doi.org/10.1007/978-3-030-32245-8_56) contains supplementary material, which is available to authorized users.

been designed to acquire part of the desired k-t measurements and then reconstruct the images by exploiting spatio-temporal redundancies within the data.

Inspired by traditional k-t methods from the area of compressed sensing [8,9,15] for accelerated dynamic MR imaging, here we propose a novel dynamic MR image reconstruction NEtwork with X-f Transform, termed k-t NEXT, which exploits the signal redundancies in both x-f domain and image domain. In particular, the proposed k-t NEXT formulates the reconstruction process in an iterative fashion, where in each iteration, it consists of two sub-modules: a xf-CNN that learns to recover the true signals from aliased signals in x-f domain, and a convolutional recurrent neural network (CRNN) that exploits spatio-temporal redundancies in image domain. The dynamic reconstruction process thus alternates between x-f space and image space, which potentially enables the network to learn complementary features simultaneously from both domains. Experiments were performed on highly undersampled short-axis cardiac cine MR scans, where we show that the proposed model outperforms the current state-of-the-art dynamic MR reconstruction methods.

1.1   Related Work

Over the years, a number of approaches have been proposed for the reconstruction of accelerated dynamic MR images. In general, these methods can be mainly divided into three categories, based on exploiting correlations in k-space, in time, and in both k-space and time [15]. The first class of approaches exploit the correlations between k-space points at the same time frame, and then reconstruct each frame independently from other time frames, such as reduced field-of-view (FOV) [6] and parallel imaging methods [3], while the second group of strategies is to exploit redundancies in time, where the missing data at a given position can be interpolated or extrapolated from the measured data at other time points, such as keyhole imaging [7] and data sharing [18]. Relevant to our method, the third type of approaches is based on exploiting correlations in both k-space and time. One of the examples is the model-based k-t BLAST and k-t SENSE method [15], which takes advantage of a-priori information about the x-f support obtained from the training stage and then to remedy the aliasing artefacts during acquisition stage. Based on that, k-t FOCUSS [8,9] then formulated the problem in a compressed sensing MRI framework, which enforced the sparsity in x-f domain for the signal recovery. Similarly, a low rank and sparse reconstruction scheme (k-t SLR) [10] was proposed to exploit correlations between the temporal profiles of the voxels by introducing non-convex spectral norms and spatio-temporal total variation norm. In more recent years, deep learning approaches have gained their popularity for MR image reconstruction [2,12,13,16]. Most approaches investigate on exploiting information in a single frame (or static image) either in image domain [4,11,14] or in k-space domain [1,5,17], where each frame (or image) is reconstructed independently. In order to exploit the temporal redundancies, Schlemper et al. [13] proposed a data sharing (DS) layer in an image space cascaded 3D convolutional network to utilise the similar information contained in neighboring k-space samples. Qin et al. [12] also proposed a bidirectional CRNN model to exploit the temporal dependencies of dynamic sequences in image domain. In contrast, our approach proposes to reconstruct the images in both x-f and image domains, where complementary information from two different domains can be fully exploited.

2   Methods

2.1   Problem Formulation

Consider a Cartesian k-space trajectory where k_x denotes the phase encoding direction, k_y denotes the readout direction, while $\sigma(x,t)$ denotes the image domain content at x and time t. The k-space measurement $v(k,t)$ is then formulated as:

$$v(k,t) = \int \sigma(x,t)e^{-j2\pi kx}dx = \int \int \rho(x,f)e^{-j2\pi(kx+ft)}dx\,df, \tag{1}$$

where $\rho(x,f)$ is the 2D spectral signal in x-f domain. This can also be represented in a matrix form: $\mathbf{v} = \mathcal{F}\rho$, in which $\mathbf{v}$ and ρ stand for the stacked k-t space measurement vectors and x-f image respectively, and $\mathcal{F}$ is the 2D Fourier transform along the x-f direction. From the perspective of compressed sensing, the problem can be formulated by exploiting the sparsity of the unknown signal:

$$\min \|\rho\|_1, \quad s.t. \ \|\mathbf{v} - \mathcal{F}\rho\|_2 \leq \epsilon, \tag{2}$$

where ϵ denotes the noise level. In k-t FOCUSS [8,9], the underdetermined inverse problem was solved via a sparse reconstruction algorithm called FOCUSS. The solution then can be expressed as the form that consists of a baseline signal $\bar{\rho}$ and its residual encoding for the n-th estimate of the x-f signal $\rho^{(n)}$:

$$\rho^{(n)} = \bar{\rho} + \text{FOCUSS}(\rho^{(n-1)} - \bar{\rho}, \rho^{(n-1)}). \tag{3}$$

Here the mathematical form of FOCUSS algorithm is omitted for simplicity. For details, please refer to [8,9].

2.2   *k-t* NEXT for Dynamic MRI Reconstruction

Motivated by k-t BLAST [15] and k-t FOCUSS [9], we propose a dynamic image reconstruction NEtwork with X-f Transform (k-t NEXT) to exploit the spatio-temporal correlations from both x-f space and image space. Specifically, k-t NEXT formulates the iterative reconstruction process in an unfolded cascading way, as it has been shown to be a powerful technique in MR reconstruction [12,13]. In each iteration, our proposed approach learns to reconstruct the true images by alternating between x-f and image spaces, so that the spatio-temporal redundancies can be jointly exploited from these two complementary domains. In particular, a xf-CNN is proposed for the recovery of signals in x-f domain

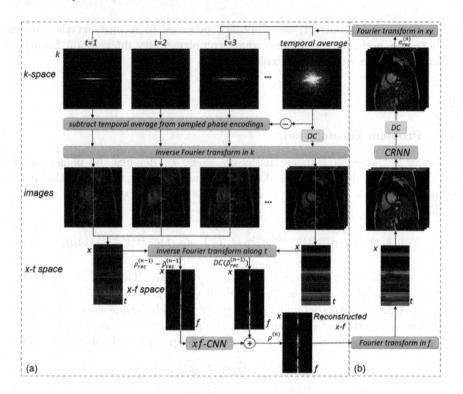

Fig. 1. The $k\text{-}t$ NEXT reconstruction diagram. True signals can be recovered by iteratively updating the reconstruction in both (a) $x\text{-}f$ and (b) image domains via learning the xf-CNN and CRNN jointly. For mathmetical notations, please refer to Eq. 4.

inspired by the traditional $k\text{-}t$ method, and a variation of the CRNN-MRI [12] network is adopted for the subsequent image space reconstruction. We can compactly represent a single iteration of the $k\text{-}t$ NEXT as follows:

$$\rho^{(n)} = \text{DC}(\bar{\rho}_{rec}^{(n-1)}) + xf\text{-CNN}(\rho_{rec}^{(n-1)} - \bar{\rho}_{rec}^{(n-1)}), \tag{4a}$$

$$\sigma_{rec}^{(n)} = \text{CRNN}(\mathcal{F}_f \rho^{(n)}; \mathbf{v}^{(0)}), \quad \rho_{rec}^{(n)} = \mathcal{F}_f^H \sigma_{rec}^{(n)}, \tag{4b}$$

where $\sigma_{rec}^{(n)} \in \mathbb{C}^D$ denotes the complex-valued reconstructed image sequence at iteration n, and $\sigma_{rec}^{(0)} = \sigma_u$ is the acquired zero-filled undersampled images. Here $D = D_x D_y T$, in which D_x and D_y are width and height of the frame and T is the number of frames. $\mathcal{F}_f$ denotes the Fourier transform along f dimension, and $\rho_{rec}^{(n)}$ is the $x\text{-}f$ spectral signal transformed from $\sigma_{rec}^{(n)}$, while $\rho^{(n)}$ stands for the intermediate reconstructed signal from xf-CNN. Also $\bar{\rho}_{rec}^{(n-1)}$ denotes the temporally averaged $x\text{-}f$ signal (see Eq. (5)), DC stands for the data consistency layer [13], and $\mathbf{v}^{(0)} \in \mathbb{C}^M$ ($M \ll D$) is the acquired raw data. An illustrative diagram of $k\text{-}t$ NEXT is shown in Fig. 1. We will introduce it in the following.

***xf*-CNN Exploiting Spatio-Temporal Correlations in *x-f* Domain.** Following the formulation in Eq. (3), here we propose to formulate the *xf*-CNN reconstruction as Eq. (4a), where instead of using model-based [15] or compressed sensing [9] algorithms to recover the true signals, we employ a stack of CNN layers to estimate the missing data based on other available points, typically within its vicinity in *x-f* space. In particular, here the *x-f* baseline signal $\bar{\rho}_{rec}^{(n)}$ is a temporal average of a sequence, i.e.,

$$\bar{\rho}_{rec}^{(n)} = \mathcal{F}^H \left[\sum_t \mathbf{v}^{(n)} ./\max(1, \sum_t \delta(\mathbf{v}^{(n)})) \right], \quad \delta(a) = \begin{cases} 0 & a = 0 \\ 1 & a \neq 0 \end{cases} \quad (5)$$

in which $\mathbf{v}^{(n)}$ is the *k*-space data that is Fourier transformed from $\sigma_{rec}^{(n)}$, and the ./ and max operation is performed element-wise. Thereby, *xf*-CNN learns to reconstruct residuals of each frame, which further exploits the signal sparsity.

The illustrative diagram of *x-f* reconstruction is shown in Fig. 1(a). Specifically, we formulate the *k-t* to *x-f* transformation process as a **x-f transform layer** in the network. In details, the *x-f* transform layer receives input from *k-t* space data. For iteration *n*, the acquired *k*-space data is firstly averaged along *t* to yield a temporal average (Eq. (5)), which is then subtracted from data at each time frame. To ensure data fidelity for the baseline estimate, here we propose to incorporate a data consistency (DC) term for $\bar{\rho}_{rec}^{(n-1)}$ at each frame separately. Then the subtracted data and temporally averaged data are inverse Fourier transformed to image space to obtain a sequence of aliased images and a data-consistent temporally averaged sequence. Each frequency-encoding position is then processed separately hereafter. The image columns from aliased images or baseline images are then gathered and inverse Fourier transformed along *t* to yield an *x-f* image, corresponding to $\rho_{rec}^{(n-1)} - \bar{\rho}_{rec}^{(n-1)}$ and DC($\bar{\rho}_{rec}^{(n-1)}$) respectively, which are then fed as inputs to *xf*-CNN for *x-f* space reconstruction (Eq. (4a)). After the signal de-aliasing in *x-f* domain, another Fourier transform along *f* is adopted to transform the estimated *x-f* signal $\rho^{(n)}$ back to dynamic image space for the subsequent image space reconstruction (Eq. (4b)).

***k-t* NEXT Exploiting Spatio-Temporal Redundancies in Complementary Domains.** Previous approaches [2] have shown that exploring cross-domain knowledge is beneficial for MR reconstruction task. Inspired by this, with the aim of exploiting redundancies in complementary domains, here we propose to learn a dynamic MR reconstruction network in both *x-f* and image spaces jointly. In particular, we employ the CRNN model for image space reconstruction due to its effectiveness in exploiting temporal redundancies with a relatively smaller network capacity [12]. Thus, in each cascade, the proposed *k-t* NEXT consists of a *xf*-CNN and a CRNN block, where it employs all 2D convolutions across spatial and temporal dimensions, in contrast to 3D convolutions used in the baseline method [13]. This enables the network to be more efficient and effective in learning useful and complementary features in *x-f*, spatial and temporal space simultaneously.

Given the training data S with undersampled data as input and fully sampled data as target, i.e., (σ_u, σ_t) in image space and (ρ_u, ρ_t) in x-f space, the network is trained end-to-end by minimising the pixel-wise mean squared error (MSE) between the reconstructed data and the ground truth fully sampled data:

$$\mathcal{L}(\boldsymbol{\theta}) = \frac{1}{n_S} \sum \left(\left\| \sigma_t - \sigma_{rec}^{(N)} \right\|_2^2 + \left\| \rho_t - \rho^{(N)} \right\|_2^2 \right), \tag{6}$$

where $\sigma_{rec}^{(N)}$ and $\rho^{(N)}$ denote the predicted image and x-f array at iteration N, i.e., the final output in image domain and x-f domain respectively, $\boldsymbol{\theta}$ is the set of network parameters, and n_S is the number of training samples.

3 Experiments and Results

3.1 Dataset and Implementation Details

The dataset used in our experiments consists of 10 fully sampled complex-valued short-axis cardiac cine MRI. Each scan contains a single slice SSFP acquisition with 30 temporal frames. The raw data has 32-channel data with sampling matrix 192×190, which was zero-filled to 256×256, and the raw multi-coil data was then reconstructed to produce a single complex-valued image. In experiments, images were transformed back to k-space to simulate a fully sampled single-coil acquisition. A shear grid k-t Cartesian sampling pattern with four central lines (see Fig. 3(b)) was employed to undersample the k-space data to generate the undersampled input image sequences. The undersampling rate mentioned is stated with respect to the matrix size of the data, which is 192×190.

In the proposed k-t NEXT, xf-CNN is composed of 5 layers of 2D CNN with a residual connection from the baseline estimate. For the CRNN model, a variation of architecture [12] is employed which consists of 4 layers of bidirectional CRNN, 1 layer of 2D CNN, a residual connection and a DC layer. We used dilated convolutions with kernel size 3×3 and dilation factor $(3, 3)$, and the number of cascade N was set to 4 for all comparison methods. For detailed network architecture, please refer to supplementary materials. The network was implemented in PyTorch. During training, ADAM optimiser was employed with a learning rate of 10^{-4}. Data augmentation was performed on-the-fly, with random rotation, scaling, and elastic transformation. All evaluations were done via a 3-fold cross validation.

3.2 Results

In experiments, we compared our proposed approach (k-t NEXT) with different dynamic MR reconstruction methods, including compressed sensing method k-t FOCUSS [9], deep learning method CRNN-MRI [12], and DS+3DCNN [13] that incorporates data sharing (DS). To investigate the effectiveness of xf-CNN, an additional baseline approach is proposed which replaces all x-f reconstruction in k-t NEXT with DS component, termed DS+CRNN. In DS methods, we set

Table 1. Comparison results of different methods on dynamic cardiac cine MRI with high undersampling rate 9 and 12. Best results are indicated in bold.

Method		*k-t* FOCUSS	CRNN-MRI	DS+3DCNN	DS+CRNN	*k-t* NEXT
Capacity		-	260,866	352,770	265,474	374,020
9×	PSNR	29.52 (1.58)	32.45 (1.33)	33.47 (1.41)	33.24 (1.38)	**34.23** (1.44)
	SSIM	0.951 (0.013)	0.969 (0.008)	0.975 (0.006)	0.975 (0.006)	**0.979** (0.005)
	HFEN	0.340 (0.033)	0.249 (0.032)	0.214 (0.026)	0.215 (0.027)	**0.196** (0.030)
12×	PSNR	28.14 (1.56)	31.30 (1.32)	32.46 (1.36)	32.34 (1.35)	**33.18** (1.40)
	SSIM	0.937 (0.016)	0.962 (0.009)	0.969 (0.007)	0.970 (0.007)	**0.975** (0.005)
	HFEN	0.382 (0.035)	0.282 (0.034)	0.242 (0.027)	0.239 (0.029)	**0.225** (0.031)

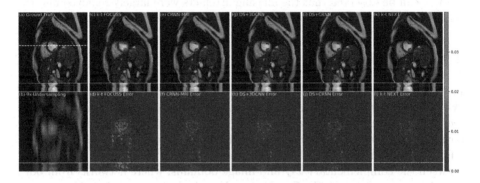

Fig. 2. Comparison results on spatial and temporal dimensions with their error maps. A dynamic video is shown in supplementary materials for better visualisation.

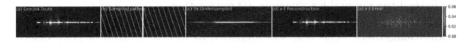

Fig. 3. Visualisation in *x-f* domain. (a) Ground Truth (b) *k-t* sampling pattern (c) 9× undersampled data (d) Reconstructed *x-f* image (e) Error between (c) and (d).

the number of neighbouring frame as $n_{adj} \in \{0, 1, ...5\}$ as in [13]. Note that for a fair comparison with our *k-t* NEXT, we modified the baseline approaches DS+3DCNN and DS+CRNN to learn the residual of a temporally averaged frame as well. Quantitative comparison results of different methods on dynamic cardiac data with undersampling rates 9 and 12 are presented in Table 1, where it compares the network capacity per cascade, peak-to-noise-ratio (PSNR), structural similarity index (SSIM) and high frequency error norm (HFEN) [12]. Networks for different undersampling factors were trained separately in this case. It can be seen that our proposed *k-t* NEXT can outperform other baseline methods by a large margin in terms of all these measures at different undersampling rates, with roughly the same level of network capacity. In particular, *k-t* NEXT performs better than its corresponding DS pair, which indicates the merits of exploiting correlations in *x-f* space and complementary domains.

Additionally, we compared the qualitative results on 9× undersampled data in Fig. 2, where it shows the reconstructed images along both spatial and temporal dimensions, as well as their corresponding error maps. It can be observed that our proposed model can faithfully recover the images with smaller errors especially around dynamic regions compared with other baseline methods. In particular, k-t NEXT produced visually sharper images than DS methods. This is reflected by the fact that, in contrast to DS approaches which fill in k-space data from neighboring frames and therefore could possibly generate averaged and smooth images, k-t NEXT directly estimates the missing data in x-f space. A visualisation of x-f reconstruction is also presented in Fig. 3, where it displays the reconstructed x-f image and its error map in comparison to the input aliased data. It can be observed that the aliasing artefacts were largely removed and the undersampled data were recovered to approximate the ground truth signals.

4   Conclusion

In this paper, we have presented a novel deep learning based method, k-t NEXT (k-t NEtwork with X-f Transform), for highly undersampled dynamic MR image reconstruction. xf-CNN is proposed to exploit correlations in k-t space via reconstructing the true signals from aliased signals in x-f domain. Based on that, k-t NEXT is then proposed to learn to iteratively recover the images by alternating between the complementary x-f and image domains, where networks from both domains were trained jointly. Experimental results have shown that the proposed k-t NEXT outperforms state-of-the-art dynamic MR reconstruction methods in terms of both quantitative and qualitative performance. For the future work, we will extend the method for dynamic 3D applications.

Acknowledgement. This work was supported by EPSRC programme grant SmartHeart (EP/P001009/1).

References

1. Akçakaya, M., Moeller, S., Weingärtner, S., et al.: Scan-specific robust artificial-neural-networks for k-space interpolation (RAKI) reconstruction: Database-free deep learning for fast imaging. Magn. Reson. Med. **81**(1), 439–453 (2019)
2. Eo, T., Jun, Y., Kim, T., et al.: KIKI-net: cross-domain convolutional neural networks for reconstructing undersampled magnetic resonance images. Magn. Reson. Med. **80**(5), 2188–2201 (2018)
3. Griswold, M.A., Jakob, P.M., Heidemann, R.M., et al.: Generalized autocalibrating partially parallel acquisitions (GRAPPA). Magn. Reson. Med. **47**(6), 1202–1210 (2002)
4. Hammernik, K., Klatzer, T., Kobler, E., et al.: Learning a variational network for reconstruction of accelerated MRI data. Magn. Reson. Med. **79**(6), 3055–3071 (2018)
5. Han, Y., Ye, J.C.: k-space deep learning for accelerated MRI. arXiv preprint arXiv:1805.03779 (2018)

6. Hu, X., Parrish, T.: Reduction of field of view for dynamic imaging. Magn. Reson. Med. **31**(6), 691–694 (1994)
7. Jones, R., Haraldseth, O., Müller, T., et al.: K-space substitution: a novel dynamic imaging technique. Magn. Reson. Med. **29**(6), 830–834 (1993)
8. Jung, H., Sung, K., Nayak, K.S., et al.: k-t FOCUSS: a general compressed sensing framework for high resolution dynamic MRI. Magn. Reson. Med. **61**(1), 103–116 (2009)
9. Jung, H., Ye, J.C., Kim, E.Y.: Improved k-t BLAST and k-t SENSE using FOCUSS. Phys. Med. Biol. **52**(11), 3201 (2007)
10. Lingala, S.G., Hu, Y., DiBella, E., et al.: Accelerated dynamic MRI exploiting sparsity and low-rank structure: k-t SLR. IEEE Trans. Med. Imaging **30**(5), 1042–1054 (2011)
11. Liu, J., Kuang, T., Zhang, X.: Image reconstruction by splitting deep learning regularization from iterative inversion. In: Frangi, A.F., Schnabel, J.A., Davatzikos, C., Alberola-López, C., Fichtinger, G. (eds.) MICCAI 2018. LNCS, vol. 11070, pp. 224–231. Springer, Cham (2018). https://doi.org/10.1007/978-3-030-00928-1_26
12. Qin, C., Schlemper, J., Caballero, J., et al.: Convolutional recurrent neural networks for dynamic MR image reconstruction. IEEE Trans. Med. Imaging **38**(1), 280–290 (2019)
13. Schlemper, J., Caballero, J., Hajnal, J.V., et al.: A deep cascade of convolutional neural networks for dynamic MR image reconstruction. IEEE Trans. Med. Imaging **37**(2), 491–503 (2018)
14. Schlemper, J., et al.: Bayesian deep learning for accelerated MR image reconstruction. In: Knoll, F., Maier, A., Rueckert, D. (eds.) MLMIR 2018. LNCS, vol. 11074, pp. 64–71. Springer, Cham (2018). https://doi.org/10.1007/978-3-030-00129-2_8
15. Tsao, J., Boesiger, P., Pruessmann, K.P.: k-t BLAST and k-t SENSE: dynamic MRI with high frame rate exploiting spatiotemporal correlations. Magn. Reson. Med. **50**(5), 1031–1042 (2003)
16. Ye, J.C., Han, Y., Cha, E.: Deep convolutional framelets: a general deep learning framework for inverse problems. SIAM J. Imaging Sci. **11**(2), 991–1048 (2018)
17. Zhang, P., Wang, F., Xu, W., et al.: Multi-channel generative adversarial network for parallel magnetic resonance image reconstruction in k-space. In: MICCAI, pp. 180–188 (2018)
18. Zhang, S., Block, K.T., Frahm, J.: Magnetic resonance imaging in real time: advances using radial FLASH. Magn. Reson. Med. **31**(1), 101–109 (2010)

Model-Based Reconstruction for Highly Accelerated First-Pass Perfusion Cardiac MRI

Teresa Correia[1]($\boxtimes$) , Torben Schneider[2], and Amedeo Chiribiri[1]

[1] School of Biomedical Engineering and Imaging Sciences, King's College London,
London, UK
teresa.correia@kcl.ac.uk
[2] Philips Healthcare, Guildford, Surrey, UK

Abstract. First-pass perfusion cardiac magnetic resonance (FPP-CMR) allows the assessment of coronary heart disease. However, conventional FPP-CMR suffers from low spatial resolution, insufficient heart coverage and requires long breath-holds. At present, perfusion abnormalities are usually identified visually by highly trained physicians. Recently, quantitative analysis of FPP-CMR has emerged as a more reliable and operator-independent approach for identifying perfusion defects. Typically, quantitative FPP-CMR first reconstructs individual dynamic images, which are then converted to contrast agent concentration, and finally, tracer-kinetic modeling is used to generate quantitative myocardial perfusion maps. Here, we propose a model-based FPP-CMR reconstruction approach, which combines image reconstruction and tracer-kinetic modeling, to better exploit the redundancies in the FPP-CMR data. We show that such synergistic approach enables very high undersampling rates at each time frame, and thus allows for much higher spatial resolution and coverage than the traditional method. Furthermore, our proposed method can be combined with respiratory motion correction and k-t undersampling to improve myocardial perfusion quantification, while substantially increasing patient comfort.

Keywords: Model-based reconstruction · Tracer-kinetic parameter mapping · Quantitative perfusion cardiac MRI

1 Introduction

Coronary artery disease (CAD) is the leading cause of death worldwide. It is usually caused by atherosclerosis, which reduces blood flow to the heart (myocardial ischemia). Positron emission tomography (PET) is the clinical reference for noninvasive myocardial perfusion quantification in patients with ischemia [1]. Nevertheless, first-pass perfusion cardiac magnetic resonance (FPP-CMR) is rapidly evolving into an essential tool for detecting myocardial perfusion deficits [1]. It has advantages, such as higher spatial resolution, no radiation exposure, wider

© Springer Nature Switzerland AG 2019
D. Shen et al. (Eds.): MICCAI 2019, LNCS 11765, pp. 514–522, 2019.
https://doi.org/10.1007/978-3-030-32245-8_57

availability and lower scan cost compared to PET. However, FPP-CMR requires ultra-fast acquisitions (to capture the first pass of a contrast bolus), Electro-cardiogram (ECG)-gating and breath-holding techniques to reduce cardiac and respiratory motion, leading to a trade-off between spatial resolution ($\sim$2.5 mm) and cardiac coverage ($\sim$3 slices) [2,3]. The diagnostic accuracy is also com-promised by respiratory induced motion artefacts (patients are often unable to breath-hold) and false-positive defects due to dark-rim artefacts [2]. Moreover, perfusion abnormalities are often identified visually, which has a prognostic value that is dependent on the level of training and experience of the operator [4].

The lack of reproducible and accurate results are the main factors limiting the wide-spread clinical adoption of FPP-CMR. Recently, quantification meth-ods have been proposed to achieve a more reliable and operator-independent assessment of myocardial perfusion in FPP-CMR [5,6]. Typically, quantitative FPP-CMR methods first involve reconstructing individual dynamic contrast-enhanced images, which are then converted to contrast agent concentration, and finally, tracer-kinetic (TK) modeling is used to generate TK parameter maps; these methods can be referred to as "indirect" methods.

Direct model-based parametric reconstruction has been used in PET [7] and few applications in dynamic contrast-enhance MR imaging [8,9] to directly obtain TK parameter maps from the acquired data. This approach showed supe-rior quantitative performance over conventional indirect quantification methods. In addition, direct model-based reconstruction approaches reduce the dimension-ality of the problem, i.e., the image reconstruction problem is reduced to finding 2–4 TK parameters maps, instead of $\sim$60 time points per pixel. Therefore, this approach provides accurate TK parameters maps, while also enabling very high acceleration factors by exploiting the redundancy of spatial information between time-points. So far, compressed sensing (CS) and parallel imaging reconstruction approaches have been used to accelerate FPP-CMR acquisitions up to $\sim$8x and achieve higher spatial resolution [2,10,11].

In this work, a DIRect QuanTitative (DIREQT) FPP-CMR reconstruction framework is proposed to directly estimate quantitative myocardial perfusion maps from undersampled data. The proposed framework was evaluated on a numerical FPP-CMR phantom and patient with suspected CAD.

2   Methods

Figure 1 shows the steps required in the conventional indirect method and gener-ation of the DIREQT forward model, which converts TK parameters to (multicoil undersampled) FPP-CMR measurements.

2.1   DIREQT Reconstruction

The proposed DIREQT method directly estimates TK parameters maps from the measured FPP-CMR data. This is achieved by inverting a forward model that includes the operations described below (indicated by the small red arrows in Fig. 1).

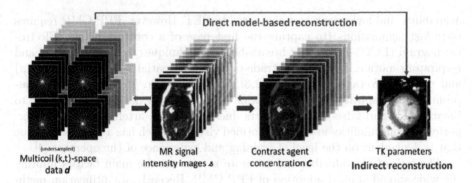

Fig. 1. Flow chart illustrating the indirect method and proposed DIREQT reconstruction to obtain TK parameters from multicoil (undersampled) data d. The indirect reconstruction consists of three steps (blue arrows): First, FPP-CMR signal intensity images s are estimated from the acquired (k, t)-space data d. Then, contrast agent concentration over time C is estimated from s. Finally, TK parameters maps are estimated from C. In the DIREQT reconstruction, TK parameters are estimated directly from the (k, t)-space data d (long red arrow) by solving an inverse problem using an iterative reconstruction scheme. The forward model used for the conversion from TK parameter maps to (k, t)-space data d is indicated by the small red arrows.

TK Parameter Maps to Contrast Agent Concentration. The Patlak model [12] is used to estimate the contrast agent concentration over time, $C(\mathbf{r}, t)$:

$$C(\mathbf{r}, t) = K^{\text{Trans}}(\mathbf{r}) \int_0^t C_{\text{AIF}}(\tau) \, d\tau + \nu_{\text{p}}(\mathbf{r}) \, C_{\text{AIF}}(t), \tag{1}$$

where $\mathbf{r} \in (x, y)$ are the image domain spatial coordinates, C_{AIF} is the arterial input function, K^{Trans} and ν_{p} are TK parameters, representing the contrast transfer coefficient and fractional plasma volume, respectively. The parameter K^{Trans} is related to vascular permeability and blood flow.

Contrast Agent Concentration to Signal Intensity. The contrast agent concentration $C(\mathbf{r}, t)$ changes T_1 according to the following equation:

$$\frac{1}{T_1(\mathbf{r}, t)} = \frac{1}{T_1(\mathbf{r}, 0)} + \gamma \, C(\mathbf{r}, t), \tag{2}$$

where $T_1(\mathbf{r}, 0)$ is the precontrast T_1 and γ is the contrast relaxivity. The dynamic contrast-enhanced image series $s(\mathbf{r}, t)$ is related to T_1 by the saturation-recovery prepared fast gradient echo signal equation:

$$s(\mathbf{r}, t) = s_0(\mathbf{r}) \left[\left(1 - e^{-T_\text{S} R_1}\right) a^{n-1} + \left(1 - e^{-T_\text{R} R_1}\right) \frac{1 - a^{n-1}}{1 - a} \right] \tag{3}$$

where $s_0(\mathbf{r})$ is proportional to the equilibrium longitudinal magnetization, T_S is the saturation time, T_R is the repetition time, n is the number of excitation pulses applied before acquiring the k-space center, $R_1 = \frac{1}{T_1}$ and $a = \cos\alpha \; e^{-T_R R_1}$, which contains the flip angle α.

Signal Intensity to Undersampled Data. The undersampled (k,t)-space data $d(\mathbf{k}, t)$ are related to $\mathfrak{s}(\mathbf{r}, t)$ as follows:

$$d(\mathbf{k}, t) = A(\mathbf{k}, t) \, \mathcal{F} \, S(\mathbf{r}) \, \mathfrak{s}(\mathbf{r}, t) \tag{4}$$

where $\mathbf{k} \in (k_x, k_y)$ represents k-space coordinates, $A(\mathbf{k}, t)$ is the (k,t)-space sampling trajectory, $\mathcal{F}$ is the Fourier transform and $S(\mathbf{r})$ are the coil sensitivities. Hence, the DIREQT forward problem is given by:

$$d(\mathbf{k}, t) = f\left(K^{\mathrm{Trans}}(\mathbf{r}), \, \nu_{\mathrm{p}}(\mathbf{r})\right) \tag{5}$$

where f is the forward model that combines Eqs. (1)–(4). Therefore, the TK parameter maps can be estimated by solving the following optimization problem:

$$\left(\hat{K}^{\mathrm{Trans}}(\mathbf{r}), \, \hat{\nu}_{\mathrm{p}}(\mathbf{r})\right) = \underset{K^{\mathrm{Trans}}(\mathbf{r}), \nu_{\mathrm{p}}(\mathbf{r})}{\arg\min} \, \left\| d(\mathbf{k}, t) - f\left(K^{\mathrm{Trans}}(\mathbf{r}), \, \nu_{\mathrm{p}}(\mathbf{r})\right) \right\|_2^2 \tag{6}$$

Spatial sparsity constrains on the TK parameter maps can be added to Eq. (6):

$$\left(\hat{K}^{\mathrm{Trans}}(\mathbf{r}), \, \hat{\nu}_{\mathrm{p}}(\mathbf{r})\right) = \underset{K^{\mathrm{Trans}}(\mathbf{r}), \nu_{\mathrm{p}}(\mathbf{r})}{\arg\min} \, \left\{ \left\| d(\mathbf{k}, t) - f\left(K^{\mathrm{Trans}}(\mathbf{r}), \, \nu_{\mathrm{p}}(\mathbf{r})\right) \right\|_2^2 \right.$$
$$\left. + \lambda_1 \left\| \nabla_{\mathrm{s}} K^{\mathrm{Trans}}(\mathbf{r}) \right\|_1 + \lambda_2 \left\| \nabla_{\mathrm{s}} \nu_{\mathrm{p}}(\mathbf{r}) \right\|_1 \right\} \tag{7}$$

where ∇_{s} is the 2D spatial finite differences operator, λ_1 and λ_2 are regularization parameters. A limited-memory BFGS quasi-Newton method can be used to solve this nonlinear inverse problem.

2.2   Indirect Reconstruction

First, individual dynamic contrast-enhanced images are reconstructed from undersampled (k,t)-space data by solving the following optimization problem:

$$\hat{\mathfrak{s}}(\mathbf{r}, t) = \underset{\mathfrak{s}(\mathbf{r}, t)}{\arg\min} \, \left\{ \left\| d(\mathbf{k}, t) - A(\mathbf{k}, t) \, \mathcal{F} \, S(\mathbf{r}) \, \mathfrak{s}(\mathbf{r}, t) \right\|_2^2 \right.$$
$$\left. + \lambda_1 \left\| \nabla_{\mathrm{s}} \mathfrak{s}(\mathbf{r}, t) \right\|_1 + \lambda_2 \left\| \nabla_t \mathfrak{s}(\mathbf{r}, t) \right\|_1 \right\} \tag{8}$$

where ∇_t is the finite differences operator along the temporal dimension. Then, the change in concentration $C(\mathbf{r}, t)$ is derived from the signal intensity, and finally, TK parameters maps are obtained from $C(\mathbf{r}, t)$, by solving the inverse problems of Eqs. (3) and (1), respectively.

2.3   Digital Phantom

Fully-sampled FPP-CMR data was generated using the MRXCAT numerical phantom [13] and the following parameters: field-of-view (FOV) = 320 × 320 × 80 mm^3, spatial resolution = 2 × 2 mm^2, slice thickness = 5 mm, $T_S/T_R/T_E$ = 150.0/2.0/1.0 ms, flip angle = 15°, contrast agent dose = 0.075 mmol/kg, contrast agent relaxivity = 5.6 L/mmol s, 6 receiver coils, 32 time frames and population average C_{AIF}. A radial k-t sampling strategy was used to undersample acquisitions by a factor of 10, 20, 30 and 40. Gaussian noise was added to each dataset to obtain a contrast-to-noise ratio (CNR) of 40. Six noise realizations were performed for each undersampling rate. DIREQT and indirect reconstructions were obtained from the undersampled datasets.

2.4   In-Vivo Experiments

A rest FPP-CMR fully-sampled acquisition was performed in one patient with suspected CAD using a dual-bolus technique with 0.0075 + 0.075 mmol/kg of Gadobutrol (Gadovist; Bayer, Germany) and a 3 T scanner (Achieva; Philips Healthcare, Netherlands). A saturation-recovery turbo field echo (TFE) ECG-triggered sequence was used to acquire a single short-axis slice in free-breathing using the following parameters: FOV = 320 × 320 mm^2, resolution = 2.8 × 2.8 mm^2, slice thickness = 10 mm, $T_S/T_R/T_E$ = 120.0/1.96/0.93 ms, flip angle = 15°, acquisition window = 224.3 ms, total acquisition time = 1 min 20 s, contrast agent relaxivity = 5.0 L/mmol s. The same radial sampling strategy used in the simulations was used to generate 20×, 30× and 40× undersampled datasets. The C_{AIF} was found using a large region of interest drawn in the left ventricle and the precontrast $T_1(\mathbf{r}, 0)$ was extracted from a T1 mapping sequence. In addition, the signal intensity was normalized to the precontrast signal.

Motion Correction The free-breathing FPP-CMR acquisition was initially reconstructed using the vendors default reconstruction. The dynamic images were used to estimate the frame-by-frame translational motion by registering every frame to the sliding average of its predecessor (±7 frames). Then, translational motion correction was performed directly in k-space by applying a linear phase shift. Finally, these motion-corrected datasets were reconstructed using the indirect and DIREQT methods.

The value of adding spatial sparsity constraints on the TK parameters maps, in the form of spatial total variation (TV) regularization (see Eq. (7)), was also tested. The regularization parameters were selected empirically for all methods. TK parameters maps obtained with the DIREQT and indirect methods were quantitatively evaluated against the reference (fully-sampled) TK parameters maps using the normalized mean square error (NMSE) and correlation coefficient (CC). Reconstructions were performed using MATLAB (MathWorks, USA) on an Intel i7-86508 @ 1.9 GHz laptop with 32 GB memory.

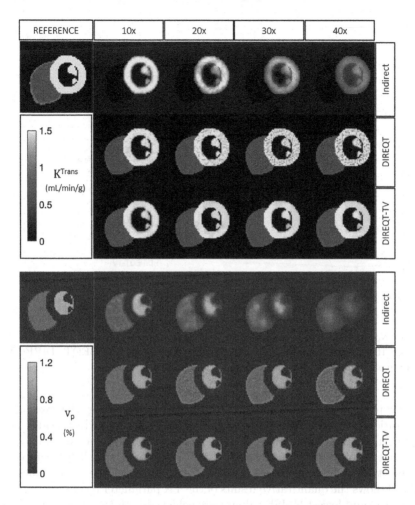

Fig. 2. Numerical phantom K^{Trans} and ν_{p} reconstructions obtained from 10×, 20×, 30× and 40× undersampled data using the indirect method, proposed DIREQT and DIREQT with TV regularization (DIREQT-TV). The reference images are displayed for comparison. The proposed DIREQT generates high-quality TK maps even at very high undersampling rates.

3   Results and Discussion

Figure 2 shows the DIREQT reconstructions, with and without TV regularization, obtained from simulated undersampled data together with the fully-sampled reference and indirect reconstructions. For the indirect method, the image quality of the TK maps at acceleration 10× is comparable to the reference images. For higher acceleration rates, the quality of the TK parameters maps rapidly deteriorates and false perfusion defects become visible. In comparison, the overall image quality of the TK parameter maps obtained with DIREQT is

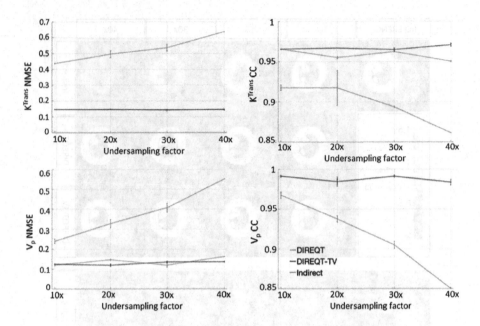

Fig. 3. Normalized mean square error (NMSE) and correlation coefficient (CC) between the reference images and TK maps obtained with DIREQT, DIREQT-TV and indirect methods.

superior to the indirect method at all levels of undersampling. However, at high acceleration rates the DIREQT problem becomes ill-posed, which leads to noise amplification. In these instances, regularization strategies can be employed to stabilize the solution. Figure 2 shows that TV regularization helps reduce noise amplification at high accelerations and it also improves the convergence rate. Figure 3 shows the quantitative results of the TK parameter reconstructions. The highest CC and lowest NMSE values were achieved with the proposed DIREQT method, indicating a better agreement with the reference images.

Finally, Fig. 4 displays the TK parameter maps estimated from fully-sampled, $20\times$, $30\times$ and $40\times$ undersampled patient data using the indirect and DIREQT methods. Note that FPP-CMR data was acquired without breath-holding, for improved patient comfort, and to minimize respiratory motion artefacts, which can greatly affect the quantification results. The proposed method yields good results even at very high acceleration rates. The total reconstruction times for the indirect and DIREQT methods were $\sim$290 s and $\sim$185 s, respectively.

The Patlak model was chosen in this work because it provides results comparable to other TK models normally used in FPP-CMR [14], such as Fermi and two-compartment model, with the advantage that it can be linearized, which simplifies calculations. However, a comparison between different TK models will be the subject of a future study. Furthermore, other regularization strategies could be employed that could further increase the robustness of the proposed

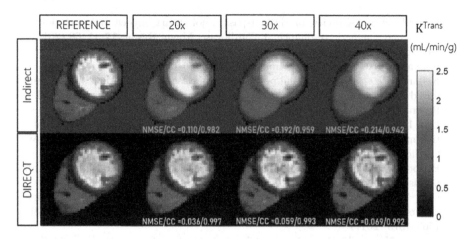

Fig. 4. Indirect and DIREQT K^{Trans} reconstructions obtained from fully-sampled (reference), 20×, 30× and 40× undersampled patient data. Normalized mean square error (NMSE) and correlation coefficient (CC) are shown in each subfigure. There is a good agreement between the fully-sampled and undersampled DIREQT K^{Trans} maps.

method against noise, pushing the acceleration further. In future studies, the DIREQT method will be evaluated in a large cohort of patients with suspected CAD using prospective undersampled acquisitions. These studies will also aim to achieve much higher spatial resolution and coverage, and hence, greater diagnostic accuracy.

4 Conclusion

A novel and highly efficient direct model-based reconstruction framework for FPP-CMR has been described. The proposed DIREQT method generates quantitative myocardial perfusion maps directly from the acquired data. Compared to conventional indirect methods, the DIREQT method improves the quantification accuracy and allows higher acceleration factors. The proposed DIREQT method can be combined with respiratory motion correction to facilitate free-breathing FPP-CMR imaging with improved spatial resolution and heart coverage.

Acknowledgements. This work was supported by the Wellcome/EPSRC CME [WT 203148/Z/16/Z] and MedIAN EPSRC [EP/N026993/1].

References

1. Heo, R., et al.: Noninvasive imaging in coronary artery disease. Semin. Nucl. Med. **44**(5), 398–409 (2014)
2. Motwani, M., et al.: Advanced cardiovascular magnetic resonance myocardial perfusion imaging: high-spatial resolution versus 3-dimensional whole-heart coverage. Circ.: Cardiovasc. Imaging **6**(4), e22 (2013)

3. Fair, M., et al.: A review of 3D first-pass, whole-heart, myocardial perfusion cardiovascular magnetic resonance. J. Cardiovasc. Magn. Reson. **17**(1), 68 (2015)
4. Sammut, E., et al.: Prognostic value of quantitative stress cardiovascular magnetic resonance. JACC Cardiovasc. Imaging **11**(5), 686–694 (2018)
5. Kellman, P., et al.: Myocardial perfusion cardiovascular magnetic resonance: optimized dual sequence and reconstruction for quantification. J. Cardiovasc. Magn. Reson. **19**(42), 1–14 (2017)
6. Hsu, L.Y., et al.: Diagnostic performance of fully automated pixel-wise quantitative myocardial perfusion imaging by cardiovascular magnetic resonance. JACC Cardiovasc. Imaging **11**(5), 697–707 (2018)
7. Petibon, Y., et al.: Direct parametric reconstruction in dynamic PET myocardial perfusion imaging: in vivo studies. Phys. Med. Biol. **62**(9), 3539 (2017)
8. Guo, Y., et al.: Direct estimation of tracer-kinetic parameter maps from highly undersampled brain dynamic contrast enhanced MRI. Magn. Reson. Med. **78**(4), 1566–1578 (2017)
9. Dikaios, N., et al.: Direct parametric reconstruction from undersampled (k, t)-space data in dynamic contrast enhanced MRI. Med. Image Anal. **18**(7), 989–1001 (2014)
10. Otazo, R., et al.: Combination of compressed sensing and parallel imaging for highly accelerated first-pass cardiac perfusion MRI. Magn. Reson. Med. **64**(3), 767–776 (2010)
11. Vitanis, V., et al.: High resolution three-dimensional cardiac perfusion imaging using compartment-based k-t principal component analysis. Magn. Reson. Med. **65**(2), 575–587 (2011)
12. Patlak, C.S., et al.: Graphical evaluation of blood-to-brain transfer constants from multiple-time uptake data. J. Cereb. Blood Flow Metab. **3**(1), 1–7 (1983)
13. Wissmann, L., et al.: MRXCAT: realistic numerical phantoms for cardiovascular magnetic resonance. J. Cardiovasc. Magn. Reson. **16**, 63 (2014)
14. Pack, N., DiBella, E.: Comparison of myocardial perfusion estimates from dynamic contrast-enhanced magnetic resonance imaging with four quantitative analysis methods. Magn. Reson. Med. **64**(1), 125–137 (2010)

Learning Shape Priors for Robust Cardiac MR Segmentation from Multi-view Images

Chen Chen[1(✉)], Carlo Biffi[1], Giacomo Tarroni[1], Steffen Petersen[2], Wenjia Bai[3,4], and Daniel Rueckert[1]

[1] Biomedical Image Analysis Group, Imperial College London, London, UK
chen.chen15@imperial.ac.uk
[2] NIHR Barts BRC, Queen Mary University of London, London, UK
[3] Data Science Institute, Imperial College London, London, UK
[4] Department of Medicine, Imperial College London, London, UK

Abstract. Cardiac MR image segmentation is essential for the morphological and functional analysis of the heart. Inspired by how experienced clinicians assess the cardiac morphology and function across multiple standard views (i.e. long- and short-axis views), we propose a novel approach which learns anatomical shape priors across different 2D standard views and leverages these priors to segment the left ventricular (LV) myocardium from short-axis MR image stacks. The proposed segmentation method has the advantage of being a 2D network but at the same time incorporates spatial context from multiple, complementary views that span a 3D space. Our method achieves accurate and robust segmentation of the myocardium across different short-axis slices (from apex to base), outperforming baseline models (e.g. 2D U-Net, 3D U-Net) while achieving higher data efficiency. Compared to the 2D U-Net, the proposed method reduces the mean Hausdorff distance (mm) from 3.24 to 2.49 on the apical slices, from 2.34 to 2.09 on the middle slices and from 3.62 to 2.76 on the basal slices on the test set, when only 10% of the training data was used.

1 Introduction

Accurate segmentation of cardiac magnetic resonance (CMR) images is fundamental for assessing cardiac morphology and diagnosing heart conditions [10]. Manual segmentation of the anatomical structures is tedious, time-consuming and prone to subjective errors, which is not suitable for large-scale studies such as UK Biobank[1] [1]. Therefore, it is essential to develop automated, fast and accurate CMR segmentation techniques.

---

[1] https://imaging.ukbiobank.ac.uk/.

Electronic supplementary material The online version of this chapter (https://doi.org/10.1007/978-3-030-32245-8_58) contains supplementary material, which is available to authorized users.

© Springer Nature Switzerland AG 2019
D. Shen et al. (Eds.): MICCAI 2019, LNCS 11765, pp. 523–531, 2019.
https://doi.org/10.1007/978-3-030-32245-8_58

Recently, convolutional neural network (CNN) based methods have achieved very good performance for cardiac image segmentation in terms of both speed and accuracy [1,2,12]. However, they may still produce sub-optimal segmentation results in some circumstances. For example, in the Automatic Cardiac Diagnosis Challenge (ACDC) [2], the top segmentation methods (all CNN-based) achieve high overall segmentation scores for mid-ventricular short-axis slices. However, they sometimes produce poor results or even fail to locate the myocardium in basal slices (due to its more complex shape) and apical slices (due to its small size). This problem is not uncommon and has been reported in the related literature [2,7,15]. Methods based on 2D networks, trained in a slice-by-slice fashion, are particularly affected by this problem since they do not incorporate spatial context from neighboring SA images or long-axis (LA) views. On the other hand, 3D networks are capable of incorporating 3D spatial information to perform the segmentation task. Yet the 3D spatial context can be affected by potential inter-slice motion artefacts [13] and the low through-plane spatial resolution in cardiac SA stacks, thus limiting their segmentation performance. Compared to 2D ones, 3D networks usually contain more parameter and are prone to over-fitting especially when the training set is limited in size since they use 3D volumes rather than 2D slices as input, significantly reducing the number of training samples.

Experienced clinicians are able to assess the cardiac morphology and function from multiple standard views, using both SA and LA images to form an understanding of the cardiac anatomy. Inspired by this, we propose a method which learns the anatomical prior knowledge across four standard views and leverages this to perform segmentation on 2D SA images. The intuition behind our work is that the representation learnt from multiple standard views is beneficial for the segmentation task on the SA slices as different views should share the same representation of the 3D anatomy if they are from the same subject.

The main contributions of this paper are the following: (a) we developed a novel autoencoder architecture (Shape MAE) which learns latent representation of cardiac shapes from multiple standard views; (b) we developed a segmentation network (multi-view U-Net, adapted from [11]), which is capable of incorporating the anatomical shape priors learned from multi-view images to guide the segmentation on SA images; (c) we assessed the segmentation accuracy and the data efficiency of the proposed segmentation method against common 2D and 3D segmentation baselines by limiting the number of training images, demonstrating that the proposed method is more robust, and less dependent on the size of training data.

Related Literature. A large number of methods have been developed to improve the robustness of the cardiac segmentation. One approach is to learn an ensemble model where the predictions of a 2D and a 3D network are combined [6]. This method is capable of producing accurate results, but has a relatively high computational cost and requires an extra post-processing step to merge the predictions from the two networks. Another approach is to incorporate cardiac anatomical prior knowledge into segmentation networks [5,9]. In [9], the learned representation of the 3D cardiac shape is employed to constrain the segmentation model to predict anatomically plausible shapes. The main bottleneck of this method is the requirement of fully annotated 3D high-resolution CMR images which are free from inter-slice motion artefacts and have high through-plane spatial resolution. However, compared to the standard 2D imaging protocol, the 3D one requires the subjects to hold their breath for a relatively long time and therefore is often not feasible for patients with cardiovascular diseases. Instead of using 3D images, we exploit *routinely acquired* 2D standard views to learn the shape representation of the cardiac structures. The learned representation is then injected into a segmentation network to improve its performance on SA CMR images. Of note, the approach in [8] also injects shape priors produced from an autoencoder into a segmentation network. However, the aim of that approach is to generate multiple segmentation hypotheses for ambiguous images, and cannot be readily employed to learn shape priors from different views to enhance cardiac segmentation.

2   Methods

The proposed method consists of two novel architectures: (1) a **shape-aware multi-view autoencoder (Shape MAE)** which aims at learning anatomical shape priors from standard cardiac acquisition planes incl. short-axis and long-axis views and (2) a **multi-view U-Net** which performs cardiac short-axis image segmentation by incorporating anatomical priors learned by Shape MAE into a modified U-Net architecture.

Shape MAE: Shape-Aware Multi-view Autoencoder. As illustrated in Fig. 1, we first present a novel architecture named shape-aware multi-view autoencoder (Shape MAE) which learns anatomical shape priors from standard cardiac views through multi-task learning. Given a source view X_i, the network learns the low-dimensional representation z_i of X_i that best reconstructs all the j target views segmentations Y_j. In this work, we employ four source views X_i ($i = 1, \ldots, 4$) which are three LA images - the two-chamber view (LA1), three-chamber view (LA2), the four-chamber view (LA3) - and one mid-ventricular slice (Mid-V) from the SA view. The target segmentations views Y_j ($j = 1, \ldots, 6$) correspond to the four previous views plus two SA slices: the apical one and the basal one. All encoders $E_i : z_i = E_i(X_i)$ and all decoders $D_j : Y_j = D_j(z_i)$ in the Shape MAE share the same architecture (see Fig. 1b). The **loss function** $\mathcal{L}_{\text{Shape MAE}}$ for the whole network is defined as follows:

$$\mathcal{L}_{\text{Shape MAE}} = \mathcal{L}_{intra} + \alpha \mathcal{L}_{inter} + \beta \mathcal{L}_{reg} \qquad (1)$$

The first two terms of Eq. 1 are defined as the cross entropy loss $\mathcal{F}$ between the predicted myocardium segmentation $\hat{Y}_{i \to j} = D_j(E_i(X_i))$ for the target view j given a source image X_i of the same subject and its ground truth segmentation Y_j. $\mathcal{L}_{intra}$ denotes the segmentation loss when the source view X_i and the target view Y_j correspond to the same view: $\mathcal{L}_{intra} = \sum_{i=1,i=j}^{4} \mathcal{F}(Y_j, \hat{Y}_{i \to j})$, whereas the second term $\mathcal{L}_{inter}$ denotes the loss when two views are different: $\mathcal{L}_{inter} = \sum_{i=1}^{4} \sum_{j=1,i \neq j}^{6} \mathcal{F}(Y_j, \hat{Y}_{i \to j})$. The third term is a regularisation term on the latent

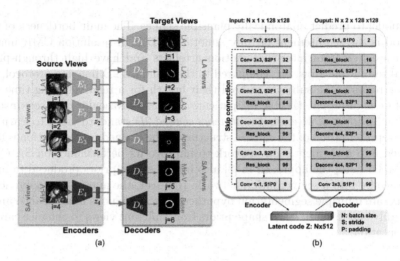

Fig. 1. (a) Overview of Shape MAE. (b) Detailed architectures of each encoder and each decoder. Each rectangle represents one or a series of convolutional (Conv) or transposed convolutional (Deconv) layers where the number in the square box represents the number of filters for each layer. A 'Res_block' (pink rectangles) consists of two convolutional layers (3×3) with a residual connection which adds its input to the features from the second layer. Instance normalisation and leaky ReLU activation are applied throughout the network. A sigmoid function is applied to the latent code z to bound its range.

representations $z_i, z_i \in Z$: $\mathcal{L}_{reg} = \frac{1}{|Z|} \sum_{i=1}^{4} ||z_i - \bar{z}||^2$, which penalises the L2 distance between z_i and $\bar{z}$, with $\bar{z} = \frac{1}{|Z|} \sum_{i=1}^{4} z_i$ being the average z for a subject. Although the latent shape codes from different views of the same subject are not directly shared, this regularisation term forces them to be close to each other. We use coefficients α and β to control the relative importance of $\mathcal{L}_{inter}$ and $\mathcal{L}_{reg}$.

The principle behind the proposed network is that different views require *independent* functions to map them to the latent space that describes **global** shape characteristics; whereas translating this latent space to another view or plane also requires a *specific* projection function. Predicting the shape of the myocardium based on the six target views instead of a single view encourages the network to learn and exploit correlations between different views, resulting in a global, view-invariant shape representation rather than a local representation for a particular view. All the encoders and the decoders in this framework are trained jointly in a multi-task learning fashion, with the benefit of avoiding overfitting and encouraging model generalisation [3].

MV U-Net: Multi-view U-Net. As shown in Fig. 2, we propose a segmentation network called multi-view U-Net (MV U-Net) based on the original U-Net [11] for cardiac SA image segmentation. The proposed network is capable of incorporating the anatomical shape priors learned by Shape MAE. Similar to the original architecture, the proposed architecture comprises 4 down-sampling

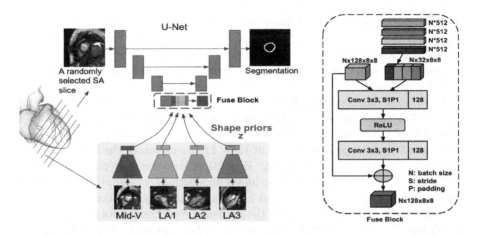

Fig. 2. (a) Overview of the proposed MV U-Net. (b) Architecture of the 'Fuse Block'. The number of shown feature map blocks of the U-Net is reduced for clarity of presentation. Batch normalisation and ReLU activations are applied throughout the network. For each subject, the shape code of each view is reshaped to $1 \times 4 \times 8 \times 8$ and then concatenated with the other three along the second axis to form an input of $1 \times 32 \times 8 \times 8$ to the Fuse Block.

blocks and 4 up-sampling blocks to learn multi-scale features. Differently from the original U-Net, we reduced the number of filters at each level by four times to account for the fact that cardiac segmentation is simpler than the lesion segmentation (with multiple candidates) which was the task that the original U-Net was applied to. In addition, a module called 'Fuse Block' is introduced in the bottleneck of the network (see Fig. 2b) to inject the latent codes into the segmentation network. This fusing approach is different from that in [8] where the latent codes are simply concatenated with U-Net activations. The proposed module consists of two convolutional (Conv) kernels (3×3) and a residual connection to combine the shape representations from different views through learnable weights. Thanks to this module, given an arbitrary short-axis image slice I^p from a subject p and its correspondent shape representations $z_1^p, z_2^p, z_3^p, z_4^p$ obtained by Shape MAE (one for each of the four standard views), the network can predict a segmentation $S^p = f_{\text{MV U-Net}}(I^p, z_1^p, z_2^p, z_3^p, z_4^p; \theta)$ by distilling the prior knowledge to the high-level features of the network, allowing it to efficiently refine the segmentations through multi-view information. The network is trained using standard training procedure with a cross entropy loss to optimise the parameters θ of MV U-Net.

3 Experiments and Results

Cardiac Multi-view Image Dataset. Experiments were performed on a dataset acquired from 734 subjects. For each subject, a stack of 2D SA slices and three orthogonal 2D LA images are available. All the LV myocardium were annotated on the SA images as well as the LA images at the end-diastolic (ED) frame using an automated method followed by manual quality control. All the images were acquired using one scanner. The spatial resolution of the images is $1.8 \times 1.8 \times 10\,\mathrm{mm}$.

In our experiments, the dataset was randomly split into two subsets: a training set (570 cases), a test set (164 cases). All LA images were registered to a template subject using rigid transformation with MIRTK toolkit[2]. All 2D SA slices have been cropped to the size of 128×128 pixels where the left ventricle is roughly in the center of every image. Benefiting from the view planning (which is a standard step during the cardiac image acquisition), we simply use the intersection point of the three orthogonal LA images on every SA slice to determine its center of the interest region. All the networks were trained for 200 epochs on an NVIDIA® GeForce® 2080 Ti, using an Adam optimizer with a batch size of 10. The learning rate for Shape MAE was set to 0.0001 whereas the learning rate for the segmentation network was set to 0.001. In our experiments, α was empirically set to 0.5 and β to 0.001 in $\mathcal{L}_{\text{Shape MAE}}$. The proposed algorithm was implemented in Pytorch.

Segmentation Results. To evaluate the segmentation accuracy, we use two measurements: the Dice score and the Hausdorff distance (HD). The proposed method is compared against: a 2D U-Net [11], a state-of-the-art 2D FCN for cardiac MR image segmentation [1], and a 3D U-Net [4]. For fairness and ease of comparison, all models were set with the same number of filters at each level (starting with 16 filters in the first layer) and trained with the same preprocessing and training schedule. For the 3D network, we resampled SA images to a voxel size of $1.8 \times 1.8 \times 1.8\,\mathrm{mm}$ and cropped each to a size of $128 \times 128 \times 64$ during pre-processing. We trained MV U-Net and the baseline networks with two settings: in one case we used **10%** of the training set, while in the other one we used **100%**. Of note, in each setting, we first trained a Shape MAE and then trained a MV U-Net where shape priors of four standard views were obtained using corresponding encoders in the Shape MAE.

Results on the test set are shown in Table 1. From the table, it can be observed that the proposed method outperforms the baseline models in both the low-data setting and the high-data setting, with improved Dice scores at the apex, middle, and base of the left ventricular myocardium. In particular, when only 10% data was used, the proposed method reduces the mean HD from 3.24 to 2.49 mm on the apical slices, from 2.34 to 2.09 on the middle slices and from 3.62 to 2.76 on the basal slices, compared to the 2D U-Net. Figure 3 shows examples of the segmentation results from all the networks where the proposed method not only produces more robust segmentation across slices compared to the results from the 2D networks, but also achieves more anatomically plausible results in comparison to the 3D one (see the red arrows in this figure). Visualization results of the segmentation networks trained in the high-data setting and Shape MAE are provided in the supplementary material.

---

[2] https://mirtk.github.io/.

Table 1. Comparison of the myocardium segmentation accuracy of the baseline models and the proposed method in terms of the mean and the standard deviation of Dice score and HD distance (mm) obtained on the test set (n = 164). The comparison has been carried out separately for apical, mid-ventricular, and basal slices.

Method	# Training subjects	Dice			HD		
		Apex	Middle	Base	Apex	Middle	Base
2D U-Net	57 (10%)	0.898 (0.090)	0.932 (0.035)	0.923 (0.077)	3.239 (6.918)	2.337 (2.913)	3.617 (9.058)
2D FCN	57 (10%)	0.873 (0.113)	0.926 (0.041)	0.919 (0.069)	3.088 (3.882)	2.317 (1.440)	2.948 (2.691)
3D U-Net	57 (10%)	0.890 (0.083)	0.923 (0.043)	0.923 (0.043)	2.839 (3.980)	3.573 (9.05)	4.469 (10.02)
MV U-Net	57 (10%)	**0.905 (0.076)**	**0.932 (0.025)**	**0.926 (0.088)**	**2.487 (3.022)**	**2.093 (0.577)**	**2.758 (3.697)**
2D U-Net	570 (100%)	0.937 (0.029)	0.955 (0.016)	0.948 (0.071)	1.917 (0.294)	1.888 (0.178)	2.327 (2.566)
2D FCN	570 (100%)	0.934 (0.032)	0.958 (0.015)	0.949 (0.078)	1.913 (0.297)	1.890 (0.347)	2.161 (1.068)
3D U-Net	570 (100%)	0.913 (0.112)	0.945 (0.078)	0.933 (0.093)	2.104 (1.24)	1.957 (0.68)	2.722 (3.57)
MV U-Net	570 (100%)	**0.938 (0.027)**	**0.958 (0.013)**	**0.952 (0.079)**	**1.903 (0.345)**	**1.874 (0.142)**	**2.146 (1.004)**

Approx. # of conv weights (million)   2D U-Net: 0.8   2D FCN: 1.0   3D U-Net: 2.5   MV U-Net: 1.2

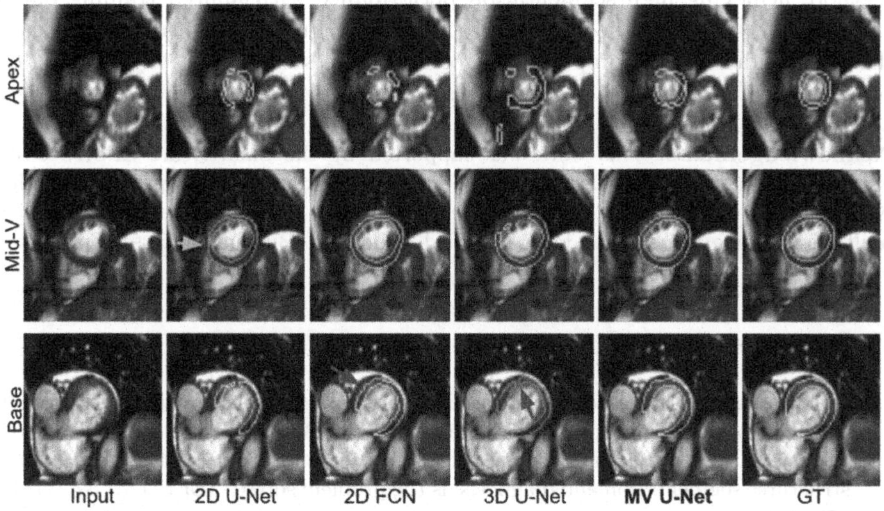

Fig. 3. Visualisation of the predicted segmentations and correspondent ground truth (GT) from the baseline models and MV U-Net (all trained with **10%** training subjects) on an apical, a mid-ventricular and a basal slice from one patient. Compared to the baseline models, MV U-Net produces more accurate segmentation with stronger spatial coherence.

4   Discussion and Conclusion

In this work, we presented a shape-aware multi-view autoencoder, a neural network capable of learning anatomical shape priors from multiple standard views, as well as a multi-view U-Net, a modification of the original U-Net architecture that incorporates the learned shape priors to improve the robustness of cardiac segmentation. In contrast to existing works which treat long-axis CMR segmentation and short-axis CMR segmentation as two separate tasks [1,14], our approach, to the best of our knowledge, is the first that exploits the spatial context from the long-axis images to guide the segmentation on the short-axis images. The reported experimental results show that the proposed segmentation method not only demonstrates superior segmentation accuracy over state-of-the-art 2D baseline methods [1,11], but also outperforms a 3D U-Net [4]. This improvement is particularly evident on the basal and apical slices in the low-data setting, as expected. When training data is limited, segmenting these challenging slices particularly benefits from the additional anatomical information extracted from the LA views and injected into the segmentation network. Of note, our approach does not require a dedicated acquisition protocol, since LA images are routinely acquired in most CMR imaging schemes. Moreover, the proposed MV U-Net maintains the computational advantage of a 2D network, using fewer parameters ($\sim$1.2 million weights) than the 3D U-Net ($\sim$2.5 million weights) during training. This advantage also contributes to the data efficiency of our method, achieving high segmentation performance with limited training data. Importantly, our method could be extended in the future to multi-structure cardiac segmentation. The proposed approach could also be potentially adopted to other medical image segmentation tasks.

Acknowledgements. This work was supported by the SmartHeart EPSRC Programme Grant (EP/P001009/1). Steffen Petersen acknowledges support from the National Institute for Health Research Barts Biomedical Research Centre. The cardiac multi-view image dataset has been provided under UK Biobank Access Application 18545.

References

1. Bai, W., et al.: Automated cardiovascular magnetic resonance image analysis with fully convolutional networks. JCMR **20**(1), 65 (2018)
2. Bernard, O., et al.: Deep learning techniques for automatic MRI cardiac multi-structures segmentation and diagnosis: is the problem solved? IEEE TMI **37**, 2514–2525 (2018)
3. Caruana, R.: Multitask learning. Mach. Learn. **28**(1), 41–75 (1997)
4. Çiçek, Ö., Abdulkadir, A., Lienkamp, S.S., Brox, T., Ronneberger, O.: 3D U-Net: learning dense volumetric segmentation from sparse annotation. In: Ourselin, S., Joskowicz, L., Sabuncu, M.R., Unal, G., Wells, W. (eds.) MICCAI 2016. LNCS, vol. 9901, pp. 424–432. Springer, Cham (2016). https://doi.org/10.1007/978-3-319-46723-8_49
5. Duan, J., et al.: Automatic 3D bi-ventricular segmentation of cardiac images by a shape-refined multi-task deep learning approach. IEEE TMI **38**, 2151–2164 (2019)
6. Isensee, F., et al.: Automatic cardiac disease assessment on cine-MRI via time-series segmentation and domain specific features. In: Pop, M., et al. (eds.) STACOM 2017. LNCS, vol. 10663, pp. 120–129. Springer, Cham (2018). https://doi.org/10.1007/978-3-319-75541-0_13
7. Khened, M., et al.: Fully convolutional multi-scale residual densenets for cardiac segmentation and automated cardiac diagnosis using ensemble of classifiers. MedIA **51**, 21–45 (2019)

8. Kohl, S., et al.: A probabilistic U-Net for segmentation of ambiguous images. In: NeuralIPS, pp. 6965–6975 (2018)
9. Oktay, O., et al.: Anatomically constrained neural networks (ACNNs): application to cardiac image enhancement and segmentation. IEEE TMI **37**(2), 384–395 (2018)
10. Petersen, S.E., et al.: Reference ranges for cardiac structure and function using cardiovascular magnetic resonance (CMR) in caucasians from the UK biobank population cohort. JCMR **19**(1), 18 (2017)
11. Ronneberger, O., Fischer, P., Brox, T.: U-Net: convolutional networks for biomedical image segmentation. In: Navab, N., Hornegger, J., Wells, W.M., Frangi, A.F. (eds.) MICCAI 2015. LNCS, vol. 9351, pp. 234–241. Springer, Cham (2015). https://doi.org/10.1007/978-3-319-24574-4_28
12. Tao, Q., et al.: Deep learning-based method for fully automatic quantification of left ventricle function from cine MR images: a multivendor, multicenter study. Radiology **290**(1), 81–88 (2018)
13. Tarroni, G., et al.: A comprehensive approach for learning-based fully-automated inter-slice motion correction for short-axis cine cardiac MR image stacks. In: Frangi, A.F., Schnabel, J.A., Davatzikos, C., Alberola-López, C., Fichtinger, G. (eds.) MICCAI 2018. LNCS, vol. 11070, pp. 268–276. Springer, Cham (2018). https://doi.org/10.1007/978-3-030-00928-1_31
14. Vigneault, D.M., et al.: Omega-Net: fully automatic, multi-view cardiac MR detection, orientation, and segmentation with deep neural networks. MedIA **48**, 95–106 (2018)
15. Zheng, Q., et al.: 3-D consistent and robust segmentation of cardiac images by deep learning with spatial propagation. IEEE TMI **37**(9), 2137–2148 (2018)

Right Ventricle Segmentation in Short-Axis MRI Using a Shape Constrained Dense Connected U-Net

Hao Yang, Zexiong Liu, and Xuan Yang[✉]

College of Computer Science and Software Engineering, Shenzhen University,
Guangdong, China
leonhyang@foxmail.com, gsunfeng@163.com, yangxuan@szu.edu.cn

Abstract. Segmentation of right ventricle (RV) in short-axis MRI is an essential step for evaluating the structure and function of RV. In this paper, a shape constrained deep learning network based on dense connectivity and dilated convolutions is proposed, which aims to strengthen feature propagation and have more diversified features through dense connections and skip connections. In the meantime, dilated convolution is used to expand the receptive fields and enhance the connectivity of segmentation results. The shape constraint of RV is introduced into the loss function to improve the prediction accuracy. Transfer learning is employed to strengthen the generalization of the network to the RV shape constraint. Finally, post-processing is performed by analysing boundary curvature of segmentation results and shape correlation of endocardium and epicardium of RV. Our network is validated on the MICCAI2012 public dataset, and the evaluation results show that our network outperforms the state-of-the-art methods in several evaluation metrics.

Keywords: RV segmentation · Convoluational neural network · Shape constraint · Short-axis MRI

1 Introduction

In recent years, evaluation of RV structure and function has got more and more attention due to its importance in most cardiac disorders, such as pulmonary hypertension and coronary heart. MRI has become a standard tool in the evaluation of the RV function. Short-axis MRI is acquired by imaging perpendicular to the long axis, which is commonly used in RV segmentation. However, automated segmentation of RV has proven more challenging to develop due to its highly variable boundary.

Recent years, with the development of machine learning techniques, machine learning based approaches are proposed to segment RV, especially the deep learning based methods. The commonly used deep learning networks can be divided

Supported by the National Natural Science Foundation of China (61871269) and the Shenzhen Fundamental Research Program (JCYJ20170818100006280).

© Springer Nature Switzerland AG 2019
D. Shen et al. (Eds.): MICCAI 2019, LNCS 11765, pp. 532–540, 2019.
https://doi.org/10.1007/978-3-030-32245-8_59

into three categories. The first one is the convolutional neural network (CNN). Luo *et al.* [5] employed two CNNs to locate the ROI of RV and segment the endocardium and epicardium of RV, respectively. Avendi *et al.* [1] combined a CNN with a stacked autoencoder to delineate an initial contour of RV, and the deformable models are further used to provide accurate RV contours. The second one is the fully convolutional neural network (FCN). Tran *et al.* [11] is the first one using the FCN for pixel-wise labelling of RV in cardiac MRI. Bai *et al.* [2] trained a FCN in a semi-supervised way to segment the RV cavity. Duan *et al.* [3] employed a FCN to predict bi-ventricles and performed the multi-atlas registration to refine the FCN results. To improve the performance of FCNs for segmentation of small objects of RV, Zhang *et al.* [12] proposed a scheme to enhance the segmentation accuracy of FCN in zooming way. The other kind of network used in RV segmentation is the U-net [10]. The U-Net is built upon the FCN and yields better segmentation in the medical image domain. Zheng *et al.* [13] employed a U-net architecture to locate ROI of RV, and modified the U-net to segment the cropped ROIs further.

In CNNs, dense connections make each layer receive all previous layers output feature maps as the input, and have advantages of feature propagation and reuse. However, dense connections between different layers are rarely used in existing networks for RV segmentation. On the other hand, prior knowledge about the shapes of the objects to be segmented can significantly improve the accuracy of segmentation results. However, how to guide RV segmentation using shape information in networks is still an open problem. In this paper, we construct a dense connected U-net and introduce the shape constraint to the network to segment RV. The contributions of our paper include: (1) Dense connections are used to strengthen feature propagation and extract more diversified feature maps from short-axis MRIs. Moreover, dilated convolution is used to expand the receptive fields of convolutions in the most coarse layer; (2) The shape constraint of RV is introduced into the loss function of the network and transfer learning is employed to train the network; (3) Post-processing of the segmentation results by analyzing the curvature of object boundaries and the relationship between endocardium and epicardium is performed. Our network is evaluated on the MICCAI2012 RV segmentation challenge (RVSC) dataset. Evaluation results show the improvement in segmentation accuracy achieved by introducing dense connectivity and shape prior to our network.

2   Methods

2.1   Network Architecture

We designed a U-net shaped network with dense connections. The architecture of the network is illustrated in Fig. 1. Our network is composed of the encoding path and the decoding path. Dense connections are introduced to the encoding path, aiming to strengthen feature propagation. All the dense blocks consist of three 3×3 convolution layers and a 1×1 convolution layer. Each 3×3 convolution layer is followed by a batch-normalization layer and a Rectified Linear Units (ReLu).

A 1×1 convolution layer is employed to descend the dimension of feature maps to the next scale. Considering the size of images we use, three dense blocks with different spatial scales are cascaded in the encoding path. Besides, zero paddings are used in all convolution layers to keep the images the same size. In the decoding path, traditional convolutions are performed to take the high dimensional features and generate a semantic segmentation result.

Moreover, to increase the receptive view of the network, dilated convolutions are employed in the lowest block. Dilated convolutions skip some points during convolution, which focus on the wider context of images and enhance the connectivity of segmentation results.

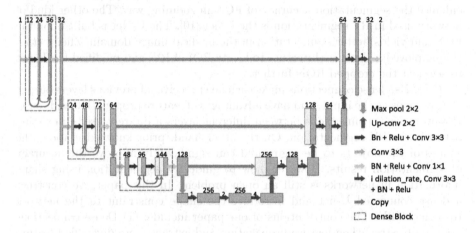

Fig. 1. The architecture of the dense connected U-net. The boxes illustrate the multi-channel feature maps with the number of channels on the top of them. The arrows denote different operations.

2.2 Shape Constrained Loss Function

It is difficult to obtain accurate RV segmentation results without utilizing any prior information about the RV chamber. As we know, traditional methods to segment RV are highly dependent on the prior information, such as active shape models (ASM), active appearance models (AAM), and atlas. Prior knowledge about the shape of RV can significantly improve the accuracy of the segmentation result. To introduce prior shape information of RV to our network, we propose a novel shape-aware loss function as:

$$L_s(y, \hat{y}) = APD\left(B(y), B(\hat{y})\right) \times \left(1 - \sum_l w_l \frac{\sum_j y_{j,l} \hat{y}_{j,l}}{\sum_j y_{j,l} + \sum_j \hat{y}_{j,l}}\right), \quad (1)$$

where y and $\hat{y}$ are the ground truth and the prediction probability map, respectively. $B(\hat{y})$ is the estimated boundary of RV using the prediction probability map $\hat{y}$, and $B(y)$ is the RV boundary of the ground truth. $y_{j,l}$ and $\hat{y}_{j,l}$ are the ground truth and the prediction probability of the jth pixel of the lth class, w_l is the loss weight to balance the classes. In our RV segmentation task, $l = 2$. The average perpendicular distance (APD) is a metric to measure the shape similarity between two contours. APD measures the distance from the automatically segmented contour to the corresponding manually drawn expert contour, averaged over all contour points. A high value implies that the two contours do not match closely. When the contour of the predicted object is not similar to the contour of the ground truth, a large penalty coefficient makes the loss function value large, and network parameters are adjusted correspondingly. Figure 2 illustrates segmentation examples before and after using the shape constraint. It can be seen that unreasonable details are generated in the segmentation results before the shape constraint is introduced, for example, the anatomical tissue on the left side of the RV is segmented as part of the RV. By introducing the shape constraint into the loss function, the accuracy of segmentation results can be improved further.

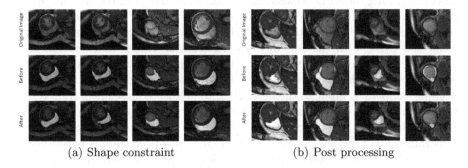

(a) Shape constraint   (b) Post processing

Fig. 2. Comparison of segmentation results before and after introducing the shape constraint to the loss function (left), and before and after post processing (right).

Equation (1) is indeed a weighted soft dice loss function using the APD as the weight coefficient. The soft dice is derived from the dice metric, which measures the overlap between two objects. The definition of the soft dice is the term in the bracket. Compared with the commonly used cross entropy, the soft dice can result in prediction probabilities with significant discrimination. Figure 3 shows the prediction probabilities of two RVs using the soft dice and the cross entropy as the loss function, respectively. It can be seen uncertain probabilities occur at the boundary of RV using the cross entropy, while there is a significant difference between probabilities of pixels locating on the RV and that locating at the background using the soft dice.

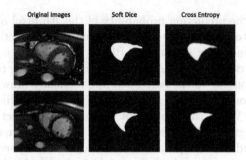

Fig. 3. Comparison of prediction probability maps using the soft dice and the cross entropy. From left to right: the original images, predication probabilites using the soft dice and that using the cross entropy.

2.3   Transfer Learning

Since computing the APD between the estimated boundary of RV and the ground truth boundary of RV is dependent on the prediction result, the network with the shape constrained loss function should be trained specially. At first, the dense connected U-net with the soft dice loss function is trained and denoted as g. The dense connected U-net with the shape constrained loss function is denoted as g_s. Suppose g_s has been trained for k iterations. In the $k + 1$th iteration, a training sample x is input to the network g_s to predicate its segmentation result, which can be used to obtain $B(\hat{y})$. The boundary of its corresponding ground truth is $B(y)$. The APD between $B(\hat{y})$ and $B(y)$ is computed. Then, the shape constrained loss function can be evaluated, and back-propagate is performed to update network parameters. The transfer learning can be performed from the first iteration. During this procedure, two strategies are employed to initialize the new network g_s. The first one is to initialize g_s randomly, and the second one is transfer learning, that is to copy parameters of g as the initial parameters of g_s. Experimental results show that transfer learning outperforms the random initialization. The reason is that the APD generated by the randomly initialized network is unreliable, which results in bad convergence of the network.

2.4   Post-processing

Post-processing is performed to improve the segmentation results further based on boundary curvature analysis. It is observed that the boundary of a good segmentation result is smooth, and the mean curvature value along the boundary is small. When the area of segmented RV of a slice is larger than that of its last slice in the 3D image, it might be a mis-segmented result. For the mis-segmentation results, the morphological operators are performed to fill gaps inside the objects and eliminate small details. Here, it is needed to emphasize that only the basal and middle ventricle of RV are processed in this way. Besides, the post-processing is performed from the basal slice to the apical slice.

Furthermore, since the myocardial wall of RV is 3−6 times thinner than the wall of LV [6], the endocardium of RV is similar to the epicardium of RV in size and shape. The relationship between endocardium and epicardium can be used to improve the segmentation results further. When the areas of the epicardium and endocardium are not similar to each other, it implies that at least one of them is a mis-segmented result. Suppose the endocardium is decided as mis-segmented, then, the epicardium is eroded to be the endocardium segmentation result. The erode size is the average perpendicular distance between the endocardium and epicardium of its last slice. If the epicardium is decided as mis-segmented, the endocardium is dilated to be the epicardium segmentation result. If both the endocardium and the epicardium are decided as mis-segmented, nothing is performed.

3   Experiment and Results

3.1   Datasets and Evaluation Metrics

The MICCAI2012 Right ventricle segmentation challenge dataset [7] is used to train and evaluate our network. The dataset consists of a training set and two test sets. The training set contains only 243 physician-segmented images from the short-axis MR images of 16 patients. We choose images of the last three patients as the validation set and the others as the training set. Two test sets contain images of 32 patients, which is used to evaluate the performance of our network. The Dice metric (DM) and Hausdorff distance (HD) are used to measure the performance of our network.

3.2   Training

Our method is developed in Keras framework with Tensorflow backend, performed on a computer with an Intel I7-8700K 3.70 GHz CPU and 11 GB graphic memory with GTX1080Ti. Adaptive Moment Estimation (ADAM) method is used to optimize our network with the initial learning rate of 0.001 and a batch size of 32, and 800 epochs is trained for the network g. The learning rate is 0.0005, and 500 epochs are trained for the network g_s using transfer learning. Data augmentation, including rotation, translation, zoom, and elastic deformation, is performed to improve the generalization ability of the network.

3.3   Results

To demonstrate the performance of dense connections and dilated convolutions in networks, five kinds of networks are compared with each other: the Dilated Dense Connected U-net with shape constraint (DDCU-sc) proposed in this paper, the Dilated Dense Connected U-net without shape constraint (DDCU), Dilated U-net, which is the modified DDCU without dense connections, Dense Connected U-net, which is the modified DDCU without dilated convolutions, and the traditional U-net. Images of the last three patients of the training set are used to validate the performance of different networks. It is needed to emphasize that the soft dice is employed as the loss function for DDCU, Dilated U-net, Dense Connected U-net, and U-net. Table 1 lists the mean DM of the validation set using four networks. It can be seen that our DDCU outperforms other networks, which implies that dense connections and dilated convolutions can improve segmentation accuracy. Furthermore, by introducing the shape constraint into the loss function, the DM using our DDCU is 0.89 for endocardium segmentation.

Table 1. The mean DM of endocardium segmentation of the validation set using different network architectures, with optimal results in bold.

Networks	Dense connections	Dilated convolutions	Shape constraints	DM
DDCU-sc	✓	✓	✓	**0.89**
DDCU	✓	✓	✗	0.88
Dilated U-net	✗	✓	✗	0.87
Dense Connected U-net	✓	✗	✗	0.84
U-net	✗	✗	✗	0.82

Furthermore, performances comparison of endocardium prediction of our proposed DDCU-sc between before and after post-processing, between using cross entropy and using soft dice loss, between transfer learning and random initialization, respectively, are provided in Table 2. The mean DM of the validation set is employed as the evaluation metric. It can be seen that post-processing improve the performance of DDCU-sc obviously. Moreover, the DDCU-sc using soft dice loss outperforms the one using cross entropy loss. Obviously, the DDCU-sc initialized by transfer learning achieves better performance than random initialization.

Table 2. Performance comparison of endocardium prediction of our proposed DDCU-sc between before and after post-processing, between using cross entropy and using soft dice loss, between transfer learning and random initialization, respectively.

Post-processing		Loss		Initilization	
Before	*After*	*Cross entropy*	*Soft dice*	*Transfer learning*	*Random*
0.8989	0.9052	0.8801	0.8845	0.8989	0.8623

By employing our shape constrained dense connected U-net network, the segmentation results of two test sets are evaluated by the LITIS lab. The reported results show the average DM of endocardium segmentation is 0.8577 (standard deviation 0.15) and 0.8736 (0.16), and the average HD is 6.73 (5.06) and 6.13 (9.47) for test1 set and test2 set, respectively. For epicardium segmentation, the average DM is 0.8891 (0.16) and 0.8966 (0.14), and the average HD is 6.75 (5.04) and 6.49 (9.44) for test1 set and test2 set, respectively. The Wilcoxon test is performed to test the dice and the HD of endocardium and epicardium segmentation results because these data do not follow a Gaussian distribution. A p value <0.005 is considered statistically significant. Test results show that the dice of endocardium segmentation comes from a population with a median greater than 0.8855, and the dice of epicardium segmentation comes from a population with a median greater than 0.9103. The HD of endocardium segmentation comes from a population with a median less than 5.43 mm, and the HD of epicardium segmentation comes from a population with a median less than 5.77 mm. The standard deviation of evaluation results implies that there are several cases that fail in achieving accurate segmentation. By observing the segmentation results, we found it is challenging to segment RVs with non-uniform intensity distribution in the endocardium. Another kind of challenging case is to segment RV in apical slices due to too small objects.

Table 3 summarizes the evaluation results of two test sets using our network, and comparison with the state-of-the-art researches. It is noted that our network outperforms previous automatic and semi-automatic methods both on endocardium and epicardium segmentation in respect of all evaluation metrics, which demonstrates the efficiency of our network.

Table 3. Comparison of RV endocardium and epicardium segmentation performance between our network and the state-of-the-art researches. Values of DM and HD are averaged over two test sets in format: mean value (±standard deviation), with optimal results in bold.

Method	A/SA^*	Dice index		Hausdorff (mm)	
		Endo	Epi	Endo	Epi
Our method	A	**0.865 ± 0.15**	**0.892 ± 0.15**	**6.435 ± 7.55**	**6.622 ± 7.52**
Avendi et al. [1]	A	0.82 ± 0.15	-	7.85 ± 4.20	-
Tran et al. [11]	A	0.84 ± 0.21	0.86 ± 0.20	8.86 ± 11.27	9.33 ± 10.79
Ringenberg et al. [9]	A	0.83 ± 0.17	-	8.89 ± 7.30	-
Luo et al. [5]	A	0.86 ± 0.09	0.84 ± 0.13	6.9 ± 2.6	8.9 ± 5.7
Guo et al. [4]	SA	0.86 ± 0.10	-	7.79 ± 5.36	-
Punithakumar et al. [8]	SA	0.84 ± 0.14	0.87 ± 0.09	7.10 ± 4.20	7.52 ± 3.89

*Automatic/Semi-Automatic

4   Conclusion

A shape constrained dense connected U-net network is proposed in this paper to segment the right ventricle automatically. Through dense connections and dilated convolutions, RV features can be extracted more efficiently and a larger receptive view can be provided. The average perpendicular distances between contours of RV and contours of ground truth are introduced to the loss function of our network to constrain the shapes of segmentation results. Evaluation results on public dataset exhibit that our proposed network achieves more accurate segmentation results, and outperforms the state-of-the-art methods in respect of dice measure and Hausdorff distance.

References

1. Avendi, M.R., Kheradvar, A., Jafarkhani, H.: Automatic segmentation of the right ventricle from cardiac MRI using a learning-based approach. Magn. Reson. Med. **78**(6), 2439–2448 (2017)
2. Bai, W., et al.: Semi-supervised learning for network-based cardiac MR image segmentation. In: Descoteaux, M., Maier-Hein, L., Franz, A., Jannin, P., Collins, D.L., Duchesne, S. (eds.) MICCAI 2017. LNCS, vol. 10434, pp. 253–260. Springer, Cham (2017). https://doi.org/10.1007/978-3-319-66185-8_29
3. Duan, J., et al.: Combining deep learning and shape priors for bi-ventricular segmentation of volumetric cardiac magnetic resonance images. In: Reuter, M., Wachinger, C., Lombaert, H., Paniagua, B., Lüthi, M., Egger, B. (eds.) ShapeMI 2018. LNCS, vol. 11167, pp. 258–267. Springer, Cham (2018). https://doi.org/10.1007/978-3-030-04747-4_24
4. Guo, Z.Z., et al.: Local motion intensity clustering (LMIC) model for segmentation of right ventricle in cardiac MRI images. IEEE J. Biomed. Health Inform. **23**, 723–730 (2018)
5. Luo, G., An, R., Wang, K., Dong, S., Zhang, H.: A deep learning network for right ventricle segmentation in short-axis MRI. In: 2016 Computing in Cardiology Conference (CinC), pp. 485–488. IEEE (2016)
6. Petitjean, C., Dacher, J.N.: A review of segmentation methods in short axis cardiac MR images. Med. Image Anal. **15**(2), 169–184 (2011)
7. Petitjean, C., et al.: Right ventricle segmentation from cardiac MRI: a collation study. Med. Image Anal. **19**(1), 187–202 (2015)
8. Punithakumar, K., Noga, M., Ayed, I.B., Boulanger, P.: Right ventricular segmentation in cardiac MRI with moving mesh correspondences. Comput. Med. Imaging Graph. **43**, 15–25 (2015)
9. Ringenberg, J., Deo, M., Devabhaktuni, V., Berenfeld, O., Boyers, P., Gold, J.: Fast, accurate, and fully automatic segmentation of the right ventricle in short-axis cardiac MRI. Comput. Med. Imaging Graph. **38**(3), 190–201 (2014)
10. Ronneberger, O., Fischer, P., Brox, T.: U-net: convolutional networks for biomedical image segmentation. In: MICCAI (2015)
11. Tran, P.V.: A fully convolutional neural network for cardiac segmentation in short-axis MRI. arXiv preprint arXiv:1604.00494 (2016)
12. Zhang, L., Karanikolas, G.V., Akçaya, M., Giannakis, G.B.: Fully automatic segmentation of the right ventricle via multi-task deep neural networks. In: 2018 IEEE International Conference on Acoustics, Speech and Signal Processing (ICASSP), pp. 6677–6681. IEEE (2018)
13. Zheng, Q., Delingette, H., Duchateau, N., Ayache, N.: 3-D consistent and robust segmentation of cardiac images by deep learning with spatial propagation. IEEE Trans. Med. Imaging **37**, 2137–2148 (2018)

Self-Supervised Learning for Cardiac MR Image Segmentation by Anatomical Position Prediction

Wenjia Bai[1,2(✉)], Chen Chen[3], Giacomo Tarroni[3], Jinming Duan[3,4],
Florian Guitton[1], Steffen E. Petersen[5], Yike Guo[1], Paul M. Matthews[2,6],
and Daniel Rueckert[3]

[1] Data Science Institute, Imperial College London, London, UK
w.bai@imperial.ac.uk
[2] Department of Medicine, Imperial College London, London, UK
[3] BioMedIA, Department of Computing, Imperial College London, London, UK
[4] School of Computer Science, University of Birmingham, Birmingham, UK
[5] NIHR Barts BRC, Queen Mary University of London, London, UK
[6] UK Dementia Research Institute, Imperial College London, London, UK

Abstract. In the recent years, convolutional neural networks have transformed the field of medical image analysis due to their capacity to learn discriminative image features for a variety of classification and regression tasks. However, successfully learning these features requires a large amount of manually annotated data, which is expensive to acquire and limited by the available resources of expert image analysts. Therefore, unsupervised, weakly-supervised and self-supervised feature learning techniques receive a lot of attention, which aim to utilise the vast amount of available data, while at the same time avoid or substantially reduce the effort of manual annotation. In this paper, we propose a novel way for training a cardiac MR image segmentation network, in which features are learnt in a self-supervised manner by predicting anatomical positions. The anatomical positions serve as a supervisory signal and do not require extra manual annotation. We demonstrate that this seemingly simple task provides a strong signal for feature learning and with self-supervised learning, we achieve a high segmentation accuracy that is better than or comparable to a U-net trained from scratch, especially at a small data setting. When only five annotated subjects are available, the proposed method improves the mean Dice metric from 0.811 to 0.852 for short-axis image segmentation, compared to the baseline U-net.

1 Introduction

Cardiac MR image segmentation plays a central role in characterising the structure and function of the heart. Quantitative phenotypes derived from the segmentations provide important biomarkers for diagnosing and managing cardiovascular diseases. In the recent years, convolutional neural networks have greatly

© Springer Nature Switzerland AG 2019
D. Shen et al. (Eds.): MICCAI 2019, LNCS 11765, pp. 541–549, 2019.
https://doi.org/10.1007/978-3-030-32245-8_60

advanced the performance of cardiac MR image segmentation due to their capacity in learning discriminative image features for the segmentation task [1–3]. Most successful methods are fully supervised and rely on a large amount of annotated data to learn the features. However, annotated medical imaging data may not always be available. The annotations are expensive to acquire and often limited by the available resource of expert image analysts. To address this challenge, we propose a novel way for training a cardiac MR image segmentation network, which formulates a self-supervised task for feature learning and alleviates the cost of data annotation.

There are two major contributions of this work. First, the proposed method learns image features from anatomical positions automatically defined by cardiac chamber view planes, which is a novel pretext task for self-supervised learning and provides a strong supervisory signal. Importantly, the chamber view plane information is freely available from standard cardiac MR scans, which means the method has the potential to be extended to a clinical setting, where a lot of unannotated MR scans stored on the PACS in hospitals can be utilised for feature learning. Second, we demonstrate the learning performance on two tasks, namely short-axis image and long-axis image segmentations. For both tasks, self-supervised learning demonstrates a strong boost to segmentation accuracy, especially at a small data setting.

Related Works: To address the challenge of limited data annotations, there is increased interest in developing methods that do not require a large amount of annotations for feature learning. Directions of research include transfer learning, domain adaptation, semi-supervised, weakly-supervised, unsupervised and self-supervised learning [4]. Here, we focus on self-supervised learning, which formulates a *pretext* task based on unannotated data for feature learning.

For natural image and video analysis problems, a number of pretext tasks have been explored, including prediction of image rotation [5], relative position [6], colorisation [7] and image impainting [8] etc. In medical imaging domain, self-supervised learning has also been explored but to a less extent. Jamaludin et al. proposed a pretext task for subject identification [9]. A Siamese network was trained to classify whether two spinal MR images came from the same subject or not. The pretrained features were used to initialise a disease grade classification network. Ross et al. defined re-colourisation of surgical videos as a pretext task and used the pretrained features to initialise a surgical instrument segmentation network [10]. Tajbakhsh et al. used rotation prediction as a pretext task and the self-learnt features were transferred to lung lobe segmentation and nodule detection tasks [11]. Different from previous works in the medical imaging domain, we propose a novel pretext task, which is to predict anatomical positions. In particular, we leverage the rich information encoded in the cardiac MR scan view planes and DICOM headers to define the anatomical positions for the task.

2   Methods

Here we describe the cardiac MR view planes, the pretext task for self-supervised learning and architectures for transferring a self-trained network to a new task.

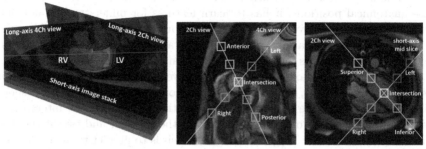

(a) Cardiac MR view planes   (b) Short-axis image   (c) Long-axis 4Ch image

Fig. 1. Cardiac MR view planes and anatomical positions. (a) Short-axis and long-axis view planes with regard to the heart. (b) Short-axis image with overlaid 2Ch and 4Ch view planes (yellow lines) and anatomical positions defined by view planes (coloured boxes). (c) Long-axis 4Ch view image with overlaid 2Ch and mid short-axis view planes and anatomical positions. (Color figure online)

Cardiac MR View Planes: A standard cardiac MR scan consists of images acquired at different angulated planes with regard to the heart, including short-axis, long-axis 2 chamber (2Ch, vertical long-axis), 4 chamber (4Ch, horizontal long-axis) and 3 chamber (3Ch) views. They are used for evaluating different anatomical regions of the heart. For example, the short-axis view shows the cross-sections of the left ventricle (LV) and right ventricle (RV). The long-axis views show the septal and lateral walls of the ventricles, as well as the atrial chambers, including the left atrium (LA) and right atrium (RA). Figure 1(a) illustrates how the short-axis and long-axis 2Ch, 4Ch views are oriented with regard to the heart.

Most previous works on cardiac MR image segmentation [1–3] consider short-axis and long-axis views separately and disregard the relative orientation of different views. Typically, images from a specific view and the corresponding label maps are used to train a segmentation network from scratch. In this work, we propose that the relative orientation of short-axis and long-axis views and the anatomical positions, defined by the view planes, can be used to formulate a pretext task for training the network in a self-supervised manner and increasing data efficiency.

Self-Supervised Learning (SSL): Figure 1(b) shows a short-axis image, with the overlaid 2Ch view and 4Ch view (yellow lines). As it shows, the 2Ch view bisects both the LV and RV, whereas the 4Ch view bisects the LV. They intersect at the LV. Along the chamber view lines, we define nine anatomical positions, represented by bounding boxes, including the intersection, two boxes on the left, two on the right, two at the anterior and two at the posterior. The orientations from left to right and from posterior to anterior are available from the DICOM headers. The pretext task is to predict the anatomical positions defined by these nine bounding boxes. The intuition here is that for the network to recognise these anatomical positions, it has to learn features for understanding not only where the left and right ventricles roughly are but also what their neighbouring regions look like. The learnt features can be transferred to a related but more demanding task, which is accurate segmentation of the ventricles.

Similarly, for a long-axis 4Ch view image, we can overlay the 2Ch view and mid short-axis view on it, shown by Fig. 1(c). Along the 2Ch view and mid short-axis view lines, we define nine anatomical positions, including the intersection, two boxes on the left, two on the right, two at the superior and two at the inferior. The pretext task for long-axis image analysis is to predict these anatomical positions. To learn from the pretext task, we train a 10-way segmentation network, which segments the nine bounding boxes and the background. A standard U-net architecture [12] is used, which consists of the encoder part, decoder part, skip connections between them and the task head (the last convolutional layer), depicted by Fig. 2(a). Cross-entropy is used as the loss function.

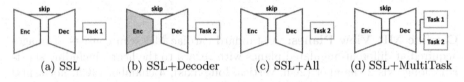

Fig. 2. Network architectures for self-supervised learning (SSL) and three different ways for transfer learning. The gray area in (b) denotes the freezed encoder.

Transfer Learning: After the network is self-trained on the pretext task (task 1), it is transferred to a new task (task 2), which is accurate segmentation of the anatomical structures, e.g. the LV cavity, myocardium and RV cavity. To achieve this, we can simply replace the head of task 1 by a new head for task 2. The task head refers to the last convolutional layer of the U-net, which is 1×1 convolution with K-channel output, K denoting the number of classes.

We investigate three different ways for transfer learning. The first way is to freeze the weights learnt at the encoder and only finetunes the decoder and task head, using the annotations for task 2. This method is named as "SSL+Decoder" and illustrated by Fig. 2(b). The second way is to finetune all the weights [4], including the encoder, decoder and task head. This method is named as "SSL+All" and illustrated by Fig. 2(c). The third way is perform multi-task learning for finetuning. Two task heads are used, one for the pretext task and the other for the new task. This is to avoid forgetting about the pretext task while learning for the new task. This method is named as "SSL+MultiTask" and illustrated by Fig. 2(d). The loss function for multi-task learning is formulated as, $L(\theta) = L_{task_1}(x, y_1|\theta) + \beta \cdot L_{task_2}(x, y_2|\theta)$, where θ denotes the network parameters, x denotes the image, y_1 denotes the label map of nine anatomical positions for task 1, y_2 denotes the label map of anatomical structures manually annotated by human experts for task 2, β denotes the weight.

3   Experiments and Results

Data: For self-supervised learning, short-axis and long-axis images of 3,825 subjects were used, acquired from the UK Biobank. The typical image dimension is 208×180, with $1.82 \times 1.82\,\mathrm{mm}^2$ in-plane resolution. The short-axis image stack consists of ~10 slices. There is 1 slice for long-axis 4Ch view and 1 slice for 2Ch view. Bounding boxes were automatically placed at nine anatomical positions on the short-axis and long-axis 4Ch view images at end-diastole (ED) and end-systole (ES). Each box was empirically set to 11×11 pixels and adjacent boxes were 30 pixels apart. For transfer learning, 200 subjects with manual annotations were used, which were randomly split into 100 subjects for training and 100 subjects for test. For short-axis images, LV, myocardium and RV were manually annotated by experienced image analysts at ED and ES frames. For long-axis 4Ch view images, LV, myocardium, RV, LA and RA were manually annotated.

Implementation: The method was implemented using Tensorflow. For self-supervised learning, the Adam optimiser was used, with a learning rate of 0.001, a batch size of 20 image slices and 50,000 iterations. For transfer learning, the same setting was used. For both cases, data augmentation was performed online, including random rotation and scaling. For multi-task transfer learning, the weight β was empirically set to 10 to emphasise the new task. As the input datasets were not consistent for the two tasks (task 1 with 3,825 subjects, task 2 with much fewer and different subjects), training was implemented as that at each iteration, task 1 was optimised for one sub-iteration, followed by optimising task 2 for β sub-iterations. Since stochastic optimisation was performed, this was approximately equivalent to assigning a weight to task 2. Training multiple tasks alternately is a commonly adopted practice for inconsistent data input [4]. We made sure that task 2 was trained for 50,000 sub-iterations to enable a fair comparison. Finally, a U-net was also trained with exactly the same setting, but initialised with random weights. This is our baseline method, "U-net-scratch".

Short-Axis Image Segmentation: We evaluated the performance on two transfer learning tasks, which are segmentations for short-axis and long-axis images. Table 1 compares the Dice metrics (averaged across LV, myocardium and RV) for short-axis image segmentation between the U-net trained from scratch and self-supervised learning methods. As it shows, even if we freeze the encoder and only tune the decoder (SSL+Decoder), we can achieve a high accuracy comparable to training a U-net from scratch. This indicates that SSL

Table 1. Comparison of the Dice metrics for short-axis image segmentation. Column 1 lists the number of training subjects and manually annotated image slices. Columns 2 to 5 report the performance of the baseline method and different self-supervised learning methods. Values are mean (standard deviation).

#subjects (#slices)	U-net-scratch	SSL+Decoder	SSL+All	SSL+MultiTask
1 (18)	0.361 (0.047)	0.515 (0.099)	0.618 (0.068)	**0.704** (0.065)
5 (102)	0.811 (0.037)	0.837 (0.048)	0.844 (0.046)	**0.852** (0.046)
10 (208)	0.859 (0.037)	0.860 (0.039)	0.873 (0.036)	**0.875** (0.036)
50 (980)	0.876 (0.035)	0.871 (0.038)	**0.884** (0.033)	0.873 (0.037)
100 (1,936)	0.886 (0.030)	0.867 (0.037)	0.883 (0.035)	**0.887** (0.031)

is able to learn good features at the encoder which are transferrable for the segmentation task. The table also shows when we tune all the weights (SSL+All and SSL+MultiTask), the segmentation accuracy is generally better than U-net-scratch, especially when the number of training subjects is small. On average, SSL+MultiTask performs the best.

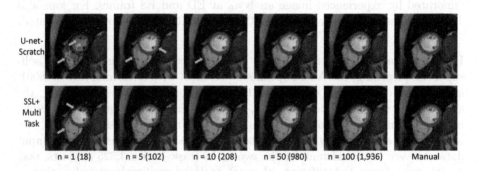

Fig. 3. Short-axis image segmentations for U-net-scratch and SSL+MultiTask with an increasing number of training subjects (slices), as well as manual segmentations. The yellow arrows indicate segmentation errors. (Color figure online)

Figure 3 visualises exemplar segmentations for U-net-scratch and SSL+ MultiTask with an increasing number of training subjects. It shows that when $n = 1$, due to the extremely small training set, U-net-scratch completely fails to segment the image. On the contrary, SSL+MultiTask is still able to segment some part of the LV and myocardium. When n increases to 5 or 10, SSL+MultiTask outperforms U-net-scratch at details, for example, without RV under-segmentation errors. However, when n increases to 50 or 100, the two methods perform similar to each other. Figure 4 plots quantitative metrics including the Dice metric and mean contour distance error for each anatomical structure for the two methods. It shows a similar trend that at a small data setting ($n \leq 10$), SSL+MultiTask outperforms U-net-scratch for all the structures. When there are more training data ($n \geq 50$), their performances become close to each other.

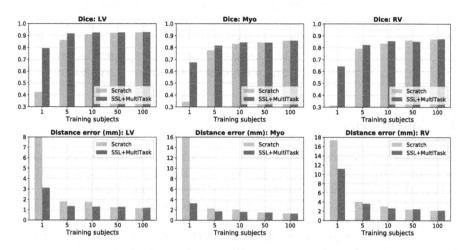

Fig. 4. Comparison of the Dice metrics and mean contour distance errors on short-axis image segmentation for U-Net-scratch and SSL+MultiTask.

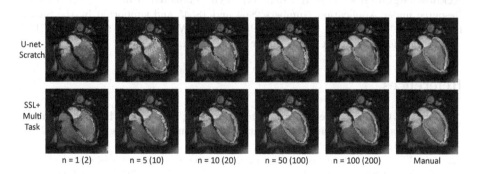

Fig. 5. Long-axis image segmentations for U-net-scratch and SSL+MultiTask with an increasing number of training subjects (slices).

Long-Axis Image Segmentation: We performed similar experiments for long-axis image segmentation. Table 2 reports the mean Dice overlap metrics. It shows that with SSL, for most of the cases, the segmentation accuracy is increased compared to U-net-scratch. Figure 5 visualises exemplar segmentation results. It demonstrates that with limited training data, SSL+MultiTask generally produces better segmentations compared to U-net-scratch.

Table 2. Comparison of Dice overlap metrics for long-axis image segmentation. Values are mean (standard deviation).

#subjects (#slices)	U-net-scratch	SSL+Decoder	SSL+All	SSL+MultiTask
1 (2)	0.678 (0.132)	0.699 (0.069)	**0.733** (0.081)	0.600 (0.122)
5 (10)	0.848 (0.080)	0.850 (0.068)	**0.875** (0.051)	0.861 (0.049)
10 (20)	0.875 (0.044)	0.888 (0.039)	**0.905** (0.039)	0.889 (0.031)
50 (100)	0.922 (0.031)	0.914 (0.035)	0.925 (0.028)	**0.926** (0.029)
100 (200)	0.930 (0.032)	0.924 (0.037)	0.933 (0.031)	**0.934** (0.029)

4   Conclusions

In this paper, we propose a novel method that leverages self-supervised learning for cardiac MR image segmentation. We formulate anatomical position prediction as the pretext task. Experiments on short-axis and long-axis image segmentation tasks demonstrate that with self-supervised learning, the proposed method outperforms a standard U-net trained from scratch at the small data setting and is of comparable performance at the large data setting. For future work, we will explore other anatomically meaningful pretext tasks to increase data efficiency in medical imaging applications.

Acknowledgements. This research has been conducted using the UK Biobank Resource under Application Numbers 2964 and 18545 and supported by the Smart-Heart EPSRC Programme Grant (EP/P001009/1). We would like to thank NVIDIA Corporation for donating a Titan Xp for this research.

References

1. Bernard, O., et al.: Deep learning techniques for automatic MRI cardiac multi-structures segmentation and diagnosis. IEEE Trans. Med. Imaging **37**(11), 2514–2525 (2018)
2. Bai, W., et al.: Automated cardiovascular magnetic resonance image analysis with fully convolutional networks. J. Cardiovasc. Magn. Reson. **20**(1), 65 (2018)
3. Tao, Q., et al.: Deep learning-based method for fully automatic quantification of left ventricle function from cine MR images. Radiology **290**(1), 81–88 (2019)
4. Doersch, C., et al.: Multi-task self-supervised visual learning. In: ICCV (2017)
5. Gidaris, S., et al.: Unsupervised representation learning by predicting image rotations. In: ICLR (2018)
6. Doersch, C., et al.: Unsupervised visual representation learning by context prediction. In: ICCV (2015)
7. Zhang, R., et al.: Colorful image colorization. In: ECCV (2016)
8. Pathak, D., et al.: Context encoders: feature learning by inpainting. In: CVPR (2016)
9. Jamaludin, A., et al.: Self-supervised learning for spinal MRIs. In: MICCAI DLMIA Workshop (2017)

10. Ross, T., et al.: Exploiting the potential of unlabeled endoscopic video data with self-supervised learning. Int. J. Comput. Assist. Radiol. Surg. **13**(6), 925–933 (2018)
11. Tajbakhsh, N., et al.: Surrogate supervision for medical image analysis: effective deep learning from limited quantities of labeled data. In: ISBI (2019)
12. Ronneberger, O., et al.: U-Net: convolutional networks for biomedical image segmentation. In: MICCAI (2015)

A Fine-Grain Error Map Prediction and Segmentation Quality Assessment Framework for Whole-Heart Segmentation

Rongzhao Zhang[✉] and Albert C. S. Chung

The Hong Kong University of Science and Technology, Hong Kong, China
{rzhangbe,achung}@cse.ust.hk

Abstract. When introducing advanced image computing algorithms, e.g., whole-heart segmentation, into clinical practice, a common suspicion is how reliable the automatically computed results are. In fact, it is important to find out the failure cases and identify the misclassified pixels so that they can be excluded or corrected for the subsequent analysis or diagnosis. However, it is not a trivial problem to predict the errors in a segmentation mask when ground truth (usually annotated by experts) is absent. In this work, we attempt to address the pixel-wise error map prediction problem and the per-case mask quality assessment problem using a unified deep learning (DL) framework. Specifically, we first formalize an error map prediction problem, then we convert it to a segmentation problem and build a DL network to tackle it. We also derive a quality indicator (QI) from a predicted error map to measure the overall quality of a segmentation mask. To evaluate the proposed framework, we perform extensive experiments on a public whole-heart segmentation dataset, i.e., *MICCAI 2017 MMWHS*. By 5-fold cross validation, we obtain an overall Dice score of 0.626 for the error map prediction task, and observe a high Pearson correlation coefficient (PCC) of 0.972 between QI and the actual segmentation accuracy (Acc), as well as a low mean absolute error (MAE) of 0.0048 between them, which evidences the efficacy of our method in both error map prediction and quality assessment.

Keywords: Error map prediction · Segmentation quality assessment · Semantic segmentation

1 Introduction

Assessing per-case image segmentation quality is an important issue when researchers want to develop a computer-aided diagnosis (CADx) system or integrate automated image analysis methods into large-scale medical studies. Since image segmentation usually serves as a low-level module in a CADx system or a clinical study pipeline, errors incurred by segmentation algorithms will be

© Springer Nature Switzerland AG 2019
D. Shen et al. (Eds.): MICCAI 2019, LNCS 11765, pp. 550–558, 2019.
https://doi.org/10.1007/978-3-030-32245-8_61

delivered or even amplified in the subsequent calculation of image-based measurements and other downstream procedures, which may result in misleading statistical conclusions or slow down the diagnosis process. Automatic quality assessment is an appealing solution to such problems, which, ideally, should not only report the per-case segmentation quality, but also highlight those misclassified pixels, so that doctors (or an automatic system) can easily verify the reliability of a segmentation result and decide whether to keep it for further analysis. Besides, an automatic pixel-wise error prediction algorithm has a great potential in medical training, where it can provide inexperienced students with fine-grain feedback by pointing out which pixels are mislabeled.

Although the quality assessment for segmentations can be done by simply comparing with experts' annotation, this method is too costly to be applied in large-scale studies or automated pipelines. In natural image analysis area, there have been a number of unsupervised image segmentation evaluation methods [7], which employ low-level features, e.g., color error, texture, entropy, and their combinations to measure a segmentation's visual consistency with human observers. However, the application of such methods in medical area remains unclear [6]. Reserve validation method [8] trains classifiers with pseudo ground truth to quantify how well a classifier performs on a target domain, but it can only give a single quality measurement for a classifier across the whole test set, which cannot meet the per-case demand of a quality assessment algorithm. Recently, Valindria *et al.* proposed reverse classification accuracy (RCA) [5,6] method which is able to evaluate the quality for each single case, but this method has high computational cost and cannot predict a fine-grain error map. Robinson *et al.* developed a deep learning model to directly regress the Dice Similarity Coefficient (DSC) of a segmentation mask, which is much faster but still can only provide an image-level measurement and requires a large-scale training set.

In this study, we build an automatic quality assessment framework that is capable of simultaneous pixel-wise and per-case evaluation for segmentation masks. Specifically, we first formally define the pixel-wise error map prediction problem, and then show the capacity of a modern deep learning (DL) model in predicting error maps for auto-generated segmentation masks. We also derive a quality indicator (QI) from the output error maps, which can measure segmentation quality in a per-case manner. To generate diverse and representative segmentation masks, we train a VoxResNet [1] and its 2D version on the training sets, and collect all their side (induced by the deep supervision [3] paths) and final outputs as sample segmentations. To demonstrate the efficacy of our method, we evaluate it on a public 3D whole-heart segmentation dataset, i.e., *MICCAI 2017 MMWHS*. The quality and quantity results of a 5-fold cross validation show that our framework is able to identify the misclassified pixels in an input mask with satisfiable accuracy. We also observe a strong correlation between QI and the actual segmentation accuracy (Acc), as well as between QI and DSC score, evidencing the capacity of our framework working as an image-level segmentation quality evaluator. To the best of our knowledge, this is the first time that the segmentation quality assessment problem is addressed in a pixel-wise manner for medical images, and we are also a pioneer who manages to predict per-case segmentation quality accurately only based on relatively small training sets (e.g., 16 training MRI scans in each fold).

2   Method

Our method is mainly composed of a mask generation part (segmentor) and an error map prediction part (error map predictor), as shown in Fig. 1(a). In this section, we will first define the error map prediction problem, then elaborate the mask generation and error map prediction methods, and finally detail the training of the proposed framework.

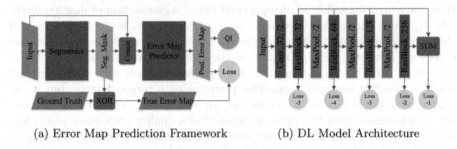

(a) Error Map Prediction Framework   (b) DL Model Architecture

Fig. 1. Flowchart of the proposed error map prediction framework and the DL model architecture (VoxResNet) employed in this paper.

2.1   Formulation of Error Map Prediction Problem

We define the error map $\mathcal{E}$ of a segmentation mask S as

$$\mathcal{E}(i) = \begin{cases} 1, & S(i) \neq GT(i), \\ 0, & S(i) = GT(i), \end{cases} \tag{1}$$

where GT is the ground truth segmentation and i specifies the pixel (voxel) location. $S(i), GT(i) \in \{0, 1, \cdots, C\}$, where C is the number of foreground classes and 0 denotes the background class. When ground truth segmentation is not available, we build a model M that is parameterized by θ to estimate the error map:

$$\widehat{\mathcal{E}} = M(I, S; \theta), \tag{2}$$

where I denotes the original image, $\widehat{\mathcal{E}}$ is the predicted error map for the segmentation mask S. Thus, given a dataset $\mathcal{D} = \{I_i, \{S_i^k\}_{k=1}^m, GT_i\}_{i=1}^N$, the error map prediction problem can be formulated as an optimization task over model parameter θ:

$$\min_{\theta} \frac{1}{mN} \sum_{i=1}^{N} \sum_{k=1}^{m} d\left(\mathcal{E}(S_i^k, GT_i), \widehat{\mathcal{E}}(I_i, S_i^k; \theta)\right), \qquad (3)$$

where N is the number of images, m is the number of generated segmentation masks for each image, $d(\cdot, \cdot)$ is a distance metric such as cross entropy, which measures the difference between the true and the predicted error maps. An example error map is shown in Fig. 2(a).

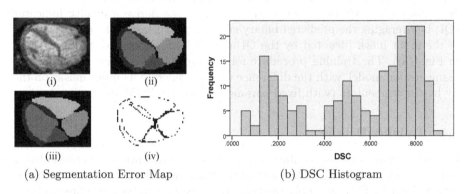

(a) Segmentation Error Map   (b) DSC Histogram

Fig. 2. (a) An example error map, where (i), (ii), (iii) and (iv) are the original image, auto-generated mask, ground truth and error map, respectively. Note that the intensity of the error map is reversed (0 for error and 1 for correct pixels) for better visualization. (b) Histogram of DSC score of the generated segmentation masks.

2.2 Mask Generation

To enable the training and evaluation of the error map predictor, we train two different CNN models on the training sets and collect all their outputs to form a mask set $\{S_i^k\}_{i,k}$. One segmentation model is VoxResNet [1], a representative and state-of-the-art CNN model designed for volumetric medical image segmentation tasks, which leverages residual connections [2] and combines multi-scale features to make a quality prediction, as schematically illustrated in Fig. 1(b). To encourage the diversity of collected masks, we also employ a 2D version of VoxResNet to perform the generation work, as it is believed that the outputs of 2D and 3D models can be significantly different since their receptive fields are distinctive. Further, the side outputs of these models, which are generated by the deep supervision pathways (corresponding to Loss-2 to Loss-5 in Fig. 1(b)), are also added to the mask collection to involve more examples with various segmentation qualities. Overall, the number of auto-generated masks for each scan is $m = 2 \times (4 + 1) = 10$, where 4 is the number of side outputs in a segmentor. The DSC score histogram of the generated segmentations is shown in Fig. 2(b).

2.3   Error Map Predictor and Quality Indicator

Since an error map has the same size as the corresponding segmentation mask
and takes 0–1 values, the error map predictor can be implemented by a binary
segmentation model. Without loss of generality, we employ another VoxResNet
to carry out the prediction, which has the same architecture as the 3D segmentor
but different input and output channels. As shown in Fig. 1(a), the error map
predictor takes the concatenation of the segmentation mask (with one-hot coding) and the original image as inputs, and output a probabilistic map indicating
the probability of each pixel being misclassified by the segmentor (then we can
get the binary error map by thresholding). Since the mean value across a true
error map is exactly the segmentation accuracy, we derive a quality indicator
(QI) by averaging the predicted binary error map to measure the overall quality
of the input mask (denoted by the QI node following the predicted error map
in Fig. 1(a)). The training procedure for the predictor is similar to a standard
segmentation model, with the difference that we generate its input masks on the
fly by the segmentors (with fixed parameters) to save RAM space.

2.4   Training Details

For the training of the segmentors, we optimize the summation of a cross entropy
(CE) loss and a multi-class Dice loss on the training set with a standard segmentation pipeline. Then we apply the trained segmentors to both training and test
sets, and collect their outputs on the training set for the subsequent training of
the predictor, and save the outputs on the test set for evaluation of the error
map predictor. In this way, both the segmentors and predictor can only access
the training set during the learning phase, and their performance are evaluated
solely on the test set. Besides, since the predictor is essentially a binary segmentation model, we optimize it by the summation of a CE loss and a binary Dice
loss (error pixels as the positive class).

3   Experiments and Results

Dataset. We evaluated our framework on a public whole-heart segmentation
dataset, i.e., *MICCAI 2017 MMWHS*[1] [9]. We employed the 20 MRI scans in
this dataset which are paired with manual annotations with 7 foreground classes.
For preprocessing, we resampled each scans to an isotropic voxel resolution of
$2 \times 2 \times 2$ mm, normalized their intensity to $[-1, 1]$ and then extracted the heart
region with a method similar to [4]. The preprocessed scans have a size of around
$120 \times 120 \times 90$. Standard data augmentation methods are applied during the
training of segmentors and the predictor, including random cropping (to a patch
size of $96 \times 96 \times 80$, or 96×96 for 2D), flipping along each axis and scaling.
For all experiments, we run 5-fold cross validations since the dataset is relatively
small.

---

[1] http://www.sdspeople.fudan.edu.cn/zhuangxiahai/0/mmwhs17/index.html.

Table 1. Error map prediction performance

Mask type	#Masks	DSC	Acc	Prec	Recl	Seg. DSC	Seg. Acc
3D final	20	0.4313	0.9757	0.3766	0.5479	0.8102	0.9816
3D-2	20	**0.8611**	0.9842	0.8132	0.9175	0.2751	0.938
3D-3	20	0.5666	0.9769	0.8133	0.6665	0.7781	0.9762
3D-4	20	0.5772	0.9676	0.4953	0.7074	0.6781	0.9674
3D-5	20	0.7421	0.9597	0.6501	0.8668	0.2387	0.932
GT	20	0.25	**0.9967**	0.25	1	1	1
3D-average	100	0.6357	0.9728	0.6297	0.7412	0.5560	0.9590
2D-average	100	0.6161	0.9691	0.5092	0.7927	0.5483	0.9647
Overall-auto	200	0.6259	0.9710	0.5695	0.7670	0.5522	0.9619
Overall-GT	220	0.5917	0.9733	0.5404	0.7881	0.5929	0.9653

Metrics. As the error map prediction problem is essentially a segmentation task, we employ common segmentation metrics to measure its performance, which include Dice similarity coefficient (DSC), accuracy (Acc), precision (Prec) and recall (Recl). Note that in the metric calculation we regard the error pixels as the positive class, though in the figures we show error pixels by low intensity for the sake of clear visualization.

Error Map Predictor. To thoroughly investigate the performance of the error map predictor, we evaluate it on different kinds of segmentation masks and report their performance in Table 1. The predictor's performance on the final outputs of the 3D VoxResNet is tagged by '3D-Final', and its side outputs are tagged by '3D-2' to '3D-5', respectively. Ground truth masks are referred to as 'GT'. We omit the detailed mask categories of 2D generators as they are similar to the 3D case, and only report their average values to save space. The last two rows show the predictor's overall performance on all masks with or without GT, respectively. We also list segmentation metrics in the table (last two columns) in order for better interpretation of the prediction results. Considering both prediction and segmentation metrics, we find that the error map predictor performs worse on those masks with better quality, and vice versa. This is because, for masks with good quality, the error regions are usually small (or thin) and near to the class boundaries (as the first case shown in Fig. 3), where it is hard to tell which pixel is wrong if GT is not available. On the other hand, low-quality masks tend to have larger error regions that do not concentrate on subtle boundaries, which can be easily identified by our error prediction model (an example is illustrated in the second row of Fig. 3). Another observation is that our error map predictor performs well for GT masks, on which the it achieves the highest prediction accuracy, i.e., 0.9967, meaning that our model can 'feel' that a GT mask is of high quality, even though it has never seen this GT mask before. Note that the prediction DSC for GT masks is low because the true error map for a GT mask

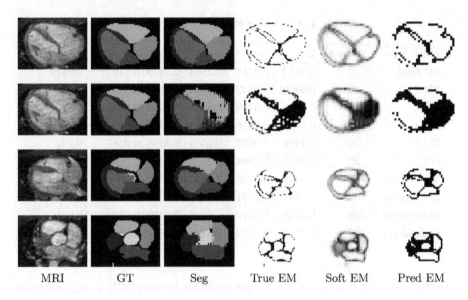

| MRI | GT | Seg | True EM | Soft EM | Pred EM |

Fig. 3. Representative error map predictions. The last two columns show the raw (probabilistic) predicted error maps and the thresholded binary maps, respectively.

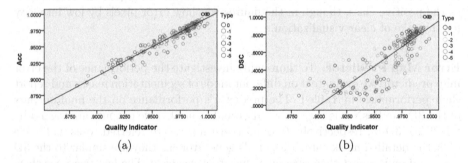

Fig. 4. Scatter plots of (a) Real Acc and QI, and (b) Real DSC and QI. Different colors denotes different mask types (0: GT; −1: final output; −2 to −5: side outputs).

is all zero, such that even a single wrong pixel will lead to a zero DSC score. Overall, our error map predictor achieves a good DSC of 0.626 (0.592 if considering GT masks), demonstrating the efficacy of the proposed error map prediction model. Qualitative results can be found in Fig. 3, where several representative error map predictions are present.

Quality Indicator. As mentioned in Sect. 2.3, we derive a QI by averaging the predicted error map. To measure how well QI can represent the segmentation quality, we compute the Pearson correlation coefficient (PCC), mean absolute error (MAE) between QI and real segmentation accuracy, as well as the PCC between QI and real DSC using all 220 masks, and the results are as follows:

$$PCC_{QI,Acc} = 0.972, \ PCC_{QI,DSC} = 0.856, \ MAE_{QI,Acc} = 0.0048, \quad (4)$$

where both correlations are significant with $p < 0.0001$. We also draw two scatter plots (QI-Acc and QI-DSC) in Fig. 4 to visualize the relationship between QI and the segmentation measurements. Considering the high PCC and low MAE between QI and Acc, as well as the strong linear relationship observed in Fig. 4(a), QI can be regarded as a precise approximator to the real segmentation accuracy, thus can work as a good segmentation quality measurement.

4 Conclusion

Per-case and fine-grain segmentation quality assessment plays a crucial role in automating the image-based pipelines in medical research or clinical diagnosis, but this area has not yet been fully studied. This work formally defines a fine-grain error map prediction problem, and attempts to address it using a DL framework. The evaluation results on a public whole-heart segmentation dataset demonstrates the efficacy of our error map predictor, and also shows that a per-case quality measurement can be derived from the predicted error maps, which approximates the real segmentation accuracy well with a small MAE. Future work will investigate the potential of error map predictors in improving segmentor's robustness, where an error map predictor can serve as a critic to regularize the segmentation model. The proposed framework is inherently generic, in which the segmentors and predictors can be replaced with different types of models (e.g., random forest), and it can be adapted to other segmentation applications easily.

References

1. Chen, H., Dou, Q., Yu, L., Qin, J., Heng, P.A.: VoxResNet: deep voxelwise residual networks for brain segmentation from 3D MR images. NeuroImage **170**, 446–455 (2018)
2. He, K., Zhang, X., Ren, S., Sun, J.: Deep residual learning for image recognition. In: Proceedings of the IEEE Conference on Computer Vision and Pattern Recognition, pp. 770–778 (2016)
3. Lee, C.Y., Xie, S., Gallagher, P., Zhang, Z., Tu, Z.: Deeply-supervised nets. In: Artificial Intelligence and Statistics, pp. 562–570 (2015)
4. Payer, C., Štern, D., Bischof, H., Urschler, M.: Multi-label whole heart segmentation using CNNs and anatomical label configurations. In: Pop, M., et al. (eds.) STACOM 2017. LNCS, vol. 10663, pp. 190–198. Springer, Cham (2018). https://doi.org/10.1007/978-3-319-75541-0_20
5. Robinson, R., et al.: Automatic quality control of cardiac MRI segmentation in large-scale population imaging. In: Descoteaux, M., Maier-Hein, L., Franz, A., Jannin, P., Collins, D.L., Duchesne, S. (eds.) MICCAI 2017. LNCS, vol. 10433, pp. 720–727. Springer, Cham (2017). https://doi.org/10.1007/978-3-319-66182-7_82

6. Valindria, V.V., et al.: Reverse classification accuracy: predicting segmentation performance in the absence of ground truth. IEEE Trans. Med. Imaging **36**(8), 1597–1606 (2017)
7. Zhang, H., Fritts, J.E., Goldman, S.A.: Image segmentation evaluation: a survey of unsupervised methods. Comput. Vis. Image Underst. **110**(2), 260–280 (2008)
8. Zhong, E., Fan, W., Yang, Q., Verscheure, O., Ren, J.: Cross validation framework to choose amongst models and datasets for transfer learning. In: Balcázar, J.L., Bonchi, F., Gionis, A., Sebag, M. (eds.) ECML PKDD 2010. LNCS (LNAI), vol. 6323, pp. 547–562. Springer, Heidelberg (2010). https://doi.org/10.1007/978-3-642-15939-8_35
9. Zhuang, X., Shen, J.: Multi-scale patch and multi-modality atlases for whole heart segmentation of MRI. Med. Image Anal. **31**, 77–87 (2016)

Cardiac Segmentation from LGE MRI Using Deep Neural Network Incorporating Shape and Spatial Priors

Qian Yue, Xinzhe Luo, Qing Ye, Lingchao Xu,
and Xiahai Zhuang[(⊠)]

School of Data Science, Fudan University, 200433 Shanghai, China
zxh@fudan.edu.cn

Abstract. Cardiac segmentation from late gadolinium enhancement MRI is an important task in clinics to identify and evaluate the infarction of myocardium. The automatic segmentation is however still challenging, due to the heterogeneous intensity distributions and indistinct boundaries in the images. In this paper, we propose a new method, based on deep neural networks (DNN), for fully automatic segmentation. The proposed network, referred to as SRSCN, comprises a shape reconstruction neural network (SRNN) and a spatial constraint network (SCN). SRNN aims to maintain a realistic shape of the resulting segmentation. It can be pre-trained by a set of label images, and then be embedded into a unified loss function as a regularization term. Hence, no manually designed feature is needed. Furthermore, SCN incorporates the spatial information of the 2D slices. It is formulated and trained with the segmentation network via the multi-task learning strategy. We evaluated the proposed method using 45 patients and compared with two state-of-the-art regularization schemes, i.e., the anatomically constraint neural network and the adversarial neural network. The results show that the proposed SRSCN outperformed the conventional schemes, and obtained a Dice score of $0.758 \pm .227$ for myocardial segmentation, which compares with $0.757 \pm .083$ from the inter-observer variations.

Keywords: LGE MRI · Shape prior · Cardiac segmentation · Deep learning

1 Introduction

Analysis of myocardial (Myo) viability is crucial to better understand the physiological and pathological processes for patients suffering from myocardial infarction (MI). Late gadolinium enhancement (LGE) MRI is a valuable tool for MI assessment, because it can visualize the important pathological information. For quantitative assessment, segmentation of the myocardium is a prerequisite.

Manual segmentation can be time-consuming and suffer from inter-observer variations, thus automating this process is desirable in the clinic. Rajchl *et al.* proposed to segment the myocardium indirectly using a multi-region approach [1]. Many automatic methods use cine MRI as prior knowledge, and the image registration techniques are applied for more accurate segmentations [2]. These methods generally require an

© Springer Nature Switzerland AG 2019
D. Shen et al. (Eds.): MICCAI 2019, LNCS 11765, pp. 559–567, 2019.
https://doi.org/10.1007/978-3-030-32245-8_62

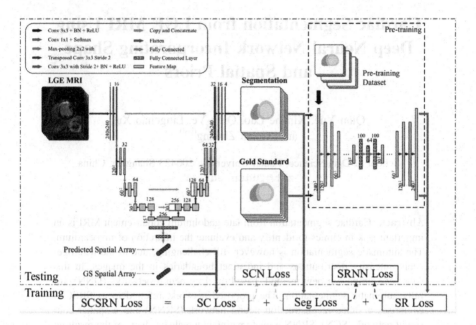

Fig. 1. Overall structure of SRSCN, whose loss comes from three parts: the segmentation loss is specially design as a function of cross entropy and Dice, the spatial constraint (SC) loss to assist segmentation, and the shape reconstruction (SR) loss for shape regularization.

accurate registration between the cine MRI and LGE MRI. However, this registration can also be challenging, considering the intra-image misalignments as well as inter-image misregistration. Therefore, manual interaction is commonly used. Liu *et al.* employed the multi-component Gaussian mixture model to automatically segment the myocardium from a single LGE MRI sequence [3]. The coupled level set is employed as a spatial constraint, which can be iteratively adapted according to the image characteristics.

Fully automated segmentation of LGE MRI is challenging due to the heterogeneous intensity distributions of images and the large shape variation of the heart. Furthermore, the annotated data are meanwhile limited; thus, the attempt to solve this problem automatically is still rarely reported. In the field of medical imaging, anatomical priors can be essential in assisting the segmentation task in the deep neural network (DNN)-based algorithms. Therefore, in this work we propose an enhanced DNN model with shape reconstruction (SR) and spatial constraint (SC) to tackle the challenging segmentation task, particularly with a small set of annotated training data. The resulting network is expected to be able to constrain the segmentation to generate results with realistic heart shapes.

We first propose a shape reconstruction neural network (SRNN). SRNN can be pre-trained by anatomical priors such as a set of label images, and it works as a shape constraint to regularize the results. Hence, SRNN can maintain a realistic heart shape of the segmentation result. Furthermore, we propose the spatial constraint network (SCN) to solve the large variation of the 2D slices across different positions of a 3D cardiac MRI. This is because the 2D slices may come from any position, from the apex to the base of the ventricles. The shape and appearance of these slices can vary considerably if they come from different positions. SCN is designed to incorporate this information. By combining the learning task of spatial information with the segmentation problem and formulating them as a two-task-learning problem, one can expect the SCN to significantly improve the general performance of the network, opposed to the separate training for the two tasks. In addition, we investigate two state-of-the-art alternatives for shape regularization, i.e. the anatomical constraint neural network (ACNN) [4] and the generative adversarial network (GAN) [5], though neither of them has been used for this segmentation task, to the best of our knowledge.

2 Method

Figure 1 presents the structure of the proposed network, i.e., SRSCN, which is based on an enhanced U-Net [6]. SRSCN includes two modules to incorporate the prior knowledge, i.e., the SR module and the SC module. The models solely combining U-Net with SR and SC are denoted as SRNN and SCN, respectively.

2.1 Architecture of the Segmentation Network

Ronneberger *et al.* proposed U-Net for medical image segmentation, which has two key modules, i.e. the feature extraction and up sampling module [6]. Based on the fully connected network (FCN), it has the advantage of utilizing multi-scale information of the images. U-Net has a symmetric pyramid structure, where an input image is compressed into higher semantic features and then unsampled to its original resolution. The combination of local and contextual information enables a good segmentation of medical images.

In our work, we adopted the Exponential Logarithmic Loss [7] as the loss function to measure the result of the segmentation. This loss function combines cross entropy and Dice score in a balanced fashion to facilitate training, and it takes the label balance into account to accelerate convergence, i.e.,

$$L_{Seg} = \lambda_{Dice}L_{Dice} + \lambda_{Cross}L_{Cross}, \tag{1}$$

where, λ_{Dice} and λ_{Cross} are the balancing parameters, respectively for the weighted Dice score term, $L_{Dice} = \boldsymbol{E}[(-\ln(Dice_i))^{\gamma_1}]$, and the weighted cross entropy term, $L_{Cross} = \boldsymbol{E}[w_l(-\ln(p_l(\boldsymbol{x})))^{\gamma_2}]$ with $\boldsymbol{x}$ the pixel position, i the label, and l the ground-truth label at $\boldsymbol{x}$; γ_1 and γ_2 are two hyperparameters that control the nonlinearities of the loss functions.

DNN, however, generally requires a large set of annotated data to train the network. With limited training data, the generalization capacity of the network could be impaired. Therefore, constraints from prior knowledge should be included to enhance the performance of the DNN.

2.2 SRNN for Prior Knowledge of Shapes

SRNN aims to learn an intermediate representation, from which the original inputs can be reconstructed. Internally, by several down sampling operations, it can compress the information or knowledge of original input into some codes acting as a compact representation of the input image. Through this information compression, features of the inputs are captured and mapped into a high-density space.

Hence, an SRNN model, pre-trained from a set of shape images, is able to function as a constraint to regularize a segmentation result into a desired realistic shape. The architecture of this SRNN is illustrated in Fig. 1, where the SR module (in dark red) is connected, as an extended network to U-Net. During the optimization process, a regularization term produced by SRNN is in charge of constraining segmentation output. The loss function for training SRNN is formulated as follows,

$$L_{SRNN} = L_{Seg} + \lambda_{SR} L_{SR}, \qquad (2)$$

where λ_{SR} is the balancing parameter; L_{SR} is the SR module loss and is defined from Frobenius norm,

$$L_{SR} = \sum_{i=1}^{n} \left\| \widehat{R}_i - R_i \right\|_F^2. \qquad (3)$$

Here, n is the number of training samples, R_i indicates the reconstructed gold standard segmentation, and $\widehat{R}_i$ denotes the reconstructed segmentation from the SRNN prediction; $\|\cdot\|_F$ is the Frobenius norm of an $m \times n$ matrix, and it is defined as the square root of the sum of the absolute squares of matrix elements.

2.3 SCN for Prior Knowledge of Spatial Constraints

The idea of utilizing spatial information comes from the fact that the shapes and appearance of the heart in the basal and apical slices can vary significantly. Therefore, we develop an SC module to include the prediction of the spatial information of each slice. At the same time, the segmentation task cooperates with spatial information prediction task, which forms a multi-task learning problem. Multi-task learning has been shown to be able to significantly improve the performance in contrast to learning each task independently, both empirically [8] and theoretically [9, 10]. This is the case not only when a few data per task are available but also when two tasks can intuitively strengthen each other.

As Fig. 1 shows, we propose the SC module (in dark blue), connected to the bottom of the U-Net, to predict the position of an LGE MRI slice. The SC loss is designed to penalize the erroneous prediction of the spatial positions,

$$L_{SC} = \sum_{i=1}^{n} \left\| \widehat{P}_i - P_i \right\|_F^2, \qquad (4)$$

where P_i is the ground truth spatial information of slice i, and $\widehat{P}_i$ is the prediction. Similarly, the SCN loss is formulated with the weighted loss terms,

$$L_{SCN} = L_{Seg} + \lambda_{SC}L_{SC}. \tag{5}$$

By incorporating SC, the network can combine two tasks, i.e., the regression of position and the segmentation of images, to form a two-task-learning problem.

2.4 The Proposed SRSCN

Finally, we combine the SRNN and SCN to obtain the SRSCN, as shown in Fig. 1, whose loss function is then defined as follows,

$$L_{SRSCN} = L_{Seg} + \lambda_{SC}L_{SC} + \lambda_{SR}L_{SR}. \tag{6}$$

These two techniques can strengthen each other and result in better segmentation. The two weights, λ_{SC} and λ_{SR}, balance the regularization effect of these two terms.

2.5 Alternative Technology for Shape Constraints

For comparisons, we further investigate the two state-of-the-art networks for shape regularization, i.e., ACNN and GAN.

ACNN takes a series of cardiac label images as the inputs [4]. Through the pre-trained auto-encoder network, the shape features are encoded as the compact codes of the network. In contrast to the proposed SRNN using the reconstruction to assist segmentation, ACNN solely uses the codes created by the encoder. Specifically, one can obtain the ACNN by replacing the regularization term in SRNN with the L2-norm between the codes coming from the segmentation result and gold standard.

GAN trains a discriminator to distinguish the authenticity of the inputs [5]. The generator of GAN is responsible for producing more realistic inputs to fool the discriminator. Integrating this idea into the segmentation task, it is quite natural to train a discriminator whose task is to identify gold standard and segmentation results. Our main purpose is to guide the segmentation network, that is U-Net to obtain better segmentation results under this regularization. Specifically, two major modifications have been performed on the U-Net to obtain the GAN-regularized U-Net segmentation. Firstly, these segmentation results to be distinguished and gold standard are fed to GAN as it plays the role of predicting a probability determining whether the current input is gold standard label or not. The Sigmoid cross entropy used for GAN penalizes this discriminator for wrong predictions. Secondly, the cost function includes a regularization term created by GAN, with fixed parameters and an input of gold standard label.

3 Experiment

3.1 Data, Experimental Setup and Implementation Details

The LGE MRI used in the study were collected from 45 patients, of which 25 patients were randomly selected for training, 5 selected for validation and 15 for testing. Note that one of the 15 test cases failed all the methods, due to the particularly poor image quality. Hence, the statistics of the results reported here exclude this outlier. To

Table 1. Segmentation performance of SRSCN for cardiac LGE MRI.

Metrics	Myo (Epi)	LV (Endo)	RV (Endo)
Dice	0.812 ± 0.105	0.915 ± 0.052	0.882 ± 0.084
ASD (mm)	1.480 ± 0.997	1.749 ± 1.512	1.619 ± 1.748
HD (mm)	11.04 ± 5.818	12.25 ± 6.455	18.07 ± 14.17

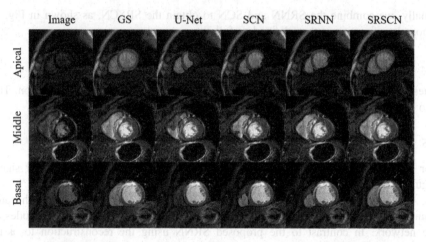

Fig. 2. Visualization of three typical slices. Here, GS denotes gold standard segmentation.

augment the training data, we registered the training images to other image spaces using a set of artificially generated rigid, affine and deformable transformations, resulting in 1,350 augmented 3D images and 20,405 2D slices.

We used Dice coefficient, average symmetric surface distance (ASD) and Hausdorff Distance (HD) as metrics for evaluation of segmentation accuracy. ASD measures the average of all the distances from points on the boundary of segmentation (Seg) to the boundary of gold standard (GS),

$$ASD = \frac{1}{|B_{Seg}| + |B_{GS}|} \times \left(\sum_{x \in B_{Seg}} d(x, B_{GS}) + \sum_{y \in B_{GS}} d(y, B_{Seg}) \right).$$

The HD metric measures how far two subsets of a metric space are from each other, $HD = \max_{x \in Seg} \min_{y \in GS} \|x - y\|$.

For SRSCN, we used 5e-4 for the weight of SRNN and 1e-6 for SCN as default. Note that it is possible to obtain better performance if an exhaustive search for the optimal value could be employed. The inputs to the networks were 2D slices of size 240×240 in pixels; the size of mini-batch was 32; the learning rate was 0.001. We trained each model for 30 epochs. GAN was trained for 10 epochs with manual monitoring of convergence, due to the particularly expensive training. The codes and models were implemented using TensorFlow [11], and the optimizer for training was

Table 2. Dice scores of the different methods from the study of shape constraints.

Methods	LV	RV	Myo	Mean
U-Net	0.816 ± 0.177	0.712 ± 0.272	0.682 ± 0.200	0.737 ± 0.216
SCN	0.885 ± 0.119	0.797 ± 0.170	0.773 ± 0.156	0.818 ± 0.148
SRNN	0.910 ± 0.051	0.825 ± 0.122	0.796 ± 0.115	0.844 ± 0.096
SRSCN	0.915 ± 0.052	0.882 ± 0.084	0.812 ± 0.105	0.870 ± 0.080
ACNN	0.913 ± 0.044	0.835 ± 0.102	0.800 ± 0.088	0.849 ± 0.078
GAN	0.885 ± 0.109	0.792 ± 0.190	0.781 ± 0.154	0.819 ± 0.151

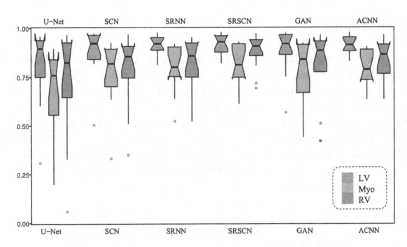

Fig. 3. Box plots of the Dice scores of the different methods.

AdamOptimizer [12]. We used one GPU of type GTX 1080ti for training and testing. Each model required 5 to 8 h to train and the testing of a subject took 2 to 3 s.

3.2 Performance of the Proposed Method

Table 1 presents the statistics of the three metrics of the proposed SRSCN. Dice score for myocardium segmentation reaches $0.812 \pm .105$, which compares the inter-observer Dice of $0.757 \pm .083$. Note that the mean Dice score drops to $0.758 \pm .227$ if the one failure case is included.

3.3 Study of Constraints

3.3.1 Ablation Study of SRSCN

The results of the ablation study are presented in Table 2. SCN outperforms U-Net by 8% in terms of generalized Dice score. SRNN further improves Dice performance by 3%. The proposed model, which consists of both of the SR and SC modules achieves more than 13% improvement. Figure 2 visualizes three typical slices, i.e. from apical, middle and basal ventricle, and Fig. 3 compares the distributions of Dice scores of different methods. The segmentation improvements are evident in the ablation study.

3.3.2   Comparisons with Two State-of-the-Art Models

Table 2 and Fig. 3 also present the segmentation results from the two state-of-the-art deep-learning-based algorithms, i.e. ACNN [4] and GAN [13]. Compared to ACNN, SRSCN obtains marginally better mean Dice; compared to GAN, it achieves more than 5% improvement. Compared to U-Net without shape regularization, SRSCN has evidently and significantly better Dice scores in all categories (p < 0.01).

4   Conclusion

In this work, we propose the SRSCN for cardiac segmentation of LGE MRI. SRSCN incorporates the shape and spatial priors via the SC and SR modules. SC module is introduced as a spatial constraint for 2D slices and is formulated in the unified loss function as a multi-task-learning problem. SR aims to maintain a realistic shape of the resulting segmentation. We have evaluated the proposed method using 45 patients, and compared it with two state-of-the-art regularization schemes, i.e., ACNN and GAN. The results have demonstrated the effectiveness of the SR and SC regularization terms, and showed the superiority of segmentation performance of the proposed SRSCN over the conventional schemes.

Acknowledgement. This work was funded by the National Natural Science Foundation of China (NSFC) grant (61971142), and the Science and Technology Commission of Shanghai Municipality grant (17JC1401600).

References

1. Rajchl, M., et al.: Interactive hierarchical-flow segmentation of scar tissue from late-enhancement cardiac MR images. IEEE Trans. Med. Imaging **33**(1), 159–172 (2014)
2. Dikici, E., O'Donnell, T., Setser, R., White, R.D.: Quantification of delayed enhancement MR images. In: Barillot, C., Haynor, David R., Hellier, P. (eds.) MICCAI 2004. LNCS, vol. 3216, pp. 250–257. Springer, Heidelberg (2004). https://doi.org/10.1007/978-3-540-30135-6_31
3. Liu, J., et al.: Myocardium segmentation from DE MR using multicomponent Gaussian mixture model and coupled level set. IEEE Trans. Biomed. Eng. **64**(11), 2650–2661 (2017)
4. Oktay, O., Ferrante, E., Kamnitsas, K., et al.: Anatomically constrained neural networks (ACNNs): application to cardiac image enhancement and segmentation. IEEE Trans. Med. Imaging **37**(2), 384–395 (2018)
5. Goodfellow, I., Pouget-Abadie, J., et al.: Generative adversarial nets. In: Advances in Neural Information Processing Systems, pp. 2672–2680 (2014)
6. Ronneberger, O., Fischer, P., Brox, T.: U-net: convolutional networks for biomedical image segmentation. In: Navab, N., Hornegger, J., Wells, W.M., Frangi, A.F. (eds.) MICCAI 2015. LNCS, vol. 9351, pp. 234–241. Springer, Cham (2015). https://doi.org/10.1007/978-3-319-24574-4_28

7. Wong, K.C.L., Moradi, M., Tang, H., Syeda-Mahmood, T.: 3D segmentation with exponential logarithmic loss for highly unbalanced object sizes. In: Frangi, A.F., Schnabel, J. A., Davatzikos, C., Alberola-López, C., Fichtinger, G. (eds.) MICCAI 2018. LNCS, vol. 11072, pp. 612–619. Springer, Cham (2018). https://doi.org/10.1007/978-3-030-00931-1_70

8. Evgeniou, T., Micchelli, C.A., Pontil, M.: Learning multiple tasks with kernel methods. J. Mach. Learn. Res. 6(Apr), 615–637 (2005)

9. Ando, R.K., Zhang, T.: A framework for learning predictive structures from multiple tasks and unlabeled data. Mach. Learn. Res. 6(Nov), 1817–1853 (2005)

10. Argyriou, A., Evgeniou, T., Pontil, M.: Multi-task feature learning. In: Advances in Neural Information Processing System, pp. 41–48 (2007)

11. Abadi, M., Barham, P., et al.: TensorFlow: a system for large-scale machine learning. arXiv preprint arXiv:1603.04467 (2016)

12. Kingma, D.P., Ba, J.: Adam: a method for stochastic optimization. arXiv preprint arXiv:1412.6980 (2014)

13. Luc, P., Couprie, C., Chintala, S., Verbeek, J.: Semantic segmentation using adversarial networks. arXiv preprint arXiv:1611.08408 (2016)

Curriculum Semi-supervised Segmentation

Hoel Kervadec[✉], Jose Dolz, Éric Granger, and Ismail Ben Ayed

ÉTS Montréal, Montréal, Canada
hoel.kervadec.1@estmtl.net

Abstract. This study investigates a curriculum-style strategy for semi-supervised CNN segmentation, which devises a regression network to learn image-level information such as the size of the target region. These regressions are used to effectively regularize the segmentation network, constraining the softmax predictions of the unlabeled images to match the inferred label distributions. Our framework is based on inequality constraints, which tolerate uncertainties in the inferred knowledge, e.g., regressed region size. It can be used for a large variety of region attributes. We evaluated our approach for left ventricle segmentation in magnetic resonance images (MRI), and compared it to standard proposal-based semi-supervision strategies. Our method achieves competitive results, leveraging unlabeled data in a more efficient manner and approaching full-supervision performance.

Keywords: Image segmentation · Semi-supervised learning · Constrained CNNs

1 Introduction

In the recent years, deep learning architectures, and particularly convolutional neural networks (CNNs), have achieved state-of-the-art performances in a breadth of visual recognition tasks. These architectures currently dominate the literature in medical image segmentation [12]. The generalization capabilities of these networks typically rely on large and annotated datasets, which, in the case of segmentation, consist of precise pixel-level annotations. Obtaining expert annotations in medical images is a costly process that also requires clinical expertise. The lack of large annotated datasets has driven research in deep segmentation models that rely on reduced supervision for training, such as weakly [8,9,11,17] or semi-supervised [1,19] learning. These strategies assume that annotations are limited or coarse, such as image-level tags [15,17], scribbles [20] or bounding-boxes [18].

In this paper, we focus on semi-supervised learning, a common scenario in medical imaging, where a small set of images are assumed to be fully annotated, but an abundance of unlabeled images is available. Recent progress of these techniques in medical image segmentation has been bolstered by deep learning [1,2,6,14,19,24]. Self-training is a common semi-supervised learning strategy, which consists of employing reliable predictions generated by a deep learning architecture to re-train

© Springer Nature Switzerland AG 2019
D. Shen et al. (Eds.): MICCAI 2019, LNCS 11765, pp. 568–576, 2019.
https://doi.org/10.1007/978-3-030-32245-8_63

it, thereby augmenting the training set with these predictions as pseudo-labels [1,17,18]. Although this approach can leverage unlabeled images, one of its main drawbacks is that early mistakes are propagated back to the network, being re-amplified during training [4,25]. Several techniques were proposed to overcome this issue, such as co-training [24] and adversarial learning [5,13,23]. Nevertheless, with these approaches, training typically involves several networks, or multiple objective functions, which might hamper the convergence of such models.

Alternatively, some weakly supervised segmentation approaches have been proposed to constrain the network predictions with global label statistics, for example, in the form of target-region size [7,8,17]. For instance, Jia et al. [7] employed an $\mathcal{L}_2$ penalty to impose equality constraints on the size of the target regions in the context of histopathology image segmentation. However, their formulation requires the exact knowledge of region size, which limits its applicability. More recently, Kervadec et al. [8] proposed using inequality constraints, which provide more flexibility, and significantly improves performance compared to cases where learning relies on partial image labels in the form of scribbles. Nevertheless, the values used to bound network predictions in [8] are derived from manual annotations, which is a limiting assumption. Another closely related work is the curriculum learning strategy proposed in the context of unsupervised domain adaptation for urban images in [22]. In this case, the authors proposed to match global label distributions over source (labelled) and target (unlabelled) images by minimizing the KL-divergence between distributions. Finally, it is worth noting that the semi-supervised learning technique in [6] embeds semantic constraints on the adjacency graph of a given region.

Inspired by this research, we propose a curriculum-style strategy for deep semi-supervised segmentation, which employs a regression network to predict image-level information such as the size of the target region. These regressions are used to effectively regularize the segmentation network, enforcing the predictions for the unlabeled images to match the inferred label distributions. Contrary to [22], our framework uses inequality constraints, which provides greater flexibility, allowing uncertainty in the inferred knowledge, e.g., regressed region size. Another important difference is that the proposed framework can be used for a large variety of region attributes (e.g., shape moments). We evaluated our approach in the task of left ventricle segmentation in magnetic resonance images (MRI), and compared it to standard proposal-based semi-supervision strategies. Our method achieves very competitive results, leveraging unlabeled data in a more efficient manner and approaching full-supervision performance. We made our code publicly available[1].

2   Self-training for Semi-supervised Segmentation

Let $X : \Omega \subset \mathbb{R}^{2,3} \rightarrow \mathbb{R}$ denotes a training image, with Ω its spatial domain. Consider a semi-supervised scenario with two subsets: $\mathcal{S} = \{(X_i, Y_i)\}_{i=1,...,n}$

---

[1] https://github.com/LIVIAETS/semi_curriculum.

which contains a set of images X_i and their corresponding pixel-wise ground-truth labels Y_i, and $\mathcal{U} = \{X_j\}_{j=1,\dots,m}$ a set of unlabeled images, with $m \gg n$. In the fully supervised setting, training is formulated as minimizing the following loss with respect to network parameters $\boldsymbol{\theta}$:

$$\mathcal{L}_Y(\boldsymbol{\theta}) = -\sum_{i\in\mathcal{S}}\sum_{p\in\Omega} Y_{i,p} \log S(X_i|\boldsymbol{\theta})_p \tag{1}$$

where $S(X_i|\boldsymbol{\theta})_p$ represents a vector of softmax probabilities generated by the CNN at each pixel p and image i. To simplify the presentation, we consider the two-region segmentation scenario (i.e., two classes), with ground-truth binary labels $Y_{i,p}$ taking values in $\{0,1\}$, 1 indicating the target region (foreground) and 0 indicating the background. However, our formulation can be easily extended to the multi-region case. Common approaches for semi-supervised segmentation [1, 15] generate fake full masks (segmentation proposals) $\tilde{Y}$ for the unlabeled images, which are then used iteratively for network training by adding a standard cross-entropy loss of the form in Eq. (1): $\min_\theta \mathcal{L}_Y(\boldsymbol{\theta}) + \mathcal{L}_{\tilde{Y}}(\boldsymbol{\theta})$. The process consists of alternating segmentation-proposal generation and updating network parameters using both labeled data and the new generated masks. Typically such proposals are refined with additional priors such as dense CRF [20]. However, errors in such proposals may mislead training as the cross-entropy loss is minimized over mislabled points and, reinforcing early mistakes during training, as is well-known in the semi-supervised learning literature [4,25].

3   Curriculum Semi-supervised Learning

The general principle of curriculum learning consists of solving easy tasks first in order to infer some necessary properties about the unlabeled images. In particular, the first task is to learn image-level properties, e.g. the size of the target region, which is easier than learning pixelwise segmentations within an exponentially large label space. Then, we use such image-level properties to facilitate segmentation via constrained CNNs. Figure 1 depicts an illustration of our curriculum semi-supervised segmentation. We first use an auxiliary network that predicts the target-region size for a given image. Particularly, we train a regression network R (with parameters $\tilde{\boldsymbol{\theta}}$) by solving the following minimization problem:

$$\min_{\tilde{\theta}} \sum_{i\in\mathcal{S}} \left(R(X_i|\tilde{\boldsymbol{\theta}}) - \sum_{p\in\Omega} Y_{i,p} \right)^2. \tag{2}$$

This amounts to minimizing the squared difference between the predicted size and the actual region size.

Now we can define our constrained-CNN segmentation problem using auxiliary size predictions $R(X_i|\tilde{\boldsymbol{\theta}})$:

$$\min_\theta \mathcal{L}_Y(\boldsymbol{\theta})$$

$$\text{s.t.}\quad \forall i \in \mathcal{U} : (1-\gamma)R(X_i|\tilde{\boldsymbol{\theta}}) \le \sum_{p\in\Omega} S(X_i|\boldsymbol{\theta})_p \le (1+\gamma)R(X_i|\tilde{\boldsymbol{\theta}}), \tag{3}$$

where the inequality constraints impose the learned image-level information (i.e., region size) on the outputs of the segmentation network for unlabeled images, and γ is a hyper-parameter controlling constraints tightness. We use a penalty-based approach [8] for handling the inequality constraints, which accommodates standard stochastic gradient descent. This amounts to replacing the constraints in (3) with the following penalty over unlabeled samples:

$$\mathcal{L}_{\mathcal{U}}(\boldsymbol{\theta}) = \sum_{i \in \mathcal{U}} \mathcal{C} \left(\sum_{p \in \Omega} S(X_i|\boldsymbol{\theta})_p \right) \tag{4}$$

$$\mathcal{C}(t) = \begin{cases} (t - (1 - \gamma)R(X_i|\tilde{\boldsymbol{\theta}}))^2 & \text{if } t \leq (1 - \gamma)R(X_i|\tilde{\boldsymbol{\theta}}) \\ (t - (1 + \gamma)R(X_i|\tilde{\boldsymbol{\theta}}))^2 & \text{if } t \geq (1 + \gamma)R(X_i|\tilde{\boldsymbol{\theta}}) \\ 0 & \text{otherwise} \end{cases} \tag{5}$$

This gives our final unconstrained optimization problem: $\min_\theta \mathcal{L}_Y(\boldsymbol{\theta}) + \lambda \mathcal{L}_{\mathcal{U}}(\boldsymbol{\theta})$, with λ a hyper-parameter controlling the relative contribution of each term.

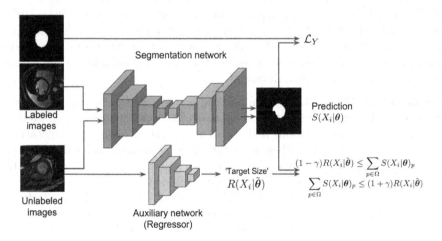

Fig. 1. Illustration of our curriculum semi-supervised segmentation strategy.

4   Experiments

4.1   Setup

Data. Our experiments focused on left ventricular endocardium segmentation. We used the training set from the publicly available data of the 2017 ACDC Challenge [3]. This set consists of 100 cine magnetic resonance (MR) exams covering well defined pathologies: dilated cardiomyopathy, hypertrophic cardiomyopathy, myocardial infarction with altered left ventricular ejection fraction and abnormal right ventricle. It also included normal subjects. Each exam only contains acquisitions at the diastolic and systolic phases. We sliced and resized the exams into 256×256 images. No additional pre-processing was performed.

Training. For the experiments, we employed 75 exams for training and the remaining 25 for validation. From the training set, we consider that n images are fully annotated and the pixel-wise annotations of the remaining $75-n$ images are unknown. The n images, and their corresponding ground truth, are employed to train both the auxiliary size predictor and the main segmentation network, in a separate way. To validate both networks, we split the validation set into two smaller subsets of 5 and 20 exams, respectively. The training set undergoes data augmentation only to train the size regressor, by flipping, mirroring and rotating (up to $45°$) the original images, obtaining a training set that is 10 times larger.

Implementation Details. We employed ResNeXt 101 [21] as the backbone architecture for our regressor model, with the squared $\mathcal{L}_2$ norm as the objective function. We trained via standard stochastic gradient descent, with a learning rate of 5×10^{-6}, a momentum of 0.9 and a weight decay of 10^{-4}, for 200 epochs. The learning rate was halved at epochs 100 and 150. We used a batch size of 10. We used ENet [16] as the segmentation network, trained with Adam [10], a learning rate of 5×10^{-4}, $\beta_1 = 0.9$ and $\beta_2 = 0.99$ for 100 epochs. The learning rate was halved if validation DSC did not improve for 20 epochs. We used a batch size of 1, and γ from Eq. (4) is set at $\gamma = 0.1$. We did not use any form of post-processing on the network output.

Comparative Methods. We compare the performance of the proposed semi-supervised curriculum segmentation approach to several models. First, we train a network using only n exams and their corresponding pixel-wise annotations, which is referred to as *FS*. Then, once this model is trained, and following standard proposal-based strategies for semi-supervision, e.g., [1], we perform the inference on the remaining $75-n$ exams, and include the CNN predictions in the training set, which serve as pseudo-labels for the non-annotated images (referred to as *Proposals*). In this particular case, the training reduces to minimizing the cross-entropy over all the pixels in the manually annotated images and over the pixels predicted as left-ventricle in the pseudo-labels. Since we investigate how to leverage unlabeled data only by learning from the subset of labeled data, we do not integrate any additional cues during training, such as Conditional Random Fields (CRF)[2]. Finally, we train a model with the exact size derived from the ground truth for each image, as in [8], which will serve as an upper bound, referred to as *Oracle*.

Evaluation. We resort to the common dice (DSC) overlap metric between the ground truth and the CNN segmentation to evaluate the performances of the segmentation models. More specifically, we report the mean and standard deviation of the validation DSC over the last 50 epochs of training.

---

[2] Note that the proposal-based methods in [1] use CRF to boost performance.

4.2   Results

We report in Table 1 and Fig. 2 the quantitative evaluation of the different segmentation models. First, we can observe that integrating the size predicted on unlabeled images by the auxiliary network improves the performance compared to solely training from labeled images. The gap is particularly significant when few annotated images are available, ranging from nearly 15 to 25% of difference in terms of DSC. As more labeled images are available, the proposed strategy still improves the performance of the fully supervised counterpart, but by a smaller margin, which goes from 1 to 3%. Compared to the *Oracle*, our method achieves comparable results as the number of training samples increases. This suggests that, when few annotated patients are available, having a better estimation of the size helps to better regularize the network. It is noteworthy to mention that in the *Oracle*, the exact size is known for each image, which results in extra supervision compared to the proposed method. The *proposals* method achieves the same or worse results than its *FS* counterpart, for all the n values evaluated. These results indicate that n patients are not sufficient to train an auxiliary network that generates usable pseudo-labels, due to the difficulty of the segmentation task. This confirms that training a network on an easier task, e.g., learning the size of the target region, can guide the training in a semi-supervised setting.

Table 1. Quantitative results for the different models. Values represent the mean Dice (and standard deviation) over the last 50 epochs.

# labeled patients	Method			
	FS	Proposals	Proposed	Oracle [8]
5	24.8 (4.9)	8.1 (0.8)	53.1 (3.0)	74.3 (2.5)
10	44.4 (8.3)	43.9 (2.9)	58.5 (3.6)	75.7 (3.9)
20	71.7 (3.2)	49.1 (5.0)	72.7 (1.6)	79.0 (2.5)
30	73.1 (1.7)	62.6 (4.4)	75.4 (1.6)	77.0 (1.9)
40	75.8 (2.4)	68.8 (5.6)	76.3 (2.1)	80.4 (2.1)
75	81.6 (1.9)	NA	NA	NA

Evolution of DSC on the validation set over training for some models is depicted in Fig. 3. From these plots, we can observe that the auxiliary network facilitates the training of a harder task, consistently achieving higher performance and better stability than its *FS* counterpart, especially when few labeled images are available. Regarding the instability of the *FS* method, it may be caused by the small number of samples employed for training, with no other source of information that regularizes the network.

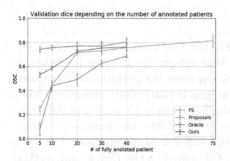

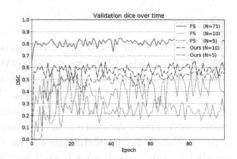

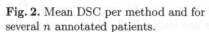

Fig. 2. Mean DSC per method and for several *n* annotated patients.

Fig. 3. Validation DSC over time, with a subset of the evaluated models.

Qualitative results are depicted in Fig. 4. Particularly, we show the prediction on the same slice with the different methods and for increasing *n*. We first observe that predictions of the *FS* model are very unstable, not clearly improving as more labeled images are included in the training, which aligns with the results found in Fig. 3. Then, the *Proposals* approach fails to generate visually acceptable segmentations, even with 30 pixel-wise labeled patients. Although

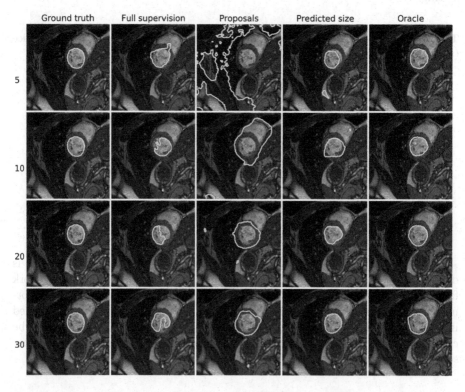

Fig. 4. Visual comparison for the different methods, with varying number of fully annotated patients used for training. Best viewed in colors

its performance improves with the number of labeled patients used in training, its results are not visually satisfying for any value of n. Our curriculum semi-supervised segmentation approach achieves decent results from $n = 5$. It only requires 20 patients to yield comparable segmentations to those of the *Oracle* and the manual ground truth.

References

1. Bai, W., et al.: Semi-supervised learning for network-based cardiac MR image segmentation. In: Descoteaux, M., Maier-Hein, L., Franz, A., Jannin, P., Collins, D.L., Duchesne, S. (eds.) MICCAI 2017. LNCS, vol. 10434, pp. 253–260. Springer, Cham (2017). https://doi.org/10.1007/978-3-319-66185-8_29
2. Baur, C., Albarqouni, S., Navab, N.: Semi-supervised deep learning for fully convolutional networks. In: Descoteaux, M., Maier-Hein, L., Franz, A., Jannin, P., Collins, D.L., Duchesne, S. (eds.) MICCAI 2017. LNCS, vol. 10435, pp. 311–319. Springer, Cham (2017). https://doi.org/10.1007/978-3-319-66179-7_36
3. Bernard, O., et al.: Deep learning techniques for automatic MRI cardiac multi-structures segmentation and diagnosis: is the problem solved? IEEE TMI **37**(11), 2514–2525 (2018)
4. Chapelle, O., Scholkopf, B., Zien, A.: Semi-supervised learning. IEEE Trans. Neural Netw. **20**(3), 542–542 (2009). (Chapelle, O. et al. (eds.) 2006) [book reviews]
5. Dong, N., Kampffmeyer, M., Liang, X., Wang, Z., Dai, W., Xing, E.: Unsupervised domain adaptation for automatic estimation of cardiothoracic ratio. In: Frangi, A.F., Schnabel, J.A., Davatzikos, C., Alberola-López, C., Fichtinger, G. (eds.) MICCAI 2018. LNCS, vol. 11071, pp. 544–552. Springer, Cham (2018). https://doi.org/10.1007/978-3-030-00934-2_61
6. Ganaye, P.-A., Sdika, M., Benoit-Cattin, H.: Semi-supervised learning for segmentation under semantic constraint. In: Frangi, A.F., Schnabel, J.A., Davatzikos, C., Alberola-López, C., Fichtinger, G. (eds.) MICCAI 2018. LNCS, vol. 11072, pp. 595–602. Springer, Cham (2018). https://doi.org/10.1007/978-3-030-00931-1_68
7. Jia, Z., Huang, X., Chang, E.I., Xu, Y.: Constrained deep weak supervision for histopathology image segmentation. IEEE TMI **36**(11), 2376–2388 (2017)
8. Kervadec, H., Dolz, J., Tang, M., Granger, E., Boykov, Y., Ben Ayed, I.: Constrained-CNN losses for weakly supervised segmentation. Med. Image Anal. **54**, 88–99 (2019)
9. Khoreva, A., Benenson, R., Hosang, J., Hein, M., Schiele, B.: Simple does it: weakly supervised instance and semantic segmentation. In: CVPR, pp. 876–885 (2017)
10. Kingma, D.P., Ba, J.: Adam: a method for stochastic optimization. arXiv preprint arXiv:1412.6980 (2014)
11. Lin, D., Dai, J., Jia, J., He, K., Sun, J.: ScribbleSup: scribble-supervised convolutional networks for semantic segmentation. In: CVPR, pp. 3159–3167 (2016)
12. Litjens, G., et al.: A survey on deep learning in medical image analysis. Med. Image Anal. **42**, 60–88 (2017)
13. Mondal, A.K., Dolz, J., Desrosiers, C.: Few-shot 3D multi-modal medical image segmentation using generative adversarial learning. arXiv:1810.12241 (2018)
14. Nie, D., Gao, Y., Wang, L., Shen, D.: ASDNet: attention based semi-supervised deep networks for medical image segmentation. In: Frangi, A.F., Schnabel, J.A., Davatzikos, C., Alberola-López, C., Fichtinger, G. (eds.) MICCAI 2018. LNCS, vol. 11073, pp. 370–378. Springer, Cham (2018). https://doi.org/10.1007/978-3-030-00937-3_43

15. Papandreou, G., Chen, L.C., Murphy, K., Yuille, A.L.: Weakly-and semi-supervised learning of a DCNN for semantic image segmentation. In: ICCV (2015)
16. Paszke, A., Chaurasia, A., Kim, S., Culurciello, E.: ENet: a deep neural network architecture for real-time semantic segmentation. arXiv preprint: arXiv:1606.02147 (2016)
17. Pathak, D., Krahenbuhl, P., Darrell, T.: Constrained convolutional neural networks for weakly supervised segmentation. In: ICCV, pp. 1796–1804 (2015)
18. Rajchl, M., et al.: DeepCut: object segmentation from bounding box annotations using convolutional neural networks. IEEE TMI 36(2), 674–683 (2017)
19. Sedai, S., Mahapatra, D., Hewavitharanage, S., Maetschke, S., Garnavi, R.: Semi-supervised segmentation of optic cup in retinal fundus images using variational autoencoder. In: Descoteaux, M., Maier-Hein, L., Franz, A., Jannin, P., Collins, D.L., Duchesne, S. (eds.) MICCAI 2017. LNCS, vol. 10434, pp. 75–82. Springer, Cham (2017). https://doi.org/10.1007/978-3-319-66185-8_9
20. Tang, M., Perazzi, F., Djelouah, A., Ben Ayed, I., et al.: On regularized losses for weakly-supervised CNN segmentation. In: ECCV, pp. 507–522 (2018)
21. Xie, S., Girshick, R., Dollár, P., Tu, Z., He, K.: Aggregated residual transformations for deep neural networks. In: CVPR, pp. 1492–1500 (2017)
22. Zhang, Y., David, P., Gong, B.: Curriculum domain adaptation for semantic segmentation of urban scenes. In: ICCV, pp. 2020–2030 (2017)
23. Zhang, Y., Yang, L., Chen, J., Fredericksen, M., Hughes, D.P., Chen, D.Z.: Deep adversarial networks for biomedical image segmentation utilizing unannotated images. In: Descoteaux, M., Maier-Hein, L., Franz, A., Jannin, P., Collins, D.L., Duchesne, S. (eds.) MICCAI 2017. LNCS, vol. 10435, pp. 408–416. Springer, Cham (2017). https://doi.org/10.1007/978-3-319-66179-7_47
24. Zhou, Y., et al.: Semi-supervised 3D abdominal multi-organ segmentation via deep multi-planar co-training. In: IEEE WACV, pp. 121–140 (2019)
25. Zhu, X., Goldberg, A.B.: Introduction to semi-supervised learning. Synth. Lect. Artif. Intell. Mach. Learn. 3(1), 1–130 (2009)

A Multi-modality Network
for Cardiomyopathy Death Risk
Prediction with CMR Images
and Clinical Information

Chaoyang Xia[1], Xiaojie Li[1], Xin Wang[2], Bin Kong[3], Yucheng Chen[4],
Youbing Yin[2], Kunlin Cao[2], Qi Song[2], Siwei Lyu[5], and Xi Wu[1(✉)]

[1] College of Computer Science, Chengdu University of Information Technology,
Chengdu, China
xi.wu@cuit.edu.cn
[2] CuraCloud Corporation, Seattle, WA 98104, USA
xinw@curacloudcorp.com
[3] University of North Carolina at Charlotte, Charlotte, USA
[4] West China Hospital, Sichuan University, Chengdu, China
chenyucheng2003@126.com
[5] SUNY Albany, Albany, USA

Abstract. Dilated Cardiomyopathy (DCM) is one of the main worldwide causes of sudden cardiac death (SCD). Early diagnostics significantly increases the chances of correct treatment and survival. However, there are no efficient methods for mortality risk prediction from learning cardiac magnetic resonance (CMR) image and clinical data due to the poor image quality and extreme imbalanced datasets. To solve this problem, we proposed an effective multi-modality network (MMNet) for mortality risk prediction in DCM, and we firstly directly optimize the AUC to train the multimodal deep learning classifier by maximizing the WMW statistic. This can achieve significant improvements in AUC, especially under the imbalanced learning problem. MMNet consists of two branches: clinical data branch and T1 mapping CMR images branch, which allows the model to learn more comprehensive features and makes a more accurate prediction. We validated our approach on a DCM dataset, which contains 450 CMR images that only holds 34 positive samples. Experimental results show that our approach archived accuracy of 98.89%, AUC of 99.61%, sensitivity of 100% and specificity of 98.8%, demonstrating the effectiveness of the proposed method.

Keywords: Dilated cardiomyopathy · Cross-modality medical data ·
AUC optimization

This study was supported by the major project of the Education Department in Sichuan (2017JQ0030 and 17ZA0063) and the National Natural Science Foundation of China (Grant No. 61602066), and in partly by the Project of Sichuan Outstanding Young Scientific and Technological Talents (19JCQN0003) and the Natural Science Foundation for Young Scientists of CUIT (J201704).
C. Xia and X. Li—Contributed equally to this work.

D. Shen et al. (Eds.): MICCAI 2019, LNCS 11765, pp. 577–585, 2019.
https://doi.org/10.1007/978-3-030-32245-8_64

1 Introduction

Dilated Cardiomyopathy (DCM) is a common chronic and life-threatening cardiopathy [5]. It can lead to cardiovascular death, progressive heart failure or sudden cardiac death (SCD). Thus, immediate emergency diagnosis of DCM is critical for life saving and later recovery. For severe cardiomyopathy patients, cardiologists may consider ventricular assist devices (VAD) or heart transplants operation in the early stage of an incident. However, both are not only expensive but also can lead to serious complications, including infection, thromboembolism, and multiple organ failure. In routine clinical diagnosis, especially for early screening and postoperative assessment, visual assessment and empirical evaluation are widely used. Nevertheless, they are subject to high inter-observer variability, and the results are subjective and non-reproducible. Furthermore, utilizing multi-modality medical data (e.g, clinical text report and magnetic resonance imaging (MRI)) to assess the accurate risk of DCM patients are even more challenging due to the complex nature of medical data (e.g., height, weight, family history of cardiopathy, blood pressure, and so on).

In this regard, automatic computer-aided diagnosis systems are highly desirable. Many attempts have been made to automatically assess the mortality risk in DCM. Traditional risk assessment approaches have been mainly based on boosted ensemble algorithms (feature selection by information gain ranking) [1,9]. However, most of these methods are based on a small subset of the clinical and imaging data. As a result, they are not able to capture sufficient information to establish intrinsic correspondences between the mortality risk and clinical and imaging data. Additionally, their performances are confined by the handcrafted descriptors. As the one of the most successful machine learning techniques today, Li et al. [7,8] provided manifold alignment and efficient boundary point detection method, which can help in the study of the characteristics of diseases. Deep learning has been successfully applied to the recognition and prediction of prostate cancer, Alzheimers disease, and vertebrae and neural foramina stenosis. In this work, we aim to propose a deep learning based framework for DCM mortality risk assessment.

Automatic assessment the mortality risk in DCM remains a challenging problem due to two main issues. First, due to the rare occurrences of death, the imaging data as well as the discrete clinical text data are highly imbalanced. Nevertheless, most of the existing classification losses such as cross entropy are not suitable for dealing with imbalanced classes. In machine learning literautre [10], many a study has suggested that compared to simple classification losses, AUC (area under the receiver operating characteristic curve) is a robust evaluation measure for classification problem. However, it is non-differentiable and not easy to compute. Therefore, directly optimize the AUC loss to train a classifier is usually impractical. Although existing sampling, adjust class weight and data enhancement have shown great success [3,12], the imbalanced learning problem is still challenging. Second, in routine clinical procedures, risk assessment of DCM is often carried out through evaluation of multi-modality image data (e.g., images and clinical text), in which one data modality is complementary to other modalities. Thus, fusing multi-modality medical data for accurate mortality risk assessment is highly desired.

In this paper, an end-to-end multimodal framework is proposed to solve the above issues. The core idea is to leverage the fused features extracted from the multi-modality data. It consists of two branches: clinical branch and image branch. The image branch is a 2D convolutional network, which extracts image features from the left ventricle T1 mapping CMR images. The clinical branch is a fully-connected network, which extracts features from clinical textual data. Afterward, these features are fused by concatenation layer for the final prediction. Furthermore, inspired by [13], we optimize the alternative Wilcoxon-Mann-Whitney (WMW) loss to directly optimize the AUC instead of other typical classification losses to address the imbalanced learning issue. Our method main contributions are as follows: (1) a multi-modal framework seamlessly fuse CMR images and clinical data features to better learn hierarchical feature representations; (2) we combine AUC optimization and multimodal framework together to train the proposed network. This approach effectively addresses the imbalanced learning issue. To the best of our knowledge, this is first work to directly use AUC to optimize complex deep neural networks.

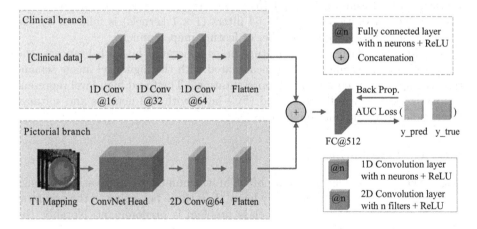

Fig. 1. The architecture of the multi-modality framework. It mainly consists of a pictorial branch and a clinical branch. The model is directly optimized by the AUC Loss.

2 Methodology

Figure 1 shows an overview of the proposed method. Our goal is to automatically generate a prediction score for the cardiac patients. A multi-modality framework is proposed to seamlessly fuse CMR images and clinical text features, thereby generating better hierarchical feature representations for accurate DCM risk assessment. Our network is able to effectively fuse the information from multi-modality medical data, helping it to generate more reliable predictions. We directly optimize the AUC loss to train the proposed network.

2.1 A Multi-Modality Network (MMNet)

As shown in Fig. 1, the proposed framework consists of two branches: the clinical branch and the pictorial branch. The clinical branch is used to extract 1D texture record features from clinical textual data. The first layers will learn the low level features with multiple 1D convolutional layers, which are followed by ReLU non-linearity activation layers. There are three convolutional layers (with 16, 32 and 64 filters) for feature extraction.

The pictorial branch automatically extract discriminative features from the CMR images. It consists of a ConNet Head (a convolutional network) and a convolutional layer. The ConvNet head is used to successively extract noisy-invariant high-level representations from the images. This is extremely important, especially when low-level features (e.g., color, texture) is not sufficient to represent the image due to various reasons (e.g., variation of image intensities). Note that our ConvNet Head is not limited to one kind of network. It can be VGG-16 [11], DenseNet-121, Inception-V3, and Xception, etc. To reduce the computational costs, a 2D convolution layer with 64 filters (1×1 kernels) is followed by the ConvNet head to reduce the number of feature map channels.

Finally, after flattening the feature maps generated by both branches, the high-level textual semantics are concatenated with the high-level image semantics, yielding the fused high-level representations. The fused high-level representations is fed into a fully connected (FC) layer with 512 neurons and softmax layer, generating the final predictions.

2.2 AUC Optimization

Due to the extremely low mortality of DCM, the number of observations belonging to the death class is significantly lower than those belonging to the non-fatal class. As a result, the imbalanced class problem is predominant. Notably, the rate of negative samples to positive samples is 12.23 in our dataset. In this situation, if the common loss functions such as cross entropy is employed to train the network, the prediction will be extremely biased. Although a very high accuracy can be obtained, the specificity is very low. Although AUC is non-differentiable and not easy to compute (it is usually used as a robust measure to evaluate the performance of classifiers), several works [13] had demonstrated that maximizing the alternative Wilcoxon-Mann-Whitney (WMW) loss is equivalent to directly optimizing AUC. Inspired by [13], we adopted the WMW loss to optimize our network. Formally,

$$
R(x_i, y_j) = \begin{cases} (-(x_i - y_j - \gamma))^p, & x_i - y_j < \gamma \\ 0, & otherwise \end{cases}
\tag{1}
$$

where the x_i is the predicted score for i^{th} positive sample, and y_j is the predicted generated for j^{th} negative sample. The margin γ and exponent p are two hyper-parameters. Finally, we directly optimize the AUC by minimizing the objective function U_R with $0 < \gamma \le 1$ and $p > 1$:

$$U_R = \sum_{i=0}^{m-1} \sum_{j=0}^{n-1} R(x_i, y_j). \tag{2}$$

Note that function R is differentiable, we can use any gradient based methods to train the MMNet.

3 Experiments

Data Acquisition and Pre-processing. Our experiments are conducted on a dataset with 450 patients, which are collected from our collaborative hospital. The clinical text reports and the incidents are provided by senior cardiologists during clinical examinations and follow-up visits. As each report belongs to a cardiomyopathy patient and each patient has several CMR images, each clinical text report corresponds to several CMR images.

All CMR images are 2D short axis cine native T1 mapping MR images. The pixel spaces of those CMR images range from $1.172 \times 1.172 \times 1.0\,\text{mm}^3$ to $1.406 \times 1.406 \times 1.0\,\text{mm}^3$. The original dimension size is $256 \times 218 \times 1$ pixels. To ensure the training datasets are one and the same common space to enable improved quantitative analysis, we resample the image to a spacing of $1.0 \times 1.0 \times 1.0\,\text{mm}^3$ to ensure isotropy and normalize the of CMR image intensities to $[-1, 1]$. The clinical text data contains extensive patient information such as family history of cardiopathy, height, weight, blood pressure. We normalize the categorical clinical textual values to $[0, 1]$.

Unfortunately, as the mortality rate is 7.5%, our dataset is extremely imbalanced. Due to the lack of positive samples, several data augmentations are applied to them to virtually enlarge the training set. These augmentations include: random rotation from 0 to 180 degrees, random vertical or horizontal flip, and random shift along the X axis or Y axis from 0 to 2%. During the augmentation process, the corresponding text data is duplicated. Four types of criteria is used to measure the performance of classifiers: (1) accuracy; (2) sensitivity; (3) specificity; (4) AUC.

Implementation Details. We adopted 5-fold cross-validation to evaluate the performances of different methods. The final evaluation score is calculated by averaging the scores of all 5 folds. We use Adam optimizer [6] with a initial learning rate of 0.003, and leave other parameters as Keras default. Our model uses batch size of 32 training with 40 epochs.

Results and Analysis. We compared our method with the signal model methods [4,11] that only using CMR images and traditional methods which only using clinical data to predict death risk. Table 1 shows the performance by traditional methods: Linear SVM, Decision Tree, Random Forest and other advanced CNN models: VGG-16 [11], ResNet-50 [4], DenseNet-121, Inception-V3, and Xception [2]. For a classifier, WMW loss aims to achieve reliable improvements in the AUC measure. In order to demonstrate the effectiveness of AUC optimization on imbalanced datasets, we also compare our framework with different loss function: BCE loss and WMW loss in deep architecture (see Table 1). Table 1 illustrates that our method in general achieve better performance than all the other methods, in terms of Accuracy, Sensitivity, Specificity and AUC, and the ROC curve for each method is shown in Fig. 2 (Left).

Table 1. Comparison of the proposed MMNet with the other advanced CNN methods of risk assessment.

Methods	Loss	Inputs	Accuracy	Sensitivity	Specificity	AUC
Linear SVM	–	Clinical	85.29%	0.0	100%	66.21%
Decision tree	–	Clinical	82.35%	0.0	100%	45.52%
Random forest	–	Clinical	85.29%	0.0	100%	63.10%
VGG-16	BCE	CMR	–	–	–	–
ResNet-50	BCE	CMR	80.67%	47.06%	83.41%	73.36%
Inception-V3	BCE	CMR	89.11%	26.47%	94.23%	73.47%
Xception	BCE	CMR	86.00%	41.18%	89.66%	78.00%
MMNet	BCE	CMR+Clinical	97.04%	100%	96.81%	99.31%
VGG-16	WMW	CMR	–	–	–	–
ResNet-50	WMW	CMR	72.00%	67.65%	72.36%	76.21%
Inception-V3	WMW	CMR	90.44%	44.12%	94.23%	75.24%
Xception	WMW	CMR	84.00%	41.18%	87.50%	78.09%
MMNet	WMW	CMR+Clinical	98.89%	100%	98.80%	99.61%

From the results of risk assessment in Table 1, we can observe three key points. First, it is difficult to train an effective classifier under imbalanced datasets. Traditional classification methods cannot identify any positive samples. Due to vanishing gradient problem, the VGG-16 cannot report valid results. Although Inception-V3 produce a high classification accuracy of 90.44%, the sensitivity actually is 44.12% and the specificity is 94.23% by contraries. This illustrates the Inception-V3 model learn too much about majority class, but it provides insufficient information about minority class. Therefore, it may predict almost every sample as majority class. Second, our proposed MMNet takes the advantage of the combined information of CMR images and clinical data, it performs much better in terms of five types of criteria than the other methods only use image information, but without clinical data. Specifically, MMNet with BCE loss achieves a classification accuracy of 97.04%, a sensitivity of 100%, a specificity of 96.81% and an AUC of 99.31%. Finally, AUC optimization is crucial for classification task when using imbalanced datasets. As shown in the rear rows in the Table 1, the MMNet with WMW loss achieve better performance than one with BCE loss. Moreover, Fig. 2 (Left) demonstrates again that our method achieves substantial improvement of the ROC curve over other advanced CNN models.

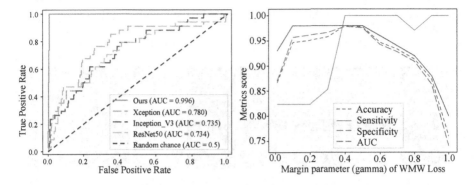

Fig. 2. Left: the ROC curves with AUC values for 5-fold cross-validation results of different methods. Right: the Accuracy, Sensitivity, Specificity and ROC curves of different γ for WMW Loss when $p = 3$ over 5-fold cross validation.

Hyper-parameter Selection. The WMW loss (Eq. (1)) has two essential hyper-parameters: the exponent p and the margin γ. Generally, we set $p = 3$ as suggested in [13]. Figure 2 (Right) shows how the average performance of our model varies with the parameter γ. As we can see, when $\gamma \leq 0.4$, our model consistently increases as γ increases. When $\gamma > 0.4$, all the metric scores in the figure start to decrease. Nevertheless, the AUC is less affected when γ is near 0.4, which demonstrates that the model has high robustness when $\gamma = 0.4$. Thus, we set $p = 3$ and $\gamma = 0.4$ in our experiment for the WMW loss.

Evaluation of the ConvNet Head. To investigate the effectiveness of using different convolutional network as ConvNet Head, we evaluate several widely used ConvNets in our framework and the results are summarized in Table 2. Experimental results show that our framework is consistent robust for various ConvNet Head.

Table 2. Comparison results of the different ConvNet as image branch heads.

Head	Accuracy	Sensitivity	Specificity	AUC
ResNet-50	99.11%	100%	99.04%	99.43%
VGG-16	99.11%	100%	99.04%	99.49%
Xception	96.22%	100%	95.91%	99.53%
Inception-V3	98.89%	100%	98.80%	99.61%

Class Activation Map (CAM). To further understand how the classifier make the predictions, we visualize the class activation map (CAM) [14] of the last convolutional layer. Two group of negative and positive examples are shown in Fig. 3. There are obvious difference on the corresponding CAMs of negative (survivors) and positive (dead) samples. We can see that the heatmap or jet color map of positive samples is more comparatively concentrated than that of negative samples.

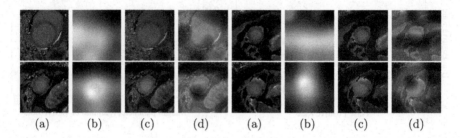

(a)   (b)   (c)   (d)   (a)   (b)   (c)   (d)

Fig. 3. Activation maps. The first row is examples of negative samples. The Second row is examples of positive samples. (a) shows the original CMR images. (b) are the activation maps, the green color indicates larger standard deviations, the pink color represents the maximum values and the white color is composed of both types. The heatmap is overlaid on the original images in (c). (d) displays heatmaps as jet color map and overlap on the original image, the red color highlights the activation region associated with the predicted class. (Color figure online)

4   Conclusion

In this paper, we proposed an effective multi-modality framework (MMNet) for mortality risk prediction in DCM. As far as we know, we are the first to directly optimize the AUC to train the multimodal deep learning classifier by maximizing the WMW statistic. This can achieve significant improvements in AUC, especially for the imbalanced learning problems. Experiment results demonstrate the superiority of the proposed method.

References

1. Afshin, M., et al.: Assessment of regional myocardial function via statistical features in MR images. In: Fichtinger, G., Martel, A., Peters, T. (eds.) MICCAI 2011. LNCS, vol. 6893, pp. 107–114. Springer, Heidelberg (2011). https://doi.org/10.1007/978-3-642-23626-6_14
2. Chollet, F.: Xception: deep learning with depthwise separable convolutions. In: CVPR, pp. 1251–1258 (2017)
3. Fadaee, M., Bisazza, A., Monz, C.: Data augmentation for low-resource neural machine translation. arXiv preprint arXiv:1705.00440 (2017)
4. He, K., Zhang, X., Ren, S., Sun, J.: Deep residual learning for image recognition. In: CVPR, pp. 770–778 (2016)

5. Jefferies, J.L., Towbin, J.A.: Dilated cardiomyopathy. Lancet **375**(9716), 752–762 (2010)
6. Kingma, D.P., Ba, J.: Adam: a method for stochastic optimization. arXiv preprint arXiv:1412.6980 (2014)
7. Li, X., Lv, J.C., Zhang, Y.: Manifold alignment based on sparse local structures of more corresponding pairs. In: Twenty-Third International Joint Conference on Artificial Intelligence (2013)
8. Li, X., Lv, J., Yi, Z.: An efficient representation-based method for boundary point and outlier detection. IEEE Trans. Neural Netw. Learn. Syst. **29**(1), 51–62 (2018)
9. Motwani, M., Dey, D., Berman, D.S., Germano, G., Achenbach, S., et al.: Machine learning for prediction of all-cause mortality in patients with suspected coronary artery disease: a 5-year multicentre prospective registry analysis. Eur. Heart J. **38**(7), 500–507 (2016)
10. Provost, F.J., Fawcett, T., Kohavi, R., et al.: The case against accuracy estimation for comparing induction algorithms. In: ICML, vol. 98, pp. 445–453 (1998)
11. Simonyan, K., Zisserman, A.: Very deep convolutional networks for large-scale image recognition. arXiv preprint arXiv:1409.1556 (2014)
12. Szegedy, C., et al.: Going deeper with convolutions. In: CVPR, pp. 1–9 (2015)
13. Yan, L., Dodier, R.H., Mozer, M., Wolniewicz, R.H.: Optimizing classifier performance via an approximation to the Wilcoxon-Mann-Whitney statistic. In: ICML, pp. 848–855 (2003)
14. Zhou, B., Khosla, A., Lapedriza, A., Oliva, A., Torralba, A.: Learning deep features for discriminative localization. In: CVPR, pp. 2921–2929 (2016)

3D Cardiac Shape Prediction with Deep Neural Networks: Simultaneous Use of Images and Patient Metadata

Rahman Attar[1,2(✉)], Marco Pereañez[1], Christopher Bowles[1],
Stefan K. Piechnik[3], Stefan Neubauer[3], Steffen E. Petersen[4],
and Alejandro F. Frangi[1,2(✉)]

[1] Center for Computational Imaging and Simulation Technologies in Biomedicine,
School of Computing, University of Leeds, Leeds, UK
[2] Biomedical Imaging Department,
Leeds Institute for Cardiovascular and Metabolic Medicine, School of Medicine,
University of Leeds, Leeds, UK
{r.attar,a.frangi}@leeds.ac.uk
[3] Oxford Center for Clinical Magnetic Resonance Research (OCMR),
Division of Cardiovascular Medicine, University of Oxford, John Radcliffe Hospital,
Oxford, UK
[4] William Harvey Research Institute, NIHR Barts Biomedical Research Unit,
Queen Mary University of London and Barts Heart Centre,
St Bartholomew's Hospital, Barts Health NHS Trust, London, UK

Abstract. Large prospective epidemiological studies acquire cardiovascular magnetic resonance (CMR) images for pre-symptomatic populations and follow these over time. To support this approach, fully automatic large-scale 3D analysis is essential. In this work, we propose a novel deep neural network using both CMR images and patient metadata to directly predict cardiac shape parameters. The proposed method uses the promising ability of statistical shape models to simplify shape complexity and variability together with the advantages of convolutional neural networks for the extraction of solid visual features. To the best of our knowledge, this is the first work that uses such an approach for 3D cardiac shape prediction. We validated our proposed CMR analytics method against a reference cohort containing 500 3D shapes of the cardiac ventricles. Our results show broadly significant agreement with the reference shapes in terms of the estimated volume of the cardiac ventricles, myocardial mass, 3D Dice, and mean and Hausdorff distance.

1 Introduction

Cardiovascular disease (CVD) is the most prevalent cause of death worldwide [1]. Early quantitative assessment of cardiac function and structure allow for proper preventive care, and early cardiovascular treatment. To support such an approach, analysis and interpretation of large-scale population-based cardiovascular

© Springer Nature Switzerland AG 2019
D. Shen et al. (Eds.): MICCAI 2019, LNCS 11765, pp. 586–594, 2019.
https://doi.org/10.1007/978-3-030-32245-8_65

magnetic resonance (CMR) imaging studies are of high importance in the medical image analysis community. This helps to identify patterns and trends across population groups, and accordingly, reveal insights into key risk factors before CVDs fully develop.

We believe that true 3D analysis is essential for the structural assessment of global and regional cardiac function. We propose a new approach that ensures the global coherence of the cardiac anatomy and naturally lends itself to further analysis in which full 3D anatomy is necessary; for example, in mechanical and flow simulations, or modelling the relationship between cardiac morphology and patient information such as: socio-demographic, lifestyle and environmental, family history, genetic, and omics data.

Though fully automatic 3D segmentation is required for further analysis, the complexity of anatomical structures and their local intensity variation across a population cohort make it challenging. Statistical 3D shape model-based approaches such as [1] have been successfully used for automatically segmenting cardiac structures and generating associated function indexes. This is mainly attributed to the inclusion of prior knowledge of the cardiac shape into the segmentation method. These segmentation approaches typically use very simple features such as gradients on intensity profiles to fit a 3D model. This is an iterative process in which the goal is to minimise the Mahalanobis distance between an intensity profile sampled at a candidate position and its corresponding intensity appearance model by deforming the shape within its range of normal variation to match the image data. On the other hand, in the last decade, fully convolutional networks (FCN) have shown great potential in image-based pattern recognition in a variety of tasks, including cardiac segmentation. However, their output results are, by nature, 2D segmentation masks for every short axis (SAX) and long axis (LAX) CMR slices. Although these 2D masks are sometimes extended via a further step of non-rigid registration to a 3D atlas to produce a 3D cardiac shape [2], this is not efficient for learning topological shape information.

In this paper, we propose to exploit image features obtained using deep FCNs trained on both SAX and LAX views, along with the rich shape priors learned using statistical shape models, to jointly and simultaneously predict the parameters of 3D cardiac shapes, instead of a pixel-wise classification across each 2D slice. Another significant aspect of this work is the integration of patient metadata into the process of shape prediction using a Multilayer Perceptron (MLP). This information, which is currently ignored in cardiac segmentation or shape generation, has been shown in different clinical studies to have an impact on cardiac morphology and structure [3]. We hope this work inspires other researchers to exploit the priors offered by patient metadata in other applications for potentially more accurate and patient-specific models.

The Contributions of this Paper are Three-Fold: we propose (1) an innovative end-to-end deep neural network that directly predicts 3D shape parameters derived from a Principal Component Analysis (PCA) space; (2) a novel approach using two CMR image views and patient metadata simultaneously to predict cardiac shape; (3) a creative loss function defined in the domain of 3D shape parameters which weights each PCA mode of variation independently, prioritising the more significant modes and leading to more accurate shape prediction.

2   Methods

2.1   Reference 3D Shapes of Cardiac Ventricles

We generated a reference cohort of 3D shapes through the non-rigid registration of a 3D biventricular model to a set of 3D points obtained from manual delineations using the Coherent Point Drift (CPD) method [4]. The 3D model is comprised of two structures; the Left Ventricle (LV) and the Right Ventricle (RV). The LV is a closed water-tight mesh comprising both endo and epicardial walls. The RV is an open mesh representing only the RV endocardium. The RV has two openings, the atrioventricular valve opening, and the pulmonary valve opening. Figure 1 shows a sample of manual 2D contours and its corresponding 3D shape obtained from the CPD method.

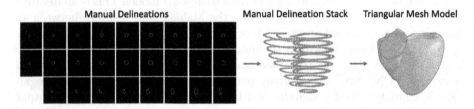

Fig. 1. An example 3D shape of cardiac ventricles constructed from a stack of 2D manual contours on SAX view slices.

2.2   Point Distribution Model (PDM)

The PDM encodes the mean and variance of the 3D cardiac shapes. The PDM is constructed during training using PCA on a set of generalised Procrustes-aligned shapes. Assume a training set of M shapes, each described by N points in $\mathcal{R}^3$, i.e., $(\mathbf{x}_j^i, \mathbf{y}_j^i, \mathbf{z}_j^i)$ with $i = 1, ..., M$ and $j = 1, ..., N$. Further, let $\mathbf{s}_i = (\mathbf{x}_1^i, \mathbf{y}_1^i, \mathbf{z}_1^i, ..., \mathbf{x}_N^i, \mathbf{y}_N^i, \mathbf{z}_N^i)^T$ be the i-th vector representing the i-th shape. Finally, let $\mathbf{S} = [\mathbf{s}^1, ..., \mathbf{s}^M]$ be the set of all training shapes in matrix form. The shape class mean and covariance of $\mathbf{S}$ is calculated as follows:

$$\bar{\mathbf{s}} = \frac{1}{M} \sum_{i=1}^{M} \mathbf{s}_i \quad \text{and} \quad \mathbf{C} = \frac{1}{M-1} \sum_{i=1}^{M} (\mathbf{s}_i - \bar{\mathbf{s}})(\mathbf{s}_i - \bar{\mathbf{s}})^T \tag{1}$$

The shape covariance is represented in a low-dimensional PCA space. This provides l eigenvectors $\boldsymbol{\Phi} = [\varphi_1 \varphi_2 ... \varphi_l]$, and corresponding eigenvalues $\boldsymbol{\Lambda} =$

$diag(\lambda_1, \lambda_2, ..., \lambda_l)$ computed through the Singular Value Decomposition of the covariance matrix. Hence, assuming the shape class follows a multi-dimensional Gaussian probability distribution, any shape in the shape class can be approximated from the following linear generative model:

$$\mathbf{s} \approx \bar{\mathbf{s}} + \mathbf{\Phi}\mathbf{b} \tag{2}$$

where $\mathbf{b}$ are shape parameters restricted to $|\mathbf{b}_i| \leq \beta\sqrt{\lambda_i}$; we typically set $\beta = 3$ to capture 99.7% of shape variability. The shape parameters of $\mathbf{s}$ can then be estimated as follows:

$$\mathbf{b} = \mathbf{\Phi}_l^T(\mathbf{s} - \bar{\mathbf{s}}). \tag{3}$$

Here, the entries of $\mathbf{b}$ are the projection coefficients of mean-centred shapes $(\mathbf{s} - \bar{\mathbf{s}})$ along the columns of $\mathbf{\Phi}$.

2.3 Images and Metadata

Each CMR image volume was pre-processed as follows. Each 9-slice SAX stack was intensity normalised by saturating the top 0.2% of intensities and scaling between 0 and 1, and spatially normalised by aligning a fixed point, defined as the average point of intersection between the three LAX views and each SAX slice, and angle, defined as the angle of the 4-chamber LAX, to a standard location and angle respectively. A 64×64 px region of interest (ROI) was then sampled from each slice at a 2 mm isotropic resolution. The corresponding 4-chamber LAX views were similarly intensity normalised, with a 80×60 px ROI sampled at the same 2 mm resolution around the point of intersection between the three LAX views and the basel SAX slice, and zero-padded to 80×80 px. Table 1 shows the summary of the metadata available for every image volume including both continuous and categorical variables. All variables were scaled to the range $[0, 1]$, including categorical variables (viz. $sex/alcohol \in (0, 1)$, $smoking \in (0, 0.5, 1)$).

2.4 Network Architecture and Loss Function

Figure 2 shows a diagram of the proposed method. The network has three inputs: SAX view images, LAX view image, and metadata. The output is the predicted shape parameters $b^P = \{b_i^P | i = 1, ..., k\}$. To train the proposed architecture, we introduce the following loss function for training:

$$\mathbf{E}(\theta) = \sum_{i=1}^{k} f(b_i^P(\theta), b_i^R) \cdot w(i, k) \quad \text{where} \quad w(i, k) = \sqrt{\frac{k - i + 1}{k}} \tag{4}$$

where k is the number of shape parameters, θ denotes the network parameters, $f(.)$ denotes the absolute error of the difference between the reference value (b_i^R) and the value $(b_i^P(\theta))$ predicted by the network. $w(.)$ denotes a weighting function depending on the importance of the $i - th$ mode of variation on shape

Table 1. Summary of the subject metadata used in this study.

Type	Metadata	Range
Continuous	Age (years)	61 ± 7
	Weight (kg)	76 ± 15
	Height (cm)	170 ± 9
	Body mass index (kg/m2)	27 ± 4
	Body surface area (m2)	1.8 ± 0.2
	Heart rate (bpm)	68 ± 11
	Diastolic blood pressure (mmHg)	79 ± 11
	Systolic blood pressure (mmHg)	139 ± 19
Categorical	Sex	Male/female
	Smoking status	Never/previous/current
	Alcohol consumed	Yes/no

prediction, i.e. it assigns a higher weight to first modes of variation in the shape's PCA space. The first modes of variations in the PCA space are critical as they are the main parameters to affect the shape structure. Predicting these accurately is, therefore, more important as they have the greatest control over the final predicted shape. Ultimately, having the mean shape, eigenvectors and predicted shape parameters, the final shape can be predicted using Eq. 2.

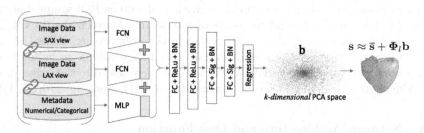

Fig. 2. The proposed method extracts a high-level representation of the image from SAX and LAX views using two FCNs, and concatenates the image features together along with the output of an MLP network applied to the metadata. Four fully connected layers with ReLU or Sigmoid activation functions and batch normalisation then produce the k parameters in PCA space which describe the 3D shape of the cardiac ventricles.

As illustrated in Fig. 3, the FCN used in this work has been adapted from the down-sampling path of a U-Net [5] architecture with an encoder depth of 2 for the LAX and 4 for the SAX images. The last layer of the FCNs have an extra convolutional layer with the kernel size of the current feature map dimensions to produce a vector of features - 1024 for SAX and 256 for LAX. The MLP has 11 inputs (size of metadata feature vector), 3 hidden layers (with 16, 32, and 64

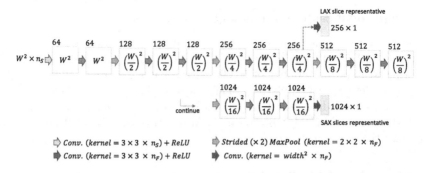

Fig. 3. The architecture of the two FCNs used in this study to obtain a vector of features representing the image information derived from the LAX and SAX views. A separate network is used for each view, with the LAX and SAX networks containing 9 and 15 layers respectively. The FCNs are composed of convolutional layers, with ReLUs and max-pooling. W is the image width and height, n_S and n_F are the number of slices in each image volume and the number of activation maps respectively.

neurons), and an output layer (with 128 neurons). ReLU is used in hidden and output layers.

The outputs of the three sub-networks are concatenated to construct one feature vector (with the size of $1024 + 256 + 128 = 1408$ neurons) that contains the behavioural, phenotypic, and demographic information derived from the metadata in addition to visual information from the imaging data. This information is fed into four fully connected layers, with ReLU (first two layers) and Sigmoid (last two layers) activation functions and batch normalisation, so that, by minimising $E(\theta)$ from Eq. 4, they produce the first k parameters in PCA space which describe the 3D shape of the cardiac ventricles. To capture 99.7% of shape variability in the training dataset we set $k = 28$ and regress only those parameters from randomly initialised weights.

3 Experiments and Results

3.1 Data and Annotations

We performed experiments on 3500 CMR image volumes from the UK Biobank (UKB) using both end-diastolic and end-systolic time points. In terms of population sample size, experimental setup, and quality control, the most reliable reference annotations of cardiovascular structure and function found in the literature are those reported by [6], in which CMR scans were manually delineated and analysed by a team of eight expert observers. These delineations were used to generate the reference 3D shapes, as explained in Sect. 2.1. The dataset was randomly split into a training (3000) and test set (500). The performance is reported on the test set with mean ± standard deviation.

3.2   Implementation and Training

The method was implemented using Python and Tensorflow. The network was trained using Adam for optimising the loss function (Eq. 4) with the learning rate of 0.001 and iteration number of 50,000 with a batch size of 10 subjects, all of which were determined empirically. There was no data augmentation. Training took ~10 h on Nvidia Tesla V100 GPUs hosted by Amazon Web Service and accessed using the MULTI-X platform [7]. At test time, it took less than a second to predict the shape parameters.

3.3   Accuracy of Predicted Shapes

Figure 4 shows some samples of ventricular shapes generated by our proposed method (in purple) overlaid with the corresponding reference shapes (in grey). It confirms that the network is capable of predicting accurate shape parameters to generate shapes very similar to the reference shapes obtained by manual delineations. To quantify the amount of similarity, we evaluated the performance of the proposed method by computing the Dice index ($\mathcal{D}$), and the mean ($\mathcal{M}$) and Hausdorff distance ($\mathcal{H}$) between reference and predicted shapes. Since this method outputs the parameters of a shape in the space, we first align the two shapes by removing their orientation and translation before computing the aforementioned metrics. $\mathcal{D}$ is between 0 and 1, with a higher $\mathcal{D}$ indicating a better match between the two shapes. $\mathcal{M}$ and $\mathcal{H}$ measure the mean and maximum distance, respectively, between the two surfaces, with a lower value indicating a better the agreement. Moreover, we report the effect of including the metadata in Table 2. As expected, the use of the metadata alongside the image information improves the network, leading to a more accurate prediction in all cardiac substructures. In addition to comparing against reference measurements, we also compare against one baseline method proposed by Attar et al. [1] in which the authors carried out 3D analysis of the UKB CMR images using a shape model-based approach where the model is fitted during an iterative process using traditional intensity profiles.

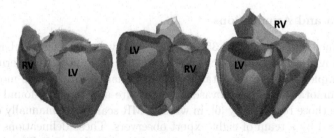

Fig. 4. Three samples of the generated 3D shapes of LV and RV. The grey shape is the reference whereas the purple shape is the predicted. (Color figure online)

Table 2. Comparison of shape prediction accuracy using only images (IMG) or images with metadata (IMG+MTDT) in terms of $\mathcal{D}$ (%), $\mathcal{M}$ (mm) and $\mathcal{H}$ (mm) for LV endo-/epicardium and RV endocardium. **Bold** indicates best performing method.

	LV endocardium			LV epicardium			RV endocardium		
	[1]	IMG	IMG+MTDT	[1]	IMG	IMG+MTDT	[1]	IMG	IMG+MTDT
$\mathcal{D}$	**0.91±0.05**	0.82±0.09	0.90±0.04	0.92±0.05	0.83±0.08	**0.93±0.05**	0.88±0.08	0.79±0.09	**0.90±0.08**
$\mathcal{M}$	1.85±0.75	3.45±0.94	**1.81±0.70**	**1.80±0.62**	3.02±0.84	1.82±0.66	2.02±0.72	3.00±0.91	**2.00±0.70**
$\mathcal{H}$	3.76±1.52	8.78±1.96	**3.11±1.49**	**3.32±1.38**	7.69±1.77	3.55±1.49	8.32±3.12	12.11±5.21	**7.05±3.03**

As shown in Table 2, $\mathcal{D}$ values show excellent agreement between reference and predicted shapes (≥ 0.90). $\mathcal{M}$ values are comparable to the in-plane pixel spacing range of 1.8 mm to 2.3 mm found in the UKB. Although $\mathcal{H}$ is larger, it is still within an acceptable range when compared with the distance range seen in [1] or [2]. Note that the performance of the proposed method on RV is consistently better than the other approaches. Furthermore, we report the absolute and relative difference of the main cardiac function indexes (viz. LV and RV volume (ml) and myocardium mass (g)) derived from the predicted and the reference shapes in Table 3. The proposed method achieved significantly lower error in volume and mass estimation, with p < 0.001 in paired t-tests.

Table 3. Comparison of the absolute and relative difference between the reference and predicted shapes. **Bold** indicates best performing method.

	Absolute difference			Relative difference (%)		
	[1]	IMG	IMG+MTDT	[1]	IMG	IMG+MTDT
LV volume	7.51 ± 5.42	9.80 ± 6.33	**6.01 ± 4.98**	9.50 ± 8.80	10.31 ± 9.45	**8.03 ± 5.05**
LV mass	8.42 ± 5.22	10.11 ± 8.14	**7.11 ± 5.14**	9.10 ± 8.01	12.03 ± 9.22	**8.12 ± 7.54**
RV volume	10.59 ± 7.16	12.62 ± ± 10.14	**9.24 ± 5.20**	11.36 ± 8.11	14.55 ± 9.89	**10.03 ± 7.00**

Overall, the proposed method (IMG+MTDT) has superior accuracy to reference shapes than [1], while being on average ~30 times faster during test time. This can be attributed to the combined use of image and patient metadata within a single network to directly predict shape parameters. The introduction of the metadata yielded a substantial positive impact on shape prediction with a ~15% average improvement across all metrics. We believe that including this information provides the network with a variable prior by allowing it to learn the likely distributions of shape parameters across different populations.

4 Conclusion

In this study, we presented a fully automatic framework capable of producing 3D cardiac shapes via the simultaneous use of images and patient metadata. We validated our workflow on a reference cohort of 500 subjects for which ground truth shapes exist with promising results. In particular, we showed a significant positive impact from including the metadata. As future work, in addition to investigating the effect of other clinical variables on shape prediction, we would like to increase the robustness of our pipeline to locate the shape in the image space, and handle severe pathological morphology, variable image quality, and alternative modalities. We also plan to explore the use of patient metadata in other deep learning applications.

Acknowledgements. RA was funded by a PhD scholarship from the School of Computing, University of Leeds. AFF is supported by the Royal Academy of Engineering Chair in Emerging Technologies Scheme (CiET1819\19) and the MedIAN Network (EP/N026993/1) funded by the Engineering and Physical Sciences Research Council (EPSRC).

References

1. Attar, R., et al.: High throughput computation of reference ranges of biventricular cardiac function on the UK biobank population cohort. In: Pop, M., et al. (eds.) STACOM 2018. LNCS, vol. 11395, pp. 114–121. Springer, Cham (2019). https://doi.org/10.1007/978-3-030-12029-0_13
2. Duan, J., et al.: Automatic 3D bi-ventricular segmentation of cardiac images by a shape-refined multi-task deep learning approach. IEEE Trans. Med. Imaging (2019)
3. Gilbert, K., et al.: Independent left ventricular morphometric atlases show consistent relationships with cardiovascular risk factors: a UK biobank study. Sci. Rep. **9**(1), 1130 (2019)
4. Myronenko, A., Song, X.: Point set registration: coherent point drift. IEEE Trans. Pattern Anal. Mach. Intell. **32**(12), 2262–2275 (2010)
5. Ronneberger, O., Fischer, P., Brox, T.: U-net: convolutional networks for biomedical image segmentation. In: Navab, N., Hornegger, J., Wells, W.M., Frangi, A.F. (eds.) MICCAI 2015. LNCS, vol. 9351, pp. 234–241. Springer, Cham (2015). https://doi.org/10.1007/978-3-319-24574-4_28
6. Petersen, S.E., et al.: Reference ranges for cardiac structure and function using cardiovascular magnetic resonance (CMR) in caucasians from the UK biobank population cohort. J. Cardiovasc. Magn. Reson. **19**(1), 18 (2017)
7. de Vila, M.H., Attar, R., Pereanez, M., Frangi, A.F.: MULTI-X, a state-of-the-art cloud-based ecosystem for biomedical research. In: 2018 IEEE International Conference on Bioinformatics and Biomedicine (BIBM), pp. 1726–1733. IEEE (2018)

Discriminative Consistent Domain Generation for Semi-supervised Learning

Jun Chen[1], Heye Zhang[2], Yanping Zhang[1($\boxtimes$)], Shu Zhao[1], Raad Mohiaddin[3,4], Tom Wong[3,4], David Firmin[3,4], Guang Yang[3,4($\boxtimes$)], and Jennifer Keegan[3,4]

[1] School of Computer Science and Technology, Anhui University, Hefei, China
zhangyp2@gmail.com
[2] School of Biomedical Engineering, Sun Yat-Sen University, Shenzhen, China
[3] Cardiovascular Research Centre, Royal Brompton Hospital, London SW3 6NP, UK
[4] National Heart and Lung Institute, Imperial College London,
London SW7 2AZ, UK
g.yang@imperial.ac.uk

Abstract. Deep learning based task systems normally rely on a large amount of manually labeled training data, which is expensive to obtain and subject to operator variations. Moreover, it does not always hold that the manually labeled data and the unlabeled data are sitting in the same distribution. In this paper, we alleviate these problems by proposing a discriminative consistent domain generation ($DCDG$) approach to achieve a semi-supervised learning. The discriminative consistent domain is achieved by a double-sided domain adaptation. The double-sided domain adaptation aims to make a fusion of the feature spaces of labeled data and unlabeled data. In this way, we can fit the differences of various distributions between labeled data and unlabeled data. In order to keep the discriminativeness of generated consistent domain for the task learning, we apply an indirect learning for the double-sided domain adaptation. Based on the generated discriminative consistent domain, we can use the unlabeled data to learn the task model along with the labeled data via a consistent image generation. We demonstrate the performance of our proposed $DCDG$ on the late gadolinium enhancement cardiac MRI (LGE-CMRI) images acquired from patients with atrial fibrillation in two clinical centers for the segmentation of the left atrium anatomy (LA) and proximal pulmonary veins (PVs). The experiments show that our semi-supervised approach achieves compelling segmentation results, which can prove the robustness of $DCDG$ for the semi-supervised learning using the unlabeled data along with labeled data acquired from a single center or multicenter studies.

J. Chen and H. Zhang—These authors contributed equally to this work.

Electronic supplementary material The online version of this chapter (https://doi.org/10.1007/978-3-030-32245-8_66) contains supplementary material, which is available to authorized users.

D. Shen et al. (Eds.): MICCAI 2019, LNCS 11765, pp. 595–604, 2019.
https://doi.org/10.1007/978-3-030-32245-8_66

1   Introduction

Fitting the possible differences of distributions between labeled data and unlabeled data is of high importance for the semi-supervised learning. The usage of unlabeled data can overcome the limitation of insufficient labeled data, which is normally a hurdle in medical image analysis problems that lack labeled data. In practice, incorporating unlabeled data may fail due to the domain shift between labeled data and unlabeled data [1].

The domain adaptation can learn generically adaptive representation domain but is subject to the limited discriminative feature domain for the task model learning. On the one hand, recent domain adaptation approaches usually introduce a discriminator to encourage data from one domain to generate a feature domain that is similar to the other one by keeping inter representation invariant between the two domains. They are based on a single adaptation direction. Thus the generated feature space is limited by one of the two domains. Because the original feature space of the other domain is lost, it can result in a reduced feature space of the two domains. On the other hand, the widespread domain adaptation approaches work with only the labeled data for the task model learning. The unlabeled data is only used to generate the domain adaptation space along with the labeled data based on an adversarial learning. Therefore, the discriminativeness of adapted features for subsequent task model still completely rely on the labeled data. Consequently, it is hard to guarantee the discriminativeness of adapted features for task learning of the unlabeled data.

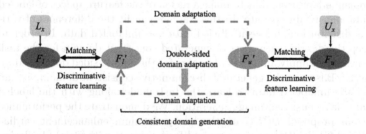

Fig. 1. Indirect double-sided domain adaptation. The labeled data (L_x) and the unlabeled data (U_x) are mapped to the adapted consistent feature domain $F(F_l$ and $F_u)$. The F is generated based on the double-sided domain adaptation via an indirect adversarial learning that the domain discriminator is applied to the feature domain F', which is obtained from the predicted label. Feature matching is then used to keep the consistence between F and F'.

In this work, we propose a discriminative consistent domain generation method based on double-sided domain adaptation (as shown in Fig. 1) to learn a task model (TM) in a semi-supervised manner. In our proposed $DCDG$, the available labeled data $L = (L_x, L_y)$ come from domain D_l and the unlabeled data $U = (U_x)$ come from domain D_u. The D_l and D_u are from the same or a similar domain. We adopt the double-sided domain adaptation to generate a consistent feature domain F that fuses the feature spaces of D_l and D_u instead of extracting the common parts of two domains or making one domain to adapt the other one. $DCDG$ shares a feature representation generator $FG \rightarrow F$ that maps L_x and U_x to the consistent feature domain F (F_l and F_u). For the purpose of discriminative feature generation, we map F to the predicted label domain via TM. Then the domain discriminator maps predicted label domain to another feature domain (F') to make an identification via indirect double-sided domain adaptation for F. During the indirect double-sided domain adaptation, the parameters of TM are fixed and we constrain F' to match the F generated by FG. We can adapt the F indirectly by adapting the F' to guarantee the discriminativeness of feature domain F for the subsequent learning of TM. During the discriminative consistent feature domain generation, we can learn the TM although there are no available labels in U_x for us to directly learn the TM. The F' is matched with F, which is produced by both the L_x and U_x. We can further map F' to the generated labeled and unlabeled data (L'_x and U'_x) to use the image consistency as the semi-supervised information to learn the TM. We demonstrate the performance of our proposed $DCDG$ for the left atrium segmentation [2,3] on a LGE-CMRI dataset, which plays an important role in the management of atrial fibrillation and myocardial infarction [4,5].

2   Method

The proposed $DCDG$ tries to generate the discriminative consistent feature domain with fused feature space from the labeled data L_x and unlabeled data

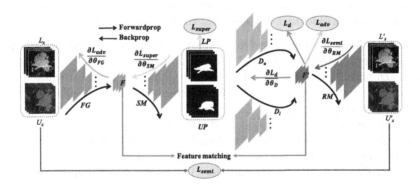

Fig. 2. Illustration of the proposed $DCDG$. L_x and U_x represent the labeled data and unlabeled data respectively. They share a common feature generator (FG) to generate the consistent features F. Then the F is mapped to the LP and UP of LA and PVs mask for L_x and U_x by the segmentation model (SM). Next, two domain discriminators with shared weights map the LP and UP to a feature domain (F') to make an identification via indirect double-sided adversarial learning for F. During the adversarial learning, the parameters of SM are fixed and we constrain F' to match the F generated by FG. Finally, the F' is mapped to the L'_x and U'_x matched with L_x and U_x.

U_x by the indirect double-sided domain adaptatipon. Meanwhile, we introduce an extra image consistent generation as the semi-supervised learning. Then the segmentation model can also be trained by the U_x along with the L_x. Detailed network configuration can be found in the supplementary materials.

Discriminative Feature Extraction via Indirect Learning. We aim to generate the consistent feature domain via double-sided domain adaptation to learn a segmentation model using both the labeled data L_x and the unlabeled data U_x. It is important to maintain the discriminativeness of feature representations for the generated consistent feature domain. Hence, we introduce the indirect learning for the discriminative feature domain extraction. In our proposed $DCDG$, we use a feature generator FG to generate the consistent feature domain F (F_l and F_u) from the L_x and U_x without using any knowledge of the source of images during testing [6]. In order to guarantee the discriminativeness of the generated features for subsequent segmentation model, we introduce the indirect domain adaptation instead of direct domain adaptation for F. We map the generated feature F to the estimated LA and PVs with probability maps (LP and UP) of L_x and U_x via the segmentation model (SM). Then the domain discriminator (D) generates the feature domain F' (F'_l and F'_u) by the final convolutional layer from LP and UP, and finally produces a scalar value to identify the F'_l and F'_u. During the indirect learning, we fix the parameters of SM and match the feature domains between F' and F via the squared L_2-norm that is defined as:

$$L_{fm} = ||F_l - F'_l||_2^2 + ||F_u - F'_u||_2^2 \tag{1}$$

where the F_l and F_u is produce by the FG (L_x) and FG (U_x) respectively. The F'_l and F'_u is produce by the final convolutional layer of the domain discriminator.

Therefore, we identify the F indirectly by identifying the F' to guarantee the discriminativeness of feature domain F for the learning of segmentation network.

Consistent Feature Domain Generation via Double-Sided Adaptation. In order to generate the consistent feature domain, we introduce two discriminators (D_l and D_u) to achieve a double-sided domain adaptation which enables the features produced by the L_x and U_x to adapt each other as shown in Fig. 2. D_l is used to encourage the L_x to generate the feature domain that is similar to the ones produced by U_x. D_u is used to force the U_x to generate the feature domain that is similar to the ones produced by L_x. Hence, a double-sided adversarial training is used to achieve the double-sided domain adaptation. During the double-sided adversarial training, for the learning of domain discriminator, F'_l is used as the *fake* feature and F'_u is used as the *real* feature to learn the D_l, while F'_l is used as the *real* feature and F'_u is used as the *fake* feature to learn the D_u simultaneously. For the learning of feature generator FG, D_l tries to identify the F'_l as *real* features and D_u tries to identify the F'_u as *real* features. In order to reduce the parameters of network, we make the D_l and D_u to share a discriminator D_{lu} to achieve the double adversarial learning directly. Inspired by this, we take the F'_l and F'_u as *real* features and *false* features respectively to directly learn the D_{lu}. When we learn the generator, the F'_l and the F'_u are assigned with the *False* label and *True* label respectively. Overall, during the double-sided adaptation, we fix the parameters of segmentation model SM and aim to optimize the following L_d and L_{adv} for learning the domain discriminator and feature generator respectively:

$$L_d(\theta_{D_{lu}}) = \sigma(D_{lu}(SM(FG(L_x))), 1) + \sigma(D_{lu}(SM(FG(U_x))), 0) \qquad (2)$$

$$L_{adv}(\theta_{FG}) = \sigma(D_{lu}(SM(FG(L_x))), 0) + \sigma(D_{lu}(SM(FG(U_x))), 1) \qquad (3)$$

where the L_x and U_x represent the input of the labeled and unlabeled data, respectively. σ is the binary cross-entropy loss. SM represents the segmentation model. During the domain adaptation, the parameters of the SM are fixed.

Semi-supervised Segmentation Model Learning. During the generation of the discriminative consistent feature domain, we learn the segmentation model SM by L_x and U_x. Since there is no available labels for U_x, U_x cannot be directly used for training the segmentation model along with the L_x. However, during the double-sided domain adaptation, we get the matched feature domains between F and F', while the F is generated from the L_x and U_x. Hence, we perform a reverse mapping (RM) that mapping the F' to the L_x' and U_x' which are matched with L_x and U_x to achieve the consistent image generation. Then the U_x can use a consistent image loss as semi-supervised loss L_{semi} to train the SM along with the supervised loss L_{super} from the L_x. Finally, we use L_x and U_x to train SM with the loss defined as follows:

$$L_{super,semi}^l(\theta_{SM}, \theta_{RM}, L_x) = ||L_x - L_x'||_2^2 + DL(LP, L_y) \qquad (4)$$

$$L_{semi}^u(\theta_{SM}, \theta_{RM}, U_x) = ||U_x - U_x'||_2^2 \qquad (5)$$

where LP is the estimated LA and PVs map. L_y is the ground truth. $|| \cdot ||_2^2$ is the squared L_2-norm. F and F' are the matched features. $DL(\cdot)$ represents the Dice loss function. We train the SM after each epoch of the domain adaptation.

Evaluation Criteria. We use the region-based metrics: the Dice coefficient $(Dice = 2\frac{|P \bigcap G|}{|P| + |G|})$ and intersection-over-union $(IoU = \frac{|P \bigcap G|}{|P \bigcup G|})$, which validate the predicted LA and PVs (P) against the ground-truth (G). And the surface-based metric of mean surface distance defined as $MSD = \frac{1}{2}[\overline{d}(S, S') + \overline{d}(S', S)]$, which $\overline{d}(S, S')$ is the mean of the distances between every surface voxel in predicted mesh S and the closest surface voxel in ground-truth mesh S'.

3   Experimental Results and Discussion

In our experiments, we used two centers dataset (detailed imaging parameters can be found in the supplementary materials) for the LA and PVs segmentation to validate the proposed $DCDG$. The final segmentation model was obtained using 'early stopping' on validation data. To demonstrate the performance of our proposed $DCDG$, we compare our proposed $DCDG$ with full supervised methods, e.g., *2D UNet* [7], *SegNet* [8] and a recent state-of-the-art 3D segmentation architecture namely 3D DenseNet [9], and also make a comparision between DCDG and a semi-supervised [10] (AR) method along with a domain adaptation [11] (ASOS) method with the single-level adversarial learning. In addition, we also compared DCDG to itself but used in a fully supervised manner, namely full supervised segmentation (FSS).

Table 1. Comparison of the performance of our proposed DCDG on C1.

Method	IoU	MSD (mm)	Dice
2D UNet	0.8695 ± 0.0294	1.1149 ± 0.4745	0.9299 ± 0.0170
SegNet	0.8418 ± 0.0265	1.2788 ± 0.2666	0.9139 ± 0.0157
3D DenseNet	0.8414 ± 0.0258	1.4548 ± 0.5463	0.9136 ± 0.0153
FSS	0.8719 ± 0.0272	1.0318 ± 0.2776	0.9314 ± 0.0157
AR (25%)	0.8215 ± 0.0330	1.5829 ± 0.4103	0.9016 ± 0.0200
ASOS (25%)	0.8252 ± 0.0312	1.5645 ± 0.4455	0.9039 ± 0.0189
DCDG (25%)	0.8474 ± 0.0338	1.2823 ± 0.3524	0.9170 ± 0.0202
AR (50%)	0.8349 ± 0.0377	1.4538 ± 0.4038	0.9096 ± 0.0288
ASOS (50%)	0.8529 ± 0.0341	1.1741 ± 0.3647	0.9203 ± 0.0184
DCDG (50%)	0.8709 ± 0.0276	1.0236 ± 0.2749	0.9307 ± 0.0161
AR (75%)	0.8541 ± 0.0255	1.1536 ± 0.3531	0.9211 ± 0.0149
ASOS (75%)	0.8602 ± 0.0238	1.1176 ± 0.2805	0.9247 ± 0.0139
DCDG (75%)	$\mathbf{0.8803 \pm 0.0188}$	$\mathbf{0.9285 \pm 0.2566}$	$\mathbf{0.9362 \pm 0.0107}$

Experiments on a Single Center Dataset. We performed multiple experiments on data with the same image domain based on different ratios of labeled data acquired at center 1 denoted as C1. The total number of C1 data is 175, in which 140 samples are randomly selected and used to train the model. We randomly selected 15 samples for model validation (7 pre-ablation and 8 post-ablation samples). We also randomly selected 20 samples for independent testing (10 pre-ablation and 10 post-ablation samples). During the experiment, we randomly selected different ratio r of labeled cases ($r = 25\%, 50\%, 75\%$) from 140 samples along with the ratio $(1 - r)$ of the unlabeled data for the semi-supervised learning of DCDG and AR, while the ASOS is learned by the labeled data of ratio r with the test data. The full supervised methods performed with the standard supervised training manner based on all the labeled data. The quantitative results are summarized in Table 1. As shown in Table 1, when we use 50% labeled data, the performance of DCDG is superior to 2D UNet, SegNet, 3D DenseNet. When we use 75% labeled data, the performance of DCDG is superior to FSS, which use 100% labeled data with fully supervised learning. Compared to those methods, we can use much less labeled data to obtain better results. It has great significance to avoid costly manual labeling when there is limited expert availability. Furthermore, compared with AR and ASOS, our proposed DCDG also achieves the best results.

Table 2. Comparison of the performance of our proposed *DCDG* on C1 and C2

Method	IoU	MSD (mm)	Dice
2D UNet	0.8125 ± 0.0355	1.7503 ± 0.6119	0.8961 ± 0.0216
SegNet	0.7420 ± 0.0474	3.1581 ± 1.4469	0.8510 ± 0.0310
3D DenseNet	0.7922 ± 0.0339	**1.1819 ± 0.4967**	0.8836 ± 0.0212
AR	0.6748 ± 0.0610	3.6165 ± 1.0855	0.8043 ± 0.0434
ASOS	0.7878 ± 0.0353	1.8757 ± 0.5038	0.8808 ± 0.0222
DCDG	**0.8315 ± 0.0254**	1.4031 ± 0.4948	**0.9078 ± 0.0151**
FSS	0.8154 ± 0.0401	2.5606 ± 2.1998	0.8978 ± 0.0245

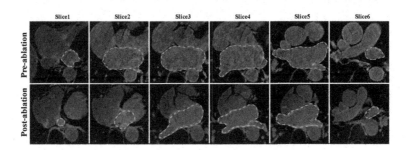

Fig. 3. Qualitative visualization of LA and PVs segmentation results compared to the manual delineation for representative slices on a pre-ablation and a post-ablation 3D LGE-CMRI images. Each estimated segmentation is represented as a dashed green contour, and its corresponding manual delineation is represented as a red contour. (Color figure online)

Experiments on a Two Center Dataset. For the experiment performed at $C1$ data was labelled as opposed to $C2$ which was unlabelled. The total number of $C2$ data is 94. We randomly selected 20 samples for testing (including 10 pre-ablation samples and 10 post-ablation samples). The remained 74 samples with no labels were used to train the *DCDG* along with the 140 samples with available labels from $C1$. We also apply the same 15 validation dataset used in the learning from the single center data to validate the segmentation model during training. For *2D UNet*, *SegNet*, *3D DenseNet* and *FSS*, supervised learning were performed on 140 samples with available labels from $C1$. As shown in Table 2, although *2D UNet*, *SegNet*, *3D DenseNet* have achieved great success in many medical image segmentation applications, they can not be directly applied to learn a good model from the distribution of one domain to the other domain thus obtained sub-performance. In addition, our *DCDG* also obtained the best results compared to the *AR* and *ASOS*. Figure 3 visually gives a further illustration to demonstrate the good performance of *DCDG*.

Model Variation Study. To verify the effectiveness of each component in our proposed *DCDG*, we perform Model variation study on $C1$ and $C2$. We take

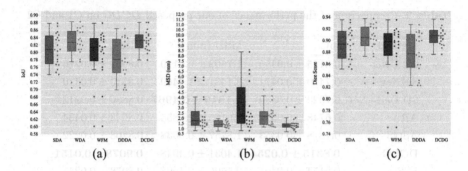

Fig. 4. Boxplots of IoU, MSD and $Dice$ evaluations for ablation tests.

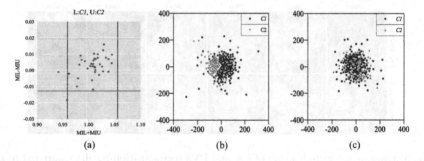

Fig. 5. (a) The stability of double-sided domain adaptation. The MIL and MIU are the mean identification value of the discriminator on labeled samples and unlabeled samples respectively after each learning of the double-sided domain adaptation. The intervals between the two vertical lines and two horizontal lines are the confidence intervals of 95% limits of agreement for MIL-MIU and MIL+MIU. (b) and (c): The t-Distributed Stochastic Neighbor Embedding (t-SNE) visualization of feature distribution on two-center data via double-sided adaptation (c) compared to the ones without adaptation (b). The red and blue points represent the samples from $C2$ and $C1$ respectively. (Color figure online)

the structure of $DCDG$ as the baseline. Then we train the model with single domain adaptation (SDA), without domain adaptation (WDA), without feature matching (WFM) and with the direct double-sided domain adaptation ($DDDA$) for F. We compare these models with the $DCDG$ and the results are shown in Fig. 4. As shown in the Fig. 4, our proposed $DCDG$ achieves the best results across these models on the measures of IoU, MSD and $Dice Score$, which proves the effectiveness of our $DCDG$.

Effectiveness of Double-Sided Domain Adaptation. In our proposed $DCDG$, the double-sided domain adaptation aims to generate the discriminative consistent feature domain. Its effectiveness can be demonstrated by the identified accuracy of discriminator for L_x and U_x. Ideally, the probability values are identified by the discriminator for L_x and U_x are both 0.5. In our experiment, we record the MIL and MIU as shown in Fig. 5(a). Ideally, the value of MIL plus

MIU is 1, while the value of MIL minus MIU is 0. In this situation, the identification values of discriminator on labeled data and unlabeled data are both 0.5, which illustrates that the model achieves the double-sided domain adaptation. As shown in Fig. 5(a), in each epoch during double-sided domain adaptation, the value of MIL plus MIU is close to 1. Meanwhile, the value of MIL minus MIU is close to 0. Furthermore, the adapted features show the fused features of L_x and U_x (Fig. 5(c)) compared to no adapted feature distribution (Fig. 5(b)).

4   Conclusion

In this paper, we proposed a discriminative consistent domain generation for the semi-supervised learning. In our proposed $DCDG$, we investigate the double-sided domain adaptation based on an indirect adversarial learning to fit the differences between labeled data and unlabeled data and generate the discriminative feature domain with fused feature space. Validation of our framework has been performed against manually delineated ground truth of the LA and PVs segmentation task. Compared to other supervised, semi-supervisd and domain adaptation methods, our $DCDG$ has demonstrated superior performance. In conclusion, our proposed $DCDG$ makes it possible to create a robust semi-supervised learning model using the unlabeled data along with labeled data collected from a single center or a multicenter studies that can be well extended to solve other medical image analysis problems.

Acknowledgments. This work was supported in part by the Young Scientists Fund of the National Natural Science Foundation of China (61602003), in part by the Natural Science Foundation of China (61771464 and U1801265) and in part by the Guangdong Science and Technology (2018A050506031 and 2019B010110001).

References

1. Patel, V.M., Gopalan, R., Li, R., Chellappa, R.: Visual domain adaptation: a survey of recent advances. IEEE Sign. Process. Mag. **32**(3), 53–69 (2015)
2. Chen, J., et al.: Multiview two-task recursive attention model for left atrium and atrial scars segmentation. In: Frangi, A.F., Schnabel, J.A., Davatzikos, C., Alberola-López, C., Fichtinger, G. (eds.) MICCAI 2018. LNCS, vol. 11071, pp. 455–463. Springer, Cham (2018). https://doi.org/10.1007/978-3-030-00934-2_51
3. Yang, G., et al.: Multiview sequential learning and dilated residual learning for a fully automatic delineation of the left atrium and pulmonary veins from late gadolinium-enhanced cardiac MRI images. In: EMBC, pp. 1123–1127 (2018)
4. Yang, G., et al.: Fully automatic segmentation and objective assessment of atrial scars for long-standing persistent atrial fibrillation patients using late gadolinium-enhanced MRI. Med. Phys. **45**(4), 1562–1576 (2018)
5. Zhang, N., et al.: Deep learning for diagnosis of chronic myocardial infarction on nonenhanced cardiac cine MRI. Radiology **291**(3), 606–617 (2019)
6. Zhang, Y., Zhang, Y., Wang, Y., Tian, Q.: Domain-Invariant Adversarial Learning for Unsupervised Domain Adaption. arXiv preprint arXiv: 1811.12751 (2018)

7. Ronneberger, O., Fischer, P., Brox, T.: U-Net: convolutional networks for biomedical image segmentation. In: Navab, N., Hornegger, J., Wells, W.M., Frangi, A.F. (eds.) MICCAI 2015. LNCS, vol. 9351, pp. 234–241. Springer, Cham (2015). https://doi.org/10.1007/978-3-319-24574-4_28

8. Badrinarayanan, V., et al.: SegNet: a deep convolutionalencoder-decoder architecture for image segmentation. IEEE Trans. Pattern Anal. Mach. Intell. **39**(12), 2481–2495 (2017)

9. Bui, T.D., Shin, J., Moon, T.: 3D densely convolution networks for volumetric segmentation. arXiv preprint arXiv: 1709.03199 (2017)

10. Koziński, M., et al.: An adversarial regularisation for semi-supervised training of structured output neural networks. arXiv preprint arXiv: 1702.02382 (2017)

11. Tsai, Y.H., et al.: Learning to adapt structured output space for semantic segmentation. In: CVPR, pp. 7472–7481 (2018)

Uncertainty-Aware Self-ensembling Model for Semi-supervised 3D Left Atrium Segmentation

Lequan Yu[1(✉)], Shujun Wang[1], Xiaomeng Li[1], Chi-Wing Fu[1],
and Pheng-Ann Heng[1,2]

[1] Department of Computer Science and Engineering,
The Chinese University of Hong Kong, Sha Tin, Hong Kong
ylqzd2011@gmail.com
[2] T Stone Robotics Institute,
The Chinese University of Hong Kong, Sha Tin, Hong Kong

Abstract. Training deep convolutional neural networks usually requires a large amount of labeled data. However, it is expensive and time-consuming to annotate data for medical image segmentation tasks. In this paper, we present a novel uncertainty-aware semi-supervised framework for left atrium segmentation from 3D MR images. Our framework can effectively leverage the unlabeled data by encouraging consistent predictions of the same input under different perturbations. Concretely, the framework consists of a student model and a teacher model, and the student model learns from the teacher model by minimizing a segmentation loss and a consistency loss with respect to the targets of the teacher model. We design a novel uncertainty-aware scheme to enable the student model to gradually learn from the meaningful and reliable targets by exploiting the uncertainty information. Experiments show that our method achieves high performance gains by incorporating the unlabeled data. Our method outperforms the state-of-the-art semi-supervised methods, demonstrating the potential of our framework for the challenging semi-supervised problems.

Keywords: Semi-supervised learning · Uncertainty estimation · Self-ensembling · Segmentation

1 Introduction

Automated segmentation of left atrium (LA) in magnetic resonance (MR) images is of great importance in promoting the treatment of atrial fibrillation. With a large amount of labeled data, deep learning has greatly advanced the segmentation of LA [15]. In the medical imaging domain, however, it is expensive and tedious to delineate reliable annotations from 3D medical images in a slice-by-slice manner by experienced experts. Since unlabeled data is generally abundant,

Code is available in https://github.com/yulequan/UA-MT.

© Springer Nature Switzerland AG 2019
D. Shen et al. (Eds.): MICCAI 2019, LNCS 11765, pp. 605–613, 2019.
https://doi.org/10.1007/978-3-030-32245-8_67

we focus on studying semi-supervised approach on LA segmentation by leveraging both limited labeled data and abundant unlabeled data.

Considerable effort has been devoted to utilizing unlabeled data to improve the segmentation performance in medical image community [1–3,7,19]. For example, Bai *et al.* [1] introduced a self-training-based method for cardiac MR image segmentation, where the network parameters and the segmentation for unlabeled data were alternatively updated. Besides, adversarial learning has been used in semi-supervised learning [6,12,18]. Zhang *et al.* [18] designed a deep adversarial network to use the unannotated images by encouraging the segmentation of unannotated images to be similar to those of the annotated ones. Another approach [12] utilized an adversarial network to select the trustworthy regions of unlabeled data to train the segmentation network. With the promising results achieved by self-ensembling methods [9,14] on semi-supervised natural image classification, Li *et al.* [10] extended the Π-model [9] with transformation consistent for semi-supervised skin lesion segmentation. Other approaches [5,13] utilized the weight-averaged consistency targets for semi-supervised MR segmentation. Although promising progress has been achieved, these methods do not consider the reliability of the targets, which may lead to meaningless guidance.

In this paper, we present a novel uncertainty-aware semi-supervised learning framework for left atrium segmentation from 3D MR images by additionally leveraging the unlabeled data. Our method encourages the segmentation predictions to be consistent under different perturbations for the same input, following the same spirit of mean teacher [14]. Specifically, we build a teacher model and a student model, where the student model learns from the teacher model by minimizing the segmentation loss on the labeled data and the consistency loss with respect to the targets from the teacher model on all input data. Without ground truth provided in the unlabeled input, the predicted target from the teacher model may be unreliable and noisy. In this regard, we design the uncertainty-aware mean teacher (UA-MT) framework, where the student model gradually learns from the meaningful and reliable targets by exploiting the uncertainty information of the teacher model. Concretely, besides generating the target outputs, the teacher model also estimates the *uncertainty* of each target prediction with Monte Carlo sampling. With the guidance of the estimated uncertainty, we filter out the unreliable predictions and preserve only the reliable ones (low uncertainty) when calculating the consistency loss. Hence, the student model is optimized with more reliable supervision and in return, encourages the teacher model to generate higher-quality targets. Our method was extensively evaluated on the dataset of MICCAI 2018 Atrial Segmentation Challenge. The results demonstrate that our semi-supervised method achieves large improvements for the LA segmentation by utilizing the unlabeled data, and also outperforms other state-of-the-art semi-supervised segmentation methods.

2   Method

Figure 1 illustrates our uncertainty-aware self-ensembling mean teacher framework (UA-MT) for semi-supervised LA segmentation. The teacher model gener-

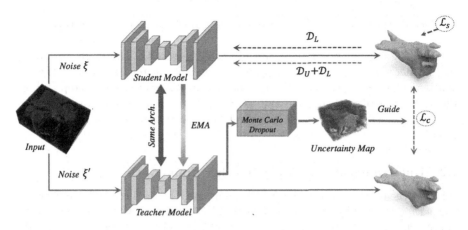

Fig. 1. The pipeline of our uncertainty-aware framework for semi-supervised segmentation. The student model is optimized by minimizing the supervised loss $\mathcal{L}_s$ on labeled data $\mathcal{D}_L$ and the consistency loss $\mathcal{L}_c$ on both unlabeled data $\mathcal{D}_U$ and labeled data $\mathcal{D}_L$. The estimated uncertainty from the teacher model guides the student to learn from the more reliable targets from the teacher.

ates targets for the student model to learn from and also estimates the uncertainty of the target. The uncertainty-guided consistency loss improves the student model and the robustness of the framework.

2.1   Semi-supervised Segmentation

We study the task of semi-supervised segmentation for 3D data, where the training set consists of N labeled data and M unlabeled data. We denote the labeled set as $\mathcal{D}_L = \{(x_i, y_i)\}_{i=1}^{N}$ and the unlabeled set as $\mathcal{D}_U = \{x_i\}_{i=N+1}^{N+M}$, where $x_i \in \mathbb{R}^{H \times W \times D}$ is the input volume and $y_i \in \{0, 1\}^{H \times W \times D}$ is the ground-truth annotations. The goal of our semi-supervised segmentation framework is to minimize the following combined objective function:

$$\min_{\theta} \sum_{i=1}^{N} \mathcal{L}_s(f(x_i; \theta), y_i) + \lambda \sum_{i=1}^{N+M} \mathcal{L}_c(f(x_i; \theta', \xi'), f(x_i; \theta, \xi)), \qquad (1)$$

where $\mathcal{L}_s$ denotes the supervised loss (*e.g.*, cross-entropy loss) to evaluate the quality of the network output on labeled inputs, and $\mathcal{L}_c$ represents the unsupervised consistency loss for measuring the consistency between the prediction of the teacher model and the student model for the same input x_i under different perturbations. Here, $f(\cdot)$ denotes the segmentation neural network; (θ', ξ') and (θ, ξ) represents the weights and different perturbation operations (*e.g.*, adding noise to input and network dropout) of the teacher and student models, respectively. λ is an ramp-up weighting coefficient that controls the trade-off between the supervised and unsupervised loss.

Recent study [9,14] show that ensembling predictions of the network at different training process can improve the quality of the predictions, and using them as the teacher predictions can improve the results. Therefore, we update the teacher's weights θ' as an *exponential moving average* (EMA) of the student's weights θ to ensemble the information in different training step [14]; see Fig. 1. Specifically, we update the teacher's weights θ'_t at training step t as: $\theta'_t = \alpha\theta'_{t-1} + (1 - \alpha)\theta_t$, where α is the EMA decay that controls the updating rate.

2.2   Uncertainty-Aware Mean Teacher Framework

Without the annotations in the unlabeled inputs, the predicted targets from the teacher model may be unreliable and noisy. Therefore, we design an uncertainty-aware scheme to enable the student model to gradually learn from the more reliable targets. Given a batch of training images, the teacher model not only generates the target predictions but also estimates the uncertainty for each target. Then the student model is optimized by the consistency loss, which focuses on only the confident targets under the guidance of the estimated uncertainty.

Uncertainty Estimation. Motivated by the uncertainty estimation in Bayesian networks, we estimate the uncertainty with the Monte Carlo Dropout [8]. In detail, we perform T stochastic forward passes on the teacher model under random dropout and input Gaussian noise for each input volume. Therefore, for each voxel in the input, we obtain a set of softmax probability vector: $\{\mathbf{p}_t\}_{t=1}^T$. We choose the predictive entropy as the metric to approximate the uncertainty, since it has a fixed range [8]. Formally, the predictive entropy can be summarized as:

$$\mu_c = \frac{1}{T}\sum_t \mathbf{p}_t^c \quad \text{and} \quad u = -\sum_c \mu_c \log\mu_c, \tag{2}$$

where $\mathbf{p}_t^c$ is the probability of the c-th class in the t-th time prediction. Note that the uncertainty is estimated in voxel level and the uncertainty of the whole volume U is $\{u\} \in \mathbb{R}^{H \times W \times D}$.

Uncertainty-Aware Consistency Loss. With the guidance of the estimated uncertainty U, we filter out the relatively unreliable (high uncertainty) predictions and select only the certain predictions as targets for the student model to learn from. In particular, for our semi-supervised segmentation task, we design the uncertainty-aware consistency loss $\mathcal{L}_c$ as the voxel-level mean squared error (MSE) loss of the teacher and student models only for the most certainty predictions:

$$\mathcal{L}_c(f', f) = \frac{\sum_v \mathbb{I}(u_v < H)\, \|f'_v - f_v\|^2}{\sum_v \mathbb{I}(u_v < H)}, \tag{3}$$

where $\mathbb{I}(\cdot)$ is the indicator function; f'_v and f_v are the predictions of teacher model and student model at the v-th voxel, respectively; u_v is the estimated uncertainty U at the v-th voxel; and H is a threshold to select the most certain targets. With our uncertainty-aware consistency loss in the training procedure, both the student and teacher can learn more reliable knowledge, which can then reduce the overall uncertainty of the model.

2.3 Technique Details

We employ V-Net [11] as our network backbone. We remove the short residual connection in each convolution block, and use a joint cross-entropy loss and dice loss [16]. To adapt the V-Net as a Bayesian network to estimate the uncertainty, two dropout layers with dropout rate 0.5 are added after the *L-Stage 5* layer and *R-Stage 1* layer of the V-Net. We turn on the dropout in the network training and uncertainty estimation, while we turn off the dropout in the testing phase, as we do not need to estimate uncertainty. We empirically set the EMA decay α as 0.99 referring to the previous work [14]. Following [9,14], we use a time-dependent Gaussian warming up function $\lambda(t) = 0.1 * e^{(-5(1-t/t_{max})^2)}$ to control the balance between the supervised loss and unsupervised consistency loss, where t denotes the current training step and t_{max} is the maximum training step. Such design can ensure that at the beginning, the objective loss is dominated by the supervised loss term and avoid the network get stuck in a degenerate solution where no meaningful target prediction of unlabeled data is obtained [9]. For the uncertainty estimation, we set $T = 8$ to balance the uncertainty estimation quality and training efficiency. We also use the same Gaussian ramp-up paradigm to ramp up the uncertainty threshold H from $\frac{3}{4}U_{max}$ to U_{max} in Eq. (3), where U_{max} is the maximum uncertainty value (*i.e.*, ln2 in our experiments). As the training continues, our method would filter out less and less data and enable the student to gradually learn from the relatively certain to uncertain cases.

3   Experiments and Results

Dataset and Pre-processing. We evaluated our method on the Atrial Segmentation Challenge dataset[1]. It provides 100 3D gadolinium-enhanced MR imaging scans (GE-MRIs) and LA segmentation mask for training and validation. These scans have an isotropic resolution of $0.625 \times 0.625 \times 0.625 \, \text{mm}^3$. We split the 100 scans into 80 scans for training and 20 scans for evaluation. All the scans were cropped centering at the heart region for better comparison of the segmentation performance of different methods, and normalized as zero mean and unit variance.

Implementation. The framework was implemented in PyTorch, using a TITAN Xp GPU. We used the SGD optimizer to update the network parameters (weight decay = 0.0001, momentum = 0.9). The initial learning rate was set as 0.01 and divided by 10 every 2500 iterations. We totally trained 6000 iterations

---

[1] http://atriaseg2018.cardiacatlas.org/.

Table 1. Comparison between our method and various methods.

Method	# scans used		Metrics			
	Labeled	Unlabeled	Dice [%]	Jaccard [%]	ASD [voxel]	95HD [voxel]
Vanilla V-Net	16	0	84.13	73.26	4.75	17.93
Bayesian V-Net	16	0	86.03	76.06	3.51	14.26
Vanilla V-Net	80	0	90.25	82.40	1.91	8.29
Bayesian V-Net	80	0	91.14	83.82	1.52	5.75
Self-training [1]	16	64	86.92	77.28	2.21	9.19
DAN [18]	16	64	87.52	78.29	2.42	9.01
ASDNet [12]	16	64	87.90	78.85	**2.08**	9.24
TCSE [10]	16	64	88.15	79.20	2.44	9.57
UA-MT-UN (ours)	16	64	88.83	80.13	3.12	10.04
UA-MT (ours)	16	64	**88.88**	**80.21**	2.26	**7.32**

as the network has converged. The batch size was 4, consisting of 2 annotated images and 2 unannotated images. We randomly cropped $112 \times 112 \times 80$ subvolumes as the network input and the final segmentation results were obtained using a sliding window strategy. We used the standard data augmentation techniques on-the-fly to avoid overfitting following [17], including randomly flipping, and rotating with 90°, 180° and 270° along the axial plane.

Evaluation of Our Semi-supervised Segmentation. We use four metrics to quantitatively evaluate our method, including Dice, Jaccard, the average surface distance (ASD), and the 95% Hausdorff Distance (95HD). Out of the 80 training scans, we use 20% (*i.e.*, 16) scans as labeled data and the remaining 64 scans as unlabeled data. Table 1 presents the segmentation performance of V-Net trained with only the labeled data (the first two rows) and our semi-supervised method (UA-MT) on the testing dataset. Compared with the Vanilla V-Net, adding dropout (Bayesian V-Net) improves the segmentation performance, and achieves an average Dice of 86.03% and Jaccard of 76.06% with only the labeled training data. By utilizing the unlabeled data, our semi-supervised framework further improves the segmentation by 4.15% Jaccrad and 2.85% Dice.

To analyze the importance of consistency loss for labeled data and unlabeled data, we conducted another experiment (UA-MT-UN) with the consistency loss only on the unlabeled data. The performance of this method is very close to UA-MT, validating that the performance of our method improves mainly due to the unlabeled data. We trained the fully supervised V-Net with all 80 labeled scans, which can be regarded as the upper-line performance. As we can see, our semi-supervised method is approaching the fully supervised ones. To validate our network backbone design, we reference the state-of-the-art challenging method [4], which used multi-task U-Net for LA segmentation. They reported a 90.10% Dice on 20 testing scans with 80 training scans. Compared with this method, we can regard our V-Net as a standard baseline model.

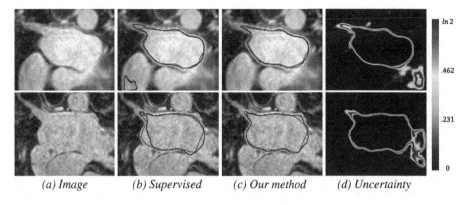

(a) Image   *(b) Supervised*   *(c) Our method*   *(d) Uncertainty*

Fig. 2. Visualization of the segmentations by different methods and the uncertainty. Blue and red colors show the predictions and ground truths, respectively. (Color figure online)

Table 2. Quantitative analysis of our method.

Method	# scans used		Metrics			
	Labeled	Unlabeled	Dice [%]	Jaccard [%]	ASD [voxel]	95HD [voxel]
MT	16	64	88.23	79.29	2.73	10.64
MT-Dice [5]	16	64	88.32	79.37	2.76	10.50
Our UA-MT	16	64	88.88	80.21	2.26	7.32
Bayesian V-Net	8	0	79.99	68.12	5.48	21.11
Our UA-MT	8	72	84.25	73.48	3.36	13.84
Bayesian V-Net	24	0	88.52	79.70	2.60	10.45
Our UA-MT	24	56	90.16	82.18	2.73	8.90

Comparison with Other Semi-supervised Methods. We implemented several state-of-the-art semi-supervised segmentation methods for comparison, including self-training based method [1], deep adversarial network (DAN) [18], adversarial learning based semi-supervised method (ASDNet) [12], and Π-Model based method (TCSE) [10]. Note that we used the same network backbone (Bayesian V-Net) in these methods for fair comparison. As shown in Table 1, compared with the self-training method, the DAN and ASDNet improve by 0.60% and 0.98% Dice, respectively, showing the effect of adversarial learning in semi-supervised learning. The ASDNet is better than DAN, since it selects the trustworthy region of unlabeled data for training the segmentation network. The self-ensembling-based methods TCSE achieve slightly better performance than ASDNet, demonstrating that perturbation-based consistency loss is helpful for the semi-supervised segmentation problem. Notably, our method (UA-MT) achieves the best performance over the state-of-the-art semi-supervised methods, except that the ASD performance is comparable with ASDNet, corroborating that our uncertainty-aware mean teacher framework has the full capability to draw out the rich information from the unlabeled data.

Analysis of Our Method. To validate the effectiveness of our uncertainty-aware scheme, we evaluate the performance of the original mean teacher method (MT) and an adapted mean teacher method (MT-Dice) with dice-loss-like consistency loss [5]. As shown in Table 2, our uncertainty-aware method outperforms both the MT model and MT-Dice model. We also investigate the impact of using different numbers of labeled scans in our semi-supervised method. As shown in Table 2, our semi-supervised method consistently improves the supervised-only V-Net (Bayesian V-Net) by utilizing the unlabeled data on both 10% (*i.e.*, 8) and 30% (*i.e.*, 24) labeled scans, demonstrating our method effectively utilizes the unlabeled data for the performance gains. In Fig. 2, we show some segmentation examples of supervised method and our semi-supervised method, and the estimated uncertainty. Compared with the supervised method, our results have higher overlap ratio with the ground truth (the second row) and produce less false positives (the first row). As shown in Fig. 2(d), the network estimates high uncertainty near the boundary and ambiguous regions of great vessels.

4   Conclusion

We present a novel uncertainty-aware semi-supervised learning method for left atrium segmentation from 3D MR images. Our method encourages the segmentation to be consistent for the same input under different perturbations to use the unlabeled data. More importantly, we explore the model uncertainty to improve the quality of the target. The comparison with other semi-supervised methods confirm the effectiveness of our method. The future works include investigating the effect of different uncertainty estimation manners and applying our framework to other semi-supervised medical image segmentation problems.

Acknowledgments. The work was partially supported by HK RGC TRS project T42-409/18-R, HK RGC project (Project No. CUHK 14225616), and in part by the T Stone Robotics Institute, The Chinese University of Hong Kong.

References

1. Bai, W., et al.: Semi-supervised learning for network-based cardiac MR image segmentation. In: Descoteaux, M., Maier-Hein, L., Franz, A., Jannin, P., Collins, D.L., Duchesne, S. (eds.) MICCAI 2017. LNCS, vol. 10434, pp. 253–260. Springer, Cham (2017). https://doi.org/10.1007/978-3-319-66185-8_29
2. Baur, C., Albarqouni, S., Navab, N.: Semi-supervised deep learning for fully convolutional networks. In: Descoteaux, M., Maier-Hein, L., Franz, A., Jannin, P., Collins, D.L., Duchesne, S. (eds.) MICCAI 2017. LNCS, vol. 10435, pp. 311–319. Springer, Cham (2017). https://doi.org/10.1007/978-3-319-66179-7_36
3. Chartsias, A., et al.: Factorised Spatial representation learning: application in semi-supervised myocardial segmentation. In: Frangi, A.F., Schnabel, J.A., Davatzikos, C., Alberola-López, C., Fichtinger, G. (eds.) MICCAI 2018. LNCS, vol. 11071, pp. 490–498. Springer, Cham (2018). https://doi.org/10.1007/978-3-030-00934-2_55
4. Chen, C., Bai, W., Rueckert, D.: Multi-task learning for left atrial segmentation on GE-MRI. arXiv preprint arXiv:1810.13205 (2018)

5. Cui, W., et al.: Semi-supervised brain lesion segmentation with an adapted mean teacher model. In: Chung, A.C.S., Gee, J.C., Yushkevich, P.A., Bao, S. (eds.) IPMI 2019. LNCS, vol. 11492, pp. 554–565. Springer, Cham (2019). https://doi.org/10.1007/978-3-030-20351-1_43

6. Dong, N., Kampffmeyer, M., Liang, X., Wang, Z., Dai, W., Xing, E.: Unsupervised domain adaptation for automatic estimation of cardiothoracic ratio. In: Frangi, A.F., Schnabel, J.A., Davatzikos, C., Alberola-López, C., Fichtinger, G. (eds.) MICCAI 2018. LNCS, vol. 11071, pp. 544–552. Springer, Cham (2018). https://doi.org/10.1007/978-3-030-00934-2_61

7. Ganaye, P.-A., Sdika, M., Benoit-Cattin, H.: Semi-supervised learning for segmentation under semantic constraint. In: Frangi, A.F., Schnabel, J.A., Davatzikos, C., Alberola-López, C., Fichtinger, G. (eds.) MICCAI 2018. LNCS, vol. 11072, pp. 595–602. Springer, Cham (2018). https://doi.org/10.1007/978-3-030-00931-1_68

8. Kendall, A., Gal, Y.: What uncertainties do we need in Bayesian deep learning for computer vision? In: NIPS, pp. 5574–5584 (2017)

9. Laine, S., Aila, T.: Temporal ensembling for semi-supervised learning. arXiv preprint (2016)

10. Li, X., Yu, L., Chen, H., Fu, C.W., Heng, P.A.: Semi-supervised skin lesion segmentation via transformation consistent self-ensembling model. BMVC (2018)

11. Milletari, F., Navab, N., Ahmadi, S.A.: V-Net: fully convolutional neural networks for volumetric medical image segmentation. In: 3DV, pp. 565–571 (2016)

12. Nie, D., Gao, Y., Wang, L., Shen, D.: ASDNet: attention based semi-supervised deep networks for medical image segmentation. In: Frangi, A.F., Schnabel, J.A., Davatzikos, C., Alberola-López, C., Fichtinger, G. (eds.) MICCAI 2018. LNCS, vol. 11073, pp. 370–378. Springer, Cham (2018). https://doi.org/10.1007/978-3-030-00937-3_43

13. Perone, C.S., Cohen-Adad, J.: Deep semi-supervised segmentation with weight-averaged consistency targets. In: Stoyanov, D., et al. (eds.) DLMIA/ML-CDS - 2018. LNCS, vol. 11045, pp. 12–19. Springer, Cham (2018). https://doi.org/10.1007/978-3-030-00889-5_2

14. Tarvainen, A., Valpola, H.: Mean teachers are better role models: weight-averaged consistency targets improve semi-supervised deep learning results. In: NIPS (2017)

15. Xiong, Z., Fedorov, V.V., Fu, X., Cheng, E., Macleod, R., Zhao, J.: Fully automatic left atrium segmentation from late gadolinium enhanced magnetic resonance imaging using a dual fully convolutional neural network. TMI **38**(2), 515–524 (2019)

16. Yang, X., Bian, C., Yu, L., Ni, D., Heng, P.-A.: Hybrid loss guided convolutional networks for whole heart parsing. In: Pop, M., et al. (eds.) STACOM 2017. LNCS, vol. 10663, pp. 215–223. Springer, Cham (2018). https://doi.org/10.1007/978-3-319-75541-0_23

17. Yu, L., et al.: Automatic 3D cardiovascular MR segmentation with densely-connected volumetric convnets. In: Descoteaux, M., Maier-Hein, L., Franz, A., Jannin, P., Collins, D.L., Duchesne, S. (eds.) MICCAI 2017. LNCS, vol. 10434, pp. 287–295. Springer, Cham (2017). https://doi.org/10.1007/978-3-319-66185-8_33

18. Zhang, Y., Yang, L., Chen, J., Fredericksen, M., Hughes, D.P., Chen, D.Z.: Deep adversarial networks for biomedical image segmentation utilizing unannotated images. In: Descoteaux, M., Maier-Hein, L., Franz, A., Jannin, P., Collins, D.L., Duchesne, S. (eds.) MICCAI 2017. LNCS, vol. 10435, pp. 408–416. Springer, Cham (2017). https://doi.org/10.1007/978-3-319-66179-7_47

19. Zhou, Y., et al.: Semi-supervised multi-organ segmentation via multi-planar co-training. arXiv preprint arXiv:1804.02586 (2018)

MSU-Net: Multiscale Statistical U-Net for Real-Time 3D Cardiac MRI Video Segmentation

Tianchen Wang[1(✉)], Jinjun Xiong[2], Xiaowei Xu[1], Meng Jiang[1], Haiyun Yuan[3], Meiping Huang[3], Jian Zhuang[3], and Yiyu Shi[1]

[1] University of Notre Dame, Notre Dame, USA
{twang9,xxu8,yshi4}@nd.edu
[2] IBM Thomas J. Watson Research Center, New York, USA
jinjun@us.ibm.com
[3] Guangdong General Hospital, Guangzhou, China
yhy_yun@163.com, huangmeipng@126.com, zhuangjian5413@tom.com

Abstract. Cardiac magnetic resonance imaging (MRI) is an essential tool for MRI-guided surgery and real-time intervention. The MRI videos are expected to be segmented on-the-fly in real practice. However, existing segmentation methods would suffer from drastic accuracy loss when modified for speedup. In this work, we propose Multiscale Statistical U-Net (MSU-Net) for real-time 3D MRI video segmentation in cardiac surgical guidance. Our idea is to model the input samples as multiscale canonical form distributions for speedup, while the spatio-temporal correlation is still fully utilized. A parallel statistical U-Net is then designed to efficiently process these distributions. The fast data sampling and efficient parallel structure of MSU-Net endorse the fast and accurate inference. Compared with vanilla U-Net and a modified state-of-the-art method GridNet, our method achieves up to 268% and 237% speedup with 1.6% and 3.6% increased Dice scores.

1 Introduction

Real-time Magnetic Resonance Imaging (MRI) techniques have been providing fast and accurate visual guidance in multiple fields. The duration of cardiac surgery (e.g., prosthetic valve implantation in the correct location at the aortic annulus) has been significantly shortened since interactive real-time MRI was getting applied [6]. Interventional real-time MRI has also been adopted for congenital, ischemic, and structural heart disease for its capacity of visualizing 3D anatomy and assessing myocardial tissue as well as local hemodynamics [2]. To achieve real-time MRI guidance, the images need to be segmented on-the-fly, at a speed of at least **30**, preferably up to 100 frames per second (FPS) [3,9].

However, performing real-time segmentation on cardiac MRI images is a challenging task. In addition to the difficult effects such as anisotropic resolution, cardiac border ambiguity and large variations among targeting objects

© Springer Nature Switzerland AG 2019
D. Shen et al. (Eds.): MICCAI 2019, LNCS 11765, pp. 614–622, 2019.
https://doi.org/10.1007/978-3-030-32245-8_68

from patients [11], the requirement of real-time fast segmentation demands a lightweight and efficient processing framework. Existing approaches used complicated neural network architectures to achieve good accuracy and were not able to make inference in real time [4,12]. Recently, Statistical Convolutional Neural Network (SCNN) was proposed to speed up conventional CNNs with little performance loss in video object detection [10]. Instead of feeding the input samples as deterministic values, SCNN used Independent Component Analysis (ICA) to extract parameterized statistical distributions in canonical form to compactly model the temporally and contextually correlated information. Then the network model propagated the distributions in canonical form more efficiently than deterministic values.

In this work, we propose Multiscale Statistical U-Net (MSU-Net) for real-time cardiac MRI segmentation. We incorporate SCNN and a new multiscale data sampling method with the U-Net to capture spatio-temporal correlation in the input data. Our model adopts a parallel architecture to efficiently propagate the multiscale distributions. Specifically, we apply ICA with multiple sets of temporal image patches to generate a cluster of canonical form distributions, each of which represents a different scale to model the input data. This multiscale sampling method can preserve the information of spatio-temporal correlations at different scales. Then we implement a number of parallel yet light-weight encoder-decoder style branches for efficient inference. Each branch propagates the specific scale of canonical form distributions. Experimental results show that our MSU-Net achieves up to 268% and 237% speedup with 1.6% and 3.6% increased Dice scores compared with vanilla U-Net and a modified state-of-the-art method GridNet [12].

2   Background

SCNN [10] was the first model that feeds CNNs with a reasonable number of statistical distributions that were decomposed from the input data. SCNN is lighter and thus of higher speed than conventional CNNs that conduct deterministic operations (such as sum and max).

SCNN applied ICA to decompose video frames that exhibit spatio-temporal correlation into canonical form distributions as follows:

$$D = a_0 + a_1 X_1 + \ldots + a_m X_m + a_r R, \tag{1}$$

where (1) D is a random multivariate signal, which in video object detection represents the same pixel across multiple frames in a snippet; (2) a_0 is the mean value of D; (3) X_i ($i \in \{1 \ldots m\}$) are additive independent subcomponents of D; (4) a_i ($i \in \{1 \ldots m\}$) are the corresponding weight act as mixing matrix; (5) R denotes uncorrelated Gaussian noise and a_r is the weight of R; (6) m is the basis dimension of the canonical form distribution.

With the help of predefined core operations (weighted *sum* and *max*) that keep their outputs still in canonical form distributions, SCNN needs little modification to the standard gradient descent based scheme. It can be trained using the same forward and back propagation procedures as conventional CNNs. At the output, the results are mixed to form a temporal feature map for each sample by plugging in the values of independent sources X_i from the ICA process. By processing multiple frames at a time through distributions, SCNN significantly speedups object detection in videos over conventional CNNs with slight accuracy degradation.

3   Method

In this section, we first present a multiscale sampling method to extract canonical form distributions from input 3D MRI videos. Then we introduce the architecture of MSU-Net and explain how it processes these distributions for real-time segmentation.

3.1   Distribution Extraction with Multiscale Data Sampling

In order to build linear distributions in parameterized canonical form (Eq. 1) via ICA, we need to decide how to properly extract samples from 3D MRI video to feed into ICA, i.e., what information each D should represent. In the approach of SCNN for video object detection [10], the video clips are resized and split into small snippets, and each distribution D models the same pixel across multiple frames in the same snippet. However, this cannot be applied to 3D MRI video directly since lots of semantic details important to segmentation would be lost. Thus, we propose to use D to represent a patch within a small range (both spatially and temporally) where strong correlation exists. Specifically, we denote the dimension of an input 3D MRI video as $[X, Y, Z, T]$, where $X - Y$ plane is the short axis plane, Z is the short axis and T is the temporal dimension. The common issues of slice shifting as well as large inter-slice gap in MRI cardiac images along short-axis (Z axis) [12] lead to minimum spatial correlation in $X - Z$ and $Y - Z$ planes. Therefore, we extract patches within the dimension $[X, Y, T]$, independent of Z.

Before extracting the patches, the 3D MRI videos are normalized first to remove offsets among videos. Each patch is then extracted using a window of size (n, n) on the $X - Y$ plane over t time steps. We call t as snippet span. We propose to allow different canonical forms to have different n and t, as such an approach covers potential spatio-temporal correlations at different scales. We call this cluster of distributions with multiple patch sizes as multiscale distributions. An example of the extraction process of multiscale distributions with different patch sizes on one slice is shown in Fig. 1(a). The patches are collected at the same position over time and fed to ICA to extract canonical form distributions. ICA has to be used because the propagation of the canonical form distributions requires all the bases to be independent. Other approahces such as PCA cannot guarantee this unless the samples follow Gaussian distributions, which is not the case in our problem. As a result, the snippet of 3D MRI video is "collapsed" into a smaller 3D image, with each voxel representing a canonical form distribution

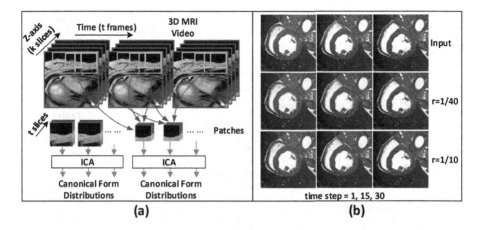

Fig. 1. (a) Illustration of multi-scale data sampling from cropped 3D MRI video. Each canonical form is extracted using the samples from the same position in the $X - Y$ plane and collected at different time steps. Different canonical forms can have different patch sizes. (b) Restored inputs with multi-scale data sampling method at different time steps (t) using different compression ratio (r). The restored inputs with r = 1/40 have more noises than those with r = 1/10.

(Eq. 1) that has both spatial and temporal correlations: with patch size (n, n, t) and predetermined independent basis dimension d, a compression ratio of $r = d/(n^2 t)$ is achieved.

To show the feasibility of the proposed data sampling, we extract the multi-scale canonical form distributions using our procedure with various compression ratio r by changing the basis dimension d with $n = 7$ and $t = 5$. The visual results along with the compression ratio are shown in Fig. 1(b). With a larger ratio (r = 1/40, smaller basis dimension of canonical form distribution), the restored video gain more noise with vague contours, which would bring obstruction to the segmentation task. With a smaller ratio (r = 1/10), the difference between the input video and the restored mixing video is negligible. Therefore, we adopt r = 1/10 as the compression ratio in our following experiments.

3.2 Real-Time Segmentation with MSU-Net

The multiscale canonical form distributions provide compact data representation for efficient processing. In this subsection, we explore a parallel structure, namely MSU-Net, that can further speedup the segmentation.

Figure 2 illustrates our MSU-Net which consists of multiple DownTubes (DTs), UpTubes (UTs), Center blocks, and a final evaluator (FE). The DTs and UTs act as the encoders and decoders in U-Net for feature propagation. Multiple DTs are built for a set of splitting patch sizes, each consisting of multiple blocks with downscaling convolution layers to perform feature downscaling and reuse. The ICA process and the corresponding mixing operations are done

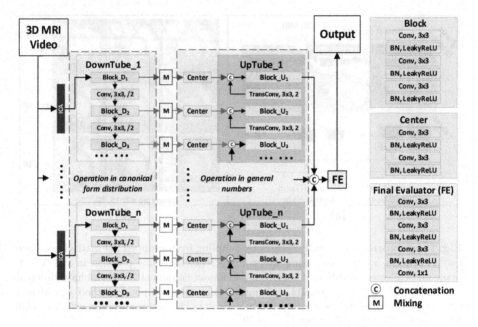

Fig. 2. The architecture of MSU-Net. The number of Blocks in DownTube/UpTube varies to accommodate the various input dimensions.

before and after the operations in DT, repsectively, and the operations in DT are performed in canonical form distributions similar to the work developed in SCNN [10]. The features in UT are propagated and upscaled with the blocks made of convolutional layers, and transposed convolutional layers, respectively. The features after each upscaling are concatenated with the one skipped from DT for feature reuse. After the outputs are obtained from UTs with various patch sizes, all features would have the same dimensions, which are then concatenated and forwarded to the final evaluator to generate the final output. The number of blocks in DT/UT varies to accommodate the input dimensions of 3D images.

4   Experiments

4.1   Experiment Setup

The evaluation task is to segment right ventricle (RV), myocardium (MYO), and left ventricle (LV) from MRI video clips in real time. We evaluate the proposed MSU-Net and competitive baselines on segmenting the RV, MYO and LV from the frames of End Diastolic (ED) and End Systolic (ES) instant. These frames were collected from the ACDC MICCAI 2017 challenge dataset [1] with additional labeling done by experience radiologists. These frames have similar properties as 3D cardiac MRI videos. The dataset has 150 exams from different patients with 100 for training and 50 for testing. The images were collected following the common clinical SSFP cine-MRI sequence with a series of short-axis slices starting from the mitral valves down to the apex of the left ventricle. We perform 5-fold cross-validation and use the Dice score to evaluate the segmentation accuracy.

We implement two versions of MSU-Net with specific snippet spans ($t = 5$ and 10, denoted as T5, T10, respectively) for evaluation. The ICA processing time is included when we evaluate the inference time of MSU-Net. Existing approaches have reported their FPS on the same dataset: ~1 [4], and 5.56 [12]. Clearly, none of them can perform real-time inference (i.e., at least 30 FPS). Therefore, we modify and rebuild these approaches to speed them up so that they can be compared with MSU-Net on a relatively fair basis. We implement a set of shallower/slimmer versions (i.e., with fewer layers/fewer channels) of the models. Specifically, we modify the 2D U-Net [7] to a shallow version with a depth of 3 and initial filter of 8 or 16. We denote them as D3+IF8 and D3+IF16, respectively. The 2D U-Net with vanilla configuration (D5+IF64) is also included. We also modify GridNet to shallower versions with a depth of 2 or 3 and initial filter of 32, denoted as D2+IF32 and D3+IF32, respectively. The vanilla version of GridNet is one of the best models in the ACDC 2017 challenge. All these methods are fully trained after modification.

In our experiments, we do not include 3D U-Net for comparison due to its excessive memory consumption, unbalanced input dimensions, and slow inference speed [4, 7]. Meanwhile we do not include lightweight networks such as ShuffleNet [5] or MobileNet [8] which is designed with small memory footprint for mobile devices in image classification/object detection rather than medical segmentation, while inference speed is not their primary concern (which mainly depends on the network depth). We have tried ShuffleNet/MobileNet in our experiment settings and the speeds are only at 8.45/11.58 FPS, which are slower than the nets we reported.

We implement MSU-Net and 2D U-Nets using PyTorch. The GridNet was implemented using TensorFlow [12]. All experiments run on a machine with 16 cores of Intel Xeon E5-2620 v4 CPU, 256G memory, and an NVIDIA GeForce GTX 1080 GPU.

4.2   Results

Table 1 presents the comparison among U-Net, GridNet, and the proposed MSU-Net on Dice score and FPS. Our MSU-Nets can achieve the fastest processing speed (highest FPS) and the best Dice score. Compared with the fastest baseline method U-Net (D3+IF8), our MSU-Net (T10) runs $1.63\times$ faster and makes an improvement of 26% on segmentation accuracy. Compared with the most accurate baseline method (with the highest Dice score) GridNet (D3+IF32), our MSU-Net (T5) can achieve a slightly higher accuracy and $2.75\times$ faster processing speed. From the table, it is clear that MSU-Nets are the only capable method to segment real-time 3D MRI videos.

Table 1. Comparison between baseline methods and our MSU-Net on Dice score and FPS for 3D MRI video segmentation. "T5"/"T10" denotes the video snippet span in MSU-Net (t = 5/t = 10). "D" and "IF" denote the depth of the network and the initial filters number of the input layer, respectively.

Methods	FPS	Dice score			
		RV	MYO	LV	Average
GridNet (D3+IF32)	15.7	.842 ± .028	.804 ± .026	.901 ± .036	.849 ± .014
U-Net (D5+IF64)	16.1	**.865 ± .036**	.761 ± .039	**.911 ± .026**	.846 ± .025
GridNet (D2+IF32)	18.2	.815 ± .025	.812 ± .014	.851 ± .033	.826 ± .011
U-Net (D3+IF16)	33.2	.564 ± .071	.738 ± .045	.767 ± .026	.690 ± .036
U-Net (D3+IF8)	43.2	.552 ± .079	.674 ± .060	.759 ± .059	.662 ± .058
MSU-Net (T5)	**43.2**	.855 ± .026	**.836 ± .022**	.897 ± .017	**.862 ± .011**
MSU-Net (T10)	**70.2**	.837 ± .034	.811 ± .049	.854 ± .040	.834 ± .020

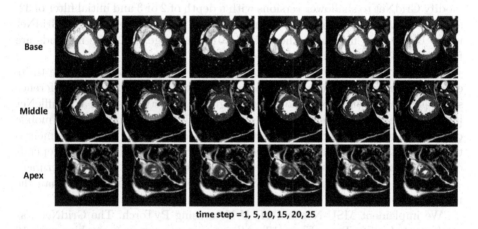

Base

Middle

Apex

time step = 1, 5, 10, 15, 20, 25

Fig. 3. The segmentation results of our method MSU-Net (T5) on the testing data. The rows indicate the slices at the base, the middle, and the apex of LV. The columns show the results at various time steps in series. RV, MYO, and LV are labeled in blue, green and red, respectively. (Color figure online)

For MSU-Net, a bigger video snippet span (T10) can obtain a faster processing speed with a slight accuracy degradation (only 0.028). However, for U-Net, when it is modified into shallow/slim versions such as U-Net (D3+IF16) and (D3+IF8) for real-time processing (≥30 FPS), the accuracy degrades significantly: We observe that the accuracy drops from 0.846 to 0.690 and 0.662, respectively. We observe the same pattern for GridNet, and conclude that MSU-Net can achieve a stable accuracy when configured for segmentation in real time.

Finally, Fig. 3 shows the examples of MSU-Net segmentation results at various time steps. Note that our MSU-Net can accurately segment the target areas. The boundaries are clearly extracted on most of the slices. In the base and middle slices, the segmentation fits the contours of targets. In some of the apex slices, the segmentation of RV (labeled in blue) is not as accurate as MYO and LV, because of the unclear boundaries between the instances.

5   Conclusions

In this paper, we proposed Multiscale Statistical U-Net (MSU-Net) for real-time 3D cardiac MRI video segmentation. Based on the scheme of Statistical Convolutional Neural Network, we model the input samples as multiscale canonical form distributions for speedup, while the spatio-temporal correlationis still fully utilized. A parallel statistical U-Net is then proposed to process these multiscale distributions efficiently. On the 3D cardiac MRI videos from the ACDC MICCAI 2017 dataset, MSU-Net achieves up to 268% and 237% speedup with 1.6% and 3.6% increased Dice scores compared with vanilla U-Net and a modified state-of-the-art method GridNet, respectively.

Acknowledgement. This work was approved by the Research Ethics Committee of Guangdong General Hospital, Gunagdong Academy of Medical Sciences with protocol No. 20140316. This work was supported by the National key Research and Development Program [2018YFC1002600], Science and Technology Planning Project of Guangdong Province, China [No. 2017A070701013, 2017B090904034, 2017030314109, and 2019B020230003], National Science Foundation grant [CCF-1919167], and Guangdong peak project [DFJH201802].

References

1. Bernard, O., et al.: Deep learning techniques for automatic MRI cardiac multi-structures segmentation and diagnosis: is the problem solved? IEEE Trans. Med. Imaging **37**(11), 2514–2525 (2018)
2. Campbell-Washburn, A.E., et al.: Real-time MRI guidance of cardiac interventions. J. Magn. Reson. Imaging **46**(4), 935–950 (2017)
3. Iltis, P.W., Frahm, J., Voit, D., Joseph, A.A., Schoonderwaldt, E., Altenmüller, E.: High-speed real-time magnetic resonance imaging of fast tongue movements in elite horn players. Quant. Imaging Med. Surg. **5**(3), 374 (2015)
4. Isensee, F., Jaeger, P.F., Full, P.M., Wolf, I., Engelhardt, S., Maier-Hein, K.H.: Automatic cardiac disease assessment on cine-MRI via time-series segmentation and domain specific features. In: Pop, M., et al. (eds.) STACOM 2017. LNCS, vol. 10663, pp. 120–129. Springer, Cham (2018). https://doi.org/10.1007/978-3-319-75541-0_13
5. Ma, N., Zhang, X., Zheng, H.T., Sun, J.: ShuffleNet V2: practical guidelines for efficient CNN architecture design. In: Proceedings of the European Conference on Computer Vision (ECCV), pp. 116–131 (2018)
6. McVeigh, E.R., et al.: Real-time interactive MRI-guided cardiac surgery: aortic valve replacement using a direct apical approach. Magn. Reson. Med.: Official J. Int. Soc. Magn. Reson. Med. **56**(5), 958–964 (2006)

7. Ronneberger, O., Fischer, P., Brox, T.: U-Net: convolutional networks for biomedical image segmentation. In: Navab, N., Hornegger, J., Wells, W.M., Frangi, A.F. (eds.) MICCAI 2015. LNCS, vol. 9351, pp. 234–241. Springer, Cham (2015). https://doi.org/10.1007/978-3-319-24574-4_28

8. Sandler, M., Howard, A., Zhu, M., Zhmoginov, A., Chen, L.C.: MobileNetV2: inverted residuals and linear bottlenecks. In: Proceedings of the IEEE Conference on Computer Vision and Pattern Recognition, pp. 4510–4520 (2018)

9. Schaetz, S., Voit, D., Frahm, J., Uecker, M.: Accelerated computing in magnetic resonance imaging: real-time imaging using nonlinear inverse reconstruction. In: Computational and Mathematical Methods in Medicine 2017 (2017)

10. Wang, T., Xiong, J., Xu, X., Shi, Y.: SCNN: a general distribution based statistical convolutional neural network with application to video object detection. arXiv preprint arXiv:1903.07663 (2019)

11. Zheng, Q., Delingette, H., Duchateau, N., Ayache, N.: 3D consistent and robust segmentation of cardiac images by deep learning with spatial propagation. IEEE Trans. Med. Imaging **37**, 2137–2148 (2018)

12. Zotti, C., Luo, Z., Lalande, A., Jodoin, P.M.: Convolutional neural network with shape prior applied to cardiac MRI segmentation. IEEE J. Biomed. Health Inf. **23**, 1119–1128 (2018)

The Domain Shift Problem of Medical Image Segmentation and Vendor-Adaptation by Unet-GAN

Wenjun Yan[1], Yuanyuan Wang[1(✉)], Shengjia Gu[2], Lu Huang[3],
Fuhua Yan[2], Liming Xia[3], and Qian Tao[4(✉)]

[1] Department of Electrical Engineering, Fudan University, Shanghai, China
yywang@fudan.edu.cn
[2] Department of Radiology, Ruijin Hospital, Shanghai Jiaotong University,
Shanghai, China
[3] Department of Radiology, Tongji Hospital,
Huazhong University of Science and Technology, Wuhan, China
[4] Department of Radiology, Leiden University Medical Center, Leiden,
The Netherlands
Q.Tao@lumc.nl

Abstract. Convolutional neural network (CNN), in particular the Unet, is a powerful method for medical image segmentation. To date Unet has demonstrated state-of-art performance in many complex medical image segmentation tasks, especially under the condition when the training and testing data share the same distribution (i.e. come from the same source domain). However, in clinical practice, medical images are acquired from different vendors and centers. The performance of a U-Net trained from a particular source domain, when transferred to a different target domain (e.g. different vendor, acquisition parameter), can drop unexpectedly. Collecting a large amount of annotation from each new domain to retrain the U-Net is expensive, tedious, and practically impossible.

In this work, we proposed a generic framework to address this problem, consisting of (1) an unpaired generative adversarial network (GAN) for vendor-adaptation, and (2) a Unet for object segmentation. In the proposed Unet-GAN architecture, GAN learns from Unet at the feature level that is segmentation-specific. We used cardiac cine MRI as the example, with three major vendors (Philips, Siemens, and GE) as three domains, while the methodology can be extended to medical images segmentation in general. The proposed method showed significant improvement of the segmentation results across vendors. The proposed Unet-GAN provides an annotation-free solution to the cross-vendor medical image segmentation problem, potentially extending a trained deep learning model to multi-center and multi-vendor use in real clinical scenario.

Keywords: Domain adaptation · Left ventricle segmentation · GAN · Unet

© Springer Nature Switzerland AG 2019
D. Shen et al. (Eds.): MICCAI 2019, LNCS 11765, pp. 623–631, 2019.
https://doi.org/10.1007/978-3-030-32245-8_69

1 Introduction

Recent years have witnessed a tremendous boost in computer vision brought by deep neural networks. Deep convolutional neural networks (CNN) have swept almost every image analysis problem since its resurgence [1, 2]. For medical image segmentation, the Unet architecture has achieved remarkable success, surpassing human in speed-accuracy balance [3, 4].

1.1 The Domain Shift Problem of CNN Segmentation

On the other hand, although CNN is argued to be biologically inspired by human vision, researchers have discovered an intriguing gap between human and computer vision. A type of domain variance can be formulated as adversarial perturbation. In tribute to the well-known Panda-Gibbon example [5], we generated adversarial examples for a well-trained Unet for the left ventricle (LV) segmentation task in magnetic resonance image (MRI). We used the fast gradient sign method: the perturbation was computed as equal to the sign of the gradient of the loss function with respect to the input. The perturbation was meant to distract the CNN in a guided manner.

Figure 1 shows two examples of such adversarial attacks. Although almost imperceptible to human eye, the minor perturbation completely misguided a well-trained CNN. In practice, such variance may also come from "distribution shift" [6], which is common when medical images come from different centers, vendors, or acquisition parameters. This leads to a major difficulty of deploying CNN in real clinical scenarios: the performance of CNN can be excellent in the test data from the same distribution, but could drop unexpectedly in unseen data from a different distribution.

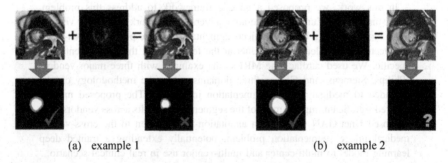

(a)   example 1   (b)   example 2

Fig. 1. Two examples to show that the trained Unet are vulnerable to the carefully calculated perturbation added to the original image. The perturbation hardly affects human vision, but leads to failure of the Unet: in the first example, the segmentation went wrong; in the second example, the segmentation completely failed.

Generalization capability of a trained CNN is of paramount importance for its utilization in clinical scenario. An intuitive solution is to include as much data as possible in training, which enlarges the scope of distribution learned by CNN. However, manual annotation of data in large amount, for every new (and unknown) distribution, is practically impossible. Data augmentation in the source domain shows not to be the ultimate solution in closing the generalization gap, since distribution shift is not accidental but systematic [7].

In this work, we proposed a generic framework to address this problem, consisting of (1) an unpaired generative adversarial network (GAN) for vendor-adaptation, and (2) a Unet for segmentation, using the LV segmentation from cine MRI as an example. We integrated the two networks in the design, and name it as *Unet-GAN*.

2 Method

LV-Unet. A supervised CNN, named LV-Unet, can be trained on the source dataset S that has sufficient annotated LV segmentation. LV-Unet follows an asymmetric encoder-decoder structure as illustrated in Fig. 2(a).

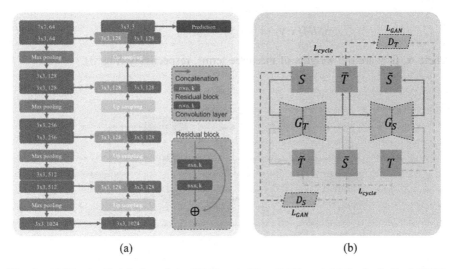

(a)   (b)

Fig. 2. (a) The detailed design of the LV-Unet in Unet-GAN, and (b) the basic CycleGAN.

CycleGAN. CycleGAN is an established architecture designed for unpaired image-to-image translation [8]. It contains two generators and two discriminators as shown in Fig. 2(b). The generators G_S and G_T play roles of translators between source and target domains. The discriminators D_S and D_T differentiate if the image is original or translated. The loss function is a composite of two losses: one is the general adversarial loss of GAN, defined as: $L_{GAN}(G_x, D_x, x, y) = E_x[\log D(x)] + E_y[1 - \log D(G(y))]$, the other is the L_2 loss defined as: $L_{cycle}(G_x, G_y, x, y) = E_{x,y}\|x - G_x(G_y(y))\|_2$, which enforces the generator to learn the representative features of a specific domain in an unpaired way. The overall loss function of CycleGAN is:

$$L(G_S, G_T, D_S, D_T) = L_{GAN}(G_S, D_S, S, T) + L_{GAN}(G_T, D_T, T, S) + \lambda[L_{cycle}(G_S, G_T, S, T)$$
$$+ L_{cycle}(G_T, G_S, T, S)]$$

$$(1)$$

Structural Similarity Index (SSIM). The structural similarity (SSIM) index is a measure to assess the quality of generated images [9]. The SSIM formula comprises of three similarity measurements between images x and y: luminance, contrast, and structure. The three measurements are expressed as follows:

$$l(x,y) = \frac{2\mu_x\mu_y + c_1}{\mu_x^2 + \mu_y^2 + c_1}, \; c(x,y) = \frac{2\sigma_x\sigma_y + c_2}{\sigma_x^2 + \sigma_y^2 + c_2}, \; s(x,y) = \frac{2\sigma_{xy} + c_3}{\sigma_x\sigma_y + c_3} \quad (2)$$

where μ_x/μ_y and σ_x^2/σ_y^2 are mean value and variance of x and y, respectively, σ_{xy} is covariance of x and y, and $c_i(i = 1, 2, 3)$ is the parameters to stabilize the dividing operation. The SSIM index is defined as the exponentially weighted combination of the three:

$$SSIM(x,y) = [l(x,y)^\alpha \cdot c(x,y)^\beta \cdot s(x,y)^\gamma] \quad (3)$$

where α, β, γ are the weights of the three terms, respectively (Fig. 3).

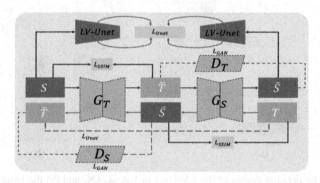

Fig. 3. The Unet-GAN architecture, which integrates Unet and CycleGAN.

Unet-GAN: Dedicated to Medical Image Segmentation Across Domains. The proposed Unet-GAN has a loss function combining information at the image and feature level:

SSIM Loss at Image Level: The original loss in CycleGAN is an image-level loss computing the mean square error (MSE) between the input image and the translated one. An inherent requirement for medical image domain adaptation is that the luminance and contrast can vary but anatomical structures should be preserved. Based on this observation, we used SSIM as a modified image loss for medical image adaptation:

the structure term of SSIM is given a much higher weight than the luminance and contrast terms. L_{SSIM} is defined as:$L_{SSIM} = E_{x,y}\|1 - SSIM(x,y)\|_2$.

Unet Loss at Feature Level: The image-level loss leads to visually similar image, but can still be vulnerable to adversarial noises. To tackle this problem, we propose a novel loss defined at the feature level. The encoder path of the LV-Unet is regarded as an effective feature extractor, highlighting features most relevant for the segmentation task. We used the output from its layers in the encoder path as feature f, and measured the MSE of features f between the original and translated image. In this way we enforce the GAN to generate images that produce the same segmentation-specific features. The new loss at feature level is called L_{Unet}:

$$L_{Unet} = E_{x,y}\|f_x - f_y\|_2 = \frac{\sum_{i=1}^{N}\left(f_{original}^{i} - f_{translated}^{i}\right)^2}{N} \tag{4}$$

The overall loss function of Unet-GAN is defined as:

$$L(G_S, G_T, D_S, D_T) = L_{GAN} + \lambda_1 L_{Unet} + \lambda_2 L_{SSIM} \tag{5}$$

Overall Workflow. The proposed framework for cross-vendor medical image segmentation consists of three steps:

1. Firstly, the Unet is trained by data from the source domain with sufficient annotation, and the performance in the test set from the same source domain is guaranteed to be up to the state-of-the-art.
2. The generators G_S, G_T and discriminators D_S, D_T in Unet-GAN are trained alternately using unannotated data from both source and target domains, using the loss function defined in the previous section, integrating the Unet features.
3. Finally, data from the target domain are first translated to the source domain by G_S, and then fed to the trained Unet for segmentation.

3 Experiments and Results

3.1 Data

The experiments involved short-axis steady-state free precession (SSFP) cine MR images of 144 subjects acquired by three major MRI machines as three domains (44 Philips samples, 50 GE samples, 50 Siemens samples). Image size varied from 256×256 to 512×512 pixels. All images were rescaled to the same in-plane resolution of 1.5×1.5 mm. Cine MR and label images were cropped at the center to a size of 192×192 for faster training and testing.

Ground truth annotation of the LV myocardium and blood pool were performed on the cine MR images by experienced radiologists. The number of available annotated images in each domain was 4823, 2084, and 2602 for Philips, GE, and Siemens, respectively. Philips data was set as the source domain to train the LV-Unet. We randomly selected 35 subjects out of 44 for training (3920 images) and the rest 9 for testing (903 images). Siemens and GE were defined as the two target domains. To train the Unet-GAN, we separated every domain into training/testing set: 3008/1815 for Philips, 1680/924 for Siemens, and 1320/764 for GE.

3.2   Experiments and Performance Evaluation

LV-Unet: We used adaptive moment estimation (Adam) optimization with learning rate of 10^{-4} and a mini-batch size of 10. The number of epochs was set to 35 when network converged and the mean Dice coefficient reached 88% on the test dataset (the state-of-art for LV segmentation [10, 11]).

Unet-GAN: We used Adam optimization with learning rate of 10^{-5}. Weighting parameters λ_1 was set to 15 and λ_2 was set to 5 empirically. As GAN is generally hard to train, we applied the early stopping strategy during training to prevent model overfitting. Two Unet-GANs were trained to translate image from one domain to another one: (1) Siemens $\rightarrow$ Philips, trained with 3008 Philips images and 1680 S images, and (2) GE $\rightarrow$ Philips, trained with 3008 Philips images and 1320 GE images.

Based on our experiments with the LV-Unet, the layers after three max-pooling operations tend to extract high-level semantic features. Therefore, we selected features from the 7th and 9th residual blocks in the LV-Unet for the Unet loss. For the SSIM loss, α, β, γ were assigned the value of 0.1, 0.1, and 1, respectively.

We performed comparative experiments to evaluate the performance improvement brought by Unet-GAN, with the follow three scenarios tested:

(1) Segment data of the target domain directly by LV-Unet trained on the *clean* source domain (i.e. original data);
(2) Segment data of the target domain by LV-Unet trained on the *polluted* source domain (i.e. original data added with random noise);
(3) First translate data of the target domain by Unet-GAN to the source domain, then segment the translated data by the LV-Unet trained on the clear source data.

The polluted Unet meant to evaluate how much systematic augmentation can address the domain shift problem, in comparison to the proposed Unet-GAN. The performance of LV segmentation was evaluated in terms of Dice overlap index between the ground truth and the segmentation results.

3.3   Results

The Dice indices resulting from the comparative experiment is reported in Table 1. Figures 4 and 5 give some examples, showing the performance degradation caused by changes of domain and the improvement brought by Unet-GAN.

Table 1. Comparison of segmentation performance of LV-Unet on datasets from different domains. Three scenarios as aforementioned are compared: clean Unet, noisy Unet, Unet-GAN.

Dice	Clean Unet	Noisy Unet	Unet-GAN
Philips (test)	0.892 ± 0.032	0.877 ± 0.034	–
Siemens	0.474 ± 0.071	0.502 ± 0.064	**0.805 ± 0.041**
GE	0.727 ± 0.042	0.813 ± 0.040	**0.867 ± 0.035**

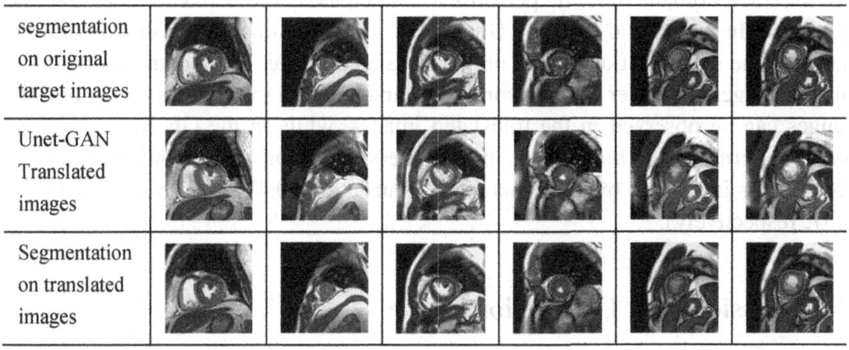

segmentation on original target images	
Unet-GAN Translated images	
Segmentation on translated images	

Fig. 4. Comparison of LV segmentation results before and after Unet-GAN translation of Siemens examples. The original and translated images were both segmented by the LV-Unet. Upper row: LV segmentation on original target images, middle row: Unet-GAN translated images to the source domain, lower row: LV segmentation on translated images, results overlaid onto the original domain.

segmentation on original target images	
Unet-GAN Translated images	
Segmentation on translated images	

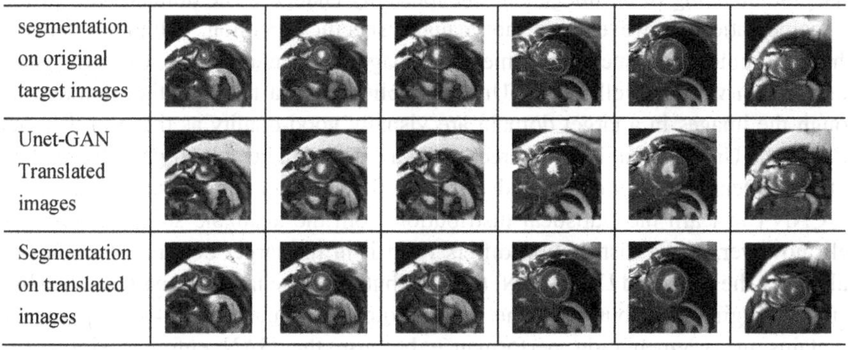

Fig. 5. Comparison of LV segmentation results before and after Unet-GAN translation of GE examples. The original and translated images were both segmented by the LV-Unet. Upper row: LV segmentation on original target images, middle row: Unet-GAN translated images to the source domain, lower row: LV segmentation on translated images, results overlaid onto the original domain.

The original LV-Unet trained on the "clean" Philips data appeared sensitive to the change of domain, and the performance drops significantly, especially on Siemens data (from 0.892 to 0.474). When trained on "polluted" Philips data with random noise, the segmentation accuracy degraded on the Philips data itself (from 0.892 to 0.877) but improved on Siemens and GE data with a small margin (0.474 to 0.502, and 0.727 to 0.813, respectively). Figures 4 and 5 provide a few examples of the vendor-adaptation results for Siemens and GE, respectively. In the first row, it can be seen while LV in the original images can be easily recognized by human eyes, the well-trained LV-Unet from another domain did not perform as anticipated, often having the LV under-segmented. In the second row, the Unet-GAN translated images are shown, and in the third row, the segmentation results on the translated images are shown (overlaid on the original images for easier comparison to the first row). In the Siemens case, brightness changes can be observed in the translated images, while in the GE case, changes are hardly discernable. In both cases, nevertheless, the final segmentation results were substantially improved by the Unet-GAN translation (0.474 to 0.805, and 0.727 to 0.867, respectively).

4   Discussion and Conclusion

In this paper, we first stated the vulnerability of CNN in medical image segmentation, a practical issue for deployment of CNNs in clinical practice. Intrigued by this problem, we proposed a network architecture combining Unet and GAN, dedicated to the medical image segmentation problems across domains (MRI vendors in this case).

The domain shift problem of CNN has been an inspiring research area in machine learning, and most studies have focused on classification, (e.g., with random-appearing noise, the labelling of an image can unexpectedly change). The domain shift problem of segmentation, however, has not caught specific attention. Although Unet has achieved tremendous success in medical image segmentation, we observed similar phenomenon when a well-trained Unet is applied to data from another domain: even though the images in a target domain are visually good-quality as those in the source domain, the Unet can fail in an unpredicted way. This can be at least partially explained by the independent and identically distribution (i.i.d.) assumption of statistical learning: the CNN can learn the statistical distribution from the available source domain very well, however, if the distribution differs from it in the target domain, it cannot generalize. By the proposed Unet-GAN, the distribution in the target domain can be shifted to fit the original distribution of the source domain, in such a way that it particularly maintains the segmentation performance because the GAN enforces similarity of segmentation-specific Unet features.

In conclusion, we proposed a network architecture called Unet-GAN, which adapts images across vendors such that a Unet trained on one vendor can generalize well to another vendor without need of new annotation. The method extends the utilization of a trained CNN to multi-center and multi-vendor use in real clinical scenario.

References

1. Long, J., Shelhamer, E., Darrell, T.: Fully convolutional networks for semantic segmentation. IEEE Trans. Pattern Anal. Mach. Intell. **39**(4), 640–651 (2014)
2. Yang, X., et al.: Towards automatic semantic segmentation in volumetric ultrasound. In: Descoteaux, M., Maier-Hein, L., Franz, A., Jannin, P., Collins, D.L., Duchesne, S. (eds.) MICCAI 2017. LNCS, vol. 10433, pp. 711–719. Springer, Cham (2017). https://doi.org/10.1007/978-3-319-66182-7_81
3. Badrinarayanan, V., Kendall, A., Cipolla, R.: SegNet: a deep convolutional encoder-decoder architecture for image segmentation. IEEE Trans. Pattern Anal. Mach. Intell. **39**(12), 2481–2495 (2017)
4. Szegedy, C., et al.: Intriguing properties of neural networks. CoRR, arXiv:1312.6199 (2013)
5. Tzeng, E., Hoffman, J., Saenko, K., Darrell, T.: Adversarial discriminative domain adaptation. In: Computer Vision and Pattern Recognition (2017)
6. Jo, J., Bengio, Y.: Measuring the tendency of CNNs to learn surface statistical regularities (2017)
7. Zhu, J.-Y., Park, T., Isola, P., Efros, A.A.: Unpaired image-to-image translation using cycle-consistent adversarial networks. In: International Conference on Computer Vision, ICCV (2017)
8. Wang, Z., Bovik, A.C., Sheikh, H.R., Simoncelli, E.P.: Image quality assessment: from error visibility to structural similarity. IEEE Trans. Image Process. **13**(4), 600–612 (2004)
9. Qin, C., et al.: Joint learning of motion estimation and segmentation for cardiac MR image sequences. In: Frangi, A.F., Schnabel, J.A., Davatzikos, C., Alberola-López, C., Fichtinger, G. (eds.) MICCAI 2018. LNCS, vol. 11071, pp. 472–480. Springer, Cham (2018). https://doi.org/10.1007/978-3-030-00934-2_53
10. Bai, W., et al.: Semi-supervised learning for network-based cardiac MR image segmentation. In: Descoteaux, M., Maier-Hein, L., Franz, A., Jannin, P., Collins, D.L., Duchesne, S. (eds.) MICCAI 2017. LNCS, vol. 10434, pp. 253–260. Springer, Cham (2017). https://doi.org/10.1007/978-3-319-66185-8_29
11. Zeiler, M.D., Fergus, R.: Visualizing and understanding convolutional networks. arXiv:1311.2901 (2013)

Cardiac MRI Segmentation with Strong Anatomical Guarantees

Nathan Painchaud[1(✉)], Youssef Skandarani[1,2], Thierry Judge[1],
Olivier Bernard[3], Alain Lalande[2], and Pierre-Marc Jodoin[1]

[1] Department of Computer Science, University of Sherbrooke, Sherbrooke, Canada
nathan.painchaud@usherbrooke.ca
[2] Université de Bourgogne Franche-Comté, Dijon, France
[3] Université de Lyon, Lyon, France

Abstract. Recent publications have shown that the segmentation accuracy of modern-day convolutional neural networks (CNN) applied on cardiac MRI can reach the inter-expert variability, a great achievement in this area of research. However, despite these successes, CNNs still produce anatomically inaccurate segmentations as they provide no guarantee on the anatomical plausibility of their outcome, even when using a shape prior. In this paper, we propose a cardiac MRI segmentation method which always produces anatomically plausible results. At the core of the method is an adversarial variational autoencoder (aVAE) whose latent space encodes a smooth manifold on which lies a large spectrum of valid cardiac shapes. This aVAE is used to automatically warp anatomically inaccurate cardiac shapes towards a close but correct shape. Our method can accommodate any cardiac segmentation method and convert its anatomically implausible results to plausible ones without affecting its overall geometric and clinical metrics. With our method, CNNs can now produce results that are both within the inter-expert variability and always anatomically plausible.

Keywords: CNN · Variational autoencoder · Cardiac MRI segmentation

1 Introduction

Magnetic Resonance Imaging (MRI) is a non-invasive imaging technique of choice to evaluate the heart. The cardiac function is typically evaluated from a series of kinetic images (cine-MRI) acquired in short-axis orientation [9]. In clinical practice, cardiac parameters are usually estimated from the knowledge of the endocardial and epicardial borders of the left ventricle (defined as the cavity (LV) and the myocardium (MYO)) and the endocardial border of the right

Electronic supplementary material The online version of this chapter (https://doi.org/10.1007/978-3-030-32245-8_70) contains supplementary material, which is available to authorized users.

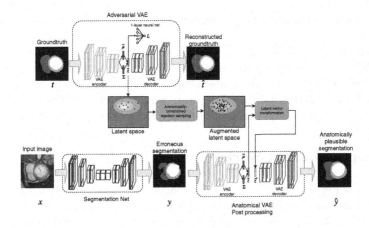

Fig. 1. Schematic representation of our method.

ventricle (RV) in end-diastolic (ED) and end-systolic (ES) phases. In the last few years, several deep learning segmentation methods (in particular CNNs) have had great success at estimating these clinical parameters [3–5,11]. Some of them provide excellent segmentation results with overall Dice index and/or Hausdorff distance within the inter- and intra-observer variations [4]. Unfortunately, these methods still generate anatomically impossible shapes like a LV connected to the background or two disconnected RV regions. Therefore, despite their excellent results on average, these methods are still unfit for day-to-day clinical use.

To reduce such errors, several papers integrate shape priors into their cardiac deep learning segmentation methods. In particular, Oktay *et al.* used an approach named anatomically constrained neural network (ACNN) [5]. Their neural network is similar to a 3D U-Net, whose segmentation output is constrained to be close to a non-linear compact representation of the underlying anatomy derived from an auto-encoder network. More recently, Zotti *et al.* proposed a method based on the grid-net architecture that embeds a cardiac shape prior to segment MR images [11]. Their shape prior encodes the probability of a 3D location point being a member of a certain class and is automatically registered with the last feature maps of their network. Finally, Duan *et al.* implemented a shape-constrained bi-ventricular segmentation strategy [3]. Their pipeline starts with a multi-task deep learning approach that aims to locate specific landmarks. These landmarks are then used to initialize atlas propagation during a refinement stage of segmentation. Although the use of an atlas improves the quality of the results, their final segmented shapes strongly depend on the accuracy of the located landmarks. From these studies, it appears that only soft constraints are currently imposed in the literature to steer the segmentation outputs towards a reference shape. As we will be shown in this paper, shape-prior methods are not immune to producing anatomically incorrect results.

Another simple way of reducing the number of anatomically inaccurate results is through the use of post-processing tools. It typically involves morphological operators or some connected component analysis to remove small isolated regions. Unfortunately, such post-processing methods cannot guarantee the anatomical plausibility of every segmentation map.

In this paper, we present the first deep learning formalism which guarantees the anatomical plausibility of cardiac shapes. Our method can be plugged to the output of any segmentation method as it would reduce to zero its number of anatomically invalid shapes while preserving the overall quality of its results.

2   Proposed Framework

As shown in Fig. 1, our method has three main blocks namely: (i) an adversarial VAE that learns a 32-dim latent representation of anatomically correct cardiac shapes, (ii) an anatomically-constrained data augmentation of the latent vectors and (iii) a post-processing VAE which converts erroneous segmentation maps into anatomically plausible ones. The anatomical guarantees that our method provides comes from a transformation function that replaces the latent vector of an anatomically erroneous shape by a close but anatomically correct one.

2.1   Cardiac MR Images and Anatomical Metrics

The goal of our method is to produce cardiac segmentation maps with strong anatomical guarantees from short-axis cine-MRI. In that perspective we defined 16 anatomical metrics that will be used to detect incorrect cardiac shapes.

We first consider any holes in the LV, the RV or the MYO, and between the LV and the MYO and between the RV and the MYO as being anatomically impossible. The presence of more than one LV, RV or MYO is also considered implausible. We also measure if the RV is disconnected from the MYO, if the LV touches the RV or the background, and if the LV, RV and MYO suffer from unusually acute concavities. The threshold beyond which a concavity is considered abnormal was defined based on the groundtruth of the ACDC training set (c.f. Sect. 3). We also implemented a circularity metric for the LV and the MYO which is the ratio of their area to that of a circle having the same perimeter. Again, the threshold for that ratio was obtained from the ACDC training set. Please note that since these metrics are not included in the loss, they do not need to be differentiable.

2.2   Adversarial Variational Autoencoder (aVAE)

VAEs [7] are encoder/decoder unsupervised learning methods used to derive a latent representation of a set of data. In our case, the encoder takes as input a cardiac segmentation map $x \in \mathbb{R}^{n \times n}$ and outputs the parameters (μ and σ) of a Gaussian probability density $q_\theta(z|x)$ where $z \in \mathbb{R}^{32}$ is a latent vector. The decoder takes in a latent variable z sampled from $q_\theta(z|x)$ and outputs $\hat{x}$, a reconstructed version of the input cardiac shape x.

In our method, we implemented an adversarial VAE (aVAE) [10] which forces the latent space to be as linear as possible. The constraint comes in the form of a single-layer neural network [1] trained simultaneously with the rest of the VAE. This neural network is used to predict the slice index of the input image x given its latent vector z using a regression loss. Since the regression's gradient signal propagates through the *encoder*, it forces it to learn a more linear (and thus less convoluted) latent space.

2.3   Anatomically-Constrained Data Augmentation

Once the aVAE is trained, every groundtruth short-axis cardiac shape is projected onto the 32d latent space. Since the ACDC dataset [4] contains a total of 1902 short axis maps, the latent space gets populated by 1902 latent vectors z. These latent vectors are "anatomically correct" since the deterministic aVAE decoder can convert them back to anatomically valid cardiac shapes. Unfortunately, these 1902 vectors are too few to densely populate the 32d manifold of anatomically correct latent vectors.

To solve that problem, we increase the number of anatomically correct latent vectors with a rejection sampling (RS) method [8]. The goal is to produce a new set of latent vectors Z' such that the distribution $P(z')$ of the newly generated samples is close to $P(z)$, the distribution from which derive the original 1902 points. RS generates a series of samples iid of $P(z)$ but based on a second and easier to sample pdf $Q(z)$. Since in our case $P(z)$ is unknown, we estimate it with a Parzen window distribution [1]. Meanwhile, $Q(z)$ is a Gaussian of mean and variance equal to the distribution of the original 1902 points. A key idea with RS is that $P(z) > MQ(z)$ where $M > 1$. Given $p(z)$ and $Q(z)$, the sampling procedure first generates a random sample z_i iid of $Q(z)$ as well as a uniform random value $u \in [0, 1]$. If $u < \frac{P(z_i)}{MQ(z_i)}$ then z_i is kept, otherwise it is rejected.

In our case, in addition to an increased number of latent vectors, we want those new vectors to correspond to anatomically correct cardiac shapes. As such, we redefine the RS criterion as follows:

$$u < \mathbb{1}\left(\operatorname{dec}(z_i)\right) \frac{P(z_i)}{MQ(z_i)} \tag{1}$$

where $\mathbb{1}\left(\operatorname{dec}(z_i)\right)$ is an indicator function which returns 1 when the decoded latent vector z_i is a valid cardiac anatomy and zero otherwise. We call this operation an *anatomically-constrained rejection sampling augmentation*. The procedure is repeated up until the desired number of samples are generated. This operation allows us to generate 4 million latent vectors which all have a valid cardiac shape, i.e. that respect all 16 metrics defined in Sect. 2.1. Images of generated samples are provided in the supplementary materials.

2.4   Latent Vector Transformation

Our system contains a post-processing VAE (at the bottom right of Fig. 1) used to convert erroneous segmentation maps into anatomically valid segmentations.

The post-processing VAE has the same architecture and the same weights as the aVAE. Thus, any erroneous segmentation map fed to the VAE *encoder* gets projected into the same latent space as that of the aVAE. Furthermore, since the VAE *decoder* is deterministic, any anatomically valid latent vector z is guaranteed to be converted into an anatomically correct cardiac shape.

The goal is to transform the latent vector z of an erroneous cardiac shape to a similar but anatomically valid latent vector z', which can be summarized as:

$$z' = \arg\min_{z'} ||z - z'||^2, \quad s.t. \ \mathbb{1}\left(\dec(z')\right) = 1. \tag{2}$$

Said otherwise, the goal is to find the anatomically valid latent vector z' that is the closest to z. Unfortunately, since $\mathbb{1}\left(\dec(z')\right) = 1$ involves the 16 non-differentiable metrics, this function cannot be minimized with a usual Lagrangian formulation. As a solution, we redefined the problem of finding z' as a problem of finding the smallest vector $\delta_{z'}$ such that $z' = z + \alpha\delta_{z'}$. In this paper, we recover $\delta_{z'}$ based on the nearest neighbor in the augmented latent space. In this way, $\delta_{z'} = (z_{N1} - z)$ where z_{N1} is the nearest neighbor of z in the augmented latent space and $\alpha \in [0, 1]$. This leads to an easier 1D optimization problem:

$$\alpha = \arg\min_{\alpha} |\alpha|, \quad s.t. \ \mathbb{1}\left(z + \alpha\delta_{z'}\right) = 1 \tag{3}$$

that we solve with a dichotomic search. At each iteration, the remaining search space of α is divided in two and the anatomical criterion $\mathbb{1}\left(\dec(z + \alpha\delta_{z'})\right) = 1$ specifies which of the upper-half or lower-half should be divided at the next iteration. Since the search space decreases exponentially fast, the optimization algorithm is stopped after five iterations, selecting the smallest alpha that validates the anatomical criterion.

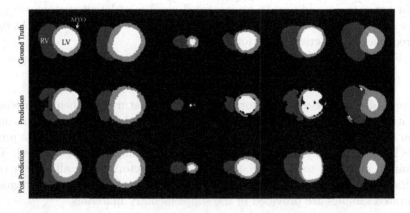

Fig. 2. Groundtruth and erroneous maps before and after our post-processing method.

2.5 Implementation Details

The *encoder* of our aVAE has ten 3×3 convolution layers with stride 2 with ELU [2] activation layers which output a 32-dim latent vector. The *decoder* follows the same architecture except for the transposed convolutions that increase the feature maps resolution. For the adversarial network, we used a single-layer neural network with an L2 regression loss. The whole network is trained end-to-end using Adam [6] with a learning rate of $6 * 10^{-5}$ and a $L2$ weight regularization with $\lambda = 0.01$. Note that the segmentation maps fed to our VAEs have a size of 256×256 and are registered so the center of the LV is in the middle of the image. This translation and rotation registration is done at runtime.

Table 1. Ablation study of our aVAE showing the average % of anatomical errors while navigating through the latent space.

AE	VAE	VAE + registered	VAE + adversarial	VAE + regist. + adv.
64.76	5.84	5.85	8.48	1.25

3 Experimental Setup and Results

3.1 Dataset, Evaluation Criteria, and Other Methods

We trained and tested our method on the 2017 ACDC dataset [4] which contains cine-MR images of 150 patients, 100 for training and 50 for testing. As shown in Fig. 2, the LV, RV and MYO of every patient has been manually segmented. We report the average 3D Dice index and Hausdorff distance (HD) for the LV, RV and MYO as well as the LV and RV ejection fraction (EF) absolute error. Since our approach can accommodate any segmentation method, we tested it on the test results reported by the ten ACDC challengers. Their methods are summarized by Bernard *et al.* [4] except for Zotti-2 [11] whose results have been uploaded recently. We also report results for the ACNN method of Oktay *et al.* [5] that uses a latent anatomical prior to train a segmentation CNN. Results from our best implementation (which involves a U-Net and our VAE) are very close to that of the original paper despite the fact that the ACDC training set is smaller than the one they used. HD values are also slightly larger since we use a 3D HD instead of a 2D HD as in the original paper.

3.2 Experimental Results

Adversarial Variational Autoencoder. We validated the design of our aVAE through the ablation study of Table 1. Since our post-processing method relies on latent vector interpolation (c.f. Eq. (3)), we computed the percentage of anatomically implausible results obtained after interpolating two valid latent vectors. To do so, we iteratively selected the groundtruth of two random slices from two random patients of the ACDC test set, encoded it to the latent space with the aVAE encoder and linearly interpolated 25 new vectors. We then converted these 25 vectors to segmentation maps with the aVAE decoder and computed their percentage of anatomical errors. We repeated that process 500 times for the aVAE with and without registration and with and without an adversarial regression loss. As can be seen, the use of registration and an adversarial regression loss reduces the percentage of anatomically implausible results down to 1.25% which is more than 4x lower than for the other configurations.

Table 2. Number of anatomically invalid segmentation results on the ACDC test set for 11 segmentation methods with and without our post-processing methods.

Submissions	Original	VAE	Nearest neighbors		
			w/o RS	w/ RS	Dicho
Zotti-2	55	16	0	0	0
Khened	55	16	0	0	0
Baumgartner	79	17	0	0	0
Zotti	82	15	0	0	0
Grinias	89	12	0	0	0
Isensee	128	21	0	0	0
Rohé	287	40	0	0	0
Wolterink	324	42	0	0	0
Jain	185	28	0	0	0
Yang	572	182	0	0	0
ACNN	139	41	0	0	0

Postprocessing Results. Results on the ACDC test set are in Tables 2 and 3. Table 2 contains the total number of slices with at least one anatomical error, Table 3 shows at the top the overall Dice index and HD and at the bottom the LV and RV EF absolute errors. Results without our post-processing are under the *Original* column. As shown, every method produces a non-negligible number of anatomical errors (the ACDC testset has a total of 1078 slices).

By feeding every erroneous segmentation map to our VAE without transforming the latent vector z, we get to drastically reduce the number of anatomical errors without affecting too much the HD, the Dice and the EF. This comes as no surprise since the VAE was trained to reproduce groundtruth (and thus anatomically correct) cardiac shapes. However, like any neural network, a basic VAE provides no guarantee on the quality of its output. To completely eliminate erroneous segmentations, we first swap erroneous latent vectors with their nearest neighbor (i.e. by fixing α to 1 in Eq. 3) using groundtruth data from the ACDC training set (i.e. 1902 short axis maps) without RS augmentation (w/o RS). While that procedure eliminated every anatomical error and did not

Table 3. [Top] Average Dice index and Hausdorff distance (in mm) and [Bottom] Average error on LV and RV ejection fraction (EF) for the ACDC test set with and without our post-processing method.

Submissions	Original	VAE	Nearest neighbors		
			w/o RS	w/ RS	Dicho
Zotti-2	.913/9.7	.910/10.1	.899/14.4	.909/11.0	.910/10.1
Khened	.915/11.3	.912/12.3	.894/15.2	.909/12.7	.912/10.9
Baumgartner	.914/10.5	.911/11.2	.889/18.2	.907/12.6	.910/10.6
Zotti	.910/9.7	.907/10.9	.878/19.6	.903/12.6	.907/11.0
Grinias	.835/15.9	.833/19.3	.752/32.5	.825/16.9	.833/15.8
Isensee	.926/9.1	.923/10.7	.881/18.4	.917/11.2	.923/9.2
Rohé	.891/12.2	.887/14.6	.756/32.2	.874/15.1	.887/12.8
Wolterink	.907/10.8	.903/13.0	.752/32.8	.887/13.5	.903/11.0
Jain	.891/12.2	.886/12.6	.820/31.9	.878/14.2	.886/11.6
Yang	.800/27.5	.752/21.7	.455/29.7	.722/11.5	.752/10.2
ACNN	.892/12.3	.886/26.2	.885/12.0	.885/12.2	.889/13.1
Zotti-2	2.54/5.11	2.63/5.12	2.49/5.57	2.58/5.18	2.62/5.18
Khened	2.39/5.24	2.41/4.96	2.70/5.36	2.63/5.07	2.42/5.27
Baumgartner	2.58/6.00	2.62/6.30	2.83/6.72	2.85/6.48	2.64/6.33
Zotti	2.98/5.48	2.98/5.42	3.06/5.72	3.10/5.71	3.06/5.59
Grinias	4.14/7.39	4.18/7.86	4.67/8.00	4.33/7.35	4.01/7.43
Isensee	2.16/4.85	2.15/4.61	2.49/5.58	2.35/4.48	2.20/4.82
Rohé	2.84/8.18	2.95/7.85	3.13/8.93	3.39/7.97	2.91/8.11
Wolterink	2.75/6.59	2.82/6.39	3.40/6.93	3.48/6.07	2.84/6.44
Jain	4.36/8.49	4.35/8.83	4.98/9.63	4.59/8.69	4.40/8.72
Yang	6.22/15.99	6.80/20.56	7.57/27.9	7.77/22.09	9.10/21.76
ACNN	2.46/3.68	2.53/4.09	2.51/3.89	2.96/3.82	2.50/3.71

change much the EF error, the Dice index and HD suffered considerably. We then tested the same method but with the latent space augmented by 4 million anatomically correct vectors (c.f. Sect. 2.3). This approach (w/ RS) also provides strong anatomical guarantees but better Dice and HD than without RS. The last column shows the results of our complete method, i.e. Eq. (3) optimized with a dichotomic search. While results are all anatomically correct, the EF error, the Dice index are almost identical to that of the original methods. The HD also never increases more than 1.3 mm, which, considering that the average voxel size is near $1.4 \times 1.4 \times 10\,\text{mm}^3$, corresponds to less than 1 pixel in the image. This shows that our approach does not degrade the overall results but only warps anatomically incorrect results towards the closest anatomically viable shape. Figure 2 shows erroneous predictions before and after our post-processing. While the correct areas are barely affected by our method, erroneous sections, big or small, get smoothly warped. Our method takes roughly 1 s to process a 2D image on a mid-end computer equipped with a Titan X GPU.

4   Conclusion

We presented a post-processing VAE which converts anatomically invalid cardiac shapes into close but correct shapes. Our method relies on 16 anatomical metrics that we use both to detect abnormalities and populate an aVAE latent space. Since those metrics are not included in the loss, they need not be differentiable. According to the inter- and intra-expert variations reported by Bernard *et al.*[4], methods such as Isensee *et al.*, Zotti-2, Khened and Baumgartner are on average as accurate as an expert and, with our post-processing method, are now guaranteed to produce anatomically plausible results.

References

1. Bishop, C.M.: Pattern Recognition and Machine Learning, 5th edn. Springer, New York (2007)
2. Clevert, D.-A., Unterthiner, T., Hochreiter, S.: Fast and accurate deep network learning by exponential linear units (ELUs). In: ICLR (2016)
3. Duan, J., Bello, G., Schlemper, J., et al.: Automatic 3D bi-ventricular segmentation of cardiac images by a shape-refined multi-task deep learning approach. IEEE TMI **38**, 2151–2164 (2019)
4. Bernard, O., et al.: Deep learning techniques for automatic MRI cardiac multi-structures segmentation and diagnosis: Is the problem solved? IEEE TMI **37**, 2514–2525 (2018)
5. Oktay, O., et al.: Anatomically constrained neural networks (ACNNs): application to cardiac image enhancement and segmentation. IEEE-TMI **37**(2), 384–395 (2017)
6. Kingma, D., Ba, J.: Adam: a method for stochastic optimization. In: ICLR (2015)
7. Kingma, D., Welling, M.: Auto-encoding variational Bayes. In: ICLR (2013)
8. Koller, D., Friedman, N.: Probabilistic Graphical Models: Principles and Techniques. MIT Press, Cambridge (2009)
9. Salerno, M., Shari, B., Arheden, B.H., et al.: Recent advances in cardiovascular magnetic resonance: techniques and applications. Circ. Card. Imaging **10**(6), e003951 (2017)
10. Makhzani, A., Shlens, J., Jaitly, N., Goodfellow, I.J.: Adversarial autoencoders. In: ICLR (2016)
11. Zotti, C., Luo, Z., Lalande, A., Jodoin, P.-M.: Convolutional neural network with shape prior applied to cardiac MRI segmentation. IEEE JBHI **23**, 1119–1128 (2018)

Decompose-and-Integrate Learning for Multi-class Segmentation in Medical Images

Yizhe Zhang[1(✉)], Michael T. C. Ying[2], and Danny Z. Chen[1]

[1] Department of Computer Science and Engineering, University of Notre Dame, Notre Dame, IN 46556, USA
yzhang29@nd.edu
[2] Department of Health Technology and Informatics, The Hong Kong Polytechnic University, Hung Hom, Hong Kong

Abstract. Segmentation maps of medical images annotated by medical experts contain rich spatial information. In this paper, we propose to decompose annotation maps to learn disentangled and richer feature transforms for segmentation problems in medical images. Our new scheme consists of two main stages: *decompose* and *integrate*. *Decompose*: by annotation map decomposition, the original segmentation problem is decomposed into multiple segmentation sub-problems; these new segmentation sub-problems are modeled by training multiple deep learning modules, each with its own set of feature transforms. *Integrate*: a procedure summarizes the solutions of the modules in the previous stage; a final solution is then formed for the original segmentation problem. Multiple ways of annotation map decomposition are presented and a new end-to-end trainable K-to-1 deep network framework is developed for implementing our proposed "decompose-and-integrate" learning scheme. In experiments, we demonstrate that our decompose-and-integrate segmentation scheme, utilizing state-of-the-art fully convolutional networks (e.g., DenseVoxNet in 3D and CUMedNet in 2D), improves segmentation performance on multiple 3D and 2D datasets. Ablation study confirms the effectiveness of our proposed learning scheme for medical images.

1 Introduction

Segmentation annotation maps are crucial for supervised training a deep learning based segmentation model. For segmentation annotation maps, besides the class label dimension, there are spatial dimensions that contain rich information of object size, shape, and between-object/between-class relations.

Previous work has proposed some methods for modifying annotation maps for training better deep learning based segmentation models. Directional map [10] was proposed to generate additional training loss based on the relative positions of the pixels to the centers of their corresponding objects. Deep watershed transform [1] provided a similar approach that converts an annotation map to

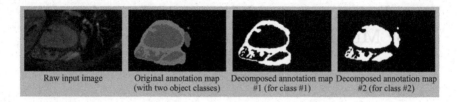

Raw input image | Original annotation map (with two object classes) | Decomposed annotation map #1 (for class #1) | Decomposed annotation map #2 (for class #2)

Fig. 1. Segmentation annotation map decomposition based on object classes.

a watershed energy map to guide the training of a segmentation model. These efforts demonstrated that changing segmentation annotation maps to include additional information (e.g., relative position, stronger instance-level information) can help train better deep learning models for segmentation tasks.

In medical image segmentation, different classes of objects often have strong locations and spatial correlations. Due to these correlations, learning representation and feature transform for one object class can often indicate the existence of some other object classes (possibly nearby). A conventional way of using multi-class annotation maps is to treat a full annotation map as a whole subject and use spatial cross-entropy loss function to compare it with the model's outputs in back propagation [3,8,13]. Due to spatial correlations among different object classes, directly using annotations of all object classes to train a deep network may cause a deep network not being able to fully explore its representation learning ability for every object class, especially for those classes with small sizes and unclear/confusing appearance. Furthermore, there may be multiple distinct structures/clusters under one class of objects, and each sub-class structure may better utilize a unique set of feature representations. In principle, we believe that modeling individual classes and sub-classes of structures or objects can encourage deep learning models to learn richer and more comprehensive feature transforms and data representations for segmentation problems.

In this paper, we propose to systematically decompose the original annotation maps to encourage deep networks to learn richer and possibly more disentangled feature transforms and representations. Our new scheme consists of two main stages: *decompose* and *integrate*. *Decompose*: by annotation map decomposition, the original segmentation problem is decomposed into multiple segmentation sub-problems (e.g., see Fig. 1); these new segmentation sub-problems are modeled by training multiple deep learning modules, each with its own set of feature transforms. *Integrate*: a procedure summarizes the solutions of the modules in the previous stage; a final solution is then formed for the original segmentation problem. This decompose-and-integrate scheme allows to explicitly enforce a deep learning model to learn representations for every object class. Besides, it can also be applied to learn feature transforms and representations for (human expert defined) meaningful sub-class data clusters and structures (see Fig. 2).

In Sect. 2, we present different ways to decompose annotation maps for different scenarios, and develop a new K-to-1 deep network model for implementing our new learning scheme. In Sect. 3, we evaluate our decompose-and-integrate

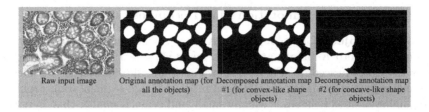

| Raw input image | Original annotation map (for all the objects) | Decomposed annotation map #1 (for convex-like shape objects) | Decomposed annotation map #2 (for concave-like shape objects) |

Fig. 2. Segmentation annotation map decomposition based on object shape property.

learning scheme utilizing multiple state-of-the-art fully convolutional networks (FCNs) on three medical image segmentation datasets, and examine several proposed annotation decomposition (AD) methods.

2 Decompose-and-Integrate Learning

Consider a K-class segmentation training dataset $\{(x_i, y_i),\ i = 1, 2, \ldots, h\}$, $x_i \in R^{m \times n}$ is a raw image, and $y_i \in \{1, 2, \ldots, K\}^{m \times n}$ is a segmentation annotation map containing all the annotations of the K classes of interest. Supervised learning for K-class segmentation tasks aims to learn a function $f \in F$ that transforms x to y. Note that each y_i can be denoted as $\{y_i^1, y_i^2, \ldots, y_i^K\}$, where $y_i^k \in \{0, 1\}^{m \times n}$ is an annotation map for object class k, for $k = 1, 2, \ldots, K$.

For a segmentation problem with two foreground object classes A and B, suppose modeling $p(y^B | x)$ for class B is more difficult than modeling $p(y^A | x)$ for class A. This means that learning a robust latent representation $R^B(x)$ for class B takes more computational effort (e.g., more training iterations/gradient descent effort) than learning a robust latent representation $R^A(x)$ for class A. Note that $R^B(x)$ and $R^A(x)$ are **not** necessarily disjoint. When $p(y^A)$ and $p(y^B)$ have moderate or high spatial correlations, using joint annotations of these two classes for training a deep learning model can lead to: (1) $p(y^A | x)$ is quite likely to be modeled using $R^A(x)$; (2) $p(y^B | x)$ would be modeled with help from $R^A(x)$, and not mainly by using $R^B(x)$; (3) $R^B(x)$ is not fully explored during model training, due to the "help" of the annotations from class A. For a better representation and feature learning performance, such "help" is undesired. Besides multi-class segmentation scenarios, when an object class has distinct meaningful underlining sub-class structures/clusters, having a separate modeling for each individual structure/cluster enforces a deep network to learn more meaningful and useful data representations and feature transforms for such a class.

Below in Sect. 2.1, we present several ways to decompose annotation maps under different scenarios. In Sect. 2.2, a new K-to-1 deep network framework is proposed for implementing our decompose-and-integrate learning scheme.

2.1   Segmentation Annotation Map Decomposition

Based on Object Classes. For a K-class segmentation problem, we can decompose y_i into K binary annotation maps y_i^k, $k = 1, 2, \ldots, K$. Algorithm 1 gives the exact procedure. Figure 1 shows an image illustration of the effect of this annotation decomposition (AD). In medical image segmentation problems, the number of object classes is usually small, and is much smaller than in natural scene images. A general guideline is that the decomposed segmentation maps and their associated extra computational costs should be under a manageable level. Table 1 shows that object-class based AD can effectively improve segmentation performance for segmentation problems with multiple foreground classes.

Algorithm 1. Object-class based annotation decomposition

1: **function** ANNOTATIONDECOMPOSITION1($y_i \in \{1, 2, \ldots, K\}^{m \times n}$)
2:     **for** $k \leftarrow 1$ to K **do**
3:         y_i^k = a new array of size $m \times n$ with all 0;
4:         y_i^k [where($y_i == k$)] $\leftarrow 1$;
5:     **return** $y_i^1, y_i^2, \ldots, y_i^K$

Based on Object Shapes. Annotation maps can also be decomposed based on different shape structures in the annotation maps. This type of decomposition can be applied to 2-class segmentation and also K-class segmentation for $K > 2$.

Shape information contains valuable cues for segmentation tasks. Decomposing annotation maps based on different object shapes can encourage a deep learning model to learn feature transforms that encode the raw images into different shape-guided representations. In histology image analysis, morphological features such as shape convexity play an important role in object detection, segmentation, and diagnosis. Thus, we propose to decompose segmentation annotation maps based on shape convexity of objects in the annotation maps. Specifically, two sub-segmentation maps are generated from an original segmentation annotation map, one containing convex-like shape objects and the other containing concave-like shape objects. This decomposition provides additional information that directly helps a learning model to perceive object information at a higher (object shape) level. The detailed procedure and image illustration are provided in Algorithm 2 and Fig. 2. In practice, we set T_{shape} as 0.9. Table 2 demonstrates the usefulness of shape based AD when segmentation problems contain objects with several shape types.

Based on Image-Level Information. Image-level information, statistics, and cues can be utilized for annotation map decomposition. For example, if images contain one or multiple foreground objects, we can decompose the segmentation maps based on the number of objects appeared in an image. As the number of objects could only be revealed at a global level or deeper layer in a deep learning model, this decomposition method pushes a learning model to be more aware of global and higher-level information when generating segmentation results.

Algorithm 2. Object-shape based annotation decomposition

1: **function** ANNOTATIONDECOMPOSITION2($y_i \in \{1, 2, \ldots, K\}^{m \times n}$, T_{shape})
2:     $y_i^{convex} \leftarrow$ a new array of size $m \times n$ with all 0;
3:     $y_i^{concave} \leftarrow$ a new array of size $m \times n$ with all 0;
4:     **for** every object p in y_i **do**
5:         Compute the convex hull p^{convex} of p
6:         $ratio = \text{size}(p)/\text{size}(p^{convex})$
7:         **if** $ratio > T_{shape}$ (p is of a convex-like shape) **then**
8:             Add object p to y_i^{convex}
9:         **else**
10:            Add object p to $y_i^{concave}$
11:    **return** y_i^{convex} and $y_i^{concave}$

Algorithm 3. Image-level information based annotation decomposition

1: **function** ANNOTATIONDECOMPOSITION3($y_i \in \{1, 2, \ldots, K\}^{m \times n}$)
2:     $y_i^{single\_obj} \leftarrow$ a new array of size $m \times n$ with all 0;
3:     $y_i^{multiple\_obj} \leftarrow$ a new array of size $m \times n$ with all 0;
4:     **if** y_i contains only one object **then**
5:         $y_i^{single\_obj} \leftarrow y_i$
6:     **if** y_i contains multiple objects **then**
7:         $y_i^{multiple\_obj} \leftarrow y_i$
8:     **return** $y_i^{single\_obj}$ and $y_i^{multiple\_obj}$

An exact annotation decomposition procedure based on the image-level number of objects is given in Algorithm 3. In Table 3, we show the effectiveness of image-level information based AD for lymph node segmentation in ultrasound images.

2.2 The K-to-1 Deep Network for Decompose-and-Integrate Learning

Suppose every original annotation map y_i, $i = 1, 2, \ldots, h$, is decomposed into K annotation maps y_i^k, $i = 1, 2, \ldots, h$ and $k = 1, 2, \ldots, K$. We aim to model each sub-segmentation problem using a deep learning segmentation module with its own set of parameters. Then another modeling procedure is applied on top of these K modules to form the final solution of the original segmentation problem.

Thus, we propose a new K-to-1 deep network framework for implementing our above decompose-and-integrate learning scheme. Figure 3 shows an overview of our K-to-1 deep network. The modules (e.g., Seg-Module 1.1, Seg-Module 2) used in this network can be changed according to the type of images (e.g., 2D or 3D images) of the specific segmentation problem. The full model can be trained in end-to-end manner. Let the function of the overall K-to-1 network be denoted as $f_{complete}$, and the function of Seg-Module 1.k be denoted as $f_{1.k}$. The overall loss for the decompose-and-integrate learning scheme is defined as:

$$\frac{1}{h} \sum_{i=1}^{h} \left(\mathcal{L}\left(f_{complete}(x_i), y_i\right) + \lambda \sum_{k=1}^{K} \mathcal{L}(f_{1.k}(x_i), y_i^k) \right) \tag{1}$$

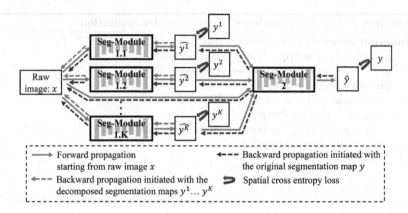

Fig. 3. The K-to-1 deep network framework for our new decompose-and-integrate learning scheme. y^k, $k = 1, 2, \ldots, K$, are decomposed segmentation annotation maps, and y is the original segmentation annotation map.

where $\mathcal{L}$ is the spatial cross entropy loss, and λ is set as simple as a normalization term $\frac{1}{K}$. We aim to minimize the above function with respect to the parameters of $f_{complete}$ and $f_{1.k}$ for $k = 1, 2, \ldots, K$.

Table 1. Comparison of segmentation results on the HVSMR dataset.

Method	Myocardium			Blood pool			Overall score
	Dice	ADB	Hausdorff	Dice	ADB	Hausdorff	
3D U-Net [5]	0.694	1.461	10.221	0.926	0.940	8.628	−0.419
VoxResNet [2]	0.774	1.026	6.572	0.929	0.981	9.966	−0.202
DenseVoxNet [12]	0.821	0.964	7.294	0.931	0.938	9.533	−0.161
Ensemble Meta-learner [13]	0.823	0.685	3.224	0.935	0.763	5.804	0.215
Class-AD + K-to-1 DenseVoxNet (**ours**)	0.839	0.744	3.500	0.941	0.658	5.973	**0.223**
Ablation study							
Large DenseVoxNet	0.804	0.847	3.980	0.935	0.756	7.706	0.079
2-stacked DenseVoxNet	0.837	0.797	3.405	0.939	0.629	7.529	0.167
K-to-1 DenseVoxNet w/o AD	0.824	0.776	3.619	0.940	0.677	6.632	0.177

3   Experiments and Results

We conduct experiments on three datasets. The 3D cardiovascular segmentation dataset [7] contains two classes of foreground objects (myocardium and great vessels), which have close spatial relations. Thus, we apply object-class based annotation decomposition (AD) to this dataset. The gland segmentation dataset [9] contains glands that have quite different shapes (from concave shape to convex shape); hence shape convexity based annotation decomposition (AD) is applied to this dataset. Our in-house lymph node dataset contains the lymph node areas of 237 patients in ultrasound images (one image may contain one or more lymph nodes). Thus, image-level information based AD is applied to this dataset.

Implementation Details. The input window size of the deep learning segmentation models we use is set as $64 \times 64 \times 64$ for 3D experiments and 192×192 for 2D experiments. During training, random cropping, rotation, and flipping are applied. Since the images in each dataset are larger than the model window size, there are virtually many more samples for model training than the number of images in each dataset. The Adam optimizer is used for model training. The mini-batch size is set as 8. The maximum number of training iteration is set to 60000. We find that usually 60000 iterations using Adam are sufficient for an FCN-type model to converge for a moderate sized training set. The learning rate is set as 0.0005 initially, and decreased to 0.00005 after 30000 iterations.

3D Cardiovascular Segmentation in MR Images. The HVSMR dataset [7] seeks to segment myocardium and great vessels (blood pool) in 3D cardiovascular MR images. The ground truth of the test data is not available to the public; the evaluations are done by submitting segmentation results to the organizers' server. We experiment with the object class based AD for this dataset. Table 1 shows that our AD combined with K-to-1 network (utilizing DenseVoxNets) achieves state-of-the-art performance on this dataset. In the ablation study part of Table 1, we compare our full model with K-to-1 network without AD, a 2-stacked DenseVoxNet, and a large-size DenseVoxNet that uses a similar amount of parameters as the K-to-1 DenseVoxNet. K-to-1 without AD is an ablation study setting in which the model architecture is the same as the K-to-1 model, but no annotation decomposition is utilized. That is, the K modules work on the same annotation map and learning task as the original map and segmentation task. The 2-stacked DenseVoxNet is a two-stage stacked DenseVoxNet. The first stage is a DenseVoxNet, and the second stage is another DenseVoxNet that takes both the raw image and the output of the first DenseVoxNet as its input. The overall ablation study results demonstrate the effectiveness of our decompose-and-integrate learning scheme.

Gland Segmentation in H&E Stained Images. This dataset [9] contains 85 training images (37 benign (BN), 48 malignant (MT)), 60 testing images (33 BN, 27 MT) in part A, and 20 testing images (4 BN, 16 MT) in part B. We modify the original CUMedNet [3] to make it deeper with two more encoding and decoding blocks (denoted as CUMedNet$^+$). We run all the experiments for the K-to-1 network and ablation study 5 times. Table 2 shows the mean performance and standard derivations. Compared with the state-of-the-art models, our AD + K-to-1 network (utilizing CUMedNet$^+$) yields considerably better segmentation results. In ablation study (the bottom part of Table 2), we compare AD + K-to-1 network with K-to-1 network without AD, a 2-stacked CUMedNet$^+$, and a large-size CUMedNet$^+$.

Lymph Node Segmentation in Ultrasound Images. We collected patients' lymph node ultrasound images. We use 137 images for model training, and 100 images for model testing. The image size is 1080×768. There is no identity

Table 2. Comparison of segmentation results on the gland segmentation dataset.

Method	F_1 score		ObjectDice		ObjectHausdorff	
	Part A	Part B	Part A	Part B	Part A	Part B
CUMedVision [4]	0.912	0.716	0.897	0.718	45.418	160.347
Multichannel2 [11]	0.893	0.843	0.908	0.833	44.129	116.821
MILD-Net [6]	0.914	0.844	**0.913**	0.836	41.54	105.89
CUMedNet [3]$^+$	0.907 ± 0.007	0.835 ± 0.009	0.893 ± 0.007	0.832 ± 0.008	49.97 ± 2.12	113.40 ± 7.22
Shape-AD + K-to-1 (ours)	**0.923 ± 0.002**	**0.861 ± 0.004**	0.910 ± 0.004	**0.846 ± 0.001**	**40.79 ± 1.72**	**101.42 ± 1.49**
Ablation study						
Large CUMedNet$^+$	0.918 ± 0.005	0.817 ± 0.021	0.903 ± 0.002	0.827 ± 0.012	43.81 ± 1.39	109.43 ± 5.39
2-stacked CUMedNet$^+$	0.914 ± 0.002	0.830 ± 0.009	0.908 ± 0.001	0.844 ± 0.002	45.32 ± 1.05	101.43 ± 2.25
K-to-1 w/o AD	0.915 ± 0.007	0.829 ± 0.008	0.898 ± 0.007	0.831 ± 0.004	45.23 ± 3.71	108.92 ± 4.74

overlap between the training data and testing data. The AD procedure follows Algorithm 3. Table 3 demonstrates that AD + K-to-1 network can effectively improve lymph node segmentation performance in ultrasound images.

Table 3. Comparison of segmentation results on the lymph node segmentation dataset.

Method	IoU	Precision	Recall	F_1 score
U-Net [8]	0.661	0.834	0.7607	0.7957
Deeper U-Net	0.7369	0.8555	0.8416	0.8485
CUMedNet [3]$^+$	0.7595	0.8472	0.8801	0.8633
Image-level-AD + K-to-1 (ours)	**0.8102**	**0.9012**	**0.8893**	**0.8952**
Ablation study				
Large CUMedNet$^+$	0.7795	0.8808	0.8714	0.8761
2-stacked CUMedNet$^+$	0.7759	0.876	0.8716	0.8738
K-to-1 w/o AD	0.7842	0.8798	0.8783	0.8790

Model Complexity and Time Cost. Because of the added K modules, in the 3D cardiovascular segmentation experiment, the K-to-1 DenseVoxNet ($K = 2$) and large DenseVoxNet are about 3 times as large as DenseVoxNet. In the gland segmentation experiment, Shape-AD + K-to-1 ($K = 2$) and large CUMedNet$^+$ are about 3 times as large as CUMedNet$^+$. In the lymph node segmentation experiment, Image-level-AD + K-to-1 ($K = 2$) and large CUMedNet$^+$ are about 3 times as large as CUMedNet$^+$. The model inference time for the K-to-1 model is shorter than what its model complexity suggests since the K modules in the first stage can be executed on GPU in parallel. Annotation decomposition, such as building the convex hull, is algorithmically fast.

4   Conclusions

In this paper, we developed a new decompose-and-integrate learning scheme for medical image segmentation. Our new learning scheme is well motivated, sound, and flexible. Comprehensive experiments on multiple datasets show that our new learning scheme is effective in learning more robust feature transforms and improving segmentation performance.

Acknowledgements. This work was supported in part by NSF grants CCF-1617735 and CNS-1629914, the Departmental General Research Fund (G-UADH; Project ID: P0008696) of the Hong Kong Polytechnic University, and the Global Collaboration Initiative (GCI) Program of the University of Notre Dame.

References

1. Bai, M., Urtasun, R.: Deep watershed transform for instance segmentation. In: CVPR, pp. 5221–5229 (2017)
2. Chen, H., Dou, Q., Yu, L., Qin, J., Heng, P.A.: VoxResNet: deep voxelwise residual networks for brain segmentation from 3D MR images. NeuroImage **170**, 446–455 (2018)
3. Chen, H., Qi, X., Cheng, J.Z., Heng, P.A.: Deep contextual networks for neuronal structure segmentation. In: AAAI, pp. 1167–1173 (2016)
4. Chen, H., Qi, X., Yu, L., Heng, P.A.: DCAN: deep contour-aware networks for accurate gland segmentation. In: CVPR, pp. 2487–2496 (2016)
5. Çiçek, Ö., Abdulkadir, A., Lienkamp, S.S., Brox, T., Ronneberger, O.: 3D U-Net: learning dense volumetric segmentation from sparse annotation. In: Ourselin, S., Joskowicz, L., Sabuncu, M.R., Unal, G., Wells, W. (eds.) MICCAI 2016. LNCS, vol. 9901, pp. 424–432. Springer, Cham (2016). https://doi.org/10.1007/978-3-319-46723-8_49
6. Graham, S., Chen, H., Dou, Q., Heng, P.A., Rajpoot, N.: MILD-Net: minimal information loss dilated network for gland instance segmentation in colon histology images. arXiv preprint arXiv:1806.01963 (2018)
7. Pace, D.F., Dalca, A.V., Geva, T., Powell, A.J., Moghari, M.H., Golland, P.: Interactive whole-heart segmentation in congenital heart disease. In: Navab, N., Hornegger, J., Wells, W.M., Frangi, A.F. (eds.) MICCAI 2015. LNCS, vol. 9351, pp. 80–88. Springer, Cham (2015). https://doi.org/10.1007/978-3-319-24574-4_10
8. Ronneberger, O., Fischer, P., Brox, T.: U-Net: convolutional networks for biomedical image segmentation. In: Navab, N., Hornegger, J., Wells, W.M., Frangi, A.F. (eds.) MICCAI 2015. LNCS, vol. 9351, pp. 234–241. Springer, Cham (2015). https://doi.org/10.1007/978-3-319-24574-4_28
9. Sirinukunwattan, K., et al.: Gland segmentation in colon histology images: the GlaS challenge contest. Med. Image Anal. **35**, 489–502 (2017)
10. Uhrig, J., Cordts, M., Franke, U., Brox, T.: Pixel-level encoding and depth layering for instance-level semantic labeling. In: German Conference on Pattern Recognition, pp. 14–25 (2016)
11. Xu, Y., et al.: Gland instance segmentation by deep multichannel neural networks. arXiv preprint arXiv:1607.04889 (2016)

12. Yu, L., et al.: Automatic 3D cardiovascular MR segmentation with densely-connected volumetric ConvNets. In: Descoteaux, M., Maier-Hein, L., Franz, A., Jannin, P., Collins, D.L., Duchesne, S. (eds.) MICCAI 2017. LNCS, vol. 10434, pp. 287–295. Springer, Cham (2017). https://doi.org/10.1007/978-3-319-66185-8_33
13. Zheng, H., et al.: A new ensemble learning framework for 3D biomedical image segmentation. arXiv preprint arXiv:1812.03945 (2018)

Missing Slice Imputation in Population CMR Imaging via Conditional Generative Adversarial Nets

Le Zhang[1,2(✉)], Marco Pereañez[3], Christopher Bowles[3], Stefan Piechnik[4],
Stefan Neubauer[4], Steffen Petersen[5], and Alejandro Frangi[3]

[1] Centre for Computational Imaging and Simulation Technologies in Biomedicine,
Department of Electronic and Electrical Engineering,
University of Sheffield, Sheffield, UK
le.zhang@sheffield.ac.uk
[2] Queen Square Institute of Neurology, University College London, London, UK
[3] Centre for Computational Imaging and Simulation Technologies in Biomedicine,
School of Computing and School of Medicine, University of Leeds, Leeds, UK
[4] Oxford Center for Clinical Magnetic Resonance Research (OCMR),
Division of Cardiovascular Medicine, John Radcliffe Hospital,
University of Oxford, Oxford, UK
[5] William Harvey Research Institute, Barts Heart Centre, Barts Health NHS Trust,
Queen Mary University of London, London, UK

Abstract. Accurate ventricular volume measurements depend on complete heart coverage in cardiac magnetic resonance (CMR) from where most immediate indicators of normal/abnormal cardiac function are available non-invasively. However, incomplete coverage, especially missing basal or apical slices in CMR sequences is insufficiently addressed in population imaging and current clinical research studies yet has important impact on volume calculation accuracy. In this work, we propose a new deep architecture, coined Missing Slice Imputation Generative Adversarial Network (MSIGAN), to learn key features of cardiac short-axis (SAX) slices across different positions, and use them as conditional variables to effectively infer missing slices in the query volumes. In MSI-GAN, the slices are first mapped to latent vectors with position features through a regression net. The latent vector corresponding to the desired position is then projected onto the slice manifold conditional on slice intensity through a generator net. The latent vector along with the slice features (*i.e.*, intensity) and desired position control the generation vs. regression. Two adversarial networks are imposed on the regressor and generator, encouraging more realistic slices. Experimental results show that our method outperforms the previous state-of-the-art in missing slice imputation for cardiac MRI.

Keywords: Deep learning · Data imputation · Generative adversarial net · Ventricular volume · MRI · Population imaging

© Springer Nature Switzerland AG 2019
D. Shen et al. (Eds.): MICCAI 2019, LNCS 11765, pp. 651–659, 2019.
https://doi.org/10.1007/978-3-030-32245-8_72

1 Introduction

Cardiac Magnetic Resonance Imaging (CMRI) can not only provide anatomical information from the heart, but also yields physiological information associated with cardiovascular diseases. Ejection fraction (EF) and cardiac output (CO) of both ventricles directly relate to the volume of these chambers, whose extents in turn defined between their basal and apical slices, are the most commonly used clinical diagnostic parameters for cardiac function. Most published studies addressing computation of EF and CO assume a complete data set in the sense all imaging planes are available for all samples. In practice, in population imaging, clinical trials, or clinical routine, this assumption may not hold as certain datasets may have missing or corrupted information due to imaging artifacts and acquisition/storage errors [10]. Additionally, many discriminative classifiers, such as SVMs, require training and testing data where a full set of features is available for every sample.

A common strategy to account for unavailable features is the removal of incomplete samples from the study cohort [9]. However, excluding data reduces not only statistical power and cause bias, but is also of ethical and financial concern as partially acquired subject data remains unused, and limits the application of such methods to similarly complete datasets. Some data imputation based methods have been proposed to deal with this problem, such as using the mean of the data or model-based missing data estimation [3]. If the missing mechanism is random, the missing variable can be imputed by the marginal distribution of the observed data using maximum likelihood estimation (MLE) [2]. The stochastic regression imputation method can better use the information provided by the data to solve the collinearity problem caused by the high correlation of predicted variables [7]. When the data missingness is non-random, the missing variable cannot be predicted from the available variables in the database alone, and there is no general method of handling missing data properly [3]. The performance of imputation approaches is ideally assessed by both the feature error and the classification accuracy on the imputed features.

In this paper, we adapt the developed generative adversarial net (GAN) to generate missing CMRI slices after applying quality control (QC). We propose a missing slice imputation based generative adversarial network (MSIGAN) model to infer missing slice features from multi-position input images. After inference, the features of the desired position and slice intensity are concatenated to generate real images in a certain position with the correct appearance. The main contributions of the MSIGAN are highlighted:

(1) A novel deep MSIGAN architecture is proposed for generating missing SAX slices for CMRI across different positions. First, a regression net learns the intrinsic features of the input slices. Conditioned on these features, and a pre-computed feature of the expected position, a generator and discriminator aim to generate the realistic image in the expected position.

(2) Given the slice features and expected position, we design a conditional generative network to infer an image matching the missing slice of the input

cardiac volume. The adversarial training mechanism and auxiliary slice position regressor is combined to achieve effective feature generation.

(3) This is the first paper to exploit deep learning methods, especially GANs, for missing slice imputation in cardiac MRI, which is an important step after QC and before quantitative medical image analysis. It can be learned once and then applied to synthesize missing slices in cases of incomplete heart coverage with no further training.

2   Methodology

2.1   Problem Formulation

The overall target of missing slice imputation (MSI) for cardiac MRI is similar to the missing data imputation problem in data mining [4]. Given a query cardiac MR volume, a regression list of slice positions in the data set is desired, followed by image synthesis to impute the query volume's missing slices. For each input 3D cardiac image $\mathbf{X}$, we aim to map it to a feature representation $\mathbf{f}$ and synthesize the missing slice $\hat{\mathbf{x}}$ using the following function:

$$\hat{\mathbf{x}} = \Gamma(series(\{\mathbf{f}_n\}_{n=1}^N)) = \Gamma(series(\mathcal{R}(\mathbf{X}) \cdot \{\Upsilon_n\}_{n=1}^N)). \tag{1}$$

where the operator $\mathcal{R}(\cdot)$ is to extract the features (i.e., intensity) of the input image $\mathbf{X}$. $\{\Upsilon_n\}_{n=1}^N$ is obtained by the regression model to identify the slice position information, like the distance to basal/or apical slice, from the cardiac volume. N is the number of slices. The operator $\Gamma(\cdot)$ denotes the transformation from the concatenated features to the inferred slice features in the cardiac volume. Finally, we can synthesize the missing slice from a certain position. Therefore, the most significant factor to achieve effective synthesis is how to design and optimize $\mathcal{R}(\cdot)$, Υ and $\Gamma(\cdot)$.

We formulate the image synthesis component for the MSI problem with these three steps: first, given an 3D cardiac volume $\mathbf{X} = \{\mathbf{x}_1, \mathbf{x}_2, ..., \mathbf{x}_n\}$ and the corresponding slice position label $\mathbf{y} = \{y_1, y_2, ..., y_n\}$, a regression net $\mathcal{R}(\cdot)$ aims to learn the cardiac intensity feature $\mathbf{f}_{int}$ and the slice position maps Υ. Then, using the feature maps for different slice positions and intensities as conditions, we aim to generate the desired slice features via $\Gamma(\cdot)$ with an adversarial training architecture. A generative net takes the intrinsic slice features (i.e., intensity), a random vector and the position feature of the desired slice as input to synthesize a cardiac cine MRI in the corresponding position within the same input volume. Finally, a discriminative net distinguishes the generated samples from the real images, and simultaneously tries to match the inferred slices with correct features and positions. The network architecture is illustrated in Fig. 1. The synthesized slices can be directly adopted for imputing the missing slice in the target CMR volume.

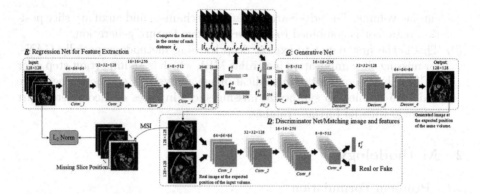

Fig. 1. Structure of the proposed MSIGAN network for cardiac missing slice imputation. The regressor R maps each slice of the input volume to a vector containing intensity and position features. The central point feature of each position cluster over the whole training set can be obtained and used for generator G. Concatenating the intensity feature and random noise to the inferred position cluster centre feature, the new latent vector FC_3 is fed to G. Both R and G are updated based on the L_2 loss between the original and synthetic volumes. The discriminative net D forces the output slice to be realistic and plausible for a given position label.

2.2   MSI Conditional GAN (MSIGAN)

Cardiac Feature Learning and Slice Position Estimation: To generate CMR slices in SAX view, a deep regression network R aims to learn CMR image features including slice position $\mathbf{f}_d$ and intensity $\mathbf{f}_{Int}$. Formally, $\mathbf{X}_S$ denotes the input cardiac image stack with full ventricular coverage. The trunk architecture of the regression net consists of 4 convolutional layers (kernel size = 5, padding = 2 and stride = 2) and 2 fully-connected layers. The Leaky-ReLU is set after each layer. We then configure two layers for learning the 256-dimensional $\mathbf{f}_{Int}$ with the intrinsic intensity features and 128-dimensional $\mathbf{f}_d$ with the inferred slice position regression separately, since we expect slice position information weakened in $\mathbf{f}_{Int}$, but strengthened in $\mathbf{f}_d$. While training the regression net, the loss function can be fast and well converged. Thus, we can easily learn each position's feature cluster from all the training data by k-means clustering, and compute the feature in the centre of each cluster, $\mathbf{f}_{dc}$, as a condition to generate slices in the missed position.

Conditional Cardiac GAN: Instead of generating real images using regular GANs, our model aims to transform the features from CMR volumes with full ventricular coverage into the query CMR volumes, which miss slices in certain positions, using a conditional generative model. The conditional generator is defined as $G: \mathbb{R}^F \times \mathbb{R}^Z \times \mathbb{R}^T \rightarrow \mathbb{R}^S$, where F is the dimension of the intrinsic cardiac intensity, Z is for random noise, T is the dimension of the inferred slice position and S is the cardiac slice. Besides, the discriminator is denoted as D: $\mathbb{R}^S \rightarrow \{0,1\} \times \prod l_i$, where $i = \{1 : \mathbf{f}_{Int}, 2 : \mathbf{f}_{dc}\}$. l_i denotes the range of each label. The optimization of the G and D can be reformulated as:

$$\mathcal{L}_D = E_{\mathbf{x} \sim p_{data}(\mathbf{x})}[\log D(\mathbf{x})] - \sum_{i=1}^{2} \|l_i - D(\mathbf{x}))\|_2^2 \qquad (2)$$

$$\mathcal{L}_G = E_{A;B;C}[\log(1 - D(G(\mathbf{f}_{dc}^T, \mathbf{z}, \mathbf{f}_{Int}^S)))], \qquad (3)$$

where $A \to \mathbf{f}_{dc}^T \sim p_{data}(\mathbf{f}_{dc}^T)$, $B \to \mathbf{z} \sim p_{\mathbf{z}}(\mathbf{z})$, and $C \to \{\mathbf{f}_{Int}^S\} \sim p_{data}(\mathbf{f}_{Int}^S)$. The input of generator G is the concatenation of $\mathbf{f}_{Int}^S, \mathbf{f}_{dc}^T$ and a random noise prior $\mathbf{z} \sim \mathcal{N}(0, 1)$. $\mathbf{f}_{Int}^S$ and can be regarded as intrinsic intensity features from the *original slices*, while $\mathbf{f}_{dc}^T$ is the *target* position feature in the centre of the cluster. A fully-connected layer is set for better fusing the three vectors and then four deconvolutional layers are adopted for generating synthesized slice samples. The architecture of the generative net is set as the reverse of the regression net R.

The discriminator D takes the generated samples and the real images in the target CMR volume as inputs. The main structure of the Discriminator has a similar structure to the regression net. To match the inferred slices with the same intensity features and correct slice position in the query volumes, we add a fully-connected layer and simultaneously optimize the whole discriminative net by slice position regression. The position label for the synthetic slice is same as the expected position label in the query volume. Batch normalization and ReLU are also adopted for all the layers in the discriminator. Meanwhile, to ensure the output slice shares the intensity of the input image (during training), the input image and output image are expected to be similar as expressed in Eq. (4), where $L(\cdot)$ denotes L_2 norm.

$$\mathcal{L}_{L2N} = L(\mathbf{x}, G(R(\mathbf{x}))) \qquad (4)$$

2.3 Optimisation

The training scheme for MSIGAN consists of three steps. In the first step, R, for slice feature learning, is trained using the deep regression net. The computed different slice position features are then obtained. Next, G is fed by the learned real position features from different cardiac volumes, which is fused with the intensity features $\mathbf{f}_{Int}^S$ and the random noise $\mathbf{z}$. Four deconvolutional layers are adopted for G to generate synthesized slice samples. Both the regressor and the generator are updated based on the L_2 loss between the input and output volumes to ensure they are similar. In the following step, the discriminative net D employs a general fully convolutional network to distinguish the real images from the generated ones. Rather than maximizing the output of the discriminator for generated data, the objective of feature matching [6] is employed to optimize G to match the statistics of features in an intermediate layer of D. The objective function is defined in the following equation:

$$\mathcal{L}_{MSI} = \min_{G} \max_{D,R} E(\log(1 - D(G(\{\mathbf{f}_{Int}^S, \mathbf{z}, \mathbf{f}_{dc}^T\})))) + \sum_{i=1}^{2} \|l_i - D(\mathbf{x})\|_2^2$$

$$+ \left\| E(D_k(\{\mathbf{f}_{Int}^S, \mathbf{f}_d^S\})) - E(D_k(G(\{\mathbf{f}_{Int}^S, \mathbf{z}, \mathbf{f}_{dc}^T\}))) \right\|_2^2 - L(\mathbf{x}, G(R(\mathbf{x}))) \tag{5}$$

where k means the kth layer in D ($k = 4$ in our setting). Moreover, D is trained with slice position regression to better match generated position features with the identity of the input volume. We apply one more *conv* layer to output the final position features. For all the *conv* layers in G and D. The conditioned G and D nets can be optimized by $\mathcal{L}_{MSI}$ to infer the missing features from query input volumes.

3 Experiments and Analysis

Materials and Position Label Generation. Quality-scored CMR data is available for circa 5,000 volunteers of the UK Biobank imaging (UKBB) resource. Following visual inspection, manual annotation for SAX images was carried out with a simple 3-grade quality score [1]. 4,280 sequences correspond to quality score 1 for both ventricles, which indicates full coverage of the heart from base to apex, and form the source datasets to construct the ground-truth distance label for our experiments. Note that having full coverage should not be confused with having the top/bottom slices corresponding exactly to base/apex [12].

The slice position labels are generated from the distances to apex point and base point. To obtain the apex point, we take last 2 apical 2D manual delineations and fit a spline curve to extrapolate the location of the apex, before measuring the distance to this point for all image slices. To obtain the base point, we use left atrium (LA) manual delineations on the 4CH long-axis image view to define the centre of the mitral valve (MV) as the base, and measure the distance from this point to all image slices. To make each slice label represent the distance to apex and base simultaneously, we normalize the distance from base to apex 1 for all cases (base as 0 and apex as 1), and label the middle slices with values equally increased from 0 to 1. For the slices above the base or below the apex, we also use the equal interval to label them.

Experimental Settings. We performed two groups of experiments in this work. In the first experiment, we aim to evaluate the quality of the images generated by MSIGAN. The averaged peak signal-to-noise ratio (PSNR) and structural similarity index (SSIM) are used to measure the image quality of the ground-truth and synthetic MR images. In the second group, we evaluate the imputed cardiac volumes with corresponding ground-truth for the tasks of LV segmentation and cardiac function measurement based on blood volumes. Four parameters are used for performance evaluation, including two commonly used indexes of the cardiac function derived from such volumes viz. stroke volume (SV) and ejection

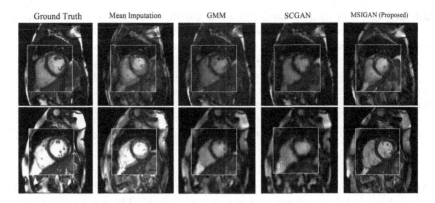

Fig. 2. Example of synthesized images (*left*) generated by Mean, GMM, SCGAN and MSIGAN, compared to the ground truths (*right*) in each pairs.

Table 1. Quantitative results for missing cardiac MRI synthesis based on PSNR and SSIM. Higher values indicate better performance. Values in brackets represent the standard deviation. Highest performing results seen in bold.

	Mean	GMM [5]	SCGAN [11]	MSIGAN (Proposed)
PSNR	20.49 ± 5.21	22.17 ± 3.75	17.49 ± 3.46	$\mathbf{24.49 \pm 3.69}$
SSIM	0.547 ± 0.21	0.686 ± 0.24	0.512 ± 1.71	$\mathbf{0.703 \pm 0.11}$

fraction (EF), and similarly report the differences between the real and imputed coverages.

Performance of Image Synthesis Model. To evaluate the quality of the images generated by MSIGAN, we first train the MSIGAN model using 3,280 complete subjects from the 4,280 cases with quality score 1 in UKBB, and test our model on the remaining 1,000 subjects. We take the 1,000 testing subjects for which the ground-truth slices are available and randomly remove slices to generate incomplete volumes, before using our MSIGAN to synthesize the missed slices. We also impute the missing slice using mean, mixture of factor analyzers based GMM model [5] and the SCGAN model [11]. Several typical images with real and synthetic slices are shown in Fig. 2. From Fig. 2, we can observe that the synthetic slices produced by MSIGAN show the best image quality against the Mean, GMM and SCGAN methods. The mean and standard deviation of PSNR and SSIM values of synthetic slice are listed in Table 1. MSIGAN significantly outperforms the other three methods based on PSNR and SSIM for missing slice synthesis. These results imply that our trained MSIGAN model is reasonable, and the synthetic cardiac MRI scans have acceptable image quality.

Results of Cardiac Functional Parameters Calculation. To assess the impact of synthetic images in real applications, such as measurement of cardiac function based on blood volumes, we design an experiment where incom-

Table 2. Effect of incomplete cardiac coverage (MBS) on the left ventricle end-diastolic volume (LVEDV), end-systolic volume (LDESV), stroke volumes (LVSV) and ejection fraction (LVEF). Values are shown as Mean ± standard deviations.

	Ground truth	Missing Basal Slice (MBS)	Effect (%)	Synthetic image	Effect (%)
LVEDV (ml)	155.8 ± 35.6	136.1 ± 33.4	−12.6%	151.7 ± 33.7	**−2.6%**
LVESV (ml)	66.8 ± 21.2	53.0 ± 19.0	−20.7%	61.3 ± 22.3	**−8.2%**
LVSV (ml)	89.1 ± 19.8	83.1 ± 19.7	−6.7%	90.4 ± 18.7	**+1.5%**
LVEF (%)	57.1 ± 0.06	61.0 ± 0.06	+6.8%	59.6 ± 0.06	**+4.4%**

plete coverage is simulated and volume differences between ground-truth, synthetic volumes and incomplete volumes are measured. The experimental results achieved by four cardiac parameters using the LV segmentation method in [8] are reported in Table 2. For this experiment, we compute blood pool volumes at the ED and ES phases, and from these, we obtain $SV = EDV - ESV$ and $EF = SV/EDV$. Then, the average volumes and indexes are computed across the sample, comparing the ground-truth, synthetic volumes and incomplete volumes. Table 2 shows that MBS reduces ED and ES volumes by an average of 12% and 20%, respectively. The synthetic values are much closer than the GT values, with 2.6% and 8.2% reduction in volumes at ED and ES phases. These results demonstrate synthetic images generated by MSIGAN are useful in population imaging applications.

4   Conclusion

In this paper, we proposed a novel deep MSIGAN to implement missing slice generation in cardiac cine MRI and contribute to the missing data imputation problem neglected by the medical imaging community. The MSI adopts a slice position regression model and an adversarial training architecture to impute missing slices based on their corresponding distances to the base and apex, considering the relationship between neighbouring slices scanned for the same subject. Extensive experimental results showed that our model could achieve satisfactory performance on missing slice generation compared to some baseline methods. Our method is also reasonable for practical applications. Only the complete images are used for learning the segmentation models. Using these synthetic slice data could further augment the training samples for improvement of the segmentation models, which will be our future work.

References

1. Carapella, V., et al.: Towards the semantic enrichment of free-text annotation of image quality assessment for UK biobank cardiac cine MRI scans. In: Carneiro, G., et al. (eds.) LABELS/DLMIA -2016. LNCS, vol. 10008, pp. 238–248. Springer, Cham (2016). https://doi.org/10.1007/978-3-319-46976-8_25

2. Dong, Y., Peng, C.Y.J.: Principled missing data methods for researchers. Springer-Plus **2**(1), 222 (2013)

3. García-Laencina, P.J., Sancho-Gómez, J.L., Figueiras-Vidal, A.R.: Pattern classification with missing data: a review. Neural Comput. Appl. **19**(2), 263–282 (2010)

4. Myrtveit, I., Stensrud, E., Olsson, U.H.: Analyzing data sets with missing data: an empirical evaluation of imputation methods and likelihood-based methods. IEEE Trans. Softw. Eng. **27**(11), 999–1013 (2001)

5. Richardson, E., Weiss, Y.: On GANs and GMMs. In: Advances in Neural Information Processing Systems, pp. 5852–5863 (2018)

6. Salimans, T., Goodfellow, I., Zaremba, W., Cheung, V., Radford, A., Chen, X.: Improved techniques for training GANs. In: Advances in Neural Information Processing Systems, pp. 2234–2242 (2016)

7. Schlomer, G.L., Bauman, S., Card, N.A.: Best practices for missing data management in counseling psychology. J. Couns. Psychol. **57**(1), 1 (2010)

8. Tran, P.V.: A fully convolutional neural network for cardiac segmentation in short-axis MRI. arXiv preprint arXiv:1604.00494 (2016)

9. Williams, D., Liao, X., Xue, Y., Carin, L., Krishnapuram, B.: On classification with incomplete data. IEEE Trans. Pattern Anal. Mach. Intell. **29**(3), 427–436 (2007)

10. Zhang, L., et al.: Automatic assessment of full left ventricular coverage in cardiac cine magnetic resonance imaging with fisher-discriminative 3-D CNN. IEEE Trans. Biomed. Eng. **66**(7), 1975–1986 (2019)

11. Zhang, L., Gooya, A., Frangi, A.F.: Semi-supervised assessment of incomplete LV Coverage in cardiac MRI using generative adversarial nets. In: Tsaftaris, S.A., Gooya, A., Frangi, A.F., Prince, J.L. (eds.) SASHIMI 2017. LNCS, vol. 10557, pp. 61–68. Springer, Cham (2017). https://doi.org/10.1007/978-3-319-68127-6_7

12. Zhang, L., Pereañez, M., Piechnik, S.K., Neubauer, S., Petersen, S.E., Frangi, A.F.: Multi-input and dataset-invariant adversarial learning (MDAL) for left and right-ventricular coverage estimation in cardiac MRI. In: Frangi, A.F., Schnabel, J.A., Davatzikos, C., Alberola-López, C., Fichtinger, G. (eds.) MICCAI 2018. LNCS, vol. 11071, pp. 481–489. Springer, Cham (2018). https://doi.org/10.1007/978-3-030-00934-2_54

Unsupervised Standard Plane Synthesis in Population Cine MRI via Cycle-Consistent Adversarial Networks

Le Zhang[1,2]([✉]), Marco Pereañez[3], Christopher Bowles[3], Stefan K. Piechnik[4],
Stefan Neubauer[4], Steffen E. Petersen[5], and Alejandro F. Frangi[3]

[1] Centre for Computational Imaging and Simulation Technologies in Biomedicine,
Department of Electronic and Electrical Engineering, University of Sheffield,
Sheffield, UK
le.zhang@sheffield.ac.uk

[2] Queen Square Institute of Neurology, University College London, London, UK

[3] Centre for Computational Imaging and Simulation Technologies in Biomedicine,
School of Computing and School of Medicine, University of Leeds, Leeds, UK

[4] Oxford Center for Clinical Magnetic Resonance Research (OCMR),
Division of Cardiovascular Medicine, John Radcliffe Hospital, University of Oxford,
Oxford, UK

[5] William Harvey Research Institute, Barts Heart Centre, Barts Health NHS Trust,
Queen Mary University of London, London, UK

Abstract. In clinical studies or population imaging settings, cardiac magnetic resonance (CMR) images may suffer from artifacts due to variability in the breath-hold position adopted by the patient during the scan. Consistent orientation of image planes with respect to the cardiac ventricles in CMR sequences forms a crucial step in the assessment of cardiac function via parameters such as the Ejection Fraction (EF) and Cardiac Output (CO) of both ventricles, which are the most immediate indicators of normal/abnormal cardiac function. In this paper, we present a novel unsupervised approach for the realistic transformation of acquired CMR images to a standard orientation using Cycle-Consistent Adversarial Networks (Cycle-GANs). We tackle this challenge by splitting the problem into two principal subtasks. First, we consider a bidirectional generator mapping between the re-oriented image and the original, hence allowing direct comparison to the input image without the need to resort to paired training data. Second, we devise a novel loss function incorporating intensity and orientation terms, and aims to produce images of high perceptual quality. Extensive experiments conducted on the CMR images in the UK Biobank dataset demonstrate that the images rendered by our model can improve the accuracy of the image derived cardiac parameters.

Keywords: Deep learning · Cycle-Consistent Adversarial Networks ·
Cardiac orientation · Ventricular volume · MRI · Population imaging

© Springer Nature Switzerland AG 2019
D. Shen et al. (Eds.): MICCAI 2019, LNCS 11765, pp. 660–668, 2019.
https://doi.org/10.1007/978-3-030-32245-8_73

1   Introduction

Cardiac anatomy and function are widely used in diagnosis and monitoring of disease progression in cardiology, with CMR imaging arguably being one of the most wide-spread techniques for clinical diagnostic imaging of the heart. CMR requires a carefully selected and consistent orientation of short-axis (SAX) image planes with respect to the cardiac ventricles, particularly the basal slice (BS) and apical slice (AS) plane which contain key anatomical structures [10]. If the plane orientation deviates significantly from expected values, local image structure may change enough to cause subsequent image feature-based algorithms to fail in localizing key features required for further morphological and functional analysis. However, it is challenging and time-consuming, even for experienced MRI operators, to manually find the correct imaging plane, particularly when it is subject to subsequent patient movement. The task is highly operator-dependent and requires a great amount of expertise. With the advent of CMRI, 2D SAX slices can be acquired quickly with little training. But the problem of locating the standard planes required for diagnostically important biometric measurements remains. There is a strong need to develop automatic methods for 2D standard plane generation from existing 2D slices to improve clinical workflow efficiency.

Image generation is a hot topic which has achieved great success on many vision tasks such as text-to-image generation [8] and image style transformation [5]. Conditional GAN [6] are more advanced image generators and more suitable for image translation tasks. It is developed by adding an input condition vector, which can include a vast amount of information, to the generator. Medical image synthesis is currently an emerging area of interest for applying the latest image generation techniques mentioned above. Zhou et al. [11] use a cycle consistency loss as a way of mapping back the initially rendered image to the original image to achieve unpaired image-to-image translation. They have shown impressive results in rendering new realistic images. Nie et al. [7] proposed a context-aware GAN by adding an image gradient difference term to the loss function of the generator, to retain the sharpness of the generated images. Dar et al. [1] utilized the image conditioned architectures Cycle-GAN and pix2pix to generate T1- from T2-weighted MR contrast and vice versa.

Inspired by this idea, we propose a fully unsupervised approach based on GANs that, given a SAX slice with incorrect plane orientation (IPO), automatically generates images under the correct orientation. To train our model using unlabeled data (*i.e.*, our training data consists of query slices and slices with correct orientation from other cardiac volumes), we propose a Cycle-GAN based architecture that aims at producing new images of high perceptual quality [2] by combining loss functions used in orientation transfer. The main contributions of the standard plane synthesis GAN (SPSGAN) are highlighted:

(1) A novel deep architecture is proposed for generating SAX slices with standard plane orientation. To achieve this, we devised a novel loss function computed over the images from a Cycle-GAN for cardiac orientation transfer.
(2) We propose a fully unsupervised strategy trained without paired training examples for image-to-image translation.

(3) This is the first paper to exploit deep learning method, especially GANs, for orientation based cardiac slice generation, which is an important step after quality control (QC) and before quantitative CMR analysis.

2 Methodology

2.1 Problem Formulation

To produce realistic standard orientation transformations of an input slice while retaining the intensity appearance, we use a single SAX slice as input and train a GAN model using an unsupervised approach. Formally, we seek to learn the mapping $(\mathbf{x}_t^i, \mathbf{f}_{\theta_o}, \mathbf{f}_{\gamma_o}) \rightarrow \mathbf{x}_o^i$ between an image $\mathbf{x}_t^i \in \mathbb{R}^{H \times W \times Z}$ in a volume with incorrect orientation $<\theta_t, \gamma_t>$ and the image $\mathbf{x}_o^i \in \mathbb{R}^{H \times W \times Z}$ of the same volume with the correct orientation $<\theta_o, \gamma_o>$. Orientations are represented by $<\theta, \gamma>$, where θ indicates the deflection angle in the xoy plane and γ indicates the deflection angle in the z direction of the 3D coordinate system. The subscripts o and t denote the correct and transformed orientations, respectively. The model is trained using an unsupervised approach with training samples $\{\mathbf{x}_o^i, \mathbf{x}_t^j\}_{i,j=1}^N$, which do not include the ground-truth image $\mathbf{x}_o^j$.

2.2 Unsupervised SPSGAN

Figure 1 shows the structure of our SPSGAN model consisting of five main modules: (1) The real orientation features $[\mathbf{f}_\theta, \mathbf{f}_\gamma]$ are learned from different cardiac volumes and concatenated with the features in the generator to better generate an image with the desired orientation. (2) A generator $G(\mathbf{x} | (\mathbf{f}_\theta, \mathbf{f}_\gamma))$ that maps one given slice under an incorrect orientation to an output slice under the standard orientation with the same cardiac identity. G is used twice in our network, first to map the input image $\mathbf{x}_{tr}^i \rightarrow \mathbf{x}_{og}^i$ and then render the latter back to the initial orientation $\mathbf{x}_{og}^i \rightarrow \hat{\mathbf{x}}_{tg}^i$; (3) A regressor R responsible of estimating the slice orientation of a given image. Note that R is different from the pre-trained regression net for feature extraction in (1); (4) A discriminator D that tries to discriminate the generated and real images; (5) A loss function that is computed without ground-truth and aims to preserve the cardiac intensity. To address this challenge, we propose a novel loss function that enforces the intensity content similarity of $\mathbf{x}_{tr}^i$ and $\hat{\mathbf{x}}_{tg}^i$, and orientation similarity between $\mathbf{x}_{og}^i$ and $\mathbf{x}_{or}^j$. In the following, we describe in detail each of the five modules.

Orientation Feature Embedding: The orientations of all volumes are linearly distributed and categorized with two parameters $<\theta, \gamma>$. Since the loss of the orientation regressor can be fast and well converged during the training process, we can easily learn each orientation feature cluster from all the training data by k-means clustering, and compute the feature in the center of the cluster as a condition to generate images in desired orientation. The feature of each orientation in an image $\mathbf{x}_t^i \in \mathbb{R}^{H \times W \times Z}$ is represented as a probability density map $\mathbf{f}$ computed over the entire image domain as:

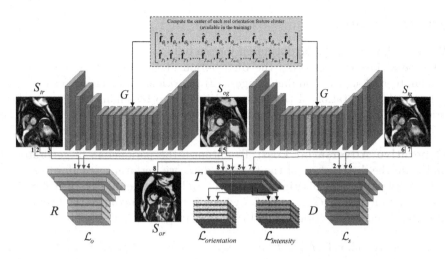

Fig. 1. The structure of our SPSGAN to generate the standard plane of the cardiac MRI in SAX view. Our model consists of five main components: a generator G, a discriminator D, an orientation regressor R, the transfer net T and the pretrained orientation features. S_{tr} is the original (IPO) image, S_{og} is the synthesized image, S_{tg} is the rendered back image, S_{or} is the image with correct orientation of different volume. Neither ground-truth image is considered.

$$\mathbf{f} = \Gamma(series(\{\mathbf{x}_n\}_{n=1}^N)) \tag{1}$$

where the operator $\Gamma(\cdot)$ is to extract the feature of the input image $\mathbf{x}$ and N is the defined number of slices.

Generator: Given an input image $\mathbf{x}$ with incorrect orientation, the generator $G(\mathbf{x}\,|(\mathbf{f}_\theta, \mathbf{f}_\gamma))$ aims to render $\mathbf{x}$ in a standard orientation with $<\theta_o, \gamma_o>$. To condition the generator with the orientation features we consider the concatenation $(\mathbf{x}, \mathbf{f}_\theta, \mathbf{f}_\gamma) \in \mathbb{R}^{H \times W \times Z}$ and feed this into a feedforward network, which generates output images of the same size as $\mathbf{x}$. To achieve improved image-to-image translation results, we adopt the network variation from [4] to construct the generator.

Image Discriminator: We adopt the PatchGAN [3] network as the discriminator $D(\mathbf{x})$, which maps from the input image $\mathbf{x}$ to a matrix $Y_s \in \mathbb{R}^{26 \times 26}$. The discriminator then classifies each 26×26 patch in an image as real or fake. Since a smaller PatchGAN can generate high perceptual quality images with fewer parameters and less time [3], we run the discriminator across the image in a convolutional manner and average all responses to provide the final output D.

Orientation Regressor: D distinguishes the generated samples from the real images. We simultaneously use an orientation regressor R to regress the inferred slice with correct orientations. R is implemented with the ResNet architecture described in [11].

2.3   Optimisation

We have three terms to be optimized for the full loss function. (1) A generative adversarial loss that enforces the distribution of the generated images to be similar to that of the training images. (2) An orientation regression loss that enforces the orientation of the generated images to be similar to the standard orientation. (3) The transfer loss that preserves the cardiac identity between the generated and the input images. Next, we will describe each of these in detail.

Generative Adversarial Loss: To optimize the parameters of generator G and learn the distribution of the training data, we perform a standard *minmax* game between G and discriminator D. G and D are jointly trained with the objective function $\mathcal{L}_s(G, D, \mathbf{x}, \mathbf{f}_\theta, \mathbf{f}_\gamma)$ where D tries to maximize the probability of correctly classifying original and rendered images while G tries to fool D.

$$\mathcal{L}_s(G, D, \mathbf{x}, \mathbf{f}_\theta, \mathbf{f}_\gamma) = E[\log D(\mathbf{x})] + E[\log(1 - D(G(\mathbf{x}\,|(\mathbf{f}_\theta, \mathbf{f}_\gamma))]] \tag{2}$$

Orientation Regression Loss: G must not only maximise the loss of D, but also must reduce the error produced by the orientation regressor R. In this way, while learning to produce realistic samples, G also learns how to generate images with the standard orientation $<\theta, \gamma>$. This loss is defined by:

$$\mathcal{L}_o(G, R, \mathbf{x}, \mathbf{f}_\theta, \mathbf{f}_\gamma) = \|R(G(\mathbf{x}\,|(\mathbf{f}_\theta, \mathbf{f}_\gamma))) - <\mathbf{f}_\theta, \mathbf{f}_\gamma>\|_2^2 \tag{3}$$

Transfer Loss: With the two previously defined losses $\mathcal{L}_s$ and $\mathcal{L}_o$, G is enforced to generate realistic slices with correct orientation. However, in the absence of ground-truth supervision, there is no constraint to ensure appearance identity. We derive inspiration from the previously introduced content-style loss to maintain high perception quality in image style transfer [2]. The loss mainly consists of two parts, one retains intensity similarity and the other transfers orientation similarity. Inspired by this idea, we define two sub-losses to maintain the identity between the input slice $\mathbf{x}_{tr}^i$ and the rendered slice $\mathbf{x}_{og}^i$.

For the intensity term, we define that G should be able to render-back the initial slice $\mathbf{x}_{tr}^i$ given the generated slice $\mathbf{x}_{og}^i$ and the original orientation features $<\mathbf{f}_{\theta_t}, \mathbf{f}_{\gamma_t}>$, that is $\hat{\mathbf{x}}_{tg}^i \approx \mathbf{x}_{tr}^i$, where $\hat{\mathbf{x}}_{tg}^i = G(G(\mathbf{x}_{tr}^i\,|(\mathbf{f}_{\theta_o}, \mathbf{f}_{\gamma_o}))\,|(\mathbf{f}_{\theta_t}, \mathbf{f}_{\gamma_t}))$. However, it is difficult to handle high frequency details by directly comparing $\mathbf{x}_{tr}^i$ and $\hat{\mathbf{x}}_{tg}^i$ using Patch-GAN at a pixel level, which will lead to overly-smoothed images. Instead, we compare them based on their intensity content. Formally, we define the intensity loss to be:

$$\mathcal{L}_{intensity} = \left\|T_l(\mathbf{x}_{tr}^i) - T_l(\mathbf{x}_{tg}^i)\right\|_2^2 \tag{4}$$

where $T_l(\cdot)$ represents the feature representation at the lth layer of the network.

In order to transfer the standard orientation information from the real slice to the synthesized one, we take over the spatial extent of the feature maps to design the feature space for capturing texture information. Previous work [2] implements this by computing the Gram matrix $\mathbf{M}^l \in \mathbb{R}^{U \times U}$, where $\mathbf{M}^l$ is the inner product between the vectorised feature maps of $\mathbf{x}_{og}^i$. The orientation loss is then computed as the mean square error between visible pairs of Gram matrices of the same joint in both images $\mathbf{x}_{og}^i$ and $\mathbf{x}_{or}^j$:

$$\mathcal{L}_{orientation} = \frac{1}{L} \sum_{l=0}^{L} \left(\frac{\mathbf{M}_{og}^{i,l} - \mathbf{M}_{or}^{j,l}}{UV} \right)^2 \tag{5}$$

where $\mathbf{M}_{og}^{i,l}$ and $\mathbf{M}_{or}^{j,l}$ are the orientation representations in the layer l of the generated and real image with standard orientation, respectively. In layer l, there is U_l feature maps each of size V_l, where V_l is the height times the width of the feature map. Finally, we define the transfer loss as the weighted sum of the intensity and orientation losses:

$$\mathcal{L}_{TS} = \mathcal{L}_{content}(T, \mathbf{x}_{tr}^i, \hat{\mathbf{x}}_{tg}^i) + \lambda \mathcal{L}_{orientation}(T, \mathbf{x}_{tr}^i, \mathbf{x}_{og}^i, \mathbf{x}_{or}^j) \tag{6}$$

where the parameter λ controls the relative importance or the two components.

Full Loss: We take the full loss as a linear combination of all previous loss terms:

$$\mathcal{L}_{SPS} = \arg \min_{G} \max_{D,R,T} \{ \mathcal{L}_s(G, D, \mathbf{x}, \mathbf{f}_\theta, \mathbf{f}_\gamma) + \alpha \mathcal{L}_o(G, R, \mathbf{x}, \mathbf{f}_\theta, \mathbf{f}_\gamma) + \mathcal{L}_{TS} \} \tag{7}$$

where α is the weighting factors for image adversarial and orientation regression loss ($\alpha = 400$ and $\lambda = 0.2$ in this work).

3   Experiments and Analysis

Materials and Evaluation Metrics: We used a series with the first 5,000 CMR subjects available from the UK Biobank (UKBB) imaging resource, with each volumetric sequence containing about 50 cardiac phases. Based on analysis of the in-plane orientation angle distribution for the 5,000 subjects for which manual segmentations are available (and therefore θ, γ can be computed), we found that θ has the median value of 132.8° and standard deviation of 8.0°, while γ has the median value of 7.1° with standard deviation of 3.9°. Among them, there are 302 cases under standard cardiac orientations ($\theta = 135°, \gamma = 0°$). The set of orientation labels were chosen from these realistic distributions and trained in a regression net to obtain the real orientation features.

Since our model is trained using the unsupervised approach and there is no ground-truth for the test images, we need to generate the slices with correct orientation as reference samples to evaluate the synthetic images. The reference images are resampled from the interpolated 3D cardiac volumes by Paraview[1]. The resampled slices are chosen with correct orientations and the same position (*i.e.*, the distance to base and apex) compared with the original images.

---

[1] https://www.paraview.org/.

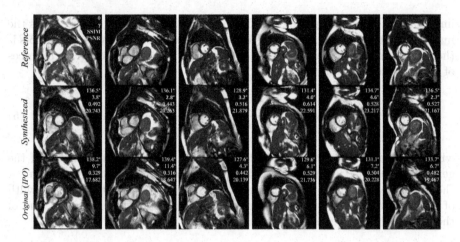

Fig. 2. Synthesized images by SPSGAN and corresponding original (IPO) images with orientation angles, PSNR and SSIM values, compared to the references.

Experimental Settings: We verify the effectiveness of the unsupervised SPS-GAN model through two groups of experiments. In the first experiment, the synthetic slice is evaluated against the reference image using rotation angles between the planes. Image similarity of the planes is also measured using peak signal-to-noise ratio (PSNR) and structural similarity (SSIM). In the second experiment, we evaluate synthetic slices against the corresponding reference slices on the tasks of LV segmentation and the measurement of cardiac function based on blood volumes. Four parameters are used for performance evaluation, including two commonly used indexes of the cardiac function derived from such volumes, stroke volume (SV) and EF, and similarly report differences between real and imputed image data.

Performance of Image Synthesis. We train the SPSGAN model using the 302 subjects with correct orientation and the same number of cases with incorrect orientations in UKBB, and test the model on another 100 subjects with incorrect orientations with comparisons to the corresponding resampled reference slices. Training images are only associated to the original slices with correct and incorrect orientations. No reference images are considered during training. Several typical images with real and synthetic slices are shown in Fig. 2. We can observe that our synthetic images show a slight difference from their corresponding original images, but similar to their corresponding reference images. This is because the local image structure in planes with different orientations will change. The orientation angles, SSIM and PSNR between synthetic, original and reference slices are also shown in Fig. 2. These results imply that our trained SPSGAN model is reasonable, and the synthetic CMR images have an acceptable representation in the standard planes.

Cardiac Functional Parameters Calculation. To assess the impact of synthetic images in real applications, such as the measurement of cardiac function

Table 1. Effect of IPO on the ED, ES, SV and EF. Values are shown as mean ± standard deviations.

	Reference image	Synthetic image	Effect (%)	IPO image	Effect (%)
LVEDV (ml)	159.6 ± 32.7	151.5 ± 34.9	−5.1%	142.9 ± 31.5	−10.5%
LVESV (ml)	72.4 ± 23.1	68.3 ± 20.3	−5.7%	64.3 ± 22.4	−11.2%
LVSV (ml)	87.2 ± 17.6	83.2 ± 18.4	−4.6%	78.6 ± 17.9	−9.9%
LVEF (%)	54.6 ± 0.08	54.9 ± 0.09	+0.5%	55.0 ± 0.08	+0.7%

based on blood volumes, we design an experiment to measure the differences between volumes derived from the reference volumes, synthetic volumes and original volumes with incorrect cardiac orientation. The experimental results across four different cardiac parameters using the LV segmentation method described in [9] are reported in Table 1. For this experiment, we compute blood pool volumes at the End-diastolic (ED) and End-systolic (ES) phases, and from these, we obtain SV and EF. The average volumes and indexes are computed across the sample, comparing the reference volumes, synthetic volumes and incomplete volumes. Table 1 shows that the incorrect plane orientation reduces ED and ES volumes by an average of 11%. In contrast, the synthetic images provide values which are much closer than the reference values, with only 5.1% and 5.7% reductions in volume at ED and ES phases. These results clearly demonstrate synthetic images generated by SPSGAN model convey relevant information and possess clinical utility.

4   Conclusion

We have presented a novel approach for generating cardiac cine MRI slices under a standard ventricle plane orientation using a GAN model that can be trained using a fully unsupervised approach. Finding the correct standard plane is highly operator-dependent and requires a great amount of expertise. To tackle this challenge, we proposed a fully unsupervised framework that aims to transfer the plane orientation and retaining the cardiac intensity of the original image without depending on the corresponding ground-truth. Extensive experimental results showed that our model could achieve satisfactory performance in standard cardiac slice generation compared to other methods. In the future, we plan to further apply our approach to other datasets and to different modalities for which supervision is not possible.

References

1. Dar, S.U., Yurt, M., Karacan, L., Erdem, A., Erdem, E., Çukur, T.: Image synthesis in multi-contrast MRI with conditional generative adversarial networks. IEEE Trans. Med. Imaging (2019)
2. Gatys, L.A., Ecker, A.S., Bethge, M.: Image style transfer using convolutional neural networks. In: Proceedings of the IEEE Conference on Computer Vision and Pattern Recognition, pp. 2414–2423 (2016)

3. Isola, P., Zhu, J.Y., Zhou, T., Efros, A.A.: Image-to-image translation with conditional adversarial networks, pp. 1125–1134 (2017)

4. Johnson, J., Alahi, A., Fei-Fei, L.: Perceptual losses for real-time style transfer and super-resolution. In: Leibe, B., Matas, J., Sebe, N., Welling, M. (eds.) ECCV 2016. LNCS, vol. 9906, pp. 694–711. Springer, Cham (2016). https://doi.org/10.1007/978-3-319-46475-6_43

5. Liu, M.Y., Tuzel, O.: Coupled generative adversarial networks. In: Advances in Neural Information Processing Systems, pp. 469–477 (2016)

6. Mirza, M., Osindero, S.: Conditional generative adversarial nets. arXiv preprint arXiv:1411.1784 (2014)

7. Nie, D., et al.: Medical image synthesis with context-aware generative adversarial networks. In: Descoteaux, M., Maier-Hein, L., Franz, A., Jannin, P., Collins, D.L., Duchesne, S. (eds.) MICCAI 2017. LNCS, vol. 10435, pp. 417–425. Springer, Cham (2017). https://doi.org/10.1007/978-3-319-66179-7_48

8. Reed, S., Akata, Z., Yan, X., Logeswaran, L., Schiele, B., Lee, H.: Generative adversarial text to image synthesis. arXiv preprint arXiv:1605.05396 (2016)

9. Tran, P.V.: A fully convolutional neural network for cardiac segmentation in short-axis MRI. arXiv preprint arXiv:1604.00494 (2016)

10. Zhang, L., et al.: Automatic assessment of full left ventricular coverage in cardiac cine magnetic resonance imaging with fisher-discriminative 3-D CNN. IEEE Trans. Biomed. Eng. **66**(7), 1975–1986 (2019)

11. Zhu, J.Y., Park, T., Isola, P., Efros, A.A.: Unpaired image-to-image translation using cycle-consistent adversarial networks. In: Proceedings of the IEEE International Conference on Computer Vision, pp. 2223–2232 (2017)

Data Efficient Unsupervised Domain Adaptation For Cross-modality Image Segmentation

Cheng Ouyang[1(✉)], Konstantinos Kamnitsas[1], Carlo Biffi[1], Jinming Duan[1,2], and Daniel Rueckert[1]

[1] Biomedical Image Analysis Group, Imperial College London, London, UK
c.ouyang@imperial.ac.uk
[2] School of Computer Science, University of Birmingham, Birmingham, UK

Abstract. Deep learning models trained on medical images from a source domain (*e.g.* imaging modality) often fail when deployed on images from a different target domain, despite imaging common anatomical structures. Deep unsupervised domain adaptation (UDA) aims to improve the performance of a deep neural network model on a target domain, using solely unlabelled target domain data and labelled source domain data. However, current state-of-the-art methods exhibit reduced performance when target data is scarce. In this work, we introduce a new data efficient UDA method for multi-domain medical image segmentation. The proposed method combines a novel VAE-based feature prior matching, which is data-efficient, and domain adversarial training to learn a shared domain-invariant latent space which is exploited during segmentation. Our method is evaluated on a public multi-modality cardiac image segmentation dataset by adapting from the labelled source domain (3D MRI) to the unlabelled target domain (3D CT). We show that by using only one single unlabelled 3D CT scan, the proposed architecture outperforms the state-of-the-art in the same setting. Finally, we perform ablation studies on prior matching and domain adversarial training to shed light on the theoretical grounding of the proposed method.

1 Introduction

Ideally, deep learning models deployed in medical imaging applications should be invariant to image appearance shifts caused by reasons such as different imaging modalities, scanning protocols or demographic properties. Unfortunately, in reality, deep learning usually suffers from the domain shift problem [1]. Given two different input domains with data X and distribution $P(X)$, $\mathcal{D}_S = \{X_S, P(X_S)\}$, $\mathcal{D}_T = \{X_T, P(X_T)\}$ and a shared label space $\mathcal{Y} = \{Y\}$, a predictive model $f(\cdot)$ which approximates $P(Y|X)$ trained on the source domain $\mathcal{D}_S$ is likely to underperform on the target domain $\mathcal{D}_T$ when the distribution of data in $\mathcal{D}_T$ is different (*e.g.* image appearance differences as described above). In this case, to transfer the source model to the target domain, target data and corresponding labels

© Springer Nature Switzerland AG 2019
D. Shen et al. (Eds.): MICCAI 2019, LNCS 11765, pp. 669–677, 2019.
https://doi.org/10.1007/978-3-030-32245-8_74

$\{(\boldsymbol{x}_T, \boldsymbol{y}_T)\}$ are necessary for supervised fine-tuning-based transfer learning. In many settings though, such as medical imaging applications, manual labelling for target images is usually prohibitively expensive or impractical. This motivates *unsupervised domain adaptation* (UDA), a methodology that seeks to learn a model that performs well in a target domain using solely **unlabelled** target domain data $\{\boldsymbol{x}_T\}$, besides any labelled data available in source domain.

UDA usually assumes an underlying domain-invariant feature space $\mathcal{Z}$, which can be projected from $\mathcal{D}_S$ and $\mathcal{D}_T$ and can be utilized for a specific task. The most popular way to perform UDA is therefore learning mappings $\{h_S(\cdot), h_T(\cdot)\}$ from $\mathcal{D}_S$ and $\mathcal{D}_T$ to $\mathcal{Z}$ by matching their distributions in $\mathcal{Z}$ under certain distance metrics (*e.g.* Jensen-Shannon distance). Using this framework, [13] proposes to minimize the Maximum Mean Discrepancy (MMD) between source and target feature representations. With recent significant advancement of generative adversarial networks (GAN), distances between source and target domain can be estimated and minimized with domain adversarial training [7,12], where the discriminator differentiates the domain of its input, while the generator generates domain-invariant representations to confuse the discriminator. Inspired by the work in [16], [8] further promotes the performance by retaining semantic information of feature maps during domain transfers, by enforcing cycle-consistencies.

Related Work: In medical image analysis, recent related works are mainly based on domain adversarial training. They are designed to mitigate domain gaps including modalities [3,4,6,15], scanning protocols [10], and cross-center differences [5]. The most recent state-of-the-art methods is *SIFA* [4], which is designed for medical image segmentation and is reported to outperform peer methods designed for natural images. It uses cycle-consistency as in [8] and further employs a synergy of image-level and feature-level domain adversarial training. However, these methods suffer from an idealized assumption that abundant target data $\{\boldsymbol{x}_T\}$ is always available, which is not always realistic in clinic practice. Current pure data-driven, adversarial UDA is sub-optimal in such low-resource setting as data-driven GANs become inaccurate with small amounts of samples.

Contributions: In this work, we for the first time investigate the challenging problem of *UDA with scarce target data* in medical image segmentation. We propose a novel data-efficient UDA method for it. We focus on mitigating domain gaps manifested by differences in image appearance, of which cross-modality difference is a typical example. To compensate for the drawback of domain adversarial training given only a small number of target samples, we propose to introduce prior regularization on a shared feature space of the source and target domain images where segmentation is operated on. By independently enforcing the prior distributions for the source features and target features to be close to a fixed prior distribution (in our case, $\mathcal{N}(0, I)$), the prior regularization serves as an additional constraint for distribution matching. This constraint is in particular data-efficient, since KL-divergences from source or target feature distributions to $\mathcal{N}(0, I)$ can be estimated analytically. To easily obtain and to fully exploit this prior matching effect, we propose to (i) combine variational

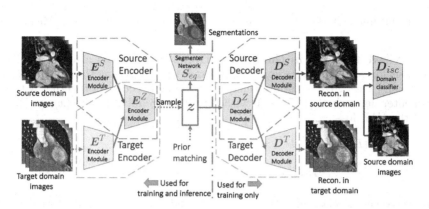

Fig. 1. Overview of the proposed architecture. A single image from the source domain or from the target domain is sent into its corresponding domain-specific encoder: $E^Z \circ E^S$ (source), or $E^Z \circ E^T$ (target). The encoder predicts the posterior of the latent feature Z in $\mathcal{Z}$. The S_{eg} then takes this as input. In training, we send the feature map to decoders $D^S \circ D^Z$ and $D^T \circ D^Z$ simultaneously to reconstruct images in both domains. The domain classifier network D_{isc} then differentiates whether its input is from the original source image set or from the outputs of the source decoder.

autoencoder (VAE), whose prior distribution of latent space can be analytically regularized, with domain adversarial training (ii) to directly operate image segmentation in this VAE latent space, for UDA in cross-modality medical image segmentation.

2   Method

Overview: The proposed method learns a feature space $\mathcal{Z} = \{Z\}$, shared by both domains $\mathcal{D}_S$, $\mathcal{D}_T$, and the mapping $h(\cdot)$'s from input images X from $\mathcal{D}_S$ or $\mathcal{D}_T$ such that $Z = h(X)$. It also learns a segmenter S_{eg} from $\mathcal{Z}$ to label space $\mathcal{Y}$. For simplicity, we use subscripts S and T to refer to the domain of an image: *e.g.* $\boldsymbol{x}_S \sim P(X_S)$, of a mapping function: *e.g.* $h_S(\cdot)$ and of a feature map sampled from its posterior in feature space: *e.g.* $\boldsymbol{z}_S \sim q(Z|\boldsymbol{x}_S)$.

The overall architecture here consists of a VAE with two domain-specific encoders and decoders, which is extended from recent work by [2], and a segmenter S_{eg} operating on the VAE's latent space $\mathcal{Z}$ which will be learned to be domain invariant. The mappings $h(\cdot)$'s are realized with two encoders of the VAE. An overview of the network structure is illustrated in Fig. 1. The posteriors $q(Z|\boldsymbol{x}_S)$ or $q(Z|\boldsymbol{x}_T)$ predicted by the source or the target encoder are modeled as multi-dimensional Gaussians $\mathcal{N}(\mu_Z, \Sigma_Z)$ with diagonal covariance matrices. To train the model, $\boldsymbol{z} \sim q(Z|\boldsymbol{x})$ is drawn at each iteration via the re-parameterization trick. It is then passed to both decoders to generate reconstructed images in two domains. Given an input $\boldsymbol{x}_S$ from $\mathcal{D}_S$, we note as $\boldsymbol{x}_{SS} = \boldsymbol{x}_{S \to S}$ the reconstructed image in the same domain and as $\boldsymbol{x}_{ST} = \boldsymbol{x}_{S \to T}$

the output image in the other domain (*vice versa* for input from $\mathcal{D}_T$). Meanwhile, z is also used as input for the segmentation network S_{eg}.

Supervised Training in the Source Domain: To obtain a source model as the basis for domain adaptation, we first train the VAE using the source encoder $h_S(\cdot) = E^Z \circ E^S : \mathcal{D}_S \to \mathcal{Z}$ and the corresponding decoder, in together with the segmenter network $S_{eg} : \mathcal{Z} \to \mathcal{Y}$ with source image-label pairs $\{(\boldsymbol{x}_S, \boldsymbol{y}_S)\}$. We have the VAE loss:

$$\mathcal{L}_{vae}^S(E^S, E^Z, D^S, D^Z) = \lambda_{rec} \mathcal{L}_{rec}^S + \lambda_{kl} \mathcal{L}_{kl}^S$$
$$= -\lambda_{rec} \mathbb{E}_{\substack{z_S \sim q(Z|\boldsymbol{x}_S) \\ \boldsymbol{x}_S \sim P(X_S)}} [\log p(\boldsymbol{x}_S|\boldsymbol{z}_S)] + \lambda_{kl} KL(q(\boldsymbol{z}_S|\boldsymbol{x}_S)||\mathcal{N}(0, I)). \quad (1)$$

To overcome the class imbalance between relatively small segmentation labels and the large background, we employ a sum of soft Dice and weighted cross-entropy (CE) losses to train S_{eg} (which is common for medical image segmentation scenarios).

$$\mathcal{L}_{Seg}^S(S_{eg}, E^Z) = \mathbb{E}_{\substack{z_S \sim q(Z|\boldsymbol{x}_S) \\ \boldsymbol{x}_S \sim P(X_S)}} [-Dice(S_{eg}(\boldsymbol{z}_S), \boldsymbol{y}_S) + CE(S_{eg}(\boldsymbol{z}_S), \boldsymbol{y}_S)]. \quad (2)$$

In the meantime we pre-train the domain classifier D_{isc} to classify whether its input is from the source training set $\{\boldsymbol{x}_S\}$ or from reconstructed $\{\boldsymbol{x}_{SS}\}$ [2]. At present, E^S, E^Z, D^Z, D^S are updated to minimize Eq. 3 and D_{isc} is updated to maximize Eq. 3.

$$\mathcal{L}_{adv}^S(E^S, E^Z, D^Z, D^S, D_{isc}) = \mathbb{E}_{\boldsymbol{x}_S \sim P(X_S)}[\log D_{isc}(\boldsymbol{x}_S)]$$
$$+ \mathbb{E}_{\boldsymbol{z}_S \sim q(Z_S|\boldsymbol{x}_S)}[\log(1 - D_{isc}(D^S(D^Z(\boldsymbol{z}_S))))]. \quad (3)$$

UDA with Prior Matching: The domain adaptation training starts after the source model is obtained. In addition to losses in Eqs. 1–3, we train the target encoding $h_T(\cdot) = E^Z \circ E^T$ and its decoding with a VAE loss. Similar to the process for the source domain, the posterior distribution $q(Z|\boldsymbol{x}_T)$ in $\mathcal{Z}$ is predicted by feeding $\boldsymbol{x}_T$'s to the target encoder. We therefore use the same form of VAE loss $\mathcal{L}_{vae}^T$ as that in $\mathcal{D}_S$ (Eq. 4). To prevent E^Z and D^Z from overfitting on small $\{\boldsymbol{x}_T\}$, only E^T and D^T are updated [2]:

$$\mathcal{L}_{vae}^T(E^T, D^T) = \lambda_{rec} \mathcal{L}_{rec}^T + \lambda_{kl} \mathcal{L}_{kl}^T. \quad (4)$$

We note that the regularizations $\mathcal{L}_{kl}^S$ and $\mathcal{L}_{kl}^T$ are particularly beneficial for data-efficient UDA. They match priors $P(Z_S)$ and $P(Z_T)$ by enforcing both priors to be close to $\mathcal{N}(0, I)$. We term this as *prior matching* effect.

UDA with Domain Adversarial Training: For domain adversarial training, we add $\boldsymbol{x}_{TS}$'s into D_{isc}'s input set as fake examples.

$$\mathcal{L}_{adv}^T(E^T, D^T, D_{isc}) = \mathbb{E}_{\boldsymbol{x}_S \sim P(X_S)}[\log D_{isc}(\boldsymbol{x}_S)] + \mathbb{E}_{\boldsymbol{x}_{TS}}[\log(1 - D_{isc}(\boldsymbol{x}_{TS}))],$$
$$\text{where } \boldsymbol{x}_{TS} = D^S(D^Z(\boldsymbol{z}_T)), \, \boldsymbol{z}_T \sim q(Z_T|\boldsymbol{x}_T), \, \boldsymbol{x}_T \sim P(X_T). \quad (5)$$

The D_{isc} therefore is trained to differentiate real source images $\{x_S\}$ against outputs of source specific decoder $\{x_{SS}\} \cup \{x_{TS}\}$.

To ensure two encoders providing aligned outputs for similar semantic information, we enforce cycle-consistency for images before and after encoding-decoding to a different domain [16]. Unlike the common practice, cycle-consistency here is only applied on $\mathcal{D}_T \rightarrow \mathcal{D}_S \rightarrow \mathcal{D}_T$ direction, since mapping a large $\{x_S\}$ to a small $\{x_T\}$ and mapping back is intuitively difficult in terms of preserving the large variety in visual appearance within $\{x_S\}$ [2]. We therefore have:

$$\mathcal{L}_{cyc}^T(E^T, D^T) = \mathbb{E}_{x_T}[\|D^T(D^Z(E^Z(E^S(x_{TS})))) - x_T\|_1],$$
$$\text{where } x_{TS} = D^S(D^Z(z_T)), \; z_T \sim q(Z_T|x_T), \; x_T \sim P(X_T). \tag{6}$$

We further propose to train S_{eg} with $\{(z_{ST}, y_S)\}$'s, where z_{ST} is sampled from posterior obtained by sending x_{ST} to the target specific encoder. This encourages S_{eg} to be robust to remaining differences between Z_T and Z_S in $\mathcal{Z}$ due to imperfections of two encoders. We term this as *task-consistency* as a straightforward analogy to cycle-consistency, which has also been independently found useful in [9].

$$\mathcal{L}_{cyc}^{task}(S_{eg}, E^Z) = \mathbb{E}_{z_{ST}}[-Dice(S_{eg}(z_{ST}), y_S) + CE(S_{eg}(z_{ST}), y_S)],$$
$$\text{where } z_{ST} \sim q(Z|x_{ST}), \; x_{ST} = D^T(D^Z(E^Z(E^S(x_S)))), \; x_S \sim P(X_S). \tag{7}$$

By summarizing Eqs. 1–7, we have the entire training objective as follows:

$$\mathcal{L} = \lambda_{rec}(\mathcal{L}_{rec}^S + \mathcal{L}_{rec}^T) + \lambda_{kl}(\mathcal{L}_{kl}^S + \mathcal{L}_{kl}^T) + \lambda_{seg}(\mathcal{L}_{seg} + \mathcal{L}_{cyc}^{task})$$
$$+ \lambda_{adv}(\mathcal{L}_{adv}^S + \mathcal{L}_{adv}^T) + \lambda_{cyc}\mathcal{L}_{cyc}^T. \tag{8}$$

Model Implementation: The network is implemented with PyTorch. E^S, E^T, D^S, D^T, D^Z and D_{isc} are configured as proposed in [2]. Although similar network structures have been used for unsupervised image translation [2,11], the effects of various implementations of VAE on their tasks are often not studied in too much details. Unlike in some of popular implementations where the posterior covariance Σ_Z is fixed to the identity matrix, in our implementation the last 2 blocks of E^Z branch out to predict μ_Z and Σ_Z maps separately. We have observed this design-of-choice yields the best performance by allowing the network to decide covariance Σ_Z for different latent features. We employed a dilated residual network (DRN-26) [14] for segmentation, with modifications on the front and the end layer configurations in adjust to our input and output sizes. We simply chose the hyper-parameters of λ_{rec}, λ_{cyc}, λ_{kl} and λ_{adv} as 1.0, 10.0, 0.1 and 1.0 as proposed in [2]. We also refer readers to the work in [11] on unsupervised image translation. Their network structure is similar to ours, and is shown to be relatively robust to different hyper-parameter selections. As $\mathcal{L}_{seg}$ and $\mathcal{L}_{cyc}^{task}$ are ordinary image segmentation losses, we simply set λ_{seg} to be 1.0, same as common practices.

3   Results

Dataset and Training Settings: Our method is tested on the *MICCAI Multi-modality Whole Heart Segmentation Challenge* [17] dataset. It contains 20 3D cardiac MRI and 20 3D CT scans from different clinical sites (note that the MR and CT images are **unpaired**). Each CT contains ∼256 coronal slices while each MRI contains ∼128 after pre-processing. We chose the MR images as the source domain with sixteen labelled scans for training, four for testing whether the training on source domain functions properly. The CT images are taken as the target with sixteen scans chosen to create a pool for random selection for training while the remaining four scans are used for testing (as in [4,6]). Assignments from each individual scan to training or testing sets are kept the same as in [4,6]. Images are reformated as 2D along the coronal plane with a size of $3 \times 256 \times 256$. Four cardiac structures including the left ventricle myocardium (LV-M), left atrium blood cavity (LA-B), left ventricle blood cavity (LV-B) and ascending aorta (A-A) constitute the segmentation labels. Small rotations, translations, shearings, elastic transformations, gamma transforms and intensity normalizations are used for data augmentation. The Dice score, and average symmetric surface distance (ASSD) of the largest 3D connected component for each label class, are employed for evaluation. See Table 1 and Fig. 2 for quantitative and qualitative results.

Table 1. Quantitative evaluations with the format $^{mean}_{(std.)}$. Postfixes **−16** or **−1** after names of each method indicate the number of unlabelled target scans used for training.

	Dice [%] ↑					ASSD [voxel] ↓				
	LV-M	LA-B	LV-B	A-A	Mean	LV-M	LA-B	LV-B	A-A	Mean
Oracle	82.35	88.45	89.28	87.92	87.0	8.20	8.26	7.08	1.61	5.74
	(2.29)	(1.92)	(3.42)	(12.33)	(7.11)	(1.16)	(2.67)	(3.08)	(1.13)	(3.34)
Unadapted	12.25	46.05	1.42	20.39	20.03	24.46	22.81	47.11	42.72	34.28
	(14.92)	(20.32)	(2.31)	(10.96)	(21.47)	(12.07)	(21.91)	(17.91)	(12.61)	(19.81)
Pnp-AdaNet-16 [6]	49.89	77.37	60.41	78.75	66.61	10.00	4.04	8.60	2.28	6.22
	(5.13)	(3.71)	(11.97)	(3.88)	(13.96)	(3.20)	(0.76)	(1.93)	(0.84)	(3.72)
SIFA-16 [4]	63.58	80.03	79.90	79.58	75.77	3.44	3.89	3.31	2.64	3.32
	(3.30)	(3.21)	(7.51)	(3.64)	(8.50)	(0.40)	(0.85)	(1.41)	(1.85)	(1.32)
Pnp-AdaNet-1 [6]	29.00	48.06	33.48	58.19	42.19	25.18	27.19	27.74	7.14	21.81
	(17.34)	(21.70)	(23.51)	(19.81)	(23.75)	(28.10)	(37.18)	(28.70)	(5.43)	(28.79)
SIFA-1 [4]	39.76	76.65	53.36	**80.27**	62.51	12.58	4.12	7.70	**2.72**	6.78
	(19.86)	**(6.29)**	(24.42)	**(5.81)**	(23.35)	(11.16)	**(1.19)**	(4.45)	**(1.07)**	(7.16)
Proposed-1	**60.21**	78.25	**71.88**	78.38	**72.18**	**7.37**	3.87	**6.44**	2.77	**5.11**
	(15.89)	(9.88)	**(17.93)**	(13.21)	**(16.31)**	**(10.87)**	(1.23)	**(2.18)**	(3.21)	**(6.09)**

Baseline and Upperbound: To illustrate the domain shift problem, we first obtained the **unadpated** baseline given by directly feeding target images to the source encoder after supervised training in the source domain. The result in Table 1 indicates that the source model completely failed on target images with

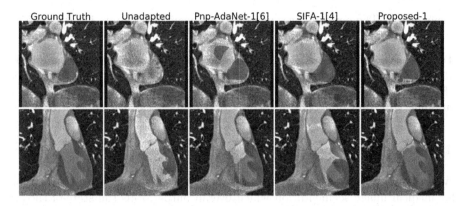

Fig. 2. Qualitative results of adaptation performances on segmentation.

a mean dice of 20.03%. We also obtained the upperbound **oracle** by supervised fine-tuning on the source model with **all sixteen** target scans and their **labels**.

Data-Efficient Domain Adaptation: To simulate the scenario where only a small number of target data is available, we here randomly draw only **one** scan from the target training pool and train the proposed data-efficient UDA. This is in drastic contrast to recent UDA works on this dataset, which use up **all sixteen** target scans for training [4,6]. To avoid being biased on one particular target training scan, the results shown on Table 1 are the averages of repeating the UDA training six times on different randomly chosen target scans. Compared with the unadapted baseline, a significant improvement by 52.15% to 72.18% in mean Dice is achieved. As shown In Fig. 2, the proposed method yields results which are visually close to the ground truth.

Comparison with the State-of-the-Art Method: Under the same experiment setting and one-scan target training sample selections, we also compared our proposed method with two recent UDA methods which are specially designed for medical images: the *Pnp-AdaNet*[1] [6] which is based on domain adversarial training [12], and the recent state-of-the-art *SIFA*[2] [4] which has been introduced in the *Introduction* section. Table 1 shows that under the same target-data scarcity scenario, the proposed method in general outperforms the other two. We also include results of both methods trained on all sixteen target scans for reference. The proposed method obtains results which are close to those of *SIFA-16*, but only require 1/16 of target data.

Ablation Studies: To highlight complementary effects of prior matching and domain adversarial training for UDA in faced of target data scarcity, we performed ablation studies by removing each of these two components separately. By removing one of prior regularization or domain adversarial training, the model

---

[1] https://github.com/carrenD/Medical-Cross-Modality-Domain-Adaptation.

[2] https://github.com/cchen-cc/SIFA.

easily overfit. The performances measured by mean Dice drop to lower than 55% and they oscillate instead of converge.

Toward Few-Shot UDA: We experimented adaptation with a few target **2D slices** by training with only 3 consecutive target slices intersecting with three of four labels. The model overfits eventually. Nevertheless, by applying early stopping after tens of epochs, it could still realize a mean Dice of over 60%.

4 Conclusion and Discussion

We present a novel data efficient unsupervised domain adaptation method for medical image segmentation which overall outperforms the state-of-the-art method given only a small target set. Unlike most of previous UDA methods which use plain encoder-decoder networks and focus on pure domain adversarial training, we demonstrate the effectiveness of VAE-based prior matching in faced of target data scarcity. Although not upperbounding them (KL-divergence does not satisfy the triangular inequality), $\mathcal{L}_{kl}^S + \mathcal{L}_{kl}^T$ provides approximations of KL-divergences between prior distributions of features from two domains, which are in principle extremely difficult to directly estimate given the small target set. By independently forcing source and target prior distributions to be close to $\mathcal{N}(0, I)$, we can match distributions between domains better. From the perspective of data augmentation, sampling from posteriors with noise augments the data. This naturally improves model robustness by introducing further variabilites and perturbations when training its downstream network components.

Our UDA work also differs from VAE-based unsupervised image translation (UIT) [2,11]. Instead of obtaining high-quality transferred images or disentangled representations for manipulation as in UIT, our method focuses on obtaining distribution-matched latent semantic features, and therefore manages to fully exploits the prior matching effect described above. Finally, we performed an extreme test on few-shot UDA with the hope to inspire future studies.

Acknowledgement. This work is supported by the EPSRC Programme Grant (EP/P001009/1).

References

1. Ben-David, S., Blitzer, J., Crammer, K., Kulesza, A., Pereira, F., Vaughan, J.W.: A theory of learning from different domains. Mach. Learn. **79**(1–2), 151–175 (2010)
2. Benaim, S., Wolf, L.: One-shot unsupervised cross domain translation. In: Advances in NeurIPS, pp. 2108–2118 (2018)
3. Cai, J., Zhang, Z., Cui, L., Zheng, Y., Yang, L.: Towards cross-modal organ translation and segmentation: a cycle-and shape-consistent generative adversarial network. Med. Image Anal. **52**, 174–184 (2019)
4. Chen, C., Dou, Q., Chen, H., Qin, J., Heng, P.A.: Synergistic image and feature adaptation: towards cross-modality domain adaptation for medical image segmentation. arXiv preprint arXiv:1901.08211 (2019)

5. Dong, N., Kampffmeyer, M., Liang, X., Wang, Z., Dai, W., Xing, E.: Unsupervised domain adaptation for automatic estimation of cardiothoracic ratio. In: Frangi, A.F., Schnabel, J.A., Davatzikos, C., Alberola-López, C., Fichtinger, G. (eds.) MICCAI 2018. LNCS, vol. 11071, pp. 544–552. Springer, Cham (2018). https://doi.org/10.1007/978-3-030-00934-2_61

6. Dou, Q., Ouyang, C., Chen, C., Chen, H., Glocker, B., Zhuang, X., Heng, P.A.: PnP-AdaNet: plug-and-play adversarial domain adaptation network with a benchmark at cross-modality cardiac segmentation. arXiv preprint arXiv:1812.07907 (2018)

7. Ganin, Y., Ustinova, E., Ajakan, H., Germain, P., Larochelle, H., Laviolette, F., Marchand, M., Lempitsky, V.: Domain-adversarial training of neural networks. J. Mach. Learn. Res. **17**(1), 2030–2096 (2016)

8. Homan, J., Tzeng, E., Park, T., Zhu, J.Y., Isola, P., Saenko, K., Efros, A.A., Darrell, T.: CyCADA: cycle-consistent adversarial domain adaptation. arXiv preprint arXiv:1711.03213 (2017)

9. Hosseini-Asl, E., Zhou, Y., Xiong, C., Socher, R.: Augmented cyclic adversarial learning for low resource domain adaptation (2018)

10. Kamnitsas, K., Baumgartner, C., Ledig, C., Newcombe, V., Simpson, J., Kane, A., Menon, D., Nori, A., Criminisi, A., Rueckert, D., Glocker, B.: Unsupervised domain adaptation in brain lesion segmentation with adversarial networks. In: Niethammer, M., Styner, M., Aylward, S., Zhu, H., Oguz, I., Yap, P.-T., Shen, D. (eds.) IPMI 2017. LNCS, vol. 10265, pp. 597–609. Springer, Cham (2017). https://doi.org/10.1007/978-3-319-59050-9_47

11. Liu, M.Y., Breuel, T., Kautz, J.: Unsupervised image-to-image translation networks. In: Advances in NIPS, pp. 700–708 (2017)

12. Tzeng, E., Hoffman, J., Saenko, K., Darrell, T.: Adversarial discriminative domain adaptation. In: Proceedings of the IEEE CVPR, pp. 7167–7176 (2017)

13. Tzeng, E., Hoffman, J., Zhang, N., Saenko, K., Darrell, T.: Deep domain confusion: Maximizing for domain invariance. arXiv preprint arXiv:1412.3474 (2014)

14. Yu, F., Koltun, V., Funkhouser, T.: Dilated residual networks. In: Proceedings of the IEEE Conference on Computer Vision and Pattern Recognition, pp. 472–480 (2017)

15. Zhang, Y., Miao, S., Mansi, T., Liao, R.: Task driven generative modeling for unsupervised domain adaptation: application to X-ray image segmentation. In: Frangi, A.F., Schnabel, J.A., Davatzikos, C., Alberola-López, C., Fichtinger, G. (eds.) MICCAI 2018. LNCS, vol. 11071, pp. 599–607. Springer, Cham (2018). https://doi.org/10.1007/978-3-030-00934-2_67

16. Zhu, J.Y., Park, T., Isola, P., Efros, A.A.: Unpaired image-to-image translation using cycle-consistent adversarial networks. In: Proceedings of the IEEE ICCV, pp. 2223–2232 (2017)

17. Zhuang, X., Shen, J.: Multi-scale patch and multi-modality atlases for whole heart segmentation of MRI. Med. Image Anal. **31**, 77–87 (2016)

Recurrent Aggregation Learning for Multi-view Echocardiographic Sequences Segmentation

Ming Li[1,2], Weiwei Zhang[1], Guang Yang[3,4], Chengjia Wang[5], Heye Zhang[6(✉)], Huafeng Liu[7], Wei Zheng[1(✉)], and Shuo Li[8]

[1] Shenzhen Institutes of Advanced Technology, Chinese Academy of Sciences, Shenzhen, China
zhengwei@siat.ac.cn
[2] Shenzhen College of Advanced Technology, University of Chinese Academy of Sciences, Shenzhen, China
[3] Cardiovascular Research Centre, Royal Brompton Hospital, London SW3 6NP, UK
[4] National Heart & Lung Institute, Imperial College London, London SW7 2AZ, UK
[5] BHF Centre for Cardiovascular Science, University of Edinburgh, Edinburgh, UK
[6] School of Biomedical Engineering, Sun Yat-Sen University, Shenzhen, China
zhangheye@mail.sysu.edu.cn
[7] Zhejiang University, Hangzhou, China
[8] Western university, London, ON, Canada

Abstract. Multi-view echocardiographic sequences segmentation is crucial for clinical diagnosis. However, this task is challenging due to limited labeled data, huge noise, and large gaps across views. Here we propose a recurrent aggregation learning method to tackle this challenging task. By pyramid ConvBlocks, multi-level and multi-scale features are extracted efficiently. Hierarchical ConvLSTMs next fuse these features and capture spatial-temporal information in multi-level and multi-scale space. We further introduce a double-branch aggregation mechanism for segmentation and classification which are mutually promoted by deep aggregation of multi-level and multi-scale features. The segmentation branch provides information to guide the classification while the classification branch affords multi-view regularization to refine segmentations and further lessen gaps across views. Our method is built as an end-to-end framework for segmentation and classification. Adequate experiments on our multi-view dataset (9000 labeled images) and the CAMUS dataset (1800 labeled images) corroborate that our method achieves not only superior segmentation and classification accuracy but also prominent temporal stability.

1 Introduction

Multi-view echocardiographic sequences delineation provides important insight for clinical diagnosis. The knowledge pattern of cardiac structures and textures associated with deforming tissues can be observed in echocardiographic sequence

© Springer Nature Switzerland AG 2019
D. Shen et al. (Eds.): MICCAI 2019, LNCS 11765, pp. 678–686, 2019.
https://doi.org/10.1007/978-3-030-32245-8_75

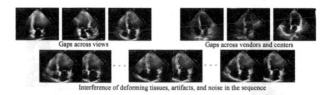

Fig. 1. Top left: multi-view samples (A2C, A3C, and A4C). Top right: A4C samples across vendors and centers. Bottom row: echocardiographic sequence

while in single frames the information is always missing and incomplete [1]. Echocardiographic sequence also permits the assessment of wall motion and identification of end-diastolic (ED) and end-systolic (ES) phases. Cardiologists usually check multi-view echocardiographic sequences in clinical decision-making [2]. The apical-2-chamber view (A2C), A3C, and A4C are the most commonly used views for the left ventricle (LV) functional assessment. Most clinical indexes of the LV (e.g., area, volume, and ejection fraction) are basically measured in these standard apical views. Segmentation of the LV is generally a prerequisite for such quantitative analysis [3]. In clinical routine, quantitative analysis of the LV still involves careful review and massive manual interpretation by experts, which is a tedious and time-consuming task. Thus, automatic methods are desired to facilitate this process. However, multi-view echocardiographic sequences segmentation remains a challenging task as illustrated in Fig. 1. First, the fuzzy border, huge noise, and abounding artifacts of echocardiographic images result in local missing and incomplete of the anatomical structures; Second, multi-view heterogeneous data varies in the anatomical structure, and image properties differ widely across vendors and centers; Third, in the sequence, artifacts and noise are much severer, and the motion of mitral valve, trabeculation, and papillary muscles also poses additional interference; Finally, limited labeled data restricts the performance of supervised learning based methods.

The application scenario of existing methods is always limited and only suitable under a specific situation. They mostly focus on specific view [4] or single frames (i.e., without considering the sequence) [5] or one single vendor and center [6]. As for sequence segmentation, existing methods try to leverage temporal information by using a deformable model combined with the optical flow [7,8] or fine-tuning pretrained CNN dynamically with first frame's label till the last frame [9]. The major downsides of these temporal methods are that they are computational cumbersome and not an end-to-end manner. The limited labeled data and specific application scenario confine the performance of existing methods and lead to the suboptimal solution.

To achieve a unified model for multi-view echocardiographic sequences segmentation, we propose a recurrent aggregation learning method (RAL). The workflow is depicted in Fig. 2. Pyramid ConvBlocks joint hierarchical ConvL-STMs are utilized to capture multi-level and multi-scale spatial-temporal information, enabling RAL the ability to harness the knowledge across heteroge-

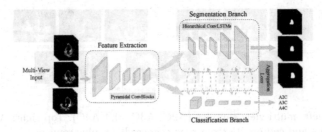

Fig. 2. Workflow overview of our method.

neous data (multi-view, multi-center, and multi-vendor). We further introduce a double-branch aggregation mechanism for segmentation and classification to lessen gaps across multi-view data. Different from existing methods, RAL fully exploits the long term spatial-temporal information in an end-to-end manner and does not depend on any deformable model or optical flow or pretrained segmentation models. RAL can accommodate heterogeneous data, not only generate accuracy segmentation results but also achieve the classification of different views at the same time and gain prominent temporal stability.

2 Method

RAL is built as an end-to-end framework and comprised of three key components: the feature extraction module, the segmentation branch, and the classification branch (as depicted in Fig. 2). The feature extraction module consists of pyramid dilated dense convolution blocks (ConvBlocks). The segmentation branch contains hierarchical recurrent architecture of multiple ConvLSTMs [10]. While the classification branch involves a series of aggregation downsample and fully connected layers.

Multi-level and Multi-scale Features Extraction. We design pyramid ConvBlocks architecture in the feature extraction module, which includes 5 ConvBlocks to extract multi-level and multi-scale features. Multi-level information provides the global geometric characteristic of the LV, while multi-scale information can help to strengthen thin and small regions, further refine the boundaries of the LV. They contribute to lessening the gap across views, vendors, and centers, increasing robustness to images conditions and the anatomical structure variations. One ConvBlock contains L densely connected dilated convolution layers as shown in Fig. 3, which can expand the receptive field and meanwhile preserve the resolution of feature maps. While the transition layer changes channels and resolution of feature maps by convolution and pooling. The feedforward information propagation from preceding l layers to $(l + 1)^{th}$ layer can be formulated as

$$y_l = D(C(y_1, y_2, ..., y_{l-1})) \tag{1}$$

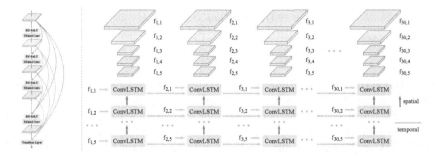

Fig. 3. Left: Dilated dense convolution block. Right: Hierarchical ConvLSTMs for spatial-temporal modeling.

where y_l are the output of the lth layer, $C(\cdot)$ refers to the concatenation of previous layers' outputs. $D(\cdot)$ is a composite function of three connected operations: batch normalization (BN), rectified linear unit (ReLU), and dilated convolution. Five ConvBlocks generate multi-level and multi-scale features $f_t = \{f_{t,1}, f_{t,2}, f_{t,3}, f_{t,4}, f_{t,5}\}$ for frame t in the sequence.

Pyramid ConvBlocks endow RAL with the superior feature extraction ability and the LV region detection capacity in multi-level and multi-scale space, further contribute to capturing the global geometric characteristic of the LV and then establishing uniform semantic features. Thus RAL can detect and extract the LV accurately and robustly from not only ED and ES frames but also other frames in the sequence where the boundary is not clear (disturbed by noise and other tissues, see sequence samples in Fig. 1).

Recurrent Features Fusion for Spatial-Temporal Modeling. For sequence segmentation, capturing the LV characteristic over time is essential for temporal stability. Recent studies based on LSTM have shown great ability to learn sequential information. Inspired by [11,12], we conduct hierarchical ConvLSTMs to exploit long term spatial-temporal modeling as depicted in Fig. 3. We add recurrence in the temporal domain to generate prediction S_t for frame t in the sequence, which carries forward the LV information from previous frames to following frames and allows the matching between consecutive frames naturally. Additionally, we also add recurrence in the spatial domain for multi-level and multi-scale features fusion, which helps to integrate multi-level and multi-scale features efficiently.

The output $y_{t,k}$ of the kth ConvLSTM at frame t depends on the following variables: (1) k^{th} level and scale feature $f_{t,k}$ from the feature extraction module; (2) the output $y_{t,k-1}$ of preceding $(k-1)^{th}$ ConvLSTM at the same frame t; (3) the output $y_{t-1,k}$ from the kth ConvLSTM of previous frame $t-1$; (4) the hidden state representation $h_{t,k-1}$ from preceding $(k-1)^{th}$ ConvLSTM at the same frame t, which is the spatial hidden state; (5) the hidden state representation $h_{t-1,k}$ from the kth ConvLSTM of previous frame $t-1$, which is the temporal hidden state. The information flow can be formulated as

$$x_{input} = [f_{t,k} \mid B(y_{t,k-1}) \mid y_{t-1,k}] \tag{2}$$

$$h_{state} = [h_{t,k-1} \mid h_{t-1,k}] \tag{3}$$

$$y_{t,k} = ConvLSTM_k(x_{input}, h_{state}) \tag{4}$$

where $B(\cdot)$ is the bilinear upsampling operator. At each time step, every ConvLSTM accepts hidden states and encoded spatial-temporal features from previous ConvLSTMs and frame, the corresponding extracted feature from the feature extraction module, it then outputs encoded spatial-temporal features to next ConvLSTM and frame. Finally, predictions S_t are generated by the last ConvLSTM at every frame.

Double-Branch Aggregation Learning. To further lessen the gaps across multi-view and refine multi-view segmentation results, we introduce a double-branch aggregation mechanism for simultaneous segmentation and classification of multi-view echocardiographic sequences as depicted in Fig. 2. Feature from the last ConvBlock is sent to the classification branch. Next, it goes through successive convolution and pooling operators to deeply aggregate with multi-level and multi-scale spatial-temporal features from the segmentation branch. Finally, the classification result is produced by fully connected layers.

Table 1. Specifications of our dataset (left) and the CAMUS dataset (right).

Vendor Machines	Patients	Sequences	Images		A2C	A3C	A4C		CAMUS	A2C	A4C	Vendor Machine
Philips EPIQ 7C	60	180	5400	Sequences	100	100	100	Images	900	900	
GE VIVID E9	20	60	1800	Training		240		Training	1600		GE VIVID E95
Philips IE33	20	60	1800	Testing		60		Testing	200		
Total	100	300	**9000**	Total		300		Total	**1800**		

The segmentation branch generates multi-view segmentations while the classification branch discriminates the specific view. They are mutually promoted by deep aggregation of multi-level and multi-scale spatial-temporal features. The segmentation branch provides multi-level and multi-scale spatial-temporal information to guide the classification while the classification branch affords multi-view discriminative regularization to refine the segmentation results and further lessen the gaps across views. This double-branch aggregation mechanism endows RAL outstanding ability to adapt complex variations of anatomical structure.

Additionally, we propose an aggregation loss to dynamically facilitate the communication between the segmentation branch and the classification branch as illustrated in Fig. 2. The aggregation loss comprises the segmentation loss and classification loss. The segmentation loss is a combination of binary cross-entropy loss and dice loss. While the classification loss is categorical cross-entropy loss. Thus the aggregation loss function can be formulated as

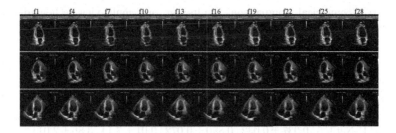

Fig. 4. The LV contours of multi-view sequences segmented by our method (red) and experts (green). Ten frames are selected from every sequence to fit the layout view. (top row: A2C; middle row: A3C; bottom row: A4C)

Table 2. Ablation results of our methods under different configurations.

Configurations	Accuracy	Dice	HD (mm)	MAD (mm)	Classification
Full	0.987 ± 0.005	0.919 ± 0.040	5.87 ± 3.46	2.90 ± 1.49	0.933
w/o classification	0.971 ± 0.008	0.910 ± 0.049	5.99 ± 3.69	3.10 ± 1.66	–
w/o ConvBlock	0.963 ± 0.015	0.907 ± 0.057	6.21 ± 4.95	3.27 ± 1.85	0.867
w/o temporal	0.955 ± 0.019	0.896 ± 0.062	6.64 ± 5.04	3.51 ± 1.93	0.917
5 w/o spatial	0.968 ± 0.011	0.911 ± 0.054	6.03 ± 4.16	3.08 ± 1.71	0.883

$$L_{segmentation} = -[G \cdot log(P) + (1 - G) \cdot log(1 - P)] + \frac{2 \cdot G \cdot P}{G + P} \tag{5}$$

$$L_{classification} = -\sum_{i=1}^{3} g_i \cdot log(p_i) \tag{6}$$

$$L_{aggregation} = \lambda_s \cdot L_{segmentation} + \lambda_c \cdot L_{classification} \tag{7}$$

where G and P denote ground truth and prediction of segmentation respectively, g and p refer to ground truth and prediction of classification separately, i indicates the type of view. Besides, λ_s and λ_c are the corresponding balance coefficients, both are chosen empirically during the training process.

3   Experiments

Datasets. To validate the efficiency of RAL, we built a large multi-view echocardiographic sequences dataset, which was acquired from three centers' various vendor machines (The Second People's Hospital of Shenzhen, The Third People's Hospital of Shenzhen, and Peking University First Hospital). We further evaluate RAL on the public CAMUS dataset [6]. Our dataset contains 300 sequences from 3 views and every sequence includes 30 frames. All 9000 frames were labeled by two experts. Figure 4 presents A2C, A3C, and A4C sequences samples segmented by RAL and experts. While the CAMUS dataset only contains manual

Table 3. Geometrical comparison results on our multi-view echocardiographic sequences dataset.

Methods	Accuracy	Dice	HD (mm)	MAD (mm)
RAL	0.987 ± 0.005	0.919 ± 0.040	5.87 ± 3.46	2.90 ± 1.49
U-Net	0.942 ± 0.030	0.883 ± 0.068	8.94 ± 6.87	3.72 ± 1.87
ACNN	0.959 ± 0.013	0.893 ± 0.061	7.70 ± 6.58	3.40 ± 1.57
U-Net++	0.937 ± 0.032	0.880 ± 0.072	9.01 ± 7.14	3.86 ± 2.01

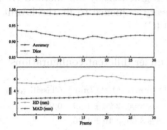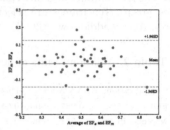

Fig. 5. Left: Mean of Accuracy, Dice, HD, and MAD at different frames of the cardiac cycle. Right: Bland-Altman analysis (EF_a and EF_m: ejection fraction calculated from automatic segmentations and manual labels)

labels at ED and ES frames, which was acquired from a single vendor and center. Table 1 shows the specifications of two datasets.

Evaluation Metrics. Accuracy, Dice, Mean Absolute Distance (MAD) and Hausdorff Distance (HD) are used to measure segmentation results. We further evaluate the segmentation performance with the ED, ES volume, and ejection fraction on the CAMUS dataset. We utilize the output of RAL to compute clinical indices according to standard guidelines [3].

Implementation Details. All images are resized to 256×256 for computational efficiency. We employ Adam with the learning rate of 0.001 as the optimizer. The dilated rates of 5 ConvBlocks are $1, 1, 2, 4, 8$ respectively, and every ConvBlock contains 6 layers. Besides, a dynamical decay mechanism is utilized to reduce the learning rate by monitoring the change of Dice. Ten-fold cross-validation was utilized to provide an unbiased estimation.

Ablation Study. We evaluate our method under different configurations to corroborate the necessity of every component in RAL. The classification branch, ConvBlock, spatial modeling and temporal modeling are removed respectively. Table 2 shows the ablation results, we can see that full RAL achieves higher mean values of Accuracy and Dice, lower mean values of HD and MAD, and lower standard deviations of all metrics compared against other configurations. RAL also achieves the best classification accuracy (0.933). Every single component brings important improvement for the LV segmentation, especially when adding recurrence in the temporal domain.

Table 4. Clinical comparison results on CAMUS dataset. (EDV: ED volume; ESV: ES volume; EF: ejection fraction; corr: Pearson correlation; mae: mean absolute error)

Methods	EDV			ESV			EF		
	corr	bias (ml)	mae (ml)	corr	bias (ml)	mae (ml)	corr	bias (%)	mae (%)
RAL	0.952	-7.5 ± 11.0	8.8	0.960	-3.8 ± 9.2	7.1	0.839	-0.9 ± 6.8	5.0
U-Net	0.954	-6.9 ± 11.8	9.8	0.964	-3.7 ± 9.0	6.8	0.823	-1.0 ± 7.1	5.3
ACNN	0.945	-6.7 ± 12.9	10.8	0.947	-4.0 ± 10.8	8.3	0.799	-0.8 ± 7.5	5.7
U-Net++	0.946	-11.4 ± 12.9	13.2	0.952	-5.7 ± 10.7	8.6	0.789	-1.8 ± 7.7	5.6

Comparison Study I: Geometrical. We compare RAL with U-Net, ACNN, and U-Net++ on our multi-view sequences dataset. As shown in Table 3, RAL outperforms other methods on all metrics, achieving the highest mean values of Accuracy (0.987) and Dice (0.919), the lowest mean values of HD (5.87 mm) and MAD (2.90 mm), and significantly lower standard deviations of all metrics. These strongly prove that RAL is able to accomplish the best region coverage, the highest contour accuracy, and the minimum distance error when processing multi-view echocardiographic sequences across multi-vendor and multi-center.

Comparison Study II: Clinical. We compare RAL with U-Net, ACNN, and U-Net++ on the CAMUS dataset to calculate clinical indices. As shown in Table 4, RAL obtained high correlation scores (0.952 for EDV, 0.960 for ESV, and 0.839 for EF), reasonably small biases and standard deviations, and relatively low mae (8.8 ml for EDV, 7.1 ml for ESV, and 5.0% for EF). Figure 5 presents a more intuitional result by Bland-Altman plot. 94% of the measurements locate in the ± 1.96 standard deviation in Bland-Altman plot. These results reveal the clinical potential of RAL.

Temporal Stability. We compute the mean of Accuracy, Dice, HD, and MAD at different frames of all echocardiographic sequences and then observe the volatility of each metric to assess the temporal stability. As shown in Fig. 5, RAL achieves stable mean values of all four metrics in the cardiac cycle, only exists moderate fluctuating in the middle of the sequence. This means spatial-temporal modeling of RAL is efficient. RAL achieves not only superior segmentation accuracy but also a good coherence of consecutive frames in the sequence.

Limitation. In Fig. 5, from ED to ES frames, we observe that Accuracy and Dice decay slightly while HD and MAD increase mildly, and all metrics keep relatively stable in the diastole but show feeblish recoverability. The sequential process carries errors forward resulting in accumulation of temporal errors in the cardiac cycle. Fortunately, the fluctuating rate is moderate and the worst results are still fairly good. This limitation could be alleviated via Bi-direction LSTM.

4   Conclusion

In this paper, we present a recurrent aggregation learning method to exploit long term spatial-temporal information for simultaneous segmentation and classification of multi-view echocardiographic sequences. Multi-level and multi-scale features are recurrently aggregated on both spatial domain and temporal domain for effective spatial-temporal modeling. A double-branch aggregation mechanism further brings multi-view discriminative regularization to refine the segmentation results. Adequate experiments of geometrical and clinical evaluation demonstrate that RAL achieves not only superior segmentation and classification accuracy, prominent temporal stability, but also high correlations on clinical indices.

Acknowledgment. This work is funded by the Shenzhen Basic Research Program (JCYJ20170818164343304, JCYJ20180507182432303).

References

1. Huang, X., et al.: Contour tracking in echocardiographic sequences via sparse representation and dictionary learning. Med. Image Anal. **18**(2), 253–271 (2014)
2. Madani, A., et al.: Fast and accurate view classification of echocardiograms using deep learning. NPJ Digital Med. **1**(1), 6 (2018)
3. Lang, R.M., et al.: Recommendations for cardiac chamber quantification by echocardiography in adults: an update from the American Society of echocardiography and the European Association of Cardiovascular Imaging. Eur. Hear. J.-Cardiovasc. Imaging **16**(3), 233–271 (2015)
4. Carneiro, G., et al.: The segmentation of the left ventricle of the heart from ultrasound data using deep learning architectures and derivative-based search methods. IEEE Trans. Image Process. **21**(3), 968–982 (2012)
5. Chen, H., Zheng, Y., Park, J.-H., Heng, P.-A., Zhou, S.K.: Iterative multi-domain regularized deep learning for anatomical structure detection and segmentation from ultrasound images. In: Ourselin, S., Joskowicz, L., Sabuncu, M.R., Unal, G., Wells, W. (eds.) MICCAI 2016. LNCS, vol. 9901, pp. 487–495. Springer, Cham (2016). https://doi.org/10.1007/978-3-319-46723-8_56
6. Leclerc, S., et al.: Deep learning for segmentation using an open large-scale dataset in 2D echocardiography. IEEE Trans. Med. Imaging (2019)
7. Pedrosa, J., et al.: Fast and fully automatic left ventricular segmentation and tracking in echocardiography using shape-based b-spline explicit active surfaces. IEEE Trans. Med. Imaging **36**(11), 2287–2296 (2017)
8. Zhang, N., et al.: Deep learning for diagnosis of chronic myocardial infarction on nonenhanced cardiac cine MRI. Radiology **291**(3), 606–617 (2019)
9. Yu, L., et al.: Segmentation of fetal left ventricle in echocardiographic sequences based on dynamic convolutional neural networks. IEEE Trans. Biomed. Eng. **64**(8), 1886–1895 (2017)
10. Xingjian, S., et al.: Convolutional LSTM network: a machine learning approach for precipitation nowcasting. In: NIPS, pp. 802–810 (2015)
11. Chen, J., et al.: Multiview two-task recursive attention model for left atrium and atrial scars segmentation. In: Frangi, A.F., Schnabel, J.A., Davatzikos, C., Alberola-López, C., Fichtinger, G. (eds.) MICCAI 2018. LNCS, vol. 11071, pp. 455–463. Springer, Cham (2018). https://doi.org/10.1007/978-3-030-00934-2_51
12. Yang, G., et al.: Multiview sequential learning and dilated residual learning for a fully automatic delineation of the left atrium and pulmonary veins from late gadolinium-enhanced cardiac MRI images. In: EMBC, pp. 1123–1127. IEEE (2018)

Echocardiography View Classification Using Quality Transfer Star Generative Adversarial Networks

Zhibin Liao[1(✉)], Mohammad H. Jafari[1], Hany Girgis[1,2], Kenneth Gin[1,2], Robert Rohling[1], Purang Abolmaesumi[1], and Teresa Tsang[1,2]

[1] The University of British Columbia, Vancouver, BC, Canada
liaoz@ece.ubc.ca
[2] Vancouver General Hospital, Vancouver, BC, Canada

Abstract. 2D echocardiography (echo) is the most widely used imaging technique to identify cardiac disease. In addition to anatomical variability in patients, the quality of acquired echo image can vary significantly depending on the ultrasound (US) machine and the experience level of the operator, where a poor image quality can affect the diagnosis. This variability can also result in reduced performance of machine learning models trained on these data. With the recent advances in generative adversarial networks (GAN), we demonstrate that it is possible to transfer the image quality of echo images to a user-defined quality level with the use of a multi-domain transfer approach referred as Star-GAN. The proposed quality transfer StarGAN (QT-StarGAN) requires no pairs of low-and high-quality echo images and incorporates the temporal information of echo images during the training phase. We evaluate the proposed approach using 16,612 echo cine series obtained from 3,157 patients. Using a standard echo view classification task, we demonstrate that the accuracy of classification is significantly improved using QT-StarGAN.

Keywords: Echocardiography · Ultrasound · Image quality · View classification · Generative network · Domain transfer · GAN

1 Introduction

2D echocardiography (echo) is the most widely used imaging technique to identify cardiac disease. Echo examination is low-cost and non-invasive, and given its portability specifically using the latest generation mobile ultrasound technology, it can be used as first line imaging for emergency diagnoses and point-of-care. The echo image quality is determined by the presence and contrast of target heart anatomies (*i.e.*, valve and chamber wall), proper centering, imaging depth, and

---

Z. Liao, M. H. Jafari and H. Girgis–Joint first authorship.
P. Abolmaesumi and T. Tsang–Joint senior authorship.

© Springer Nature Switzerland AG 2019
D. Shen et al. (Eds.): MICCAI 2019, LNCS 11765, pp. 687–695, 2019.
https://doi.org/10.1007/978-3-030-32245-8_76

imaging gain settings [6]. Hence, in addition to inter-patient anatomical variations, the experience level of a sonographer and the imaging system itself are the main factors contributing to echo image quality.

To improve quality, conventional methods have investigated speckle reduction, and contrast and edge enhancements [5,19,24], which are difficult to generalize across patients and imaging systems. With the increasing popularity of deep learning in medical imaging, neural networks-based image de-nosing and super-resolution methods have been shown to improve image quality of CT and PET [2,13]. However, these methods typically require paired source and target domain images (*i.e.*, low and high quality counterparts showing the exact patient anatomy) to train the transfer model, which is virtually impossible to obtain during echo acquisition given above-mentioned factors contributing to variations in image quality. Nevertheless, deep neural networks have been used to assess ultrasound image quality [1,20,21] with the supervision of expert labels.

Image quality transfer task can be viewed as an image-to-image translation problem conditioned on the quality attribute. For echo images, the difficulty mainly stems from the limited availability of source and target image pairs. The recently proposed Cycle-Consistent GAN (CycleGAN) [23] enforces the image transfer consistency in a GAN framework to avoid the need for image pairs. CycleGAN has fixed source and target domains; thus, multiple CycleGAN models are needed for multi-domain transfer. StarGAN [4] combines the CycleGAN and conditional GAN [12] to encapsulate multi-domain transfer in one model.

In this paper, we propose an echo image quality transfer network, trained with echo images and corresponding quality labels, which enables the translation of echo images towards a user-defined quality level. To achieve this, we first start with StarGAN [4]. We demonstrate that using the original StarGAN structure to transfer image quality leads to significant reconstruction artifacts. To alleviate this, we present several critical modifications to StarGAN's generator and discriminator networks and introduce Quality Transfer StarGAN (QT-StarGAN), which can produce images that are visually very close to clinically obtained data. For quantitative evaluation, we use echo view classification task as a testbed, and demonstrate that our proposed QT-StarGAN results in significantly improved classification accuracy.

2   Dataset

To collect the gold standard labels, a cardiologist with 30 years clinical experience was given the task to assign the quality assessment and also the view classification labels for a total of 16,612 echo cine series from 3,157 unique patients.[1] The training, validation and test sets were split with a 6:2:2 ratio at the patient level. Each echo series contained 40–70 image frames. For each cine series, all

---

[1] 14 standard cardiac views: see the 13 class labels in Fig. 5(b) and due to the extreme similarity, PSAX-{M, PM} views are combined as one class. This dataset was collected from Vancouver General Hospital PACS system, under the approvals from the institutional Medical Research Ethics Board and the Information Privacy Office.

image frames inherit the assigned labels. The quality labels were defined in four coarse quality categories: *Poor* (0%–25%), *Fair* (25%–50%), *Good* (50%–75%), and *Excellent* (75%–100%), with the percentages reference to the lowest to highest image qualities within each category. The dataset quality distribution is 8%, 38%, 35% and 19% from *Poor* to *Excellent*. Given that our goal is to freely transfer the echo image quality to any level between 0% to 100%, we modify the aleatoric uncertainty modelling method proposed by [14,16] to directly supervise the training of a numerical quality estimation module.

3 Methodology

Let us note the collected dataset as $\mathcal{D} = \{\mathbf{x}_i, q_i, v_i\}_{i=1}^{|\mathcal{D}|}$, where $\mathbf{x}_i$ is a 2D echo image, $q_i \in \mathcal{C} = \{c : Poor, \ldots, Excellent\}$ and $v_i \in \{AP2, \ldots, SUPRA\}$ are the corresponding image quality and view classification labels, and $\mathbf{q}_i$ and $\mathbf{v}_i$ are vectors representing the one-hot version of respective label. For simplifying the notations, images $\mathbf{x}_{i-1}$ and $\mathbf{x}_{i+1}$ in the dataset represent the previous and the next frames of $\mathbf{x}_i$ from one echo cine series, where the special cases of boundary frame samples are not discussed.

The QT-StarGAN is constructed by a generator G and a discriminator D, and the network architecture can be view in Fig. 1. An image $\tilde{\mathbf{x}}_i = G(\mathbf{x}_i, t_i)$ is generated by forwarding $\mathbf{x}_i$ and a user-defined target quality level $t_i \in (0,1]$. The quality estimation branch D_q needs to handle the fine-grained numerical quality level t_i for $\tilde{\mathbf{x}}_i$ and the coarse categorical quality labels q_i for $\mathbf{x}_i$. By following Kendall and Gal [14], our D_q emits two numerical outputs $D_{q^\mu}, D_{q^\sigma} \in (0,1]$ to model the quality level as a Gaussian distribution $\mathcal{N}(D_{q^\mu}, D_{q^\sigma})$, instead of a typical regression module with only a numerical output. To accept the one-hot categorical target label $\mathbf{q}_i$, we compute the probability distribution $\mathbf{p}_i$ of each coarse quality class using the Gaussian Cumulative Density Function (CDF):

$$\mathrm{cdf}(z) = \frac{1}{2}\Big(1 + \mathrm{erf}\Big(\frac{z - D_{q^\mu}(\mathbf{x})}{D_{q^\sigma}(\mathbf{x})\sqrt{2}}\Big)\Big),$$

$$p_c^* = \mathrm{cdf}(u_c) - \mathrm{cdf}(l_c), \text{ and, } p_c = \frac{p_c^*}{\sum_{c \in C} p_c^*}, \tag{1}$$

where erf(.) denotes the error function, l_c and u_c are the respective lower and upper bound for c, and the subscript i is dropped for clarity. For training with the fine-grained numerical value t_i, only the $D_{q^\mu}(\tilde{\mathbf{x}}_i)$ is trained with the mean absolute loss function. Hence, the loss function for D_q is defined as:

$$\ell_q(\mathbf{x}_i) = H(\mathbf{q}_i, \mathbf{p}_i) + \lambda_t |t_i - D_{q^\mu}(\tilde{\mathbf{x}}_i)|, \tag{2}$$

where $H(.,.)$ represents the cross-entropy loss, $\mathbf{p}_i = [p_{c,i}]_{c \in \mathcal{C}}^{\mathrm{T}}$ denotes an one-hot vector of the probability distribution, and $\lambda_t = 10$ is determined by grid search.

The second job of D is to make sure that appearance of $\tilde{\mathbf{x}}_i$ is close to a real 2D echo image. This is commonly achieved by following the adversarial training [7]: $\ell_{adv} = \log D_{adv}(\mathbf{x}_i) + \log\big(1 - D_{adv}(1 - \tilde{\mathbf{x}}_i)\big)$. The original StarGAN

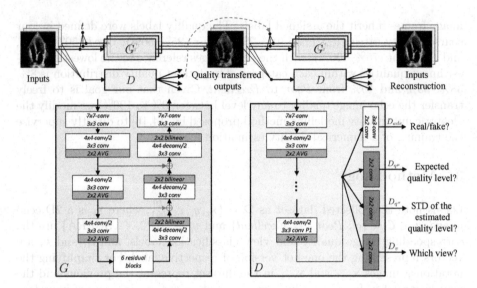

Fig. 1. The network structure of the proposed QT-StarGAN (c3). "/#" denotes the stride other than 1. The green blocks represent the added layers; the red connections represent the introduced parameter-free skip connections; and the blue dotted connection represents the use of D estimated quality level of the original images for transferring the generated images back to the original quality level. (Color figure online)

model implements the Wasserstein GAN objective [3] with gradient penalty [8] to improve the training stability, which is unchanged in our network:

$$\ell_{adv}(\mathbf{x}_i) = D_{adv}(\mathbf{x}_i) - D_{adv}(\tilde{\mathbf{x}}_i) - \lambda_{gp}(\|\nabla D_{adv}(\hat{\mathbf{x}}_i)\|_2 - 1)^2, \qquad (3)$$

where D_{adv} represents the second output branch of D, $\hat{\mathbf{x}}_i$ denotes a sample uniformly drawn from a straight line between $\mathbf{x}_i$ and $\tilde{\mathbf{x}}_i$, and $\lambda_{gp} = 10$ is a weighting factor determined by [4].

Here, we add a regularization loss to D to ensure $\tilde{\mathbf{x}}_i$ can preserve the correct heart anatomical patterns that are necessary to fulfill the view classification task, via a third output branch D_v:

$$\ell_v(\mathbf{x}_i) = H(\mathbf{v}_i, D_v(\mathbf{x}_i)) + H(\mathbf{v}_i, D_v(\tilde{\mathbf{x}}_i)). \qquad (4)$$

Finally, the generator should be able to re-generate $\mathbf{x}_i$, given $\tilde{\mathbf{x}}_i$ and q_i, following the cycle consistent reconstruction [15,23]. Since q_i is categorical, we replace q_i with $D_{q_\mu}(\mathbf{x}_i)$ (treated as a constant in the computation graph):

$$\ell_{rec}(\mathbf{x}_i) = |\mathbf{x}_i - G(\tilde{\mathbf{x}}_i, D_{q_\mu}(\mathbf{x}_i))|. \qquad (5)$$

Therefore, the overall training objective combines the above loss components:

$$\ell(\mathbf{x}_i) = \frac{1}{|\mathcal{D}|} \sum_{i=1}^{|\mathcal{D}|} \left(\lambda_q \ell_q(\mathbf{x}_i) + \ell_{adv}(\mathbf{x}_i) + \lambda_v \ell_v(\mathbf{x}_i) + \lambda_{rec} \ell_{rec}(\mathbf{x}_i)\right), \qquad (6)$$

where we find $\lambda_q = \lambda_v = 1$, and $\lambda_{rec} = 10$ yield the optimal performance.

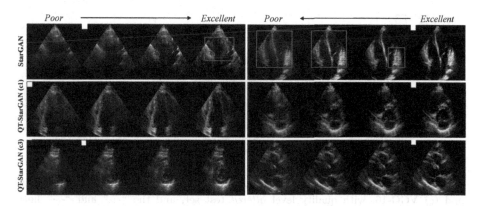

Fig. 2. Examples of quality level altered images generated by StarGAN, QT-StarGAN (c1), QT-StarGAN (c3), with red boxes indicating the reconstruction artifacts. The sub-images with a white square on the top-left corner are the original images before the translation. (Color figure online)

3.1 Network Modifications

In the original StarGAN network, G is in a form of auto-encoder with a series of down-sampling convolution (conv) layers (contraction path), a series of residual layers (feature tuning path), and a series of up-sampling deconvolution (deconv) layers (expansion path), and D is a multi-layer conv network.

Bilinear Up-Sampling and Skip Connection: Using the original StarGAN network, we observe that the generated images can contain visually noticeable artifacts (see the first row of Fig. 2). These artifacts have grid appearance patterns, which is a result of using deconv layers with stride 2 to up-sample the spatial size of the feature tensor. Hence, we replaced the deconv layers with bilinear up-sampling layer followed by conv layer with stride 1 during the up-sampling phase. Motivated by U-Net [17] and ResNet [9] designs, we added two parameter-free skip-addition shortcuts, allowing a chance for the high-frequency information to be utilized in image generation. These two network modifications (NM) have been illustrated in Fig. 1 with the combined improvements shown as StarGAN+NM in Fig. 3.

Temporal Discriminator: While keeping G on single frame generation, we extend a temporal window of three frames for D to allow temporal information to aid to the optimization of the objectives. In Fig. 2, we show examples of the single-frame and three-frame variations of QT-StarGAN as QT-StarGAN (c1)/(c3), respectively. This modification is simply an alteration to the input of D to a stack of three frames, noted as $D(\{\mathbf{z}_{i-1}, \mathbf{z}_i, \mathbf{z}_{i+1}\})$ for $\mathbf{z} \in \{\mathbf{x}, \tilde{\mathbf{x}}, \hat{\mathbf{x}}\}$, where the respective task labels remain the same for all three frames.

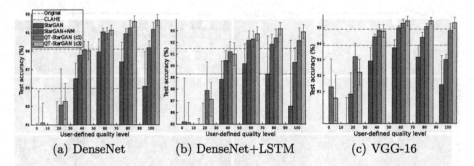

(a) DenseNet　　　　(b) DenseNet+LSTM　　　　(c) VGG-16

Fig. 3. The view classification performance on (a) DenseNet, (b) DenseNet+LSTM, and (c) VGG-16, with quality level *altered* test set, and the "- -" and "- ·" lines indicate the classification performance with the *original* test set and CLAHE *altered* test set [24], respectively. Sub-figures share the same legend.

4   Experiments and Discussion

For quantitative evaluation, we compare a state-of-the-art view classification model proposed by Zhang *et al.* [22] (*i.e.*, a VGG-16 [18] network), a point-of-care mobile ultrasound view classification and quality assessment model [20] (*i.e.*, a lightweight DenseNet [11] + LSTM [10] model), a standalone DenseNet extracted from the above DenseNet+LSTM model, and an contrast enhancement method CLAHE [24]. For standardization, we uniformly adjusted the input size of the deep models to 128 × 128 to match the image size of QT-StarGAN. D_{q^μ} and D_{q^σ} modules are also integrated in the deep models to estimate image quality level. For statistically analyzing the view classification performance of the quality transferred images, we trained five instances for each quality transfer model and each view classification model, paired to generate the following experiment results. At last, Eq. (1) is applied to handle the categorical quality labels for all listed quality transfer models.

It can be observed in Fig. 3: (1) StarGAN exhibits a performance drop at high target qualities (which can be related to the artifacts shown in Fig. 2); (2) the network modifications in StarGAN+NM (*i.e.*, QT-StarGAN (c1) without ℓ_v) can lead to significant improvement in view classification accuracy; (3) the further addition of ℓ_v in QT-StarGAN (c1) can alleviate the performance drop problem at high target qualities; and, (4) the benefit of the temporal discriminator can be observed with the improved view classification accuracy of c3 *vs.* c1.

From Fig. 4, we observe a phenomenon that the estimated quality from the view classification model does not always match the user defined quality level. We suspect that this due to the correlation between the defined echo image quality and ultrasound imaging parameters such as the imaging depth and proper centering. From Fig. 2, we see that QT-StarGAN is able to alter the image contrast by enhancing the anatomical edges and changing the speckle patterns over the quality translation, while the imaging depth and centering are preserved. As a result, QT-StarGAN cannot fully adjust the image quality level to a user-

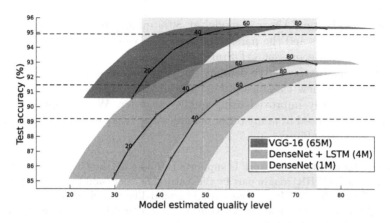

Fig. 4. The mean (the values on the black lines) and STD (the horizontal slice width of the polygon) of target quality level *vs.* view classification model estimated quality level after transfer by QT-StarGAN (c3). The gray background area indicates the mean and STD of the *original* test set. "# M" indicates the number of model parameters.

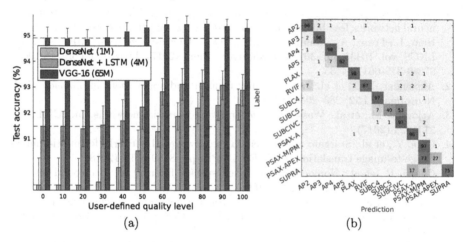

Fig. 5. (a) The performance of QT-StarGAN (c3) by only transfer the test images that with estimated image quality lower than the user-defined quality level; and (b) the *normalized* confusion matrix (in %) of QT-StarGAN (c3) at 80% quality.

defined value. Intuitively for echo imaging analysis tasks such as view classification, transferring the quality to a lower level does not have any value except providing extra training samples to regularize the model.

In Fig. 5(a), we only transfer the images with the estimated quality lower than the user-defined level, which improves classification accuracy with statistical significance at above 60% user-defined quality level for DenseNet and DenseNet+LSTM, and at 80% quality for VGG-16. Finally in Fig. 5(b), we observe the QT-StarGAN (c3) model at 80% quality majorly confuses within the subcostal views and the parasteral short axis views.

In summary, we present QT-StarGAN to transfer echo image quality by a user-defined quality level. We demonstrate the effectiveness of this network by testing the echo view classification accuracy, where the classification accuracy can be significantly improved using quality transfer. We anticipate that QT-StarGAN can be used in many other classification tasks to reduce the impact of image quality variability.

Acknowledgements. This work is supported in part by the Canadian Institutes of Health Research (CIHR) and in part by the Natural Sciences and Engineering Research Council of Canada (NSERC). The authors would like to acknowledge the support provided by Dale Hawley and the Vancouver Coastal Health in providing us with the anonymized, de-identified data.

References

1. Abdi, A.H., et al.: Quality assessment of echocardiographic cine using recurrent neural networks: feasibility on five standard view planes. In: Descoteaux, M., Maier-Hein, L., Franz, A., Jannin, P., Collins, D.L., Duchesne, S. (eds.) MICCAI 2017. LNCS, vol. 10435, pp. 302–310. Springer, Cham (2017). https://doi.org/10.1007/978-3-319-66179-7_35
2. Alexander, D.C., et al.: Image quality transfer and applications in diffusion MRI. NeuroImage **152**, 283–298 (2017)
3. Arjovsky, M., et al.: Wasserstein generative adversarial networks. In: ICML, pp. 214–223 (2017)
4. Choi, Y., et al.: Stargan: unified generative adversarial networks for multi-domain image-to-image translation. In: IEEE CVPR, pp. 8789–8797 (2018)
5. Coupé, P., et al.: Nonlocal means-based speckle filtering for ultrasound images. IEEE TIP **18**(10), 2221–2229 (2009)
6. Gaudet, J., et al.: Focused critical care echocardiography: development and evaluation of an image acquisition assessment tool. Crit. Care Med. **44**(6), e329–e335 (2016)
7. Goodfellow, I., et al.: Generative adversarial nets. In: NIPS, pp. 2672–2680 (2014)
8. Gulrajani, I., et al.: Improved training of wasserstein gans. In: NIPS, pp. 5767–5777 (2017)
9. He, K., et al.: Deep residual learning for image recognition. In: CVPR, pp. 770–778 (2016)
10. Hochreiter, S., Schmidhuber, J.: Long short-term memory. Neural Comput. **9**(8), 1735–1780 (1997)
11. Huang, G., et al.: Densely connected convolutional networks. In: IEEE CVPR, vol. 1–2, p. 3 (2017)
12. Isola, P., et al.: Image-to-image translation with conditional adversarial networks. In: IEEE CVPR, pp. 1125–1134 (2017)
13. Kang, E., et al.: A deep CNN using directional wavelets for low-dose X-ray CT reconstruction. Med. Phys. **44**(10), 360–375 (2017)
14. Kendall, A., Gal, Y.: What uncertainties do we need in Bayesian deep learning for computer vision? In: NIPS, pp. 5574–5584 (2017)

15. Kim, T., et al.: Learning to discover cross-domain relations with generative adversarial networks. In: ICML, pp. 1857–1865. JMLR. org (2017).
16. Nix, D.A., Weigend, A.S.: Estimating the mean and variance of the target probability distribution. In: Neural Networks, vol. 1, pp. 55–60. IEEE (1994)
17. Ronneberger, O., Fischer, P., Brox, T.: U-Net: convolutional networks for biomedical image segmentation. In: Navab, N., Hornegger, J., Wells, W.M., Frangi, A.F. (eds.) MICCAI 2015. LNCS, vol. 9351, pp. 234–241. Springer, Cham (2015). https://doi.org/10.1007/978-3-319-24574-4_28
18. Simonyan, K., Zisserman, A.: Very deep convolutional networks for large-scale image recognition. In: ICLR, pp. 1–14 (2015)
19. Tsantis, S., et al.: Multiresolution edge detection using enhanced fuzzy c-means clustering for ultrasound image speckle reduction. Medical Physics 41(7), 72903-1-11 (2014)
20. Van Woudenberg, N., et al.: Quantitative echocardiography: real-time quality estimation and view classification implemented on a mobile android device. In: Stoyanov, D., et al. (eds.) POCUS/BIVPCS/CuRIOUS/CPM -2018. LNCS, vol. 11042, pp. 74–81. Springer, Cham (2018). https://doi.org/10.1007/978-3-030-01045-4_9
21. Wu, L., et al.: FUIQA: fetal ultrasound image quality assessment with deep convolutional networks. IEEE Trans. Cybern. 47(5), 1336–1349 (2017)
22. Zhang, J., et al.: Fully automated echocardiogram interpretation in clinical practice: feasibility and diagnostic accuracy. Circulation 138(16), 1623–1635 (2018)
23. Zhu, J.Y., et al.: Unpaired image-to-image translation using cycle-consistent adversarial networks. In: IEEE ICCV, pp. 2223–2232 (2017)
24. Zuiderveld, K.: Contrast limited adaptive histogram equalization. In: Graphics Gems IV, pp. 474–485. Academic Press Professional Inc. (1994)

Dual-View Joint Estimation of Left Ventricular Ejection Fraction with Uncertainty Modelling in Echocardiograms

Delaram Behnami[1]($\boxtimes$), Zhibin Liao[1], Hany Girgis[1,2], Christina Luong[1,2], Robert Rohling[1], Ken Gin[1,2], Teresa Tsang[1,2], and Purang Abolmaesumi[1]

[1] University of British Columbia, Vancouver, Canada
delaramb@ece.ubc.ca
[2] Vancouver General Hospital, Vancouver, BC, Canada

Abstract. Echocardiography (echo) is a standard-of-care imaging technique for characterizing heart function and structure. Left ventricular ejection fraction (EF) is the single most commonly measured cardiac metric and a powerful prognostic indicator of cardiac events. In two-dimensional transthoracic echo, EF is measured via (1) segmentation of left ventricle on multiple cross-sectional 2D views; and/or (2) visual assessment of echo cines. However, due to high inter- and intra-observer in both approaches, robust EF estimation has proven challenging. In this paper, we propose a dual-stream multi-tasking network for segmentation-free joint estimation of both segmentation- and visual assessment-based EF, across two echo views. To account for variability in EF labels, we introduce an uncertainty modelling layer, which enables the network to inherently capture the variability in expert-annotated clinical labels, of both regression and classification types. We trained a model on 1,751 apical two- and four-chamber pairs of echo cine loops and their corresponding EF labels, and achieved an R^2 of 0.90, mean absolute error of 4.5%, and classification accuracy of 91% on a test set of 430 patients. Our proposed framework (1) requires no segmentation; (2) provides estimates for four clinical EF measurements derived from the two views; (3) recognizes the inherent uncertainties in echo measurements and encodes it; (4) provides measurements with corresponding uncertainties, which may help increase the interpretability and adoption of computer-generated clinical measurements. The proposed framework can be used as a generic approach for deriving other cardiac function parameters from echo.

D. Behnami, Z. Liao, and H. Girgis—Joint first authors.
T. Tsang, and P. Abolmaesumi—Joint senior authors.

Electronic supplementary material The online version of this chapter (https://doi.org/10.1007/978-3-030-32245-8_77) contains supplementary material, which is available to authorized users.

D. Shen et al. (Eds.): MICCAI 2019, LNCS 11765, pp. 696–704, 2019.
https://doi.org/10.1007/978-3-030-32245-8_77

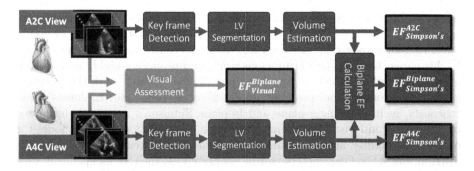

Fig. 1. The clinical workflow for EF assessment. The dark and light purple paths in the workflow illustrate the Simpson's and visual assessment methods, respectively. (Heart schematics: courtesy of 123 Sonography) (Color figure online).

1 Introduction

Heart disease is the global leading cause of death [8]. Echocardiography (echo) is the most frequent imaging technique used for diagnosis and management of heart disease [2,9]. One of the most important clinical measurements of an echo exam is left ventricular ejection fraction (EF), which evaluates the systolic performance of the heart, that is, the strength of contractile function. In 2D echo, EF is calculated through the biplane Simpson's method of disks, which is the current standard-of-care. The Simpson's method involves measuring the minimum, *i.e.*, end-systolic (ESV), and maximum, *i.e.*, end-diastolic (EDV), volumes of the LV by estimating the LV surface area in two standard 2D echo views, referred to as apical two-chamber (A2C) and apical four-chamber (A4C). The accuracy of Simpson's method is highly dependent on accurate (a) selection of end-diastolic (ED) and end-systolic (ES) frames; and (b) segmentation of the LV endocardium, in both apical windows. The alternative technique for volumetric estimation of EF in clinics is visual assessment of echo cine series. This approach is commonly used by experienced echocardiographers, who after years of practice, can subjectively estimate EF accurately. Visual assessment is also robust to segmentation and frame selection errors. Figure 1 demonstrates the clinical workflow for measuring EF using these methods. Nevertheless, both methods suffer from high inter- and intra-observer variability, making EF estimation challenging [2]. Factors contributing to such variability in EF labels include: (1) low inherent image quality in echo; (2) inaccurate segmentation or key frame detection; and (3) errors due to volume estimation from 2D images.

Several works have previously attempted LV segmentation for EF assessment [4,7,11,16,17]. Other related works include three-way classification of EF using residual networks [10], and segmentation-free estimation of EF in cardiac magnetic resonance (CMR) images [3,5,12,15]. We previously proposed direct estimation of EF in echo cine series using 2D convolutional networks (CNNs) for frame-level feature extraction and recurrent neural networks (RNNs) for temporal embedding of the videos [1]. However, given significant observer variability affecting gold-standard labels, accurate estimation of EF has proven challenging. In this paper, we build on our previous work, and propose a highly accurate EF estimation method based on very large and diverse dataset, with the following key contributions: (1) our proposed approach can estimate four EF labels simultaneously, including single plane and bi-plane Simpson's measurements based on regression and visual assessment based on classification; (2) we model the observer variability and uncertainties in clinical measurements as a Gaussian distribution, whose parameters can be separately learned as independent variables in neural networks. We empirically show that uncertainty modelling in clinical measurements can improve the robustness of the EF estimation framework. Moreover, providing such critical computer-generated clinical measurements in terms of a distribution, rather than a single value, may help improve the interpretability and adoption of machine learning techniques by the clinicians.

2   Materials and Methods

2.1   Uncertainty Modelling

The inherent low quality of clinical images and variability in the ground truth labels leads to an inherent uncertainty, referred to as *aleatoric* uncertainty [6]. In learning-based approaches, this type of uncertainty cannot be resolved simply by acquiring more data and increasing the number of training samples. To model such uncertainty in a supervised learning framework, we define the clinical measurement as a random sample drawn from a distribution of *expert-annotated* labels. Formally, let $(\mathbf{x}_i, \mathbf{y}_i)$ denote the i-th datum, where $\mathbf{x}_i$ represents the input data used for deriving the measurement $\mathbf{y}_i$. We can define $\mathbf{y}_i$ as an observation made from the possible distribution $\mathbf{d}_i$; $\mathbf{y}_i \leftarrow \mathbf{d}_i$. In this paper, we characterize $\mathbf{d}_i$ as a normal distribution with the mean $\mu(\mathbf{x}_i)$ and standard deviation function $\sigma(\mathbf{x}_i)$. The parameters of the distribution $\mathbf{d}_i$ can be learned using a neural network with weights denoted by $\mathbf{W}_\mu$ and $\mathbf{W}_\sigma$. The observation distribution can then be expressed as $\mathbf{d}_i \sim \mathcal{N}\big(\mu(\mathbf{x}_i; \mathbf{W}_\mu), \sigma^2(\mathbf{x}_i; \mathbf{W}_\sigma)\big)$. For simplicity, let $\mathbf{W} = \mathbf{W}_\mu \cup \mathbf{W}_\sigma$. By modelling the observation as a Gaussian distribution, we can now use the Gaussian probability density function (PDF) to compute the likelihood of the expert distribution $\mathbf{d}_i$. The Gaussian PDF can hence be computed as:

$$p(\mathbf{d}_i | \mathbf{x}_i, \mathbf{W}) = \frac{1}{\sqrt{2\pi\sigma^2(\mathbf{x}_i)}} \exp\big(\frac{-||y_i - \mu(\mathbf{x}_i)||^2}{2\sigma^2(\mathbf{x}_i)}\big). \tag{1}$$

We can estimate $\mathbf{W}$ by optimizing the negative log-likelihood (NLL):

$$-\ln\big(p(\mathbf{d}_i | \mathbf{x}_i, \mathbf{W})\big) = \frac{1}{2}\big(\frac{||\mathbf{y}_i - \mu(\mathbf{x}_i)||^2}{\sigma^2(\mathbf{x}_i)} + \ln\sigma^2(\mathbf{x}_i)\big). \tag{2}$$

R^2	$EF^{A2C}_{Simpson's}$	$EF^{A4C}_{Simpson's}$	$EF^{Biplane}_{Simpson's}$	$EF^{Biplane}_{Visual}$
$EF^{A2C}_{Simpson's}$	1.00	0.58	0.88	0.79
$EF^{A4C}_{Simpson's}$	0.58	1.00	0.88	0.80
$EF^{Biplane}_{Simpson's}$	0.88	0.88	1.00	0.90
$EF^{Biplane}_{Visual}$	0.79	0.80	0.90	1.00

(a)

$EF^{Biplane}_{Simpson's}$ Class c^j	l_{c^j}	u_{c^j}	LV Function Diagnosis
1	0.0	0.20	Severe dysfunction
2	0.20	0.40	Moderate dysfunction
3	0.40	0.55	Mild Dysfunction
4	0.55	0.80	Normal Function

(b)

Fig. 2. A closer look at the EF dataset and labels. The variability and inherent aleatoric uncertainty in the four EF measurements is highlighted in (a) in terms of agreement between the four labels in terms of R^2 scores (as low as 0.58 for $EF^{A2C}_{Simpson's}$ and $EF^{A4C}_{Simpson's}$). A break-down of the categorical $EF^{Biplane}_{Visual}$ labels is provided in (b) (Color figure online).

For learning the discrete classification labels used in categorical grading of clinical measurements, we can extend the uncertainty modelling framework by computing the class likelihood from the Gaussian cumulative density function (CDF). The Gaussian CDF for z becomes:

$$\Phi(z) = \frac{1}{2}\left(1 + \mathrm{erf}\left(\frac{z - \mu(\mathbf{x}_i)}{\sigma(\mathbf{x}_i)\sqrt{2}}\right)\right), \tag{3}$$

where the error function is $\mathrm{erf}(z) = \frac{2}{\sqrt{\pi}} \int_0^z \exp(-t^2)dt$. The likelihood that a prediction $\hat{\mathbf{y}}_i$ is made from an expert-annotated class c^j can thus be computed, based on the class interval defined by $(l_{c^j}$ and $u_{c^j}]$ over the regression space:

$$p(c^j|\mathbf{x}_i, \mathbf{W}) = p(\hat{\mathbf{y}}_i \in (l_{c^j}, u_{c^j}]|\mathbf{x}_i, \mathbf{W}) = \Phi(u_{c^j}) - \Phi(l_{c^j}). \tag{4}$$

Model parameters $\mathbf{W}$ can be learned by minimizing a classification loss, *e.g.*, the categorical cross-entropy (CCE) loss ℓ_{CCE}.

2.2 EF Dataset

The dataset used for this study was obtained through Vancouver Coastal Health. It consists of echo cine series in various cardiac views (input data), as well as the diagnostic reports created by examining echocardiographers, which list several echo quantities including four EF-related measurements. Following the notation from the previous section, we define i-th datum $(\mathbf{x}_i, \mathbf{y}_i)$, where $\mathbf{x}_i$ represents the input echo cine series required for EF assessment (A2C and A4C) for the i-th exam. Similarly, $\mathbf{y}_i$ denotes the corresponding ground truth expert-annotated EF measurement, and $y_i \in [0, 1]$, since EF is expressed as a percentage:

$$(\mathbf{x}_i, \mathbf{y}_i) = \left(\{\mathbf{V}_i^{A2C}, \mathbf{V}_i^{A4C}\}, \{\mathbf{EF}^{A2C}_{i,Simpson's}, \mathbf{EF}^{A4C}_{i,Simpson's}, \mathbf{EF}^{Biplane}_{i,Simpson's}, \mathbf{EF}^{Biplane}_{i,Visual}\right).$$

The superscript and subscript represent the measurement method and the corresponding required views for measurement, respectively. Hence, $\mathbf{V}_i^v$ denotes the cine series captured in the view $v = \{A2C, A4C\}$, and consists of a stack of F gray-scale echo frames $I_{i,f}^v$ of height and width H × W for $f = 1 : F$. Biplane measurements correspond with both A2C and A4C cine series. The Simpson's labels were acquired by expert echocardiographers via segmentation of LV in the ED and ES frames. These are continuous (regression) labels within the range 0%–100%. $\mathbf{EF}_{\text{Visual}}^{\text{Biplane}}$ labels are categorical and were visually estimated directly from the cine series of A2C and A4C views, without any LV delineation, by expert clinicians. Figure 2(a) shows the coefficients of determination (R^2 scores) for the combinations of the four EF labels, and highlights the clinical aleatoric uncertainty in measuring EF in echo. A breakdown of the categorical EF labels is provided in Fig. 2(b) for the classification of $\mathbf{EF}_{\text{Visual}}^{\text{Biplane}}$. The interval $(\mathbf{l}_{c^j}, \mathbf{u}_{c^j}]$ is defined over the regression space for class $c^{j=1:4}$. Throughout this paper, the colors blue and red are used for inputs and outputs associated with A2C and A4C, respectively.

2.3   Network Architecture

An overview of the proposed model is depicted in Fig. 3.

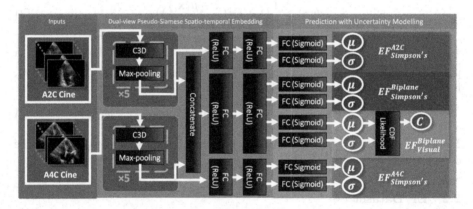

Fig. 3. The proposed architecture for dual-view cine-based joint estimation of four EF labels with uncertainty modelling, which characterizes each prediction as $\mathcal{N}(\mu, \sigma)$.

Spatio-Temporal Feature Embedding (STFE): In order to encode the cine loops, we first extract spatio-temporal features by applying 3D convolution (C3D) in the STFE block. C3D-based structures have proven promising for video analysis tasks [13], and despite being computationally expensive, are feasible for analyzing relatively short echo cine series, which capture a few heart beats. In this approach, the input video is represented as a stack of 2D video frames, creating a 3D tensor, consisting of two spatial and one temporal dimensions; H × W × F. The STFE block contains five $(3, 3, 3)$ C3D and $(2, 2, 2)$ max-pooling layers.

Label	R^2	*MAE*
$EF^{A2C}_{Simpson's}$	0.82	5.6%
$EF^{A4C}_{Simpson's}$	0.87	5.1%
$EF^{Biplane}_{Simpson's}$	0.90	4.5%

(a)

	Severe	Moderate	Mild	Normal
Normal	0	1	13	119
Mild	1	2	184	10
Moderate	0	75	2	3
Severe	16	2	2	0
$EF^{Biplane}_{Simpson's}$	Severe	Moderate	Mild	Normal

(b)

Fig. 4. (a) Quantitative test results ($N = 430$) for regression of $\mathbf{EF}^{A2C}_{Simpson's}$, $\mathbf{EF}^{A4C}_{Simpson's}$, $\mathbf{EF}^{Biplane}_{Simpson's}$, and (b) confusion matrix for classification of $\mathbf{EF}^{Biplane}_{Visual}$.

Pseudo-siamese Multi-tasking Structure: The network consists of two streams, designated for A2C and A4C cine series. A pseudo-siamese structure is utilized, in that, the streams have the similar architecture, but the parameters are not coupled. The spatio-temporal feature vectors obtained are merged after the STFE block through a concatenation layer. The outputs are the four aforementioned EF labels. $\mathbf{EF}^{A2C}_{Simpson's}$ and $\mathbf{EF}^{A4C}_{Simpson's}$ are linked to the input A2C and A4C cine series, respectively. The other two outputs $\mathbf{EF}^{Biplane}_{Visual}$ and $\mathbf{EF}^{Biplane}_{Simpson's}$ are linked to both A2C and A4C views as they involve biplane measurements. The model is trained by jointly minimizing the loss for the four EF labels:

$$\ell_{total} = \ell_{reg}\mathbf{EF}^{A2C}_{i,Simpson's} + \ell_{reg}\mathbf{EF}^{A4C}_{i,Simpson's} + \ell_{reg}\mathbf{EF}^{Biplane}_{i,Simpson's} + \ell_{CCE}\mathbf{EF}^{Biplane}_{i,Visual}. \quad (5)$$

3   Experiments and Results

Data Preparation: We obtained a dataset of size $N = 2,181$ patients consisting of clinical echo cine series $\mathbf{x}_i$ and the four corresponding ground truth expert-generated EF labels ($\mathbf{y}_i$ for $i = 1 : N$). The dataset is diverse, and includes patients with a wide range of EF (see Fig. 4(b)), and echo series acquired using machines manufactured by different vendors (mainly GE and Philips). No demographic restrictions were used for selecting the dataset. A2C and A4C cine loops were extracted using an echo view classifier [14]. Figure 2(a) shows the correlation of the four EF labels in terms of R^2 scores to highlight the variability in these clinical measurements.

Training: The proposed network as well as the uncertainty modelling layer were implemented in Keras with TensorFlow backend. We automatically cropped the images around the ultrasound beam and uniformly down-sampled the cine series to tensors of dimensions $H \times W \times F = 128 \times 128 \times 15$ on the fly, where the F frames were sampled uniformly from one full cardiac cycle in each video. The network

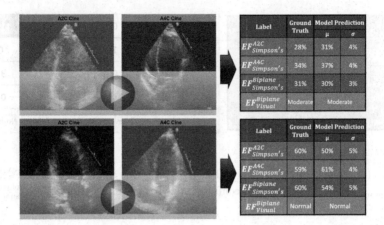

Fig. 5. Results on two test samples: the network inputs cine loops (videos on the left), expert-annotated ground labels, and the network's predictions, expressed in terms of (μ, σ) in the tables (see supplementary material). (To play the videos, open the PDF in Adobe Acrobat, Internet Explorer or other PDF viewers, enable Flash Player, and click on the snapshots.)

was hence trained end-to-end from scratch on an Nvidia Tesla GPU. Adaptive moment (Adam) optimization was used, with the learning rate of $\alpha = 1e^{-4}$, which was found experimentally. To account for the imbalanced distribution of samples, for each sample, we assigned weights inversely proportional to the frequency of the $\mathbf{EF}^{A2C}_{Simpson's}$ class to which they belonged. In order to prevent model over-fitting, heavy data augmentation was performed by applying random gamma intensity transformations, rotation, zoom and cropping, on the fly during training. Similarly, the starting point of the cine series were selected randomly during training to ensure the invariance of the visual assessment model with respect to cardiac phase. Regularization was applied on the weight decay.

Model Performance: A randomly drawn 20%-portion of the dataset was set aside as test data for evaluation of the proposed model. Quantitative results obtained are listed in Fig. 4(a) in terms of R^2 score and mean absolute error (MAE) for regression of the Simpson's labels. For the four-class classification, an accuracy of 91.4% was obtained. The confusion matrix obtained on the test set is shown in Fig. 4(b). Class confusion occurs mainly for adjacent classes. Figure 5 demonstrates a sample set of A2C and A4C videos, as well as the corresponding labels and prediction.

4   Discussion and Conclusion

In this paper, we introduced a dual-stream, multi-output network for joint estimation of regression and classification clinical EF labels in echo video data. We incorporated the uncertainties in the individual measurements by modelling the

EF measurements as a random variable drawn from a normal distribution, whose mean and standard deviation describe the predicted clinical measurement, and the aleatoric uncertainties, respectively. The advantages of the proposed uncertainty modelling are two-fold. From a technical standpoint, modelling the observation as a distribution $\mathcal{N}(\mu, \sigma)$ by decoupling μ and σ allows the model to better capture the inherent and inevitable variability in the observation, leading to better convergence in training, and subsequently, better model performance. From a clinical perspective, providing the clinician with computer-generated EF measurements, expressed in terms of $EF \pm \sigma$, is beneficial because it gives the user more context regarding the reliability of the model's predictions, and improves the interpretability of the machine learning solution, which can in turn, increase the clinicians' confidence in integrating the technology in their workflow.

Our proposed solution achieves accuracy superior to automatic cine-based literature [1], and comparable to semi-automatic segmentation-based works [5,10], with the key added advantage that it can estimate four EF parameters simultaneously while explicitly modelling the label uncertainty. We observed that the network performed better EF prediction in biplane compared to single-plane analysis. This is consistent with our previous findings [1] as well as the clinical literature [2]. In this paper, we focused on C3D neural networks for spatio-temporal feature learning as they have proven more successful for video analysis compared to architectures that relied on RNNs [1,10,13] for aggregating frame-level features and temporal embedding. We also found these architectures were notably easier to train compared to RNN-based ones. Furthermore, features acquired by purely convolutional layers can be visualized and interpreted more intuitively compared to networks that contain recurrent layers. Interpretability of unsupervised features computed by neural networks plays a key role in integration of automatic technologies. In conclusion, we demonstrated that robust visual segmentation-free volumetric assessment of EF is feasible with deep learning. Nevertheless, quality of the echo images still plays a crucial role in reliability of the proposed solution. Future work involves incorporating quality scores [14] as inputs to the EF measurement framework.

This work is supported in part by the Canadian Institutes of Health Research (CIHR) and in part by the Natural Sciences and Engineering Research Council of Canada (NSERC). The authors would like to acknowledge the support provided by Dale Hawley and the Vancouver Coastal Health in providing us with the anonymized, de-identified data.

References

1. Behnami, D., et al.: Automatic detection of patients with a high risk of systolic cardiac failure in echocardiography. In: Stoyanov, D., et al. (eds.) DLMIA/ML-CDS -2018. LNCS, vol. 11045, pp. 65–73. Springer, Cham (2018). https://doi.org/10.1007/978-3-030-00889-5_8
2. Foley, T.A., et al.: Measuring left ventricular ejection fraction-techniques and potential pitfalls. Eur. Cardiol. 8(2), 108–114 (2012)

3. Gu, B., Shan, Y., Sheng, V.S., et al.: Sparse regression with output correlation for cardiac ejection fraction estimation. Inf. Sci. **423**, 303–312 (2018)
4. Jafari, M.H., et al.: A unified framework integrating recurrent fully-convolutional networks and optical flow for segmentation of the left ventricle in echocardiography data. In: Stoyanov, D., et al. (eds.) DLMIA/ML-CDS -2018. LNCS, vol. 11045, pp. 29–37. Springer, Cham (2018). https://doi.org/10.1007/978-3-030-00889-5_4
5. Kabani, A.W., El-Sakka, M.R.: Ejection fraction estimation using a wide convolutional neural network. In: Karray, F., Campilho, A., Cheriet, F. (eds.) ICIAR 2017. LNCS, vol. 10317, pp. 87–96. Springer, Cham (2017). https://doi.org/10.1007/978-3-319-59876-5_11
6. Kendall, A., Gal, Y.: What uncertainties do we need in Bayesian deep learning for computer vision? In: NIPS, pp. 5574–5584 (2017)
7. Leclerc, S., Grenier, T., Espinosa, F., et al.: A fully automatic and multi-structural segmentation of the left ventricle and the myocardium on highly heterogeneous 2D echocardiographic data. In: 2017 IEEE International Ultrasonics Symposium (IUS), pp. 1–4. IEEE (2017)
8. Organization, W.H.: Global health observatory (GHO) data (2017). http://www.who.int/gho/mortality_burden_disease/causes_death/top_10/en/
9. Potter, E., Marwick, T.H.: Assessment of left ventricular function by echocardiography: the case for routinely adding global longitudinal strain to ejection fraction. JACC Cardiovasc. Imaging **11**(2), 260–274 (2018)
10. Silva, J.F., Silva, J.M., Guerra, A., et al.: Ejection fraction classification in transthoracic echocardiography using a deep learning approach. In: CBMS, pp. 123–128. IEEE (2018)
11. Smistad, E., Østvik, A., et al.: 2D left ventricle segmentation using deep learning. In: Ultrasonics, pp. 1–4. IEEE (2017)
12. Tan, L.K., Liew, Y.M., Lim, E., McLaughlin, R.A.: Cardiac left ventricle segmentation using convolutional neural network regression. In: 2016 IEEE EMBS Conference on Biomedical Engineering and Sciences (IECBES), pp. 490–493. IEEE (2016)
13. Tran, D., Wang, H., Torresani, L., et al.: A closer look at spatiotemporal convolutions for action recognition. In: CVPR, pp. 6450–6459 (2018)
14. Vaseli, H., et al.: Designing lightweight deep learning models for echocardiography view classification. In: Medical Imaging 2019: Image-Guided Procedures, Robotic Interventions, and Modeling, vol. 10951, p. 109510F. International Society for Optics and Photonics (2019)
15. Xue, W., Lum, A., Mercado, A., Landis, M., Warrington, J., Li, S.: Full quantification of left ventricle via deep multitask learning network respecting intra- and inter-task relatedness. In: Descoteaux, M., Maier-Hein, L., Franz, A., Jannin, P., Collins, D.L., Duchesne, S. (eds.) MICCAI 2017. LNCS, vol. 10435, pp. 276–284. Springer, Cham (2017). https://doi.org/10.1007/978-3-319-66179-7_32
16. Zhang, J., Gajjala, S., Agrawal, P., et al.: A web-deployed computer vision pipeline for automated determination of cardiac structure and function and detection of disease by two-dimensional echocardiography. arXiv:1706.07342 (2017)
17. Zhuang, X., et al.: Evaluation of algorithms for multi-modality whole heart segmentation: an open-access grand challenge. arXiv preprint. arXiv:1902.07880 (2019)

Frame Rate Up-Conversion in Echocardiography Using a Conditioned Variational Autoencoder and Generative Adversarial Model

Fatemeh Taheri Dezaki[1(✉)], Hany Girgis[2], Robert Rohling[1], Ken Gin[2], Purang Abolmaesumi[1], and Teresa Tsang[2]

[1] The University of British Columbia, Vancouver, BC, Canada
fatemeht@ece.ubc.ca
[2] Vancouver General Hospital's Cardiology Laboratory, Vancouver, BC, Canada

Abstract. Accurate detection of heart-related diseases in echocardiography (echo) often requires determining the performance of cardiac valves or contractile events such as strain at a high temporal resolution. In high-end cart-based imaging systems, this is achieved by increasing the frame rate using specialized beamforming and imaging hardware, or by limiting the imaging field of view (FOV). In point-of-care imaging, such a high frame rate imaging technology is currently unavailable. In this paper, we propose a new frame rate up-conversion technique, as a post-processing step during or after the echo acquisition. The proposed technique takes advantage of both variational autoencoders (VAE) and generative adversarial networks (GAN), and produces realistic frames at a high frame rate that can be used to augment conventional imaging. The proposed technique is robust to variations in heart rate since its latent space not only uses immediate previous frames, but it also takes into account the appearance of end-diastolic and end-systolic frames in its estimation. Our results show that the proposed technique can increase the frame rate by at least 5 times without any requirement for limiting the imaging FOV.

Keywords: Ultrasound imaging · Frame rate · Temporal resolution

1 Introduction

Echo imaging is based on the acoustic pulse-echo measurement: an ultrasound pulse is transmitted, and echo signals are subsequently received. Temporal Resolution (TR) is the ability to locate moving structures at anytime accurately and

---

F. T. Dezaki and H. Girgis—Joint first authors.
P. Abolmaesumi and T. Tsang—Joint senior authors.

Electronic supplementary material The online version of this chapter (https://doi.org/10.1007/978-3-030-32245-8_78) contains supplementary material, which is available to authorized users.

© Springer Nature Switzerland AG 2019
D. Shen et al. (Eds.): MICCAI 2019, LNCS 11765, pp. 705–713, 2019.
https://doi.org/10.1007/978-3-030-32245-8_78

is determined by imaging frame rate (FR). More images per second improve TR. In high-end cart-based imaging systems, the frame rate is increased by using specialized beamforming and imaging hardware, or by limiting the imaging field-of-view. In mobile point-of-care imaging, given cost, memory storage, and limitations in computation power and data transmission, full field-of-view high frame rate imaging technology is currently unavailable.

Traditional 2-dimensional (2D) echo imaging is on the basis of a TR of less than 100 Hz. Although these frame rates are adequate to assess cardiac morphology and certain functional aspects, they do not allow the resolution of all mechanical events, as some of them are very short-lived [1]. High frame rates enable us to see rapidly moving structures (such as valves) without motion artifacts and also perform velocity and deformation analysis (*i.e.*, tissue Doppler).

There are two sets of approaches to increase the frame rate in echocardiography. The first one is based on acquisition schemes, while the second one is based on post-processing techniques.

In the first sets of approaches, several technical advances in cardiac ultrasound allow data to be acquired at a very high frame rate. The main drawback of such high frame rate data acquisition is that it typically has resulted in image quality degradation [1], and increased hardware complexity [2]. Retrospective gating [3], plane wave/diverging wave imaging [4], and multi-line transmit systems [5] are among the methods in ultrafast imaging. In point-of-care imaging, such a high frame rate imaging technology is currently unavailable. In the second sets of approaches, various post-processing methods have been developed to avoid the computational costs and complex hardware requirements associated with acquisition schemes. The imaging process remains the same as traditional echo imaging with standard clinical echocardiography equipment, and the frame rate up-conversion (FRUC) is done in the processing time. FRUC is a technique that increases the frame rate of the video by inserting newly generated frames into the original sequence.

Several FRUC algorithms have been proposed that use motion estimation and dictionary learning [2,6,7]. Deep learning has been also used for future frame prediction in computer vision [8,9]. The most recent methods use variational auto-encoders to reduce image reconstruction artifacts [10] and adversarial loss [11] to obtain more realistic results.

In this paper, we propose the first deep-learning-based solution for frame rate up-conversion in echocardiography that can be used to augment conventional imaging without the need of specialized beamforming and imaging hardware, or limiting the imaging field of view. It should be noted that our design is robust to variations in heart rate. The proposed technique takes advantage of both variational autoencoders (VAE) and generative adversarial networks (GAN), and conditions the latent space of the VAE through taking into account not only the immediate previous frames but also the appearance of end-diastolic and end-systolic frames. Using data from 3,112 patient studies, we demonstrate that the proposed technique can increase the frame rate by 5 times without compromising the imaging FOV, and generate realistic images that are visually indistinguishable from clinically acquired echo data.

2   Methods

We start by explaining how our model generates new echo cine frames, before detailing the training procedure. The future frame $\hat{x}_t$ is synthesized based on a latent variable z_{t-1} and the previous frame $\hat{x}_{t-1}$. This process is shown in the red box in Fig. 1. The latent variable z_{t-1} is sampled from a prior distribution $p(z_{t-1})$ that is learned during the training procedure. The previous frame $\hat{x}_{t-1}$ can be either a ground-truth frame (for the initial frames) or the last predicted frame. The recurrent generator network G predicts sequence of future frames $\hat{x}_{1:T}$ using convolutional Long Short Term Memory (LSTM) [12]. As shown in Fig. 2, predicted pixel-space transformations between current frame and its next frame are convolved with the input image to generate the next frame. The training procedure is illustrated in the black box in Fig. 1, and discussed in detail in the following sections.

2.1   Variational Autoencoders

To address the challenge of mapping from a high-dimensional input to a high-dimensional output distribution, learning a low-dimensional latent code to represent aspects of the possible outputs not contained in the input image is of great help. Intuitively, the latent codes encapsulate any ambiguous or stochastic events that might affect the future. The predictions are conditioned on a set of c context frames, $x_{t-c}, ..., x_{t-1}$ ($c = 1$ for conditioning on one frame). Our goal is to sample from $p(x_t|x_{t-c:t-1}, z_{t-c:t-1})$, which is intractable as it involves marginalizing over the latent variables. We instead maximize the variational lower bound as in the variational autoencoder [13]. To encode any transitional information between consecutive frames, the encoder E is conditioned on x_{t-1} and x_t. Moreover, to encode the volume changes of the cardiac chambers during a cycle, the encoder is conditioned on end diastolic (ED) and end systolic (ES) frames. This is a conditional version of variational autoencoder, which embed ground truth frames in the latent code z_{t-1}. During training, the latent code is sampled from a Gaussian distribution $\mathcal{N}(\mu_{z_{t-1}}, \sigma^2_{z_{t-1}})$ using a reparameterization approach [13]. The reconstruction loss is as follows:

$$\mathcal{L}_R(G, E) = \mathbb{E}_{x_{0:T},\, z_t \sim E(x_{t-1}, x_t, x_{ED}, x_{ES})|_{t=0}^{t=T-1}} \left[\sum_{t=1}^{T} ||x_t - G(x_0, z_{0:t-1})||_1 \right]. \quad (1)$$

A regularization term encourages the approximate posterior to be close to the prior distribution:

$$\mathcal{L}_{KL}(E) = \mathbb{E}_{x_{0:T}} \left[\sum_{t=1}^{T} \mathcal{D}_{KL}\big(E(x_{t-1}, x_t, x_{ED}, x_{ES})||p(z_{t-1})\big) \right]. \quad (2)$$

2.2   Generative Adversarial Networks

We can enforce our model to generate sharper and more realistic frames with the help of GANs. Given a discriminator network D that is trained to distinguish

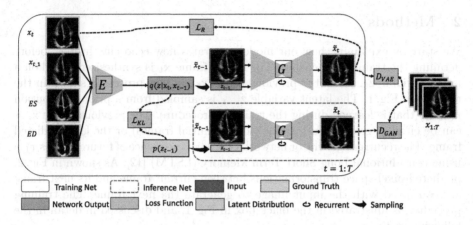

Fig. 1. Frame rate up-conversion network.

between generated videos $\hat{x}_{1:T}$ from real videos $x_{1:T}$, the generator can be trained to match the distribution of real echo cines using the binary cross-entropy loss:

$$\mathcal{L}_{GAN}(G, D) = \mathbb{E}_{\mathbf{x}_{1:T}} \left[log D(\mathbf{x}_{0:T-1}) \right] + \mathbb{E}_{\mathbf{x}_{1:T}, \ \mathbf{z}_t \sim p(\mathbf{z}_t)|_{t=0}^{T-1}} [log(1 - D(G(\mathbf{x}_0, \mathbf{z}_{0:T-1})))]. \tag{3}$$

2.3 Complementary Effect of VAE and GAN

GAN models are capable of generating natural videos under the guidance of learned discriminator networks. However, GANs suffer from the mode collapse [14], which can lead to the generator producing limited varieties of samples, by finding the most realistic image from the discriminator perspective. In other words, $\hat{x}$ will be independent of $\mathbf{z}$. On the other hand, VAEs encourage latent variables to be meaningful so that they can make accurate predictions at training time. However, latent variables used in VAEs are the encoding of the ground truth images, unlike GANs which are trained with completely random variables. Moreover, the discriminator D does not see results sampled from the prior during training. To combine both approaches (Shown in Fig. 1), another discriminator network D_{VAE} can be introduced to improve the performance of the generator [11]. Note that the same generator network with shared weights is used at every time step. The latent variables in this approach are sampled from the VAE's latent distribution $q(\mathbf{z}_t | \mathbf{x}_t, \mathbf{x}_{t-1})$:

$$\mathcal{L}_{GAN}^{VAE}(G, D_{VAE}) = \mathbb{E}_{\mathbf{x}_{1:T}} \left[log D_{VAE}(\mathbf{x}_{0:T-1}) \right]$$
$$+ \mathbb{E}_{\mathbf{x}_{1:T}, \ \mathbf{z}_t \sim q(\mathbf{z}_t | \mathbf{x}_t, \mathbf{x}_{t-1}, \mathbf{x}_{ED}, \mathbf{x}_{ES})} [log(1 - D_{VAE}(G(\mathbf{x}_0, \mathbf{z}_{0:T-1})))]. \tag{4}$$

Therefore, the final objective of the echo cine series prediction is:

$$G^*, E^* = \arg \max_{G, E} \max_{D, D_{VAE}} \lambda_R \mathcal{L}_R(G, E) + \lambda_{KL} \mathcal{L}_{KL}(E) + \mathcal{L}_{GAN}(G, D)$$
$$+ \mathcal{L}_{GAN}^{VAE}(G, E, D_{VAE}), \tag{5}$$

where λ_R and λ_{KL} control the relative importance of each term.

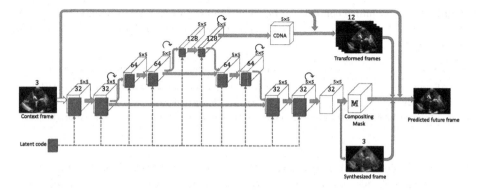

Fig. 2. The detailed generator network.

2.4   Network Architecture

Figure 2 depicts our generator network G. The network is inspired from the architecture proposed by [8], *i.e.*, convolutional dynamic neural advection (CDNA). The sequence of future frames is predicted by feeding the latent variable z_{t-1} and the previous frame $\hat{x}_{t-1}$ (either the ground truth or the previous prediction frame). Latent codes are concatenated along the channel dimension of all the convolutional layers of the network. Each convolutional layer is followed by instance normalization [15] and rectified linear (ReLU) activations [16]. Convolutional LSTMs are used to model motion. For each time step prediction, the network predicts four convolutional kernels to produce a set of transformed frames. The network also predicts a synthesized frame and a compositing mask by passing the final layer output through two convolutional layers with sigmoid and softmax activation functions, respectively. Finally, these sets of transformed frames along with the synthesized and previous frames are merged by the mask.

The encoder E is a standard convolutional network except that the two input images and ED and ES frames are concatenated along the channel dimension. The architecture is the same as the one used in [14]. As for the architecture of the discriminator, we used a 3D convolutional neural network using all the T frames. Both the discriminators, D and D_{VAE}, have the same architecture with separate weights. The architecture is inspired from the one used in [14] except that the 2D convolution filters are inflated to 3D ones.

3   Experiments and Results

We carried out experiments on a set of 2D apical 4 chambers (AP4) cine series collected from the Picture Archiving and Communication System at Vancouver General Hospital, with ethics approval of the Clinical Medical Research Ethics Board, in consultation with the Information Privacy Office. Data set consists of 3,112 individual patient studies. Experiments were run by randomly dividing these cases into mutually exclusive patients, such that 75% of the cases

Table 1. Performance comparison between the proposed, VAE-only and VAE+GAN techniques. The results show that the proposed method performs the best since it provides the lowest LPIPS and the highest SSIM.

Method	LPIPS ($\downarrow$)	MSE ($\downarrow$)	PSNR ($\uparrow$)	SSIM ($\uparrow$)
VAE-only [10]	0.266 (0.044)	**0.006 (0.002)**	**22.67 (1.20)**	0.65 (0.043)
VAE+GAN	0.115 (0.016)	0.009 (0.002)	20.67 (1.08)	0.66 (0.045)
Conditioned VAE+GAN (proposed)	**0.096 (0.016)**	0.007 (0.002)	21.65 (1.36)	**0.68 (0.053)**

were available for training and validation, and 25% for test. These clinical echo cine series included various heart rates (*i.e.*, from 47 to 104 beats per minute). Location of the ES and ED frames in a cardiac cycle is recorded by an expert sonographer. Each cine is temporally down-sampled by a factor of 5, and the model is trained to reconstruct the original cine series.

Evaluating the performance of video prediction is a common challenge. The standard quantitative metrics are mean-squared error (MSE), peak signal-to-noise ratio (PSNR) and structural similarity (SSIM). Although these standard metrics provide a way to benchmark the proposed method against its counterparts, often, they do not correlate properly with the human preference [17]. Therefore, we also use the learned perceptual image distance metric (LPIPS) [17] to evaluate our method. The LPIPS is calculated by $\mathcal{L}_2$ distance between deep features of images. Deep features are extracted by employing pre-trained AlexNet.

Table 1 benchmarks the performance of the proposed method against the VAE-only and VAE+GAN techniques. First, we compared the performance of the three methods, including the proposed method by considering the MSE and PSNR metrics. As reported in Table 1, the VAE-only technique achieves the lowest MSE and highest PSNR. Although this result may imply that the VAE-only technique performs better than others, it produces blurry and unrealistic images. A sample result is shown in Fig. 3. This means that the MSE and PSNR metrics are not good candidates in this application. The reason that the MSE and PSNR of the proposed and VAE+GAN techniques are larger than those of the VAE-only is that the GAN gives priority to matching joint distributions of pixels, but not the per-pixel similarity. Our experiments have shown that the LPIPS corresponds better to human preferences and it is also discussed in [17]. Therefore, to fairly compare the proposed technique against its counterparts, the LPIPS and SSIM metrics must be taken into consideration. As shown in the table, the proposed technique provides the lowest LPIPS and the highest SSIM. This means that it outperforms the VAE-only and VAE+GAN techniques.

Figure 4 shows a more detailed comparison between the proposed and VAE+GAN techniques. In this figure, the average LPIPS, MSE, PSNR and SSIM metrics are plotted against the time step. As illustrated, all four metrics are improved when the proposed technique is employed. This happens since the proposed technique conditions the latent space of the VAE through the use of the appearance of ED and ES frames. Apart from what technique is used to

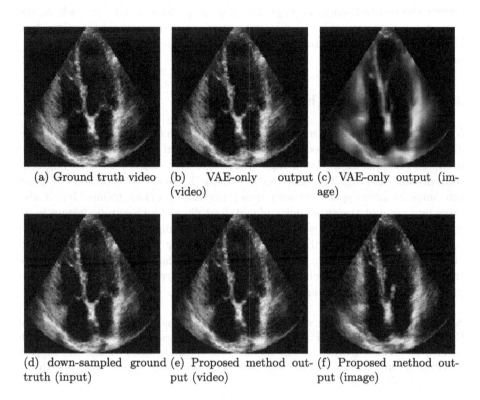

(a) Ground truth video   (b)   VAE-only   output (c) VAE-only output (im-
                            (video)   age)

(d) down-sampled ground (e) Proposed method out- (f) Proposed method out-
truth (input)   put (video)   put (image)

Fig. 3. Qualitative visualization: the prediction of our proposed model in comparison
with the VAE-only model. The VAE-only model generates blurry and unrealistic images
(video clip 3b and Fig. 3c). In contrast, the proposed method generates images that
are visually indistinguishable from real images (video clip 3e and Fig. 3f). Click the
image to play the video clip (see supplementary material).

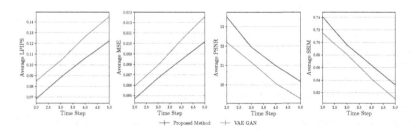

Fig. 4. Detailed comparison between the proposed and VAE+GAN techniques. From
the LPIPS, MSE, PSNR and SSIM point of views, the proposed technique exceeds its
counterpart.

predict the future frames, we expect to see the performance to degrade as the time step is increased. This phenomenon applies to the proposed technique too; however, the rate of performance degradation is slower compared to that of its counterpart.

4   Conclusion and Future Works

In this paper, we proposed a new frame rate up-conversion technique for echocardiography. The proposed technique takes advantage of both VAE and GAN, and produces realistic frames at a high frame rate that can be used to augment conventional imaging. The proposed technique is robust to variations in heart rate since its latent space not only uses immediate previous frames, but it also takes into account the appearance of end-diastolic and end-systolic frames in its estimation. Our results show that the proposed technique can increase the frame rate by at least 5 times without any requirement for limiting the imaging field of view. Our comparison to state-of-the-art using a large patient dataset shows that the proposed approach can reconstruct rapid events in echo, such as the motion of valves, at high temporal resolution.

Acknowledgements. This work is supported in part by the Canadian Institutes of Health Research (CIHR) and in part by the Natural Sciences and Engineering Research Council of Canada (NSERC). The authors would like to acknowledge the support provided by Dale Hawley and the Vancouver Coastal Health in providing us with the anonymized, deidentified data.

References

1. Cikes, M., Tong, L., et al.: Ultrafast cardiac ultrasound imaging: technical principles, applications, and clinical benefits. JACC Cardiovasc. Imaging **7**(8), 812–823 (2014)
2. Gifani, P., Behnam, H., et al.: Temporal super resolution enhancement of echocardiographic images based on sparse representation. IEEE Trans. Ultrason. Ferroelectr. Freq. Control **63**(1), 6–19 (2016)
3. Provost, J., Lee, W.N., et al.: Electromechanical wave imaging of normal and ischemic hearts in vivo. IEEE Trans. Med. Imaging **29**(3), 625–635 (2010)
4. Papadacci, C., Pernot, M., et al.: High-contrast ultrafast imaging of the heart. IEEE Trans. Ultrason. Ferroelectr. Freq. Control. **61**(2), 288–301 (2014)
5. Tong, L., Ramalli, A., et al.: Multi-transmit beam forming for fast cardiac imaging–experimental validation and in vivo application. IEEE Trans. Med. Imaging **33**(6), 1205–1219 (2014)
6. Contijoch, F., Fernandez-de Manuel, L., et al.: Increasing temporal resolution of 3D transesophageal ultrasound by rigid body registration of sequential, temporally offset sequences. In: 2010 IEEE International Symposium on Biomedical Imaging: From Nano to Macro, pp. 328–331. IEEE (2010)
7. Perrin, D.P., Vasilyev, N.V., et al.: Temporal enhancement of 3D echocardiography by frame reordering. JACC Cardiovasc. Imaging **5**(3), 300–304 (2012)

8. Srivastava, N., Mansimov, E., Salakhudinov, R.: Unsupervised learning of video representations using LSTMS. In: International Conference on Machine Learning, pp. 843–852 (2015)
9. Finn, C., Goodfellow, I., Levine, S.: Unsupervised learning for physical interaction through video prediction. In: NIPS, pp. 64–72 (2016)
10. Babaeizadeh, M., Finn, C., et al.: Stochastic variational video prediction. arXiv preprint. arXiv:1710.11252 (2017)
11. Lee, A.X., Zhang, R., Ebert, F., Abbeel, P., Finn, C., Levine, S.: Stochastic adversarial video prediction. arXiv preprint. arXiv:1804.01523 (2018)
12. Xingjian, S., Chen, Z., et al.: Convolutional LSTM network: a machine learning approach for precipitation nowcasting. In: NIPS, pp. 802–810 (2015)
13. Kingma, D.P., Welling, M.: Auto-encoding variational bayes. arXiv preprint. arXiv:1312.6114 (2013)
14. Zhu, J.Y., Zhang, R., et al.: Toward multimodal image-to-image translation. In: NIPS, pp. 465–476 (2017)
15. Ulyanov, D., Vedaldi, A., Lempitsky, V.: Instance normalization: the missing ingredient for fast stylization. arXiv preprint. arXiv:1607.08022 (2016)
16. Nair, V., Hinton, G.E.: Rectified linear units improve restricted Boltzmann machines. In: ICML, pp. 807–814 (2010)
17. Zhang, R., Isola, P., et al.: The unreasonable effectiveness of deep features as a perceptual metric. In: CVPR, pp. 586–595 (2018)

Annotation-Free Cardiac Vessel Segmentation via Knowledge Transfer from Retinal Images

Fei Yu[1], Jie Zhao[2], Yanjun Gong[3], Zhi Wang[3], Yuxi Li[3], Fan Yang[3],
Bin Dong[1,2,4], Quanzheng Li[2,5], and Li Zhang[1,2(✉)]

[1] Center for Data Science, Peking University, Beijing 100871, China
zhangli_pku@pku.edu.cn
[2] Center for Data Science in Health and Medicine, Peking University,
Beijing 100871, China
[3] Department of Cardiology, Peking University First Hospital, Beijing 100034, China
[4] Beijing International Center for Mathematical Research (BICMR),
Peking University, Beijing 100871, China
[5] MGH/BWH Center for Clinical Data Science, Boston, MA 02115, USA

Abstract. Segmenting coronary arteries is challenging, as classic unsupervised methods fail to produce satisfactory results and modern supervised learning (deep learning) requires manual annotation which is often time-consuming and can some time be infeasible. To solve this problem, we propose a knowledge transfer based shape-consistent generative adversarial network (SC-GAN), which is an annotation-free approach that uses the knowledge from publicly available annotated fundus dataset to segment coronary arteries. The proposed network is trained in an end-to-end fashion, generating and segmenting synthetic images that maintain the background of coronary angiography and preserve the vascular structures of retinal vessels and coronary arteries. We train and evaluate the proposed model on a dataset of 1092 digital subtraction angiography images, and experiments demonstrate the supreme accuracy of the proposed method on coronary arteries segmentation.

Keywords: Coronary artery segmentation · Knowledge transfer · Generative adversarial network · Deep learning

1 Introduction

Quantitative measurement of coronary arteries in medical images is important for the diagnosis, prevention and therapeutic evaluation of related diseases including hypertension, myocardial infarction, and coronary atherosclerotic disease. In the diagnosis of coronary diseases, digital subtraction angiography (DSA) has been widely used and considered the "gold standard". To quantitatively segment blood vessels in DSA, researchers have developed automated methods including region growing, level sets, and Hessian analysis [1,11].

However, due to the complexity of the vascular morphology, these unsupervised methods are difficult to obtain a clinically satisfactory segmentation of coronary arteries. On the other hand, supervised learning such as deep neural networks (DNNs) can produce better segmentation results but relies heavily on pixel-level image annotation, which is often expensive, time-consuming, and even impossible to access especially for coronary artery segmentation.

To solve the problem of the lack of DSA vessel annotation, we aim to apply a strategy to transfer the knowledge of retinal vessel segmentation to the coronary artery segmentation. The researchers have established and validated a number of public retinal vessel segmentation datasets, including DRIVE [12], STARE [4], and RITE [5]. Due to the significant differences between their anatomical regions, traditional transfer methods are not suitable. Therefore, we present a novel knowledge transfer based adversarial model containing three parts called generator, discriminator, and segmentor. Training of the model contains three major steps: (1) Frangi vessel analysis [2] is used to segment the coronary artery in the DSA images roughly. (2) The adversarial training between generator and discriminator allows the model to fuse the fundus image and the DSA image. (3) A synthetic label is then created by computing the union of rough coronary artery segmentation and retinal vessel annotation. Moreover, a shape-consistent scheme is used to ensure the shape consistency of synthetic images and synthetic annotations. The fused image and corresponding synthetic label are used to train the segmentor. The supreme accuracy demonstrates the effectiveness of our methods, which improves the accuracy of coronary artery segmentation by using the knowledge of fundus segmentation without additional manual annotation of the DSA images. The ideas of knowledge transfer and data fusion in this paper have many other application scenarios, including cell segmentation, neural segmentation, and airway segmentation. As long as the object structures in the two datasets are similar, we can use the knowledge from the annotated dataset to guide the analysis of the unannotated one.

Our work relates closely to the recent rise of knowledge transfer techniques. In the field of natural image analysis, Domain-Adversarial Neural Network (DANN) transfers the feature distribution to solve the domain-shift problem [3]. Cycle-GAN introduces a cycle consistency loss and achieves unpaired image-to-image translation [17]. AdaptSegNet adopts adversarial learning in the output space and receives favorably accuracy and visual quality [13]. In the field of medical image analysis, many studies have been dedicated to exploring cross-modality translation with GAN [10]. Using synthetic data to overcome insufficient labeled data is also an active research area. For example, using synthetic data as augmented training data can help lesion segmentation [7] and cardiovascular volumes segmentation [16]. These methods show that knowledge transfer is effective for the same anatomical region, and our work contributes by accomplishing knowledge transfer between two different anatomical regions.

2   Methods

In this section, we show two models based on knowledge transfer. The first one is the GAN model with a constraint of shape consistency (SC-GAN) proposed in this work. Then, to verify the necessity of fusion, we show another simpler model. It adopts from Mixup [15], which is to train the U-Net model by computing an average of the fundus image and the DSA image (Add U-Net).

2.1   SC-GAN

Figure 1 shows the training and test processes of the proposed model. During the training process, the generator, discriminator, and segmentor are trained simultaneously. In the test process, only the trained segmentor is needed to segment coronary arteries, which requires much less memory and inference time than training. In the previously reported knowledge transfer between different modalities within the same anatomy, the foreground and the background can be reasonably registered. In our task, however, the foreground and background of the images are completely mismatched. So we have designed a shape-consistent scheme that allows the generator and discriminator to complete the knowledge transfer of foreground and background respectively. In the following subsections, we will discuss the model's architectures and the objective functions in detail.

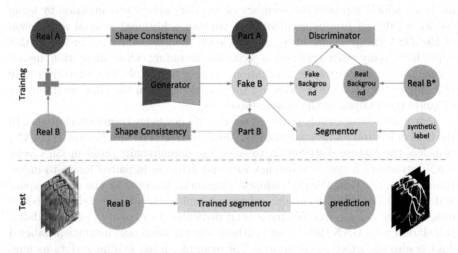

Fig. 1. The illustration of the proposed SC-GAN, an end-to-end approach for coronary artery segmentation requiring no new manual annotations.

Generator: As shown in Fig. 1, the generator uses U-Net as its network backbone. The input of the generator is an average of the fundus image (Real A) and the DSA image (Real B). The output is a synthetic image (Fake B) with the same dimensions as the input. To ensure that the Fake B has both retinal vessels and coronary arteries, we extract the two vascular regions (Part A and Part B) in Fake B using manual annotation of retinal vessels and Frangi segmentation of DSA images. A shape-consistent loss ($l1$ loss) is then used to regularize the content of the vessel regions in Fake B to be consistent with the corresponding regions in the original images,

$$\mathcal{L}_{shape_A}(G) = \mathbb{E}_{A \sim p_{data}(A), B \sim p_{data}(B)}[|||label_A * (G(A+B) - A)||_1] \quad (1)$$

$$\mathcal{L}_{shape_B}(G) = \mathbb{E}_{A \sim p_{data}(A), B \sim p_{data}(B)}[|||label_B * (G(A+B) - B)||_1] \quad (2)$$

where A represents the fundus image, B represents the DSA image, and $label_A$ and $label_B$ are the retinal vessel annotation and the Frangi segmentation results, respectively.

Discriminator: We expect that the background of Fake B is sufficiently similar to the background of a DSA image, so we first use the annotations and Frangi analysis results to mask out the vascular regions and extract the background in the generated and real DSA images,

$$Fake_{bg} = \neg(label_A \cup label_B) * G(A+B) \quad (3)$$

$$Real_{bg} = \neg(label_A \cup label_B) * B^* \quad (4)$$

where B^* (Real B^* in Fig. 1) represents a randomly chosen DSA image before the injection of the contrast medium, which guarantees a vessel-free background. For the structure of the discriminator, we adopt PatchGAN [17]. The adversarial loss between the generator and the discriminator can be expressed as,

$$\mathcal{L}_{GAN}(G, D) = \mathbb{E}_{B^* \sim p_{data}(B^*)}[logD(Real_{bg})]$$
$$+ \mathbb{E}_{A \sim p_{data}(A), B \sim p_{data}(B)}[log(1 - D(Fake_{bg}))] \quad (5)$$

Segmentor: The main structure of the segmentor is also a U-Net. We use MultiLabelSoftMarginLoss [9] as the objective function of the segmentor:

$$\mathcal{L}_{seg}(S) = -(y(i)log[\frac{exp(\hat{y}(i))}{1 + exp(\hat{y}(i))}] + (1 - y(i))log[\frac{1}{1 + exp(\hat{y}(i))}]) \quad (6)$$

where $\hat{y}$ is the prediction and y the synthetic label.

Therefore, the final objective function of our proposed model is,

$$\mathcal{L}(G, D, S) = \mathcal{L}_{GAN}(G, D) + \mathcal{L}_{seg}(S) + \lambda\mathcal{L}_{shape_A}(G) + \mu\mathcal{L}_{shape_B}(G) \quad (7)$$

where λ and μ control the relative importance of the objectives. During training, we set $\lambda = 100, \mu = 50$.

The model uses instance normalization [14] instead of batch normalization [6], the generator uses ReLU and the discriminator uses LeakyReLU as activations.

2.2 Add U-Net

Figure 2 shows the overall structure of Add U-Net. Referring to Mixup, the model takes the average of the fundus image (Real A) and the DSA image (Real B). The manual annotation of retinal vessels and the Frangi analysis results of the DSA image are combined to obtain the label of the added image. We then train a U-Net with such added images and annotations. An independent DSA dataset is used to evaluate the trained U-Net.

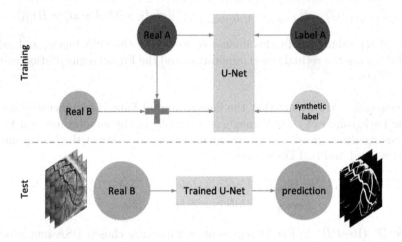

Fig. 2. The illustration of Add U-Net, where the input is an average of fundus photography and DSA image.

3   Experiments

In this section, to evaluate the effectiveness of our proposed SC-GAN, we compare the segmentation of four methods: **(1) Frangi Algorithm.** Multi-scale Frangi vessel analysis is used to segment coronary arteries. **(2) Classic U-Net.** A U-Net model is trained using Frangi Algorithm results as the learning targets. **(3) Add U-Net.** A U-Net model is trained using an average of fundus photographies and DSA images. **(4) SC-GAN.** The proposed shape-consistent GAN. We also compare the synthetic results of SC-GAN and Cycle-GAN [17]. The data and experiment details are presented below.

Data: We use the DRIVE [12] dataset as the source domain of knowledge transfer. The DRIVE dataset includes 40 fundus images with manually annotated retinal vessels. We also collect 1092 coronary angiographies (DSA) with no annotations as the target domain of knowledge transfer. Several preprocessing approaches are performed on the fundus images, including color to grayscale transform, median-filtering and contrast-limited adaptive histogram equalization [18]. Finally, we resize all images into the same size of 512×512 and randomly choose 256×256 patches as inputs of the models.

Experiment Details: In all experiments, 50% of DSA images are randomly selected as training set, 20% are validation set and 30% are test set. Meanwhile, we use the Adam solver [8] with a learning rate of 2e−4. After training for 50 epochs, we decrease the learning rate linearly for 50 epochs till 0.

4 Results

In this section, we briefly report the evaluation results in two aspects: (1) Images synthesis and (2) Images segmentation.

Images Synthesis: Figure 3 shows some examples of the fundus, DSA, and synthetic image patches. Compared to the results of Cycle-GAN [17], the synthetic images from our proposed SC-GAN have more realistic DSA background and also preserve the vascular structures corresponding to the labels (see the columns (c) and (d) in Fig. 3).

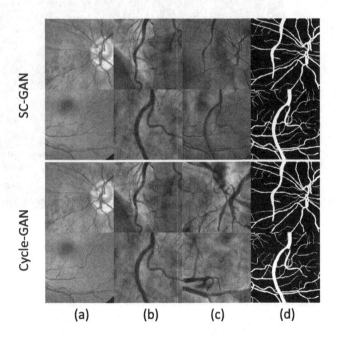

Fig. 3. Comparison of SC-GAN and Cycle-GAN. (a) Fundus patches, (b) DSA patches, (c) synthetic images, (d) synthetic labels.

Images Segmentation: We annotate 30% of the DSA dataset (328 out of 1092 images) and evaluate our proposed model on it. Table 1 compares the performance of different methods. As the baseline method of this article, the Frangi algorithm has a Dice score of 0.636 ± 0.046. If the result of the Frangi algorithm is used as an annotation to train a U-Net (Classic U-Net), the Dice score reduces to 0.589 ± 0.049. Both Add U-Net and SC-GAN have higher Dice scores (0.742 ± 0.048 and 0.824 ± 0.026). And SC-GAN also outperforms the other methods in terms of accuracy and recall. Figure 4 shows some typical examples in the test set. Columns (d–e) show better results than columns (b–c), indicating that knowledge transfer effectively enhances the identification of small blood vessels. By comparing the results of Add U-Net and SC-GAN, we can also find that GAN is better than an average in terms of the quality of knowledge transfer.

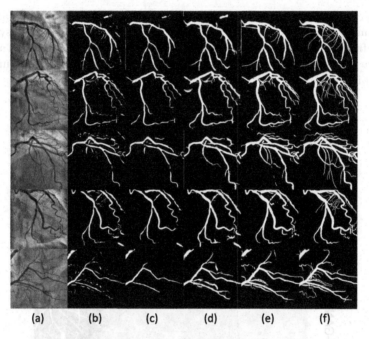

Fig. 4. Examples of different vessel segmentation methods. (a) Original images, (b) Frangi algorithm, (c) Classic U-Net, (d) Add U-Net, (e) Proposed SC-GAN, (f) Ground truth.

Table 1. Quantitative performance of different vessel segmentation methods.

Methods	Frangi Algorithm	Classic U-Net	Add U-Net	**Proposed**
Accuracy	0.927 ± 0.014	0.921 ± 0.015	0.940 ± 0.012	$\mathbf{0.953 \pm 0.009}$
Precision	0.943 ± 0.057	$\mathbf{0.975 \pm 0.052}$	0.864 ± 0.078	0.820 ± 0.031
Recall	0.481 ± 0.048	0.423 ± 0.047	0.653 ± 0.050	$\mathbf{0.829 \pm 0.039}$
Dice Coefficient	0.636 ± 0.046	0.589 ± 0.049	0.742 ± 0.048	$\mathbf{0.824 \pm 0.026}$

5   Discussion

In this paper, we proposed a shape-consistent GAN model (SC-GAN) for coronary artery segmentation, which was able to transfer the knowledge of the segmentation on public fundus dataset to an unlabeled DSA dataset. Experimental results demonstrated that SC-GAN obtained an obvious superior performance on coronary arteries segmentation. Despite the promising results, our method has several limitations and requires further investigation: 1. How well does the method perform on other datasets; 2. Although the segmentor is light-weighted in test, training SC-GAN is much more complex than in a classic supervised deep model. In future work, we will further test the proposed SC-GAN on other application scenarios and simplify the training process.

Acknowledgments. This work was supported by National Key R&D Program of China (No. 2018YFC0910700); The National Natural Science Foundation of China (NSFC) under Grants 81801778, 11831002; Beijing Natural Science Foundation (Z180001).

References

1. Adams, R., Bischof, L.: Seeded region growing. IEEE Trans. Pattern Anal. Mach. Intell. **16**(6), 641–647 (1994)
2. Frangi, A.F., Niessen, W.J., Vincken, K.L., Viergever, M.A.: Multiscale vessel enhancement filtering. In: Wells, W.M., Colchester, A., Delp, S. (eds.) MICCAI 1998. LNCS, vol. 1496, pp. 130–137. Springer, Heidelberg (1998). https://doi.org/10.1007/BFb0056195
3. Ganin, Y., et al.: Domain-adversarial training of neural networks. J. Mach. Learn. Res. **17**(1), 2030–2096 (2016)
4. Hoover, A., Goldbaum, M.: Locating the optic nerve in a retinal image using the fuzzy convergence of the blood vessels. IEEE Trans. Med. Imaging **22**(8), 951–958 (2003)
5. Hu, Q., Abràmoff, M.D., Garvin, M.K.: Automated separation of binary overlapping trees in low-contrast color retinal images. In: Mori, K., Sakuma, I., Sato, Y., Barillot, C., Navab, N. (eds.) MICCAI 2013. LNCS, vol. 8150, pp. 436–443. Springer, Heidelberg (2013). https://doi.org/10.1007/978-3-642-40763-5_54
6. Ioffe, S., Szegedy, C.: Batch normalization: accelerating deep network training by reducing internal covariate shift. In: International Conference on Machine Learning, pp. 448–456 (2015)
7. Kamnitsas, K., et al.: Unsupervised domain adaptation in brain lesion segmentation with adversarial networks. In: Niethammer, M., et al. (eds.) IPMI 2017. LNCS, vol. 10265, pp. 597–609. Springer, Cham (2017). https://doi.org/10.1007/978-3-319-59050-9_47
8. Kingma, D.P., Ba, J.: Adam: a method for stochastic optimization. arXiv preprint arXiv:1412.6980 (2014)
9. Lapin, M., Hein, M., Schiele, B.: Analysis and optimization of loss functions for multiclass, top-k, and multilabel classification. IEEE Trans. Pattern Anal. Mach. Intell. **40**(7), 1533–1554 (2018)

10. Nie, D., et al.: Medical image synthesis with context-aware generative adversarial networks. In: Descoteaux, M., Maier-Hein, L., Franz, A., Jannin, P., Collins, D.L., Duchesne, S. (eds.) MICCAI 2017. LNCS, vol. 10435, pp. 417–425. Springer, Cham (2017). https://doi.org/10.1007/978-3-319-66179-7_48

11. Osher, S., Sethian, J.A.: Fronts propagating with curvature-dependent speed: algorithms based on Hamilton-Jacobi formulations. J. Comput. Phys. **79**(1), 12–49 (1988)

12. Staal, J., Abràmoff, M.D., Niemeijer, M., Viergever, M.A., Van Ginneken, B.: Ridge-based vessel segmentation in color images of the retina. IEEE Trans. Med. Imaging **23**(4), 501–509 (2004)

13. Tsai, Y.H., Hung, W.C., Schulter, S., Sohn, K., Yang, M.H., Chandraker, M.: Learning to adapt structured output space for semantic segmentation. In: Proceedings of the IEEE Conference on Computer Vision and Pattern Recognition, pp. 7472–7481 (2018)

14. Ulyanov, D., Vedaldi, A., Lempitsky, V.: Instance normalization: The missing ingredient for fast stylization. arXiv preprint arXiv:1607.08022 (2016)

15. Zhang, H., Cisse, M., Dauphin, Y.N., Lopez-Paz, D.: mixup: Beyond empirical risk minimization. arXiv preprint arXiv:1710.09412 (2017)

16. Zhang, Z., Yang, L., Zheng, Y.: Translating and segmenting multimodal medical volumes with cycle-and shape-consistency generative adversarial network. In: Proceedings of the IEEE Conference on Computer Vision and Pattern Recognition, pp. 9242–9251 (2018)

17. Zhu, J.Y., Park, T., Isola, P., Efros, A.A.: Unpaired image-to-image translation using cycle-consistent adversarial networks. In: Proceedings of the IEEE International Conference on Computer Vision, pp. 2223–2232 (2017)

18. Zuiderveld, K.: Contrast limited adaptive histogram equalization. In: Graphics Gems IV, pp. 474–485. Academic Press Professional, Inc. (1994)

DeepAAA: Clinically Applicable and Generalizable Detection of Abdominal Aortic Aneurysm Using Deep Learning

Jen-Tang Lu[1], Rupert Brooks[4], Stefan Hahn[4], Jin Chen[4], Varun Buch[1(✉)],
Gopal Kotecha[1], Katherine P. Andriole[1,3], Brian Ghoshhajra[2], Joel Pinto[4],
Paul Vozila[4], Mark Michalski[1], and Neil A. Tenenholtz[1]

[1] MGH and BWH Center for Clinical Data Science, Boston, USA
varun.buch@mgh.harvard.edu
[2] Massachusetts General Hospital (MGH), Boston, USA
[3] Brigham and Women's Hospital (BWH), Boston, USA
[4] Nuance Communications Inc., Burlington, USA

Abstract. We propose a deep learning-based technique for detection and quantification of abdominal aortic aneurysms (AAAs). The condition, which leads to more than 10,000 deaths per year in the United States, is asymptomatic, often detected incidentally, and often missed by radiologists. Our model architecture is a modified 3D U-Net combined with ellipse fitting that performs aorta segmentation and AAA detection. The study uses 321 abdominal-pelvic CT examinations performed by Massachusetts General Hospital Department of Radiology for training and validation. The model is then further tested for generalizability on a separate set of 57 examinations with differing patient demographics and acquisition characteristics than the original dataset. DeepAAA achieves high performance on both sets of data (sensitivity/specificity 0.91/0.95 and 0.85/1.0 respectively), on contrast and non-contrast CT scans and works with image volumes with varying numbers of images. We find that DeepAAA exceeds literature-reported performance of radiologists on incidental AAA detection. It is expected that the model can serve as an effective background detector in routine CT examinations to prevent incidental AAAs from being missed.

Keywords: Segmentation · Aorta · Aneurysm · Deep learning · U-Net

1 Introduction

Abdominal aortic aneurysms (AAAs), an enlargement or widening of the abdominal aorta, commonly occurs in males older than 65 years with a prevalence of 4

Electronic supplementary material The online version of this chapter (https:// doi.org/10.1007/978-3-030-32245-8_80) contains supplementary material, which is available to authorized users.

© Springer Nature Switzerland AG 2019
D. Shen et al. (Eds.): MICCAI 2019, LNCS 11765, pp. 723–731, 2019.
https://doi.org/10.1007/978-3-030-32245-8_80

to 8% [5]. Untreated aneurysms tend to grow and eventually may rupture with mortality rates exceeding 90%. As most AAAs are asymptomatic until critical bleeding, incidental finding of AAAs becomes critical. However, on routine abdominal computed tomography (CT) exams, only 65% of AAAs are incidentally identified [2]. This low reporting rate makes it difficult to provide timely intervention for patients. Indeed, it is common for AAAs to be first diagnosed at a point where a patient is already at risk for rupture [7]. Furthermore, in routine clinical practice, the size of AAAs is determined by manual measurement of the maximal aortic diameter, which is time-consuming and prone to high inter-reader variability.

Consequently, a variety of computer-aided diagnosis techniques have been proposed over the past decade for automated aorta segmentation. Many of these previous aids used classical computer vision techniques that required prior knowledge, such as external seed points for initialization [3]. Driven by the ever-increasing capability of deep learning, neural networks have recently been used for aorta segmentation on CT angiography [6]. However, these previous deep learning algorithms focused only on CT exams with contrast, while incidental identification of AAAs on scans without contrast is equally important but more challenging. Additionally, most of the previous works concentrated on the task of automated aortic segmentation [6,9,11], but there are very few studies investigating the more applied task of AAA detection, which has much greater clinical relevance than purely performing segmentation alone.

In this paper, we demonstrate a deep-learning solution (DeepAAA) for automated aorta segmentation and AAA detection on both contrast and non-contrast CT series. Specifically, we develop a variant of a 3D U-Net [1] for aorta segmentation on abdominal CT scans. The proposed method handles series with varying numbers of images. We then apply ellipse fitting to the segmented aortic contours and estimate the largest aortic diameter. DeepAAA is a general solution, achieving a high detection rate for AAAs on both contrast and non-contrast CT scans and working with variable image resolutions and slice thicknesses. Furthermore, our solution demonstrates strong generalizability and performance relative to literature-reported values for radiologist sensitivity at AAA detection.

2   Cohort and Annotation

Image data consisted of contrast and non-contrast CT examinations of the abdomen and pelvis performed between January 2005 and April 2017 by Massachusetts General Hospital Department of Radiology. The investigators obtained local Institutional Review Board approval for the project and selected two datasets from the database. The two datasets differ in terms of their capture dates and imaging equipment used as characterized in Table 1.

2.1   Primary Data Set

The primary dataset was used for the training and initial validation of the model and contained 321 studies (223 unique patients). These were selected based on a

Table 1. Comparison between primary and additional validation data sets

Characteristics:	Primary data set	Additional validation set
Number of studies	321	57
Dates captured	2005–2007 (90%)	2012–2016 (85%)
Imaging equipment	A 96% B 4%	A 61% B 26%
manufacturer		C 8% D 5%
Contrast %	48%	51%
Presence of AAA %	77%	51%
Mean age (by study)	70 years	72 years
Gender (by study)	68% male, 32% female	68% male, 32% female
Data labelling method:		
Max. aortic diameter	Manual segmentation	Sourced from reports
Presence/absence of AAA	3.0 cm threshold applied to segmentation	Sourced from reports

keyword search of study reports ensuring a mixture of positive and negative cases of AAA. The query was biased to largely include studies captured between 2005 and 2007. Of the studies selected, there were 217 (67.6%) males and 104 (32.4%) females with a mean age of 70.3 years; 153 (47.7%) CT scans with contrast and 168 (52.3%) without; 247 (76.9%) studies with AAA present and 74 (23.1%) without AAA. For each study, the axial series was used for aorta segmentation and AAA detection. Slice thickness of the images ranged from 2 to 10 mm, while the number of images for each series varied from 40 to 384.

To generate a ground-truth aortic segmentation, the abdominal aorta was manually contoured on the axial scans slice-by-slice until the aortic bifurcation. Each study was annotated by 1 to 4 CT technologists under supervision of 2 radiologists. Based on the clinical definition [2], the presence of AAA was determined by applying a 3.0 cm threshold to the maximum aortic diameter as defined by the manual segmentations.

As many exams were annotated by multiple annotators, a partial assessment of inter-rater variability was possible. Of the 153 contrast studies, 124 were annotated by at least 2 independent technologists, leading to 517 pairwise comparisons. The non-contrast data, however, contained only 10 studies where more than one segmentation was performed, resulting in only 16 pairwise comparisons. The average inter-rater Dice on contrast series was 0.95 ± 0.03, while on noncontrast series, it was 0.90 ± 0.08. Given the small number of samples, the inter-rater variability on non-contrast data should not be considered definitive but suggests roughly similar levels of agreement. For the subsequent analysis, one reference segmentation per dataset was selected randomly as ground truth.

2.2   Additional Validation Set

An additional validation set was used to test the robustness of the model to changes in imaging equipment, imaging department capture protocols, and patient demographics. All of these factors may vary significantly over time at a single site, and thus, we selected 57 studies (57 unique patients) predominantly captured between 2012 and 2016 for this dataset. The studies were selected to include a mixture of positive and negative cases of AAA through keyword search of study reports. All negative studies were manually verified to not contain a AAA. To assess the model against radiologist-reported ground truth and validate post-processing stages which generate the AAA measurement, the maximum aortic diameter and presence of AAA was sourced from radiology reporting rather than being derived from manual segmentations (as was done for the primary data set).

3   Methods

We achieve AAA detection via two sequential steps: (1) aorta segmentation (2) aorta contour fitting for the estimation of the largest cross-sectional diameter. For abdominal aortic segmentation, we developed a variant of a 3D U-Net [1] which accepts series with varying numbers of images. As discussed in Sect. 2, our dataset contained a wide distribution of image counts and slice thicknesses as abdominal studies may also cover other regions of the body, including the pelvis or thorax. It is thus essential to develop an algorithm adapts to variability along the axial dimension. The 3D U-Net architecture we used contained 4 down/upsampling modules (plus the bottleneck layer), 2 convolutional layers per module, and 32 initial features in the network. The convolutional kernel size was $3 \times 3 \times 3$ in both the downsampling and upsampling path, while the 3D pooling kernels were $2 \times 2 \times 1$ to preserve image count. Batch normalization was applied before each ReLU activation, and dropout regularization was utilized at the bottleneck layer with a dropout rate of 0.2. A $1 \times 1 \times 1$ convolutional layer with softmax activation over two classes (background and aorta) was applied at the output layer and thresholded at 0.5 to generate the binary aorta mask.

The model was trained with the RMSprop optimizer using a learning rate of 0.0001. Weights selected for evaluation were those that minimized the loss on the validation set, which were not in general the last epoch weights. The loss function was a smoothed negative Dice coefficient:

$$D = -\frac{2\sum_{i=1}^{N} p_i g_i + 1}{\sum_{i=1}^{N} p_i + \sum_{i=1}^{N} g_i + 1} \tag{1}$$

similar, but not identical, to that used in [8]. The summation is over all N voxels in a scan, p_i is the predicted aorta probability and g_i is the ground truth classification for voxel i. The additional ones in the numerator and denominator avoid division by zero and yield a perfect score for a correct, empty segmentation.

Table 2. Results of 5-fold cross-validation. Delta is predicted minus reference largest diameter. Standard deviations combined using pooled variance.

Fold	N	Mean Dice	Mean Delta (mm)
0	64	0.887 ± 0.121	-0.4 ± 8.5
1	64	0.893 ± 0.107	-0.7 ± 5.4
2	64	0.894 ± 0.060	-3.2 ± 6.0
3	64	0.883 ± 0.126	-2.7 ± 6.3
4	63	0.877 ± 0.127	0.8 ± 9.5
All[a]	319	0.887 ± 0.111	-1.3 ± 7.3

[a]Total is not 321 as two datasets were excluded
due to truncated images. They were retained in
the generation of the full model.

In order to build a general AAA detector that worked with both contrast and non-contrast CT scans, we mixed both types of CT images for model training. All the experiments were implemented utilizing the Keras deep learning library with the Tensorflow backend on NVIDIA DGX-1 Volta.

After aorta segmentation, we applied ellipse fitting [4] image-by-image to the contours of the aorta. The largest aortic diameters (d) were thus assigned by the long axis of the ellipses. For the regions where the aorta was not parallel to the axial CT scans, angle correction was applied to retrieve the true aorta diameter, i.e. $d \cos \theta$, where θ was the angle between the secant plane of the aorta and the axial scan. Based on the definition of AAA, predicted positives were the studies where the largest diameter of the aorta segment was greater than 3 cm. We then compared the predicted results with the ground truth annotations.

4   Results

4.1   Training and Cross-validation on Primary Data Set

To assess model validity and repeatability, the primary dataset was divided into 5 folds such that no patient was repeated between folds. Cross validation was performed by selecting folds $\{n, n + 1, n + 2\}$ mod 5 as training, $n + 3$ mod 5 as validation and the remaining fold as test for $n \in \{0..5\}$. For each combination, the weights with the best validation score after 100 epochs were selected.

Inference on each test study was evaluated in terms of Dice score relative to the reference segmentation and in terms of the maximum diameter of the aorta evaluated on the inferred segmentation versus the same calculation on the reference segmentation. The detailed results of this cross validation are presented in Table 2. Over the 5 folds, the average Dice score ranged from 0.883 to 0.894, with a average Dice score of 0.887 ± 0.111. The estimate of the diameter is consistently within one standard deviation of zero. There may be a slight bias towards smaller diameter, as 4 of the 5 folds had negative means but this bias is small with overall mean -1.3 mm ± 7.3.

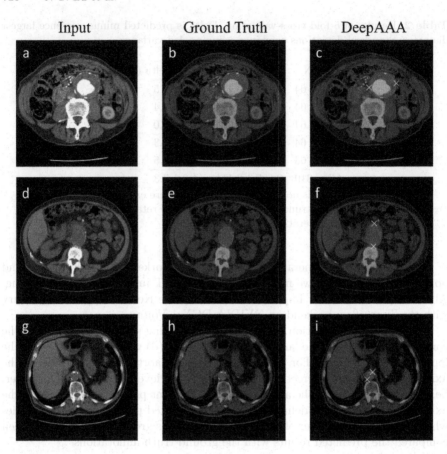

Fig. 1. DeepAAA aorta segmentation (red overlay) and the largest aortic diameter estimation (yellow crosses, the long axis of ellipse fitting [green curves] of the aorta segment): (a–c) Aneurysm with thrombus on contrast CT. (d–f) Large aneurysm on non-contrast CT where aortic boundary is hard to segment. (g–i) normal aorta. (Color figure online)

For a final set of weights, the complete primary dataset was randomly split into training (80%), validation (10%), and test sets (10%). Training was performed for 300 epochs and the weights with lowest validation loss were selected.

As shown in Fig. 1, DeepAAA successfully segments the aorta on both contrast and non-contrast CT images, and works well with more challenging cases where blood-clots are present or the aortic boundary is unclear in the images. We achieve high performance on aortic segmentation with an average Dice coefficient of 0.91, which yields high sensitivity (0.91) and high specificity (0.95) on AAA detection (Table 3). We further examine the error in the largest aortic diameter measurement $(d_{pred} - d_{true})$. We find that the algorithm tends to underestimate the aorta size, but the 2.02 mm average discrepancy is well within the 10 mm gradations on which clinical decisions are generally based.

Table 3. Performance of DeepAAA on segmentation and detection

Dataset	CT type	Segmentation		Detection of AAA	
		Dice	Mean Delta (mm)	Sensitivity	Specificity
Primary	Contrast	0.89 ± 0.05	-2.67 ± 2.62	0.89	0.94
	Non-contrast	0.90 ± 0.05	-1.36 ± 4.30	0.92	0.95
	Overall	$\mathbf{0.90 \pm 0.05}$	$\mathbf{-2.02 \pm 3.62}$	**0.91**	**0.95**
Additional validation set			$\mathbf{-0.6 \pm 3.0}$	**0.85**	**1.00**

4.2 Testing Model Robustness on the Additional Validation Set

Using the final model trained in Sect. 4.1, we performed inference on studies from the additional validation set described in Sect. 2.2. Each study was labelled for the presence of a AAA via the radiology report, and for those studies with positive findings, the maximum aortic diameter was also extracted.

For each study, the model's outputs were compared to the study labels and the model's overall performance was measured in terms of sensitivity/specificity for detecting AAA and mean error in the maximum diameter. Table 3, last row, summarizes these results, along with a comparison to the model's performance on the held-out test set for the same metrics. During the process we noted that some studies in this additional validation set extended into thoracic anatomy, and model inference of this region was removed manually in post-processing.

5 Discussion

While AAAs are rarely missed when the leading indication for a study, the rate of detection significantly decreases when the AAA is an incidental finding. DeepAAA aims to provide a "second set of eyes" and reduce the rate of missed incidental findings. Therefore, to properly contextualize model performance, it is important to quantify this rate of misdiagnosis. Claridge et al., in a retrospective analysis of 3246 abdominal CT scans and their reports, found that only 65% of AAAs were detected by radiologists [2]. DeepAAA exceeds the sensitivity they found (Table 4) while achieving a high specificity (Table 3) and localizes the suspected AAA for radiologist confirmation. Thus, a parallel read from our algorithm could potentially provide a significant reduction in missed AAAs and offer significant clinical value, enabling early detection and treatment of AAA.

Many observers have noted that machine learning models applied to radiology may not generalize well [10]. Changing the equipment used to capture input images and changing the demographics of the underlying patient cohorts tend to reduce model performance. This lack of generalizability would significantly hamper a model's clinical utility because deployment at sites other than where the model was trained may result in surprising under-performance. To test Deep-AAA's ability to generalize, we simulated a significant change in input data by creating a second cohort of validation data (Sect. 2.2) acquired from different

Table 4. Comparison between DeepAAA and literature reported performance of radiologists on AAA reporting for routine abdominal CT according to aneurysm size

Method	30–39 mm	40–49 mm	≥50 mm
DeepAAA sensitivity	**0.68**	**1.00**	**1.00**
Radiologists' sensitivity [2]	0.52	0.87	1.00

patients using different equipment more than five years after the original training data were acquired. The model showed higher specificity (100%) and reduced mean error in diameter prediction with only slightly lower sensitivity (85%) - essentially demonstrating that the model is robust and has not over-fit to any cohort- or equipment-related idiosyncrasies of the original training data.

Future work would involve extending the DeepAAA model beyond the abdominal region to include segmentation of the thoracic aorta. Thoracic aortic aneurysms (TAA), although not nearly as prevalent as AAA, are still a significant source of mortality and generally affect a younger population. In addition, models to predict AAA growth or rupture would be of significant clinical value in guiding more targeted surveillance programs and therapy.

References

1. Çiçek, Ö., Abdulkadir, A., Lienkamp, S.S., Brox, T., Ronneberger, O.: 3D U-Net: learning dense volumetric segmentation from sparse annotation. In: Ourselin, S., Joskowicz, L., Sabuncu, M.R., Unal, G., Wells, W. (eds.) MICCAI 2016. LNCS, vol. 9901, pp. 424–432. Springer, Cham (2016). https://doi.org/10.1007/978-3-319-46723-8_49
2. Claridge, R., Arnold, S., Morrison, N., van Rij, A.M.: Measuring abdominal aortic diameters in routine abdominal computed tomography scans and implications for abdominal aortic aneurysm screening. J. Vasc. Surg. **65**(6), 1637–1642 (2017). https://doi.org/10.1016/j.jvs.2016.11.044
3. de Bruijne, M., van Ginneken, B., Viergever, M., Niessen, W.: Interactive segmentation of abdominal aortic aneurysms in CTA images. Med. Image Anal. **8**(2), 127–138 (2004). https://doi.org/10.1016/j.media.2004.01.001
4. Fitzgibbon, A.W., Pilu, M., Fisher, R.B.: Direct least squares fitting of ellipses. In: Proceedings of 13th International Conference on Pattern Recognition, vol. 1, pp. 253–257, August 1996. https://doi.org/10.1109/ICPR.1996.546029
5. Lindholt, J., Juul, S., Fasting, H., Henneberg, E.: Screening for abdominal aortic aneurysms: single centre randomised controlled trial. BMJ **330**(7494), 750 (2005). https://doi.org/10.1136/bmj.38369.620162.82
6. López-Linares, K., et al.: Fully automatic detection and segmentation of abdominal aortic thrombus in post-operative CTA images using deep convolutional neural networks. Med. Image Anal. **46**, 202–214 (2018). https://doi.org/10.1016/j.media.2018.03.010
7. Mell, M.W., Hlatky, M.A., Shreibati, J.B., Dalman, R.L., Baker, L.C.: Late diagnosis of abdominal aortic aneurysms substantiates underutilization of abdominal aortic aneurysm screening for Medicare beneficiaries. J. Vasc. Surg. **57**(6), 1519–1523 (2013). https://doi.org/10.1016/j.jvs.2012.12.034

8. Milletari, F., Navab, N., Ahmadi, S.A.: V-Net: fully convolutional neural networks for volumetric medical image segmentation. In: 4th International Conference on 3D Vision (3DV), pp. 565–571 (2016)

9. Siriapisith, T., Kusakunniran, W., Haddawy, P.: Outer wall segmentation of abdominal aortic aneurysm by variable neighborhood search through intensity and gradient spaces. J. Digit. Imaging **31**(4), 490–504 (2018). https://doi.org/10.1007/s10278-018-0049-z

10. Zech, J.R., Badgeley, M.A., Liu, M., Costa, A.B., Titano, J.J., Oermann, E.K.: Variable generalization performance of a deep learning model to detect pneumonia in chest radiographs: a cross-sectional study. PLoS Med. **15**(11), 1–17 (2018). https://doi.org/10.1371/journal.pmed.1002683

11. Zhuge, F., Rubin, G.D., Sun, S., Napel, S.: An abdominal aortic aneurysm segmentation method: level set with region and statistical information. Med. Phys. **33**(5), 1440–1453 (2006). https://doi.org/10.1118/1.2193247

Texture-Based Classification of Significant Stenosis in CCTA Multi-view Images of Coronary Arteries

Antonio Tejero-de-Pablos[1,2]([⊠]) [iD], Kaikai Huang[1,2], Hiroaki Yamane[1,2], Yusuke Kurose[1,2], Yusuke Mukuta[1,2], Junichi Iho[3], Youji Tokunaga[3], Makoto Horie[3], Keisuke Nishizawa[3], Yusaku Hayashi[3], Yasushi Koyama[2,3], and Tatsuya Harada[1,2]

[1] The University of Tokyo, Bunkyo, Tokyo 113-8654, Japan
{antonio-t,huang,kurose,mukuta,harada}@mi.t.u-tokyo.ac.jp
[2] RIKEN Center for Advanced Intelligence Project, Chuo, Tokyo 103-0027, Japan
hiroaki.yamane@riken.jp
[3] Sakurabashi Watanabe Hospital, Kita, Osaka 530-0001, Japan
{j_iho,y_tokunaga,m_horie,k_nishizawa,yu_hayashi,
y_koyama}@watanabe-hsp.or.jp

Abstract. A stenosis is a coronary artery disease (CAD) that poses a high risk to the patient's life by narrowing or blocking completely the vessel. Critical luminal narrowings (i.e. significant stenoses) require urgent intervention, and thus, detecting these cases among all stenoses is vitally important. The performance of previous methods for automatically classifying significant stenosis is limited by the use of hand-crafted features or generic features that cannot represent properly the characteristics of this CAD. In this paper, we present a novel method for automatic classification of significant stenosis from coronary CT angiography scans (CCTA). Our method leverages a state-of-the-art feature extractor for texture classification that describe effectively the appearance of significant stenosis. We extract features from curved planar reformation (CPR) views of the coronary arteries: axial, sagittal, coronal, and two orthogonal diagonal-views. The final decision is made by an ensemble of the classification probabilities of each view, similar to the procedure radiologists follow in the diagnosis of significant stenosis. We evaluate our method using a CCTA-CPR dataset of 57 patients with ground truth annotations provided by three experienced experts (significant stenosis if luminal narrowing $\geq$50%). The results of our cross-validated experiments show state-of-the-art classification performance.

Keywords: Significant stenosis · Texture classification · CCTA-CPR multi-view

1 Introduction

Coronary artery disease (CAD) is one of the main causes of death worldwide. Stenosis is a CAD that narrows the artery lumen, thus, obstructing the normal

© Springer Nature Switzerland AG 2019
D. Shen et al. (Eds.): MICCAI 2019, LNCS 11765, pp. 732–740, 2019.
https://doi.org/10.1007/978-3-030-32245-8_81

flow of blood. Stenoses are due to the presence of plaques in the artery walls, and they are related to other heart diseases, so many researchers and radiologists dedicate their efforts to achieve an accurate diagnosis. Previous studies showed that Coronary Computed Tomography Angiography (CCTA) is a valid alternative to direct invasive anigiography for detecting lesions in the coronaries, such as stenosis [3]. However, manually analyzing CCTA volumes of images is time-consuming and a burden to radiologists. An automatic method capable of accurately classifying clinically-relevant stenoses (obstruction >50%) could support radiologists and provide a second opinion for diagnosis. Current automatic vessel extraction technologies are able to provide the centerline paths of the coronary arteries given a CCTA volume of the heart. From this path, a Curved Planar Reformation (CPR) volume of each artery can be obtained. This volume is used by radiologists to look for stenosis from different points of view (e.g., cross-section, longitudinal, etc.).

Several works that use CPR images have been proposed in order to automatically detect significant stenosis. One approach involves explicitly segmenting or estimating the lumen area of the cross-section views of the artery to detect narrowings [5–7]. These methods require annotations with the lumen area size on each image, which are costly, and thus, hard to obtain. Other works use handcrafted features extracted from CPR volumes [1,4,11,15]. These methods use the intensity (i.e., Hounsfield Unit, HU) values from a cylindrical region fitted to the artery, and use a classifier for detecting plaques and significant stenosis. While performing classification on the HU values directly may suffice to classify calcified plaques, it causes a high false positive rate [11], that is, stenoses that are non-significant are classified as significant. This is because, although plaques cause stenoses, not all of them are significant. Similarly, lumen segmentation-based methods may suffer from stenosis overestimation depending on the accuracy of the segmentation [7].

The most recent works in CAD diagnosis [8,9], instead of applying ad-hoc rules on the CCTA intensity values directly, they use more sophisticated methods based on convolutional neural networks (CNN) and other deep-learning techniques. Convolutional neural networks (CNN) automatically extract features that represent contours and shapes, which are useful for image classification. In [14], CNN features are extracted from the myocardium in CCTA images to detect signs of ischemia. This method allows predicting potential stenoses in the coronary arteries, but cannot detect their location. In [13], a recurrent convolutional neural network (R-CNN) for feature extraction and significant stenosis classification in CPR volumes is proposed. This method's input is an entire CPR volumetric segment, which requires a larger network than a feature extraction network for images. Thus, a non-public dataset of 166 patients is used to train the R-CNN. Unfortunately, gathering such a number of patients suffering significant stenoses is not always feasible; in such cases, simpler but more efficient networks are preferred. A deep network pretrained with a large-scale dataset provides multi-purpose features that allow solving a variety of classification problems, including CAD [9]. In recent years, more sophisticated image classification methods that use pretrained models have been proposed. In [2], texture images (e.g., fabric, carpet, marbled) are classified using pretrained CNN features. In order to adapt the features to their task, authors propose applying a Fisher vector (FV) encoding, which allows describing regions of arbitrary shapes and sizes.

In this paper, we present a novel method for automatic significant stenosis classification. Given the arbitrary shapes and sizes of significant stenosis, we propose approaching this task as a texture classification problem in a novel way, obtaining a state-of-the-art accuracy. (1) We leverage pretrained CNN features, and adapt them with a FV encoding, which is more advantageous for describing texture-like patterns instead of objects. (2) Also, instead of inputting an entire CPR volume, we approach significant stenosis classification as a combination of classification in multiple key views, similarly to the diagnosis procedure followed by radiologists. A similar multiview approach proved superior to a 3D CNN for plaque classification [12]. Because of these points, our method is highly efficient, and can be successfully trained with a limited amount of data. Finally, we provide an analysis of the extracted features, and a discussion on the usefulness of a multiview approach for stenosis classification.

2   Texture-Based Classification of Significant Stenosis in Multi-view CCTA Images

Our method classifies a set of multiple views from a CCTA-CPR segment of a coronary artery into *significant stenosis* or *non-significant stenosis*. For that, we leverage an image feature descriptor used for texture classification tasks, FV-CNN [2]. By applying a Fisher vector (FV) encoding to the general-purpose features of a pretrained convolutional neural network (CNN), local features are pooled densely while global spatial information is removed, making features more suitable at describing textures (e.g., regions of arbitrary shapes and sizes) than objects. Since FV estimates feature distributions from data of different domains, FV-CNN features transfer across general images and medical images. Besides, by using a pretrained CNN, a large-scale annotated dataset of CCTA scans is not required to successfully train our method.

Figure 1 shows an overview of the proposed method. We perform a central crop along the longitudinal axis of the CCTA-CPR volume (from 512×512 to 192×192 voxels in our case), in order to remove irrelevant information while keeping all artery voxels. Then, the volume is partitioned into T segments, so each segment is N slices long. The number N is chosen so segments are cubes (same width, height and depth in millimeters). From an input segment, five key views are generated and classified. First, image features are extracted from an input view using a pretrained CNN. Then, the dimension of the features is reduced with principal components analysis (PCA) and encoded using FV. A support vector machine (SVM) outputs the probability of the input view of containing a significant stenosis. Last, the probabilities of all views are combined in an ensemble to decide if the input section significant stenosis.

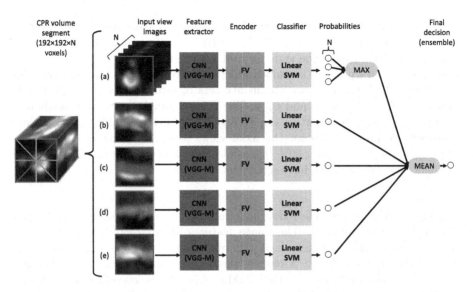

Fig. 1. Overview of the proposed method. From an input CPR volume segment, five key views are employed: (a) axial, (b) sagittal, (c) coronal, (d) diagonal$_1$ and (e) diagonal$_2$. We use a texture classification-based approach (FV-CNN [2]), in which the extracted features are encoded, and the classifier provides the probability of significant stenosis. An ensemble of all views outputs the probability of significant stenosis in the segment.

Unlike other methods, we use multiple views of the same coronary artery segment for significant stenosis classification. Although using a 3D CNN to classify an entire CPR volumetric section is another possible approach [13], it requires a large dataset in order to be trained. Thus, we propose an efficient multi-view approach capable of providing a good performance even with smaller datasets. Figure 1 shows our axial view (cross-section) and four longitudinal views (projections in the sagittal axis, coronal axis and diagonal axes). We selected them since they are the key views inspected by radiologists in manual diagnosis. Axial instances (a) are individual slices of the input CPR volume segment. The remaining views (b–e) are a concatenation of the voxels in the corresponding planes, resized to 192 × 192 using bicubic interpolation. The value of each voxel in an instance view is a Hounsfield Unit (HU), as in the original CCTA scan.

The instances in our dataset are divided in two splits, train and test. Due to the circular symmetry of CPR cross-sections, we perform data augmentation in the axial instances of the train set; more concretely, 90° rotations and horizontal flips. Image features are extracted from each instance by leveraging a pretrained CNN. In our implementation, we use the VGG-M model [10], which admits three-channel input images. Thus, we replicate our one-dimensional (HU value) instances three times in the channel dimension. Then, we apply PCA dimensionality reduction, to retain the most representative features, which are encoded using FV. The FV encoder is trained in an unsupervised way, by dedicating a subset of the training split of the dataset to learn the PCA projection and a Gaussian mixture model (GMM) of the CNN features. The encoded features of the instances in the training split are used to train a linear SVM until convergence. This pipeline is trained independently for each view, and thus, for an input CPR segment t, we obtain five sets of significant stenosis probabilities: p_{axi}^t, p_{sag}^t, p_{cor}^t, $p_{dia_1}^t$ and $p_{dia_2}^t$. The way of combining these probabilities into $p_{ensemble}^t$ is by calculating the average of the five. A single input segment t outputs N probabilities for the axial view, so $p_{axi}^t = max(p_{axi_1}^t \ldots p_{axi_N}^t)$. If $p_{ensemble}^t$ is greater than 50% (threshold determined empirically), the artery segment t is considered to have significant stenosis.

Implementation details. The following parameters were selected empirically after thorough experimentation. The image features are extracted from the *conv5* layer of a VGG-M model pretrained with ImageNet, as in the original method for texture classification [2]. PCA reduces the dimensionality of the image features to 128. FV uses 64 Gaussians in the GMM to generate the encoding. The GMM is trained using one-fourth of the instances in the training split (randomly chosen). The hyperparameter of the SVM is $C = 1$.

3 Evaluation

3.1 Dataset

We evaluated our method with a non-public dataset of CCTA scans of 57 patients (70 significant stenoses in total). From each scan, the CPR volumes for the LAD, LCX and RCA coronary arteries were extracted. The distance between voxels in the same CPR slice is $\delta_1 = 0.06$ mm, and the distance between slices is $\delta_2 = 0.8$ mm. Thus, the depth of an input segment is $N = 15$ ($N = 192 \times \delta_1/\delta_2 = 14.4 \approx 15$). Our dataset contains a total of 47590 instances for the axial view (after data augmentation), and 2611 instances for each of the longitudinal views. Each slice (axial view instances) of the CPR volume was provided an annotation by three experienced radiologists, i.e., $l_{axi_n}^t \in \{1,0\}$ as *significant stenosis* or *non-significant stenosis* respectively. Since instances in the longitudinal views comprise N slices, their annotation is calculated as $max(l_{axi_1}^t \ldots l_{axi_N}^t)$ among the annotations of the slices included in the segment. When training the proposed method, due to the strong imbalance between classes, we randomly choose a number of *non-significant stenosis* instances equal to the number of *significant stenosis* instances.

3.2 Experimental Results

We use a leave-one-out (LOO) cross-validation strategy, in which one patient is reserved for evaluation while the rest are used for training. This is repeated for all patients and the final score is the average of all iterations. If the prediction and the annotation match, the input segment is a true positive (TP)

in the case of *significant stenosis* or true negative (TN) for *non-significant stenosis*. A misclassification is a false negative (FN) for *significant stenosis* or false positive (FP) for *non-significant stenosis*. The evaluation metrics used are sensitivity $(Se \equiv TP/TP+FN)$, specificity $(Sp \equiv TN/TN+FP)$, and accuracy $(Acc \equiv TP+TN/TP+FN+TN+FP)$.

Table 1. Significant stenosis classification performance of our method (**in bold**), and indirect comparison with the state of the art (different datasets and evaluation strategies). Results marked as (—) were not provided in the original paper.

Method	Se	Sp	Acc	Dataset
(a) Axial view	84.2	65.94	67.64	57 patients (70 significant stenosis)
(b) Sagittal view	81.97	77.19	77.7	
(c) Coronal view	75.62	75.79	76.15	
(d) Diagonal$_1$ view	68.34	78.64	78.57	
(e) Diagonal$_2$ view	68.36	74.75	74.92	
Multiview ensemble	**90**	**79.84**	**80.54**	
Recurrent CNN [13]	—	—	80	163 patients (161 significant stenosis)
Healthy lumen estimation [6]	90	85	—	150 patients (—)

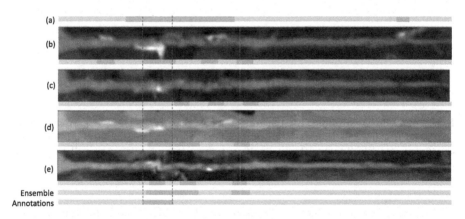

Fig. 2. Classification results along the longitudinal views of an artery. Sections classified as significant stenosis are in red, for our key views (a–e, see Table 1), the final ensemble, and the ground truth annotations. (Color figure online)

Table 1 shows a summary of the results, compared to two other state-of-the-art works in significant stenosis classification from CCTA-CPR images. Since the dataset, annotations and evaluation strategy used in those works is different from ours, this comparison only provides an indication of the performance of our method. Although each individual view is not enough to achieve state-of-the-art performance, our ensemble is able to classify significant stenosis with high accuracy. The reason is because significant stenosis that cannot be detected in one view, can likely be detected in one or more of the other views. Figure 2 shows the classification results along the longitudinal views of an artery. Our method successfully classifies segments containing significant stenosis. Using several views adds robustness against outliers, and positives hidden from a certain view. With this multiview ensemble approach, we can increase the classification accuracy without increasing the complexity of the method. Thus, our method does not require large datasets to be successfully trained.

Our performance is comparable with state-of-the-art methods in significant stenosis classification: a recurrent CNN [13][1] and a lumen area estimator [6]. However, the number of trainable parameters in [13] makes their method unsuitable for reduced datasets such as ours. Also, the method in [6] yields a higher specificity, that is, a better classification of non-significant stenosis. This is because their annotations include the ground-truth size of the lumen area of the artery, which serves as a reference to discriminate *significant* vs *non-significant* stenoses. However, such annotations are costly, and thus, hardly available.

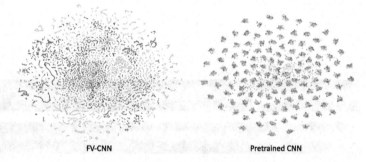

FV-CNN   Pretrained CNN

Fig. 3. FV-CNN encoding vs. pretrained CNN features. Features extracted from CCTA-CPR using a method for texture classification (left) generate distributions where significant stenosis (blue) and non-significant stenosis (red) are more easily separable. (Color figure online)

We visualized the effect of the employed FV-CNN encoding, when applied to CCTA-CPR images of coronary arteries with stenosis. Figure 3 shows a comparison between regular pretrained CNN features and ours. We used tSNE to reduce the feature space to two dimensions for the sake of visualization. FV-CNN, used originally for texture classification, provides a feature distribution where significant stenosis (blue) is more clearly separated[2].

---

[1] Authors consider *no stenosis* and *non-significant stenosis* as two different classes.
[2] The clusters in the CNN features are tSNE artifacts, with no particular meaning.

4   Discussion and Conclusions

We proposed a novel method for classification of significant stenosis in coronary arteries. We applied a feature encoding approach used for texture classification, in order to obtain features capable of describing regions of arbitrary shapes and sizes. We extract features and classify segments of five views (Fig. 1): (a) axial, (b) sagittal, (c) coronal, (d) diagonal$_1$ and (e) diagonal$_2$. Although we tried different combinations of views in our ensemble, including the common axial-sagittal-coronal triplanar view, the best performance was obtained by employing all five of them. When manually checking for significant stenosis, radiologists also evaluate diagonal views, as they may contain further cues for diagnosis; this coincides with our results. Overall, our results show a high sensitivity and specificity, which allows for a practical use assisting radiologists in detecting significant stenosis.

A limitation of the present work is that it does not take specific measures against bifurcations and other artifacts prone to false-positive results. Also, unlike [13], we do not consider the influence of the type of plaque causing the stenosis. This is partially intentional, since the presence of plaques not always indicates *significant* stenoses.

To summarize, in this paper, we successfully proposed utilizing several views, similarly to the process radiologists follow to manually detect significant stenosis. In future work, this methodology will be further explored by combining different views at the feature extraction level instead of at the classification level. We also leveraged a texture-based feature encoding method, which yielded promising results in our task. In future work, similar encodings will be further explored in related tasks, such as plaque classification in coronary arteries.

References

1. Cetin, S., Unal, G.: Automatic detection of coronary artery stenosis in CTA based on vessel intensity and geometric features. In: Proceedings of the MICCAI Workshop. 3D Cardiovascular Imaging (2012)
2. Cimpoi, M., Maji, S., Vedaldi, A.: Deep filter banks for texture recognition and segmentation. In: Proceedings of the IEEE Conference on Computer Vision and Pattern Recognition, pp. 3828–3836 (2015)
3. Dewey, M., Rutsch, W., Schnapauff, D., Teige, F., Hamm, B.: Coronary artery stenosis quantification using multislice computed tomography. Invest. Radiol. **42**(2), 78–84 (2007)
4. Duval, M., Ouzeau, E., Precioso, F., Matuszewski, B.: Coronary artery stenoses detection with random forest. In: Proceedings of the MICCAI Workshop, 3D Cardiovascular Imaging (2012)
5. Kelm, B.M., et al.: Detection, grading and classification of coronary stenoses in computed tomography angiography. In: Fichtinger, G., Martel, A., Peters, T. (eds.) MICCAI 2011. LNCS, vol. 6893, pp. 25–32. Springer, Heidelberg (2011). https://doi.org/10.1007/978-3-642-23626-6_4

6. Sankaran, S., Schaap, M., Hunley, S.C., Min, J.K., Taylor, C.A., Grady, L.: HALE: healthy area of lumen estimation for vessel stenosis quantification. In: Ourselin, S., Joskowicz, L., Sabuncu, M.R., Unal, G., Wells, W. (eds.) MICCAI 2016. LNCS, vol. 9902, pp. 380–387. Springer, Cham (2016). https://doi.org/10.1007/978-3-319-46726-9_44

7. Shahzad, R., et al.: Automatic segmentation, detection and quantification of coronary artery stenoses on CTA. Int. J. Cardiovasc. Imaging **29**(8), 1847–1859 (2013)

8. Shen, D., Wu, G., Suk, H.I.: Deep learning in medical image analysis. Annu. Rev. Biomed. Eng. **19**, 221–248 (2017)

9. Shin, H.C., et al.: Deep convolutional neural networks for computer-aided detection: CNN architectures, dataset characteristics and transfer learning. IEEE Trans. Med. Imaging **35**(5), 1285–1298 (2016)

10. Simonyan, K., Zisserman, A.: Very deep convolutional networks for largescale image recognition. In: Proceedings of the International Conference on Learning Representations, pp. 1–14 (2015)

11. Tessmann, M., Vega-Higuera, F., Fritz, D., Scheuering, M., Greiner, G.: Multiscale feature extraction for learning-based classification of coronary artery stenosis. In: Proceedings of the SPIE Medical Imaging: Computer-Aided Diagnosis, pp. 726002:1–726002:8 (2009)

12. Wolterink, J.M., Leiner, T., de Vos, B.D., van Hamersvelt, R.W., Viergever, M.A., Išgum, I.: Automatic coronary artery calcium scoring in cardiac CT angiography using paired convolutional neural networks. Med. Image Anal. **34**, 123–136 (2016)

13. Zreik, M., van Hamersvelt, R.W., Wolterink, J.M., Leiner, T., Viergever, M.A., Išgum, I.: A recurrent CNN for automatic detection and classification of coronary artery plaque and stenosis in coronary CT angiography. IEEE Trans. Med. Imaging **1**(1), 1–11 (2018)

14. Zreik, M., et al.: Deep learning analysis of the myocardium in coronary CT angiography for identification of patients with functionally significant coronary artery stenosis. Med. Image Anal. **44**, 72–85 (2018)

15. Zuluaga, M.A., Magnin, I.E., Hernández-Hoyos, M., Delgado-Leyton, E.J., Lozano, F., Orkisz, M.: Automatic detection of abnormal vascular cross-sections based on density level detection and support vector machines. Int. J. Comput. Assist. Radiol. Surg. **6**(2), 163–174 (2011)

Fourier Spectral Dynamic Data Assimilation: Interlacing CFD with 4D Flow MRI

Taha Sabri Koltukluoğlu$^{(\boxtimes)}$ (iD)

Seminar for Applied Mathematics, ETH, Zurich, Switzerland
koltukluoglu@gmail.com

Abstract. Most data assimilation studies, incorporating observations into computational blood flow simulations, have approached the problem exploiting the traditional mathematical formulation in the time domain, an approach that incurs huge computational cost. In this work, a new method is introduced to perform variational adjoint-based dynamic data assimilation. The work aims to combine the superiority of computational fluid dynamics with the advantages of phase-contrast magnetic resonance imaging and simultaneously taking into account the dynamic nature of the heart beat. In contrast to the traditional time-stepping schemes, the novel approach relies on the harmonically balanced momentum equations expressed in the frequency domain, while the combination of the corresponding solutions yields the periodic solution of the original problem. This work enables accurate characterization of the dynamic flow field in quite feasible and practicable wall clock times, which are otherwise difficult to be achieved using currently available dynamic data assimilation strategies.

1 Introduction

In time dependent adjoint-based inverse problems, all trajectories of the state variables from the original problem must be solved and stored in the memory, in order to solve the adjoint equations. The space needed for the memory is proportional to the run-time of the forward solution. In spite of ever increasing memory capabilities of large clusters, the practical application of the traditional adjoint formulation is quite limited. Certain algorithms, known as checkpointing, have been proposed to manage the difficulties with the storage requirements [1,3,8]. When using such algorithms, however, the direct problem must be solved several times in order to evaluate the adjoint problem. This process must then be repeated at each single iteration of the optimization process.

There has been an attempt to perform variational adjoint-based dynamic data assimilation (DA) in computational hemodynamics [2]. However, the authors were forced to extremely reduce the size of the problem (in such a way, that no checkpointing algorithms were required) by considering a coarse mesh and a time step of 0.004625 s. Using such time steps, however, accurate flow simulations cannot be expected at the aortic root and the ascending aorta, where

© Springer Nature Switzerland AG 2019
D. Shen et al. (Eds.): MICCAI 2019, LNCS 11765, pp. 741–749, 2019.
https://doi.org/10.1007/978-3-030-32245-8_82

the Reynolds numbers grow large. In addition, finer mesh sizes are required for reasonable evaluation of clinically relevant parameters such as the wall shear stresses (WSSs). The size-related limitations were also mentioned by the authors in their work. Especially for convection dominated problems with large Reynolds numbers, using the traditional time-stepping schemes to perform dynamic DA is absolutely impracticable and nearly impossible or difficult to be achieved.

In this work, a new method is proposed to perform variational adjoint-based dynamic data assimilation. In contrast to the traditional time-stepping schemes, the novel approach relies on the harmonically balanced momentum equations (see [6]) for the time discretization, which are expressed in the frequency domain. The combination of the corresponding solutions in the frequency domain yields the periodic solution of the original problem. Hereinafter, the new method will be referred as the Fourier spectral dynamic data assimilation (FS-DDA). This work enables accurate characterization of the dynamic flow field in quite feasible and practicable wall clock times (WCT), which are otherwise difficult or impossible to be achieved using currently available DA strategies. The method naturally avoids storage related problems, and hence, the application of additional algorithms (such as checkpointing) are not required. Further, the work addresses the limited resolution of MR velocity encoding in shear layers and aims to interlace phase-contrast magnetic resonance imaging (4D flow MRI) with computational fluid dynamics (CFD) to enable the evaluation of clinically relevant parameters. Compared to the raw measurements, the proposed approach significantly improves the reconstructed flow field at the aortic root, which is one of the most important clinically relevant locations where flow disturbances can easily lead to pathological modifications of the arterial wall. Thus the new method has a great potential for revealing clinically relevant hemodynamic phenomena.

2   Mathematical Optimization

An unsteady incompressible flow of a Newtonian fluid is considered in the time interval $\mathbb{T} := [0; T]$ through an open set Ω with boundary $\partial\Omega = \Gamma_i \cup \Gamma_o \cup \Gamma_w$. Let $\Omega \supset \Omega_s := \{x \in \Omega \mid \|x - y\| \geq s \,(\mathrm{mm}) \,\forall y \in \Gamma_w\}$ be a contracted subdomain with boundary $\partial\Omega_s = \Gamma_{si} \cup \Gamma_{so} \cup \Gamma_{sw}$, where $\Gamma_{si} \subset \Gamma_i$ and $\Gamma_{so} \subset \Gamma_o$ (see Fig. 1). The fluid flow is stimulated by some T-periodic inflow data prescribed at Γ_i, which is characterized by the T-periodic function $g(t, x) = g(t + mT, x) : \mathbb{T} \times \Gamma_i \rightarrow \mathbb{R}^3$ with $m \in \mathbb{N}$. Let $H^1(\Omega)$ be the space of square integrable vector functions with first derivatives also square integrable in Ω, whereas $L^2(\Omega)$ is the space of square integrable scalar functions in Ω. The blood flow velocity $u \in \mathcal{U}$ with $\mathcal{U} = \{v \in H^1(\Omega) \mid v|_{\Gamma_w} = \mathbf{0}\}$ is a solution of the incompressible Navier-Stokes equations, which can be expressed in the Euler-Lagrangian formulation as a set of equations for momentum $\rho\left[\partial_t u + (\nabla u)u\right] - \mu\Delta u + \nabla p = \mathbf{0}$ and continuity $\operatorname{div} u = 0$ in $\mathbb{T} \times \Omega$ (along with inflow $u = g$ on $\mathbb{T} \times \Gamma_i$), where $p \in L^2(\Omega)$ and (ρ, μ) are the density and dynamic viscosity of the fluid.

In [6], the harmonic balance (HB) approach has been employed for an approximation of the velocity field in time, which relies on the degree-n Fourier polynomial $u \approx \tilde{u}(t, x) = \hat{u}_{c_0}(x) + \sum_{k=1}^{n} \left[\hat{u}_{c_k}(x)\cos(k\omega t) + \hat{u}_{s_k}(x)\sin(k\omega t)\right]$, where

$\widehat{u}_{c_k}$ for $k = 0 \cdots n$ and $\widehat{u}_{s_k}$ for $k = 1 \cdots n$ form the discrete spectrum of $\tilde{u}$ and $\omega = \frac{2\pi}{T}$ is the angular frequency. Let $\tilde{u}^j := \tilde{u}(t_j, x)$ and $p^j := p(t_j, x)$. Inserting the approximation $\tilde{u}$ into the momentum equation and employing a collocation approach using equidistant time instants $t_j := \frac{jT}{N}$ for $j = 1, \cdots, N = 2n + 1$ results in the following harmonically balanced momentum equations,

$$\rho \left[\sum_{i=1}^{N} \tilde{u}^i c_{ij} + (\nabla \tilde{u}^j) \tilde{u}^j \right] - \mu \Delta \tilde{u}^j + \nabla p^j = \mathbf{0}, \qquad j = 1, 2, \cdots, N. \quad (1)$$

The expression $c_{ij} = \frac{2\omega}{N} \sum_{k=1}^{n} k \sin(k\omega(t_i - t_j))$ follows from the application of cosine and sine transforms (DFT) for the discrete spectrum. Equations in (1) are expressed in the frequency domain in terms of the time domain state variables $\tilde{u}^j$ and p^j at each time t_j. Detailed derivations can be found in [6].

In this work, a new method is introduced by incorporating the harmonically balanced momentum equations (1) into an optimal boundary control study and performing a variational adjoint-based data assimilation using 4D flow MRI data. As such, let us first express the harmonically balanced incompressible Navier-Stokes equations in the variational formulation as follows: Find $(u, p, r) \in \mathcal{U} \times L^2(\Omega) \times H^{-\frac{1}{2}}(\Gamma_i)$ such that $\forall (\hat{u}^j, \hat{p}^j, \hat{r}^j) \in \mathcal{U} \times L^2(\Omega) \times H^{-\frac{1}{2}}(\Gamma_i)$ it holds

$$\int_{\Omega} \left[\rho \left(\sum_{i=1}^{N} \tilde{u}^i c_{ij} + (\nabla u^j) u^j \right) \cdot \hat{u}^j + 2\mu \nabla^s u^j \cdot \nabla^s \hat{u}^j - p^j \operatorname{div} \hat{u}^j - \hat{p}^j \operatorname{div} u^j \right] d\Omega$$

$$= \int_{\Gamma_i} \hat{r}^j \cdot (u^j - g^j) \, d\Gamma + \int_{\Gamma_i} (r^j \cdot \hat{u}^j) \, d\Gamma \ , \quad j = 1, 2, \cdots, N, \quad (2)$$

where $\nabla^s(\cdot) = [\nabla(\cdot) + (\nabla(\cdot))^T]/2$ is the strain rate tensor and $H^{-\frac{1}{2}}(\Gamma_i)$ is the dual space of $H_{00}^{\frac{1}{2}}(\Gamma_i) = \left\{ g \in H^{\frac{1}{2}}(\Gamma_i) \mid g|_{\gamma_i} = 0 \right\}$.

Assuming that some T-periodic observations $u_{\text{obs}}^j \in \Omega$ are available at equidistantly spaced discrete time instants t_j. The optimal control problem aims at finding the velocity fields u^j, such that the sum of the misfits between each u_{obs}^j and u^j is minimized based on some cost function $\mathcal{O}_\Omega$. At the same time, the problem is constrained such that u^j are solutions of Eq. (2). Let β and β_1 be arbitrary parameters for a Tikhonov regularization, whereas ∇_τ denotes the surface gradient and α is a positive real number. The flow-matching problem reads

$\mathcal{O}_\Omega(u(g), g, u_{\text{obs}}) = \frac{\alpha}{2} \sum_j \left(\int_{\Omega_s} |u^j(g) - u_{\text{obs}}^j|^2 \, d\Omega + \int_{\Gamma_{si} \cup \Gamma_{so}} |u^j(g) - u_{\text{obs}}^j|^2 \, d\Gamma \right)$
$+ \sum_j \left(\frac{\beta}{2} \int_{\Gamma_i} |g^j|^2 \, d\Gamma + \frac{\beta_1}{2} \int_{\Gamma_i} |\nabla_\tau g^j|^2 \, d\Gamma \right)$, where Ω_s, Γ_{si} and Γ_{so} are the trust regions of experimental observations (see Fig. 1). The terms with the regularization parameters prevent the control function to grow unboundedly and enforce a certain regularity over the control. The choices of these terms were also motivated in [5]. Further, the choices of the terms for performing the flow-matching both in a part of the domain (in Ω_s) and in parts over the boundaries (on Γ_{si} and Γ_{so}) has been investigated in [7]. Regarding the flow-matching problem, the existence of optimal boundary control has been provided in [4].

The constrained optimization can be cast as a saddle point problem by introducing a Lagrangian functional: $\mathscr{L}_\Omega(g, u, p, r, \lambda_u, \lambda_p, \lambda_r) = \mathscr{O}_\Omega(u, g, u_{\mathbf{obs}}) - \sum_j \int_{\Gamma_i} \lambda_r^j \cdot (u^j - g^j)\, d\Gamma - \sum_j \int_{\Gamma_i} r^j \cdot \lambda_u^j\, d\Gamma + \sum_j \int_\Omega \left[\rho\left(\sum_{i=1}^N u^i c_{ij} + (\nabla u^j)u^j \right) \cdot \lambda_u^j + 2\mu \nabla^s u^j \cdot \nabla^s \lambda_u^j - p^j \operatorname{div} \lambda_u^j - \lambda_p^j \operatorname{div} u^j \right] d\Omega$. The necessary condition for having a minimum at g is provided by the Gâteaux derivative of $\mathscr{O}_\Omega$ with respect to perturbation in g. This information is contained in the critical points of the Lagrangian $\mathscr{L}_\Omega$, expressed in variational formulation for $j = 1 \cdots N$ as follows:

Direct Problem $\mathscr{P}_{\mathrm{sta}}^j(g^j, u^i)$: For $g^j \in H_{00}^{\frac{1}{2}}(\Gamma_i)$ and $u^i \in \mathcal{U}$, where $i = 1, \cdots, N$ with $i \neq j$, determine $(u^j, p^j, r^j) \in \mathcal{U} \times L^2(\Omega) \times H^{-\frac{1}{2}}(\Gamma_i)$ such that

$$\left\langle \frac{\partial \mathscr{L}_\Omega}{\partial \lambda_u^j}, \hat{\lambda}_u^j \right\rangle = \int_\Omega \left[\rho\left(\sum_{i=1}^N u^i c_{ij} + (\nabla u^j)u^j \right) \cdot \hat{\lambda}_u^j + 2\mu \nabla^s u^j \cdot \nabla^s \hat{\lambda}_u^j - p^j \operatorname{div} \hat{\lambda}_u^j \right] d\Omega$$
$$- \int_{\Gamma_i} r^j \cdot \hat{\lambda}_u^j \, d\Gamma = 0 \qquad \forall \hat{\lambda}_u^j \in \mathcal{U}, \tag{3}$$

$$\left\langle \frac{\partial \mathscr{L}_\Omega}{\partial \lambda_p^j}, \hat{\lambda}_p^j \right\rangle = - \int_\Omega \hat{\lambda}_p^j \operatorname{div} u^j \, d\Omega = 0 \qquad \forall \hat{\lambda}_p^j \in L^2(\Omega), \tag{4}$$

$$\left\langle \frac{\partial \mathscr{L}_\Omega}{\partial \lambda_r^j}, \hat{\lambda}_r^j \right\rangle = - \int_{\Gamma_i} \hat{\lambda}_r^j \cdot (u^j - g^j) \, d\Gamma = 0 \qquad \forall \hat{\lambda}_r^j \in H^{-\frac{1}{2}}(\Gamma_i). \tag{5}$$

Adjoint Problem $\mathscr{P}_{\mathrm{adj}}^j(u^j, u_{\mathbf{obs}}^j)$: For u^j, solution of (3)–(5), and $u_{\mathbf{obs}}^j$, determine $(\lambda_u^j, \lambda_p^j, \lambda_r^j) \in \mathcal{U} \times L^2(\Omega) \times H^{-\frac{1}{2}}(\Gamma_i)$ such that

$$\left\langle \frac{\partial \mathscr{L}_\Omega}{\partial u^j}, \hat{u}^j \right\rangle = \int_{\Gamma_o \cup \Gamma_i} \left[\alpha\, (\chi_{\Gamma_{so}} + \chi_{\Gamma_{si}})(u^j - u_{\mathbf{obs}}^j) \cdot \hat{u}^j \right] d\Gamma - \int_{\Gamma_i} (\lambda_r^j \cdot \hat{u}^j) \, d\Gamma$$

$$+ \int_\Omega \left[\alpha \chi_{\Omega_s}(u^j - u_{\mathbf{obs}}^j) \cdot \hat{u}^j + \rho\left(\sum_{i=1}^N c_{ji} \hat{u}^j + (\nabla \hat{u}^j)u^j + (\nabla u^j)\hat{u}^j \right) \cdot \lambda_u^j \right.$$

$$\left. + 2\mu \nabla^s \hat{u}^j \cdot \nabla^s \lambda_u^j - \lambda_p^j \operatorname{div} \hat{u}^j \right] d\Omega = 0 \qquad \forall \hat{u}^j \in \mathcal{U}, \tag{6}$$

$$\left\langle \frac{\partial \mathscr{L}_\Omega}{\partial p^j}, \hat{p}^j \right\rangle = - \int_\Omega \hat{p}^j \operatorname{div} \lambda_u^j \, d\Omega = 0 \qquad \forall \hat{p}^j \in L^2(\Omega), \tag{7}$$

$$\left\langle \frac{\partial \mathscr{L}_\Omega}{\partial r^j}, \hat{r}^j \right\rangle = - \int_{\Gamma_i} \hat{r}^j \cdot \lambda_u^j \, d\Gamma = 0 \qquad \forall \hat{r}^j \in H^{-\frac{1}{2}}(\Gamma_i), \tag{8}$$

where χ_{Ω_s}, $\chi_{\Gamma_{si}}$ and $\chi_{\Gamma_{so}}$ are the characteristic functions.

Optimality Condition $\mathscr{P}_{\mathrm{opt}}^j(\lambda_r^j)$: For λ_r^j, solution of (6)–(8), determine $g^j \in H_{00}^{\frac{1}{2}}(\Gamma_i)$ such that $\forall \hat{g}^j \in H^{\frac{1}{2}}(\Gamma_i)$ it holds

$$\left\langle \frac{\partial \mathscr{L}_\Omega}{\partial g^j}, \hat{g}^j \right\rangle = \int_{\Gamma_i} \left[\beta g^j \cdot \hat{g}^j + \beta_1 \nabla_\tau g^j \cdot \nabla_\tau \hat{g}^j + \lambda_r^j \cdot \hat{g}^j \right] d\Gamma = 0. \tag{9}$$

2.1 Gradient Descent Algorithm for Dynamic Data Assimilation

A descent-like iterative algorithm was employed to iteratively solve the nonlinear system of coupled variational equations $\mathscr{P}^j_{\mathrm{sta}}$, $\mathscr{P}^j_{\mathrm{adj}}$ and $\mathscr{P}^j_{\mathrm{opt}}$. This procedure is described in Algorithm 1. The fields $(\cdot)^{\{k\}}$ correspond to the fields $(\cdot)$ at the k-th iteration. The parameters σ^j, being adjusted dynamically, represent the step sizes for the j-th HB iteration of each optimization procedure. A tolerance parameter ξ is prescribed to test for convergence and exit the algorithm, if necessary. Spatial discretization of the equations described in the present section and the numerical methods applied to solve the aforementioned problems are as presented in [6].

Algorithm 1. Multiple steepest descent optimization with dynamic step sizes

---

   Input : $\alpha, \beta, \beta_1 > 0$, n ▷ Optimization parameters and harmonics n

        $(u^j)^{\{0\}}, (g^j)^{\{0\}}, (p^j)^{\{0\}}, u^j_{\mathbf{obs}}$ ▷ Initial guesses $(\cdot)^{\{0\}}$ and target fields

   Output : $(u^j)^{\{k\}}$, $(p^j)^{\{k\}}$ ▷ Flow fields at last iteration k

1: **procedure** DYNAMICDATAASSIMILATION$(u^{\{0\}}, g^{\{0\}}, u_{\mathbf{obs}}, N)$

2:    $\xi \leftarrow 10^{-8}$, $k \leftarrow 0$ and $\sigma^j \leftarrow 1$ for $j = 1, 2, \cdots, N$

3:    **for** $j \leftarrow 1, N$ **do**

4:       $((u^j)^{\{k\}}, \cdot, \cdot) \leftarrow \mathscr{P}^j_{\mathrm{sta\text{-}lin}}((u^j)^{\{0\}}, (g^j)^{\{0\}}, u^i)$ ▷ Evaluate (3)–(5)

5:       update u^i using new $(u^j)^{\{k\}}$ for $i = j$

6:    $cost^{\{k\}} \leftarrow \mathscr{O}_\Omega(u^{\{k\}}, g^{\{0\}}, u_{\mathbf{obs}})$ ▷ Evaluate cost function $\mathscr{O}_\Omega$

7:    **for** $k \leftarrow 1, \infty$ **do**

8:       $converged \leftarrow$ **true**

9:       **for** $j \leftarrow 1, N$ **do**

10:          $(\cdot, \cdot, (\lambda^j_r)^{\{k\}}) \leftarrow \mathscr{P}^j_{\mathrm{adj}}((u^j)^{\{k-1\}}, u^j_{\mathbf{obs}})$ ▷ Evaluate (6)–(8)

11:          $(s^j)^{\{k\}} \leftarrow \beta_1 \triangle_\tau (g^j)^{\{k-1\}} - \beta(g^j)^{\{k-1\}} - (\lambda^j_r)^{\{k\}}$ ▷ Steepest descent

12:          **repeat**

13:             $(g^j)^{\{k\}} \leftarrow (g^j)^{\{k-1\}} + \sigma^j (s^j)^{\{k\}}$ ▷ Update control using σ^j

14:             $((u^j)^{\{k\}}, \cdot, \cdot) \leftarrow \mathscr{P}^j_{\mathrm{sta\text{-}lin}}((u^j)^{\{k-1\}}, (g^j)^{\{k\}}, u^i)$

15:             $cost^{\{k\}} \leftarrow \mathscr{O}_{\mathrm{T}}(u^{\{k\}}, g^{\{k\}}, u_{\mathbf{obs}})$

16:             **if** $cost^{\{k\}} \geq cost^{\{k-1\}}$ **then** $\sigma^j \leftarrow 0.5\sigma^j$

17:          **until** $cost^{\{k\}} < cost^{\{k-1\}}$

18:          **if** $(|cost^{\{k\}} - cost^{\{k-1\}}|)/(cost^{\{k\}}) > \xi$ **then**

19:             $\sigma^j \leftarrow 1.5\sigma^j$ & $converged \leftarrow$ **false**

20:          update u^i using new $(u^j)^{\{k\}}$ for $i = j$

21:       **if** $(converged)$ **then return** $(u^j)^{\{k\}}$, $(p^j)^{\{k\}}$ for $j = 1 \cdots N$

---

3   Validation

Numerical computations are performed using computational mesh geometries denoted as $\mathbf{M_2}$, $\mathbf{M_4}$ and $\mathbf{M_7}$, with different numbers of cells, 215 000, 440 000 and 750 000 respectively. The mesh $\mathbf{M_7}$ will be referred to as the world domain, whereas the meshes $\mathbf{M_2}$ and $\mathbf{M_4}$ represent the MRI and CFD domains respectively. In the present section, a reference solution was numerically generated in the world domain $\mathbf{M_7}$, as described in [6], to serve as the ground truth for validation purposes. To test the proposed FS-DDA approach, $n = 12$ number of modes were considered, at which the HB treatment has proven to be satisfactorily accurate [6]. First, the reference solution in the world domain (mesh $\mathbf{M_7}$) was sampled at $N = 2n+1 = 25$ equidistantly placed time instants and the samples were mapped into the MRI domain (mesh $\mathbf{M_2}$) using linear interpolation. Second, an artificial noise with an isotropic VENC of 0.75 m/s and an SNR of 10 (see [7] for more details) was added to the flow fields in the MRI domain and the noisy samples were then mapped from $\mathbf{M_2}$ into the CFD domain $\mathbf{M_4}$, where the computational simulations were performed. Figure 1 illustrates these steps.

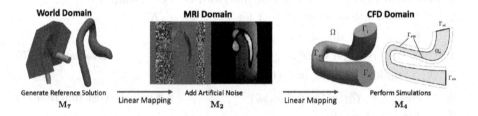

Fig. 1. Preparations for the validation of the proposed approach

Let u_{snr} denote the noisy field in $\mathbf{M_4}$. For FS-DDA, Algorithm 1 was executed with input parameters $(u^{\{0\}} = u_{\mathrm{snr}},\ g^{\{0\}} = u_{\mathrm{snr}}$ on $\Gamma_i,\ u_{\mathrm{obs}} = u_{\mathrm{snr}},\ N = 25)$ resulting in the flow field $u_{\mathrm{hb}}^{\mathrm{opt}}$ (adopting HB into optimization). Flow matching was performed in Ω_2, a contracted domain at a distance of at least 2 mm from Γ_w. Optimization parameters α, β and β_1 were set to 1, 10^{-5} and 10^{-8} respectively. In addition, the HB method was employed as a forward simulation without adopting the assimilation process, resulting in the flow field u_{hb}. Both computed fields are compared with a reference solution (ground truth data u_r) in terms of normalized root mean square error $\mathrm{nRMSE}^X(u_c, u_r) =$ $\left(\frac{100}{\operatorname*{avr}_{T,X}|u_r|}\right)\sqrt{\frac{1}{V_X \cdot T}\int_{\mathbb{T}}\int_X |u_c - u_r|^2\, dX\, dt}$, where X is a domain with volume V_X,

and the flow direction error $\mathrm{FDE}^X(u_c, u_r) = \sqrt{\frac{1}{V_X \cdot T}\int_{\mathbb{T}}\int_X \left(1 - \frac{u_c \cdot u_r}{|u_c||u_r|}\right)^2\, dX\, dt}$.

For the clinically relevant parameters, we are interested in the performance of the solvers at near-wall locations and in the close proximity of the inlet. Hence, for the evaluation of the errors nRMSE^X and FDE^X, we define the domain $X = E_2^4 \subset \Omega$, which is within 4cm proximity of the inlet and within a distance of 2 mm from the wall boundary. In addition, the errors were also evaluated in Ω. Under these conditions, the numerical results are as follows:

(x, y)	$\text{nRMSE}^{E_2^4}(x, y)$	$\text{FDE}^{E_2^4}(x, y)$	$\text{nRMSE}^{\Omega}(x, y)$	$\text{FDE}^{\Omega}(x, y)$
(u_{snr}, u_r)	16.76%	0.367	6.90%	0.166
(u_{hb}, u_r)	3.75%	0.095	1.66%	0.042
$(u_{\text{hb}}^{\text{opt}}, u_r)$	2.39%	0.055	1.59%	0.027

It can be observed that, compared with the results obtained from the HB method as a forward simulation, there is a significant improvement in the outcome provided by FS-DDA in the close proximity of the inlet. This is a remarkable finding for the improvement of the flow field, especially at the aortic root. The optimization process lasted for 54 iterations and the WCT was 943 s.

Dynamic Data Assimilation Using 4D Flow MRI Acquisition. For the optimal control problem, the proposed approach was tested in a realistic scenario using flow data gathered from real 4D flow MRI scans, as described in [6]. It is worth mentioning that the preprocessing steps detailed in [7], were also applied in the present section. This includes a projection of the observed flow field over a divergence-free space, which is useful in two ways. First, it recovers back the solenoidal property of the flow field, which is usually lost after the application of both the outlier detection scheme and the immediate mapping of the observations from MRI domain into the computational mesh domain (see [7]). Secondly, it allows to start the computations with a solenoidal initial guess.

Flow patterns obtained from both methods, FS-DDA and HB, were first compared with the MRI data by visual inspection. Figure 2 shows the magnitudes of the velocity fields, obtained from the noisy MRI measurements (in the middle) and from the computations using both the FS-DDA method (on the left) and the HB method (on the right) respectively. The presented slices correspond to the time instant at peak systole. One slice was placed at the aortic root and was oriented such that the velocity profiles in the close proximity of the inlet are clearly visible. Another slice was placed at the aortic arch to additionally illustrate the obtained flow patterns at a moderate distance from the inlet. It can be observed that the noise-free flow field obtained from the assimilation process is fairly close to the noisy flow field measured with 4D flow MRI, whereas the flow field obtained from a conventional forward simulation (without the optimization of the velocity components), is largely different compared to the measurements.

Since the observations are obtained from real 4D flow MRI acquisition, the obtained noisy flow field cannot be regarded as the ground truth. Therefore, the flow fields obtained from both methods were quantitatively compared with each other to demonstrate the extent of their difference from each other. In the whole domain, Ω, evaluation of the errors yielded $\text{nRMSE}^{\Omega}(u_{\text{hb}}, u_{\text{hb}}^{\text{opt}}) = 21.66\%$ and $\text{FDE}^{\Omega}(u_{\text{hb}}, u_{\text{hb}}^{\text{opt}}) = 0.229$, whereas in the close proximity of the inlet and at near-wall locations, the errors were $\text{nRMSE}^{E_2^4}(u_{\text{hb}}, u_{\text{hb}}^{\text{opt}}) = 30.08\%$ and $\text{FDE}^{E_2^4}(u_{\text{hb}}, u_{\text{hb}}^{\text{opt}}) = 0.314$. Notably, the better qualitative agreement between the observations and the optimized solution, along with the quantitatively significant differences between the optimized solution and the predictions from conventional forwards CFD simulation, support the fact that the optimization delivers a better solution when compared with the conventional CFD approach.

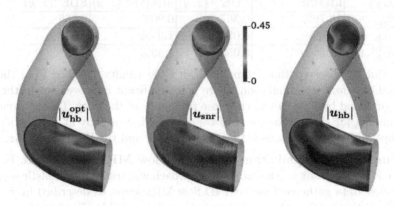

Fig. 2. Slices for the magnitudes of different velocity fields at the aortic root and arch.

4   Conclusion

This work has introduced the Fourier spectral dynamic data assimilation approach as a new method for an inverse problem to perform variational adjoint-based assimilation for pulsatile blood flow simulations. The method is being reported for the first time in computational hemodynamics and brings remarkable improvement in terms of computational effort without exhibiting deterioration of the approximate solution. This work enables accurate characterization of the dynamic flow field in quite feasible and practicable wall clock times, which are otherwise difficult or impossible to be achieved using currently available dynamic data assimilation strategies relying on traditional time-stepping schemes.

The proposed algorithm was examined in detail to estimate the efficiency of the methodology for reconstructing the blood flow at the aortic root and in near-wall regions. The new method proved to deliver physically consistent flow fields, with substantial reduction of noise present in the 4D flow MRI measurements, outperforming the predictive capabilities of conventional CFD approaches. The flow field is considerably improved at the aortic root, which is one of the most important clinically relevant locations for the development of pathological alterations of the anatomical structures underlying the arterial wall.

This work does not include the deformation of the arterial walls but is a starting point for the adaptation of contact modelling approaches for fluid-structure interaction studies. Hence, this investigation is the first of a series that will address the deformation and dynamic response of the arterial walls. The novel approach provides a systematic strategy to improve the model predictions regarding clinically relevant hemodynamic data, such as the wall shear stresses, and reveals a great potential for clinical applicability.

References

1. Aupy, G., Herrmann, J.: Periodicity in optimal hierarchical checkpointing schemes for adjoint computations. Optim. Methods Softw. **32**(3), 594–624 (2017). https://doi.org/10.1080/10556788.2016.1230612

2. Funke, S.W., Nordaas, M., Evju, Ø., Alnæs, M.S., Mardal, K.A.: Variational data assimilation for transient blood flow simulations: cerebral aneurysms as an illustrative example. Int. J. Numer. Method. Biomed. Eng. **35**(1), e3152 (2019). https://doi.org/10.1002/cnm.3152

3. Griewank, A., Walther, A.: Algorithm 799: revolve: an implementation of checkpointing for the reverse or adjoint mode of computational differentiation. ACM Trans. Math. Softw. **26**(1), 19–45 (2000). https://doi.org/10.1145/347837.347846

4. Guerra, T., Sequeira, A., Tiago, J.: Existence of optimal boundary control for the navier-stokes equations with mixed boundary conditions. Port. Math. **72**(1), 267–283 (2015). https://doi.org/10.4171/PM/1968

5. Gunzburger, M.D., Manservisi, S.: The velocity tracking problem for navier-stokes flows with boundary control. SIAM J. Control Optim. **39**(2), 594–634 (2000). https://doi.org/10.1137/S0363012999353771

6. Koltukluoğlu, T.S.: Harmonic balance techniques in cardiovascular fluid mechanics. In: Shen, D., et al. (ed.) Medical Image Computing and Computer-Assisted Intervention, vol. 11765, pp. 486–494 (2019)

7. Koltukluoğlu, T.S., Blanco, P.J.: Boundary control in computational haemodynamics. J. Fluid Mech. **847**, 329–364 (2018). https://doi.org/10.1017/jfm.2018.329

8. Wang, Q., Moin, P., Iaccarino, G.: Minimal repetition dynamic checkpointing algorithm for unsteady adjoint calculation. SIAM J. Sci. Comput. **31**(4), 2549–2567 (2009). https://doi.org/10.1137/080727890

Quality Control-Driven Image Segmentation Towards Reliable Automatic Image Analysis in Large-Scale Cardiovascular Magnetic Resonance Aortic Cine Imaging

Evan Hann[1]([⊠]) [ID], Luca Biasiolli[1], Qiang Zhang[1], Iulia A. Popescu[1],
Konrad Werys[1], Elena Lukaschuk[1], Valentina Carapella[1],
Jose M. Paiva[2], Nay Aung[2], Jennifer J. Rayner[1], Kenneth Fung[2],
Henrike Puchta[1], Mihir M. Sanghvi[2], Niall O. Moon[1],
Katharine E. Thomas[1], Vanessa M. Ferreira[1], Steffen E. Petersen[2],
Stefan Neubauer[1], and Stefan K. Piechnik[1]

[1] Oxford Centre for Clinical Magnetic Resonance Research (OCMR),
Radcliffe Department of Medicine, University of Oxford, Oxford, UK
evan.hann@cardiov.ox.ac.uk
[2] William Harvey Research Institute, NIHR Barts Biomedical Research Centre,
Queen Mary University of London, London, UK

Abstract. Recent progress in fully-automated image segmentation has enabled efficient extraction of clinical parameters in large-scale clinical imaging studies, reducing laborious manual processing. However, the current state-of-the-art automatic image segmentation may still fail, especially when it comes to atypical cases. Visual inspection of segmentation quality is often required, thus diminishing the improvements in efficiency. This drives an increasing need to enhance the overall data processing pipeline with robust automatic quality scoring, especially for clinical applications. We present a novel quality control-driven (QCD) framework to provide reliable segmentation using a set of different neural networks. In contrast to the prior segmentation and quality scoring methods, the proposed framework automatically selects the optimal segmentation on-the-fly from the multiple candidate segmentations available, directly utilizing the inherent Dice similarity coefficient (DSC) predictions. We trained and evaluated the framework on a large-scale cardiovascular magnetic resonance aortic cine image sequences from the UK Biobank Study. The framework achieved segmentation accuracy of mean DSC at 0.966, mean prediction error of DSC within 0.015, and mean error in estimating lumen area ≤ 17.6 mm^2 for both ascending aorta and proximal descending aorta. This novel QCD framework successfully integrates the automatic image segmentation along with detection of critical errors on a per-case basis, paving the way towards reliable fully-automatic extraction of clinical parameters for large-scale imaging studies.

Keywords: Quality control · Segmentation · Convolutional neural networks

© Springer Nature Switzerland AG 2019
D. Shen et al. (Eds.): MICCAI 2019, LNCS 11765, pp. 750–758, 2019.
https://doi.org/10.1007/978-3-030-32245-8_83

1 Introduction

Aortic distensibility (AoD) is a clinical parameter which measures the bio-elastic function of the aorta. It can serve as an independent predictor for cardiovascular morbidity and mortality [1]. In current clinical practice, this requires cardiovascular magnetic resonance (CMR) transaxial cine images at the level of the pulmonary artery, with manual contouring of the cross-sectional lumen area of the ascending aorta (AA) and the proximal descending aorta (PDA) over a cardiac cycle, from diastole to systole.

Manual segmentation is time-consuming, labor-intensive, and subject to inter and intra-observer variability, especially in large-scale imaging studies, such as the UK Biobank (UKBB), aiming to acquire CMR images from 100,000 participants [2]. Large-scale studies can benefit from automated image segmentation, achieve not only efficient image segmentation, but also improved consistency and objectivity for diagnosis.

However, the issue of quality control needs to be addressed before deployment of automated segmentation to large-scale imaging studies and clinical applications. The current state-of-the-art segmentation methods can still fail [3], especially in cases affected by poor image quality or pathologies. It is important to detect any critical inaccuracies, which can potentially lead to misdiagnosis or incorrect research conclusion. Current clinical practice of segmentation quality control requires visual inspection, which diminishes the benefits of efficiency brought forth by automated segmentation. This poses a demand for automated quality control to be integrated in fully-automated image analysis pipelines, to efficiently and reliably extract clinical parameters.

1.1 Related Works

Fully-automatic aortic image segmentation methods without quality control have been proposed [4, 5]. A recurrent neural network (RNN) in [4] was trained on 400 scans with label propagation and weighted loss technique to mitigate the sparse annotation problem, as only systolic and diastolic frames were manually annotated in each image sequence. Subsequently, the trained RNN was evaluated in a small-scale dataset of 100 scans. Another approach was proposed in [5] using random forest (RF) localization of the aorta, with a large-scale (3900 image sequences) evaluation. First, potential locations of AA and PDA were detected using Circular Hough Transform (CHT), followed by RF classifications based on 18 spatial, intensity, and shape features to select the most probable locations of AA and PDA. This fully-automatic localization method can initialize semi-automatic segmentation methods. It was tested in the UKBB imaging study to achieve detection accuracy over 99% for both AA and PDA. However, neither approach included a quality control mechanism to predict the accuracy of segmentations.

Automatic Dice metrics predictions have been proposed to address the segmentation quality control in the absence of manual segmentation. Kohlberger et al. [6] proposed an automated quality scoring of segmentation using machine learning with 42 handcrafted features evaluated against Dice similarity coefficient (DSC). More recently, a framework based on Reverse Classification Accuracy (RCA) [7, 8] was proposed to predict DSC and other metrics for CMR image segmentation. The RCA framework requires registration of the input image and the corresponding segmentation to a database of reference images, with available ground truth segmentations. Robinson et al. [9] proposed a simple CNN-based method trained to predict the DSC of segmentations generated by RF-based algorithms. Another CNN-based framework [10] was proposed to predict segmentation DSC using Monte Carlo sampling. With the use of random dropout unit at test time, the CNN generates several different segmentations for the same input to predict segmentation quality. However, in these prior works, DSC predictions have not been used to optimize segmentation performance.

1.2   Contributions

In this work, we present a novel quality control-driven (QCD) image analysis framework, which utilizes multiple neural networks to integrate segmentation and quality scoring on a per-case basis. The QCD framework automatically selects of the best final segmentation from multiple candidate models based on accurate DSC predictions, rather than only passive reporting as in [6–10]. We evaluate the effectiveness of QCD on a large-scale dataset of aortic cine image sequences from the UKBB imaging study.

2   Methods and Material

2.1   Candidate Segmentation Models

Multiple Convolutional Neural Networks: U-Nets [11], with different depths, are implemented to perform image segmentations of AA and PDA. In this work, we use 6 U-Nets with number of skip connections from 1 to 6 (U-Net 1 to U-Net 6 in Fig. 1B). Such differences in the hyperparameters are intended to introduce variation in segmentation performance, which is exploited for segmentation quality control.

Combined Segmentations: Statistical rank filters are used to combine multiple U-Net segmentations to generate additional segmentations (Fig. 1D) for improved robustness at small additional computation cost. In contrast to a typical rank filter which processes a single image, the rank filters used in this work are applied in a pixel-wise fashion across all 6 U-Net segmentations, such that

$$CS_t(u, v) = \begin{cases} 1, & \sum_{net \in Nets} S_{net}(u, v) \geq t \\ 0, & otherwise. \end{cases} \tag{1}$$

where CS_t is a combined segmentation with thresholding parameter $t \in \{1, 2, \ldots, 6\}$, S_{net} is the segmentation output by a U-Net net, and (u, v) is a pixel in the segmentation. Hence, for each input of aortic image, there are in total 12 candidate segmentations including U-Nets and combined segmentations for each aorta section.

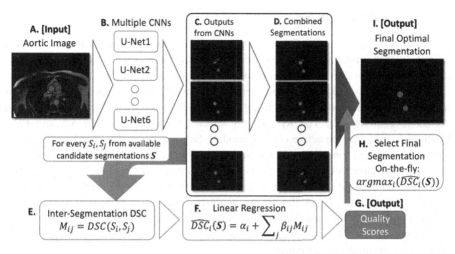

Fig. 1. The overview of the quality control-driven (QCD) framework, which feeds the same aortic CMR image frame (A) to multiple convolutional neural networks (U-Net 1–6) (B). Multiple segmentations (C) generated by the U-Nets are summed up and thresholded to form additional combined segmentations (D). The inter-segmentation DSC matrix (E) is calculated among all segmentation candidates, and fed into a previously established regression model (F) to obtain individual DSC prediction (G) for each candidate. The segmentation with the highest predicted DSC (H) among the candidates is selected on-the-fly as the final segmentation (I).

2.2 Quality Scoring and Quality Control-Driven Segmentation

Automatic Quality Scoring predicts $DSC(\cdot, S_{GT})$ by comparing multiple candidate segmentations S (Fig. 1C and D) in the absence of the manual segmentation S_{GT}. For each segmentation S_i, DSCs with other candidates S_j of the same input are calculated to form the inter-segmentation DSC matrix $M_{ij} = DSC(S_i, S_j)$ (Fig. 1E), and then used to predict $DSC(S_i, S_{GT})$ through multiple linear regression $\widehat{DSC}_i(S) = \alpha_i + \sum_j \beta_{ij} M_{ij}$ (Fig. 1F), where regression parameters α_i and β_{ij} are optimized for each segmentation model i using the training data. The prediction exploits differences among candidate segmentations, which tend to diverge in more difficult cases (e.g. affected by poor image quality), for which lower predicted DSCs are anticipated. In contrast, a higher predicted DSC is expected when there is higher agreement among candidates.

Quality Control-Driven Segmentation uses the DSC prediction to select the best final segmentation (Fig. 1I). For each aorta section in an aortic image frame, 12 candidate segmentations are generated. Each of these candidates is assigned a predicted DSC through the automatic quality scoring. Then, the framework selects the final segmentation with the highest predicted DSC (Fig. 1H) from all candidates S on-the-fly: $argmax_i\left(\widehat{DSC}_i(S)\right)$. This is to further improve accuracy and robustness of segmentation by choosing the predicted best on a per-case basis.

2.3   Data and Annotations

The dataset comprises of 5028 CMR aortic cine image sequences acquired in the UKBB. In each image sequence, 100 frames across a cardiac cycle were acquired, with pixel dimension of 240×196 and resolution of 1.58×1.58 mm^2.

The manually-validated segmentations of AA and PDA were generated prior to this work in a semi-automatic fashion using both random forest (RF) localization [5] and 2D active contour [12]. The RF method selected the most probable AA and PDA locations to initialize the active contour models. Segmentations generated by the active contours were then visually validated and manually corrected by 13 image analysts.

Due to the large volume of the dataset (502,800 image frames in total), only frames at systole and diastole ($\sim$15 out of 100 frames) were manually validated and corrected to reduce the workload on the image analysts. This presents a sparse annotation problem, similar to that reported in [4]. To mitigate this problem, all generated segmentations are used to train the QCD framework, but only manually-validated segmentations are used for evaluation.

2.4   Evaluation

The objectives of the evaluation are 3-fold: (1) to evaluate the segmentation accuracy of all segmentation models, including the QCD segmentation, using Dice metrics (DSC); (2) to evaluate the accuracy of quality scoring on all candidate segmentations, with varying quality, using mean absolute error (MAE) and Pearson correlation (r) between the ground truth DSC and the predicted DSC; (3) to evaluate the accuracy of segmentation, quality scoring, and clinical parameter estimation using a large-scale testing dataset, 10 times larger than the training dataset. Agreement in aortic lumen area (number of pixels in segmentation scaled by pixel spacing) estimated with automated and manual annotations is evaluated in terms of MAE. The evaluation is performed in the validation dataset (400 image sequences) for objectives 1 and 2, and the testing dataset (4228 image sequences) for objective 3.

3   Experiments and Results

3.1   Implementation

The framework was implemented in Python, with TensorFlow. Similar to [4], 400 CMR image sequences were used to train the framework. Each of the 6 U-Nets was independently trained in a batch size of 50 frames for 201,200 iterations. The training took 71 h in total on a desktop computer with a Nvidia Titan X GPU. On average, the framework took 67 s to segment and quality score cine of 100 cine frames.

3.2   Performance of Segmentation Models

All segmentation models were evaluated for DSC performance in the validation dataset (Table 1). QCD achieved the highest DSC for AA (0.967) and PDA (0.966) segmentation. Similar segmentation accuracy was also achieved by CS3, which was selected by QCD as the best candidate over 60% of the cases. In addition, CS2-5 obtained higher DSCs than any individual U-Nets, showing the benefit of combing multiple neural networks. Moreover, the results (Table 1) showed that QCD obtained the highest percentages ($\geq 99.7\%$) of segmentations achieving DSC over 0.9, offering additional robustness by selecting the best candidate segmentation on a per-case basis. QCD had the best overall segmentation performance in the validation data.

3.3   Quality Scoring of Segmentations

The segmentation quality scoring was evaluated for all candidate segmentations in the validation dataset. The results showed high agreement between DSC and predicted DSC for both AA and PDA segmentation, with MAE of 0.009 for AA and 0.012 for PDA, and Pearson correlations of over 0.9 for both AA and PDA. The scatter plots (Fig. 2) showed that DSC and predicted DSC met along the identity lines, indicating accurate DSC predictions for segmentations of varying quality.

Table 1. Mean DSC between manual and automatic segmentation, with percentages of segmentations achieving DSC over 0.9, for each model evaluated in the validation data

Model	Mean DSC		Percentage of DSC > 0.9	
	AA	PDA	AA	PDA
U-Net 1	0.918	0.926	77.4	83.7
U-Net 2	0.949	0.957	97.5	98.9
U-Net 3	0.954	0.961	99.4	99.3
U-Net 4	0.951	0.955	98.8	98.7
U-Net 5	0.953	0.955	99.4	98.5
U-Net 6	0.953	0.956	99.5	99.0
CS1	0.937	0.942	93.7	92.5
CS2	0.964	0.964	98.8	99.2
CS3	**0.967**	**0.966**	99.6	99.6
CS4	0.966	**0.966**	99.6	99.6
CS5	0.958	0.962	99.3	99.4
CS6	0.924	0.934	85.8	90.3
QCD	**0.967**	**0.966**	**99.9**	**99.7**

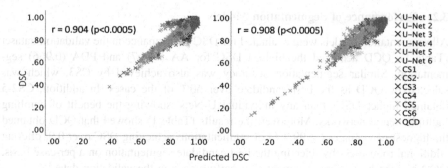

Fig. 2. Scatter plots of predicted DSC (x-axis) and DSC (y-axis) for AA (left) and PDA (right) in the validation data, with correlation coefficients (r), and p-values for all data points reported. Overall good DSC prediction for all candidate segmentations, with varying quality. Low DSC scores of poor segmentations output by U-Net 1 and CS6 were accurately predicted.

3.4 Large-Scale Testing

The QCD framework was tested on 4228 image sequences and performed as consistently in the large-scale dataset as in the smaller validation dataset. The segmentation performance, with mean DSC of 0.966 for both AA and PDA (Table 2), was comparable to the validation results. The lumen area estimation was in high agreement with the manual annotations with MAE less than 17.6 mm^2 for both AA and PDA (Table 2). Two examples of lumen area curves are shown in Fig. 3. Both curves show consistent lumen area estimation with manual annotations at systole and diastole. In addition, Fig. 4 shows an example in the testing data to demonstrate how differences in candidate segmentations influence the DSC predictions in the QCD framework.

Table 2. Evaluation results of QCD framework in the test dataset of 4228 image sequences

Label	Mean DSC	MAE in DSC prediction	MAE in lumen area (mm^2)
AA	0.966	0.011	17.6
PDA	0.966	0.015	10.5

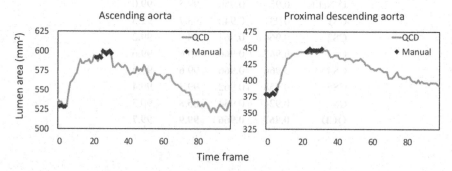

Fig. 3. Lumen area curves for AA (left) and PDA (right) estimated by QCD (blue), compared with manually validated ground truth (red; only in end-diastolic and end-systolic frames). (Color figure online)

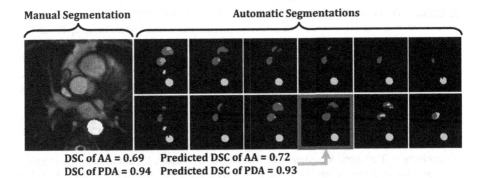

Fig. 4. Example of a poorly-planned aortic cine image (too far below the main pulmonary artery). Manual segmentation (left large panel), with multiple automatic candidate segmentations of AA (red masks) and PDA (blue masks) are shown. For the final selected segmentation (outlined in red), the predicted DSC of AA segmentation is low (0.72) due to apparent differences among candidate segmentations, as AA was affected by poor image quality; most of the automatic segmentation includes parts of the right ventricle. In contrast, PDA was less affected; the predicted DSC was higher (0.93), as there was higher agreement among candidate models. (Color figure online)

4 Conclusions

In this paper, we presented a novel quality control-driven segmentation framework comprising of different neural networks. In the absence of manual annotations, the framework exploits differences among candidate segmentations to predict Dice metrics (DSC), which are exploited to select the optimal final segmentation on a per-case basis on-the-fly. Evaluated on a large-scale dataset of aortic cine images, the framework achieved high accuracy in segmentation, quality scoring, and lumen area estimation. This paves the way for fully-automated image analysis pipeline for reliable extraction of clinical parameters for large-scale clinical studies. Future work will cover a wider range of applications in multiple organs and imaging modalities.

Acknowledgements. This study was supported by the National Institute for Health Research (NIHR) Oxford Biomedical Research Centre at The Oxford University Hospitals, University of Oxford, UK. Authors acknowledge support from the British Heart Foundation Centre of Research Excellence, and donation of GPU from NVIDIA Corp.

References

1. Redheuil, A., et al.: Proximal aortic distensibility is an independent predictor of all-cause mortality and incident CV events: the MESA study. J. Am. Coll. Cardiol. **64**, 2619–2629 (2014). https://doi.org/10.1016/j.jacc.2014.09.060
2. Petersen, S.E., et al.: Imaging in population science: cardiovascular magnetic resonance in 100,000 participants of UK Biobank - rationale, challenges and approaches. J. Cardiovasc. Magn. Reson. **50**, 46 (2013). https://doi.org/10.1186/1532-429X-15-46

758   E. Hann et al.

3. Bernard, O., et al.: Deep learning techniques for automatic MRI cardiac multi-structures segmentation and diagnosis: is the problem solved? IEEE Trans. Med. Imaging **37**, 2514–2525 (2018). https://doi.org/10.1109/TMI.2018.2837502

4. Bai, W., et al.: Recurrent neural networks for aortic image sequence segmentation with sparse annotations. In: Frangi, A.F., Schnabel, J.A., Davatzikos, C., Alberola-López, C., Fichtinger, G. (eds.) MICCAI 2018. LNCS, vol. 11073, pp. 586–594. Springer, Cham (2018). https://doi.org/10.1007/978-3-030-00937-3_67

5. Biasiolli, L., et al.: Automated localization and quality control of the aorta in cine CMR can significantly accelerate processing of the UK Biobank population data. PLoS One **14**, e0212272 (2019). https://doi.org/10.1371/journal.pone.0212272

6. Kohlberger, T., Singh, V., Alvino, C., Bahlmann, C., Grady, L.: Evaluating segmentation error without ground truth. In: Ayache, N., Delingette, H., Golland, P., Mori, K. (eds.) MICCAI 2012. LNCS, vol. 7510, pp. 528–536. Springer, Heidelberg (2012). https://doi.org/10.1007/978-3-642-33415-3_65

7. Robinson, R., Valindria, V.V., Bai, W., Suzuki, H., Matthews, P.M., Page, C., Rueckert, D., Glocker, B.: Automatic quality control of cardiac MRI segmentation in large-scale population imaging. In: Descoteaux, M., Maier-Hein, L., Franz, A., Jannin, P., Collins, D.L., Duchesne, S. (eds.) MICCAI 2017. LNCS, vol. 10433, pp. 720–727. Springer, Cham (2017). https://doi.org/10.1007/978-3-319-66182-7_82

8. Robinson, R., et al.: Automated quality control in image segmentation: application to the UK Biobank cardiac MR imaging study. J. Cardiovasc. Magn. Reson. **21**, 18 (2019). https://doi.org/10.1186/s12968-019-0523-x

9. Robinson, R., et al.: Subject-level prediction of segmentation failure using real-time convolutional neural nets. In: MIDL, pp. 3–5 (2018)

10. Roy, A.G., Conjeti, S., Navab, N., Wachinger, C.: Inherent brain segmentation quality control from fully ConvNet Monte Carlo sampling. In: Frangi, A.F., Schnabel, J.A., Davatzikos, C., Alberola-López, C., Fichtinger, G. (eds.) MICCAI 2018. LNCS, vol. 11070, pp. 664–672. Springer, Cham (2018). https://doi.org/10.1007/978-3-030-00928-1_75

11. Ronneberger, O., Fischer, P., Brox, T.: U-Net: convolutional networks for biomedical image segmentation. In: Navab, N., Hornegger, J., Wells, W.M., Frangi, A.F. (eds.) MICCAI 2015. LNCS, vol. 9351, pp. 234–241. Springer, Cham (2015). https://doi.org/10.1007/978-3-319-24574-4_28

12. Kass, M., Witkin, A., Terzopoulos, D.: Snakes: active contour models. Int. J. Comput. Vis. **1**, 321–331 (1988). https://doi.org/10.1007/BF00133570

HFA-Net: 3D Cardiovascular Image Segmentation with Asymmetrical Pooling and Content-Aware Fusion

Hao Zheng$^{(\boxtimes)}$, Lin Yang, Jun Han, Yizhe Zhang, Peixian Liang, Zhuo Zhao, Chaoli Wang, and Danny Z. Chen

Department of Computer Science and Engineering, University of Notre Dame, Notre Dame, IN 46556, USA
hzheng3@nd.edu

Abstract. Automatic and accurate cardiovascular image segmentation is important in clinical applications. However, due to ambiguous borders and subtle structures (e.g., thin myocardium), parsing fine-grained structures in 3D cardiovascular images is very challenging. In this paper, we propose a novel deep *heterogeneous feature aggregation network* (HFA-Net) to fully exploit complementary information from multiple views of 3D cardiac data. First, we utilize asymmetrical 3D kernels and pooling to obtain heterogeneous features in parallel encoding paths. Thus, from a specific view, distinguishable features are extracted and indispensable contextual information is kept (rather than quickly diminished after symmetrical convolution and pooling operations). Then, we employ a content-aware multi-planar fusion module to aggregate meaningful features to boost segmentation performance. Further, to reduce the model size, we devise a new DenseVoxNet model by sparsifying residual connections, which can be trained in an end-to-end manner. We show the effectiveness of our new HFA-Net on the 2016 HVSMR and 2017 MM-WHS CT datasets, achieving state-of-the-art performance. In addition, HFA-Net obtains competitive results on the 2017 AAPM CT dataset, especially on segmenting subtle structures among multi-objects with large variations, illustrating the robustness of our new segmentation approach.

1 Introduction

Cardiovascular diseases are a leading cause of death globally. Segmenting the whole heart in cardiovascular images is a prerequisite for morphological and pathological analysis, disease diagnosis, and surgical planning [6]. However, automatic and accurate cardiovascular image segmentation remains very challenging due to large variations in different subjects, missing/ambiguous borders, and inhomogeneous appearance and image quality (e.g., see Fig. 1(a, b)).

Electronic supplementary material The online version of this chapter (https://doi.org/10.1007/978-3-030-32245-8_84) contains supplementary material, which is available to authorized users.

D. Shen et al. (Eds.): MICCAI 2019, LNCS 11765, pp. 759–767, 2019.
https://doi.org/10.1007/978-3-030-32245-8_84

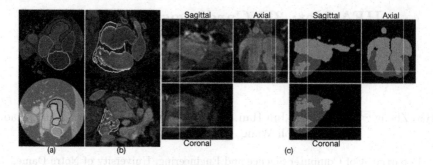

Fig. 1. Examples of cardiovascular images from (a) the MM-WHS CT dataset [14] in the axial plane and (b) the HVSMR dataset [6] in the sagittal plane. (c) Myocardium boundaries in the axial plane are easier to recognize.

Recent studies showed that deep learning based methods [2–4,11,12] can learn robust contextual and semantic features and achieve state-of-the-art segmentation performance. 3D fully convolutional networks (FCNs) are a mainstream approach for cardiac segmentation due to their ability to integrate both inter- and intra-slice information in 3D images. However, two key factors have not been well explored: (1) the imaging qualities in different anatomical planes are not the same, and thus the degrees of segmentation difficulty from different views are unequal; (2) subtle structures (e.g., myocardium, pulmonary artery) have different orientations in different anatomical planes. Symmetrical convolutional and pooling operations may cause quick diminishment of subtle structures or boundaries, incurring segmentation errors. As shown in Fig. 1(c), myocardium boundaries in the axial plane are easier to recognize; with asymmetrical pooling along the longitudinal axis, more complementary inter-slice information can be kept which in return benefits segmentation in the axial plane.

Many recent studies tried to tackle the anisotropic issue of 3D biomedical images. But still, they could not segment myocardium or pulmonary artery well. Known methods that explored anisotropic 3D kernels in FCNs can be categorized into two types. (1) The methods in [2,8] focused on designing repeatable cell structures and replaced all 3D convolutions systematically, called *short-range asymmetrical cell*. However, symmetrical pooling was used and deep features were fused periodically (with distinctive features vanishing quickly). (2) The methods in [3,5] dealt with the anisotropic problem in 3D images using 2D FCNs to extract intra-slice features and 3D FCNs to aggregate inter-slice features. But, they did not exploit the fact that complementary information in the other planes (xz- and yz-planes) can also benefit the xy-plane, especially in less anisotropic 3D data (e.g., when the spacing resolution in the z-axis is only 3–5× larger than that of the x- and y-axes).

To address the above two key factors, we propose a new *heterogeneous feature aggregation network* (HFA-Net), which is able to fully exploit complementary information in multiple views of 3D cardiac images and aggregate heterogeneous features to boost segmentation performance. To handle the issue in [2,8], we

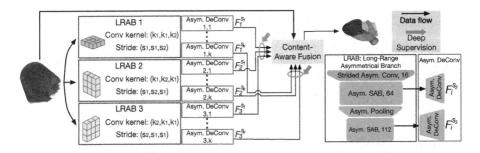

Fig. 2. An overview of our new HFA-Net framework.

utilize long-range asymmetrical branches to maintain distinguishable features associated with a specific view. Besides asymmetrical convolutional operations, we also apply asymmetrical pooling operations to maintain spatial resolution in the other planes. To address the issue in [3,5], we utilize parallel encoding paths to extract heterogeneous features from multiple geometric views of the 3D data (i.e., the axial, coronal, and sagittal planes). There is a good chance that an object can be distinguished from at least one of the geometric views. Thus, we encourage richer contextual and semantic features to be extracted. Further, to improve the parameter-performance efficiency and reduce GPU memory usage, we devise a sparsified densely-connected convolutional block for our model, and our HFA-Net thus designed can be trained end-to-end.

Experiments on three public challenge datasets [6,10,14] show that our new method achieves competitive segmentation results over state-of-the-art methods.

2   Method

Our HFA-Net has three main components (see Fig. 2): (1) Long-range asymmetrical branches (LRABs) that preserve subtle structures via asymmetrical convolutions and poolings; (2) a content-aware fusion module (CAFM) that combines multiple asymmetrical branches together, utilizing both raw images and feature maps from LRABs; (3) a new 3D sparse aggregation block (SAB) to reduce GPU memory usage and enable end-to-end training of the entire network.

2.1   Long-Range Asymmetric Branch (LRAB)

A straightforward way to exploit multiple geometric views of 3D images is to replace conventional 3D convolutional (Conv) layers by *short-range asymmetrical cell* (SRAC) [2,8]. As shown in Fig. 3(a), a 3D Conv kernel is decomposed into m parallel streams, each having n pseudo 2D kernels and a corresponding orthogonal pseudo 1D kernel. But, the typical decompositions they exploited are $\{m = 1, 2; n = 1, 2\}$, which may not make the best out of all geometric properties of 3D data. Further, such SRAC only governs the specific layer-wise computation but neglects the outer branch/network level which controls spatial resolution

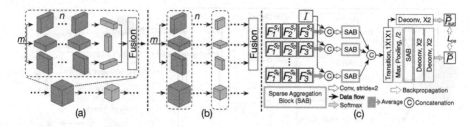

Fig. 3. (a) Short-Range Asymmetric Cell; (b) Long-Range Asymmetric Branch; (c) Content-Aware Fusion Module. I: raw image; $F_i^{s_j}$: feature maps (see Sect. 2.2).

changes. Most importantly, feature maps are added together periodically after each SRAC, which causes homogeneous feature maps in deeper layers and that parallel streams do not benefit richer feature extraction anymore. To address these issues, our method aims to fully exploit all the three orthogonal views and encourage extracting heterogeneous features from different scales. For this goal, we need to carefully design both the layer-level and branch-level operations.

Notation. We denote a 3D Conv layer as $\text{Conv}(\mathcal{K}_{k_1,k_2,k_3}/\mathcal{S}_{s_1,s_2,s_3})$, where k_i and s_i are the kernel size and stride step size in each direction. Conventionally, $k_1 = k_2 = k_3$ and $s_1 = s_2 = s_3$. A 3D kernel $\mathcal{K}_{3,3,3}$ can be decomposed into an SRAC (with $m = 1$ and $n = 1$) by $\mathcal{K}_{3,3,1} \otimes \mathcal{K}_{1,1,3}$, $\mathcal{K}_{3,1,3} \otimes \mathcal{K}_{1,3,1}$, or $\mathcal{K}_{1,3,3} \otimes \mathcal{K}_{3,1,1}$, where $\otimes$ is convolution. Similarly, we denote a 3D deconvolutional (DeConv) layer as $\text{DeConv}(\mathcal{K}_{k_1,k_2,k_3} \times \mathcal{S}_{s_1,s_2,s_3})$. A pooling layer is denoted as $\mathcal{P}_{s_1,s_2,s_3}$.

Figure 3(b) shows the concept of our *long-range asymmetrical branch* (LRAB). We utilize three LRABs ($m = 3$) to operate on three orthogonal geometric views separately, thus increasing the independency among m parallel encoding paths. The original symmetrical $\text{Conv}(\mathcal{K}_{k_a,k_a,k_a}/\mathcal{S}_{s_a,s_a,s_a})$ is replaced by an asymmetrical counterpart in each branch (i.e., $(\mathcal{K}_{k_a,k_a,1}/\mathcal{S}_{s_a,s_a,1})$, $(\mathcal{K}_{k_a,1,k_a}/\mathcal{S}_{s_a,1,s_a})$, or $(\mathcal{K}_{1,k_a,k_a}/\mathcal{S}_{1,s_a,s_a})$). Also, the consecutive 3D Conv kernel $(\mathcal{K}_{k_b,k_b,k_b}/\mathcal{S}_{s_b,s_b,s_b})$ is decomposed in the same orientation in each branch. Besides, since in each LRAB, Conv kernels are along the same orientation, conventional symmetrical pooling is no longer suitable (otherwise, inter-slice features may vanish quickly before being extracted). In our problem, cardiovascular segmentation is highly challenging especially due to the missing/ambiguous boundaries between the regions of interest and background or among various sub-structures. Thus, asymmetrical pooling (i.e., $\mathcal{P}_{s,s,1}$, $\mathcal{P}_{s,1,s}$, or $\mathcal{P}_{1,s,s}$) is utilized to maintain spatial resolution in the orthogonal direction so that there is a bigger chance that subtle distinguishable features can be kept in at least one of the geometric views.

For example, a $T \times T \times T$ tensor after three $\mathcal{P}_{2,2,2}$ becomes a $\frac{T}{8} \times \frac{T}{8} \times \frac{T}{8}$ tensor but becomes $\frac{T}{8} \times \frac{T}{8} \times T$ after three $\mathcal{P}_{2,2,1}$. Hence, additional information of subtle structures along the z-axis is kept and will be utilized by subsequent processing. Observe that the designs in [3,5] can be viewed as special cases of our LRAB since these methods only used (pre-trained) 2D FCN to extract deep feature maps from 3D data slice by slice independently with $m = 1$. Thus, our method is more cautious in heterogeneous feature aggregation. Specifically, as shown in Fig. 2, our first LRAB is composed of stacking layers of $\text{Conv}(\mathcal{K}_{3,3,1}/\mathcal{S}_{2,2,1})$, $\text{SAB}(\mathcal{K}_{3,3,1}/\mathcal{S}_{1,1,1})$, $\mathcal{P}_{2,2,1}$, and $\text{SAB}(\mathcal{K}_{3,3,1}/\mathcal{S}_{1,1,1})$, where $\text{SAB}(\mathcal{K}_{3,3,1}/\mathcal{S}_{1,1,1})$ refers to sparse aggregation block (SAB) composed of stacked $\text{Conv}(\mathcal{K}_{3,3,1}/\mathcal{S}_{1,1,1})$. We will present SAB in Sect. 2.3. In the ith LRAB, feature maps from different scales $(s_j, j = 1, 2, \ldots, k)$ are recovered by asymmetrical DeConv layers accordingly, denoted by $F_i^{s_j}$. We will discuss how to aggregate useful information from these heterogeneous feature maps in Sect. 2.2.

2.2   Content-Aware Fusion Module (CAFM)

To maximally exploit the extracted heterogeneous features maps $F_i^{S_j}$ from parallel LRABs, we need to selectively leverage the correct information and suppress the incorrect one. It is quite possible that each voxel is correctly classified in at least one geometric view; thus, a key challenge is how to deal with agreement and disagreement in different views. For this, we present a content-aware fusion module (CAFM, see Fig. 3(c)) to generate aggregated deep features.

The input of CAFM includes two parts: a raw image I and heterogeneous feature maps $F_i^{S_j}$ of the same shape, where i is for the ith LRAB and S_j is for the selected scales in LRABs. HFA-Net has $m = 3$ LRABs; thus $i \in \{1, 2, 3\}$. There are three scales in each LRAB and we choose the last two scales; thus $j \in \{2, 3\}$. To recover the asymmetrical feature maps to the original resolution of the input image I, we use asymmetrical DeConv accordingly (e.g., we use stacked $\{\text{DeConv}(\mathcal{K}_{4,4,1} \times \mathcal{S}_{2,2,1}), \text{DeConv}(\mathcal{K}_{4,4,1} \times \mathcal{S}_{2,2,1})\}$ to obtain $F_1^{S_3}$ for the 1st LRAB). Then we average the feature maps from the same scale but different branches together to obtain hierarchical features $F^{S_j} = \frac{1}{m} \sum_{i=1}^{m} F_i^{S_j}$. This averaging provides a compact representation of all $F_i^{S_j}$'s while still showing the image areas where the heterogeneous features have agreement or disagreement. Next, each F^{S_j} is concatenated with the raw image I and fed to an encoder SAB, and all the intermediate feature maps are integrated in the middle of CAFM for extracting better representations. The raw image I provides a reference for helping further find detailed features and guide the feature aggregation process.

The loss function is computed as $\ell(X, Y; \theta) = \ell_{mse}(\widetilde{P}, Y) + \lambda_1 \ell_{mse}(\widetilde{P}_{aux}, Y) + \sum_i \sum_j \lambda_{ij} \ell_{mse}(S(F_i^{S_j}), Y)$, where Y is the corresponding ground truth of each training sample X, ℓ_{mse} is the multi-class cross-entropy loss and $S(\cdot)$ is the softmax function. See supplementary material for more details on HFA-Net.

2.3   Sparse Aggregation Block (SAB)

DenseVoxNet [11] is a state-of-the-art model for cardiovascular image segmentation, built on DenseBlock with dense residual connections. It aggregates all the previously computed features to each subsequent layer, computed as $x_\ell = H_\ell([x_0, x_1, \ldots, x_{\ell-1}])$, where x_0 is the input, x_ℓ is the output of layer ℓ, $[\cdot]$ is the concatenation operation, and $H_\ell(\cdot)$ is a composite of operations such

Table 1. Datasets and training details. "GT = ✗": the ground truth of the data is kept by the organizers for fair comparison. The initial learning rate $L_r = 5 \times 10^{-4}$.

Dataset	Train		Test		# Class	Optimizer	# Iter.	Learning rate policy
	# stack	GT	# stack	GT				
2016 HVSMR [6]	10	✓	10	✗	2	Adam: $\beta_1 = 0.9$, $\beta_2 = 0.999$, $\epsilon = $ 1e-10	45,000	$L_r \times (1 - \frac{iter}{\#iter})^{0.9}$
2017 MM-WHS CT [14]	16	✓	4	✓	7		60,000	
2017 AAPM CT [10]	36	✓	12	✗	5		60,000	

as Conv, Pooling, BN, and ReLU. The dense connections help transfer useful features from shallower to deeper layers, and in turn, allow each shallow layer to receive direct supervision signal, thus alleviating the gradient vanishment issue in training deep ConvNets and achieving better parameter-performance efficiency.

However, for a DenseBlock of depth N, the number of skip connections and parameters grows quadratically asymptotically (i.e., $O(N^2)$). This means that each layer generates only a few new outputs to an ever-widening concatenation of previously seen feature representations. Thus, it is hard for the model to make full use of all the parameters and dense skip connections [13].

To further ease the training of our HFA-Net, we devise a new sparsified densely-connected convolutional block, called sparse aggregation block (SAB), to improve parameter-performance efficiency. The output x_ℓ of layer ℓ is computed as $x_\ell = H_\ell([x_{\ell-c^0}, x_{\ell-c^1}, x_{\ell-c^2}, x_{\ell-c^3}, \ldots, x_{\ell-c^k}])$, where $c > 1$ is an integer and $k \geq 0$ is the largest integer such that $c^k \leq \ell$. For an SAB of total depth N, this sparse aggregation introduces no more than $\log_c(N)$ incoming links per layer, for a total of $O(N \log(N))$ connections and parameters. We use $c = 2$ and $N = 12$ in all experiments. See supplementary material for more details.

3   Experiments and Results

Three 3D Datasets. (1) The **2016 HVSMR dataset** [6] aims to segment myocardium and great vessels (blood pool) in cardiovascular MRIs. The results are evaluated using three criteria: Dice coefficient, average surface distance (ADB), and symmetric Hausdorff distance. A score $S = \sum_{class}(\frac{1}{2}Dice - \frac{1}{4}ADB - \frac{1}{30}Hausdorff)$ is used to measure the overall accuracy of the results and for ranking. (2) The **2017 MM-WHS CT dataset** [14] aims to segment seven cardiac structures (the left/right ventricle blood cavity (LV/RV), left/right atrium blood cavity (LA/RA), myocardium of the left ventricle (LV-myo), ascending aorta (AO), and pulmonary artery (PA)). Following the setting in [1], we randomly split the dataset into the training (16 subjects) and testing (4 subjects) sets, which are fixed throughout all experiments. (3) The **2017 AAPM CT dataset** [10] aims to segment five thoracic structures (esophagus, spinal cord, left/right lung, and heart); esophagus and spinal cord are highly difficult cases.

Table 2. Segmentation results on the 2016 HVSMR dataset (top), 2017 MM-WHS CT dataset (middle), and 2017 CT AAPM dataset (bottom).

Method	Myocardium			Blood pool			Overall score
	Dice	ADB [mm]	Hausdorff [mm]	Dice	ADB [mm]	Hausdorff [mm]	
Shahzad et al. [9]	0.747	1.099	5.091	0.885	1.553	9.408	-0.330
3D Unet [4]	0.762	0.943	5.618	0.932	0.826	7.015	-0.016
DVN [11]	0.821	0.964	7.294	0.931	0.938	9.533	-0.161
DVN (ours)	0.829	0.701	3.431	0.933	0.921	8.489	0.078
S-DVN	0.822	0.689	3.729	0.936	0.900	8.770	0.065
Gonda et al. [2]	0.793	0.783	4.002	0.934	0.853	7.043	0.087
Li et al. [3]	0.802	0.876	4.243	0.930	0.978	7.481	0.012
HFA-Net	**0.837**	**0.627**	**3.301**	**0.942**	**0.751**	**5.875**	**0.239**

Model	Metrics	Structures							mean
		LV	RV	LA	RA	LV-myo	AO	PA	
Payer et al. [7]	Dice	0.918	0.909	0.929	0.888	0.881	0.933	**0.840**	0.900
Dou et al. [1]	Dice	0.888	-	0.891	-	0.733	0.813	-	-
DVN	Dice	0.942	0.891	**0.933**	0.879	0.908	0.959	0.824	0.905
	Jacard	0.891	0.806	**0.874**	0.786	0.832	0.922	0.713	0.832
	ADB[voxel]	0.084	**0.448**	0.199	0.459	**0.180**	0.132	1.710	0.459
	Hausdorff[voxel]	**6.752**	39.156	71.189	101.570	**35.422**	27.810	59.982	48.840
S-DVN	Dice	0.929	0.890	0.914	**0.899**	0.895	0.956	0.828	0.902
	Jaccard	0.870	0.805	0.843	**0.817**	0.811	0.916	0.718	0.826
	ADB[voxel]	0.610	0.666	1.384	**0.307**	0.362	0.210	0.733	
	Hausdorff[voxel]	21.214	55.473	85.726	73.757	62.053	80.511	77.181	65.131
HFA-Net	Dice	**0.946**	**0.893**	0.925	0.897	**0.910**	**0.964**	0.830	**0.909**
	Jaccard	**0.898**	**0.810**	0.861	0.816	**0.836**	**0.930**	0.722	**0.839**
	ADB[voxel]	**0.076**	0.562	0.210	0.334	0.225	**0.103**	1.685	**0.456**
	Hausdorff[voxel]	7.148	**33.128**	42.173	22.903	36.954	**12.075**	37.845	27.461

Model	Metrics	Structures					mean
		Esophagus	Spinal Cord	Lung_R	Lung_L	Heart	
DVN [4]	Dice	0.676	0.851	0.960	0.960	0.917	0.873
	ADB[mm]	2.227	0.867	**1.212**	1.295	2.418	1.604
	Hausdorff[mm]	7.748	2.298	**3.938**	4.100	6.781	4.973
HFA-Net	Dice	**0.697**	**0.874**	**0.962**	**0.964**	**0.920**	**0.883**
	ADB[mm]	**1.974**	**0.766**	1.266	**0.967**	**2.336**	**1.462**
	Hausdorff[mm]	**5.883**	**2.190**	4.149	**3.370**	**6.557**	**4.430**

Implementation Details. Our proposed method is implemented with Python using the TensorFlow framework and trained on an NVIDIA Tesla V100 graphics card with 32GB GPU memory. All the models are initialized using a Gaussian distribution and trained with the "poly" learning rate policy. We perform data augmentation to reduce overfitting. More details can be found in Table 1.

Quantitative Results. Table 2 (top) shows quantitative comparison of HFA-Net against other methods from the 2016 HVSMR Challenge Leaderboard, including a conventional atlas-based method [9] and 3D FCN based methods [4,11]. First, our re-implementation of DVN achieves the state-of-the-art performance and our S-DVN with SAB achieves competitive results while reducing the number of parameters by ~60% (4.3M *vs.* 1.6M). Second, recall the two types of the known anisotropic 3D methods (see Sect. 1). We choose at least one typical method from each type for comparison. The method [2] is based on the short-range asymmetrical cell design, which utilizes 3D kernel decomposition on the orthogonal planes to predict a class label for each voxel. The method [3] extracts features from the *xy*-plane by a 2D FCN and applies a 3D FCN to fuse inter-slice information. Our HFA-Net outperforms these methods across nearly all the metrics with a very high overall score of 0.239. The results for the 2017 MM-WHS CT dataset are given in Table 2 (middle). First, our baselines (DVN and S-DVN) already achieve better results than the known state-of-the-art

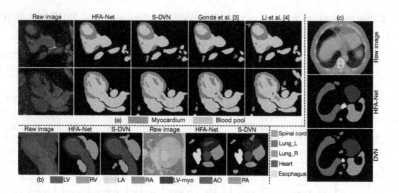

Fig. 4. Visual qualitative results: the 2016 HVSMR dataset (a), 2017 MM-WHS CT dataset (b), and 2017 CT AAPM dataset (c) (some errors marked by magenta arrows).

methods [1,7]. Second, our HFA-Net further improves the accuracy on most the categories across nearly all the metrics, especially for subtle structures such as LV-myo and AO. To further show that our method is robust and effective in delineating subtle structures, we experiment with HFA-Net on the 2017 AAPM CT dataset. Quantitative results in Table 2 (bottom) show promising performance gain, especially for esophagus and spinal cord (2% gain in Dice coefficient).

Qualitative Results. As shown in Fig. 4, our HFA-Net attains better results and shows a strong capability of delineating missing/ambiguous boundaries. More qualitative results can be found in supplementary material.

4   Conclusions

In this paper, we presented a new deep *heterogeneous feature aggregation network* (HFA-Net) for cardiovascular segmentation in 3D CT/MR images. Our proposed HFA-Net extracts rich heterogeneous features using long-range asymmetrical branches and aggregates diverse contextual and semantic deep features using a content-aware fusion module. Sparse aggregation block is utilized to give HFA-Net a better parameter-performance efficiency. Comprehensive experiments on three open challenge datasets demonstrated the efficacy of our new method.

Acknowledgement. This research was supported in part by the U.S. National Science Foundation through grants IIS-1455886, CCF-1617735, CNS-1629914, DUE-1833129 and NIH grant R01 DE027677-01.

References

1. Dou, Q., Ouyang, C., Chen, C., Chen, H., Heng, P.A.: Unsupervised cross-modality domain adaptation of ConvNets for biomedical image segmentations with adversarial loss. In: Twenty-Seventh International Joint Conference on Artificial Intelligence, pp. 691–697 (2018)
2. Gonda, F., Wei, D., Parag, T., Pfister, H.: Parallel separable 3D convolution for video and volumetric data understanding. arXiv preprint arXiv:1809.04096 (2018)
3. Li, X., Chen, H., Qi, X., Dou, Q., Fu, C.W., Heng, P.A.: H-DenseUNet: hybrid densely connected UNet for liver and tumor segmentation from CT volumes. IEEE Trans. Med. Imaging **37**(12), 2663–2674 (2018)
4. Liang, P., Chen, J., Zheng, H., Yang, L., Zhang, Y., Chen, D.Z.: Cascade decoder: a universal decoding method for biomedical image segmentation. IEEE ISBI **2019**, 339–342 (2019)
5. Liu, S., et al.: 3D anisotropic hybrid network: transferring convolutional features from 2D images to 3D anisotropic volumes. In: Frangi, A.F., Schnabel, J.A., Davatzikos, C., Alberola-López, C., Fichtinger, G. (eds.) MICCAI 2018. LNCS, vol. 11071, pp. 851–858. Springer, Cham (2018). https://doi.org/10.1007/978-3-030-00934-2_94
6. Pace, D.F., Dalca, A.V., Geva, T., Powell, A.J., Moghari, M.H., Golland, P.: Interactive whole-heart segmentation in congenital heart disease. In: Navab, N., Hornegger, J., Wells, W.M., Frangi, A.F. (eds.) MICCAI 2015. LNCS, vol. 9351, pp. 80–88. Springer, Cham (2015). https://doi.org/10.1007/978-3-319-24574-4_10
7. Payer, C., Štern, D., Bischof, H., Urschler, M.: Multi-label whole heart segmentation using CNNs and anatomical label configurations. In: Pop, M., et al. (eds.) STACOM 2017. LNCS, vol. 10663, pp. 190–198. Springer, Cham (2018). https://doi.org/10.1007/978-3-319-75541-0_20
8. Qiu, Z., Yao, T., Mei, T.: Learning spatio-temporal representation with pseudo-3D residual networks. In: ICCV, pp. 5533–5541 (2017)
9. Shahzad, R., Gao, S., Tao, Q., Dzyubachyk, O., van der Geest, R.: Automated cardiovascular segmentation in patients with congenital heart disease from 3D CMR scans: combining multi-atlases and level-sets. In: Zuluaga, M.A., Bhatia, K., Kainz, B., Moghari, M.H., Pace, D.F. (eds.) RAMBO/HVSMR -2016. LNCS, vol. 10129, pp. 147–155. Springer, Cham (2017). https://doi.org/10.1007/978-3-319-52280-7_15
10. Yang, J., et al.: Lung CT segmentation challenge 2017 – the cancer imaging archive (2017). http://doi.org/10.7937/k9/tcia.2017.3r3fvz08
11. Yu, L., et al.: Automatic 3D cardiovascular MR segmentation with densely-connected volumetric ConvNets. In: Descoteaux, M., Maier-Hein, L., Franz, A., Jannin, P., Collins, D.L., Duchesne, S. (eds.) MICCAI 2017. LNCS, vol. 10434, pp. 287–295. Springer, Cham (2017). https://doi.org/10.1007/978-3-319-66185-8_33
12. Zheng, H., et al.: A new ensemble learning framework for 3D biomedical image segmentation. In: Thirty-Third AAAI Conference on Artificial Intelligence (2019)
13. Zhu, L., Deng, R., Maire, M., Deng, Z., Mori, G., Tan, P.: Sparsely aggregated convolutional networks. In: ECCV, pp. 186–201 (2018)
14. Zhuang, X., Shen, J.: Multi-scale patch and multi-modality atlases for whole heart segmentation of MRI. Med. Image Anal. **31**, 77–87 (2016)

Spectral CT Based Training Dataset Generation and Augmentation for Conventional CT Vascular Segmentation

Pierre-Jean Lartaud[1,2]($\boxtimes$), Aymeric Rouchaud[3], Jean-Michel Rouet[1], Olivier Nempont[1], and Loic Boussel[2,3]

[1] Philips Research France, Suresnes, France
pierre-jean.lartaud@creatis.insa-lyon.fr
[2] CREATIS UMR5220, INSERM U1044, INSA,
Université de Lyon, Lyon, France
[3] Radiology Department, Hôpital Croix-Rousse, Hospices Civils de Lyon,
Lyon, France

Abstract. Deep learning has proved to be a very efficient tool for organs automated segmentation in CT scans. However, variation of iodine contrast agent concentration within the vascular system or organs is a major source of variation in image contrast. This requires building large databases representative of the important differences in contrast enhancement across CT studies. Furthermore, creating a low- or non-enhanced annotated database is still a very laborious task as semi-automatic segmentation software and even expert eyes often fail to find structures' edges on low contrast images.

In this study, we aim to develop a new deep-learning network training approach based on spectral data augmentation using dual energy spectral CT (Philips iQon) images as training dataset. Indeed this new generation of CT scanners allows generating, from a single scan, virtual non-contrast images (VNC), corresponding to unenhanced CT images on conventional CT scanners, and virtual mono-energetic (monoE) images at different kV, that mimics low (at high kV) to high (at low kV) iodine-based contrast-enhanced studies. An experienced radiologist can then segment the target structures on highly contrasted low kV monoE with a semi-automatic tool (ISP, Philips) yielding ground truth for both monoE and VNC images.

As an illustration, we trained a 3D U-net convolutional neural network for aorta segmentation on conventional CT images. In addition to greatly facilitate the creation of an annotated non-contrast CT database, we demonstrate through multiple training experiments that using a variable proportion of VNC and randomly chosen monoE kV levels during the data augmentation process allows training networks that are able to segment target structures regardless of their level of contrast enhancement.

Keywords: Data augmentation · Spectral CT · Dataset generation · Deep learning · Aorta · Segmentation · Non-contrast CT · Convolutional neural network (CNN)

© Springer Nature Switzerland AG 2019
D. Shen et al. (Eds.): MICCAI 2019, LNCS 11765, pp. 768–775, 2019.
https://doi.org/10.1007/978-3-030-32245-8_85

1 Introduction

In the recent years, deep learning has become a popular method for organs segmentation in the literature. In particular, CNN achieved state of the art performances for multiple CT segmentation tasks [1]. The current interactive semi-automatic segmentation tools facilitate the creation of the large annotated datasets needed for both training and validation of neural networks. However, non-contrast CT images still prove to be difficult to work with, especially in the cardiovascular area. Indeed, automated and semi-automated segmentation tools often fail due to the image low contrast. Creating large enough training and validation datasets using basic manual segmentation tools is thus extremely difficult and time consuming. Consequently, only a few deep learning cardio-vascular segmentation applications were proposed on these images (excluding calcium detection) [2, 3].

Moreover, the large range of indications and protocols in CT imaging induce huge variations in images. Both the amount of iodinated agent injected during the examination and the timing between injection and images acquisition greatly vary depending of the clinical indication of the CT scan, to highlight the anatomical structures of interest. To diagnose pulmonary embolism (PE), pulmonary arteries must be strongly enhanced and the CT acquisition is thus started early after the beginning of the contrast agent IV injection. On the other hand, in oncologic chest-abdomen-pelvis CT scans (CAP), a global enhancement of the vessels and the tissues is mandatory. The acquisition is therefore started later after the beginning of the injection. In other conditions, such as emphysema evaluation, no contrast agent is used. A large training dataset is consequently mandatory to account for all these conditions. Examples of these images are visible on Fig. 4.

Spectral dual energy CT, the new generation of CT scanners, allows dynamic generation of virtual non-contrast images (VNC), corresponding to unenhanced CT images on conventional CT scanners, and virtual mono-energetic (monoE) images at different kV, that mimics low (at high kV) to high (at low kV) iodine-based contrast-enhanced studies [4] and thus the different scanning conditions described above.

We therefore propose a new method to easily and quickly create non-contrast CT datasets for organ segmentation, and innovative training augmentation strategies to allow our network to segment scans with imaging protocols not present in the training dataset.

To assess our hypothesis, we developed a 3D Unet [5] convolutional neural network to segment the aorta, from the aortic valve to the aortic bifurcation. Aorta is a challenging task to illustrate our method: according to the imaging protocol, the contrast along the vessel varies greatly. Furthermore, some portions of it near the heart and through the abdominal area are complex to segment, regardless of the method used [6, 7].

This paper is organized as follows: Sect. 2 provides a detailed description of the proposed method to generate labeled databases from Spectral CT data. In Sect. 3, we present and discuss validation results on clinical CT scans.

2 Material and Methods

2.1 Dual CT Images Reconstruction

Dual CT is a recently developed technology that allows new image reconstruction approaches. In this study, we used the clinically available Philips iQon spectral CT. This system is based on dual-layer detectors technology [8]. During the scan low energy X-rays are absorbed by the first layer of detectors, then high energy ones by the second layer. The simultaneous recording of these two energies allows differentiation of materials, according to their energy attenuation characteristics [4]. Iodine and water maps can then be reconstructed, where intensity of a pixel ties to the material concentration in the patient. From these two materials maps, virtual non-contrast (VNC) images can be computed [4] through the subtraction of iodine map, and yield similar readings to traditional non-contrast CT. Mono-energetic (monoE) images can be reconstructed from the water and iodine map as followed:

$$monoE_{KV} = I_{iodine} \times \mu^{kV}_{m\,iodine} + I_{H2O} \times \mu^{kV}_{m\,H2O}, \tag{1}$$

where I_{iodine} and I_{H20} are the iodine and water maps, in g cm^{-3}, $\mu^{kV}_{m\,iodine}$ and $\mu^{kV}_{m\,H20}$ the mass attenuation coefficients at kV energy, in cm^2 g^{-1} [9]. Since low-energy X rays are easily absorbed within the patient, low-energy monoE will be more contrasted than high energy ones, as illustrated on Fig. 1.

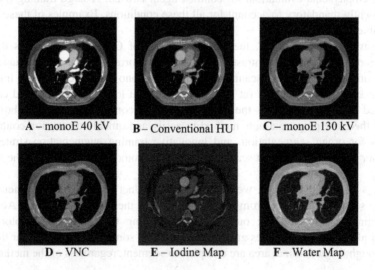

A – monoE 40 kV	**B** – Conventional HU	**C** – monoE 130 kV
D – VNC	**E** – Iodine Map	**F** – Water Map

Fig. 1. Example of images reconstructed from spectral CT. A [600–1600] window is applied to monoE, conventional and VNC images.

2.2   Training and Augmentation Strategies

To assess the benefit of spectral CT images training approach in comparison with standard CT training approach, we develop five different strategies, displayed in Table 1. We first trained our network with conventional contrast enhanced HU images and VNC (equivalent to non-contrast) as these images could be produced and segmented, although with more difficulties, on a standard CT.

Table 1. Training strategies of the Unet

Strategy	Training dataset augmentation
HU-VNC	70% HU images, 30% VNC
rME-VNC	70% of random energy monoE (range [54–100] kV), 30% of VNC
VNCo	100% VNC images only
rMEo	100% random energy monoE (range [54–100] kV) only
bdME-VNC	70% blended monoE, 30% VNC

Regarding the spectral approach, as the difference in contrast agent concentration is a major source of variation across CT exams, we use random monoE to simulate global changes in agent concentration.

We first trained a single network with both random monoE and VNC termed as rME-VNC. We then trained two separates networks one with MonoE only (rMEo) one with VNC only (VNCo), to check if two specialized solutions would outperform a generalist one.

Finally, we trained a last strategy based on blend of MonoE images. Indeed, we thought that rME-VNC's augmentation process would not fully deal with the spatial inhomogeneity of contrast medium within the vessels. Depending on the injection protocol, contrast medium may indeed be present in only a specific part of the vasculature. To simulate this inhomogeneity and especially to generate a wider range of relative contrast between the target object and neighboring vessels, we use distinct random monoE for the target structure and for the rest of the image:

$$BdME = GT \times monoE1 + (1 - GT) \times monoE2, \tag{2}$$

where *GT* is the binary segmentation mask of the target structure, and *BdME* the blended monoE images. In bdME-VNC, the training is performed using blended monoE generated on the fly as illustrated in Fig. 2.

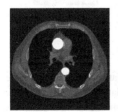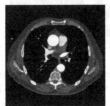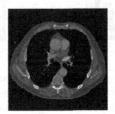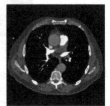

Fig. 2. Different blended monoE reconstructions from a single spectral CT slice.

2.3   Experimental Setup

We trained a state-of-the-art 3D-Unet convolutional neural network [5] on $(80 \times 80 \times 80)$ random patches, with five resolution layers. These layers consists of three $(3 \times 3 \times 3)$ convolutions activated by a rectified linear unit (ReLU), and a max pooling. Along each successive layers, the number of features channels doubles, starting from 16 up to 256.

Our training dataset consisted of 150 randomly selected patients, scanned with iQon spectral CT, including dissections and aneurysms. For each scans, standard HU images, VNC, iodine and water maps were collected. An experienced radiologist R1 generated a ground truth (GT) segmentation of the aorta on HU images for every scans, with a semi-automatic tool (Philips ISP). Aortic calcifications and dissections were included.

For our validation dataset, we collected 50 contrast-enhanced scans including 20 CAP CT performed for oncology workup and 30 PE CT, and 20 non-contrast CT scans. These scans were performed on five different conventional CT scanners in four hospitals, among the recent admissions. As for the training dataset, radiologist R1 segmented the aorta. A manual segmentation tool (3D Slicer) was used for the non-contrast CT scans. Mean time to segment one patient of this dataset was 48 min for non-contrast images, and 12 min for enhanced CT scans.

Sørensen-Dice coefficient was calculated for every strategies, on every CT protocols, on full volume for each patients. Since the training dataset includes only VNC, iodine and water maps and GT, every needed monoE were dynamically reconstructed during training, according to Eq. (1). No post-treatment was added to the network

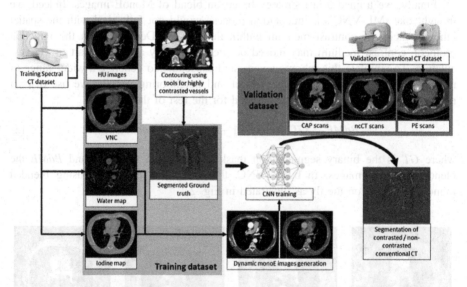

Fig. 3. Global training process workflow. Depending on the training strategy, UH, VNC, iodine and water images are provided to the network as training data. The two later are used to generate monoE as described before. Manual segmentation is provided as a ground truth to the network. Validation is performed using images acquired with conventional CT scanners.

prediction. To study the accuracy of our validation ground truths, a second experienced radiologist R2 segmented independently half of the dataset (25 enhanced, 10 non-contrast CT). The whole training and validation process is summarized in Fig. 3.

3 Results and Discussion

The 3D Unet was able to segment the aorta on every studied protocols. Typical examples of segmentations are provided in Fig. 4. The detailed segmentation performances of each training strategy by images type are shown on Fig. 5. It demonstrates that all the strategies based on spectral data augmentation and including VNC images outperformed the strategy involving only conventional non-spectral images (HU-VNC). Indeed, with our best spectral-based training strategy (bdME-VNC) we obtained an overall mean dice of 0.941 ± 0.011 (max 0.964, min 0.910) when the conventional based strategy only reached a mean dice of 0.933 ± 0.027 (max 0.960, min 0,765). One should note that the results of bdME-VNC are also favorably comparable to other studies on non-contrast CT aorta segmentation [6, 7].

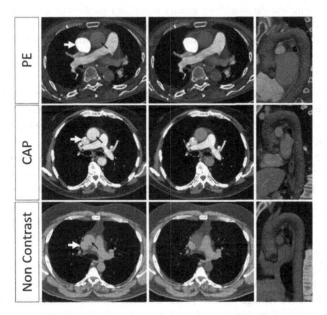

Fig. 4. Segmentation of PE, CAP and non-contrast CT scans. From left to right: original axial slice, bdME-VNC approach result (red overlay), 3D rendering of the segmentation result. The superior vena cave (white arrow) shows a very different contrast with ascending thoracic aorta (black arrow) across protocols. (Color figure online)

When comparing the spectral strategies themselves, it is notable that bdME-VNC over performed rME-VNC in all the situations, particularly on PE images, the most difficult case. Indeed, PE was not part of the training dataset and the inversion of

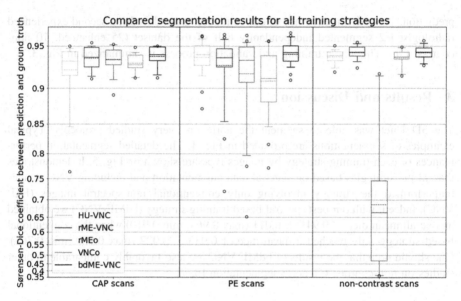

Fig. 5. Dice coefficient calculated on ground truths and predictions for CAP, PE and non-contrast CT scans, for each experiments. The boxes show the 25th and 75th percentile (interquartile) ranges. Median/average values are shown as a horizontal solid/dotted line within the boxes.

contrast between the aorta and the superior vena cava in comparison with CAP or non-contrast enhanced images prove to be complex for the networks. Nevertheless a mean dice of 0.94 was reached, underlying the fact that this strategy allows training of much more versatile networks, without the need of an extended dataset.

Excluding rMEo, which was not trained on VNC images, all results of non-contrast CT segmentations are over 0.91 of dice, thus proving that inclusion of non-contrast images in the training dataset is mandatory to obtain acceptable results during inference on such images. Furthermore it confirms that VNC image scan be used to learn to segment unenhanced images. However it should be noted that VNCo, trained only on VNC images, got the lowest score on non-contrast validation dataset. This may be due to true non-contrast images being acquired with a wide photon energy spectrum (from 80 to 140 kVp), where VNC are generated to correspond to a mean energy value of 70 kVp. Due to these variations, some spectral contrast may appear in true non-contrast images, while VNC images show more uniform contrast within the vessels. This emphasis the need of building combined dataset including contrast and non-contrast images to increase the variability of situations provided to the network during the learning phase.

Finally, results of bdME-VNC are particularly encouraging when compared to the inter-operators study. Indeed, it reveals that the mean dice value for enhanced images between the two operators' segmentation reaches 0.930 ± 0.015, with a maximum value of 0.957 and minimum of 0.900. Results on non-contrast images were a bit lower, with a mean value of 0.923 ± 0.015, maximum of 0.940 and minimum 0.898.

Most of the radiologists' disagreements are located along the edges of the vessel and near the heart, which is very similar to the typical prediction errors of our networks. The high agreement between our operators is eased by the aorta size and the operators' background, both experienced radiologists.

However, due to the validation dataset being of only 20 to 30 patients per image protocol, we cannot validate a true statistical difference between those training strategies.

4   Conclusion

In this paper, we demonstrate the effectiveness of our spectral approach for creating training datasets of contrast and non-contrast images for structures segmentation.

Data augmentation techniques with monoE and VNC helped to create a more versatile network with a reduced dataset, and showed more accurate results than a network trained on conventional images only. Following developments will include segmentation of others structures or organs such as the heart. The spectral approach may be extended in the future, especially using materials maps. With an adequate postprocessing, the proposed approach may become an efficient tool for fast segmentation on a large range of CT image protocols in clinical routine.

References

1. Maier, A., Syben, C., Lasser, T., Riess, C.: A gentle introduction to deep learning in medical image processing. Zeitschrift für Medizinische Physik **29**(2), 86–101 (2019)
2. Commandeur, F., et al.: Deep learning for quantification of epicardial and thoracic adipose tissue from non-contrast CT. IEEE Trans. Med. Imaging **37**(8), 1835–1846 (2018)
3. Singh, G., et al.: Machine learning in cardiac CT: basic concepts and contemporary data. J. Cardiovasc. Comput. Tomogr. **12**(3), 192–201 (2018)
4. Silva, A.C., Morse, B.G., Hara, A.K., Paden, R.G., Hongo, N., Pavlicek, W.: Dual-energy (spectral) CT: applications in abdominal imaging. RadioGraphics **31**(4), 1031–1046 (2011)
5. Ronneberger, O., Fischer, P., Brox, T.: U-Net: convolutional networks for biomedical image segmentation. In: Navab, N., Hornegger, J., Wells, W.M., Frangi, A.F. (eds.) MICCAI 2015. LNCS, vol. 9351, pp. 234–241. Springer, Cham (2015). https://doi.org/10.1007/978-3-319-24574-4_28
6. Xie, Y., Padgett, J., Biancardi, A.M., Reeves, A.P.: Automated aorta segmentation in low-dose chest CT images. Int. J. Comput. Assist. Radiol. Surg. **9**(2), 211–219 (2014)
7. Trullo, R., Petitjean, C., Nie, D., Shen, D., Ruan, S.: Joint segmentation of multiple thoracic organs in CT images with two collaborative deep architectures. In: Cardoso, M.J., et al. (eds.) DLMIA/ML-CDS -2017. LNCS, vol. 10553, pp. 21–29. Springer, Cham (2017). https://doi.org/10.1007/978-3-319-67558-9_3
8. Aran, S., Shaqdan, K.W., Abujudeh, H.H.: Dual-energy computed tomography (DECT) in emergency radiology: basic principles, techniques, and limitations. Emerg. Radiol. **21**(4), 391–405 (2014)
9. NIST XCOM photon cross-sections database. https://www.nist.gov/pml/xcom-photon-cross-sections-database. Accessed 31 Mar 2019

Context-Aware Inductive Bias Learning for Vessel Border Detection in Multi-modal Intracoronary Imaging

Zhifan Gao[1] and Shuo Li[1,2,3]($\boxtimes$)

[1] Department of Medical Biophysics, Western University, London, Canada
slishuo@gmail.com
[2] Department of Medical Imaging, Western University, London, Canada
[3] Digital Imaging Group of London, London, Canada

Abstract. Multi-modal intracoronary imaging (visualize the inner structure of coronary arteries) has been proved to have great ability to help the coronary disease diagnosis in recent studies. However, no reported success on detecting all clinically-valuable vessel borders in multi-modal image analysis, because of the varied environment where the vessels are located in, i.e. inconsistent image appearance and tissue morphologies. This challenges the multi-modal vessel border detection, which is difficultly addressed by the hand-engineering feature extraction in existing single-mode methods. We propose a context-aware inductive bias learning approach to enable the detection of three vessel borders in multi-modal intracoronary imaging, i.e. the lumen and media-adventitia borders in intravascular ultrasound (IVUS), and the lumen border in optical coherence tomography (OCT). Our approach exploits the detection process of one vessel border as a model constraint to another vessel border based on the vessel contextual information. It is specified by an elaborately-designed semantic-fusion multi-task neural network, which exploits the similarly semantic information and different environment information to lead the mutual regularization among different vessel border detection tasks. The extensive experiments show the effectiveness of our approach by the highly overlapping degree with the ground truth and the superiority to six state-of-the-art single-mode vessel border detection methods.

1 Introduction

Vessel border detection is of importance in the multi-modal intracoronary image analysis [1–5]. The intracoronary imaging is the catheter-based interventional imaging technique for visualizing the inner tissue morphologies of coronary arteries (see Fig. 1). Recent studies have demonstrated the potential clinical improvement when replacing the single-mode intracoronary imaging by the multiple modalities, mainly including intravascular ultrasound (IVUS) and optical coherence tomography (OCT) [6]. This is because the multi-modal images can provide more comprehensive observations of coronary disease, and thus improve

© Springer Nature Switzerland AG 2019
D. Shen et al. (Eds.): MICCAI 2019, LNCS 11765, pp. 776–784, 2019.
https://doi.org/10.1007/978-3-030-32245-8_86

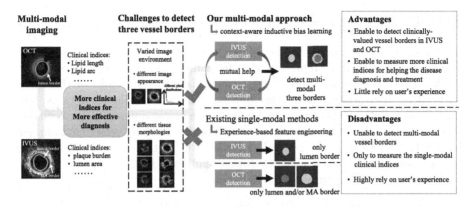

Fig. 1. The proposed approach provide a clinical tool to detect the vessel borders in multi-modal intracoronary imaging (i.e. IVUS and OCT). It can benefit the multi-modal diagnosis and treatment of coronary disease with respect to the existing single-mode methods.

the effectiveness of the clinical protocols designed based on these observations in the diagnosis and treatment. As the first step of the multi-modal intracoronary image processing, detecting the vessel borders can help the subsequent analysis of the key clinical indicators of atherosclerosis like plaque burden [7]. Moreover, it is necessary to detect the three vessel borders from different imaging modality, i.e. the lumen and media-adventitia (MA) borders in IVUS and the lumen border in OCT, rather apply the vessel borders from one imaging modality to another for analyzing coronary disease. This results from the fact that the vessels displays in different imaging modalities have incompatible degrees to deviate from the histological results [8]. However, the manual delineation of the three vessel borders is a labor-intensive work for clinicians. This motivates the requirement of the automatic and accurate vessel border detection method.

It is very challenging to develop the vessel border detection method for multi-modal intracoronary images. This challenge originates from the fact that the vessel borders are located in the varied image environment (i.e. image appearance and tissue morphologies may be varied in different intracornary images). Thus, there is no reported success on detecting all clinically-valuable vessel borders in multi-modal images to our best knowledge. Moreover, this challenges the experience-based hand-crafted features extracted in the existing single-mode methods, because they are sensitive to the varied environment. This indicates that the design experience of the single-mode methods are difficult to adapt the multi-modal images. For example, the catheter artifacts shows different sizes and morphologies between IVUS and OCT images. Thus, the catheter remove based on its experienced knowledge (e.g. set the catheter size by a fixed value [9]) is difficult to perform well both in these two imaging modalities. Accordingly, the environment-insensitive vessel feature representation is required in the multi-modal detection method.

In this paper, we propose a context-aware inductive bias (CIB) learning approach to accurately detect the vessel borders in multi-modal intracoronary images as a novel clinical tool (see Fig. 1). The CIB learns the environment-insensitive vessel feature representation from multi-modal images by minimizing the average generalization ability among the detection tasks of three vessel borders. Specifically, through the mutual constraints of the three tasks, CIB exploits the related vessel contextual information across different detection tasks to improve the detection accuracy, as well as the different vessel environment information to improve the generalization ability. To this end, CIB is specified by an elaborately-designed semantic-fusion multi-task neural network.

Our contributions can be summarized as:

1. To the best of our knowledge, for the first time the vessel border detection enabled in both IVUS (lumen and media-adventitia borders) and OCT (lumen border) images is achieved as a clinical tool, which reduces the burden on clinicians in the vessel border delineation during the multi-modal intracoronary diagnosis and treatment of atherosclerosis disease.
2. Our context-aware inductive bias learning approach provides a way to extract the contextual information insensitive to the varied image environment, which enables the border detection of the contextual-related objects in the multi-modal images under inconsistent image appearance and object morphologies.
3. Our semantic-fusion multi-task neural network provides an elaborately-designed architecture, which can effectively extract the semantic information of objects in single modality, enrich the high-level features with local detailed information, and mutually constrain the multi-modal semantic information of objects.

2 Context-Aware Inductive Bias Learning

The proposed CIB is specified by a elaborately-designed semantic-fusion multi-task neural network to solve the vessel border detection problem in multi-modal intracoronary imaging by learning the environment-insensitive feature representation (see Fig. 2). First, it proposes the cross-task feature fusion module to integrate the vessel semantic features from different tasks for learning the environment-insensitive information about the vessel contextual relatedness and the environment variation. Second, it proposes the cross-level feature fusion module to combine the low-level and high-level features for enhancing the high-level feature map with the local detailed information. Third, it proposes the pyramidal dilated dense convolution (PDDC) module to capture the global contextual information while preserving the local high-resolution information for effectively extracting the semantic features. In addition, it exploits a specially-designed loss function for optimizing the CIB from the aspects of the overlapping degree and absolute error.

2.1   Problem Formulation of CIB

The CIB formulates the vessel border detection in multi-modal intracoronary imaging as an inductive bias learning problem [10], including three task: lumen border detection in OCT (**Task 1**), lumen border detection in IVUS (**Task 2**), and MA border detection in IVUS (**Task 3**). The inductive bias learning aims to find optimal hypotheses $\mathbf{h}^* = \{h_1^*, ..., h_N^*\}$ for each of N tasks ($N = 3$) from an appropriate hypothesis space H^* in a hypothesis space family $\mathcal{H}$ under the appropriate inductive bias. For CIB, the proposed detection problem can be formulated by $\hat{y} = h(f(x))$. f is the function from the input image x to the represented feature ϕ, i.e. $\phi = f(x)$. The hypotheses h is the functions from ϕ to the output results $\hat{y}$. The hypothesis space H is the set of all possible functions g. The hypothesis space family $\mathcal{H}$ is the set of all possible functions f. The inductive bias denotes the mutual constraints in the three tasks. Then, the optimization of CIB is achieved by minimizing the empirical error $\hat{e}_z$ on the training dataset $z = (x, y)$, and formulated as

$$
\mathbf{h}^* = \arg\min_{\mathbf{h} \in H^*} \hat{e}_z(\mathbf{h}) = \arg\min_{\mathbf{h} \in H^*} \frac{1}{N} \sum_{i=1}^{N} \frac{1}{M} \sum_{j=1}^{M} L(h_i(\phi_{ij}), y_{ij})
$$

$$
H^* = \arg\min_{H \in \mathcal{H}} \frac{1}{N} \sum_{i=1}^{N} \inf_{\mathbf{h} \in H} \hat{e}_{z_i}(\mathbf{h})
$$

(1)

where y is the detection labels, z_i is the training data in the ith task, M is the number of training data in each task, and L is the loss function. As regards the diverse image appearance and tissue morphologies in IVUS and OCT, the CIB relies on the exploit of the related contextual information in the three tasks, as well as their environment difference. Accordingly, the CIB elaborately designs a semantic-fusion multi-task neural network (detailed in Sect. 2.2) to solve Eq. (1).

2.2   Semantic-Fusion Multi-task Neural Network for Accurate Vessel Border Detection

The CIB proposes a semantic-fusion multi-task neural network architecture to learn the vessel feature representation that insensitive to the varied environment in different tasks, with three core components: cross-task feature fusion, cross-level feature fusion and PDDC (see Fig. 2).

Cross-Task Feature Fusion for Learning the Relatedness of Semantic Information in Multiple Tasks. The three tasks are related in the contextual level because (1) Task 1 and Task 2 focus on the same semantic meaning (denote the lumen regions in the coronary); (2) Task 2 and Task 3 focus on the related semantic meaning (the lumen region and MA region both in IVUS) owing to their anatomical relationship; (3) Task 2 can be a bridge to connect Task 1 and Task 3. Accordingly, the cross-task feature fusion is specially designed as

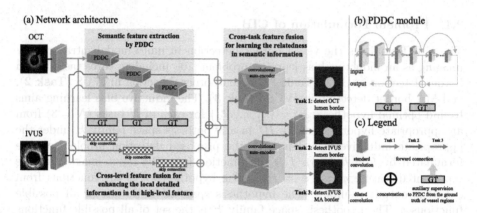

Fig. 2. Network architecture of our approach. Three contributions include the cross-task feature fusion for learning the related semantic information, cross-level feature fusion for enhancing the local detailed information in the high-level feature, and the PDDC for effectively extracting the semantic information. (Color figure online)

Fig. 2(a). It separately fuses the high-level features between Task 1 and Task 2 and those between Task 2 and Task 3. This high-level feature fusion is implemented by the convolutional auto-encoder with six layers (blue cuboid in Fig. 2a), which encodes the high-level feature maps in different tasks into a latent-space representation, and reconstructs the output from this representation. Thus, the proposed network can learn from diverse but related high-level information for improving the detection accuracy. It also considers the cross-task difference of the environment information as the regularization to each task for improving the generalization ability [11].

Cross-Level Feature Fusion for Enhancing the Local Detailed Information in the High-Level Feature. There exists the gap between the semantic information and detailed information which suppresses the effectiveness of the feature fusion [12]. The low-level features are difficult to provide sufficient high-resolution semantic guidance owing to noise corruption when fusing it with high-level features. The high-level features lack detailed information to infer the accurate semantic borders. Accordingly, the cross-level feature fusion feeds the semantic information to the low-level features by the auxiliary supervision to the feature maps in the PDDC module (the black arrows in Fig. 2a) in each task. Then, it feeds the detailed information to the high-level features by the skip connection (the blue dashed arrows in Fig. 2a). This module can increase the detailed information in the high-level features for reducing the loss of vessel border details in the cross-task feature fusion.

PDDC for Effectively Extracting the Semantic Information. The traditional forward structure of the neural network is inappropriate to extract the vessel borders with largely varied sizes and morphologies in the IVUS/OCT images.

In the high-level feature representation, the traditional network structure has the receptive field with relatively fixed size, and thus can just well response to the lumen/MA regions having similar size with the receptive field. In addition, the resolution of the feature map in the high-level network layers are largely reduced with the forward propagation because of the some operators such as pooling. This resolution loss can affect the morphology recovery of the lumen/MA borders. Thus, the proposed PDDC module aims to extract the semantic information of size-varied vessel regions while preserving the boundary-detailed information (the green cuboid in Fig. 2a). First, it uses the pyramid structure with dilated convolution kernel to rapidly increase the size of the receptive field for obtaining the semantic information (see Fig. 2b). Every three dilated convolution layers in order are considered as a group. Totally three groups are configured. The dilated rate for all groups are 2, 2 and 4, respectively. Then, PDDC constructs the dense connection within every group for preserving the high-resolution information in the high-level features.

Loss Function. We propose a specially-designed loss function L to simultaneously measure the overlapping degree and the absolute error between the regions within the detected vessel border and the ground truth. It is defined by $L = \sum_i F_1(I^i) + F_2(I^i)$. I^i is the output image of the ith task. F_1 is the generalized Dice index:

$$F_1 = 1 - 2\frac{\alpha\sum_{p=1}^{W}\sum_{q=1}^{H} I_{p,q}^i G_{p,q}^i + \beta\sum_{p=1}^{W}\sum_{q=1}^{H}(1 - I_{p,q}^i)(1 - G_{p,q}^i)}{\alpha\sum_{p=1}^{W}\sum_{q=1}^{H}(I_{p,q}^i + G_{p,q}^i) + \beta\sum_{p=1}^{W}\sum_{q=1}^{H}(2 - I_{p,q}^i - G_{p,q}^i)} \quad (2)$$

where G^i is ground truth. I^i and G^i have same image size ($W \times H$). $I_{p,q}^i$ and $G_{p,q}^i$ are the intensity value of the pixel at (p,q) in I^i and G^i, respectively. α and β are two parameters formulated as $\alpha = (\sum_{p=1}^{W}\sum_{q=1}^{H} G_{p,q}^i)^{-1}$, $\beta = (\sum_{p=1}^{W}\sum_{q=1}^{H}(1 - G_{p,q}^i))^{-1}$. F_2 is the modified mean absolute errors, formulated as $F_2 = \sum_{p=1}^{W}\sum_{q=1}^{H}\ln(1 + e^{|G_{p,q}^i - I_{p,q}^i|})$.

Network Training. The stochastic gradient descent is used with the momentum 0.9 as the optimization algorithm. The iteration number is 30 epochs. The learning rate is 0.1 at the initial time, 0.01 after 10 epochs, and 0.001 after 20 epochs. The training phase uses 70% images in the dataset. All input images are resized to 256×256 for training and testing.

3   Experiments and Results

Experiment Setup. We have collected 914 IVUS images and 914 OCT images for evaluating our approach. One cardiologist collected all IVUS images by a commercially available machine (In-Vision Gold, Volcano) using a 20-MHz solid-state IVUS catheter (EagleEye Volcano) and an automatic pullback device

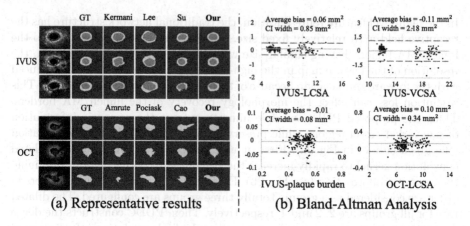

(a) Representative results   (b) Bland-Altman Analysis

Fig. 3. (a) More accurate detected borders than the comparative methods shown in the representative images. "GT" is the ground truth. (b) High agreement between our approach and the ground truth by the Bland-Altman analysis.

Table 1. Better performance than six state-of-the-art single-mode methods on Jaccard index, Dice index, Hausdorff distance (HD) and root mean square error (RMSE).

Method	Task	Jaccard	Dice	HD (mm)	RMSE (mm)
Kermani et al. [13]	IVUS lumen	0.67	0.80	0.74 ± 0.11	0.44 ± 0.06
	IVUS MA	0.81	0.89	0.54 ± 0.13	0.27 ± 0.05
Lee et al. [14]	IVUS lumen	0.85	0.92	0.21 ± 0.02	0.13 ± 0.02
	IVUS MA	0.86	0.92	0.31 ± 0.44	0.17 ± 0.05
Su et al. [2]	IVUS lumen	0.88	0.90	0.46 ± 0.02	0.13 ± 0.02
	IVUS MA	0.87	0.90	0.52 ± 0.62	0.10 ± 0.04
Amrute et al. [15]	OCT lumen	0.44	0.57	1.93 ± 0.56	0.12 ± 0.20
Pociask et al. [9]	OCT lumen	0.94	0.96	0.33 ± 0.33	0.07 ± 0.06
Cao et al. [1]	OCT lumen	0.76	0.86	2.72 ± 0.28	0.53 ± 0.10
Our approach	IVUS lumen	**0.95**	**0.97**	$\mathbf{0.15 \pm 0.08}$	$\mathbf{0.04 \pm 0.03}$
	IVUS MA	**0.95**	**0.98**	$\mathbf{0.24 \pm 0.40}$	$\mathbf{0.05 \pm 0.03}$
	OCT lumen	**0.97**	**0.98**	$\mathbf{0.09 \pm 0.18}$	$\mathbf{0.04 \pm 0.04}$

(R-100, Volcano, USA) relative to the proximal reference at a pullback speed of 0.5 mm/s. Another cardiologist collected all OCT images by OCT Illumien Optis, with catheter (dragonfly duo) at a pullback speed of 36 mm/s. The ground truth of all vessel borders are delineated by an experienced medical physician. All of the codes used in this study were implemented by TensorFlow on a NVIDIA Titan V GPU. Then, we use five evaluation methods to assess the performance of the proposed approach, including Bland-Altman analysis, Jaccard index, Dice index, Hausdorff distance, and root mean square error (RMSE). Finally, we compared our framework with six state-of-the-art single-mode methods, where three methods [2,13,14] concern the detection of lumen and MA borders in IVUS images, and the other three methods [1,9,15] concern the lumen border detection in OCT images.

High Performance with Respect to the Ground Truth (GT). (1) Fig. 3(a) visually shows the accuracy of the vessel borders detected by our approach on the representative images. (2) Table 1 presents that the detected lumen and MA region are highly overlapped with GT (Jaccard index $\geqslant 0.95$ and Dice index $\geqslant 0.97$). (3) Table 1 also presents the high closeness of the detected lumen and MA borders with GT (Hausdorff distance $\leqslant 0.24$ mm and RMSE $\leqslant 0.05$ mm). (4) Fig. 3(b) shows the high agreement on four clinical indices based on the detection results, including lumen cross-sectional area (LCSA), vessel cross-sectional area (VCSA) and plaque burden for IVUS, as well as the LCSA for OCT. By the Bland-Altman analysis, the average bias of our approach with GT are not greater than 0.11 for LCSA and VCSA, and equals 0.01 for plaque burden. The percentages of the scatter points falling within the 95% confidence interval are greater than 0.94.

Superiority to Six State-of-the-Art Single-Mode Methods. Table 1 shows the vessels detected by our approach with respect to GT have higher overlapping degree (Jaccard and Dice index increase 0.03–0.53 and 0.02–0.41) and closer border (Hausdorff distance and RMSE decrease 0.06–2.63 mm and 0.03–0.49 mm).

4   Conclusion

In this study, we have proposed a context-aware inductive bias learning approach as a novel clinical tool for the first time to detect vessel borders in multi-modal intracoronary imaging. It is instantiated by a semantic-fusion multi-task neural network architecture that can learn from the related semantic information and varied environment information of the three vessel borders. The extensive experiments demonstrates the effectiveness of our approach and its superiority to the six state-of-the-art single-mode vessel border detection methods.

Acknowledgement. We gratefully acknowledge the support of NVIDIA Corporation with the donation of the Titan V GPU used for this research.

References

1. Cao, Y., et al.: Automatic side branch ostium detection and main vascular segmentation in intravascular optical coherence tomography images. IEEE J. Biomed. Health Inf. **22**(5), 1531–1539 (2018)
2. Su, S., et al.: An artificial neural network method for lumen and media-adventitia border detection in IVUS. Comput. Med. Imaging Graph. **57**(4), 29–39 (2017)

3. Xu, C., et al.: Direct delineation of myocardial infarction without contrast agents using a joint motion feature learning architecture. Med. Image Anal. **50**, 82–94 (2018)

4. Zhao, S., et al.: Robust segmentation of intima-media borders with different morphologies and dynamics during the cardiac cycle. IEEE J. Biomed. Health Inf. **22**(5), 1571–1582 (2018)

5. Zhao, R., et al.: Weakly-supervised simultaneous evidence identification and segmentation for automated glaucoma diagnosis. In: AAAI, pp. 1571–1582 (2019)

6. Paulo, M., et al.: Combined use of OCT and IVUS in spontaneous coronary artery dissection. JACC: Cardiovasc. Imaging **6**(7), 830–832 (2013)

7. Fujii, K., et al.: Accuracy of OCT, grayscale IVUS, and their combination for the diagnosis of coronary TCFA: an ex vivo validation study. JACC: Cardiovasc. Imaging **8**(4), 451–460 (2015)

8. Waggoner, J., et al.: How do OCT and IVUS differ? A comparison and assessment of these modern imaging modalities. Card. Interv. Today **3**, 46–52 (2011)

9. Pociask, E., et al.: Fully automated lumen segmentation method for intracoronary optical coherence tomography. J. Healthc. Eng. **2018**, 1–13 (2018)

10. Baxter, J.: A model of inductive bias learning. J. Artif. Intell. Res. **12**, 149–198 (2000)

11. Ruder, S.: An overview of multi-task learning in deep neural networks. Computing Research Repository arXiv:abs/1706.05098 (2017)

12. Zhang, Z., et al.: ExFuse: enhancing feature fusion for semantic segmentation. In: Ferrari, V., Hebert, M., Sminchisescu, C., Weiss, Y. (eds.) ECCV 2018. LNCS, vol. 11214, pp. 273–288. Springer, Cham (2018). https://doi.org/10.1007/978-3-030-01249-6_17

13. Kermani, A., et al.: A new nonparametric statistical approach to detect lumen and Media-Adventitia borders in intravascular ultrasound frames. Comput. Biol. Med. **104**(1), 10–28 (2019)

14. Lee, J.H., et al.: Segmentation of the lumen and media-adventitial borders in intravascular ultrasound images using a geometric deformable model. IET Image Proc. **12**(10), 1881–1891 (2018)

15. Amrute, J.M., et al.: Polymeric endovascular strut and lumen detection algorithm for intracoronary optical coherence tomography images. J. Biomed. Opt. **23**(3), 1–14 (2018)

Growth, Development, Atrophy, and Progression

Neural Parameters Estimation for Brain Tumor Growth Modeling

Ivan Ezhov[1(✉)], Jana Lipkova[1], Suprosanna Shit[1], Florian Kofler[1],
Nore Collomb[2], Benjamin Lemasson[2], Emmanuel Barbier[2], and Bjoern Menze[1]

[1] Department of Informatics, Technical University of Munich, Munich, Germany
ivan.ezhov@tum.de
[2] Grenoble Institut des Neurosciences, University Grenoble Alpes, Grenoble, France

Abstract. Understanding the dynamics of brain tumor progression is
essential for optimal treatment planning. Cast in a mathematical formulation, it is typically viewed as evaluation of a system of partial differential equations, wherein the physiological processes that govern the growth
of the tumor are considered. To personalize the model, i.e. find a relevant
set of parameters, with respect to the tumor dynamics of a particular
patient, the model is informed from empirical data, e.g., medical images
obtained from diagnostic modalities, such as magnetic-resonance imaging. Existing model-observation coupling schemes require a large number
of forward integrations of the biophysical model and rely on simplifying
assumption on the functional form, linking output of the model with
the image information. In this work, we propose a learning-based technique for the estimation of tumor growth model parameters from medical
scans. The technique allows for explicit evaluation of the posterior distribution of the parameters by sequentially training a mixture-density
network, relaxing the constraint on the functional form and reducing the
number of samples necessary to propagate through the forward model
for the estimation. We test the method on synthetic and real scans of
rats injected with brain tumors to calibrate the model and to predict
tumor progression.

1 Introduction

Modeling brain tumor progression holds a promise of optimizing clinical treatment planning. An appropriate tumor model, personalised with respect to the
patient-specific growth dynamics, could quantify clinically relevant information -
the tumor's morphology and its character of evolution [1]. Existing mathematical
description of the pathophysiological system spans from the intracellular level of
gene expression to the macroscopic level of bio-mechanical tumor-tissue interaction. The latter is the scale at which the medical imaging analysis is typically
carried out as this is the scale where medical scans are most interpretative.

Among the family of macroscopic models, the reaction-diffusion class of equations [2] is most widely adopted to characterize information visible on medical

---

I. Ezhov and J. Lipkova—The authors contributed equally to the work.

© Springer Nature Switzerland AG 2019
D. Shen et al. (Eds.): MICCAI 2019, LNCS 11765, pp. 787–795, 2019.
https://doi.org/10.1007/978-3-030-32245-8_87

scans. Under such equations the evolution of tumor cell density is tracked by considering tumor-relevant physiological processes, such as proliferation of cancerous cells, i.e. increase of the cells number due to its division, and the cells' migration into surrounding tissue. Various approaches have been developed to link the output of the model, the distribution of the cell density, with the tumor visible on images [1,3–9]. Methods as in [5] make a certain assumption on the cell density along visible tumor outlines and fit the model output to image observation that includes lesion growth and tissue displacement. The model adjustment, realized by means of a PDE-constrained optimisation scheme, allows to obtain a point estimate of free model parameters. Bayesian methods [1,7–9] cast the problem in a probabilistic formulation and provide estimation of the parameters along with confidence intervals via Markov Chain Monte Carlo (MCMC) sampling. The authors of [7] rely on the travelling wave formulation of [4] together with a Bayesian parameter estimation. In [1,9], authors construct a probabilistic graphical model wherein the probability of imaging signal is defined to be dependent on the biophysical model's output. For magnetic-resonance images (MRI), the probability of observing abnormality is defined as a logistic sigmoid function of the tumor cell density. Phenomenological introduction of the functional form leaves the question whether it possesses a capacity to approximate the mapping between cell density and the imaging information. Also, generating samples from the posterior distribution as with the MCMC methods requires large number of evaluations of the forward model, which can be of the order 10–100 thousand evaluations [1,9]. This results in an expensive computational cost, impeding clinical validation of more complex models and eventually the approach's adoptability to a routine daily use within clinical settings.

In this paper, we adopt methodological advances in the estimation of forward model parameters, relying on learning-based strategy [10,11]. The technique allows for explicit evaluation of the distribution over the parameters by training a mixture-density network (MDN) [12]. The MDN, modeled as a feedforward fully-connected network, maps the output of the model to parameters of the distribution in a non-linear fashion. As theoretical works [13] prove, such a network can serve as a universal function approximation, thus relaxing the necessity of introducing an explicit form for the likelihood, relating the model output and imaging data. In summary, the contributions of this paper are threefold: (1) We make the technique applicable to PDE-based tumor growth models, (2) We validate our method on synthetic and real data of rats implanted with cancer cell lines, using two time points for the model initialization and calibration, (3) We demonstrate that the technique provides more accurate parametric estimations and requires less forward model's samples as compared to explicit Bayesian formulation even with highly efficient MCMC sampling method.

2   Method

Tumor Growth Model. We base our forward model on the reaction-diffusion equation, describing the tumor progression via spatial and temporal evolution of the cancerous cell density. Particularly, a special type of the reaction-diffusion formalism, the Fisher-Kolmogorov equation, is used:

$$\frac{\partial u}{\partial t} = \nabla(\mathbf{D}\nabla u) + \rho u(1 - u), \quad in \quad \Omega \tag{1}$$

$$\mathbf{n} \cdot \nabla u = 0, \quad in \quad \Gamma_\Omega. \tag{2}$$

Equation (1) considers two pathophysiological processes: the logistic proliferation of the cells and its diffusion into neighbouring tissue. u denotes the tumor cell density in the volume of the brain Ω, $\mathbf{D}$ is the diffusion tensor and ρ denotes tumor proliferation rate. The diffusion is assumed to be heterogeneous: with different degree of infiltration in the white and the grey matters, and restricted in the ventricles area. We impose no-flux boundary condition Eq. (2), $\mathbf{n}$ denotes the unit vector orthogonal to the boundary of the simulation domain Γ_Ω and ∇ is the gradient operator. We performed experiments with two variants of the model initialization: as a seed point at a fixed location $\mathbf{r}^*$ ($u(\mathbf{r}, 0) = u_0$ if $\mathbf{r} = \mathbf{r}*$, $u(\mathbf{r}, 0) = 0$ elsewhere), and as an approximation of the cell density distribution, obtained from an image observation at the first monitoring time point ($u(\mathbf{r}, 0) = u_0(\mathbf{r})$).

Linking Tumor Model and Image Observation. We calibrate the model parameters from image observations in the form of 3D binary tumor segmentations, obtained from MRI modalities. Two MRI modalities, T1-gadolinium hyper-intensities (featuring active tumor core) and T2-hyper-intensities (featuring whole tumor), were used in order to better describe the right tumor morphology. To make the output of the model consistent with the segmentations we make a physiologically plausible assumption that regions of abnormalities visible on the images correspond to regions of high cell infiltration. Respecting the assumption, we introduce two additional parameters u^{T1}, u^{T2} for thresholding the simulated cell density profile, leading to isolines of the tumor cell density that we assume to match outlines of the tumor visible in a given modality. The thresholded binary volumes are combined by element-wise summation to form a 3D label map.

Neural Parameters Inference. We can view the forward model's output X – the 3D label map – as a sample from a likelihood distribution $p(X|\theta)$ conditioned on a set of parameters $\theta = \{D, \rho, u^{T1}, u^{T2}\}$. The distribution $p(X|\theta)$ cannot be in general evaluated, but its samples are readily available from the tumor model. Given an observation X_{obs} – segmentations of the tumor in the MRI modalities (summed element-wise), our goal is to infer the posterior distribution of the tumor model parameters, using the Bayes rule: $p(\theta|X_{obs}) \propto p(X_{obs}|\theta)p(\theta)$.

In [1,9], the likelihood is approximated by Bernoulli distribution with the parameter of the distribution defined as logistic sigmoid function. In our work, for inference of the forward model's parameters, we adopt a methodology that allows to learn a nonlinear mapping from the output of the model directly to posterior distribution over its parameters [10]. The inference is based on the neural posterior estimation (NPE), wherein an approximated posterior $q_\phi(\theta|X)$, modeled as a mixture density network, converges to the true posterior $p(\theta|X)$ (via the Kullback-Leibler divergence minimization) by iteratively performing the following steps illustrated in Fig. 1:

(1) [*Blue box*] Pairs $\{\theta_i, X_i\}_{i=1}^N$ are generated to form a training dataset. First, the <u>tumor simulator</u> parameters $\{D_i, \rho_i\}$ are sampled from a prior $p(\theta)$ distribution (which is uniform at the first iteration step $s = 1$) and corresponding simulation is propagated until the fixed time point t^* to obtain the 3D cell density profile u_i. Then, u_i is transformed to obtain binary segmentation masks, using the other two sampled parameters $\{u_i^{T1}, u_i^{T2}\}$. Together, the segmentation masks form X_i.

(2) [*Yellow box*] The MDN is trained by taking X_i as input and outputting parameters $\alpha_k^s, \boldsymbol{\mu}_k^s, \boldsymbol{\Sigma}_k^s$ of a <u>mixture of Gaussians</u> $q_{\phi^s}(\theta|X) = \sum_k \alpha_k^s N(\theta|\boldsymbol{\mu}_k^s, \boldsymbol{\Sigma}_k^s)$ of K components. The objective of the approximated posterior $q_{\phi^s}(\theta|X)$ training is to maximize the total log-loss, $L(\phi^s) = \sum_i log(q_{\phi^s}(\theta_i|X_i))$.

(3) [*Orange box*] The trained MDN is used to <u>infer observation specific parameters</u> of the Gaussian mixture $\alpha_{obs}^s, \boldsymbol{\mu}_{obs}^s, \boldsymbol{\Sigma}_{obs}^s$ by evaluating $q_{\phi^s}(\theta|X = X_{obs})$ at the observation X_{obs} - the label map, obtained from MRI segmentations at t^*.

(4) [*Red box*] Finally, the observation specific parameters are used to <u>update estimation of the posterior</u> $p^s(\theta|X_{obs}) = q_{\phi^s}(\theta|X = X_{obs}; \alpha_{obs}^s, \boldsymbol{\mu}_{obs}^s, \boldsymbol{\Sigma}_{obs}^s)$, which then used as a proposal distribution for sampling model parameters during the next iteration.

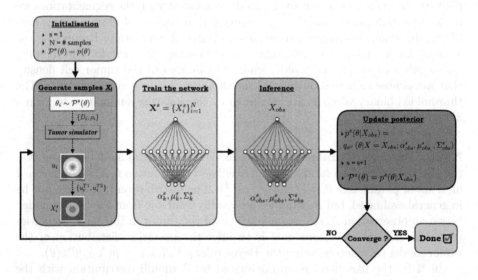

Fig. 1. The neural posterior estimator. At the heart of it is a mixture density network that maps input data to closed form estimates of the model parameters. It guides the patient-specific simulation of the tumor growth in an efficient iterative fashion.

During successive iterations all the four steps are identical except the step 2, that requires modification of the training objective. To compensate for the fact that we sample from the proposal distribution, the objective function is weighted by a ratio between the prior and proposal distributions $p(\theta_i)/p^s(\theta_i|X_{obs})$ [10]:

$$L(\phi^s) = \sum_i \frac{p(\theta_i)}{p^s(\theta_i|X_{obs})} log(q_{\phi^s}(\theta_i|X_i)) \tag{3}$$

Implementation. We implement the tumor simulator using 3D extension of the multi-resolution adaptive grid solver [14], allowing for high-parallelization. The typical execution time is 20–40 s with 8 CPU cores. The architecture of the neural estimator represents a feedforward fully-connected network with a single hidden layer of 100 units with *tanh* as an activation function. We initialize the weights of the network with He-normal [15] at the first iteration and use the weights trained at the iteration step s for initialization at the s+1 step. The latter allows to implicitly reuse the samples from previous iterations: for memory efficiency, it is desirable to avoid having to store and reuse directly old samples since we are dealing with 3D volumes. The network was trained using the Adam optimizer [16] for 100 epochs at each iteration. For each subject *a separate network is employed*. We run the experiments on NVIDIA Quadro P6000 GPU.

3   Experiments

Data. In our experiments, we use synthetic and real data of human glioma cells injected in the rat brain. For producing the synthetic data, we simulate a 3D tumor in the anatomy, obtained from rats brain atlas. We initialize the tumor as a seed point at a fixed location with the diffusion coefficient in the white matter D_w = 0.02 [mm^2/day] greater than in the grey matter $D_w = 10D_g$, and proliferation rate $\rho = 0.6$ [1/day]. To generate tumor segmentations masks, we threshold the simulated normalized cell density profile at $u^{T1} = 0.7$ and $u^{T2} = 0.25$ for T1 and T2 modalities, respectively, at a single calibration time point ($t^* = $ day 9). The day 11 is used for the model validation. The real data were obtained by injecting F98 tumor cell lines in rats brain. The tumor progression was monitored at several time points from day 9 to day 16, using T1w, T2w, and DWI imaging modalities. The images were expert-annotated. Since the initial condition of tumor location and shape is unknown in the real rats due to the injection, we made use of the DWI modality at the first monitoring time point (day 9) for model initialization. The apparent diffusion coefficient (ADC), calculated from the DWI, can be considered to be inversely proportional to the tumor cell density [17]. We used the ADC, confined within the T2w segmentation volume, as initial condition (in the late time states of tumor progression, the complex tumor microenvironment, hypoxia and necrosis complicate the simple inversely proportional relation). The binary segmentations from the T1w and T2w at the next time point ($t^* = $ day 11) are used for inference of the model parameters, and at the following days (14 and 16) we validate the model predictions, Fig. 3.

Results on Synthetic Data. For a sensitivity analysis of the inference, experiments on the synthetic data were first performed. In Fig. 2 we show a pairwise correlation of the forward model parameters $\{D, \rho, u^{T1}, u^{T2}\}$ obtained with the neural posterior estimator and the explicit Bayesian inference with MCMC sampling from [1]. For both methods, 1000 samples were used for the inference. Depicted by red stars and orange vertical lines are ground truth (gt) data. The proposed method provides the maximum a posteriori estimation (MAP) for all the parameters in a close agreement with the gt data. In consistency with [1],

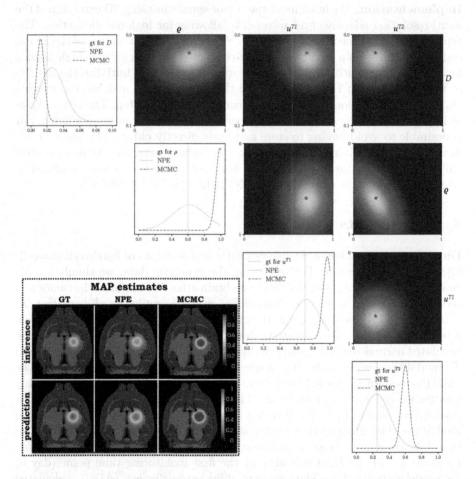

Fig. 2. Posterior distribution of the tumor growth model's parameters inferred for the synthetic rats data: 1D distributions along the diagonal (for the NPE and MCMC methods) and 2D marginals (for the NPE) elsewhere. Depicted by red stars and orange vertical lines are ground truth data. Tumors simulated in the rats brain atlas using the ground truth parameters, and MAP parametric estimates obtained by the NPE and MCMC-based methods are shown on the inset. The top row depicts 2D slices of the cell density profile at the inference time point (day 9), and the bottom row - at the prediction time point (day 11). (Color figure online)

for the MCMC, based on the likelihood formulation as a logistic sigmoid, the information in the form of binary segmentations is not sufficient to recover the gt parameters. At the same time, the NPE is more computationally efficient, since we observe accurate estimates after running 4 iterations of the posterior update, whereas the MCMC-based method requires about 20 sampling generations for convergence. This is attributed to (a) sampling from a range of the parametric space more relevant to the observation after each iteration, (b) efficient use of the samples as the technique does not imply any rejection thereof. The inset on the Fig. 2 shows the tumor cell density computed with the MAP parametric estimations from each method, in comparison with the ground truth data.

Results on Real Data. We validated the method on two real rat cases. Figure 3 shows the tumor cell distributions for one of the rats, simulated using the inferred MAP estimates, at the calibration time point (day 11) and at the validation points (days 14 and 16).The volume dynamics of T2 tumor segmentations for

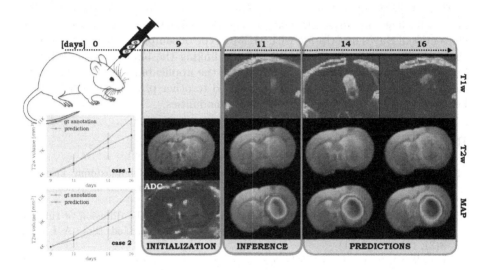

Fig. 3. Data preparation and results of the inference for the real rat cases. After the injection of cancer lines, the rats are monitored at four time points by means of the T1w, T2w and DWI modalities. The inverse ADC from the DWI at day 9 serves as an initial condition for the tumor model. The model parameters are inferred from the binary segmentations, obtained from the T1w and T2w scans at day 11. The model predictions, simulated using MAP estimations of the D, ρ parameters, are validated at days 14 and 16. In the bottom row, the predicted tumor cell density profiles, overlayed on the T2w, are shown. In the middle row, the pink outlines are boundaries of the T2w segmentations. The inset shows volume dynamics of the T2w binary segmentations, obtained from the annotation and predicted by the model, for two rats (the rat case 1 corresponds to the scans shown above). The inferred parametric uncertainties were propagated through the model to obtain mean and standard deviation (blue bars) of the dynamics. (Color figure online)

both rats, calculated from the annotation and predicted by the model, is shown on the inset. The predicted segmentations were obtained by thresholding the simulated cell density profile at the inferred u^{T2} level. While the volumes are in good agreement at the calibration time (an indication of plausible parametric inference), the model prediction underestimates the real tumor dynamics at the validation points. This can be attributed to simplifying assumptions of the Fisher-Kolmogorov model, such as constant proliferation and diffusion for all time points, which limit model's ability to describe the nonlinear character of the real tumor progression. As the proposed inference scheme opens an avenue for efficient parametric estimation, we will test more complicated tumor growth formalisms, e.g., accounting for tissue displacement and microenvironmental influence, in future work.

4   Conclusion

We present an approach for inferring parameters of a tumor model from information available on medical scans relying on a learning-based strategy. The approach allows for more efficient parametric estimation, as compared to the conventional Bayes description with MCMC type of sampling, and exempts from the necessity to introduce an explicit form, linking the biophysical model with image observation. Despite we demonstrate the applicability of the method to tumor modeling, the method can be adopted to other physical modeling problems that require calibration from imaging modalities.

References

1. Lipkova, J., et al.: Personalized radiotherapy design for Glioblastoma: integrating mathematical tumor models, multimodal scans and Bayesian inference. IEEE Trans. Med. Imaging **38**, 1875–1884 (2019)
2. Chaplain, M., Stuart, A.M.: A mathematical model for the diffusion of tumour angiogenesis factor into the surrounding host tissue. Math. Med. Biol.: A J. IMA **8**(3), 191–220 (1991)
3. Unkelbach, J., et al.: Radiotherapy planning for glioblastoma based on a tumor growth model: improving target volume delineation. Phys. Med. Biol. **59**(3), 747–770 (2014)
4. Konukoglu, E., et al.: Image guided personalization of reaction-diffusion type tumor growth models using modified anisotropic eikonal equations. IEEE Trans. Med. Imaging **29**(1), 77–95 (2010)
5. Hogea, C., et al.: An image-driven parameter estimation problem for a reaction-diffusion glioma growth model with mass effects. J. Math. Biol. **56**(6), 793–825 (2008)
6. Rockne, R., et al.: A patient-specific computational model of hypoxia-modulated radiation resistance in glioblastoma using 18F-FMISO-PET. JRS Interface **12**, 20141174 (2015)
7. Lê, M., et al.: Bayesian personalization of brain tumor growth model. In: Navab, N., Hornegger, J., Wells, W.M., Frangi, A.F. (eds.) MICCAI 2015. LNCS, vol. 9350, pp. 424–432. Springer, Cham (2015). https://doi.org/10.1007/978-3-319-24571-3_51

8. Hawkins-Daarud, A., et al.: Quantifying uncertainty and robustness in a biomathematical model-based patient-specific response metric for glioblastoma. JCO Clin. Cancer Inf. **3**, 1–8 (2019)

9. Menze, B.H., et al.: A generative approach for image-based modeling of tumor growth. In: Székely, G., Hahn, H.K. (eds.) IPMI 2011. LNCS, vol. 6801, pp. 735–747. Springer, Heidelberg (2011). https://doi.org/10.1007/978-3-642-22092-0_60

10. Lueckmann, J.M., et al.: Flexible statistical inference for mechanistic models of neural dynamics. In: NeurIPS, pp. 1289–1299 (2017)

11. Papamakarios, G., Murray, I.: Fast ϵ-free inference of simulation models with Bayesian conditional density estimation. In: NeurIPS, pp. 1028–1036 (2016)

12. Bishop, C.M.: Mixture density networks. Technical report (1994)

13. Hornik, K.: Approximation capabilities of multilayer feedforward networks. Neural Netw. **4**(2), 251–257 (1991)

14. Rossinelli, D., et al.: MRAG-I2D: multi-resolution adapted grids for remeshed vortex methods on multicore architectures. J. Comput. Phys. **288**, 1–18 (2015)

15. He, K., et al.: Delving deep into rectifiers: surpassing human-level performance on ImageNet classification. In: ICCV, pp. 1026–1034 (2015)

16. Kingma, D.P., Ba, J.: Adam: a method for stochastic optimization. In: 3rd International Conference on Learning Representations, ICLR 2015, San Diego, CA, USA, 7–9 May 2015, Conference Track Proceedings (2015)

17. Surov, A., et al.: Correlation between apparent diffusion coefficient and cellularity is different in several tumors: a meta-analysis. Oncotarget **8**(35), 59492–59499 (2017)

Learning-Guided Infinite Network Atlas Selection for Predicting Longitudinal Brain Network Evolution from a Single Observation

Baha Eddine Ezzine[1,2] and Islem Rekik[1(✉)]

[1] BASIRA Lab, Faculty of Computer and Informatics,
Istanbul Technical University, Istanbul, Turkey
[2] National Engineering School of Sousse (ENISo),
University of Sousse, Sousse, Tunisia
irekik@itu.edu.tr
http://basira-lab.com

Abstract. Building accurate predictive models to foresee the temporal evolution of diverse medical data representations derived from healthy or disordered brain images will enable a formidable, yet challenging, leap forward in the fields of neuroscience and neuro-disorders. However, such models remain very scarce. Existing landmark works on predicting follow-up medical data from a single observation have a few drawbacks. First, these were developed only for predicting brain shapes or images, while brain network representations remain untapped. Second, the bulk of such models lies in the selection of reliable atlases in the baseline domain, which act as proxies for the follow-up domains where the missing data live. However, current atlas selection strategies for prediction suffer from two major limitations: (i) they are selected based on their proximity to the testing sample using a *pre-defined* distance, which might not be robust to outliers and constrains the locality of the high-dimensional data to a fixed bandwidth, and (ii) atlases are selected *independently of one another*, which overlooks how the importance of an individual atlas is influenced by all the other atlases in the set. To address these limitations, we propose LINAs, the first framework for *predicting brain network evolution from a single timepoint* using learning-guided infinite network atlas selection in two steps. First, we learn how to select the best atlases in an *unsupervised* manner by learning an adjacency graph which encodes the pairwise similarities between all atlases. The relevance score of an atlas is estimated using all possible infinite paths connecting it to other atlases in the set, quantifying its representativeness and centrality. Second, we propose to individualize the atlas score to the testing sample by a *supervised* re-weighting strategy. Our comprehensive experiments on healthy and disordered brain networks demonstrate the outperformance of LINAs in comparison with its variants as well as state-of-the-art methods. LINAs presents the first step towards building connectome evolution models that can be leveraged for developing precision medicine.

This work was supported by Bilimsel Araştırma Projeleri (BAP) fund from Istanbul Technical University.

1   Introduction

The proliferation of longitudinal neuroimaging datasets presents formidable opportunities to build predictive methods that *learn* how to foresee data driven from brain images such as magnetic resonance imaging (MRI) based on *a single observation*. Despite their scarcity, such models provide unparalleled opportunities for predicting brain developmental [1] and aging [2] trajectories in both health and disease. In particular, accurate and effective predictive methods estimating the evolution trajectory of a specific brain disorder can help monitor the disorder in a very early stage. In fact, preventive treatment is more likely to succeed the earlier the disorder is detected, requiring subjects to wait for multiple measurements at different timepoints may hinder their treatment and recovery processes. Seminal works on predicting the spatiotemporal (i.e., 4D) trajectory of brain data from baseline mainly focused on predicting the evolution of shapes (e.g., cortical surface) in healthy infants [1] or MR images to improve the diagnosis of demented patients [2], overlooking a fundamental representation of the brain construct: networks (or connectomes) [3]. **To the best of our knowledge, no existing works attempted to solve the problem of brain network evolution prediction from baseline.** Despite their high-dimensionality, brain images or shapes present simple representations of the brain where regions of interest (ROIs) are investigated independently, whereas the brain network representation allows to examine the brain as a complex interconnected system, where *the relationship or connection* between brain regions becomes the feature of interest (Fig. 1).

Brain atlas selection has been an active field of research in developing MRI-based classification methods where single-atlas or multi-atlas based morphometric representations of brain structures are extracted [4–7], to name a few. These can serve as prior knowledge to *guide* predictive models and more recently the training of deep learning architectures for automatic brain labeling [8]. In particular, to solve the problem of learning how to map high-dimensional baseline data to high-dimensional follow-up data in the temporal domain, existing predictive frameworks [1,2] relied on selecting the best baseline atlases that act as proxies linking the baseline domain to the follow-up domains for the pre-

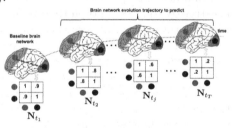

Fig. 1. *Prediction of brain network evolution trajectory from a single timepoint t_1.* In this illustration, we sketch the scenario where the connection in a brain network composed of $n_r = 2$ regions of interest (ROIs) weakens over time. This connection weakening can be explained by a normal evolution due to neural pruning during postnatal development or cognitive decline during normal aging or pathological evolution due to a particular brain disorder – to give a few possible scenarios.

diction task in hand. This essential step is rooted in the following assumption: *if one can learn how to identify the best representative atlases for a given testing subject at baseline timepoint, one can use a weighted average of their corresponding follow-up atlases to predict the missing follow-up data.* To relax this strong assumption, a few works [1] integrated an *atlas individualization* step, where the testing subject is used to locally morph the selected atlases in the baseline domain to enhance atlas-testing subjects' similarity. Next, by applying those individualizing local morphing actions to the follow-up atlases, the target missing data is predicted. However, existing atlas selection strategies for prediction suffer from two major limitations: (i) they are selected based on their proximity to the testing sample using a pre-defined distance, which might not be robust to outliers and constrains the locality of the high-dimensional data to a fixed bandwidth, and (ii) atlases are selected independently while overlooking how the importance of an individual atlas is influenced by all the other atlases in the set.

To address all these limitations, given a specific testing baseline network, we first aim to learn how to select the optimal subset of m out of n network atlases where $m \ll n$, which is an NP-hard problem since we need to evaluate C_m^n combinations of atlases. Hence, suboptimal search strategies are desired. Inspired by the vibrant field of feature selection, we leverage the idea presented in the work of Roffo *et al.* [9] where a filter-based feature selection method is designed for classification purposes by learning how to rank features based on infinite possible paths connecting them to subsets of features on a graph modeling the relationship between pairs of features. Although compelling, such method cannot handle features drawn from different distributions as it uses a *fixed* similarity measure defined using the variance and correlation of pairs of features. To address this first limitation, we propose a multiple kernel-based network atlas manifold learning strategy to *learn* a graph that models the similarity between network atlases while capturing their underlying statistical distributions with potential different bandwidths. Up to this point, all previous steps are implemented in an unsupervised manner, where network atlases are ranked based on the learned manifold where they are nested. To *individualize* our network atlas selection strategy for prediction, we propose a supervised atlas reweighting strategy, where we weigh the unsupervised learned score assigned to a particular atlas by its distance from the baseline testing network. This defines our learning-guided infinite network atlas selection (LINAs) framework for network evolution prediction from baseline.

The main contributions of our method are four-fold:

1. *On a conceptual level.* LINAs is the first framework that predicts the evolution of brain networks from a single observation.
2. *On a methodological level.* LINAs proposes a novel unsupervised infinite atlas ranking strategy based on atlas manifold learning, further boosted by a an individualization step for the target prediction task.
3. *On an clinical and translational levels.* This is the first framework to predict both disordered and normal brain evolution over time. It can be integrated in the clinical routine for *early* brain disorder diagnosis and treatment planning.

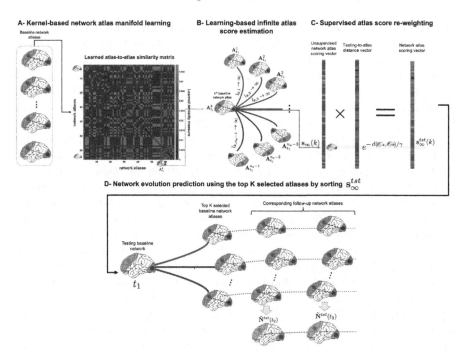

Fig. 2. *Proposed LINAs steps for predicting brain network evolution trajectory from a single observation at baseline t_1.* **(A)** *Network atlas-to-atlas relationship learning.* Using multiple kernel learning to model the relationship between a set of n_a network atlases using manifold learning. **(B)** *Unsupervised network atlas ranking in relation to other atlases.* Proposed infinite network atlas selection for identifying the most representative network atlases in an unsupervised manner, where each baseline network atlas $\mathbf{A}_{t_1}^k$ is assigned a ranking score $\mathbf{s}_\infty(k)$. **(C)** *Network atlas score individualization.* The distance between the target baseline testing network $\mathbf{N}_{t_1}^{tst}$ and each network atlas $\mathbf{A}_{t_1}^k$ is used to weigh each $\mathbf{s}_\infty(k)$ to produce the final score $\mathbf{s}_\infty^{tst}(k)$ for atlas selection. **(D)** *Prediction step.* All network atlases are sorted by decreasing scores and the top K baseline network atlases are then selected for prediction. By averaging their corresponding observations at follow-up timepoints, the testing network evolution trajectory is predicted.

4. *On a generic level.* LINAs can be also utilized to improve conventional image and shape-based evolution prediction frameworks as it nicely models the relationship among atlases to boost prediction accuracy.

2 Proposed Method

In the following, we present the main steps of LINAs for predicting longitudinal brain network evolution from a single timepoint. Matrices are denoted by bold-face capital letters, e.g., $\mathbf{X}$, and scalars are denoted by lowercase letters, e.g., x. We denote the transpose operator as $\mathbf{X}^T$. Figure 2 presents a unified view for the proposed LINAs framework in four major steps, which will be detailed below.

Overview of Prediction Network Evolution Framework from Baseline
$\mathbf{N}(t_1)$. Suppose we have n_a training subjects, each subject has T brain networks
$\mathbf{N}^{tr}(t_i)$ acquired at multiple times points t_i, $i \in \{1, 2, \ldots, T\}$. Given an unseen
testing subject with a baseline network $\mathbf{N}^{tst}(t_1)$, we aim to predict its evolution
network trajectory $\{\tilde{\mathbf{N}}^{tst}(t_2), \ldots, \tilde{\mathbf{N}}^{tst}(t_T)\}$ at available training observations.
To do so, conventional predictive methods [1,2] assumed that if one can iden-
tify the top K most similar network atlases $\{\mathbf{A}_{t_1}^1, \ldots, \mathbf{A}_{t_1}^K\}$ to the target testing
subject at baseline t_1, then a weighted average of their evolution trajectories
for $t \in \{2, \ldots, T\}$ at follow-up observations can be used as a first estimate of
the testing network evolution trajectory. In this setting, all training samples are
considered as potential atlases. Next, an individualization step can be used to
further refine the predicted evolution trajectory by further investigating the relationship between (i) the baseline testing network and (ii) each of the top selected
baseline atlases [2] or their average $\bar{\mathbf{A}}_{t_1}$ as in [1]. As illustrated in Fig. 2, this
conventional strategy only explores the relationship between the baseline atlases
and the target baseline testing network, while overlooking the relationship among
atlases. This could include redundant information from similar atlases that are
very closely nested around the testing baseline sample, thereby decreasing the
representativeness of the selected atlas set for the target prediction task. Besides,
not selecting irrelevant, redundant, or noisy atlases might be challenging in such
case since the unique pairwise relationship that is deployed for atlas selection
solely involves the testing baseline sample – as opposed to exploring all possible interactions among atlases. To address this *first* limitation, we propose a
variant of infinite feature selection method [9], where a single feature in our
case becomes a high-dimensional sample (or atlas), thereby generalizing [9] to
high-dimensional data.

Proposed Infinite Sample Selection (ISS). In this section, we present the
possibility of learning how to rank samples (in our case network atlases) in
an *unsupervised* manner according to the scale of their representativeness and
centrality with regard to other samples in the set. Note that this is an NP hard
problem, which motivates us to adopt the infinite feature selection algorithm
[9] to efficiently explore this large search space of samples. The core idea is
to propose to model the relationship between samples using a graph, where
nodes are ranked according to their individuality or representativeness as well
as centrality (or importance) in relation to other nodes. In particular, given a set
of n_a baseline network atlases $\{\mathbf{A}_{t_1}^1, \ldots, \mathbf{A}_{t_1}^{n_a}\}$, we aim to estimate a score for each
atlas in the set. To do so, first we define a graph $G_a = (V_a, E_a)$, with n_a nodes
and where the weights of each edges are mapped onto an atlas-to-atlas adjacency
matrix $\mathbf{S}$. The pairwise similarity between two atlases $\mathbf{A}_{t_1}^i$ and $\mathbf{A}_{t_1}^j$ is defined as
follows: $\mathbf{S}(i,j) = \alpha\sigma_{ij} + (1-\alpha)c_{ij}$, where α denotes a loading coefficient. c_{ij} is 1
minus the Pearson correlation coefficient between the statistical distributions of
brain connections in atlases $\mathbf{A}_{t_1}^i$ and $\mathbf{A}_{t_1}^j$. $\sigma_{ij} = max(\sigma_i, \sigma_j)$, where σ_i denotes
the standard deviation of feature values (or connectivities) belonging to $\mathbf{A}^i$.

Next, we define a baseline path γ_{ij} of length l connecting two nodes $\mathbf{A}_{t_1}^i$ and
$\mathbf{A}_{t_1}^j$, with a joint energy $\mathcal{E}_{\gamma_{ij}} = \prod_{k=0}^{l-1} \mathbf{S}(k, k+1)$ including all pairwise energies
of all nodes composing γ_{ij}. The score of a single atlas $\mathbf{A}_{t_1}^i$ can then be defined in

terms of all possible paths of length l connecting it to all other nodes in the graph as follows: $\mathbf{s}_l(i) = \sum_{j \in V} \mathbf{S}^l(i,j)$, where $\mathbf{S}^l$ denotes the lth power iteration of $\mathbf{S}$. Imagine that we try all possible infinite paths connecting $\mathbf{A}^i_{t_1}$ to other atlases. This allows to circumvent the computational complexity of computing $\mathbf{s}_l$ and leads us to define a new 'infinite' score: $\mathbf{s}_{l \to \infty} = \sum_{l=1}^{\infty} \mathbf{s}_l(i)$. By introducing a real-valued factor $r \in]0,1]$ into the infinite score equation as $\sum_{l=1}^{\infty} r^l \mathbf{s}_l(i)$, computing $\mathbf{s}_{l \to \infty}$ elegantly boils down to computing the convergence property of the geometric power series of matrix $r\mathbf{S}$ [9]:

$$\mathbf{s}_\infty(i) = ((\mathbf{I}_{n_a} - r\mathbf{S})^{-1} - \mathbf{I}_{n_a}))_i,$$ where $\mathbf{I}_{n_a}$ denotes the identify matrix of size n_a by n_a. This can be intuitively explained in the light of graph centrality measures, which quantify the number of times a node is visited on any possible path passing through it.

Although elegant, this approach has two major limitations: (1) the predefined fixed similarity measure might fail to capture sample distribution with various bandwidths and the nonlinear relationship in the data; (2) the atlas ranking is conducted in a fully unsupervised manner where the testing baseline network does not *supervise* the scoring of the most relevant atlases for predicting its evolution trajectory. To address these limitations, we propose a *learning-guided infinite network atlas selection strategy*, which learns the similarity between atlases while capturing their potential disparity in distribution, and leverages the baseline testing network to individualize and further refine the learned unsupervised scores of the baseline network atlases.

Proposed LINAs. Figure 2 presents a unified view for the proposed LINAs framework, which we detail below.

Multi-Kernel Based Network Atlas Manifold Learning Step. Instead of predefining the network atlas adjacency matrix $\mathbf{S}$, we extend the recently developed multi-kernel manifold learning (MKML) approach proposed in [10] to our aim. Specifically, [10] proposes to learn the manifold by learning the weights $\{w_k\}_{k=1}^{n_k}$ associated with a set of Gaussian kernels $\{\mathbf{K}_k\}_{k=1}^{n_k}$ with different bandwidths that can capture the diverse statistical characteristics of the input data. The learned manifold also addresses the challenge of high levels of dropout events by employing a rank constraint in the learned cell-to-cell similarity.

Each Gaussian kernel is defined as: $\mathbf{K}(\mathbf{a}^i, \mathbf{a}^j) = \frac{1}{\epsilon_{ij}\sqrt{2\pi}} e^{(-\frac{|\mathbf{a}^i - \mathbf{a}^j|^2}{2\epsilon_{ij}^2})}$, where $\mathbf{a}^i$ and $\mathbf{a}^j$ denote the feature vectors of the i-th and j-th network atlas respectively and ϵ_{ij} is defined as: $\epsilon_{ij} = \sigma(\mu_i + \mu_j)/2$, where σ is a tuning parameter and $\mu_i = \frac{\sum_{l \in KNN(\mathbf{a}^i)} |\mathbf{a}^i - \mathbf{a}^j|}{k}$, where $KNN(\mathbf{a}^i)$ represents the top k neighboring subjects of subject i. The weighted kernels are then averaged to produce the target similarity matrix $\mathbf{S}$. These are estimated along with an $n_a \times n_c$ latent matrix $\mathbf{L}$ capturing n_c inherent distribution of the data by solving the following optimization problem:

$$\min_{\mathbf{S}, \mathbf{L}, \mathbf{w}} \sum_{i,j,k} -w_k \mathbf{K}_k(\mathbf{a}^i, \mathbf{a}^j)\mathbf{S}_{ij} + \beta||\mathbf{S}||_F^2 + \eta \mathrm{tr}(\mathbf{L}^T(\mathbf{I}_{n_a} - \mathbf{S})\mathbf{L}) + \rho \sum_k w_k \log w_k$$

Subject to: $\sum_k w_k = 1, w_k \geq 0, \mathbf{L}^T\mathbf{L} = \mathbf{I}_{n_c}, \sum_j \mathbf{S}_{ij} = 1,$ and $\mathbf{S}_{ij} \geq 0, \forall(i,j).$

The first term refers to the relation between the similarity and the kernel distance with weights w_l between two network atlases. The second term denotes a regularization term that avoids over-fitting the model to the data. The learned similarity $\mathbf{S}$ should be small if the distance between a pair of networks is large. The matrix $(\mathbf{I}_{n_a} - \mathbf{S})$ denotes the graph Laplacian. The last term imposes constraints on the kernel weights to avoid selection of a single kernel. An alternating convex optimization is adopted where each variable is optimized while fixing the other variables until convergence [10].

Supervised Network Atlas Reweighting Strategy. All previous steps completely overlook the existing baseline testing network $\mathbf{N}^{tst}(t_1)$, which can be leveraged to build the predictive framework. To do so, we propose a novel weighted score for each baseline network atlas $\mathbf{A}_{t_1}^k$, which is individualized by the distance between the testing baseline network and the network atlas as follows:

$$\mathbf{s}_\infty^{tst}(k) = \mathbf{s}_\infty(k) \times e^{-||\mathbf{N}^{tst}(t_1) - \mathbf{A}_{t_1}^k||_2/\theta}$$

LINAS-Based Brain Network Prediction Step. In the last step, following the ranking of n_a network atlases, we select the top K baseline network atlases with the highest scores $\mathbf{s}_\infty^{tst}$. By retrieving their follow-up network evolution trajectories and averaging them as sketched in Fig. 2D, we obtain the predicted trajectory for the target testing subject.

3   Results and Discussion

Evaluation Dataset. We used leave-one-out cross validation to evaluate the proposed network evolution prediction framework on 67 subjects (35 diagnosed with Alzheimer's disease and 32 diagnosed with late mild cognitive impairment) from ADNI GO public dataset[1], each with two structural T1-w MR images acquired at baseline and 6-month follow-up. We used FreeSurfer to reconstruct both right and left cortical hemispheres for each subject from T1-w MRI. Next, we parcellated each cortical hemisphere into 35 cortical ROIs using Desikan-Killiany Atlas. For each subject, we constructed morphological brain networks (MBN) at each timepoint using the methodology introduced in [11–13] using mean cortical thickness measure, where the morphological connectivity strength between two regions is defined as the absolute difference between the average cortical thickness in each region.

Parameter Setting. For fair comparison across all methods, we fixed the number of the selected network atlases $K = 5$. The regularization factor r for infinite network atlas selection was defined as $r = 0.9/\rho(\mathbf{S})$, as recommended [9] for convergence, leaving it fixed for all experiments. ρ denotes the spectral radius of $\mathbf{S}$. For MKML parameters, we tested LINAs using $n_c = 2$ and $n_c = 3$ clusters due to the small sample size. We used $n_k = 21$ kernels, where each kernel was

---

[1] http://adni.loni.usc.edu.

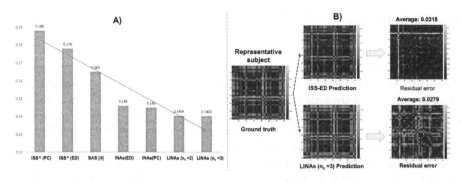

Fig. 3. (A) *Prediction accuracy using mean absolute error (MAE).* **ISS:** infinite sample selection, a generalized version of [9]* to high dimensional data. **ED:** Euclidean distance. **PC:** Pearson Correlation. **SAS:** supervised atlas selection [2]. **INAs:** a variant of LINAs discarding the atlas-to-atlas similarity learning component. n_c: number of clusters set for multi-kernel manifold learning. (B) *Comparison between the ground truth and predicted target networks for a representative subjects by LINAs and ISS-ED comparison method.* **ISS:** infinite sample selection, a generalized version of [9]* to high dimensional data, where sample-to-sample similarity is defined by exponentiating their negative Euclidean distance. We display the residual matrices computed using element-wise absolute difference between ground truth and predicted networks. We scale each graph differently for the best display effect.

determined by a set of bandwidths ($\sigma = 1 : 0.25 : 2.5$), number of top KNN neighbors in fixed to 10. We set $\theta = 1$ for infinite network atlas score reweighing.

Comparison Methods and Evaluation. We benchmarked LINAs against two baseline methods and its variant (INAs) which discards the atlas-to-atlas similarity learning component. The first comparison method is ISS using Pearson Correlation or Euclidean distance to predefine **S**. The second comparison method is supervised atlas selection (SAS) developed in [2], where the atlas selection is supervised not only by the testing subject but also its label (healthy or disordered); however, it does not investigate inter-atlas relationships. Figure 3A displays the results and shows the outperformance of LINAs for both $n_c = \{2, 3\}$ in comparison to other approaches. We also display in Fig. 3B the predicted brain networks at the follow-up timepoint using LINAs and ISS-ED approaches, along with the residual network (i.e., the absolute difference between the ground truth network and predicted one). Clearly LINAs produced follow-up networks with least residuals, and which resemble most the ground truth observations. Reproducing our results in large-scale multimodal connectomic datasets is our future research direction.

4   Conclusion

We proposed the first framework for predicting brain network evolution over time from a single observation using learning-guided infinite network atlas selection (LINAs). Our method achieved the best prediction results on our dataset. This is a first step towards building predictive intelligence in the brain connectomics research field, which might help develop precision medicine. However, there are few aspects that need to be considered when generalizing LINAs to (i) large connectomic datasets and (ii) multimodal datasets. First, when scaling our approach to a large dataset, the number of clusters for capturing the heterogeneity of network atlas distribution needs to be tuned automatically. A nested cross-validation can be used to solve this issue. Second, evaluating our method on functional connectomes might be challenging when handling negative connections. Hence, it needs to be further refined to meet this challenge and generalize to all multimodal connectomic brain networks (not only structural and morphological). In our future work, we will further extend LINAs to handle negative correlations in functional networks and evaluate the potential of predicted evolution trajectories in boosting the accuracy of diagnosing various brain disorders.

References

1. Rekik, I., Li, G., Yap, P., Chen, G., Lin, W., Shen, D.: Joint prediction of longitudinal development of cortical surfaces and white matter fibers from neonatal MRI. NeuroImage **152**, 411–424 (2017)
2. Gafuroğlu, C., Rekik, I., et al.: Joint prediction and classification of brain image evolution trajectories from baseline brain image with application to early dementia. In: International Conference on Medical Image Computing and Computer-Assisted Intervention, pp. 437–445 (2018)
3. Soussia, M., Rekik, I.: A review on image-and network-based brain data analysis techniques for Alzheimer's disease diagnosis reveals a gap in developing predictive methods for prognosis. arXiv preprint arXiv:1808.01951 (2018)
4. Cuingnet, R., et al.: Automatic classification of patients with Alzheimer's disease from structural MRI: a comparison of ten methods using the adni database. NeuroImage **56**, 766–781 (2011)
5. Liu, M., Zhang, D., Shen, D., Initiative, A.D.N.: Hierarchical fusion of features and classifier decisions for Alzheimer's disease diagnosis. Hum. Brain Mapp. **35**, 1305–1319 (2014)
6. Koikkalainen, J., et al.: Multi-template tensor-based morphometry: application to analysis of Alzheimer's disease. NeuroImage **56**, 1134–1144 (2011)
7. Min, R., Wu, G., Cheng, J., Wang, Q., Shen, D., Alzheimer's Disease Neuroimaging Initiative: Multi-atlas based representations for Alzheimer's disease diagnosis. Hum. Brain Mapp. **35**, 5052–5070 (2014)
8. Fang, L., et al.: Automatic brain labeling via multi-atlas guided fully convolutional networks. Med. Image Anal. **51**, 157–168 (2018)
9. Roffo, G., Melzi, S., Cristani, M.: Infinite feature selection. In: Proceedings of the IEEE International Conference on Computer Vision, pp. 4202–4210 (2015)

10. Wang, B., Zhu, J., Pierson, E., Ramazzotti, D., Batzoglou, S.: Visualization and analysis of single-cell RNA-seq data by kernel-based similarity learning. Nature **70**, 869–79 (2017)

11. Mahjoub, I., Mahjoub, M.A., Rekik, I.: Brain multiplexes reveal morphological connectional biomarkers fingerprinting late brain dementia states. Sci. Rep. **8**, 4103 (2018)

12. Soussia, M., Rekik, I.: Unsupervised manifold learning using high-order morphological brain networks derived from T1-w MRI for autism diagnosis. Front. Neuroinform. **12**, 70 (2018)

13. Lisowska, A., Rekik, I.: ADNI: joint pairing and structured mapping of convolutional brain morphological multiplexes for early dementia diagnosis. Brain Connect. **9**, 22–36 (2019)

Deep Probabilistic Modeling of Glioma Growth

Jens Petersen[1,2,3(✉)], Paul F. Jäger[1], Fabian Isensee[1], Simon A. A. Kohl[1],
Ulf Neuberger[2], Wolfgang Wick[4], Jürgen Debus[5,6,7], Sabine Heiland[2],
Martin Bendszus[2], Philipp Kickingereder[2], and Klaus H. Maier-Hein[1]

[1] Division of Medical Image Computing, German Cancer Research Center,
Heidelberg, Germany
jens.petersen@dkfz.de
[2] Department of Neuroradiology, Heidelberg University Hospital,
Heidelberg, Germany
[3] Department of Physics and Astronomy, Heidelberg University,
Heidelberg, Germany
[4] Department of Neurooncology, Heidelberg University Hospital,
Heidelberg, Germany
[5] Division of Molecular and Translational Radiation Oncology,
Heidelberg Institute of Radiation Oncology (HIRO), Heidelberg, Germany
[6] Heidelberg Ion-Beam Therapy Center (HIT), Heidelberg University Hospital,
Heidelberg, Germany
[7] Clinical Cooperation Unit Radiation Oncology, German Cancer Research Center,
Heidelberg, Germany

Abstract. Existing approaches to modeling the dynamics of brain
tumor growth, specifically glioma, employ biologically inspired models
of cell diffusion, using image data to estimate the associated parameters. In this work, we propose an alternative approach based on recent
advances in probabilistic segmentation and representation learning that
implicitly learns growth dynamics directly from data without an underlying explicit model. We present evidence that our approach is able to
learn a distribution of plausible future tumor appearances conditioned
on past observations of the same tumor.

Keywords: Glioma growth · Generative modeling · Probabilistic
segmentation

1 Introduction

Glial tumors, especially high grade ones known as glioblastoma multiforme
(GBM), are associated with highly irregular growth patterns, involving multiple tissue types for which the change in composition is notoriously difficult to
predict. While the prognosis for patients is generally poor, with a median survival of 15–16 months given standard of care treatment for GBM, a considerable

S. A. A. Kohl—Now with DeepMind and the Karlsruhe Institute of Technology.

D. Shen et al. (Eds.): MICCAI 2019, LNCS 11765, pp. 806–814, 2019.
https://doi.org/10.1007/978-3-030-32245-8_89

number of patients with high grade glioma survive multiple years after diagnosis [2]. An important factor for this is radiotherapy, which could benefit greatly from a better understanding of growth dynamics.

Most existing approaches that model the growth of glioma do this using variants of the reaction-diffusion equation on the basis of DTI data, e.g. [3,11], but also multi-modal data [7,10], a very recent example being [6] (for works from before 2011 we refer the reader to [9]).

In this work, we propose to learn growth dynamics directly from annotated MR image data, without specifying an explicit model, leveraging recent developments in deep generative models [5]. We further assume that imaging is ambiguous with respect to the underlying disease (an assumption shared e.g. in [6,10]), which is reflected in our approach in that it doesn't predict a single growth estimate (as is done e.g in [1,13] on a per-pixel level) but instead estimates a distribution of plausible changes for a given tumor. In plain words, we're not interested in the question "How much will the tumor grow (or shrink)?" but instead "If the tumor were to grow (or shrink), what would it look like?". From a clinical perspective, this is relevant for example in radiation therapy, where a margin of possible infiltration around the tumor will also be irradiated. This is currently done in a rather crude fashion by isotropically expanding the tumor's outline [8], thus more informed estimates of growth patterns could help spare healthy tissue. Our contributions are the following:

- We frame tumor growth modeling as a model-free learning problem, so that all dynamics are inferred directly from data.
- We present evidence that our approach learns a distribution of plausible growth trajectories, conditioned on previous observations of the same tumor.
- We provide source code: https://github.com/jenspetersen/probabilistic-unet.

2 Methods

The underlying hypothesis of our approach is that tumor growth is at least in part stochastic so that it's not possible to predict a single correct growth trajectory in time from image data alone. Hence, our aim is to *model a distribution of possible changes* of a tumor given the current and in our case one previous observation. We achieve this by training a model to reproduce true samples of observed growth trajectories—with shape and extent of the tumor being represented as multi-class segmentation maps—and using variational inference to allow the model to automatically recognize and account for ambiguity in the task.

2.1 Data

We work with an in-house dataset containing a total of 199 longitudinal MRI scans from 38 patients suffering from glioma (15 lower grade glioma and 23 glioblastoma), with a median of 96 days between scans and 5 scans per patient.

Patients have undergone different forms of treatment, a fact that we deliberately neglect by declaring it an additional source of ambiguity in the dataset. Each scan consists of 4 contrasts: native T1 (T1n), postcontrast T1 (T1ce), T2 (T2) and fluid-attenuated inversion recovery (FLAIR). All contrasts and time steps for a given patient are skull-stripped, registered to T1 space and resampled to isotropic 1 mm resolution [4]. For intensity normalization, we only employ basic z-score normalization. Ground truth segmentations of edema, enhancing tumor and necrosis were created semi-automatically by an expert radiologist.

2.2 Model

Our model along with the training procedure, based on a probabilistic segmentation approach [5], are visualized in Fig. 1. The architecture comprises three components: 1. A U-Net [12] to map scans from present and past to future tumor appearance. 2. A fully convolutional encoder that maps scans from present and past to an N-dimensional diagonal Gaussian (the *prior*; we choose $N = 3$). 3. An encoder with the same architecture that maps scans from present and past as well as the ground truth segmentation from the future to another diagonal Gaussian (the *posterior*; $N = 3$). During training we sample from the posterior and concatenate the sample to the activations of the last decoder block in the U-Net, so as to condition the softmax predictions on the sample. We employ multi-class cross entropy as the segmentation loss and use the Kullback-Leiber divergence to force prior and posterior towards each other, so that at test time— when a ground truth segmentation is no longer available—the predicted prior is as close as possible to the unknown posterior. This objective is the well known *evidence lower bound* used in variational inference.

The described training scheme will give rise to the following desirable properties: (1) The model will learn to represent the task's intrinsic ambiguity in the Gaussian latent space, in our case different plausible future tumor shapes and sizes, as we show in Sect. 3. (2) At test time we can sample multiple consistent hypotheses from the latent space (as seen in Fig. 2), and select those that match desired criteria (e.g. tumor volume increases by 20%).

We train with data augmentation (using https://github.com/MIC-DKFZ/batchgenerators) on patches of size 112^3, but evaluate on full sized scans of 192^3. For details on optimization and associated hyperparameters we refer to the provided source code (https://github.com/jenspetersen/probabilistic-unet).

2.3 Experiments and Evaluation

We seek to show that our approach learns meaningful future tumor appearances instead of just segmentation variants of the present input. For this reason we construct a baseline that is restricted to learning the latter.

Let A denote past, B present and C future. Our model is trained and evaluated for triples $AB \rightarrow C$ (that we will refer to as cases), as shown in Fig. 1. An upper bound on performance is given by a regular probabilistic segmentation model that is trained and evaluated with tuples $C \rightarrow C$. This is essentially a

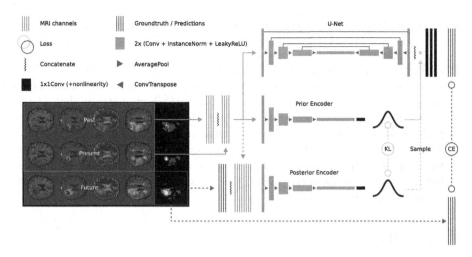

Fig. 1. The architecture employed in this work. Following the approach in [5], a U-Net [12] is augmented with two additional encoders, one for the prior and one for the posterior. The prior encoder maps the inputs of present and past scans to an N-dimensional diagonal Gaussian while the posterior does the same with additional access to the ground truth segmentation from the future. During training, a sample from the posterior is injected into the U-Net after the last decoder block to produce an output that is conditioned on the posterior. During testing the posterior is unavailable and samples can only be drawn from the prior. A KL divergence loss is used to force prior and posterior towards each other while cross entropy is used as segmentation loss. Dashed lines indicate paths that only apply during training.

model that has complete knowledge of the future and just needs to segment it. At the same time, a model trained on $B \to B$ but evaluated on $B \to C$ can serve as a lower bound to our model trained on $AB \to C$. If our performance matches that of the lower bound, we have learned to produce plausible segmentations for the current time step, but not the future.

We split our subjects randomly into 5 groups and perform 5-fold cross validation, i.e. we train on 4 subsets and predict the remaining one. For many triples, the real change between time steps is small, which makes it hard to show that our approach actually learns meaningful change. As a consequence we define two groups to report results for:

1. **Large Change:** The 10% of cases with the most pronounced change in terms of whole tumor Dice overlap, resulting in a threshold of 0.48 and 13 cases.
2. **Moderate Change:** The cases with larger than mean change (0.70), but not in top 10%, resulting in 44 cases.

We are not interested in predictive capabilities, so it makes little sense to look at the overlap of the prior mean predictions with the future ground truth (our approach performs not much better than the lower bound here). We report metrics that are representative of our model's desired capabilities, (1) a clinically relevant question, i.e. what the tumor will look like for a given expected size, and (2) how well the model is able to represent large changes in its latent space:

1. **Query Volume Dice:** We take samples from a grid around the prior mean (-3σ to $+3\sigma$ in steps of 1σ) and select the segmentation for which the whole tumor volume (i.e. all tumor classes contribute) best matches that of the ground truth. If our approach is able to model future appearances, it should perform better than the lower bound with increasing real change.
2. **Surprise:** This is the KL divergence the model assigns for a given combination of past & present scans and future ground truth. A lower KL divergence between prior and posterior means the model deems the combination more realistic, i.e. it is less *surprised*.

3   Results

3.1   Qualitative Results

We first present several qualitative examples, selected to illustrate the types of changes our approach is able to represent.

Figure 2(a) shows three cases with outlines for the prior mean (solid purple) prediction as well as the sample from the prior (dotted purple) that best matches the volume of the real future (red). The similarity of the latter two in the first two columns indicates that our model is able to represent both strong growth and strong reduction in size well. It can also be seen that the mean prediction closely matches the current state of the tumor, which is unsurprising, because small changes occur most frequently. The third column is illustrative of a general limitation of our model: encoding into the latent space removes all spatial resolution, so tumors that both shrink and grow in different locations (e.g. with multiple foci) are not represented in the current setup.

Figure 2(b) illustrates how the learned latent space represents semantically meaningful continuous variations: Dimension 2 changes the size of just the enhancing tumor while dimension 1 changes the size of the tumor core (enhancing tumor and necrosis combined). The third axis that is not shown encodes variation in the size of the edema, meaning that the model automatically learned to separate the contributions of the different tumor regions. Most importantly, all variations seem plausible. Note that while a reduction in necrosis is biologically implausible in a treatment-naive context, it might very well occur under treatment like in our dataset.

3.2   Quantitative Results

In this section we compare our approach with an upper bound and a lower bound. These are given by a regular probabilistic U-Net [5] trained for segmentation with (upper bound) and without (lower bound) knowledge of the future and both evaluated with respect to future ground truth.

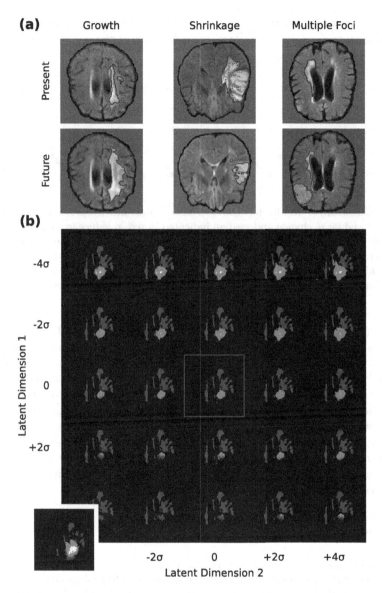

Fig. 2. Qualitative Examples: (a) Prior mean prediction (solid purple) and sample with best volume match (dashed purple) as well as future ground truth (red) overlaid on FLAIR. The approach is able to model growth or shrinkage, but is unable to represent tumors with both growth and shrinkage in different locations (for multiple foci, dotted and solid overlap). (b) Regular grid samples from prior, with mean highlighted in red and ground truth inlay in bottom left corner (unrelated to (a)). The learned latent space separates class contributions, dimension 1 seems to encode tumor core size (enhancing tumor and necrosis) while dimension 2 encodes enhancing tumor size (note how necrosis is virtually constant in the top row). The third latent dimension, not shown here, captures small variations in edema size. Purple – Edema, Orange – Enhancing Tumor, Yellow – Necrosis (Color figure online)

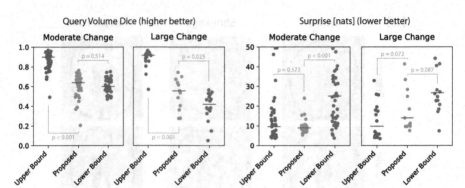

Fig. 3. Quantitative results for *Query Volume Dice* and *Surprise*, for groups with moderate and large change and median indicated in red, p-values from Wilcoxon ranksum test. For large changes, our approach can represent the future much better than the lower bound. The low surprise in our model indicates that our model's learned prior assigns higher likelihood than the lower bound to the real future tumor appearance, leveraging temporal information from previous scans. (Color figure online)

Figure 3 shows median results for two different metrics and both moderate change and large change. *Query Volume Dice* represents the clinically motivated question of estimating spatial extent for a given change in size (e.g. for radiation therapy). Particularly for cases with large change our approach outperforms the lower bound. At the same time, the *Surprise*, a measure of how close estimated prior and posterior are for a given set of inputs and future ground truth, is on par with the upper bound for cases with moderate change and still much lower than the lower bound's for large change cases. For reference, in VAEs this usually comes at the cost of poor reconstruction, but the reconstruction loss (i.e. segmentation cross entropy, not shown) is also much lower for our approach compared to the lower bound in both cases.

4   Discussion

In this work we investigated whether glioma growth dynamics can be learned directly from data without an underlying explicit biological model, instead relying on probabilistic segmentation to model distributions of future tumor appearances.

Our results indicate that this is indeed possible. We showed quantitatively that our approach can represent large variations in the inferred distributions and that these learned distributions model growth trajectories instead of just segmentation variants for a known input. Qualitative examples show overall realistic growth as well as shrinkage patterns. Compared to existing work, our approach relies on a very different hypothesis, so we elected to present metrics that evaluate our desired goals, but are unfortunately unsuitable for quantitative comparison with classical methods.

Our work has a number of shortcomings we'd like to explicitly address. While our dataset is larger than what is usually presented in the literature on glioma growth, our method clearly requires more data than existing ones that are based on explicit biological diffusion models. Without a doubt the dataset is too small to be representative of all plausible growth variations. We were also unable to apply our approach on more than two input time steps, because this reduced the amount of available training instances too drastically. As we pointed out, our model is also unable (and not designed) to predict a single correct growth trajectory. It is further unable to resolve spatially varying growth for a single tumor, likely because we employ a simple global latent space. On the other hand, more complex models would again require more data. Finally, it would be desirable to represent time continuously instead of working with discrete steps.

Contrasting the above, we also see some advantages that our approach offers. The ability to sample consistent hypotheses from the latent space, as opposed to just having pixel-wise probability estimates, lends itself to answering clinically motivated questions, e.g. exploring only samples that correspond to strong growth or those that produce predictions where a certain region is or is not affected by the tumor. We further don't rely on imaging modalities like DTI that are not typically acquired in clinical routine. It would in fact be interesting to explore if our approach can benefit from including the latter.

Overall we feel our work opens up a promising new avenue of approaching glioma growth and tumor growth in general. We are confident that much larger datasets will become available in the future that will allow our method to further improve. Most importantly, our work is entirely complementary with respect to diffusion-based models, and combining them should be exciting to explore.

References

1. Akbari, H., et al.: Imaging surrogates of infiltration obtained via multiparametric imaging pattern analysis predict subsequent location of recurrence of glioblastoma. Neurosurgery **78**(4), 572–580 (2016)
2. Bi, W.L., Beroukhim, R.: Beating the odds: extreme long-term survival with glioblastoma. Neuro-Oncology **16**(9), 1159–1160 (2014)
3. Engwer, C., Hillen, T., Knappitsch, M., Surulescu, C.: Glioma follow white matter tracts: a multiscale DTI-based model. J. Math. Biol. **71**(3), 551–582 (2015)
4. Jenkinson, M., Beckmann, C.F., Behrens, T.E.J., Woolrich, M.W., Smith, S.M.: FSL. NeuroImage **62**(2), 782–790 (2012)
5. Kohl, S.A.A., et al.: A probabilistic U-net for segmentation of ambiguous images. In: NeurIPS, vol. 31 (2018)
6. Lipkova, J., et al.: Personalized radiotherapy design for glioblastoma: integrating mathematical tumor models, multimodal scans and Bayesian inference. IEEE Trans. Med. Imaging **38**, 1875–1884 (2019)
7. Lê, M., et al.: Personalized radiotherapy planning based on a computational tumor growth model. IEEE Trans. Med. Imaging **36**(3), 815–825 (2017)
8. Mann, J., Ramakrishna, R., Magge, R., Wernicke, A.G.: Advances in radiotherapy for glioblastoma. Front. Neurol. **8**, 748 (2018)

9. Menze, B.H., Stretton, E., Konukoglu, E., Ayache, N.: Image-based modeling of tumor growth in patients with glioma. In: Optimal Control Image Processing, p. 12 (2011)
10. Menze, B.H., et al.: A generative approach for image-based modeling of tumor growth. Inf. Process. Med. Imaging **22**, 735–747 (2011)
11. Mosayebi, P., Cobzas, D., Murtha, A., Jagersand, M.: Tumor invasion margin on the Riemannian space of brain fibers. Med. Image Anal. **16**(2), 361–373 (2012)
12. Ronneberger, O., Fischer, P., Brox, T.: U-Net: convolutional networks for biomedical image segmentation. In: Navab, N., Hornegger, J., Wells, W.M., Frangi, A.F. (eds.) MICCAI 2015. LNCS, vol. 9351, pp. 234–241. Springer, Cham (2015). https://doi.org/10.1007/978-3-319-24574-4_28
13. Zhang, L., Lu, L., Summers, R.M., Kebebew, E., Yao, J.: Convolutional invasion and expansion networks for tumor growth prediction. IEEE Trans. Med. Imaging **37**(2), 638–648 (2018)

Surface-Volume Consistent Construction of Longitudinal Atlases for the Early Developing Brain

Sahar Ahmad, Zhengwang Wu, Gang Li, Li Wang, Weili Lin,
Pew-Thian Yap[(✉)], Dinggang Shen[(✉)], and the UNC/UMN Baby Connectome
Project Consortium

Department of Radiology and Biomedical Research Imaging Center (BRIC),
University of North Carolina, Chapel Hill, USA
{ptyap,dgshen}@med.unc.edu

Abstract. Infant brain atlases are essential for characterizing structural changes in the developing brain. Volumetric and cortical atlases are typically constructed independently, potentially causing discrepancies between tissue boundaries and cortical surfaces. In this paper, we present a method for surface-volume consistent construction of longitudinal brain atlases of infants from 2 weeks to 12 months of age. We first construct the 12-month atlas via groupwise surface-constrained volumetric registration. The longitudinal displacements of each subject with respect to different time points are then transported parallelly to the 12-month atlas space. The 12-month cortico-volumetric atlas is finally warped temporally to each month prior to the 12th month using the transported displacements. Experimental results indicate that the longitudinal atlases generated are consistent in terms of tissue boundaries and cortical surfaces, hence allowing joint surface-volume analysis to be performed in a common space.

Keywords: Infant brain atlas · Cortical surface · Neurodevelopment · Longitudinal trajectory

1 Introduction

A brain atlas is an anatomical representation of the brain, encapsulating population-wise brain features. Infant atlases are constructed to capture normative growth trajectories that are essential for understanding brain maturation during infancy and for early diagnosis of neurodevelopmental abnormalities [6]. Volumetric atlases facilitate the analysis of cortical and subcortical structures whereas cortical atlases provide additional information for studying cortical attributes, such as thickness, curvature, and convexity, as well as cortico-cortical connectivity [8,13,15].

Existing research focuses on constructing either volumetric or cortical atlases. For instance, Serag *et al.* [11] constructed spatio-temporal volumetric brain

© Springer Nature Switzerland AG 2019
D. Shen et al. (Eds.): MICCAI 2019, LNCS 11765, pp. 815–822, 2019.
https://doi.org/10.1007/978-3-030-32245-8_90

atlases of infants scanned between 28 and 44 weeks of age. Shi *et al.* [12] constructed a volumetric neonatal atlas using unbiased group-wise registration and patch-based sparse representation. Zhang *et al.* [17] constructed a volumetric neonatal brain atlas by combining spatial and frequency information using patch-based sparse representation. Bozek *et al.* [2] constructed neonatal cortical surface atlases for nine time points between 36–44 weeks of age. Multimodal surface matching [10] was used to align the features on the cortical surface and then temporal adaptive kernel regression was employed to generate the atlases. Li *et al.* [7] constructed infant cortical surface atlases for seven time points between 1- and 24-months of age using longitudinally consistent and unbiased group-wise registration.

Volumetric and cortical atlases are typically constructed independently, causing the following problems: (i) Misalignment of tissue boundaries in the volumetric atlas, and the pial and white matter surfaces of the cortical atlas. (ii) Blurred cortical structures in the volumetric atlas due to not using the geometry of the cortical surfaces in guiding registration. (iii) Cortical surface registration disregarding the image volume results in deformations that will unrealistically deform the brain. (iv) The volumetric and surface atlases do not reside in the same space, complicating concurrent analysis of the two entities. (v) Alignment inconsistency and inaccuracy can diminish the detectability of true but subtle longitudinal changes.

To overcome these problems, we present in this paper a method to construct longitudinal surface-volume consistent atlases for infants from 2 weeks to 12 months of age. We construct the cortical and volumetric atlases simultaneously, such that the boundaries of white matter (WM), gray matter (GM), and cerebrospinal fluid (CSF) are consistently aligned, in both volumetric and surface spaces. This allows surface and volumetric analyses to be conducted consistently in a single atlas space.

2   Methods

Our surface-volume consistent atlas construction method consists of two steps (see Fig. 1) (i) Construct the cortico-volumetric atlas at the 12-month time point; and (ii) Construct longitudinal month-specific cortico-volumetric atlases prior to the 12th month via parallel transport of displacement fields.

2.1   Construction of 12-Month Atlas

Groupwise Surface-Constrained Volumetric Registration – We first construct the 12-month atlas via group-wise registration using subjects scanned at either 11, 12 or 13 months of age. Group-wise registration simultaneously registers all the images to a hidden common space by (i) selecting as reference the image with the minimum dissimilarity to the other images and (ii) iteratively updating the reference by averaging all the images registered to it. The registration of infant brain MR images is challenging owing to the dramatic contrast

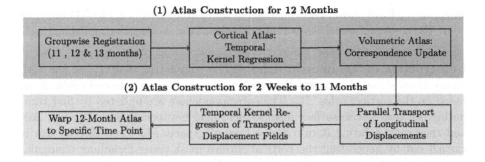

Fig. 1. Construction of cortico-volumetric atlases.

changes during the first year of life. To overcome this problem, we propose to register the segmented tissue maps instead of the intensity images. We use a surface-constrained dynamic elasticity model (SCDEM) [1] as the underlying transformation model for cross-sectional group-wise registration. The SCDEM registration algorithm determines the volumetric displacement field ϕ that matches a pair of images, constrained by the surface displacement field ψ computed as vertex-wise displacements between cortical surfaces given by Spherical Demons [16]. The volumetric displacement field is estimated using the following hyperbolic wave equation:

$$\alpha \nabla^2 \phi(x) + \alpha \nabla(\nabla \cdot \phi(x)) + \beta f^v(x) + \gamma f^s(x) = \frac{\partial^2 \phi(x)}{\partial t^2}, \tag{1}$$

where the volumetric force field f^v measures the discrepancies between the warped and reference segmented tissue maps. The surface force field f^s is computed as the error between the surface displacement field estimated by ϕ and the pre-computed surface displacement field ψ. α, β, and γ are parameters that control the smoothness of the displacement field, and the contributions of f^v and f^s, respectively. The two force fields recede gradually and eventually balance the smoothness terms in (1), causing the displacement field to converge. Once the dataset has been registered in a group-wise manner, the aligned cortical surfaces and segmented tissue maps are subsequently used to compute the 12-month cortico-volumetric atlas.

Construction of Cortical Atlas – The cortical surface atlas at the 12th month (366 days) is constructed via temporal kernel regression. Let $\{S_i | i = 1, \ldots, N\}$ be the cortical surface (left/right, white matter/pial) of the i-th subject scanned at t_i days. Let $\hat{S}_i$ be the corresponding cortical surface registered as described in the previous step. The cortical surface atlas A_{12}^s is obtained by weighted averaging of the vertex coordinates:

$$A_{12}^s = \frac{\sum_{i=1}^{N} w_i \hat{S}_i}{\sum_{i=1}^{N} w_i} \quad \text{with} \quad w_i = \frac{1}{\sigma \sqrt{2\pi}} \exp \left(\frac{-(t_i - 366)^2}{2\sigma^2} \right), \tag{2}$$

where $\sigma^2 = 15.25$ days. The constructed cortical surface atlas will be used to guide the construction of the volumetric atlas.

Construction of Volumetric Atlas – The volumetric atlas A_{12}^{v} at the 12th month is constructed by correcting the alignment of the segmented tissue maps based on the cortical atlas A_{12}^{s}. The correspondences are updated by first computing the vertex-wise surface displacement field between $\hat{S}_i$ and A_{12}^{s}, $i.e.$, $\Delta\psi$, and then extrapolating it over the volumetric space. More specifically, this is carried out by generating the cortical surface mesh using Delaunay triangulation and then, for each voxel location x, finding the mesh triangle, with vertices $\{y_j | j = 1, \ldots, 3\}$, that contains the voxel. The corrective volumetric displacement field $\Delta\phi(x)$ is computed from the surface transformation $\Delta\psi$ using Gaussian interpolation:

$$\Delta\phi(x) = \frac{\sum_{j=1}^{3} w_j \Delta\psi(y_j)}{\sum_{j=1}^{3} w_j} \quad \text{with} \quad w_j = \frac{1}{\sigma_g \sqrt{2\pi}} \exp\left(\frac{-\|x - y_j\|^2}{2\sigma_g^2}\right), \quad (3)$$

where $\sigma_g^2 = 9$ is set to ensure that the displacement at the tissue interfaces is smooth. This correspondence update step ensures that the segmented tissue maps are well-aligned with the cortical atlas. After warping each segmented tissue map with its respective final displacement field $\phi + \Delta\phi$, the volumetric atlas is computed via majority-voting fusion. The atlases at other time points are constructed based on A_{12}^{v} and A_{12}^{s}.

2.2 Construction of Longitudinal Atlases

Age-dependent cortico-volumetric atlases prior to the 12th month are constructed by determining the longitudinal change of each subject with respect to either 11-, 12- or 13-month scan of the subject (see Fig. 2) and then transporting this change to the 12-month atlas space. The within-subject longitudinal changes are represented by longitudinal displacement fields estimated via SCDEM intra-subject registration.

Parallel Transport of Longitudinal Displacements – Each longitudinal displacement field encodes the within-subject growth from an earlier time t_i' to time t_i. To characterize growth without the confound of inter-subject variability, the longitudinal displacement fields of each subject are normalized by parallel transport to the common space defined by the 12-month atlas (A_{12}^{v}). The 12-month atlas is warped by the inverse of the averaged transported displacement fields to construct the atlas at each time point. Figure 2 shows the longitudinal displacement fields $\phi^{t_i' \to t_i}$ and the cross-sectional displacement field $\phi^{t_i \to A_{12}^{\mathrm{v}}}$ of the i-th subject. Parallel transport is implemented by reorienting the displacement vectors [5,9] using the Jacobian matrix of cross-sectional deformation field $\Phi^{t_i \to A_{12}^{\mathrm{v}}} = x + \phi^{t_i \to A_{12}^{\mathrm{v}}}$, which is computed as $J_i = D\Phi^{t_i \to A_{12}^{\mathrm{v}}}$. The transported longitudinal displacement field is given as $J_i \phi^{t_i' \to t_i}$.

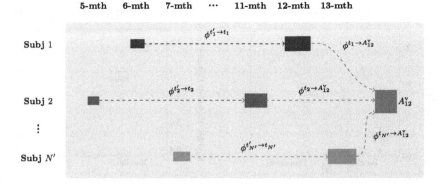

Fig. 2. Longitudinal and cross-sectional displacements used to construct the 6-month atlas via parallel transport

Temporal Kernel Regression of Transported Displacements – The displacement field from time t to the 12th month time point, $\varphi^{t \to A_{12}^{\vee}}$, is generated via weight averaging of the transported longitudinal displacement fields:

$$\varphi^{t \to A_{12}^{\vee}} = \frac{\sum_{i=1}^{N'} w_i' w_i \, J_i \phi^{t_i' \to t_i}}{\sum_{i=1}^{N'} w_i' w_i}, \tag{4}$$

where N' is the total number of subjects used to construct the month-specific atlases and,

$$w_i' = \frac{1}{\sigma \sqrt{2\pi}} \exp\left(\frac{-(t_i' - t)^2}{2\sigma^2}\right), \quad w_i = \frac{1}{\sigma \sqrt{2\pi}} \exp\left(\frac{-(t_i - 366)^2}{2\sigma^2}\right). \tag{5}$$

The inverse of the computed displacement field $\varphi^{t \to A_{12}^{\vee}}$ is used to warp the 12-month cortico-volumetric atlas to time t.

3   Results

The dataset consisted of T1- and T2-weighted images of 29 infant subjects enrolled as part of the UNC/UMN baby connectome project (BCP). The subjects were divided into three cohorts according to their first scheduled visits: 2 weeks, 1 month and 2 months. These subjects were scanned every three months, using a 3T Siemens Prisma MRI scanner with $320 \times 320 \times 208$ voxels and $0.8\,\mathrm{mm}^3$ resolution. The images were segmented into WM, GM, and CSF and the cortical surfaces were reconstructed. 34 cortical ROIs were also delineated for evaluation, by first parcellating the cortical surfaces using FreeSurfer [3] and then labeling each voxel in the GM cortical ribbon according to the cortical surface vertex nearest to the voxel.

We compared our results with those generated using diffeomorphic demons [14] (*i.e.*, the baseline method) instead of SCDEM registration. Figure 4 shows

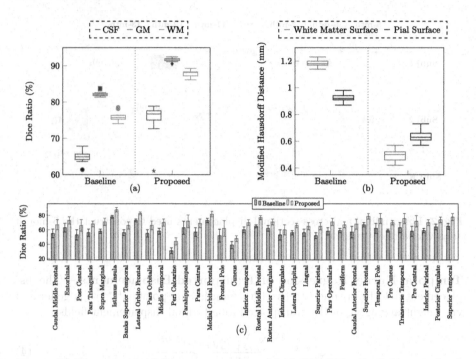

Fig. 3. (a) Dice ratios for different tissue types. (b) Modified Hausdorff distance (mm) for the cortical surfaces. (c) Dice ratios for cortical ROIs. All results are statistically significant ($p < 0.01$, paired t-test)

the results in terms of consistency between the cortical surfaces and volumetric atlases for all thirteen time points. These results indicate that the corticovolumetric atlases constructed by our method are more consistent than the baseline method. The baseline method shows greater discrepancies at the gray-white matter interface, which is more convoluted than the pial surface. From Fig. 4, it is evident that the atlases constructed by the proposed method preserve more cortical details. Figure 3 shows the quantitative results in terms of Dice ratio over different tissue types and cortical ROIs, and a modified Hausdorff distance [4] for surfaces. These metrics were computed between the 11-, 12- and 13-month registered volumes and surfaces, and the 12-month atlases constructed by the two methods. The improvements given by the proposed method, quantified using these metrics, are statistically significant ($p < 0.01$).

4 Conclusion

In this paper, we proposed a novel method for consistent construction of corticovolumetric atlases for the infant brain. The results show that the cortical surface and volumetric atlases constructed by our method are consistent and preserve more anatomical details.

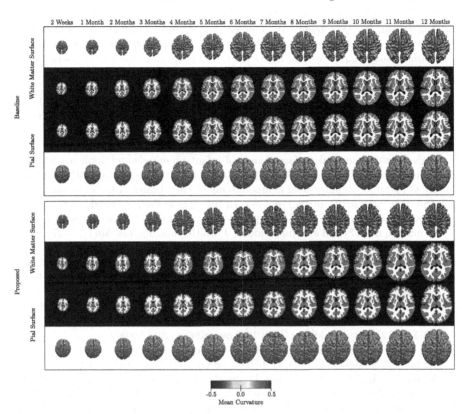

Fig. 4. Cortical surface atlases overlaid onto the volumetric atlases constructed by the proposed and baseline methods

Acknowledgment. This work utilizes approaches developed in part by NIH grants (AG053867, EB008374, MH107815, MH116225, MH117943, 1U01MH110274) and the efforts of the UNC/UMN Baby Connectome Project Consortium.

References

1. Ahmad, S., et al.: Surface-constrained volumetric registration for the early developing brain. Med. Image Anal. **58**, 101540 (2019). https://doi.org/10.1016/j.media.2019.101540
2. Bozek, J., et al.: Construction of a neonatal cortical surface atlas using multimodal surface matching in the developing human connectome project. NeuroImage **179**, 11–29 (2018). https://doi.org/10.1016/j.neuroimage.2018.06.018
3. Dale, A.M., Fischl, B., Sereno, M.I.: Cortical surface-based analysis: I. Segmentation surface reconstruction. NeuroImage **9**(2), 179–194 (1999). https://doi.org/10.1006/nimg.1998.0395
4. Dubuisson, M.P., Jain, A.K.: A modified Hausdorff distance for object matching. In: Proceedings of 12th International Conference on Pattern Recognition, vol. 1, pp. 566–568 (1994). https://doi.org/10.1109/ICPR.1994.576361

5. Duchateau, N., De Craene, M., Pennec, X., Merino, B., Sitges, M., Bijnens, B.: Which reorientation framework for the atlas-based comparison of motion from cardiac image sequences? In: Durrleman, S., Fletcher, T., Gerig, G., Niethammer, M. (eds.) STIA 2012. LNCS, vol. 7570, pp. 25–37. Springer, Heidelberg (2012). https://doi.org/10.1007/978-3-642-33555-6_3

6. Gilmore, J.H., et al.: Longitudinal development of cortical and subcortical gray matter from birth to 2 years. Cereb. Cortex **22**(11), 2478–2485 (2012). https://doi.org/10.1093/cercor/bhr327

7. Li, G., Wang, L., Shi, F., Gilmore, J.H., Lin, W., Shen, D.: Construction of 4D high-definition cortical surface atlases of infants: methods and applications. Med. Image Anal. **25**(1), 22–36 (2015). https://doi.org/10.1016/j.media.2015.04.005

8. Li, G., et al.: Computational neuroanatomy of baby brains: a review. NeuroImage **185**, 906–925 (2019). https://doi.org/10.1016/j.neuroimage.2018.03.042

9. Lorenzi, M., Pennec, X.: Efficient parallel transport of deformations in time series of images: from Schild's to pole ladder. J. Math. Imaging Vis. **50**(1), 5–17 (2014). https://doi.org/10.1007/s10851-013-0470-3

10. Robinson, E.C., et al.: Multimodal surface matching with higher-order smoothness constraints. NeuroImage **167**, 453–465 (2018). https://doi.org/10.1016/j.neuroimage.2017.10.037

11. Serag, A., et al.: Construction of a consistent high-definition spatio-temporal atlas of the developing brain using adaptive kernel regression. NeuroImage **59**(3), 2255–2265 (2012). https://doi.org/10.1016/j.neuroimage.2011.09.062

12. Shi, F., et al.: Neonatal atlas construction using sparse representation. Hum. Brain Mapp. **35**(9), 4663–4677 (2014). https://doi.org/10.1002/hbm.22502

13. Wong, K.C.L., Moradi, M., Tang, H., Syeda-Mahmood, T.: 3D segmentation with exponential logarithmic loss for highly unbalanced object sizes. In: Frangi, A.F., Schnabel, J.A., Davatzikos, C., Alberola-López, C., Fichtinger, G. (eds.) MICCAI 2018. LNCS, vol. 11072, pp. 612–619. Springer, Cham (2018). https://doi.org/10.1007/978-3-030-00931-1_70

14. Vercauteren, T., Pennec, X., Perchant, A., Ayache, N.: Diffeomorphic demons: efficient non-parametric image registration. NeuroImage **45**(Suppl. 1), S61–S72 (2009). https://doi.org/10.1016/j.neuroimage.2008.10.040

15. Wright, R., et al.: Construction of a fetal spatio-temporal cortical surface atlas from in utero MRI: application of spectral surface matching. NeuroImage **120**, 467–480 (2015). https://doi.org/10.1016/j.neuroimage.2015.05.087

16. Yeo, B.T.T., Sabuncu, M.R., Vercauteren, T., Ayache, N., Fischl, B., Golland, P.: Spherical demons: fast diffeomorphic landmark-free surface registration. IEEE Trans. Med. Imaging **29**(3), 650–668 (2010). https://doi.org/10.1109/TMI.2009.2030797

17. Zhang, Y., Shi, F., Yap, P.T., Shen, D.: Detail-preserving construction of neonatal brain atlases in space-frequency domain. Hum. Brain Mapp. **37**(6), 2133–2150 (2016). https://doi.org/10.1002/hbm.23160

Variational AutoEncoder for Regression: Application to Brain Aging Analysis

Qingyu Zhao[1]([✉]), Ehsan Adeli[1], Nicolas Honnorat[2], Tuo Leng[1,3], and Kilian M. Pohl[1,2]

[1] Department of Psychiatry and Behavioral Sciences, Stanford University, Stanford, USA
qingyuz@stanford.edu
[2] Center of Health Sciences, SRI International, Menlo Park, USA
[3] School of Computer Engineering and Sciences, Shanghai University, Shanghai, China

Abstract. While unsupervised variational autoencoders (VAE) have become a powerful tool in neuroimage analysis, their application to supervised learning is under-explored. We aim to close this gap by proposing a unified probabilistic model for learning the latent space of imaging data and performing supervised regression. Based on recent advances in learning disentangled representations, the novel generative process explicitly models the conditional distribution of latent representations with respect to the regression target variable. Performing a variational inference procedure on this model leads to joint regularization between the VAE and a neural-network regressor. In predicting the age of 245 subjects from their structural Magnetic Resonance (MR) images, our model is more accurate than state-of-the-art methods when applied to either region-of-interest (ROI) measurements or raw 3D volume images. More importantly, unlike simple feed-forward neural-networks, disentanglement of age in latent representations allows for intuitive interpretation of the structural developmental patterns of the human brain.

1 Introduction

Generative models in combination with neural networks, such as *variational autoencoders* (VAE), are often used to learn complex distributions underlying imaging data [1]. VAE assumes each training sample is generated from a latent representation, which is sampled from a prior Gaussian distribution through a neural-network, i.e., a decoder. Inferring the network parameters involves a variational procedure leading to an encoder network, which aims to find the posterior distribution of each training sample in the latent space. As an unsupervised learning framework, VAE has successfully been applied to several problems in neuroimaging, such as denoising [1], abnormality detection [2] or clustering tasks [3]. However, the use of VAE is still under-explored in the context of supervised regression; i.e., regression aims to predict a scalar outcome from an image based on a given set of training pairs. For instance in neuroimage analysis, the scalar

© Springer Nature Switzerland AG 2019
D. Shen et al. (Eds.): MICCAI 2019, LNCS 11765, pp. 823–831, 2019.
https://doi.org/10.1007/978-3-030-32245-8_91

could be a binary variable indicating if a subject belongs to the control or a disease group or a continuous variable encoding the age of a subject.

Several attempts have been made to integrate regression models into the VAE framework by directly performing regression analysis on the latent representations learned by the encoder [4,5]. These works, however, still segregate the regression model from the autoencoder in a way that the regression needs to be trained by a separate objective function. To close the gap between the two models, we leverage recent advances in learning *disentangled latent representations* [6,7]. In the latent space, a representation is considered disentangled if changes along one dimension of that space are explained by a specific factor of variation (e.g., age), while being relatively invariant to other factors (e.g., sex, race) [6]. Herein, we adopt a similar notion to define a unified model combining regression and autoencoding. We then test the model for predicting the age of a subject solely based on its structural MR image.

Unlike a traditional VAE relying on a single latent Gaussian to capture all the variance in brain appearance, our novel generative age-predictor explicitly formulates the conditional distribution of latent representations on age while being agnostic to the other variables. Inference of model parameters leads to a combination between a traditional VAE network that models latent representations of brain images, and a regressor network that aims to predict age. Unlike the traditional VAE, our model is able to disentangle a specific dimension from the latent space such that traversing along that dimension leads to age-specific distribution of latent representations. We show that through this mechanism the VAE and the regressor networks regularize each other during the training process to achieve more accurate age prediction.

Next, we introduce the proposed VAE-based regression model in Sect. 2. Section 3 describes the experiments of age prediction for 245 healthy subjects based on their structural T1-weighted MR images. We implement the model using two network architectures: a multi-layer perception for imaging measurements and a convolutional neural network for 3D volume images. Both implementations achieve more accurate predictions compared to several traditional methods. Finally, we show that the learned age-disentangled generative model provides an intuitive interpretation and visualization of the developmental pattern in brain appearance, which is an essential yet challenging task in most existing deep learning frameworks.

2   VAE for Regression

Figure 1 provides an overview of the model with blue blocks representing the generative model and red blocks the inference model.

The Generative Model. Let $\mathbf{X} = \{\boldsymbol{x}^{(1)}, ..., \boldsymbol{x}^{(n)}\}$ be a training dataset containing structural 3D MR images of n subjects, and $\{\boldsymbol{c}^{(1)}, ..., \boldsymbol{c}^{(n)}\}$ be their age. We assume each MR image $\boldsymbol{x}$ is associated with a latent representation $\boldsymbol{z} \in \mathbb{R}^M$, which is dependent on c. Then the likelihood distribution underlying each training image $\boldsymbol{x}$ is $p(\boldsymbol{x}) = \int_{z,c} p(\boldsymbol{x}, \boldsymbol{z}, c)$, and the generative process of $\boldsymbol{x}$ reads

$p(\boldsymbol{x}, \boldsymbol{z}, \boldsymbol{c}) = p(\boldsymbol{x}|\boldsymbol{z})p(\boldsymbol{z}|\boldsymbol{c})p(\boldsymbol{c})$, where $p(c)$ is a prior on age. In a standard VAE setting [8], the 'decoder' $p(\boldsymbol{x}|\boldsymbol{z})$ is parameterized by a neural network f with generative parameters θ, i.e., $p(\boldsymbol{x}|\boldsymbol{z}) \sim \mathcal{N}(\boldsymbol{x}; f(\boldsymbol{z};\theta), \mathbf{I})^1$. Different from the traditional VAE is the modeling of latent representations. Instead of using a single Gaussian prior to generate $\boldsymbol{z}$, we explicitly condition $\boldsymbol{z}$ on age c, such that the conditional distribution $p(\boldsymbol{z}|c)$ captures an age-specific prior on latent representations. We call $p(\boldsymbol{z}|c)$ a *latent generator*, from which one can sample latent representations for a given age. We further assume the non-linearity of this generative model can be fully captured by the decoder network $p(\boldsymbol{x}|\boldsymbol{z})$, such that a linear model would suffice to parameterize the generator: $p(\boldsymbol{z}|c) \sim \mathcal{N}(\boldsymbol{z}; \boldsymbol{u}^{\mathrm{T}}c, \sigma^2\mathbf{I})$, $\boldsymbol{u}^{\mathrm{T}}\boldsymbol{u} = 1$. With this construction we can see that $\boldsymbol{u}$ is essentially the disentangled dimension [6] associated with age; traversing along $\boldsymbol{u}$ yields age-specific latent representations. Note this model does not reduce the latent space to 1D but rather links one dimension of the space to age.

Inference Procedure. The parameters of the above generative model can be estimated via maximum likelihood estimation (MLE) i.e., by maximizing the sum of log likelihood $\sum_{i=1}^{N} \log p(\boldsymbol{x}^{(i)})$. For such an optimization, we adopt a standard procedure of variational inference and introduce an auxiliary function $q(\boldsymbol{z}^{(i)}, c^{(i)}|\boldsymbol{x}^{(i)})$ to approximate the true posterior $p(\boldsymbol{z}^{(i)}, c^{(i)}|\boldsymbol{x}^{(i)})$. In the following we omit index i for convenience. In so doing, $\log p(\boldsymbol{x})$ can be rewritten as the sum of the KL-divergence D_{KL} between $q(\boldsymbol{z}, c|\boldsymbol{x})$ and $p(\boldsymbol{z}, c|\boldsymbol{x})$ and the 'variational lower-bound' $\mathcal{L}(\boldsymbol{x})$:

$$\log p(\boldsymbol{x}) = D_{KL}\left(q(\boldsymbol{z}, c|\boldsymbol{x}) \;||\; p(\boldsymbol{z}, c|\boldsymbol{x})\right) + \mathcal{L}(\boldsymbol{x}). \tag{1}$$

Based on the mean-field theory, we further assume $q(\boldsymbol{z}, c|\boldsymbol{x}) = q(\boldsymbol{z}|\boldsymbol{x})q(c|\boldsymbol{x})$. Then the lower-bound can be derived as

$$\begin{aligned} \mathcal{L}(\boldsymbol{x}) := & - D_{KL}\left(q(c|\boldsymbol{x}) \;||\; p(c)\right) \\ & + \mathbb{E}_{q(\boldsymbol{z}|\boldsymbol{x})}\left[\log p(\boldsymbol{x}|\boldsymbol{z})\right] - \mathbb{E}_{q(c|\boldsymbol{x})}\left[D_{KL}\left(q(\boldsymbol{z}|\boldsymbol{x}) \;||\; p(\boldsymbol{z}|c)\right)\right] \end{aligned} \tag{2}$$

In the above equation, we formulate $q(c|\boldsymbol{x})$ as a univariate Gaussian $q(c|\boldsymbol{x}) \sim \mathcal{N}(c; f(\boldsymbol{x}; \phi_c), g(\boldsymbol{x}; \phi_c)^2)$, where ϕ_c are the parameters of the inference networks. We can see that $q(c|\boldsymbol{x})$ is essentially a regular feed-forward regression network with an additional output being the uncertainty (i.e., standard deviation) of the prediction. In this work we call $q(c|\boldsymbol{x})$ a *probabilistic regressor*. In an unsupervised setting, the KL-divergence of Eq. (2) regularizes the prediction of c with a prior. However, in our supervised setting this term can be simply replaced by $\log q(c|\boldsymbol{x})$ as the ground-truth of c is known for each training sample [9,10]^2.

Similar to a traditional VAE, the remaining part of the inference involves the construction of a *probabilistic encoder* $q(\boldsymbol{z}|\boldsymbol{x})$, which maps the input image

---

^{1} When $\boldsymbol{x}$ is binary, a Bernoulli distribution can define $p(\boldsymbol{x}|\boldsymbol{z}) \sim \mathrm{Ber}(\boldsymbol{x}; f(\boldsymbol{z};\theta))$.

^{2} In a semi-supervised setting where no informative prior in present, $\mathbb{H}(q(c|\boldsymbol{x}))$, i.e., the entropy of $q(c|\boldsymbol{x})$, is commonly used to replace the last term of Eq. 2 for samples with unknown c [9,10].

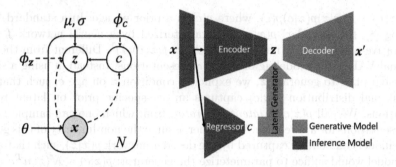

Fig. 1. Probabilistic (left) and graphical (right) diagrams of the VAE-based regression model. Each image x is assumed to be generated from its representation z, which is dependent on age c (blue blocks). The inference model (red blocks) constructs a probabilistic encoder for determining the latent representation and a probabilistic regressor for predicting age. (Color figure online)

x to a posterior multivariate Gaussian distribution in the latent space $q(z|x) \sim \mathcal{N}(z; f(x; \phi_z), g(x; \phi_z)^2 \mathbf{I})$. Then the second term of Eq. (2) encourages the decoded reconstruction from the latent representation to resemble the input [8]. The third term of of Eq. (2) encourages the posterior $q(z|x)$ to resemble the age-specific prior $p(z|c)$. This is the main mechanism for linking latent representations with age prediction: on the one hand, latent representations generated from the predicted c have to resemble the latent representation of the input image and on the other hand, age-linked variation in the latent space is encouraged to follow a direction defined by u. We used the SGVB estimator with the reparametrization trick [8] to optimize the expectation in the last two terms of Eq. (2).

Lastly, it has been shown that the supervised training of end-to-end feedforward neural networks often suffers from over-fitting problems, whereas unsupervised autoencoders can often learn robust and meaningful intermediate features that are transferable to supervised tasks [11]. By combining the two frameworks, our model therefore allows for the sharing of low-level features (e.g., by convolutional layers) jointly learned by the autoencoder and regressor.

3   Experiments

Understanding structural changes of the human brain as part of normal aging is an important topic in neuroscience. One emerging approach for such analysis is to learn a model that predicts age from brain MR images and then to interpret the patterns learned by the model. We tested the accuracy of the proposed regression model in predicting age from MRI based on two implementations[3]: the first implementation was based on a multi-layer perceptron neural network

---

[3] Implementation based on `Tensorflow 1.7.0`, `keras 2.2.2`. Source code available at https://github.com/QingyuZhao/VAE-for-Regression.

(all densely connected layers) applied to ROI-wise brain measurements while the second implementation was based on convolutional neural networks (CNN) applied to 3D volume images focusing on the ventricular area. Both implementations were cross-validated on a dataset consisting of T1-weighted MR images of 245 healthy subjects (122/123 women/men; ages 18 to 86) [12]. There was no group-level age difference between females and males ($p = 0.51$, two-sample t-test).

3.1   Age Prediction Based on ROI Measures

With respect to the perceptron neural network, the input of the encoder were the z-scores of 299 ROI measurements generated by applying FreeSurfer (V 5.3.0) to the skull-stripped MR image of each subject [12]. The measurements consisted of the mean curvature, surface area, gray matter volume, and average thickness of 34 bilateral cortical ROIs, the volumes of 8 bilateral subcortical ROIs, the volumes of 5 subregions of the corpus callosum, the volume of all white matter hypointensities, the left and right lateral and third ventricles, and the supratentorial volume (svol).

The input to the encoder was first densely connected to 2 intermediate layers of dimension (128, 32) with `tanh` as the activation function. The resulting feature was then separately connected to two layers of dimension 8 yielding the mean and diagonal covariance of the latent representation. The regressor shared the 2 intermediate layers of the encoder (Fig. 1b) and produced the mean and standard deviation for the predicted age. The decoder took the latent representation as input and used an inverse structure of the encoder for reconstruction.

3.2   Age Prediction Based on 3D MR Images

Taking advantage of recent advances in deep learning, the second implementation was build upon convolutional neural networks that directly took 3D images as input. All skull-stripped T1 images were registered to the SRI24 atlas space and down-sampled to 2 mm isotropic voxel size. Since it has been well established that the ventricular volume significantly increases with age [13], we then tested if the model would learn this structural change in predicting age. To do this, each image was cropped to a 64 * 48 * 32 volume containing the ventricle region and was normalized to have zero mean and unit variance. This smaller field of view allowed for faster and more robust training of the following CNN model on limited sample size (N = 245). Specifically, the encoder consisted of 3 stacks of 3 * 3 * 3 convolutional layers with rectified linear unit (ReLU) activation and 2 * 2 * 2 max pooling layers. The sizes of feature banks in the convolutional layers were (16, 32, 64) respectively.

Similar to the previous implementation, the extracted features were fed into 2 densely connected layers of dimension (64, 32) with `tanh` activation function. The final dimension of latent space was 16. The regressor shared the convolutional layers of the encoder and also had 2 densely connected layers of (64, 32). The decoder had an inverse structure of the encoder and used `Upsampling3D` as the inverse operation of max pooling. Since the CNN-based implementation had substantially more model parameters to determine than the first implementation, L2 regularization was applied to all densely connected layers.

Table 1. Age prediction accuracy of different methods based on ROI measurements and 3D volume images of ventricle.

		LR	Lasso	RR	SVR	GBT	K-NN	NN	Ours
ROI measures	R2	0.107	0.532	0.336	0.311	0.64	0.535	0.563	**0.666**
	rMSE	14.6	10.5	12.6	12.8	9.3	10.5	10.3	**9.0**
3D volume	R2	0.737	0.67	0.737	0.737	0.719	0.549	0.79	**0.808**
	rMSE	7.8	9.0	7.8	7.8	8.2	10.5	7.0	**6.9**

3.3 Measuring Accuracy

The accuracy of each implementation was reported based on a 5-fold cross-validation measuring the R2 score (coefficient of determination, proportion of the variance in age that is predictable from the model) and root mean squared error (rMSE). The outcome of each approach was compared to 7 other regression methods, of which 6 were non-neural-network methods as implemented in *scikit-learn* 0.19.1: linear regression (LR), Lasso, Ridge regression (RR), support vector regression (SVR), gradient-boosted tree (GBT), k-nearest neighbour regression (K-NN). The last approach was a single neural-network regressor (NN), i.e., the component corresponding to $q(c|\boldsymbol{x})$ without estimating standard deviation.

With respect to the ROI-based experiments, optimal hyperparameters of the scikit-learn methods (except for LR) were determined through a 10-fold inner cross-validation (an overall nested cross-validation). Specifically, we searched $\alpha \in \{0.01, 0.05, 0.1, 0.2\}$ for Lasso, $C \in \{1, 10, ..., 10^3\}, \gamma \in \{10^{-2}, ..., 10^2\}$ for SVR, $N \in \{10, 50, 100, 500\}$ for GBT, $\alpha \in \{10^{-3}, ..., 10^4\}, \gamma \in \{10^{-2}, ..., 10^2\}$ for RR, and $N \in \{1, 5, 10, 50\}$ for K-NN.

With respect to the 3D-image-based experiments, nested cross-validation was extremely slow for certain methods (e.g. GBT, CNN), so we simply repeated the outer 5-fold cross-validation using the hyperparameters defined in the above search space and reported the best accuracy. The search space of the L2 regularization for NN and our method was $\lambda = \{0, .001, .01, .1, 1\}$.

3.4 Results

As Table 1 shows, age prediction based on 3D images of ventricle was generally more accurate than on ROI measurements. The two neural-network-based predictions were the most accurate in terms of R2 and rMSE. Figure 3 shows the predicted age (in the 5 testing folds) estimated by our model versus ground-truth. The best prediction was achieved by our model applied to the 3D ventricle images, which yielded a 6.9-year rMSE. In the ROI-based experiment, our model was significantly more accurate ($p < 0.0001$, two-sample t-test) than the regular neural-network regressor (NN), which indicates the integration of VAE for modeling latent representations could regularize the feed-forward regressor network. In the 3D-image-based experiment, our model was more accurate than NN either with (Table 1) or without L2 regularization (when $\lambda = 0$, our model and NN yielded R2 of 0.761 and 0.745 respectively). Even though this improvement was not as significant as in the ROI-based experiment, our model enabled direct visualization of brain developmental patterns.

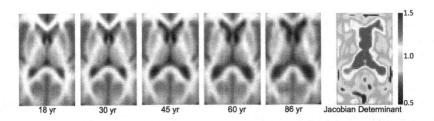

Fig. 2. Left: brain images reconstructed from age-specific latent representations. Right: Jacobian determinant map derived from the registration between the 18 year old brain and the 86 year old brain. The major expanding region is located on the ventricle.

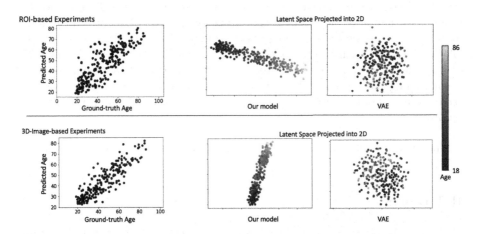

Fig. 3. Upper row: results of ROI-based experiments. Lower row: results of 3D-image-based experiments. Left: predictions made by our model vs. ground-truth. Middle: latent representations estimated by our model. Right: latent representations estimated by traditional VAE.

Indeed, despite the tremendous success of deep learning in various applications, interpretability of the black-box CNN remains an open research topic.

Most existing solutions can only produce a 'heat map' indicating the location of voxels that contribute to faithful prediction, but this does not yield any semantic meaning of the learned features that can improve mechanistic understanding of the brain. Thanks to the generative modelling, our formulation provides an alternative way for interpreting the aging pattern captured by the CNN. Specifically, Fig. 2 shows the simulated 'mean brain images' at different ages by decoding age-specific latent representations $\{z = u^{\mathrm{T}}c | c \in [18, 86]\}$, i.e., mean of the latent generator $p(z|c)$. We can clearly observe that the pattern learned by the model for age prediction was mainly linked to the enlargement of ventricle. This result is consistent with current understanding of the structural development of the brain.

Lastly, we show in Fig. 3 that the dimension related to age was disentangled from the latent space. In both ROI-based and image-based experiments, we trained our model on the entire dataset. The resulting latent representations were transformed from the latent space to a 2D plane via TSNE and color-coded by the ground-truth age. We observe that one direction of variation is associated with age, whereas the unsupervised training of traditional VAE does not lead to clear disentanglement.

4   Conclusion and Discussion

In this paper, we introduced a generic regression model based on the variational autoencoder framework and applied it to the problem of age prediction from structural MR images. The novel generative process enabled the disentanglement of age as a factor of variation in the latent space. This did not only produce more accurate prediction than a regular feed-forward regressor network, but also allowed for synthesizing age-dependent brains that facilitated the identification of brain aging pattern. Future direction of this work includes simultaneously disentangling more demographics factors of interest, e.g. sex, disease group, to study compounding effects, e.g. age-by-sex effects or accelerated aging caused by disease.

Acknowledgements. This research was supported in part by NIH grants AA017347, AA005965, AA010723, and MH113406.

References

1. Benou, A., Veksler, R., Friedman, A., Riklin Raviv, T.: De-noising of contrast-enhanced MRI sequences by an ensemble of expert deep neural networks. In: Carneiro, G., et al. (eds.) LABELS/DLMIA -2016. LNCS, vol. 10008, pp. 95–110. Springer, Cham (2016). https://doi.org/10.1007/978-3-319-46976-8_11
2. Baur, C., Wiestler, B., Albarqouni, S., Navab, N.: Deep autoencoding models for unsupervised anomaly segmentation in brain MR images. In: Crimi, A., Bakas, S., Kuijf, H., Keyvan, F., Reyes, M., van Walsum, T. (eds.) BrainLes 2018. LNCS, vol. 11383, pp. 161–169. Springer, Cham (2019). https://doi.org/10.1007/978-3-030-11723-8_16

3. Zhao, Q., Honnorat, N., Adeli, E., Pfefferbaum, A., Sullivan, E.V., Pohl, K.M.: Variational autoencoder with truncated mixture of gaussians for functional connectivity analysis. In: Chung, A.C.S., Gee, J.C., Yushkevich, P.A., Bao, S. (eds.) IPMI 2019. LNCS, vol. 11492, pp. 867–879. Springer, Cham (2019). https://doi.org/10.1007/978-3-030-20351-1_68

4. Yoo, Y., et al.: Variational autoencoded regression: high dimensional regression of visual data on complex manifold. In: CVPR (2017)

5. Chen, L., et al.: Deep autoencoding models for unsupervised anomaly segmentation in brain MR images. Inf. Sci. **428**, 49–61 (2018)

6. Higgins, I., et al.: Beta-VAE: learning basic visual concepts with a constrained variational framework. In: ICLR (2017)

7. Kim, H., Mnih, A.: Disentangling by factorising. In: ICML (2018)

8. Kingma, D., Welling, M.: Auto-encoding variational bayes. In: ICLR (2013)

9. Kingma, D.P., Rezende, D.J., Mohamed, S., Welling, M.: Semi-supervised learning with deep generative models. In: NeurIPS (2014)

10. Nalisnick, E., Smyth, P.: Stick-breaking variational autoencoders. In: ICLR (2017)

11. Zhuang, F., Cheng, X., Luo, P., Pan, S.J., He, Q.: Supervised representation learning: transfer learning with deep autoencoders. In: IJCAI (2015)

12. Adeli, E., et al.: Chained regularization for identifying brain patterns specific to HIV infection. Neuroimage **183**, 425–437 (2018)

13. Kaye, J., DeCarli, C., Luxenberg, J., Rapoport, S.: The significance of age-related enlargement of the cerebral ventricles in healthy men and women measured by quantitative computed X-ray tomography. J. Am. Geriatr. Soc. **40**(3), 225–231 (1992)

Early Development of Infant Brain Complex Network

Weixiong Jiang, Han Zhang$^{(\boxtimes)}$, Li-Ming Hsu, Dan Hu, Guoshi Li,
Ye Wu, and Dinggang Shen$^{(\boxtimes)}$

Department of Radiology and BRIC, University of North Carolina at Chapel Hill,
Chapel Hill, NC 27599, USA
{hanzhang, dgshen}@med.unc.edu

Abstract. The infant brain experiences explosive growth in the first few years of life. The developing topology of the functional network mirrors the emergence of complex cognitive functions. However, early development of brain topological properties in infants is still largely unclear due to the dearth of high-quality longitudinal infant functional MRI (fMRI) data. In this study, we employed advanced methods to investigate the developmental trajectories of various network features on high-resolution, longitudinal fMRI data of infants from birth to 2 years of age. The developmental trajectories of various global and nodal metrics were evaluated with linear mixed-effect modeling. We then investigated the association between these developmental trajectories and the visual reception ability, an important skill that could shape the future development of other cognitive functions. Four global metrics (shortest path length, global efficiency, local efficiency, and sigma (i.e., small-worldness)) showed significant developmental changes to facilitate more efficient information processing. Significant developmental changes were also found in the nodal characters with a prominent spatial specificity, and some brain regions showed increasing importance along the development. Most importantly, different associations between developmental trajectories in both global and nodal network characters and varied visual reception ability were revealed. This is the first longitudinal study on the early development of the brain functional connectome and its potential relationship to the individual variability of the visual abilities. These findings provide valuable knowledge for better understanding of normative and abnormal neurodevelopment in the first few years of life.

Keywords: Development · Complex network · Graph theory · Infant ·
Resting-state fMRI · Longitudinal · Visual reception

1 Introduction

The infant brain develops at an astonishing speed in the first two years, experiencing unprecedented changes in functional separation and integration. Developmental network neuroscience studies of infants have revealed several important early topological

Electronic supplementary material The online version of this chapter (https://doi.org/10.1007/978-3-030-32245-8_92) contains supplementary material, which is available to authorized users.

D. Shen et al. (Eds.): MICCAI 2019, LNCS 11765, pp. 832–840, 2019.
https://doi.org/10.1007/978-3-030-32245-8_92

property changes [1]. The infant brain network has been found to continuously reorganize with a small number of connections rewired toward more efficient organizations [2, 3]. Specifically, changes in functional interactions are believed to mediate emerging complex cognitive functions in early life after birth [4]. A recent study on network development during the first postnatal year found that the brain network was gradually subdivided into more modules, with increasing connector hubs and decreasing provincial hubs [5]. However, the previous studies usually investigated a few network metrics with small sample sizes in a cross-sectional manner. Therefore, applying advanced and comprehensive analytical methods on high-quality longitudinal data would greatly help investigate early development trajectory of the infant brain.

In the early brain development, the visual reception is a pivotal cognitive skill, which plays a critical role in the later behavioral and cognitive development and may largely shape the intellectual quotient and social/academic performance. To the best of our knowledge, there is no study on such an essential effect investigating how the individual difference in visual reception shape early developmental trajectories of the brain network properties. To this end, we used a large cohort of high-quality longitudinal infant resting-state functional MRI (rs-fMRI) data with unprecedentedly high spatial and temporal resolutions to comprehensively investigate longitudinal developmental trajectories of various graph-theoretical properties, as well as the possible effect of different visual reception abilities on the early brain functional development.

2   Materials and Methods

2.1   Data Acquisition and Preprocessing

All imaging data were collected by UNC/UMN Baby Connectome Project (BCP), which utilized a multiband sequence to yield high-quality high-resolution rs-fMRI data (temporal resolution = 0.8 s, and spatial resolution = 2 mm isotropic) during natural sleeping. After removing the data with bad registration or large head motion, 692 rs-fMRI data were included in this study (age ranging from 6 to 882 days).

We preprocessed the rs-fMRI data with a state-of-the-art, infant-dedicated, and accelerated longitudinal design pipeline. Except adopting several processing steps from the HCP pipeline, we especially used the following strategies to preprocess the data: (1) One-time resampling and denoising completed in each subject's native space; (2) Deep learning-based infant-dedicated segmentation for better spatial registration; and (3) Automatic deep learning-based noisy component removal for fast and robust rs-fMRI denoising.

To evaluate visual reception ability of the infants, Mullen Scales of Early Learning (MSEL) was deployed for each subject at each visit. The MSEL is appropriate for evaluating the cognitive performance of young children from birth to 68 months of age [6]. Visual reception ability is expressed by its age-normalized domain-specific T scores (with a mean of 50 and a standard deviation of 7.5). The visual reception score was chosen because there is a consensus that early visual reception skill could largely shape other important cognitive functions, such as memory and attention. For the infants with multiple scans and multiple MSEL assessments at different age time points, the last T-score based visual reception ability is chosen.

2.2 Brain Network Construction

A total of 112 cortical and subcortical brain regions (nodes) as defined with the Harvard-Oxford atlas were used to construct brain functional networks. The regional averaged rs-fMRI time series were used to build a 112×112 pairwise functional connectivity (FC) matrix for each data based on Pearson correlation. The derived FC matrices were further thresholded into different densities, ranging from 5% to 50% with a step of 1%. At each density setting, binary FC networks were obtained. The density range was based on the common practice in the literature where graph theoretical analysis is carried out [7].

2.3 Global and Nodal Graph Metrics of Infant Brain Functional Connectome

We investigated a series of graph theory-based global and nodal connectomic metrics to evaluate the network small-worldness and modular organization, network segregation and integration, assortative and hierarchical organizations, and nodal centrality measurements. The global metrics quantify the characteristics of the entire brain as an entity. In this study, eight global metrics were included: small-worldness (including clustering coefficient, characteristic path length, and sigma, an index characterizing the tradeoff between high local clustering and short path length), global efficiency, local efficiency, assortativity, synchronization, and hierarchy.

Five nodal metrics of each node (brain region) were estimated, including nodal centrality, betweenness centrality, nodal efficiency, nodal clustering coefficient, and nodal local efficiency. The details of the mathematical calculations of all these used graph theoretical metrics can be found in [7, 8]. To ensure the results are not biased by a single threshold in network binarization, we used the area under the receiver operating characteristic (ROC) curve (AUC) of each metric for the following analysis. To obtain higher reliability, the results of different resting-state imaging sessions or different phase encoding directions on the same day were merged by averaging their corresponding properties [7].

2.4 Characterization of Longitudinal Development Trajectories

The development trajectories of the global/nodal metrics were quantitatively analyzed using a linear mixed-effect regression (LMER). Three models were used to characterize different shapes of developmental trajectories, including a linear, log-linear (exponential), and a quadratic model as defined by Eqs. 1–3.

$$y_{ij} = \beta_0 + \beta_1 (\text{day}_{ij}) + (b_{0i} + b_{1i}(\text{day}_{ij}) + \varepsilon_{ij}) \tag{1}$$

$$y_{ij} = \beta_0 + \beta_1 (\log(\text{day}_{ij})) + (b_{0i} + b_{1i}(\log(\text{day}_{ij})) + \varepsilon_{ij}) \tag{2}$$

$$y_{ij} = \beta_0 + \beta_1\left(\mathrm{day}_{ij}\right) + \beta_2\left(\mathrm{day}_{ij}^2\right) + \left(b_{0i} + b_{1i}\left(\mathrm{day}_{ij}\right) + \varepsilon_{ij}\right) \qquad (3)$$

In each LMER, each global/nodal metric was modeled as the dependent variable y_{ij}, where i represents subject ($i = 1, 2, \ldots, N$) and j for age time-points ($j = 1, 2, \ldots, n_i$). The age, log(age), or age^2 in days was entered as independent variables, respectively. Random intercept and subject effects were included in each LMER. Akaike information criterion (AIC) was adopted for the model selection of the three models [9]. For all the LMER, the significance level was set to be $p < 0.05$ after false discovery rate (FDR) correction.

To further detect major spatiotemporal developmental patterns according to the different developmental properties (linear or nonlinear increase/decrease) across all the five nodal metrics, we further implemented a clustering analysis (using k-means clustering) for all the brain regions, which was repeated 100 times to account for the stochastic effect of the clustering algorithm used [10]. The consensus result over those iterations was obtained by using consensus partitions [11].

2.5 Association Between Visual Reception Ability and Network Development

To investigate the effect of visual reception on the developmental trajectories of both global and nodal network metrics, the visual reception ability was included as an additional static variable in the Eq. 1 (similarly for Eqs. 2 and 3), as below:

$$\begin{aligned} y_{ij} = &\beta_0 + \beta_1\left(\mathrm{day}_{ij}\right) + \beta_2(\mathrm{visual\_reception}_i) + \beta_3\left(\mathrm{day}_{ij} \cdot \mathrm{visual\_reception}_i\right) \\ &+ \left(b_{0i} + b_{1i}\left(\mathrm{day}_{ij}\right) + \varepsilon_{ij}\right) \end{aligned} \qquad (4)$$

where the visual reception ability was divided into three levels, i.e., high (>60), average (40–60), and low (<40) according to their visual reception scores. For nodal network metrics, we mainly focused on the 26 visual function-related brain regions as it is assumed that visual reception ability shape the developmental patterns of the visual areas. The significance level was set to be $p < 0.05$, FDR corrected. Since most of our infant rs-fMRI data were collected between 5 and 15 months old (67% of all the rs-fMRI data), the aforementioned association analysis was evaluated based on the data of this age range.

2.6 Cross-Sectional Relationship Between Global Metrics and Visual Reception Ability

As the visual reception ability can be regarded as a trait of a subject, it is essential to conduct a cross-sectional style of analysis, linking such an ability with the network metrics across different infants. Specifically, for each subject, we first chose each of the resultant global network metrics calculated based on the rs-fMRI data collected on the same day as the last Mullen data collection and then conducted a multiple linear regression (MLR) according to Eq. 5:

$$y_i = \beta_0 + \beta_1(\text{site}_i) + \beta_2(\text{gender}_i) + \beta_3(\text{day}_i) + \beta_4(\text{visual\_reception}_i) \qquad (5)$$

where each global metric was modeled as a dependent variable, and the visual reception ability was entered as an independent variable. We also included other confounding covariates, including the imaging site, gender, and age. The significance level was set to be $p < 0.05$, FDR corrected.

3   Results

3.1   Development of the Global Network Metrics

Four global network metrics showed significant development trajectories ($p < 0.05$, FDR corrected), such as sigma, shortest path length, global efficiency, and local efficiency (Fig. 1, also see Table S1 in the Supplemental Material). The sigma and global efficiency had increased development trajectories, while the shortest path length had a reversed trend. Interestingly, the local efficiency had a significant quadratic trajectory, peaking at the age of 368 days.

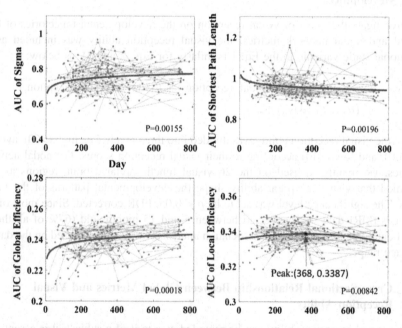

Fig. 1. The global metrics with significant development trajectories.

3.2   Development of the Nodal Network Metrics

With a prominent spatial specificity, different brain regions had significantly different developmental trajectories, indicating a spatiotemporal heterogeneity in early brain functional development (Fig. 2). Among them, the regions with significantly increased

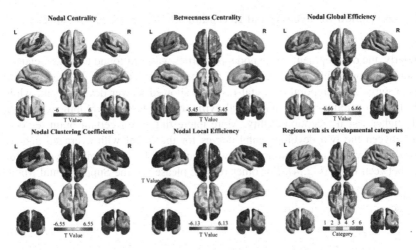

Fig. 2. Longitudinal development of five nodal network metrics. The regions were assigned with one of the six development categories according to their developmental trajectories.

development trajectories in terms of degree centrality, betweenness centrality, and nodal efficiency are mainly located symmetrically in the frontal pole, precentral/postcentral gyrus, superior occipital cortex, precuneus, posterior cingulate gyrus, and temporal cortex. On the other hand, these areas showed decreased development trajectories in nodal clustering coefficient and nodal local efficiency. According to the clustering results, we identified six categories of brain regions, each having similar developmental patterns of the five nodal properties (Fig. 2, lower right).

3.3   Association Between Visual Reception Ability and Global Property Development

The results showed slight differences in the developmental trajectory of three global network characters among the infants with different visual reception abilities (Fig. 3). For small-worldness and global efficiency, the subjects with lower-than-average visual reception abilities had a slower development, while the subjects with higher-than-average visual reception abilities had a faster development. For local efficiency, a similar trend was also observed (Fig. 3).

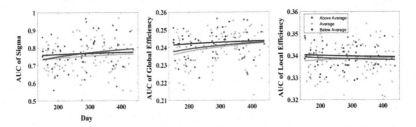

Fig. 3. Three global network properties with slightly different trajectories for infants with different levels of visual reception ability.

3.4   Association Between Visual Reception Ability and Nodal Property Development

Similarly, the development of the nodal properties was also found to be associated with visual reception ability (Fig. 4). Taking betweenness centrality as an example, the left lingual gyrus and temporal occipital fusiform showed slower development, while the right lateral occipital cortex and lingual gyrus showed faster development for subjects with higher visual reception ability. More interestingly, for certain brain regions, the gap between the two developmental curves for the infant with averaged and lower-than-average visual reception abilities were quite stable, indicating a systemic difference between them (Fig. 4). For other results, please see the Supplemental Materials.

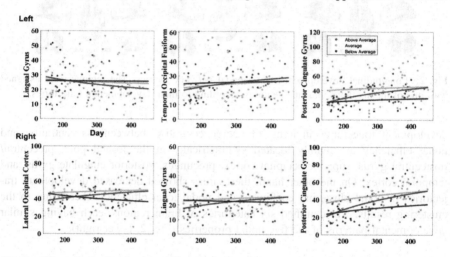

Fig. 4. Effect of visual reception ability on the development of visual-related nodal properties.

3.5   Cross-Sectional Relationship Between Global Metrics and Visual Reception Ability

In the cross-sectional analysis, two significant relationships were found between two global properties (the shorted path length and hierarchy) and visual reception ability (Fig. 5).

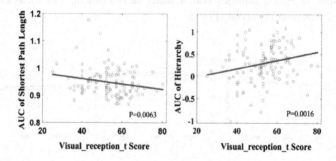

Fig. 5. Significant correlation between shortest path length/hierarchy and visual reception ability ($p < 0.05$, FDR corrected).

4 Discussion and Conclusions

In this study, we investigated infant brain development of the graph-theoretical features comprehensively and systematically. We revealed first-ever evidence on how varied visual reception levels could affect early developmental trajectories. Based on the different developmental trajectories of the nodal properties, we found different categories including the brain regions from the different functional networks, indicating a complex spatiotemporal development in the first two years of age. We revealed possible trait-related network properties, with smaller shortest path length and higher hierarchy corresponding to higher visual receptive performance. The results jointly suggest a highly complex, spatiotemporally heterogeneous development of brain functional connectome in neonates and infants. With development, the brain functional network may become more and more optimized to support more efficient information exchanges and more complex cognitive and behavioral functions [12, 13]. In summary, this study provides a thorough report on the normative network developmental trajectories, which could serve as a reference for charting the normative development and for detecting early neurodevelopmental disorders.

Acknowledgments. This work utilizes approaches developed by an NIH grant (1U01MH110274) and the efforts of the UNC/UMN Baby Connectome Project (BCP) Consortium. This work was also supported in part by an NIH grant MH117943.

References

1. Zhao, T., Xu, Y., He, Y.: Graph theoretical modeling of baby brain networks. Neuroimage **185**, 711–727 (2019)
2. Thomason, M.E., Grove, L.E., Lozon Jr., T.A., Vila, A.M., Ye, Y., et al.: Age-related increases in long-range connectivity in fetal functional neural connectivity networks in utero. Dev. Cogn. Neurosci. **11**, 96–104 (2015)
3. Cao, M., Huang, H., He, Y.: Developmental connectomics from infancy through early childhood. Trends Neurosci. **40**, 494–506 (2017)
4. Cohen, J.R., D'Esposito, M.: The segregation and integration of distinct brain networks and their relationship to cognition. J. Neurosci. **36**, 12083–12094 (2016)
5. Wen, X.Y., Zhang, H., Li, G., Liu, M.X., Yin, W.Y., et al.: First-year development of modules and hubs in infant brain functional networks. Neuroimage **185**, 222–235 (2019)
6. Yitzhak, N., Harel, A., Yaari, M., Friedlander, E., Yirmiya, N.: The Mullen scales of early learning: ceiling effects among preschool children. Eur. J. Dev. Psychol. **13**, 138–151 (2016)
7. Cao, H., McEwen, S.C., Forsyth, J.K., Gee, D.G., Bearden, C.E., et al.: Toward leveraging human connectomic data in large consortia: generalizability of fMRI-based brain graphs across sites, sessions, and paradigms. Cereb. Cort **29**, 1263–1279 (2019)
8. Rubinov, M., Sporns, O.: Complex network measures of brain connectivity: uses and interpretations. Neuroimage **52**, 1059–1069 (2010)
9. King, T.: Longitudinal data analysis for the behavioral sciences using R. Int. J. Lang. Commun. Disord. **51**, 355 (2016)
10. Medaglia, J.D., Satterthwaite, T.D., Kelkar, A., Ciric, R., Moore, T.M., et al.: Brain state expression and transitions are related to complex executive cognition in normative neurodevelopment. Neuroimage **166**, 293–306 (2018)

11. Bassett, D.S., Yang, M., Wymbs, N.F., Grafton, S.T.: Learning-induced autonomy of sensorimotor systems. Nat. Neurosci. **18**, 744–751 (2015)
12. Wang, J., Zuo, X., Dai, Z., Xia, M., Zhao, Z., et al.: Disrupted functional brain connectome in individuals at risk for Alzheimer's disease. Biol. Psychiatry **73**, 472–481 (2013)
13. Zhang, H., Shen, D., Lin, W.: Resting-state functional MRI studies on infant brains: a decade of gap-filling efforts. NeuroImage **185**, 664–684 (2019)

Revealing Developmental Regionalization of Infant Cerebral Cortex Based on Multiple Cortical Properties

Fan Wang[1], Chunfeng Lian[1], Zhengwang Wu[1], Li Wang[1], Weili Lin[1], John H. Gilmore[2], Dinggang Shen[1], and Gang Li[1(✉)]

[1] Department of Radiology and BRIC,
University of North Carolina at Chapel Hill, Chapel Hill, NC, USA
gang_li@med.unc.edu
[2] Department of Psychiatry, University of North Carolina at Chapel Hill,
Chapel Hill, NC, USA

Abstract. The human brain develops dynamically and regionally heterogeneously during the first two postnatal years. Cortical developmental regionalization, i.e., the landscape of cortical heterogeneity in development, reflects the organization of underlying microstructures, which are closely related to the functional principles of the cortex. Therefore, prospecting early cortical developmental regionalization can provide neurobiologically meaningful units for precise region localization, which will advance our understanding on brain development in this critical period. However, due to the absence of dedicated computational tools and large-scale datasets, our knowledge on early cortical developmental regionalization still remains intact. To fill both the methodological and knowledge gaps, we propose to explore the cortical developmental regionalization using a novel method based on nonnegative matrix factorization (NMF), due to its ability in analyzing complex high-dimensional data by representing data using several bases in a data-driven way. Specifically, a novel multi-view NMF (MV-NMF) method is proposed, in which multiple distinct and complementary cortical properties (i.e., multiple views) are jointly considered to provide comprehensive observation of cortical regionalization process. To ensure the sparsity of the discovered regions, an orthogonal constraint defined in Stiefel manifold is imposed in our MV-NMF method. Meanwhile, a graph-induced constraint is also included to improve the compactness of the discovered regions. Capitalizing on an unprecedentedly large dataset with 1,560 longitudinal MRI scans from 887 infants, we delineate the first neurobiologically meaningful representation of early cortical regionalization, providing a valuable reference for brain development studies.

1 Introduction

The human brain undergoes a protracted course of development after birth, while maintains an exceptionally high rate of development in the first two years [1, 2]. There is a growing consensus that early development strongly affects brain cognition and function throughout the entire lifespan, suggesting that exploring the early brain

© Springer Nature Switzerland AG 2019
D. Shen et al. (Eds.): MICCAI 2019, LNCS 11765, pp. 841–849, 2019.
https://doi.org/10.1007/978-3-030-32245-8_93

developmental patterns is of great importance in understanding both ordered and disordered brains [1, 3]. Due to the non-uniformities in underlying cortical microstructures, which are closely related to functional principles of the cortex, the infant cerebral cortex grows in regionally heterogeneous manners, thus forming a unique landscape of cortical developmental regionalization. Prospecting such developmental regionalization could potentially provide neurobiologically meaningful units to facilitate precise region localization, inter-subject and inter-study comparison, and effective feature reduction for early brain disorder identification [4], thus advancing our understanding on brain development in this critical early period. However, due to the absence of dedicated computational tools and large-scale datasets, our knowledge of such infantile cortical developmental regionalization still remains intact.

To fill the methodological gap and hence to advance our knowledge towards this critical early postnatal period, we are motivated to explore cortical developmental regionalization in the first two postnatal years, by leveraging a novel multi-view nonnegative matrix factorization (MV-NMF) method and an unprecedentedly large-scale infant MRI dataset. The utilization of NMF to analyze complex high-dimensional cortical data is mainly motivated by three reasons. (1) It can naturally discover different groups of vertices varying in similar manners across different subjects and ages, thus providing a part-based cortical representation to facilitate the interpretability of the cortical regionalization. (2) By varying the desired number of output components/parts, NMF can reveal the regionalization at different resolutions in a hierarchical manner. (3) It is more flexible than other development-based analyses [5], as there is no strict requirement of longitudinal data with multiple time points. On the other hand, the motivation to use multiple views, i.e., multiple cortical attributes (e.g., cortical thickness and surface area), is to provide comprehensive and complementary characterizations of the cortical regionalization process, as different cortical attributes have distinct neurobiological mechanisms and thus reflect distinct aspects of the regionalization progress.

Therefore, in our proposed MV-NMF method, we minimize an objective function to jointly decompose multi-view data matrices (of cortical attributes) for grouping cortical vertices into hierarchical regions. Specifically, apart from the conventional reconstruction error in each view, a multi-view regularization is included in our objective function to iteratively fuse multi-view information to encourage the consistency of regionalization results between different views. To improve the sparsity of the discovered regions, the orthogonal constraint is effectively imposed during the alternative optimization procedure by computing the gradient in the Stiefel manifold [6]. Moreover, a graph-induced regularization is also incorporated in our objective function to further improve the compactness of the results. The proposed MV-NMF method has been applied to an unprecedentedly large dataset with 1,560 longitudinal MRI scans from 887 typically developing infants. The revealed landscape of early cortical regionalization provides a reliable reference for studying early postnatal cortical organization and progression.

2 Materials and Methods

2.1 Dataset and Image Processing

Totally 1,560 longitudinal MRI scans were collected from 887 typically developing infants (466 males/421 females) with age at scan ranging from 0.2 months to 29.3 months. Using a Siemens 3T head-only scanner, T1w images with the resolution of $1 \times 1 \times 1$ mm^3 were acquired with the parameters: TR = 1,900 ms, TE = 4.38 ms, inversion time = 1,100 ms, and flip angle = 7°. T2w images with the resolution of $1.25 \times 1.25 \times 1.95$ mm^3 were acquired with the parameters: TR = 7,380 ms, TE = 119 ms, and flip angle = 150°.

All MR images were preprocessed following a standard procedure [7], including skull stripping, cerebellum and brain stem removal, intensity inhomogeneity correction, rigid alignment of each scan to the age-matched infant brain atlas, tissue segmentation, non-cortical structure masking and filling, and left-right hemisphere separation. Inner and outer cortical surfaces were reconstructed for each hemisphere and mapped onto a spherical space. To establish cortical correspondences across subjects and ages, we employed a longitudinally consistent registration strategy. Specifically, first, for each subject, longitudinal cortical correspondences were established by spherical registration of surfaces at the early time points to the corresponding surface at the last time point [8]. Then, inter-subject cortical correspondences were established by groupwise registration of all spherical cortical surfaces at the last time point. All cortical surfaces were finally resampled to a standard mesh tessellation, and computed with surface area and cortical thickness for each vertex [8], which will be used as cortical attributes for discovering cortical developmental regionalization.

2.2 Nonnegative Matrix Factorization (NMF)

In a data-driven way, the NMF method approximates complex high-dimensional data by representing them as the linear combinations of limited bases, with each basis corresponding to a part/component. Taking cortical thickness as an example, the data matrix $X \in \mathbb{R}^{M \times N}$ is a large nonnegative matrix constructed by cortical thickness values from all scans (data samples), where M and N are the numbers of vertices and scans, respectively. Each column of X includes cortical thickness values from one scan. The NMF method decomposes X into two smaller non-negative matrices, i.e., the bases matrix $W \in \mathbb{R}^{M \times K}$ and the coefficients matrix $H \in \mathbb{R}^{K \times N}$, by satisfying $X \approx WH$. The number of bases (components/parts) should be small, i.e., $K \ll M$ and $K \ll N$. As a result, each column of W is a basis that represents one distinct region/part, which indicates a group of cortical vertices jointly developing across subjects and ages. Each data sample (i.e., each column in X) can be approximately reconstructed by a linear combination of bases from W, using the corresponding column from H as the coefficients. By minimizing the Frobenius norm of the reconstruction error $||X - WH||_F^2$, W and H can be found through an iterative multiplication [9].

2.3 Multi-View NMF

Multiple cortical attributes, e.g., cortical thickness, surface area and myelin content, have distinct biological mechanisms and provide rich complementary information on cortical development, thus improving the reliability and meaningfulness of discovered basis matrices. Hence, we propose a multi-view NMF (MV-NMF) framework, with each view corresponding to a cortical attribute, to discover early cortical developmental regionalization. Besides the multi-view regularization, our MV-NMF also imposes an orthogonal constraint by computing the true gradient in an orthogonal parameter space, namely Stiefel manifold. To further improve the compactness of the final solutions, a graph regularization is also included.

Objective Function. Let $X_v \in \mathbb{R}^{M \times N_v}$ be the data matrix for the v-th view in total V views, while $W_v \in \mathbb{R}^{M \times K}$ and $H_v \in \mathbb{R}^{K \times N_v}$ denote, respectively, the basis and coefficient matrices decomposed from X_v. Scalar N_v is the total number of samples in the v-th view. The objective function of our MV-NMF method is defined as

$$\mathcal{J} = \min_{\substack{W_v, H_v \geq 0 \\ W_v^T W_v = I}} \frac{1}{2} \sum_{v=1...V} \lambda_v ||X_v - W_v H_v||_F^2 + \mathcal{R}_{MV} + \alpha \cdot \mathcal{R}_G. \tag{1}$$

Herein, alongside the reconstruction error in the first term, we introduce two additional terms, i.e., the multi-view regularization $\mathcal{R}_{MV}$ and the graph-based regularization $\mathcal{R}_G$. Parameters λ_v and α control the influences of their corresponding terms.

The multi-view regularization is defined as

$$\mathcal{R}_{MV} = \frac{1}{2} \sum_{u=1...V} \sum_{v=1...V} \theta_{uv} ||W_u - W_v||_F^2, \tag{2}$$

which aims to minimize the dissimilarity between the bases of different views. Parameter θ_{uv} controls the influence of the inconsistency between any two paired views.

The graph-based regularization $\mathcal{R}_G$ is introduced to improve the compactness and remove small artifacts of discovered regions. Denoting matrix A as a symmetric adjacent matrix, which defines the one-ring connections of vertices on the cortical surface. Matrix D is a diagonal matrix, where each element D_{ii} represents the sum of the i-th row (or column) of A. Let $Tr(\cdot)$ denote the trace of a matrix, the graph-based regularization is defined in terms of the graph Laplacian [10], i.e.,

$$\mathcal{R}_G = \frac{1}{2} \sum_{v=1...V} Tr(W_v^T (A - D) W_v)). \tag{3}$$

Updating Rule. First, the partial gradient of $\mathcal{J}$ toward H_v is found to be

$$\nabla_{H_v} \mathcal{J} = -\lambda_v W_v^T X_v + \lambda_v W_v^T W_v H_v. \tag{4}$$

Thus, it is straightforward to have the form of updating rule for $\boldsymbol{H}_v$, with $\odot$ representing the elementwise multiplication:

$$\boldsymbol{H}_v \leftarrow \boldsymbol{H}_v \odot \frac{\boldsymbol{W}_v^T \boldsymbol{X}_v}{\boldsymbol{W}_v^T \boldsymbol{W}_v \boldsymbol{H}_v}. \tag{5}$$

To update $\boldsymbol{W}_v$, we first compute the corresponding partial gradient:

$$\nabla_{\boldsymbol{W}_v} \mathcal{J} = -\lambda_v \boldsymbol{X}_v \boldsymbol{H}_v^T - \sum_{u=1\ldots V} \theta_{uv} \boldsymbol{W}_u + \sum_{u=1\ldots V} \theta_{uv} \boldsymbol{W}_v + \lambda_v \boldsymbol{W}_v \boldsymbol{H}_v \boldsymbol{H}_v^T + \alpha(\boldsymbol{A} - \boldsymbol{D})\boldsymbol{W}_v. \tag{6}$$

Then, in Stiefel manifold, which is a parameter space with the orthogonality constraint $\boldsymbol{W}_v^T \boldsymbol{W}_v = \boldsymbol{I}$, the *true* gradient $\tilde{\nabla}_{\boldsymbol{W}_v} \mathcal{J}$ (with orthogonality) [6] is computed by

$$\begin{aligned}
\tilde{\nabla}_{\boldsymbol{W}_v} \mathcal{J} &= \nabla_{\boldsymbol{W}_v} \mathcal{J} - \boldsymbol{W}_v [\nabla_{\boldsymbol{W}_v} \mathcal{J}]^T \boldsymbol{W}_v \\
&= \left[\lambda_v \boldsymbol{W}_v \boldsymbol{H}_v \boldsymbol{X}_v^T \boldsymbol{W}_v + \sum_{u=1,\ldots,V} \theta_{uv} \boldsymbol{W}_v \boldsymbol{W}_u^T \boldsymbol{W}_v + \alpha \boldsymbol{D} \boldsymbol{W}_v + \alpha \boldsymbol{W}_v \boldsymbol{W}_v^T \boldsymbol{A} \boldsymbol{W}_v \right] \\
&\quad - \left[\lambda_v \boldsymbol{X}_v \boldsymbol{H}_v^T + \sum_{u=1,\ldots,V} \theta_{uv} \boldsymbol{W}_u + \alpha \boldsymbol{A} \boldsymbol{W}_v + \alpha \boldsymbol{W}_v \boldsymbol{W}_v^T \boldsymbol{D} \boldsymbol{W}_v \right].
\end{aligned} \tag{7}$$

Accordingly, the multiplicative update rule for $\boldsymbol{W}_v$ is of the form

$$\boldsymbol{W}_v \leftarrow \boldsymbol{W}_v \odot \frac{\lambda_v \boldsymbol{X}_v \boldsymbol{H}_v^T + \sum_{u=1}^{V} \theta_{uv} \boldsymbol{W}_u + \alpha \boldsymbol{A} \boldsymbol{W}_v + \alpha \boldsymbol{W}_v \boldsymbol{W}_v^T \boldsymbol{D} \boldsymbol{W}_v}{\lambda_v \boldsymbol{W}_v \boldsymbol{H}_v \boldsymbol{X}_v^T \boldsymbol{W}_v + \sum_{u=1}^{V} \theta_{uv} \boldsymbol{W}_v \boldsymbol{W}_u^T \boldsymbol{W}_v + \alpha \boldsymbol{D} \boldsymbol{W}_v + \alpha \boldsymbol{W}_v \boldsymbol{W}_v^T \boldsymbol{A} \boldsymbol{W}_v}. \tag{8}$$

Iterative Optimization. To generate meaningful solutions, an appropriate initialization for NMF-based methods is necessary. Many single-view NMF methods employ the *nndsvd* initialization method [11], which has shown faster reduction of the residual error than random initialization. Herein, we also apply *nndsvd* algorithm for initialization, but with some modifications to adapt our proposed multi-view scheme. Specifically, we first obtain initializations from each view separately, which encode the potential jointly developing vertices on each view. Second, we explicitly look for the intersections from the initializations of different views to generate new components in the initialization, since their intersections encode the potential jointly developing vertices on all views. Third, according to the desired number of initialization components, the smallest components are removed. In this way, the multi-view NMF scheme can be appropriately initialized. The optimal bases matrices $\boldsymbol{W}_v$ and coefficients matrices $\boldsymbol{H}_v$ of each view were obtained by iteratively calling Eqs. (8) and (5). The final regions discovered using MV-NMF were the average of regions from different views.

3 Experiments

In this paper, *cortical thickness* and *surface area* were used in our MV-NMF scheme to explore cortical regionalization, since they are two important cortical morphological attributes with distinct neurobiological/genetic mechanisms and growth patterns during infancy [4]. The data matrix of each view is normalized so that each column averages to 1. In our experiments, parameters of the proposed MV-NMF method were empirically set as: $\lambda_1 = \lambda_2 = 1$, $\theta_{uv} = 1000$, and $\alpha = 500$.

Effectiveness of MV-NMF. To integrate information from multiple views, one straightforward solution is to concatenate the multiple data matrices into a single matrix. Specifically, assume $X_1 \in \mathbb{R}^{M \times N_1}$ and $X_2 \in \mathbb{R}^{M \times N_2}$ are two data matrices in term of cortical thickness and surface area, respectively. One can directly concatenate X_1 and X_2 (as $[X_1, X_2]$), and then apply the conventional NMF on the concatenated big matrix for exploring cortical regionalization. We refer this method as rig-NMF, since it rigidly imposes the bases from different views to be identical. Hence, we compared the rig-NMF with our MV-NMF using the same data and initialization. For a fair comparison, we employed an orthogonal projective version of NMF [9] for the rig-NMF method, given its state-of-the-art performance with high orthogonality and compactness [12].

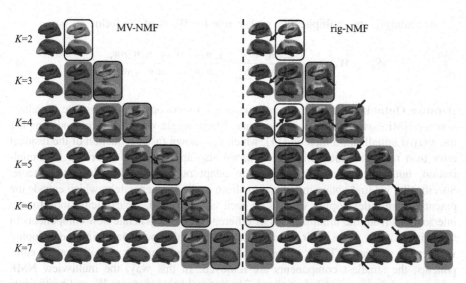

Fig. 1. The layers of hierarchical structures obtained by MV-NMF and rig-NMF, by increasing the component number K from 2 to 7. The inconsistent borders across different layers are pointed out with blue arrows. (Color figure online)

We assume that the effectiveness of a method can be reflected by the border consistency of its discovered regionalization across different resolutions. That is, if a border is more consistently preserved along the change of K (i.e., the number of output components), the result is more likely to reflect the stable hierarchical regionalization of the underlying microstructures. Accordingly, by increasing K from 2 to 7, the border consistencies obtained by rig-NMF and our MV-NMF are compared in Fig. 1. Note that, each component highlighted by black block in a specific row (e.g., $K = 2$) means that it is hierarchically decomposed into two finer components in the next row (e.g., $K = 3$). Based on the inconsistent borders pointed by blue arrows, it can be observed that our MV-NMF discovers borders with higher consistency, indicating the effectiveness and rationality of our MV-NMF.

Robustness of MV-NMF. The proposed MV-NMF does not require different views to have the same number of samples. To show the robustness of the MV-NMF, we designed an imbalanced testing dataset, where we randomly removed half of the cortical thickness samples to check if our method can still produce similar results as using all samples. This situation could happen when estimated cortical thickness values are not reliable for some subjects, since cortical thickness (between 1 and 5 mm) is much more sensitive to cortical surface reconstruction results, compared to surface area. This process was repeated five times. By calculating the Dice coefficient between each imbalanced test and the case of using all samples, we finally summarized the mean Dice coefficients at different numbers of components in Fig. 2(a). It can be observed that, compared with rig-NMF, our MV-NMF yields similar performance when K is between 2 and 8, but much better performance when K is larger. Across all resolutions, the Dice coefficients of our MV-NMF are always larger than 0.9, demonstrating the robustness of our proposed method.

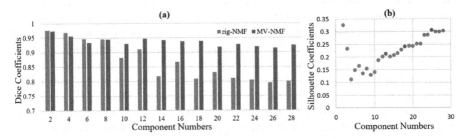

Fig. 2. (a) Mean Dice coefficients by performing five times imbalanced sample test. (b) Silhouette coefficients in terms of different resolutions. $K = 13, 25$ are local peaks. $K = 18$ shows a start of a plateau (i.e., $K = 18$ to 22).

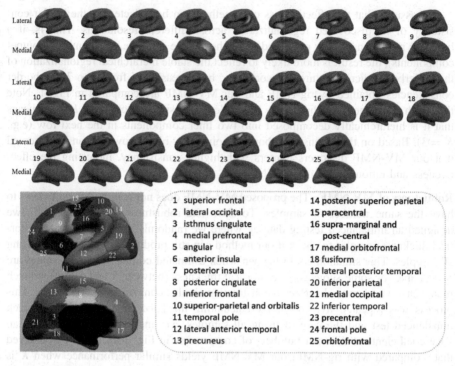

Fig. 3. The 25 regions and their topography with sharp boundaries.

Determination of Resolution K. Whereas MV-NMF provides hierarchical regions while increasing the resolution, we need to select some representative resolutions for the best representation of the studied data. To this end, a silhouette value was computed for each resolution K. It measures the intra-region similarity against inter-regions similarity. High silhouette values indicate better results. In each view, the similarity of two vertices i and j is evaluated using the correlation coefficient between $X_v(i, \cdot)$ and $X_v(j, \cdot)$. The multi-view silhouette value is the average of the values from all views, as shown in Fig. 2(b). Naturally, higher resolutions lead to higher silhouette values. Yet we can still observe local peaks, such as for $K = 13$ and 25. Meanwhile, when resolution increases from 18 to 22, a plateau is shown. We thus chose 13, 18, and 25 as the most appropriate resolutions for the landscape of early cortical regionalization.

Discovered Regions. Although 13, 18 and 25 are all shown to be appropriate resolutions, we prefer relatively finer ones when considering network/region-based analyses. Figure 3 shows the discovered regions with $K = 25$ and their topography with sharp boundaries, which correspond well with existing neuroscience knowledge according to the name of each region given in the figure. Besides, these regions are also consistent with previous findings. For example, regions 2, 11, 13, 15, 17, 18, 21, 22 and 25 are found in the genetic-based cortical topography [4]. Regions 2, 6, 7, 11, 13, 14, 15, 18, 23, 24 are found in the cortical thickness based remodeling patterns in adolescents [12].

4   Conclusion

We have proposed a novel multi-view NMF scheme to jointly consider cortical thickness and surface area for exploring the early cortical developmental regionalization. Capitalizing on an unprecedentedly large infant MRI dataset, we have provided valuable references of region topography that encodes multi-view cortical developmental patterns. Our discovered regionalizatoin reflects co-developing vertices across ages and subjects on multi-views, which differs markedly from previous cortical atlases. These references will later be publicly released to facilitate other infant-related studies, thus boosting our knowledge in the early brain development. As an important future work, we will include more cortical attributes to discover regionalization patterns based on more than two views, which will provide more insights into early brain development.

Acknowledgement. This work was supported in part by NIH grants (MH107815, MH116225, and MH117943).

References

1. Fjell, A.M., Grydeland, H., Krogsrud, S.K., et al.: Development and aging of cortical thickness correspond to genetic organization patterns. PNAS **112**, 15462–15467 (2015)
2. Li, G., Wang, L., Yap, P.-T., et al.: Computational neuroanatomy of baby brains: a review. NeuroImage **185**, 906–925 (2019)
3. Eickhoff, S.B., Constable, R.T., Yeo, B.T.: Topographic organization of the cerebral cortex and brain cartography. NeuroImage **170**, 332–347 (2018)
4. Chen, C.-H., Fiecas, M., Gutierrez, E., et al.: Genetic topography of brain morphology. PNAS **110**, 17089–17094 (2013)
5. Li, G., Wang, L., Shi, F., Lin, W., Shen, D.: Constructing 4D infant cortical surface atlases based on dynamic developmental trajectories of the cortex. In: Golland, P., Hata, N., Barillot, C., Hornegger, J., Howe, R. (eds.) MICCAI 2014. LNCS, vol. 8675, pp. 89–96. Springer, Cham (2014). https://doi.org/10.1007/978-3-319-10443-0_12
6. Choi, S.: Algorithms for orthogonal nonnegative matrix factorization. In: IJCNN 2008, pp. 1828–1832. IEEE (2008)
7. Li, G., Nie, J., Wang, L., et al.: Mapping region-specific longitudinal cortical surface expansion from birth to 2 years of age. Cereb. Cortex **23**, 2724–2733 (2013)
8. Yeo, B.T., Sabuncu, M.R., Vercauteren, T., et al.: Spherical demons: fast diffeomorphic landmark-free surface registration. IEEE TMI **29**, 650–668 (2010)
9. Yang, Z., Oja, E.: Linear and nonlinear projective nonnegative matrix factorization. IEEE TNN **21**, 734–749 (2010)
10. Cai, D., He, X., Han, J., et al.: Graph regularized nonnegative matrix factorization for data representation. IEEE TPAMI **33**, 1548–1560 (2011)
11. Boutsidis, C., Gallopoulos, E.: SVD based initialization: a head start for nonnegative matrix factorization. Pattern Recogn. **41**, 1350–1362 (2008)
12. Sotiras, A., Toledo, J.B., Gur, R.E., et al.: Patterns of coordinated cortical remodeling during adolescence and their associations with functional specialization and evolutionary expansion. PNAS **114**, 3527–3532 (2017)

Continually Modeling Alzheimer's Disease Progression via Deep Multi-order Preserving Weight Consolidation

Jie Zhang and Yalin Wang[✉]

School of Computing, Informatics, and Decision Systems Engineering,
Arizona State University, Tempe, AZ, USA
{jiezhang.joena,ylwang}@asu.edu

Abstract. Alzheimer's disease (AD) is the most common type of dementia. Identifying biomarkers that can track AD at early stages is crucial for therapy to be successful. Many researchers have developed models to predict cognitive impairments by employing valuable longitudinal imaging information along the progression of the disease. However, previous methods model the problem either in the isolated single-task mode or multi-task batch mode, which ignores the fact that the longitudinal data always arrive in a continuous time sequence and, in reality, there are rich types of longitudinal data to apply our learned model to. To this end, we continually model the AD progression in time sequence via a proposed novel Deep Multi-order Preserving Weight Consolidation (DMoPWC) to simultaneously (1) discover the inter and inner relations among different cognitive measures at different time points and utilize such relations to enhance the learning of associations between imaging features and clinical scores; (2) continually learn new longitudinal patients' images to overcome forgetting the previously learned knowledge without access to the old data. Moreover, inspired by recent breakthroughs of Recurrent Neural Network, we consider time-order knowledge to further reinforce the statistical power of DMoPWC and ensure features at a particular time will be temporally ahead of the features at its subsequential times. Empirical studies on the longitudinal brain image dataset demonstrate that DMoPWC achieves superior performance over other AD prognosis algorithms.

1 Introduction

Alzheimer's disease (AD), the most common type of dementia, is a slowly progressive neurodegenerative disorder and leads to memory loss increased and cognitive function reduced. An accurate prediction of related cognitive decline is crucial and would facilitate optimal decision-making for clinicians and patients.

Y. Wang—The research was supported in part by NIH (RF1AG051710, R01EB025032 and U54EB020403). We gratefully acknowledge the support of NVIDIA Corporation with the donation of the Tesla K40 GPU used for this research.

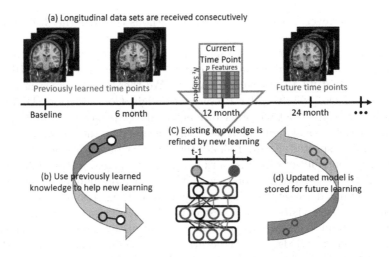

Fig. 1. Overview of proposed continual longitudinal feature learning framework.

Many researchers have studied the cognitive progression by brain magnetic resonance imaging (MRI), and their works demonstrate great potentials to use MRI biomarkers to predict cognitive decline presymptomatically in a sufficiently rapid and rigorous manner.

Traditional machine learning algorithms have been widely applied to AD progression modeling. Prior researches either predict the target clinical scores at the isolated single time point [8] or develop joint analysis schemes on multiple time points [13]. Recently, deep neural networks have brought breakthroughs in modeling AD progression. Suk *et al.* [9] proposed deep multi-task neural network while Wang *et al.* [11] modeled the problem via a recurrent neural network (RNN). Although the RNN learns the data in time order, it does not take into account that the longitudinal image data are obtained in a continuous sequence rather than a uniform batch (e.g., the MR images are taken at different time points, not at only one time point). It motivates us to develop a system to mimic how doctors monitor and prognosticate the AD progression.

In real-world disease diagnosis applications, different batches of data arrive periodically (e.g., monthly, seasonally, or yearly) with the data distribution changing over time rather than all data coming together. This presents an opportunity for continual learning, whose primary goal is to learn consecutive tasks without forgetting the knowledge learned in the past (e.g., with less longitudinal data) and leverage the previous knowledge to achieve artificial general intelligence. A straightforward way is to fine-tune the deep model for every new data set; however, this can cause "catastrophic forgetting" – a phenomenon where training a model with new tasks interferes the previously learned old knowledge – leading to performance degradation or even overwriting of the old knowledge by the new ones or the model fails to adapt new tasks, bias towards the old knowledge. Many approaches [4,5] have been proposed to overcome the "catastrophic forgetting", however, none of the existing methods consider the discriminative weight subset by incorporating inherent correlations between old tasks and new tasks. Besides, it is important to respect the valuable temporal information from the longitudinal data coming in time order (e.g., patient's 3-month MR image comes in front of its 12-month MR image). We therefore design a novel algorithm termed Deep Multi-order Preserving Weight Consolidation (DMoPWC) to continually learn the time-order of longitudinal sequence without losing statistical power on less longitudinal data and ensure that the old and new tasks correlation is respected. Figure 1 shows the overview of the DMoPWC.

The key contributions of this work can be summarized in threefold. Firstly, we formulate the AD progression in a continual learning manner which respects the longitudinal data sets coming in sequence and ensures equally prediction accuracy for future visits. To the best of our knowledge, it is the first learning model which models disease progression in a continually sequential manner and accumulate the knowledge for predicting future cognitive decline. Secondly, to overcome "catastrophic forgetting" for the old learned time points' information, we propose a novel DMoPWC—it considers the discriminative weight subset by incorporating inherent correlations between old and new time points' information and learns the task-specific patient's information from the new time point. Thirdly, we consider time order knowledge to guarantee features at the certain time point to be temporally ahead of those of succeeding time points. Our extensive experimental results show the superiority of the proposed algorithm.

2   Method

2.1   Problem Definition and Preliminaries

We define the problem as follows—there will be an unknown number of MR images belonging to different tasks (time points) with unknown distributions, arriving in sequence. The task can be a single task or multiple tasks (e.g., patients' images from a single time point or multiple time points). Our goal is to learn a deep model in such a continual learning scenario without "catastrophic forgetting". At the testing time, the task at time point t will be given and we aim to test the future clinical scores for time point $t + 1$. Given a sequence of T tasks, task at time point $t = 1, 2, \cdots, T$ with N_t images comes with dataset $\mathbf{D}_t = \{\mathbf{x}_i^t, y_i^t\}_{i=1}^{N_t}$. Specifically, for task t, y_i^t is the ground truth of the clinical scores for the i-th subject $\mathbf{x}_i^t \in \mathbb{R}^p$ at time point t. We denote the training data matrix by $\mathbf{X}^t$ for $\mathbf{D}_t$, i.e., $\mathbf{X}^t = (\mathbf{x}_1^t, \cdots, \mathbf{x}_{N_t}^t)$. When the dataset of time point t comes, all the previous training time points' datasets $\mathbf{D}_1, \cdots, \mathbf{D}_{t-1}$ are not available any more, but the deep model parameters with L layers $\theta^{t-1} = \{\theta_l^{t-1}\}_{l=1}^L$ can be accessed. The problem at time point t when given data $\mathbf{D}_t$ can be defined as follows:

$$\min_{\theta^t} \mathcal{L}_t(\theta^t | \theta^{t-1}, \mathbf{D}_t) + \lambda \Omega(\theta^t), \ t = 1, \cdots, T \tag{1}$$

where $\mathcal{L}_t$ is the loss function of solving θ^t, and θ^t is the model parameters for time point t. $\Omega(\cdot)$ includes one or more sparsity-inducing norms and λ is a non-negative parameter.

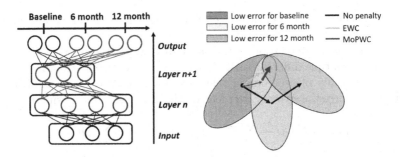

Fig. 2. Graphical illustration of the proposed Deep Multi-order Preserving Weight Consolidation (DMoPWC). DMoPWC first learns a model on baseline data (blue), then updates it after observing 6-month data (yellow) and finally updates the updated model after learning 12-month data (green). The thicker red arrow denotes larger time-order penalty on later time point. DMoPWC can keep most previously learned knowledge comparing with EWC and fine-tuning. (Color figure online)

Elastic Weight Consolidation (EWC) [4] is proposed to solve the above problem (1) that consists of a quadratic penalty on the difference between the parameter θ^t and θ^{t-1} to slow down the "catastrophic forgetting" for previously learned time point information. The posterior distribution $p(\theta^t|\mathbf{D}_t)$ is used to describe the problem by the Bayes' rule, $\log p(\theta^t|\mathbf{D}_t) = \log p(\mathbf{D}_t|\theta^t) + \log p(\theta^t|\mathbf{D}_{t-1}) - \log p(\mathbf{D}_t)$, where the posterior probability $\log p(\theta^t|\mathbf{D}_{t-1})$ embeds all the information from task $t-1$. EWC approximates it as a Gaussian distribution with mean of parameter $\bar{\theta}^{t-1}$ and a diagonal matrix I of the Fisher Information matrix $\mathbb{F}$. The Fisher information matrix $\mathbb{F}$ is computed by

$$\mathbb{F}_i^t = I(\theta^t)_{ii} = E_x\left[\left(\frac{\partial}{\partial\theta_i^t}\log p(\mathbf{D}_t|\theta^t)\right)^2 \Big|\theta^t\right]. \tag{2}$$

Therefore, the problem of EWC at time point t can be rewritten as follows:

$$\min_{\theta^t} \quad \mathcal{L}_t(\theta^t) + \frac{\lambda_1}{2}\sum_i \mathbb{F}_i^{t-1}(\theta_i^t - \bar{\theta}_i^{t-1})^2, \tag{3}$$

where λ_1 denotes how important the time point $t-1$ data is compared to time point t data and i labels each weight (layer) of the parameter θ.

2.2 Multi-order Preserving Weight Consolidation

The main problem of Eq. (3) is that it only enforces time point t data close to time point $t-1$ data. This will ignore the patient's inherent correlations within time point t and the same patient's information between previous time point knowledge and time point t and such relationship might potentially help improve the statistical power and overcome "catastrophic forgetting" on the previously learned time points' information. Learning multiple related time points' data jointly can improve performance relative to learn each time point data separately [1] when the two time points' data are related. One appealing property of the $l_{2,1}$-norm regularization is that it shares similar parameter sparsity patterns among multiple different tasks. Therefore, a new formulation, Eq. (4), may improve the ability of overcoming "catastrophic forgetting" from multiple time points and enforce the sparsity over features for multiple subjects simultaneously,

$$\min_{\theta^t} \mathcal{L}_t(\theta^t) + \frac{\lambda_1}{2} \sum_i \mathbb{F}_i^{t-1}(\theta_i^t - \bar{\theta}_i^{t-1})^2 + \lambda_2 \sum_i ||\theta_i^t||_{2,1}, \tag{4}$$

where λ_2 is the non-negative regularization parameter and $||\theta_i^t||_{2,1} = \sum_j ||\theta_{i,j}^t||_2$ is to learn the related representations and j presents j-th subject (row).

Specifically, we further consider some critical parameters which have better representation power to a subset of the specific time point. It has been shown that l_1 sparse norm [6] can identify informative longitudinal phenotypic biomarkers that are related to pathological changes of AD in brain image analysis. To this end, we propose to learn the discriminative new task-specific parameters while learning task relatedness among multi-time points multiple subjects and the objective function for time point t becomes:

$$\min_{\theta^t} \quad \mathcal{L}_t(\theta^t) + \frac{\lambda_1}{2} \sum_i \mathbb{F}_i^{t-1}(\theta_i^t - \bar{\theta}_i^{t-1})^2 + \lambda_2 \sum_i ||\theta_i^t||_{2,1} + \lambda_3 ||\theta^t||_1, \tag{5}$$

where λ_3 is the non-negative regularization parameter. Equation (5) studies the discriminative task-specific weight subset with inherent correlations among multi-time points multiple subjects while keeping previously learned knowledge via weight consolidation.

How to utilize the time ordering imaging information remains an open problem. We thus introduce a novel time-order preserving criteria to enrich Eq. (5), which is to prevent the time point t information θ^t from being temporally in front of the time point $t-1$ information of θ^{t-1}. For instance, for longitudinal data, we know that 3-month visit is behind baseline visit and 12-month visit is behind 3-month visit and baseline visit (See Fig. 1). In other words, the model observes the same temporal order as the input longitudinal time series. Thus, we introduce the expression, $w^t||\theta^t - \theta^{t-1}||_2^2$, where w^t represents the temporal order weight function for time point t. Therefore, $w^{t-1}\theta^{t-1} < w^t\theta^t$ represents the approximated temporal order of the time point t. In this work, we choose a simple element-wise linear form of the weight function $\mathbf{W}$ to reflect the longitudinal time ordering information as $\mathbf{W} = [\frac{1}{T}, \frac{2}{T}, \cdots, \frac{t}{T}, \cdots, \frac{T-1}{T}, 1]$.

Therefore, the final objective function of the proposed Deep Multi-order Preserving Weight Consolidation (DMoPWC) will become

$$\min_{\theta^t} \mathcal{L}_t(\theta^t) + \frac{\lambda_1}{2} \sum_i \mathbb{F}_i^{t-1}(\theta_i^t - \bar{\theta}_i^{t-1})^2 + \lambda_2 \sum_i ||\theta_i^t||_{2,1} + \lambda_3 ||\theta^t||_1 + \lambda_4 w^t ||\theta^t - \theta^{t-1}||_2^2, \tag{6}$$

where λ_4 is a non-negative parameter. Figure 2 shows the geometric illustration of DMoP WC, it shows that our model can learn the most common sub-area

---

Algorithm 1. Deep Multi-order Preserving Weight Consolidation (DMoPWC)

   Input   : Longitudinal dataset $\mathbf{D}_1, \cdots, \mathbf{D}_T; \lambda_1, \lambda_2, \lambda_3, \lambda_4$
   Output: θ^T

1 **begin**
2   **for** $t = 1 \rightarrow T$ **do**
3   **if** $t = 1$ **then**
4   Train an initial network with weights θ^1 by using Eq. 1 on dataset $\mathbf{D}_1$.
5   Computer Fisher information matrix $\mathbb{F}_i^1$ by using Eq. 2 on dataset $\mathbf{D}_1$.

6   **else**
7   According to $\mathbb{F}_i^{t-1}$ and θ^{t-1}, optimize θ^t by using Eq. 6 and dataset $\mathbf{D}_t$.
8   Computer Fisher information matrix $\mathbb{F}_i^t$ by using Eq. 2 on dataset $\mathbf{D}_t$.

(three colors' overlapping area) among three time points' data and preserve time-order in sequence comparing with EWC (two colors' overlapping area) and fine-tuning. The left figure in Fig. 2 illustrates our model has the same model size across multi-time points learning.

3 Experiments

Datasets. We evaluate our DMoPWC algorithm on the entire ADNI-1 cohort [3]. We study seven time points structural MR images. Responses are MMSE and ADAS-Cog scores, coming from seven different time points: baseline, M06, M12, M18, M24, M36 and M48. The sample sizes corresponding to seven time points are 837, 733, 728, 326, 641, 454 and 251. Specifically, we remove 25 subjects without MMSE and ADAS-cog from the baseline data and we use 812 subjects instead. The hippocampal surface multivariate morphometry statistics (MMS) [12] are utilized as learning features, consist of surface multivariate tensor-based morphometry, which is computed from the conformal grid and describes surface deformation on a local surface region, and radial distance, which measures the surface deformation along the surface normal direction. We use FIRST[1] to segment hippocampi from MR images and follow the same protocol as Shi *et al.* [7] and extract vertex-wise hippocampal morphometry features on every pair of hippocampal surfaces. As a result, each subject $\mathbf{x}_i^t$ has $p = 120,000$ features in total. In the prediction, we use the current time point data to predict future clinical score, e.g., we study baseline MR images and predict 12-month MMSE/ADAS-cog.

Network Settings. We use a two-layer fully-connected neural network of 100-100 units with ReLU activations as our initial network. All comparison algorithms are trained on a single Nvidia TITAN X GPU. All models and algorithms are implemented using Tensorflow[2] library.[3]

---

[1] https://fsl.fmrib.ox.ac.uk/fsl/fslwiki/FIRST.

[2] https://www.tensorflow.org/.

[3] The source code of DMoPWC is available at https://github.com/zj00377/DMopWC.

Hyperparameter Settings. All hyper-parameters in DMoPWC are optimized using grid-search and the best results for each model are reported. The SGD optimizer is used with a learning rate of 0.001 and we set batch size of 256 with 1400 iterations, $\lambda_1 = 15$, $\lambda_2 = 0.0001$, $\lambda_3 = 0.15$ and $\lambda_4 = 0.5$ on MMSE and $\lambda_1 = 13$, $\lambda_2 = 0.015$, $\lambda_3 = 0.00001$ and $\lambda_4 = 0.1$ on ADAS-cog. We use 200 subjects to compute Fisher $\mathbb{F}^t$.

Evaluation Methods. In order to evaluate the proposed model, we randomly split the data into training and testing sets using a 9:1 ratio and repeat this procedure 20 times to avoid data bias. We report the mean and standard deviation of these 20 different splits. Lastly, we evaluate the regression performance by using weighted Correlation (wCC), Pearson Correlation Coefficient (PCC) for overall measures and root Mean Square Error (rMSE) for task-specific measures. The three measures are defined as $wCC = \frac{\sum_{t=1}^{T} Corr(\mathbf{Y}_t, \hat{\mathbf{Y}}_t) N_t}{\sum_{t=1}^{T} N_t}$,

$PCC = \frac{\sum_{i=1}^{N_{total}} (\mathbf{Y}_i - \bar{\mathbf{Y}})(\hat{\mathbf{Y}}_i - \bar{\hat{\mathbf{Y}}})}{\sqrt{\sum_i (\mathbf{Y}_i - \bar{\mathbf{Y}})^2} \sqrt{\sum_i (\hat{\mathbf{Y}}_i - \bar{\hat{\mathbf{Y}}})^2}}$ and $rMSE = \sqrt{\frac{\|\mathbf{Y}_t - \hat{\mathbf{Y}}_t\|_2^2}{N_t}}$, where $Corr$ is the correlation coefficient between two vectors and N_t is the number of subjects of task t. $\mathbf{Y}_t$ and $\hat{\mathbf{Y}}_t$ are the ground truth of targets and the corresponding prediction at time point t while $\bar{\mathbf{Y}}$ and $\bar{\hat{\mathbf{Y}}}$ are the mean value of $\mathbf{Y}$ and $\hat{\mathbf{Y}}$, respectively.

Comparison Methods. We compare our algorithm with three groups of methods: single-task regression methods: (1) LASSO [10] and (2) Ridge regression [2]; multi-task regression methods: (1) L21: multi-task $\ell_{2,1}$-norm regularization with least square loss [6]. (2) cFSGL: convex fused sparse group Lasso [13]. (3) MSMT: multi-soure multi-target dictionary learning [12]; deep learning methods: (1) SN: Fine-Tuning (No penalty). (2) EWC [4]: elastic weight consolidation. (3) DMoPWC: the proposed algorithm. For linear regression methods, cross-validation is used to select the model parameters in the training data and the same training datasets with MMS features are used to predict its two time points later clinical scores. We use the same patch set of [12] as input. For deep learning methods, we use the same settings for the initial model and the sequential data is used to predict its future two-time-points later clinical scores.

Performance Comparisons. We report the results of DMoPWC and other methods on the prediction model of MMSE on ADNI-I dataset in Table 1. The proposed approach DMoPWC outperforms single-task and multi-task regression methods. For multi-task methods, we observe that dictionary learning method obtains better results than others. We also notice that the deep learning models strongly improve the prediction results over linear regressions. The proposed DMoPWC has better performance than SN because the retraining of SN does not consider the knowledge of previous time points. SN has better performance than EWC and DMoPWC on M12 due to random initialization of the weights of deep neural networks on baseline data, but M12 values of three methods are really close comparing with other time points. However, EWC has the worse performance than SN on most time points while DMoPWC significantly improve EWC because it studies the time-order information along with common weight subset and discriminative new time point features while keeping the old time

Table 1. The prediction results of MMSE on ADNI-I dataset.

Methods	wCC	PCC	M12	M18	M24	M36	M48
Lasso	0.40 ± 0.09	0.46 ± 0.07	4.04 ± 0.77	3.46 ± 0.97	5.53 ± 0.86	4.39 ± 0.74	4.73 ± 1.49
Ridge	0.41 ± 0.07	0.40 ± 0.08	4.26 ± 0.56	3.56 ± 0.93	5.05 ± 0.54	4.21 ± 0.47	3.62 ± 0.91
L21	0.57 ± 0.01	0.59 ± 0.03	3.32 ± 0.63	4.75 ± 0.75	4.64 ± 0.88	4.08 ± 1.01	3.11 ± 1.05
cFSGL	0.72 ± 0.03	0.73 ± 0.04	2.67 ± 0.32	3.40 ± 0.99	3.64 ± 0.71	2.98 ± 0.81	2.60 ± 1.13
MSMT	0.73 ± 0.02	0.74 ± 0.03	2.61 ± 0.55	3.37 ± 1.01	3.66 ± 0.78	2.73 ± 1.09	2.52 ± 1.20
SN	0.72 ± 0.05	0.68 ± 0.04	**2.54 ± 0.23**	2.05 ± 0.15	2.09 ± 0.26	2.32 ± 0.23	2.21 ± 0.13
EWC	0.71 ± 0.09	0.69 ± 0.06	2.60 ± 0.33	2.41 ± 0.28	1.98 ± 0.41	2.93 ± 0.22	2.65 ± 0.39
DMoPWC	**0.76 ± 0.04**	**0.75 ± 0.03**	2.58 ± 0.24	**1.75 ± 0.30**	**1.90 ± 0.26**	**2.30 ± 0.19**	**2.03 ± 0.12**

Table 2. The prediction results of ADAS-cog on ADNI-I dataset.

Methods	wCC	PCC	M12	M18	M24	M36	M48
Lasso	0.49 ± 0.05	0.53 ± 0.09	6.81 ± 1.03	6.87 ± 0.74	7.62 ± 0.87	8.08 ± 1.39	6.55 ± 1.34
Ridge	0.46 ± 0.07	0.49 ± 0.08	7.68 ± 0.96	6.89 ± 1.69	7.84 ± 1.54	8.59 ± 0.62	6.64 ± 1.58
L21	0.53 ± 0.07	0.59 ± 0.03	6.40 ± 0.51	6.95 ± 0.88	8.07 ± 0.67	8.00 ± 1.04	5.92 ± 0.60
cFSGL	0.73 ± 0.04	0.71 ± 0.07	5.32 ± 0.97	5.27 ± 0.66	6.79 ± 1.00	6.34 ± 1.11	5.61 ± 0.82
MSMT	0.77 ± 0.02	0.74 ± 0.05	5.18 ± 0.88	**4.64 ± 1.12**	6.76 ± 1.35	6.78 ± 1.54	**5.27 ± 1.76**
SN	0.72 ± 0.04	0.70 ± 0.05	5.18 ± 0.59	5.31 ± 0.67	5.68 ± 0.65	5.87 ± 0.69	5.95 ± 0.23
EWC	0.75 ± 0.06	0.70 ± 0.06	5.22 ± 0.47	5.24 ± 0.81	5.55 ± 0.12	5.78 ± 0.18	5.94 ± 0.43
DMoPWC	**0.78 ± 0.03**	**0.75 ± 0.04**	**5.18 ± 0.26**	5.19 ± 0.25	**5.40 ± 0.21**	**5.66 ± 0.23**	5.71 ± 0.10

points' knowledge. Moreover, DMoPWC can make equally prediction accuracy no matter how many visits the patients have made because of the online continual learning process.

We follow the same experimental settings in the MMSE study and explore the prediction model by ADAS-cog scores and report the performance in Table 2. We can observe that the best performance of predicting scores of ADAS-Cog is achieved by DMoPWC in three time points. MSMT has smallest rMSE on M18 and M48 because of the fluctuation of scores when the available amount of data becomes less. However, after DMoPWC dealing with temporary sequence information, the results are more linear, reasonable and accurate on all time points. We also find out that the proposed DMoPWC has much more improvement on M24 and M36 than MMSE prediction. Since we keep the previous time points' knowledge, the later time points do not have bias comparing with linear regression algorithms.

Effect of Time-Order Preserving Term. We compare the effectiveness of the time-order preserving term against the DMoPWC without order-preserving (oP) term. Figure 3 shows the comparison results. DMoPWC achieves better rMSE performance than DMoPWC w/o oP, which demonstrates DMoPWC further improves the results by considering the time order

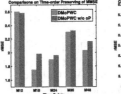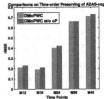

Fig. 3. Comparisons on time-order preserving term of rMSE performance on ADNI-I Dataset.

smoothness problem in longitudinal dataset, especially DMoPWC significantly improves the result of M48. This may be due to the baseline data has less correlation with later time points' data and DMoPWC w/o oP assumes each time point has the same correlation for the later time points and the results show the oP term offers a unique perspective on prognosis with longitudinal data.

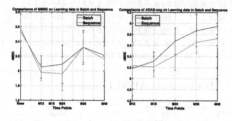

Comparisons of Learning Data in Batch Mode and Sequential Mode. We study the difference between learning longitudinal data in batch mode and sequential mode in Fig. 4 in terms of rMSE on MMSE and ADS-cog. We can observe that the performance of learning sequential longitudinal data is better than learning all data in batch. It may be partly due to the fact that the model will keep the previous time points' knowledge and learn the new time point information to improve future results when we learn the longitudinal data via continual learning. However, learning all images together ignores the relationship of early time points and cannot leverage such knowledge to boost the later time points' prediction results.

Fig. 4. Comparisons of rMSE performance on MMSE and ADAS-cog when learn data in batch and sequential mode.

Future Works. In the future, we will investigate DMoPWC with few-shot training data to further improve the performance of current continual learning framework.

References

1. Evgeniou, T., Pontil, M.: Regularized multi-task learning. In: International Conference On Knowledge Discovery and Data Mining (SIGKDD), pp. 109–117. ACM (2004)
2. Hoerl, A.E., Kennard, R.W.: Ridge regression: biased estimation for nonorthogonal problems. Technometrics **12**(1), 55–67 (1970)
3. Jack Jr., C.R., et al.: The Alzheimer's disease neuroimaging initiative (ADNI): MRI methods. J. Magn. Reson. Imaging: Off. J. Int. Soc. Magn. Reson. Med. **27**(4), 685–691 (2008)
4. Kirkpatrick, J., et al.: Overcoming catastrophic forgetting in neural networks. PNAS **114**, 3521–3526 (2017)
5. Li, Z., Hoiem, D.: Learning without forgetting. IEEE Trans. Pattern Anal. Mach. Intell. **40**, 2935–2947 (2017)
6. Liu, M., Zhang, D., Shen, D.: Identifying informative imaging biomarkers via tree structured sparse learning for ad diagnosis. Neuroinformatics **12**(3), 381–394 (2014)
7. Shi, J., Thompson, P.M., Gutman, B., Wang, Y.: Surface fluid registration of conformal representation: application to detect disease burden and genetic influence on hippocampus. NeuroImage **78**, 111–134 (2013)
8. Stonnington, C.M., Chu, C., Klöppel, S., Jack Jr., C.R., Ashburner, J., Frackowiak, R.S.: Predicting clinical scores from magnetic resonance scans in Alzheimer's disease. Neuroimage **51**(4), 1405–1413 (2010)

9. Suk, H.I., Lee, S.W., Shen, D.: Deep sparse multi-task learning for feature selection in Alzheimer's disease diagnosis. Brain Struct. Funct. **221**(5), 2569–2587 (2016)
10. Tibshirani, R.: Regression shrinkage and selection via the lasso. J. Roy. Stat. Soc. Ser. B (Methodol.) **58**, 267–288 (1996)
11. Wang, T., Qiu, R.G., Yu, M.: Predictive modeling of the progression of Alzheimer's Disease with recurrent neural networks. Sci. Rep. (Nat. Publ. Group) **8**, 1–12 (2018)
12. Zhang, J., Li, Q., Caselli, R.J., Thompson, P.M., Ye, J., Wang, Y.: Multi-source multi-target dictionary learning for prediction of cognitive decline. In: Niethammer, M., et al. (eds.) IPMI 2017. LNCS, vol. 10265, pp. 184–197. Springer, Cham (2017). https://doi.org/10.1007/978-3-319-59050-9_15
13. Zhou, J., Liu, J., Narayan, V.A., Ye, J.: Modeling disease progression via multi-task learning. NeuroImage **78**, 233–248 (2013)

Disease Knowledge Transfer Across Neurodegenerative Diseases

Răzvan V. Marinescu[1,2](✉), Marco Lorenzi[5], Stefano B. Blumberg[1],
Alexandra L. Young[1], Pere Planell-Morell[1], Neil P. Oxtoby[1],
Arman Eshaghi[1,3], Keir X. Yong[4], Sebastian J. Crutch[4], Polina Golland[2],
Daniel C. Alexander[1], and for the Alzheimer's Disease Neuroimaging Initiative

[1] Centre for Medical Image Computing, University College London, London, UK
[2] Computer Science and Artificial Intelligence Laboratory, MIT, Cambridge, USA
razvan@csail.mit.edu
[3] Queen Square MS Centre, UCL Institute of Neurology, London, UK
[4] Dementia Research Centre, University College London, London, UK
[5] University of Côte d'Azur, Inria Sophia Antipolis, Valbonne, France

Abstract. We introduce Disease Knowledge Transfer (DKT), a novel technique for transferring biomarker information between related neurodegenerative diseases. DKT infers robust multimodal biomarker trajectories in rare neurodegenerative diseases even when only limited, unimodal data is available, by transferring information from larger multimodal datasets from common neurodegenerative diseases. DKT is a joint-disease generative model of biomarker progressions, which exploits biomarker relationships that are shared across diseases. Our proposed method allows, for the first time, the estimation of plausible *multimodal* biomarker trajectories in Posterior Cortical Atrophy (PCA), a rare neurodegenerative disease where only unimodal MRI data is available. For this we train DKT on a combined dataset containing subjects with two distinct diseases and sizes of data available: (1) a larger, multimodal typical AD (tAD) dataset from the TADPOLE Challenge, and (2) a smaller unimodal Posterior Cortical Atrophy (PCA) dataset from the Dementia Research Centre (DRC), for which only a limited number of Magnetic Resonance Imaging (MRI) scans are available. Although validation is challenging due to lack of data in PCA, we validate DKT on synthetic data and two patient datasets (TADPOLE and PCA cohorts), showing it can estimate the ground truth parameters in the simulation and predict unseen biomarkers on the two patient datasets. While we demonstrated DKT on Alzheimer's variants, we note DKT is generalisable to other forms of related neurodegenerative diseases. Source code for DKT is available online: https://github.com/mrazvan22/dkt.

Keywords: Disease progression modelling · Transfer learning ·
Manifold learning · Alzheimer's disease · Posterior Cortical Atrophy

Electronic supplementary material The online version of this chapter (https://doi.org/10.1007/978-3-030-32245-8_95) contains supplementary material, which is available to authorized users.

1   Introduction

The estimation of accurate biomarker signatures in Alzheimer's disease (AD) and related neurodegenerative diseases is crucial for understanding underlying disease mechanisms, predicting subjects' progressions, and enrichment in clinical trials. Recently, data-driven disease progression models were proposed to reconstruct long term biomarker signatures from collections of short term individual measurements [1,2]. When applied to large datasets of typical AD, disease progression models have shown important benefits in understanding the earliest events in the AD cascade [1], quantifying biomarkers' heterogeneity [3] and they showed improved predictions over standard approaches [1]. However, by necessity these models require large datasets – in addition they should be both multimodal and longitudinal. Such data is not always available in rare neurodegenerative diseases. In particular, most datasets for rare neurodegenerative diseases come from local clinical centres, are unimodal (e.g. MRI only) and limited both cross-sectionally and longitudinally – this makes the application of disease progression models extremely difficult. Moreover, such a model estimated from common diseases such as typical AD may not generalise to specific variants. For example, in Posterior Cortical Atrophy (PCA) – a neurodegenerative syndrome causing visual disruption – posterior regions such as the occipital lobe are affected early, instead of the hippocampus and temporal regions in typical AD.

The problem of limited data in medical imaging has so far been addressed through transfer learning methods. These were successfully used to improve the accuracy of AD diagnosis [4] or prediction of MCI conversion [5], but have two key limitations. First, they use deep learning or other machine learning methods, which are not easily interpretable and don't allow us to understand underlying disease mechanisms that are either specific to rare diseases, or shared across related diseases. Secondly, these models cannot be used to forecast the future evolution of subjects at risk of disease, which is important for selecting the right subjects in clinical trials.

We propose Disease Knowledge Transfer (DKT), a generative model that estimates continuous multimodal biomarker progressions for multiple diseases simultaneously – including rare neurodegenerative diseases – and which inherently performs transfer learning between the modelled phenotypes. This is achieved by exploiting biomarker relationships that are shared across diseases, whilst accounting for differences in the spatial distribution of brain pathology. DKT is interpretable, which allows us to understand underlying disease mechanisms, and can also predict the future evolution of subjects at risk of diseases. We apply DKT on Alzheimer's variants and demonstrate its ability to predict non-MRI trajectories for patients with Posterior Cortical Atrophy, in lack of such data. This is done by fitting DKT to two datasets simultaneously: (1) the TADPOLE Challenge [6] dataset containing subjects from the Alzheimer's Disease Neuroimaging Initiative (ADNI) with MRI, FDG-PET, DTI, AV45 and AV1451 scans and (2) MRI scans from patients with Posterior Cortical Atrophy from the Dementia Research Centre (DRC), UK. We finally validate DKT on three datasets: (1) simulated data with known ground truth, (2) TADPOLE sub-populations with different progressions and (3) 20 DTI scans from controls and PCA patients from our clinical center.

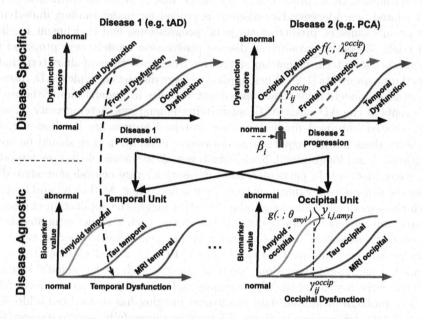

Fig. 1. Diagram of the proposed DKT framework. We assume that each disease can be modelled as the evolution of abstract dysfunction scores (Y-axis, top row), each one related to different brain regions. Each region-specific dysfunction score then further models (X-axis, bottom row) the progression of several multimodal biomarkers within that same region. For instance, the temporal dysfunction, modelled as a biomarker in the disease specific model (top row), is the X-axis in the disease agnostic model (temporal unit, bottom row), which aggregates together abnormality from amyloid, tau and MR imaging within the temporal lobe. The biomarker relationships within the bottom units are assumed to be disease agnostic and shared across all diseases modelled. Knowledge transfer between the two diseases can then be achieved via the disease-agnostic units. Mathematical notation from Sect. 2 is shown in red to ease understanding.

2   Method

Figure 1 shows the diagram of the DKT framework. We assume that the progression of each disease can be modelled as a unique evolution of dysfunction trajectories representing region-specific multimodal pathology, further modelled as the progression of several biomarkers within that same region, but acquired using different modalities (Fig. 1 bottom). Each group of biomarkers in the bottom row will be called a *disease-agnostic unit* or simply *agnostic unit*, because biomarker dynamics here are assumed to be shared across all diseases modelled.

The assumption that the dynamics of some biomarkers are disease-agnostic (i.e. shared across diseases), is key to DKT. We can make this assumption for two reasons. First, pathology in many related neurodegenerative diseases (e.g. Alzheimer's variants) is hypothesised to share the same underlying mechanisms (e.g. amyloid and tau accumulation), and within one region, such mechanisms lead to similar pathology dynamics across all the disease variants modelled [7], with the key difference that distinct brain regions are affected at different times and with different pathology rates and extent, likely caused by selective vulnerability of networks within these regions [8]. Secondly, even if the diseases share different upstream mechanisms (e.g. amyloid vs tau accumulation), downstream biomarkers measuring hypometabolism, white matter degradation and atrophy are likely to follow the same pathological cascade and will have similar dynamics.

We now model the biomarker dynamics that are specific to each disease, by mapping the subjects' disease stages to dysfunction scores. We assume that each subject i at each visit j has an underlying disease stage $s_{ij} = \beta_i + m_{ij}$, where m_{ij} represents the months since baseline visit for subject i at visit j and β_i represents the time shift of subject i. We then assume that each subject i at visit j has a dysfunction score γ_{ij}^l corresponding to multimodal pathology in brain region l, which is a function of its disease stage:

$$\gamma_{ij}^l = f(\beta_i + m_{ij}; \lambda_{d_i}^l) \tag{1}$$

where f is a smooth monotonic function mapping each disease stage to a dysfunction score, having parameters $\lambda_{d_i}^l$ corresponding to agnostic unit $l \in \Lambda$, where Λ is the set of all agnostic units. Moreover, $d_i \in \mathbb{D}$ represents the index of the disease corresponding to subject i, where $\mathbb{D}$ is the set of all diseases modelled. For example, MCI and tAD subjects from ADNI as well as tAD subjects from the DRC cohort can all be assigned $d_i = 1$, while PCA subjects can be assigned $d_i = 2$. We implement f as a parametric sigmoidal curve similar to [2], to enable a robust optimisation and because this accounts for floor and ceiling effects present in AD biomarkers – the monotonicity of this sigmoidal family is also very appropriate for many neurodegenerative diseases due to irreversability.

We further model the biomarker dynamics that are disease-agnostic, by constructing the mapping from the dysfunction scores γ_{ij}^l to the biomarker measurements. We assume a set of given biomarker measurements $Y = [y_{ijk}|(i,j,k) \in \Omega]$ for subject i at visit j in biomarker k, where Ω is the set of available biomarker measurements. We further denote by θ_k the trajectory parameters for biomarker $k \in K$ within its agnostic unit $\psi(k)$, where $\psi: \{1, ..., K\} \to \Lambda$ maps each biomarker k to a unique agnostic unit $l \in \Lambda$. These definitions allow us to formulate the likelihood for a single measurement y_{ijk} as follows:

$$p(y_{ijk}|\theta_k, \lambda_{d_i}^{\psi(k)}, \beta_i, \epsilon_k) = N(y_{ijk}|g(\gamma_{ij}^{\psi(k)}; \theta_k), \epsilon_k) \tag{2}$$

where $g(.\,; \theta_k)$ represents the trajectory of biomarker k within agnostic unit $\psi(k)$, with parameters θ_k, and is again implemented using a sigmoidal function for reasons outlined above. Parameters $\lambda_{d_i}^{\psi(k)}$ are used to define $\gamma_{ij}^{\psi(k)}$ based on Eq. 1, where agnostic unit l is now referred to as $\psi(k)$, to clarify this is the unit where biomarker k has been allocated. Variable ϵ_k denotes the variance of measurements for biomarker k.

We extend the above model to multiple subjects, visits and biomarkers to get the full model likelihood:

$$p(\boldsymbol{y}|\theta, \lambda, \beta, \epsilon) = \prod_{(i,j,k) \in \Omega} p(y_{ijk}|\theta_k, \lambda_{d_i}^{\psi(k)}, \beta_i) \tag{3}$$

where $\boldsymbol{y} = [y_{ijk}|\forall (i,j,k) \in \Omega]$ is the vector of all biomarker measurements, while $\boldsymbol{\theta} = [\theta_1, ..., \theta_K]$ represents the stacked parameters for the trajectories of biomarkers in agnostic units, $\boldsymbol{\lambda} = [\lambda_d^l|l \in \Lambda, d \in \mathbb{D}]$ are the parameters of the dysfunction trajectories within the disease models, $\boldsymbol{\beta} = [\beta_1, ..., \beta_N]$ are the subject-specific time shifts and $\boldsymbol{\epsilon} = [\epsilon_k|k \in K]$ estimates measurement noise.

We estimate the model parameters $[\boldsymbol{\theta}, \boldsymbol{\lambda}, \boldsymbol{\beta}, \boldsymbol{\epsilon}]$ using loopy belief propagation – see algorithm in supplementary material. One key advantage of DKT is that the subject's time shift β_i can be estimated using only a subset (e.g. MRI) of the subject's data – the model can then infer the missing modalities (e.g. non-MRI) using Eq. 3.

2.1   Generating Synthetic Data

We first test DKT on synthetic data, to assess its performance against known ground truth. More precisely, we generate data that follows the DKT model exactly, and test DKT's ability to recover biomarker trajectories and subject time-shifts. We generate synthetic data from two diseases (50 subjects with "*synthetic PCA*" and 100 subjects with "*synthetic AD*") using the parameters from the bottom-left table in Fig. 2, emulating the TADPOLE and DRC cohorts – see supplementary material for full details. The six biomarkers (k_1-k_6) have been *a-priori* allocated to two agnostic units l_0 and l_1. To simulate the lack of multimodal data in the synthetic PCA subjects, we discarded the data from biomarkers k_0, k_1, k_4 and k_5 for all these subjects.

2.2   Data Acquisition and Preprocessing

We trained DKT on ADNI data from the TADPOLE challenge [6], since it contained a large number of multimodal biomarkers already pre-processed and aggregated into one table. From the TADPOLE dataset we selected a subset of 230 subjects which had an MRI scan and at least one FDG PET, AV45, AV1451 or DTI scan. In order to model another disease, we further included MRI scans from 76 PCA subjects from the DRC cohort, along with scans from 67 tAD and 87 age-matched controls.

For both datasets, we computed multimodal biomarker measurements corresponding to each brain lobe: MRI volumes using the Freesurfer software, FDG-, AV45- and AV1451-PET standardised uptake value ratios (SUVR) extracted with the standard ADNI pipeline, and DTI fractional anisotropy (FA) measures from adjacent white-matter regions. For every lobe, we regressed out the following covariates: age, gender, total intracranial volume (TIV) and dataset (ADNI vs DRC). Finally, biomarkers were normalized to the $[0, 1]$ range.

3 Results on Synthetic and Patient Datasets

Results on synthetic data in the presence of ground truth (Fig. 2) suggest that DKT can robustly estimate the trajectory parameters (MAE < 0.058) as well as the subject-specific time-shifts ($R^2 > 0.98$). While some errors in trajectory estimation can be noticed, these are due to the informed priors on the model parameters in order to ensure identifiability and convergence of parameters.

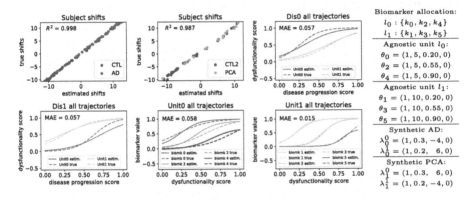

Fig. 2. Comparison between true and DKT-estimated subject time-shifts and biomarker trajectories. (top-left/top-middle) Scatter plots of the true shifts (y-axis) against estimated shifts (x-axis), for the 'synthetic AD' and 'synthetic PCA' diseases. We then show the DKT-estimated and true trajectories of the agnostic units within the 'synthetic AD' disease (top-right, "Dis0") and the 'synthetic PCA' disease (bottom-left, "Dis1"). Finally, we also show the biomarker trajectories within unit 0 (bottom-center) and unit 1 (bottom-right). Parameters used for generating the trajectory shapes are shown in the table on the right.

We then apply DKT to real patient data, with the aim of transferring multi-modal biomarker trajectories from tAD to PCA. The inferred PCA trajectories, shown in Fig. 3, recapitulate known patterns in PCA [9], where posterior regions such as occipital and parietal lobes are predominantly affected in later stages. As opposed to typical AD, we find that the hippocampus is affected later on, further suggesting the model did not transfer too much tAD specific information. Here, we demonstrate the possibility of inferring plausible non-MRI biomarkers in a rare neurodegenerative disease, in lack of such data for these subjects. As far as we are aware, this is the first time a continuous signature of non-MRI biomarkers is estimated for PCA, due to its rarity and lack of data.

3.1   Validation on DTI Data in tAD and PCA

We further validated DKT by predicting unseen DTI data from two patient datasets: (1) TADPOLE subjects with a different progression from the training subjects, and (2) a separate test set of 20 DTI scans from controls and PCA patients from the DRC – full demographics are given in the supplementary material. To split TADPOLE into subgroups with different progression, we used the SuStaIn model by [3], which resulted into three subgroups: hippocampal, cortical and subcortical, with prominent early atrophy in the hippocampus, cortical and subcortical regions respectively. To evaluate prediction accuracy, we computed the rank correlation between the DKT-predicted biomarker values and the measured values in the test data. We compute the rank correlation instead of mean squared error as it is not susceptible to systemic biases of the models when predicting "unseen data" in a certain disease.

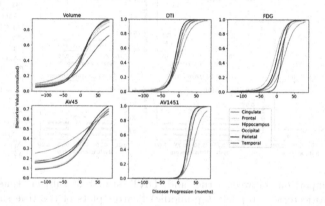

Fig. 3. Estimated trajectories for the PCA cohort. The only data that were available were the MRI volumetric data. The dynamics of the other biomarkers has been inferred by the model using data from typical AD, and taking into account the different spatial distribution of pathology in PCA vs tAD.

Validation results are shown in Table 1, for hippocampal to cortical TADPOLE subgroups (other pairs of subgroups not shown due to lack of space) as well as PCA subjects. When predicting missing DTI markers of the TADPOLE cortical subgroup as well as PCA subjects from the DRC cohort (Table 1), the DKT correlations are generally high for the cingulate, hippocampus and parietal, and lower for the frontal lobe. DKT also shows favourable performance compared to four other models: the latent-stage model from [2], a multivariate Gaussian Process model with RBF kernel that predicts a DTI ROI marker from multiple MRI markers, as well as cubic spline and linear models that predict a regional DTI biomarker directly from its corresponding MRI marker. In particular for predicting DTI FA in the parietal and temporal lobes, DKT has significantly better predictions that almost all methods tested.

Table 1. Performance evaluation of DKT and four other statistical models of decreasing complexity. We show the rank correlation between predicted biomarkers and measured biomarkers in (top) TADPOLE subgroups and (bottom) PCA. (*) Statistically significant difference in the performance of DKT vs the other models, based on a two-tailed t-test, Bonferroni corrected.

Model	Cingulate	Frontal	Hippocam.	Occipital	Parietal	Temporal
	TADPOLE: Hippocampal subgroup to Cortical subgroup					
DKT (ours)	0.56 ± 0.23	$\mathbf{0.35 \pm 0.17}$	$\mathbf{0.58 \pm 0.14}$	-0.10 ± 0.29	$\mathbf{0.71 \pm 0.11}$	$\mathbf{0.34 \pm 0.26}$
Latent stage	0.44 ± 0.25	0.34 ± 0.21	$0.34 \pm 0.24*$	$\mathbf{-0.07 \pm 0.22}$	0.64 ± 0.16	$0.08 \pm 0.24*$
Multivariate	$\mathbf{0.60 \pm 0.18}$	$0.11 \pm 0.22*$	$0.12 \pm 0.29*$	-0.22 ± 0.22	$-0.44 \pm 0.14*$	$-0.32 \pm 0.29*$
Spline	$-0.24 \pm 0.25*$	$-0.06 \pm 0.27*$	0.58 ± 0.17	-0.16 ± 0.27	$0.23 \pm 0.25*$	$0.10 \pm 0.25*$
Linear	$-0.24 \pm 0.25*$	$0.20 \pm 0.25*$	0.58 ± 0.17	-0.16 ± 0.27	$0.23 \pm 0.25*$	$0.13 \pm 0.23*$
	Typical Alzheimer's to Posterior Cortical Atrophy					
DKT (ours)	0.77 ± 0.11	0.39 ± 0.26	0.75 ± 0.09	0.60 ± 0.14	$\mathbf{0.55 \pm 0.24}$	$\mathbf{0.35 \pm 0.22}$
Latent stage	$\mathbf{0.80 \pm 0.09}$	$\mathbf{0.53 \pm 0.17}$	$\mathbf{0.80 \pm 0.12}$	0.56 ± 0.18	0.50 ± 0.21	0.32 ± 0.24
Multivariate	0.73 ± 0.09	0.45 ± 0.22	0.71 ± 0.08	$-0.28 \pm 0.21*$	0.53 ± 0.22	$0.25 \pm 0.23*$
Spline	$0.52 \pm 0.20*$	$-0.03 \pm 0.35*$	$0.66 \pm 0.11*$	$0.09 \pm 0.25*$	0.53 ± 0.20	$0.30 \pm 0.21*$
Linear	$0.52 \pm 0.20*$	0.34 ± 0.27	$0.66 \pm 0.11*$	$\mathbf{0.64 \pm 0.17}$	0.54 ± 0.22	$0.30 \pm 0.21*$

4 Discussion

In this work we made initial steps at the challenging problem of transfer learning between different neurodegenerative diseases. Our proposed DKT method enabled the estimation of quantitative non-MRI trajectories in a rare disease (PCA) where very limited data was available. To our knowledge, this is the first time a multimodal continuous signature is derived for PCA, as the only other longitudinal study of PCA only computed atrophy measures from MRI scans [10]. Our work has however several limitations, which can be addressed in future research: (1) to account for population heterogeneity, DKT can be easily extended to include subject-specific effects; (2) improved schemes for biomarker allocation to agnostic units can take connectivity into account, or derive it from the data automatically; (3) DKT can be further validated on more complex synthetic experiments with a range of datasets generated with different parameters.

Acknowledgements. This work was supported by the EPSRC Centre For Doctoral Training in Medical Imaging with grant EP/L016478/1 and in part by the Neuroimaging Analysis Center through NIH grant NIH NIBIB NAC P41EB015902. Data collection and sharing for this project was funded by the Alzheimer's Disease Neuroimaging Initiative (ADNI) (National Institutes of Health Grant U01 AG024904) and DOD ADNI (Department of Defense award number W81XWH-12-2-0012). The Dementia Research Centre is an ARUK coordination center.

References

1. Oxtoby, N.P., et al.: Data-driven models of dominantly-inherited Alzheimer's disease progression. Brain **141**(5), 1529–1544 (2018)
2. Jedynak, B.M., et al.: A computational neurodegenerative disease progression score: method and results with the Alzheimer's disease neuroimaging initiative cohort. Neuroimage **63**(3), 1478–1486 (2012)
3. Young, A.L., et al.: Uncovering the heterogeneity and temporal complexity of neurodegenerative diseases with subtype and stage inference. Nature Commun. **9**(1), 4273 (2018)
4. Hon, M., Khan, N.: Towards Alzheimer's disease classification through transfer learning. arXiv preprint arXiv:1711.11117 (2017)
5. Cheng, B., Liu, M., Zhang, D., Munsell, B.C., Shen, D.: Domain transfer learning for MCI conversion prediction. IEEE Trans. Biomed. Eng. **62**(7), 1805–1817 (2015)
6. Marinescu, R.V., et al.: TADPOLE challenge: prediction of longitudinal evolution in Alzheimer's disease (2018). arXiv:1805.03909
7. Jack Jr., C.R., et al.: Hypothetical model of dynamic biomarkers of the Alzheimer's pathological cascade. Lancet Neurol. **9**(1), 119–128 (2010)
8. Seeley, W.W., Crawford, R.K., Zhou, J., Miller, B.L., Greicius, M.D.: Neurodegenerative diseases target large-scale human brain networks. Neuron **62**(1), 42–52 (2009)
9. Crutch, S.J., Lehmann, M., Schott, J.M., Rabinovici, G.D., Rossor, M.N., Fox, N.C.: Posterior cortical atrophy. Lancet Neurol. **11**(2), 170–178 (2012)
10. Lehmann, M., et al.: Cortical thickness and voxel-based morphometry in posterior cortical atrophy and typical Alzheimer's disease. Neurobiol. Aging **32**(8), 1466–1476 (2011)

Correction to: Automatic Segmentation of Vestibular Schwannoma from T2-Weighted MRI by Deep Spatial Attention with Hardness-Weighted Loss

Guotai Wang, Jonathan Shapey, Wenqi Li, Reuben Dorent,
Alexis Dimitriadis, Sotirios Bisdas, Ian Paddick, Robert Bradford,
Shaoting Zhang, Sébastien Ourselin, and Tom Vercauteren

Correction to:
**Chapter "Automatic Segmentation of Vestibular Schwannoma
from T2-Weighted MRI by Deep Spatial Attention
with Hardness-Weighted Loss" in: D. Shen et al. (Eds.):**
Medical Image Computing and Computer Assisted
Intervention – MICCAI 2019, **LNCS 11765,**
https://doi.org/10.1007/978-3-030-32245-8_30

The original version of this chapter was revised. An author's name was misspelled. The name has been corrected to Alexis Dimitriadis.

The updated version of this chapter can be found at
https://doi.org/10.1007/978-3-030-32245-8_30

Springer Nature Switzerland AG 2021
D. Shen et al. (Eds.): MICCAI 2019, LNCS 11765, p. C1, 2021.
https://doi.org/10.1007/978-3-030-32245-8_96

Author Index

Printed in the United States
by Baker & Taylor Publisher Services